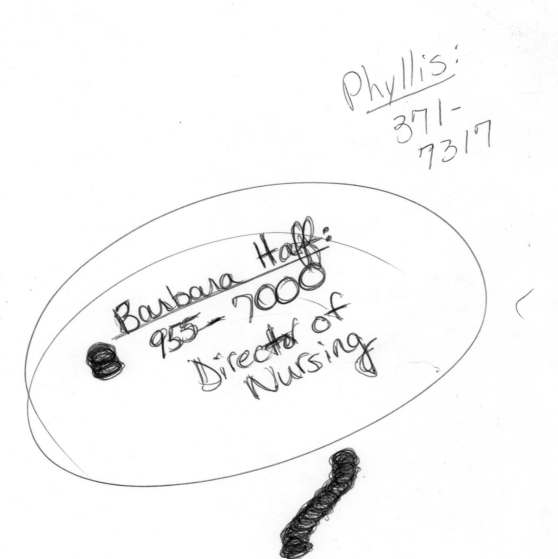

Introductory Medical–Surgical Nursing

Jeanne C. Scherer, RN, MS

Instructor
Former Assistant Director and Medical–Surgical Coordinator
Sisters of Charity Hospital
School of Nursing
Buffalo, New York

Introductory Medical–Surgical Nursing

FIFTH EDITION

J.B. LIPPINCOTT COMPANY

Philadelphia   *New York*   *St. Louis*   *London*   *Sydney*   *Tokyo*

Acquisitions Editor: *David P. Carroll*
Coordinating Editorial Assistant: *Amy R. Stonehouse*
Project Editor: *Grace R. Caputo*
Indexer: *Julia Figures*
Design Coordinator: *Ellen C. Dawson*
Designer: *Patti Maddaloni*
Interior Cover Designer: *Anne O'Donnell*
Production Manager: *Helen Ewan*
Production Coordinator: *Pamela Milcos*
Compositor: *Tapsco, Inc.*
Printer/Binder: *Courier Westford, Inc.*

5th Edition

1 3 5 6 4 2

Library of Congress Cataloging-in-Publication Data

Scherer, Jeanne C.
    Introductory medical-surgical nursing/Jeanne C. Scherer.—5th ed.
        p.   cm.
    Includes bibliographical references.
    Includes index.
    ISBN 0-397-54755-2:
    1. Nursing. 2. Surgical nursing. I. Title.
    [DNLM: 1. Nursing Care. WY 150 S326i]
RT41.S38   1991
610.73—dc20
DNLM/DLC
for Library of Congress   90-6507
                                                                     CIP

Any procedure or practice described in this book should be applied by the health care practitioner under appropriate supervision in accordance with professional standards of care used with regard to the unique circumstances that apply in each practice situation. Care has been taken to confirm the accuracy of information presented and to describe generally accepted practices. However, the author, editors, and publisher cannot accept any responsibility for errors or omissions or for any consequences from application of the information in this book and make no warranty, express or implied, with respect to the contents of the book.

Every effort has been made to ensure drug selections and dosages are in accordance with current recommendations and practice. Because of ongoing research, changes in government regulations, and the constant flow of information on drug therapy, reactions, and interactions, the reader is cautioned to check the package insert for each drug for indications, dosages, warnings, and precautions, particularly if the drug is new or infrequently used.

Preface

To those familiar with *Introductory Medical–Surgical Nursing,* this fifth edition should appear as virtually a new text. Many disorders have been added, and all material from the fourth edition has been thoroughly revised and updated. Moreover, the emphasis of the fifth edition encompasses both basic knowledge of commonly encountered disorders and clinical practice. Finally, the revised design of the book presents a format that is clear and consistent throughout, providing the reader with easy access to information about a specific disorder or group of disorders.

Introductory Medical–Surgical Nursing is divided into units according to body systems. Each unit begins with a general review of anatomy and physiology that is followed by a discussion of patient assessment. The common diagnostic and laboratory tests performed for disorders that pertain to that particular body system are described. The remaining material in the unit covers medical and surgical disorders with emphasis on symptoms, diagnosis, and treatment. Many disorders are grouped together to form a focal point for the nursing process that follows. Each chapter is prefaced with objectives that are student and instructor oriented. The reader may view the objectives as a guide to the learning experience; the instructor may use the objectives as the goals of a particular unit of study.

One of the major areas of revision is the use of the Nursing Process format throughout the *entire* textbook. Set off in a different typeface, these sections fall within discussions of disorders and disease states and provide guidance in assessing the patient (Assessment), in establishing nursing diagnoses (Nursing Diagnosis), in effecting nursing intervention (Planning and Implementation), and in evaluating patient response (Evaluation). With a few exceptions, all diseases and disorders—either as single entities or as a group—are presented in the Nursing Process sections.

The reader should use the material given in the Nursing Diagnosis sections as a guideline, because each patient is different and may require a greater or lesser number of nursing diagnoses than are given in the text. The relation of a nursing diagnosis to a patient's specific problem also may vary, requiring a different formulation than given here.

Discussion of patient management in the Planning and Implementation sections begins with a summary of patient-oriented goals and major goals of nursing management. Specific information that pertains to the nursing diagnoses as well as additional material not covered by the NANDA-approved nursing diagnoses is then presented. Emphasis is placed on patient teaching as an integral part of the nursing process.

Nursing Care Plans are used to illustrate the nursing management of some of the major disorders. Charts and tables that summarize points of patient assessment and nursing management add to the information in the text. Moreover, the use of lists throughout the text enables the reader to locate essential information easily.

Relevant nutrition, pharmacologic, and gerontologic considerations are listed at the end of most chapters to emphasize important points of nursing management. In addition, the annotated bibliography for each chapter provides a list of references commonly found in libraries at schools of nursing. The bibliography is realistic and provides the user with references that enhance the material in the text. A glossary of medical terms and an appendix of common laboratory values also are included in this edition.

A separate workbook has been designed for use with this text. All questions contained in the *Student Work Manual for Introductory Medical–Surgical Nursing* have been taken directly from this textbook.

Whereas the discussions of disorders in *Introductory Medical–Surgical Nursing* provide a basic understanding of the diseases and disorders encountered in a general hospital setting, the Nursing Process sections should assist the reader in identifying and using the major principles of patient management. Thus, with its emphasis on basic knowledge of common medical and surgical disorders as well as on clinical practice, *Introductory Medical–Surgical Nursing* provides a ready resource for aiding the reader in transferring the knowledge learned in the classroom into practicable nursing intervention in the clinical setting.

JEANNE C. SCHERER, RN, MS

Acknowledgment

Many persons were involved in the production of this book. The establishment of guidelines came from Diana Intenzo, Executive Editor. To David Carroll, Acquisitions Editor, I owe thanks for his encouragement, patience, advice, and invaluable assistance with the development and organization of the manuscript. To Larry Bryant, Director of Electronic Text Management, I give special thanks for help with the computerization of the manuscript and especially for his ability to magically turn the complicated into simple by striking a few keys. I also thank Grace Caputo, Project Editor, who contributed in many ways to the content and format of the manuscript and who eased me painlessly through the final stages of production. Last, but never least, is the author's mainstay, the manuscript editor. I am grateful to Barbara Hodgson and Rosina Miller for their skillful editing of the book.

I also thank Robert L. Bork, DDS, for supplying information on dentistry and dental problems, especially information on the temporomandibular joint. Internist Rodolfo L. Villacorta, MD, graciously answered my questions about many medical disorders. Ophthalmologist Karen R. Schoene, MD, provided information on eye disorders as well as recent developments in cataract surgery.

Finally, special recognition must go to those wonderful people called patients who are always a part of any nursing textbook.

Contents

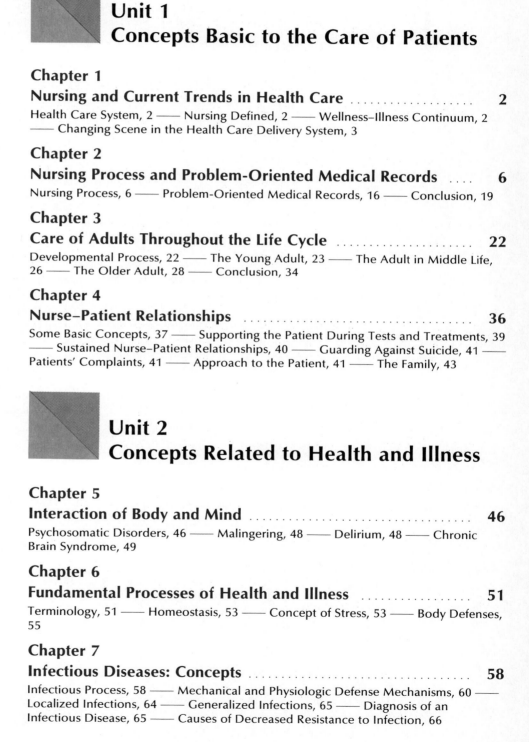

Unit 3
Medical–Surgical Nursing Interventions

Unit 4
Oncologic Nursing

Unit 5
The Respiratory System

Unit 6
The Cardiovascular System

Unit 7
The Hematopoietic and Lymphatic Systems

Unit 8
The Nervous System

Unit 9
The Special Senses

Unit 10
The Gastrointestinal Tract and Accessory Structures

Unit 11
The Endocrine System

Unit 12
Disturbances of Sexual Structures or Reproductive Function

Unit 13
The Urinary Tract

Unit 14
Orthopedic and Connective Tissue Disorders

Unit 15
The Integumentary System

Introductory Medical–Surgical Nursing

Concepts Basic to the Care of Patients

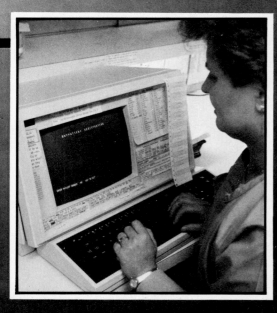

Unit 1

Chapter 1
Nursing and Current Trends in Health Care

On completion of this chapter the reader will:

- Describe and discuss the health care system
- Give a definition of nursing
- Discuss the wellness–illness continuum
- Discuss the changing scene in the health care delivery system
- Describe and discuss the purpose of HMOs
- Discuss the positive and negative aspects of DRGs
- Discuss the relevance of computers in medicine

HEALTH CARE SYSTEM

The health care system consists of a group of individuals with specific functions. The members of the health care system include both highly trained professionals, such as physicians, nurses, dietitians, and pharmacists, and other individuals who have had limited but necessary health care training, such as nursing assistants. All members of the health care system assist people with problems of health and illness. Thus, a patient with severe emphysema receives care by members of the health care system, as does a person without any detectable illness who has a yearly physical examination and evaluation. The health care system, then, is concerned with those who are ill, but it also is concerned with promoting health or wellness for all people.

NURSING DEFINED

Nursing is as difficult to define today as it was during the time of Florence Nightingale; nursing authorities themselves do not agree on an exact definition. Nursing has been described as an art and a science that encompasses the application of a professional service based on a scientific body of knowledge. Newer definitions of nursing encompass a holistic concept of humans, incorporating physical, emotional, social, and intellectual needs while stressing the importance of health maintenance as well as the treatment of illness.

A *holistic* approach is one that considers the physical, emotional, social, intellectual, and economic needs of the patient. This concept prompts all members of the health care delivery system to consider not only a person's physical needs, which had been the primary focus of health professionals, but also his or her other needs, which often are equally important.

WELLNESS–ILLNESS CONTINUUM

In the Preamble of the Constitution of the World Health Organization (WHO), health, or wellness, is defined as a "state of complete physical, mental and social well being and not merely the absence of disease and infirmity," but this definition does not account for any variation in the degree of wellness or illness. Because variation in the degrees of wellness (or health) and illness often exists, the wellness–illness continuum concept has been developed. This concept views wellness and illness on a graduated continuum, a scale on which a person's health status may range anywhere from complete health to serious illness or impending death. Thus, at any given time, a person may not be completely well or completely ill, and may simultaneously possess varying degrees of wellness and illness. For example, a person infected with a viral cold is neither completely well nor completely ill because not all body systems are affected by the infection. This person, then, could be considered to possess varying degrees of wellness and illness simultaneously. If the infection were to cause additional problems, such as a secondary bacterial infection, a movement occurs in the wellness–illness continuum toward more serious illness and, in effect, less wellness. As the viral infection is controlled by the body's natural defense mechanisms and the secondary infection is controlled with antibiotics, a shift occurs once again in the wellness–illness continuum as a result of a decrease in the seriousness of the illness and a movement toward wellness.

This concept of varying degrees of wellness and illness has changed the health care delivery system. Instead of focusing primarily on the treatment of illness, as was done in the past, greater emphasis is placed on *health maintenance*, in effect, the prevention of illness. Although not all illnesses can be prevented, many can. Smoking can cause emphysema; by not smoking, a person can decrease the chance of developing this illness. Health maintenance also includes attaining and maintaining an optimal state of wellness. Although the optimal state of wellness differs from one person to another, each person has a potential for optimal wellness. For example, patients with arthritis, a disease that cannot be cured, have a chronic illness. Treatment is aimed at decreasing the level of illness (eg, treatment or control of disease), preventing further disability, and helping them move toward an optimal level of physical, emotional, social, and intellectual wellness.

The importance of health maintenance is expressed not only by the medical profession, but also by federal, state, and local governments that monitor health problems, pass and enact laws relevant to health, and develop programs aimed at improving the general health of the population. Recognition of the importance of health maintenance has prompted programs such as those that provide adequate nutrition for the underprivileged, low-income housing, immunization programs for children, and health education for laypeople, including school-aged children.

Special interest groups such as the American Heart Association and the American Cancer Society provide the medical profession and laypeople with pertinent health maintenance information. Television, newspaper, and radio advertisements and programs provide health information as well as warnings of potential or actual health problems. Programs such as those that provide for blood pressure or diabetes screening have helped in the early detection of health problems. The greatest emphases of many programs are on health maintenance and the early recognition of illness.

CHANGING SCENE IN THE HEALTH CARE DELIVERY SYSTEM

The changing health needs of the general population have prompted some revisions in health care delivery. With a greater number of people living beyond age 70, need is increased for more nursing homes, hospital-based skilled nursing facilities, home health care agencies, senior citizen complexes, and funds for health care. Shifts in the population from urban to suburban areas have created greater concentrations of low-income groups in the cities. This development, in turn, has resulted in the recognition of the need for radical changes, such as improved housing, food programs designed to improve nutrition, health screening and educational programs for high-risk groups, and an increased number of health care facilities in a concentrated urban area.

The general economy also has affected health care delivery. When the unemployment or inflation rate rises, more of the general population is unable to afford adequate health care. The responsibility for paying for health care is then shifted from the individual to federal, state, and local agencies. For many reasons, health care costs have increased rapidly, a trend that has demonstrated a need for reevaluation of the health care delivery system. Although many methods of reducing health care costs have been explored, and in some cases instituted, it is imperative that the cost of health care be reduced.

Although there is no one answer to this problem, one approach has been to look for ways to increase the efficiency of health care delivery and thereby reduce its costs. Another method of reducing health care costs involves placing more emphasis on health maintenance. Even though programs for health maintenance are expensive, the treatment of illness appears to be even costlier.

Health Maintenance Organizations

Health maintenance organizations (HMOs) are a recent entry in the health care delivery system. HMOs, whose prototypes were groups such as the Kaiser-Permanente Foundation and the Ross-Loos plan, provide both ambulatory services and inpatient care. Although some groups have their own small hospitals, others rely on community hospitals for inpatient care.

HMOs are essentially group insurance plans, with the subscriber and usually members of the subscriber's family covered by a prepaid fee. Some HMOs allow people who are over age 65 to subscribe to their programs on an individual basis. The major emphasis of HMOs is on the delivery of comprehensive health care that meets the needs of the whole person and the family. This holistic approach encompasses the maintenance of health as well as the treatment of illness. The financial viability of HMOs is based on the ability of the group plan to keep the subscriber healthy and out of the hospital by means of periodic screening, health education, and preventive services.

Diagnostic Related Groups

Because of the rising costs of the health care delivery system, a method has been developed to cut the costs of Medicare and insurance payments. Under this plan, a predetermined amount of money is paid for hospital care of the patient in any one of some 467 diagnostic related groups (DRGs). The cost of hospitalization for a patient who requires a longer hospital stay than that specified under this plan is borne by the hospital.

Many questions have been raised by DRGs. Because no payment is received for a hospital stay that extends beyond the time stated by the plan, some hospitals may be unable to bear the financial burden of maintaining patients who require longer hospitalizations. This, in turn, may result in adverse effects on the health care delivery system. Problems that have occurred with this plan include the bankruptcy of smaller hospitals, reductions in hospital staff, increased patient or work loads for hospital personnel, and elimination of some supervisory positions. One serious consequence of DRGs is the premature discharge of patients who require hospitalization beyond the time designated by

the DRG. When a patient who still requires skilled care or supervision is discharged because payment does not cover extended hospitalization, a burden is imposed on the family and potential ethical and legal problems are raised. Hospitals are faced with a dilemma: financially, they may not be able to afford to keep the patient beyond the time for which they have been reimbursed by Medicare or insurance plans; morally, they must consider the serious consequences of discharging some of these patients before they are completely well.

However negative this scenario may sound, DRGs also have positive effects. Hospitals are forced to review and reevaluate the costs, efficiency, and effectiveness of their health care delivery, to become more cost conscious, and to reduce any abuses in the payment system.

Computers in Medicine

Computers have entered the lives of most people. Not only are computers used for nursing education and hospital administrative tasks, but they also are used in patient care. Hospitals with a mainframe computer (which stores a large volume of information) and computer terminals (which allow entering and retrieval of information) are able to reduce bookkeeping costs as well as improve departmental effectiveness and decrease personnel work loads. The computer can be used to schedule admissions, monitor supplies in various departments such as dietary and pharmacy, transmit data between hospital departments, schedule surgery, record and report laboratory data, and keep patient records. Computers also are used in the radiol-

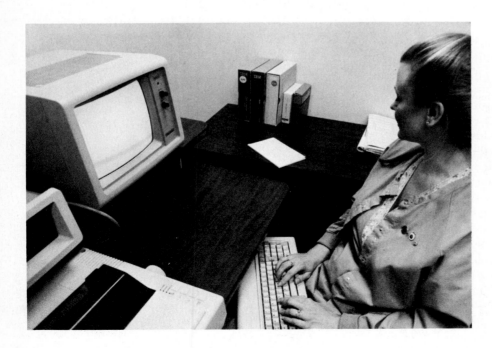

Figure 1–1. Computer terminals in nursing stations provide instantaneous retrieval of information. (Photograph by D. Atkinson).

ogy department for image enhancement, as in computed tomographic scans, and in surgical procedures such as stereotactic surgery.

Computer terminals in nursing stations can increase the effectiveness of patient care by reducing the time involved in record keeping (Fig. 1-1). Patient care plans, physician's orders and progress notes, nursing assessments, data such as vital signs and weight, nursing procedures, and patient discharge summaries can be entered in a computer terminal if the mainframe has been programmed to accept this type of data. All patient data stored in the computer can be made available instantly. The immediate retrieval of data can be of particular importance in emergency situations. Computers also can be used to monitor telemetry electrocardiograms and intravenous infusions, provide drug information such as adverse reactions or drug interactions, and calculate drug dosages.

Agencies involved in donor organ procurement use computers. Because the time of donor organ viability is short, rapid retrieval of information is essential.

When a person becomes a candidate for organ transplantation, his or her name and other vital information are entered into a computer. When a donor organ becomes available, the computer is immediately able to match the organ, the organ size, and tissue typing to a list of potential recipients. The use of a computer markedly reduces the time spent in searching records and increases the time available for transportation and transplantation of the donated organ.

Although the human element is still necessary for the final decision on the data presented, the computer is a valuable tool in the field of medicine because of its vast storage capacity in a limited space and its capability for the rapid retrieval and transmission of information within the hospital. Data also can be transmitted to other hospitals and information sent from a hospital to a company or agency such as a pharmaceutical supply house or an insurance company being billed for patient care. The transmission of data to areas outside the hospital usually is accomplished through a telephone network.

Suggested Readings

☐ Ellis JR, Hartley CL. Nursing in today's world: challenges, issues and trends. 3rd ed. Philadelphia: JB Lippincott, 1988. *(In-depth coverage of subject matter)*

☐ Grobe SJ. Computer primer and resource: a guide for nurses. Philadelphia: JB Lippincott, 1984. *(Additional coverage of subject matter)*

☐ Saba V, McCormick K. Essentials of computers for nurses. Philadelphia: JB Lippincott, 1986. *(Additional coverage of subject matter)*

☐ Skiba DJ, Slichter M. Of bits and bytes. Am J Nurs January 1984;84:102. *(Additional coverage of subject matter)*

☐ Veatch R, Fry ST. Case studies in nursing ethics. Philadelphia: JB Lippincott, 1987. *(In-depth coverage of subject matter)*

Chapter 2

Nursing Process and Problem-Oriented Medical Records

On completion of this chapter the reader will:

■ Name the four parts of the nursing process

■ State the rationale for the use of the nursing process

■ Differentiate between subjective and objective data

■ Describe the collection of objective data by means of a physical assessment

■ Briefly explain and discuss *nursing diagnosis*

■ List and describe the five components of POMR

NURSING PROCESS

The nursing process is a framework for nursing action. This process consists of four essential parts: *assessment, planning, implementation,* and *evaluation.* Some authorities include the formation of a nursing diagnosis as a fifth part of the nursing process.

The nursing process is used to develop and implement an orderly, systematic plan of management (or care) that meets the needs of a specific patient. The various elements of the nursing process enable the nurse to do the following:

■ Identify the needs of the individual patient and his or her family
■ Establish priorities and goals
■ Carry out a plan of care and develop alternative plans of action in response to the patient's changing needs
■ Evaluate the results of nursing intervention

Although the four steps of the nursing process may seem somewhat difficult and cumbersome to use, they have applications not only in nursing but also in everyday life. For example, imagine sitting in a restaurant and looking at the menu (assessment). You then choose only those foods that are low in calories (planning). The waitress takes your order (implementation), and, while eating the food, you decide whether it is good (evaluation).

Assessment

Assessment is the systematic collection and analysis of subjective and objective data (facts). This information is collected to provide a data base, and is analyzed by the nurse to identify the problems that can be resolved or alleviated by nursing actions.

Subjective data are supplied by the patient, and include the patient's description of symptoms and feelings about the current illness. This information may be obtained from the family as well as from the patient or from the family alone when the patient is unable to communicate. *Objective data* are gathered by the nurse and other members of the health care team by means of observation and inspection (eg, physical examination, laboratory tests, other diagnostic studies, and ongoing observation of the patient).

Data base (or baseline data) is a term used to describe all the information obtained during the initial interview, examination, or contact with the patient. The data base is an integral part of the assessment process; it is the source from which the patient's initial and ongoing problem list is compiled. It also is essential to have baseline data as a standard of comparison during the patient's physical and mental status examinations. A change in the patient's status usually initiates a change in the patient's management. When no information (eg, no data base) is available for comparison, a serious problem can be overlooked. For example, a patient's blood pressure may measure 110/84 mmHg, which is within the normal range. If this patient's blood pressure had been 160/90 mmHg for the past 10 years as well as at the time of admission to the hospital, however, a reading of 110/84 mmHg would be cause for concern.

Collection of Subjective Data: The Interview

The initial interview, conducted when the patient is admitted to the hospital, provides information about the patient and his or her family for the data base. To illustrate, during the interview, the patient may describe the pain in the left leg as "deep and burning." This description becomes the data base for future evaluation of the patient's pain and for determining whether the quality and type of pain have remained the same or have changed.

In some hospitals, all or part of the subjective data are collected systematically by means of a printed form or guideline. If a printed interview guide is not available, it is helpful to develop a basic format for conducting the interview and collecting data.

The interview may be divided into three parts: the preinterview period, the interview, and the postinterview period (Chart 2-1).

Preinterview Period

Before the interview, the nurse should define, whenever possible, the areas to be explored, even when a printed interview guide or form is used. Some areas, such as a drug and allergy history, apply to most patients, whereas other areas that need to be explored often depend on such factors as the patient's age and sex and the reason for admission to the hospital.

Interview Period

During the interview, relevant information about the patient and the family is collected. The categories or areas that may be included in an interview are listed in

Chart 2-2. These general areas need not be covered in this order. Under certain conditions, it may be necessary to include information not specified in Chart 2-2 or listed on an interview form or guide. What is important is the nurse's ability to plan before the interview what areas are to be covered and to adapt and change them during the interview as the need arises.

At the start of the interview, the nurse must establish rapport with the patient or the family. Making the patient feel relaxed and at ease not only facilitates the exchange of information but also establishes a bond between the patient and those concerned with caring for the patient. The patient should be addressed by name, and the nurse should clearly state his or her own name at the beginning of the interview. In addition, sitting next to the patient's bed rather than standing at the bedside creates an atmosphere of ease and relaxation.

The next step is to explain the purpose of the interview. Although no general statements are applicable to all situations, the nurse should tell the patient that the information obtained during the interview will be used in planning care. The patient should also be told that all information obtained, although shared and used by members of the health care team, will be kept confidential. In some instances, the patient may request that certain information be kept from family members; this request should be recorded in the Kardex or on the patient's chart as well as mentioned to all members of the health care team.

Questions asked during an interview may be taken from a printed form or question guide or from notes prepared by the nurse before the interview. When printed forms are used, the nurse may present one question after another, rather mechanically, so that the interview seems stilted. To avoid this effect, the nurse

---

Chart 2-1. Three Parts of the Interview

Preinterview Period
☐ Define (or list) the areas to be explored.

Interview
☐ Establish rapport.
☐ Explain the purpose of the interview.
☐ Present questions.
☐ Terminate the interview.

Postinterview Period
☐ Sort out and analyze data to be used in planning care.

Chart 2-2. Interview Guide for the Collection of Subjective Data

Psychosocial History
☐ Age, sex, marital status, number of children, occupation, education, religious affiliation, living accommodations

Medical and Surgical History
☐ Prior medical problems, previous operations, drug history (including alcohol use, smoking habits), allergy history (drug, food, environment), dental history, physicians consulted for specific problems

Symptoms and Problems Before Admission

Symptoms and Problems at the Time of the Interview

should review the major parts of the form before the interview.

The information obtained during the interview can be divided into four areas: (1) psychosocial history, (2) medical and surgical history, (3) symptoms and problems before admission, and (4) current symptoms and problems (see Chart 2-2).

PSYCHOSOCIAL HISTORY. Part of the psychosocial history, such as age, occupation, and religious affiliation, may be obtained from the patient's chart. Some of the information obtained from the chart may have to be clarified. If, for example, the patient is a factory worker, the nurse may find it necessary to ask about exposure to hazardous chemicals, dusts, and other pollutants, the occurrence of past job injuries (if any), and the exact type of work performed. This type of information may be relevant, and may assist in formulating a diagnosis as well as affect the patient's care plan.

MEDICAL AND SURGICAL HISTORY. Some of the information related to the patient's medical and surgical history may be obtained from the chart. All prior operations, including minor surgery, should be explored in depth. Information about past operations should include the type of surgery, the year it was performed, the name of the hospital where it was performed, the name of the surgeon, and whether recovery from the surgery was uneventful or accompanied by complications. Depending on the patient and the information offered, it may be necessary to ask additional questions about a particular operation.

Past medical problems also necessitate extensive review. Questions should include the type of problem, the name of the physician who treated the problem, the treatment prescribed, whether hospitalization was required, and whether the problem still exists. As with the surgical history, questions directed to areas other than those mentioned may be necessary.

A drug history should be obtained in this part of the interview. It should include information on the use of prescription drugs as well as nonprescription (over-the-counter) drugs. Related to this history is the use of alcohol and tobacco. The drug history also should include questions about allergies to drugs as well as to foods (if so, which ones) and environmental factors (eg, flowers, trees, dusts, soaps, animals). When a patient offers information about an allergy to a drug, it is important to learn the name of the drug. If the patient or family cannot remember the name of the drug, an effort should be made to obtain the name from another source, such as the physician who prescribed the drug or past hospital records if the allergy occurred while the patient was hospitalized.

SYMPTOMS AND PROBLEMS. The patient should be encouraged to describe all symptoms or problems that were present before admission as well as those cur-

rently being experienced. Once a symptom or problem is mentioned, questions related to that symptom or problem are asked. For example, the patient may describe the abdominal pain experienced for the past several weeks. The nurse then directs the questioning to such areas as how long the pain lasts, what causes the pain, and what makes it better or worse. If the patient has had pain since admission to the hospital, questions are asked so that the current pain is compared with the pain experienced hours, days, or weeks before admission.

OTHER CONSIDERATIONS. Questions should be presented clearly, and the use of medical terms should be avoided. The patient should be given ample time to answer each question and not be rushed. It also is important to establish good eye contact with the patient and to glance at the printed form only when recording data or determining the next area of the interview. Observing the patient in this way enables the nurse to collect objective data such as facial expression, the tendency to hold the area of the body where pain is occurring, and other physical mannerisms.

The time required to conduct an initial interview varies. The patient's willingness to cooperate and ability to be interviewed are contributing factors. Realistically, not all patients can be interviewed extensively because of their age, mental capacity, or illness, or for other reasons. In addition, a patient may be uncooperative or may object to what he or she perceives to be an invasion of privacy. Each circumstance is different, and there is no one method of handling any problem that may arise. If one member of the nursing staff is unable to conduct an interview with a particular patient, another nurse may be more successful in establishing rapport with that patient. Another alternative is to present the problem during a team conference. Other members of the health care team may be able to offer one or more solutions.

There is no one way to terminate an interview. Summarizing the acquired information and thanking the patient for cooperating is one effective way of ending the interview. The summary should be a brief, general statement about the information obtained during the interview.

Postinterview Period

The collection of subjective data by means of an interview is an ongoing process. The initial interview provides a data base that can be expanded or changed. For example, several days after the initial interview, a patient may offer new information or recall information that was forgotten. New information often leads to further questions. Although the inquiry at this time is brief compared with the initial interview, it is still part of the interviewing process.

Collection of Objective Data: The Physical Examination

The second part of the assessment process is the collection of objective data by means of physical examination. The examination usually is conducted by following one of two methods: the systems method or the head-to-toe method. When the systems method is used, each body system (eg, respiratory, cardiac, genitourinary) is appraised separately. With the head-to-toe method, the examination begins at the head and ends at the feet. The head-to-toe method, with variations that may be mandated by the patient's general physical condition or symptoms, is normally used during the initial assessment. The systems method is used when it is necessary to investigate specific body systems. In some instances, parts of both methods may be used in the same physical examination.

Four basic processes are used during physical examination: inspection, palpation, auscultation, and percussion.

INSPECTION. To inspect means to look at; inspection, then, is that part of the physical examination that involves looking at the patient. A general inspection or appraisal made at the time of initial patient contact can provide an overall view of the patient. Inspection also is used when examining a specific part, such as looking at the skin of the legs for lesions or dryness, or examining the nail beds for cyanosis (bluish discoloration of the skin, nail beds, or mucous membranes because of oxygen deficiency).

PALPATION. To palpate is to feel. Some structures, such as the lymph nodes and the thyroid glands, are not visible, and therefore are felt, or palpated. Palpation may reveal the size of the structure as well as its general characteristics, such as smooth, nodular (having or resembling small nodes), firm, soft, fixed, or movable. Palpation also detects abnormal structures or occurrences, such as tumors, or fluid in a cavity. Some sounds may be felt through the fingers. They include some types of heart murmurs, murmurs within blood vessels such as the carotid arteries (thrills), voice resonance in the chest, and pulmonary sounds such as crackles, or rales (abnormal sound heard in the chest caused by air passing over secretions in the bronchi). Palpation also may produce pain or tenderness in a certain area, for example, the tenderness that may be elicited with palpation in acute appendicitis.

AUSCULTATION. Auscultation means listening. A stethoscope is used to auscultate certain body organs and structures, such as the heart, lungs, intestines, and major arteries. Some of the sounds perceived by auscultation are normal, for example, peristalsis (wave-like movements of the intestines). Other sounds detected by auscultation may be abnormal. The absence of sound in some organs or structures also may be abnormal, for example, the absence of peristalsis in the intestines. To recognize pathologic (or abnormal) sounds, it is necessary to know the normal sounds of the organ or structure that is being auscultated.

When an abnormal sound is heard, it is important to describe the sound. Some of the descriptive terms that may be used are *high-pitched, low-pitched, harsh, blowing, crackling, loud, distant,* and *soft.* How frequently the sound occurs also may be important (eg, the number of peristaltic sounds per minute when auscultating the abdomen).

PERCUSSION. Percussion is the delivery of a force to elicit a sound. The middle finger of one hand is placed over the area to be percussed; the remaining fingers of the hand should not touch the area. The middle finger is then tapped just below the nail bed by the middle finger of the other hand. The motion is in the wrist, not in the finger, and the blow delivered by the finger is direct. One or two taps are delivered, and then the finger touching the skin surface is moved to another area. The areas that are percussed are the chest (or thorax) and the abdomen.

Percussion may be used to determine the size of an organ, such as the heart or liver, or to produce a sound (resonance) over an area. A dull sound produced by percussion over a specific area of the chest wall might indicate pleural effusion (escape of fluid into the pleural cavity), whereas a general hyperresonance of the chest might be noted in emphysema (changes in the lung characterized by overdistention of alveolar sacs, rupture of alveolar walls, and destruction of the alveolar capillary bed). When performing this technique, it is important to note the type of sound produced: flatness (a soft, higher-pitched sound of relatively short duration), dullness (a medium-intensity sound of medium duration), resonance (a loud sound, lower in pitch and of long duration), hyperresonance (a loud sound, very low in pitch and of long duration), and tympany (a loud sound, distinguished by its drumlike quality).

General Appraisal

The first part of the physical examination is a general appraisal. This appraisal is made at the time of the initial patient contact, and includes observation of the patient's general physical appearance; awareness and orientation; mood; dress, grooming, and personal hygiene; odor; tone of voice and speech patterns; facial expressions; emotional state; posture; body movements, facial expressions, or speech that may indicate pain, discomfort, or a disease process (eg, the tremors of parkinsonism); and overt physical problems, such as lack of movement of a part of the body, difficulty breathing, jaundice (yellow coloration of the skin or the sclera of the eyes), cyanosis, and the wearing of prosthetic devices. During a general appraisal, the patient may be weighed and his or her vital signs may be measured (which also can be done when the respiratory and cardiovascular systems are assessed). In some instances, the patient's height may be measured.

Skin and Related Structures

The skin is inspected for the following: dryness; texture; elasticity; evidence of a loss of subcutaneous tissue; scars; lesions such as a rash, petechiae (hemorrhagic spots on the skin), warts, moles, tumors, ecchymosis (bleeding into the skin or mucous membrane that produces blue-black discoloration), crusts, scales, and ulcers; temperature; presence of edema (swelling caused by the collection of fluid in the tissues); color changes such as jaundice or cyanosis; and pigmentation. When applicable, the size and shape of skin lesions are noted.

The general shape of the fingernails and toenails is noted, and they are examined for clubbing (a curving of the nails caused by enlargement of the soft tissues) or spooning (a concave nail curve). The nails and nail beds are examined for cyanosis, and the nail edges for inflammation or infection. The presence of prominent horizontal or vertical ridges in the nails is noted and recorded.

The hair is examined for texture, color, and distribution. Areas of hair loss are noted. This assessment may be performed when the head and neck are examined. The skin also may be inspected when other body areas, such as the thorax or abdomen, are examined.

Head and Neck

Assessment of the head and neck may begin with the scalp and hair. The scalp is inspected as well as palpated for irregularities, lesions, excessive tenderness, excessive dandruff, and irregular patches of hair loss. The shape and size of the head are noted.

The face is inspected for any changes or abnormalities such as enlargement of the forehead, color changes or pigmentation, excessive hair growth or lack of facial hair, and lesions.

The external structures of the eye (upper and lower lids, eyelashes, cornea, conjunctiva, iris, and pupil) are inspected for infection or inflammation. Any lesions of these structures also are noted. The size and equality of the pupils and their reaction to light are determined. The ability to follow a moving object with the eyes, without turning the head, tests the integrity of the muscles of the eye. The cornea and anterior chambers of the eye are examined for changes, such as opacities or scarring, and the color of the sclera and conjunctiva is noted. If the examiner is skilled in the use of an ophthalmoscope, the structures of the internal eye may be examined. The patient's visual acuity may be tested, especially if an eye disease or disorder is present.

The lips are examined for lesions, peeling, or evidence of injury. The corners of the mouth are inspected for lesions or breaks in the skin. If the patient is wearing full dentures or a partial plate or bridge, these should be removed (if possible) before inspection of the oral cavity. A tongue depressor and flashlight are used to inspect the structures of the oral cavity. The general condition of the teeth and gums is noted, as well as the presence of broken or jagged teeth and inflammation, bleeding, or swelling of gum tissue. The tongue is examined for any abnormalities. The patient is asked to stick out his or her tongue and to move it from side to side. The floor of the mouth, the hard palate, and the buccal areas are inspected for lesions, color changes, and other abnormalities. The oral pharynx is inspected for inflammation, symmetry, and enlargement or displacement of structures such as the tonsils and uvula.

The external ear (the earlobe, auricle, and surrounding tissues in front of and behind the ear) is examined for inflammation, swelling, drainage, crusting, scaling, rash, or other superficial lesions. The areas around the ear are palpated for tenderness or pain. Using an otoscope, the external auditory (ear) canal may be examined for inflammation, infection, drainage, wax, and foreign objects. A general hearing test may be performed by determining the patient's ability to hear a whisper or the ticking of a watch or clock.

The neck is palpated for the presence of nodes, thyroid enlargement, and the position of the trachea (which should be midline). The left and then the right carotid arteries are palpated, with the examiner noting any difference between the two sides as well as any unusual vibrations in either or both arteries. The neck veins are inspected for distention when the patient is in a sitting position.

Thorax and Lungs

The skin of the chest is inspected for color and lesions such as rash, scaling, and scars. A general inspection of the thorax is made to determine symmetry and musculature. At this time the axilla (armpit) is palpated for lymph node enlargement. The breathing pattern is observed with the patient in a sitting position. Normally, the thoracic muscles control breathing; in some people, however, the abdominal muscles are used as accessory muscles when breathing. The intercostal spaces (between the ribs) are observed for bulging during expiration, which may indicate expiratory airflow obstruction such as is seen in emphysema. Retraction of the intercostal spaces during inspiration may indicate respiratory obstruction. If retraction is noted on one side only, this may indicate a hemothorax (blood in the pleural cavity), a pneumothorax (air in the pleural cavity), or some other lung disorder. At this time the respiratory rate and depth are noted. If the respiratory rate is irregular, the pattern of irregularity should be noted.

The thorax also may be percussed to determine whether areas of dullness, hyperresonance, or tympany are present. Auscultation of the chest for breath sounds is performed to assess the flow of air throughout the lung fields. When auscultating the thorax, the anterior, posterior, and lateral areas of the chest wall are examined. The patient is instructed to breathe normally through the mouth. Abnormal sounds that may be heard include crackles and wheezes. Crackles (also called *rales*) are fine or coarse intermittent sounds that occur when (abnormally) deflated airways are reinflated during inspiration. Wheezes are whistling sounds produced by the passage of air through a narrowed bronchus; although usually expiratory, they may occur on either inspiration or expiration. A loud gurgling or bubbling sound on inspiration and expiration may be heard in patients with pulmonary edema or in the moribund patient.

Vocal resonance may be determined by having the patient repeat the word *ninety-nine* while the examiner listens to various areas of the chest. A decrease in resonance may be heard in emphysema, whereas an absence of resonance over a certain part of the lung fields may indicate pneumothorax or atelectasis (partial or total collapse of the lung).

The female breasts also may be examined during the chest assessment. The skin of the breasts is inspected for abnormal changes such as dimpling and inflammation and for localized changes in texture. The nipples are inspected for color, discharge, and inversion as well as for similarity in size and shape. The breasts are then palpated for masses. The male breasts also are inspected and palpated for masses.

Cardiovascular System

The heart may be assessed during the examination of the thorax and lungs; other assessments of the cardiovascular system such as palpation of peripheral pulses and inspection of the extremities for varicose veins may be performed when those areas are examined.

Examination of the heart includes the measurement of the blood pressure in both arms while the patient is in a standing position, a sitting position, and a lying position; the radial pulse rate; the apical pulse rate (obtained by auscultation); and the auscultation of heart sounds. It takes considerable experience to interpret correctly the various normal sounds and to identify abnormal sounds of the cardiac cycle.

The size of the heart may be determined by percussing the anterior thorax. Normally, only the left border of the heart can be located by percussion because the right border lies under the sternum. Enlargement of the heart that extends beyond the right sternal border,

as well as left-sided enlargement, can be detected by percussion. This maneuver also requires practice before accurate results can be obtained.

Abdomen

With the patient in a supine position, the abdomen is inspected for the presence of scars resulting from surgery or an injury, rashes or other skin lesions, and evidence of rapid weight loss. The color of the skin is noted, since jaundice may first be detected in the skin of the abdomen as well as the sclerae of the eyes. The skin is then gently pinched between the thumb and index finger. When released, it should quickly return to its normal position. Tenting of the skin after release indicates a lack of elasticity, which may be seen if the patient is dehydrated. The abdomen is then inspected for any visible masses, which may be seen in the patient with a hernia or a large abdominal tumor.

The abdomen is then auscultated for peristalsis. Decreased or absent peristalsis may indicate peritonitis (inflammation of the peritoneum) or a paralytic ileus (paralysis of the intestines). High-pitched tinkling sounds indicate intestinal obstruction. Auscultation of the abdomen also may reveal abnormal aortic sounds, which may indicate an aortic aneurysm (abnormal dilatation of a blood vessel caused by a defect or weakness in the vessel wall).

The size of abdominal organs such as the liver, spleen, and urinary bladder can be determined by percussion. A normal-sized spleen cannot be percussed, but sometimes enlargement can be detected by percussion. This also applies to the bladder, which can be percussed only when it is distended. Abdominal percussion also can detect the presence of ascites (fluid in the abdomen).

Palpation is used to detect tenderness, pain, muscle resistance or rigidity, abdominal masses, and enlargement or distention of the bladder, spleen, kidneys, or abdominal aorta. It also can be used to determine the size of some abdominal organs such as the liver. Hernias may be located by palpation. All tender areas are noted. Extremely tender areas may be checked for rebound tenderness, which is pain that is noted when the fingers are suddenly released after deep palpation of an area. The abdomen of the obese patient may be difficult to palpate for the location of organs or masses.

Rectum

The anus is examined for the presence of external hemorrhoids and fissures (grooves or cracks). The skin around the anus is inspected for inflammation, infection, or other skin problems such as a rash or excoriation (abrasion of the outer layer of the skin). A digital examination of the rectum is used to detect rectal tumors and enlargement of the prostate in male patients. A stool sample obtained from the gloved finger used to examine the rectum may be checked for the presence of blood.

Genitalia

An assessment of the genitalia may be performed by the experienced examiner. Examination of the male genitalia includes inspection of the penis for lesions such as venereal warts (condylomata acuminata), the chancre of syphilis, carcinoma, and genital herpes. The urethral meatus is inspected for anatomic placement and evidence of discharge or drainage. A smear or culture may be taken if urethral discharge is noted. In uncircumcised patients, the foreskin may be retracted for inspection of the urethral meatus and glans penis. The scrotum is visually examined for inflammation, enlargement, and the presence of nodules or other lesions. It is then palpated for normal placement of the scrotal structures (testes and epididymis) as well as for identification of any abnormalities such as a testicular tumor or a scrotal hernia.

Examination of the female genitalia begins with inspection of the external structures (labia, clitoris, urethral orifice, and vaginal opening) for inflammation, ulcerations, swelling, or evidence of a profuse vaginal discharge. A vaginal speculum may be inserted to provide a direct view of the vaginal wall and the cervix. A sample of purulent material (if present) may be collected for culture and the cervix may be scraped for a Papanicolaou (Pap) smear while the speculum is in place. A bimanual pelvic examination may be performed by the physician to determine the size, shape, and placement of the cervix, uterus, and ovaries and to detect any abnormalities such as tumors or severe pain on palpation.

Extremities

The arms usually are examined when the thorax is assessed, but they also may be examined at the same time as the legs. Examination of the extremities includes inspection of the skin for evidence of lesions such as rashes, plaques, and skin tumors as well as for any other overt skin changes such as discoloration and varicose veins. Palpation of the peripheral arteries of the arms (brachial and radial) and legs (dorsalis pedis, posterior tibial, popliteal, and femoral) can detect any changes in arterial blood flow. Absence of a peripheral pulse may indicate arterial obstruction. The extremities (especially the legs) also are inspected for edema.

Musculoskeletal System

The patient should be directed to walk (if able) in a straight line for a short distance. Swaying, limping, inability to lift the feet off the floor with each step (eg, a shuffling gait), or a tendency to drift toward one side should be noted. Any unusual walking movement should be accurately described and recorded.

The shoulder, elbow, wrist, finger, hip, knee, and ankle joints are evaluated for range of motion. All but the hip joint also can be inspected for enlargement, inflammation, and joint deformity. Palpation (gentle pressure) of the joint is used to detect tenderness or pain.

The muscles of some areas usually are inspected during the examination of that area, for example, inspection of the intercostal muscles during the examination of the thorax or the muscles of the legs during the examination of the extremities. The muscles are inspected for signs of atrophy, which may result from disuse or a neurologic disorder.

Neurologic Characteristics

The extent of a neurologic examination depends on the patient's symptoms. In some instances, only neurologic screening is necessary. The patient with a suspected or known neurologic disorder requires a more extensive examination.

The mental status evaluation includes observation of the patient's general appearance and grooming habits, level of consciousness, intellectual function and competence, thought processes, emotional state, and memory. An evaluation of cerebral function may be made periodically during the physical examination, but it also may be conducted as a separate examination, especially when an abnormality of cerebral function is noted. The patient with a history of psychosis or with a disorder such as severe anxiety or depression may require an in-depth psychological evaluation.

Speech is a higher cerebral function that may be evaluated if the patient exhibits difficulty during the initial interview or any part of the physical examination. Speech abnormalities include aphasia (inability to use or understand spoken and written language) and dysphasia (impairment in speech usually caused by a brain lesion). Abnormal speech patterns include scanning speech (poorly coordinated speech with an abnormal separation of word syllables that may be seen in patients with multiple sclerosis or other neurologic disorders), monotone speech, slurred speech, and hoarseness. Stuttering and lisps also may be noted, but they usually are not considered pathologic.

Evaluation of sensory integrity includes tests for the perception of pain, heat, cold, light touch, and vibration and for proprioception. Proprioception (or position sense) is the ability of the brain to sense the position of the body or its parts when the eyes are closed.

Tests to assess the motor system include those that evaluate the patient's gait, reflexes, cranial nerves, muscle strength and activity, and muscle coordination.

The gait may be evaluated by having the patient walk normally. This may be followed by having the patient walk a straight line in a heel-to-toe manner (eg, placing the heel of the one foot against the toes of the other to take a step). A percussion (or reflex) hammer is used to check the reflexes. The reflexes usually evaluated are the knee reflex, the biceps and triceps reflexes, the abdominal reflexes, and the ankle reflexes. The response to percussion is graded on a scale of 0 to 4, with 0 indicating no response and 4 indicating hyperactive response. The plantar response (or reflex) is tested by stroking the lateral aspect of the sole from the heel to the toes with a moderately sharp object or the pointed handle of the reflex hammer. Normally, the toes curl downward toward the sole. An abnormal response (also called a positive Babinski) consists of dorsiflexion of the great toe and fanning of the other toes.

The 12 cranial nerves may be assessed during examination of the head and neck or during a neurologic examination. Testing the integrity of these nerves includes tests for smell (cranial nerve I, the olfactory nerve); visual acuity (cranial nerve II, the optic nerve); pupil size, constriction, and reaction to light and extraocular movements (cranial nerves III, IV, and VI, the oculomotor, trochlear, and abducens nerves); facial sensation, chewing, and corneal reflex (cranial nerve V, the trigeminal nerve); facial muscles and taste on the anterior two thirds of the tongue (cranial nerve VII, the facial nerve); hearing (cranial nerve VIII, the auditory nerve); taste on the posterior one third of the tongue, gag reflex, and quality of speech (cranial nerves IX and X, the glossopharyngeal and vagus nerves); movement of the trapezius muscles (cranial nerve XI, the spinal accessory nerve); and movement of the tongue (cranial nerve XII, the hypoglossal nerve).

Muscle strength is tested by having the patient push against an object (such as the nurse's hand). When evaluating muscle strength of the hands and arms, the patient is asked to grip the examiner's hand. Muscle strength may be highly variable, depending on the patient's age and sex as well as other factors. The strength of one muscle group is compared with that of the other; for example, the grip of the left hand is compared with that of the right. When performing this maneuver, it is important to know whether the patient is left-handed or right-handed, because the dominant side usually is stronger. Muscle activity of the limbs and trunk is determined by inspecting these areas and noting signs of muscle wasting (atrophy) or abnormal muscle movements such as tremors or fasciculations (involuntary contractions of independent muscle fibers).

Muscle coordination is tested at the time the patient's gait is observed. Additional testing may include the Romberg test for ataxia or muscle incoordination resulting from cerebellar disease. For this test, the patient is instructed to stand with the feet together, first with the eyes open and then with the eyes closed. Only minimal swaying should be noted. Falling or severe swaying with an impending loss of balance is abnormal. Muscle coordination also may be tested by having the patient rapidly perform repetitive movements such as tapping on the thigh or touching each finger to the thumb in sequence.

After collecting subjective and objective data from the patient, additional information may be obtained from the patient's family or friends. In some instances, such as an emergency admission by means of an ambulance, those in attendance at the time of transportation and admission may supply informative data. If the patient has had prior hospital admissions, those records may be obtained for additional information.

Analysis of Data

The data collected during the interview and the physical examination must be sorted and analyzed. Actual or potential problems are identified and then ranked according to priority. Analysis of the data also may identify the need for more information, from the patient, the family, or other sources.

Nursing Diagnosis

After the data are analyzed, the patient's unmet needs (or the patient's problems) are identified and the nursing diagnosis is formulated. The nursing diagnosis is not a medical diagnosis, but a description of the patient's problems and their probable or actual related causes, based on the subjective and objective data in the data base. The nursing diagnosis identifies those problems that can be solved or prevented by means of *independent nursing actions*. Independent nursing actions are those actions that do not require a physician's order and may be legally performed by a nurse. Two examples of independent nursing actions are feeding a patient and helping a patient get out of bed.

The North American Nursing Diagnosis Association (NANDA) has approved a list of diagnostic categories to be used in formulating a nursing diagnosis. Although this list may be incomplete and require further revision and refinement, it does provide a workable tool for nurses. Most authorities believe that the NANDA categories should be used whenever possible. When a patient problem does not fit into any of the categories accepted by NANDA, the nurse can use her or his own terminology when stating a nursing diagnosis.

An example of a nursing diagnosis is anxiety (the patient's problem) related to fear that a biopsy of the patient's breast might indicate that the lump in her breast is cancerous (cause of the problem). The anxiety caused by the possibility that a breast biopsy might reveal cancer may be more extensive, but it may have been the only cause uncovered during the assessment of this particular patient. Another example of a nursing diagnosis is constipation (the patient's problem) related to decreased fluid intake, lack of bulk foods in the diet, and lack of exercise (cause of the problem). In this example, the cause of the problem was revealed during the patient history, when constipation was stated as a problem by the patient, followed by questions regarding food and fluid intake, and exercise. Constipation also may be caused by an obstructive intestinal lesion, but the causes, as stated in the example, were the ones uncovered during the collection of subjective data.

Planning

A plan of action, or patient care plan, must be developed to meet the needs identified during the assessment phase. The patient care plan is a method of developing and providing quality care based on an individual patient's unique needs or problems. The nursing care plan involves the following:

■ Establishing priorities of care derived from the nursing diagnosis
■ Identifying short- and long-term goals
■ Formulating nursing actions required to attain the identified goals (nursing interventions)

Establishing Priorities of Care

To establish a priority means to rank a group of statements with the most important, serious, or immediate statement placed first, followed by the remainder of the statements in *descending* order of importance. Priorities of care are not stationary, and may change from day to day or even hour to hour. When a priority does need to be altered, the change usually is based on ongoing nursing assessments and the development of one or more new nursing diagnoses.

To set priorities of care, the nurse must look at (or analyze) the nursing diagnoses and decide which diagnosis should receive the highest priority. In most instances, the nursing diagnosis with the highest priority is the most serious or immediate problem that has been identified during the assessment phase. On occasion, there may be two or more nursing diagnoses that have equal priority at the highest, middle, or lowest level of the rank.

Identifying Short- and Long-Term Goals

Planning includes the identification and formulation of short- and long-term goals, which may also be stated as behavioral objectives or patient outcomes. These goals arise from the nursing diagnosis. An example of a *short-term goal* is the prevention of hypostatic pneumonia in a patient who has returned from surgery after cholecystectomy (removal of the gallbladder). Stated as a behavioral objective or patient outcome, this goal may be written as follows: The patient will demonstrate deep-breathing and coughing exercises during the preoperative period and perform these exercises during the postoperative period. *How* this goal will be accomplished represents the statement of a plan of nursing actions that will be required to attain this goal. In the example cited, hypostatic pneumonia can be prevented by (1) providing preoperative explanation and demonstration of deep-breathing and coughing exercises, (2) having the patient demonstrate these exercises during the preoperative period, (3) encouraging the patient to breathe deeply and cough every 2 hours during the (immediate) postoperative period, and (4) changing the patient's position every 2 hours during the postoperative period.

Long-term goals (or desired behaviors or outcomes) usually extend throughout the patient's hospitalization. In many instances, long-term goals also extend into the posthospitalization period. An example of a long-term goal for the patient with a cerebrovascular accident (CVA, or stroke) is the return of (full or partial) function to a paralyzed limb. One plan of action is to institute active and passive exercises of the affected (paralyzed) and unaffected sides. The realization of this or any long-term goal may take many weeks, and even extend beyond the period of hospitalization. In formulating a plan of action, members of the health care team are actively employed in the achievement of this long-term goal while the patient is in the hospital. Continuation of the original plan of action constitutes an important part of discharge planning and might include teaching the patient and the family the techniques of active and passive exercises.

The formulation of short- and long-term goals and the statement of patient outcomes must be *realistic*. Setting unattainable goals defeats the purpose of setting goals and creates frustration for the patient, the patient's family, and the health care team.

Formulating Nursing Actions

Once a problem is identified, a plan of action is put in writing (documentation) and the information communicated to all of the nursing personnel and other health care team members on all three shifts. This communication establishes a continuity of care.

Figure 2-1 is a sample of one type of nursing care plan. The patient's problem, the expected patient outcome (or goal), and the nursing approach (or nursing orders) are stated, a target date is set, and the actual outcome is recorded. The target date provides a

Name: *Mrs. Rita Willard* **Age:** *68* **Date of admission:** *11/10/91*
Diagnosis on admission: *CVA c̄ left-sided weakness   10/26/91*
Nursing diagnosis *Fecal incontinence, distortion of cerebration, immobility*
Goals: *Fecal continence c̄ bowel training program, orientation, increased mobility*

Date	Problem	Expected patient outcome	Target date	Nursing orders	Outcome
1/10/91	1. Fecal incontinence → CVA	Will move bowel movement each am	12/1/91	1. Offer extra fluids during day at intervals (q2-3h). Insert Dulcolax suppository ordered by M.D. daily at 8 am. Turn on side, place disposable pads under buttocks. Check q15M for comfort of position, B.M. Explain procedure each time. Offer encouragement.	12/3/91 — Has had daily B.M. between 9-10 am. most days since 11/26/91
11/10/91	2. Distortion of cerebration CVA disoriented to time, place. Disruption of sleep pattern (awake at night).	2. Will be oriented to (approximate) date, month, year.	12/10/91	2. Place calendar on wall at foot of bed; change date daily. All personnel introduce themselves by name each time entering room. Repeat day, date several X's daily.	12/6/91 Oriented to year, month. Recognizes and calls by name some nursing personnel.
		2. Will remain awake during most of day.	11/24/91	2. Provide frequent stimuli to help remain awake. Spread out patient care activities during day to provide stimulation and prevent prolonged periods of sleep. To dayroom in wheelchair 3 pm (with other patients). Encourage communication with others.	11/24/91 Remains awake for longer periods during day; sleeps 3-4 hrs. (uninterrupted) during night.
11/10/91	3. Immobility → CVA (at home kept in bed 24 hr./day).	3. Will become physically mobile by being out of bed in chair + moving to other area outside of room.	11/11/91	3. OOB in chair T.I.D. (physician's order) 10 am, 3 pm, 6 pm. Take to dayroom 3 pm-wheelchair. Encourage observation of outside by placing near window. Encourage communication with other pts.	11/12/91 3. Tolerates being OOB. 11/20/91 Staying OOB for longer periods. 11/24/91 3. Using left arm-hand more often when OOB.

Figure 2–1. Sample nursing care plan.

time limit for the anticipated patient outcome. If the outcome is not achieved by this date, the stated outcomes, approaches, and target date should be reevaluated to identify such factors as unrealistic goals, the development of other problems that interfere with goal attainment, one or more inappropriate approaches, or a need to change the target date. Reevaluation of the plan, and in some instances reassessment of the patient's problem, should point out the error and provide information for revision of the plan.

Alternative Plans of Action

Planning also may include the selection of alternative plans of action to meet established goals. Alternatives may be selected during the initial stages of planning, or they may be formulated when the original plan of action has been ineffective. For example, the original plan of action for the patient with a hip prosthesis is to return the patient to the home environment and to arrange biweekly outpatient visits to the hospital's physical therapy department. Alternative plans could include having the patient admitted to an ambulatory care facility with physical therapy services or arranging for a licensed physical therapist to visit the patient's home twice a week.

Short- and long-term goals, as well as alternative plans of action, may change. A goal that is stated on the day of admission to a hospital unit may need to be changed as the patient's needs and problems change. Planning is an ongoing process that starts at the time of the initial assessment and continues throughout the hospitalization period.

Implementation

Implementing, or carrying out, a plan of action is the natural outgrowth of the assessment and planning phases of the nursing process. Implementation may involve one or many members of the health care team, depending on the plan of action. For example, changing the patient's position in bed may require only one or two members of the health care team, whereas bringing about a partial or total return of function to a paralyzed limb requires the efforts of many members of the health care team—the physician, the nursing staff, the physical therapist, and so on.

Implementation also may include the patient, the patient's family, and, at times, the community. Using the patient with a paralysis caused by a cerebrovascular accident as an example, the plan of action may include teaching the patient and the family the basics of active and passive exercises. The community's role with respect to this particular patient may be the loan of devices such as a cane or a walker. In essence, all are involved in the implementation of a plan of care.

The final step in the implementation phase of the nursing process is the accurate recording of the patient's response to the nursing actions that have been carried out. This step is essential in maintaining open lines of communication among members of the health care team. A well-documented nursing care plan that clearly states what nursing actions are to be carried out, who is responsible for doing them, and how the patient responds is helpful to all members of the health care team as well as to the patient in their care.

Evaluation

Evaluation is a decision-making process by which members of the health care team, either as individuals or as a group, compare the results of the implementation phase with the stated goals.

If a stated goal was not reached, the following questions might be asked:

1. Did the assessment result in a correct identification and statement of the problem?
2. Was the planning realistic and effective?
3. Was the implementation effective?

Some of the causes of failure of one or more parts of the nursing process are the following:

1. The problem was incorrectly identified.
2. Information obtained during the assessment was incomplete or in error.
3. The goal was unrealistic.
4. The goal was not changed when the patient's needs changed.
5. The plan of action was incorrectly implemented.
6. The plan of action was not made known to or carried out by all members of the health care team.

Evaluation, then, enables members of the health care team to measure the quality of care that has been given. It is thus related to the concepts of quality assurance and professional accountability associated with current Medicare and Medicaid guidelines. The evaluation process also enables health care team members to restate goals or outcomes or to select alternative plans of action when the actual outcome does not correspond to the stated goals.

PROBLEM-ORIENTED MEDICAL RECORDS

The four parts of the nursing process—assessment, planning, implementation, and evaluation—require written documentation. Traditionally, patient care has been documented on the patient's record (chart) by physicians, nurses, and other members of the health care team, each using different sections of the chart. Thus, a chart contains the physician's order sheets, the nurse's notations, laboratory data, the physician's progress sheets, and so on. This method is called *source-oriented record keeping.*

Many hospitals now use a different method of documentation—*problem-oriented medical records* (POMRs). This system focuses on the patient's problems rather than on the personnel who are recording the information.

The POMR has five components: (1) the data base, (2) a list of patient problems, (3) an initial plan of management (or patient care plan), (4) progress notes, and (5) discharge summary.

Data Base

All of the information that has been collected about the patient is included in the data base—the subjective data gathered in the patient history and interview and the objective data produced by the physical examination, various laboratory tests and diagnostic studies, and ongoing observation of the patient.

Patient Problem List

The patient's problems, which are identified from the initial assessment (interview, physical appraisal, and so on), are listed on the patient's chart or Kardex. These problems are designated by numbers and are then referred to by number throughout the patient's record. In addition to the patient's medical problems, the problem list may include other relevant problems such as the following:

■ Social problems (eg, alcoholism or drug abuse in a patient or family member)
■ Health hazards (eg, cigarette smoking and working conditions)
■ Psychiatric problems (eg, acute depression)
■ Emotional problems (eg, adaptation to illness or disability)

Active as well as inactive problems are listed on the record. The problem list is updated as the patient's condition changes and as more information becomes available.

An example of how active and inactive (or resolved) problems may be written is shown in Figure 2-2. The patient in this example was admitted to the hospital complaining of rectal bleeding accompanied by constipation, and pain or discomfort on defecation. The patient was told by her physician that she has hemorrhoids that require surgery.

The patient's primary problem is written as "rectal bleeding → (resulting from) hemorrhoids." Two or more spaces or lines may be left blank after entering the primary problem to leave room for additional entries that relate to this problem. An entry identifying the surgery performed for correction of the primary problem was made 2 days later on one of the lines below the primary problem.

Constipation, and pain or discomfort on defecation were, according to the patient, caused by hemorrhoids. These active problems are identified as 1A and 1B. Additional information obtained during the initial assessment identified two active problems: diabetes mellitus and arthritis. These problems are assigned numbers 2 and 4, respectively. Although each active problem is given a number, this number is not necessarily an indication of the seriousness of the problem. The primary problem is listed first and additional

Name: *Janet Arnold*

Date	#	Active problems	Date resolved	Inactive or resolved problems
8/4	1	Rectal bleeding → hemorrhoids	8/6	
		8/6 Hemorrhoidectomy		
		A. Constipation		
		B. Pain/discomfort on defecation		
8/4	2	Diabetes mellitus – onset 1981		
8/4	3	Frequent noncompliance with prescribed diet		
8/4	4	Arthritis – onset about 1979		
8/4	5			Appendicitis/appendectomy 1964
8/4	6	——————→		Endometriosis/panhysterectomy 1983

Figure 2-2 Patient problem list.

Name: *Janet Arnold*

Date:	#	Plan of care	Time
8/4	2	*Urine for glucose & ketones*	*7:30 am, 11:30 pm,*
			4:30 pm, hs.
8/4	2	*Observe for signs of hypoglycemia*	*Throughout day, evening.*
8/4	3	*Note any pain or difficulty on ambulation.*	
8/6	1	*Control pain.*	*q 4h prn*
8/6	1	*Inspect perianal area & pack for signs of bleeding.*	*q 2-4h*
8/7	1	*Vital signs q 8h*	*Once per shift*
8/8	1	*Warm sitz bath*	*9/2-8*
8/8	3	*Encourage compliance with prescribed diabetic diet.*	

Figure 2-3 Patient care plan.

problems may be entered without concern for placing them in order of importance.

The surgical history included two surgeries, an appendectomy and a panhysterectomy. Both are *resolved* or inactive problems but are part of the patient's health history. When a resolved problem is identified during the initial assessment, an arrow is drawn through the active column leading to the entry made in the inactive column. Whenever a change occurs or new information becomes available, it is entered in the appropriate column. Although the format for listing and updating patient problems may vary, information similar to that described here usually is included when POMR is used.

Patient Care Plan

A plan of care or patient management is based on the identification of the patient's problems. Included in the plan of management are the treatment (or plan of care), patient (or family) education, and short- and long-term goals.

Figure 2-3 shows part of a plan of care for the patient with rectal bleeding. The numbers correlate each entry with a specific patient problem. As each new problem is identified or when a change occurs, the plan of care is updated. In this example, additions are made when the patient is scheduled for surgery as well as after surgery. Entries on the plan of care that have been carried out or are no longer in effect are deleted by drawing a line through them.

Some care plans provide a column to note the time of day when a single entry in the plan is carried out. In some instances, the space may be left blank, indicating that this particular task does not conform to a time schedule.

Figure 2-4 shows the patient education plan—in this instance, the discharge teaching plan. Again, the

Name: *Janet Arnold*

#	Discharge teaching plan
1	*Continue sitz baths at home.*
1	*Avoid rubbing rectal area with toilet tissue.*
1	*Report any problem to physician.*
1	*Do not self-medicate for future constipation (if it occurs).*
1	*Keep physician's follow-up appointments.*
4	*Check with physician about use of aspirin for arthritis.*
2	*Review diet, medication (oral hypoglycemic agent), general health principles.*
3	*Encourage compliance with prescribed diet; review options allowed in food exchange lists.*

Figure 2-4. Discharge teaching plan.

numbers correlate each entry with a specific patient problem. The entries may be written by the physician, as is the first entry regarding sitz baths, or by the nurse. If there is a question about the areas to be included in a teaching plan, the physician should be consulted.

The elements shown in Figures 2-2 through 2-4 may be incorporated in a single form or used in various combinations, according to hospital policy.

Progress Notes

Changes that evolve during the period of hospitalization are recorded in the progress notes and may be written in narrative form or on flowcharts. In the POMR system, the progress notes have a specific format that is referred to by the acronyms SOAP, SOAPIE, or SOAPIER (Fig. 2-5). The initials represent the following:

S   subjective data
O   objective data
A   assessment
P   plan
I   implementation of the plan

E   evaluation
R   revision of the plan (if necessary)

Discharge Summary

When the patient is ready for discharge, a summary of what has been done is written on the POMR discharge summary sheet (Fig. 2-6). This summary briefly states each problem and relates how the problem was solved or not solved. Note that the SOAPIER format is used in writing the discharge summary.

CONCLUSION

The nursing process is a framework that enables the health care team, as individuals or as a group, to provide effective patient care. It includes the patient (or client), the family, the community, and the activities of all members of the health care team.

The nursing process is a sensible, effective approach to patient care, one that benefits both patient and nurse. Once it is understood and practiced, many

---

Name: *Janet Arnold*

Date Time	#	Problem	Progress notes
8/5/91 4:30 pm	2	*Diabetes mellitus*	S– *"I felt lightheaded and dizzy and had to get back to bed."* O– *P. 102, R. 26, BP 110/91. Skin cool, no profuse diaphoresis, is alert.* A *Possible early hypoglycemic reaction.* P *Contact intern, stay with patient, observe for additional symptoms.* I– *Intern notified at 4:40 pm. Saw patient at 5 pm.* E *Symptoms relieved after administration of orange juice 200 ml at 5:10 pm.* *B. Ward RN*

Figure 2–5. Nurse's progress notes. A revision (R) of the plan was not necessary in this example.

Name: *Janet Arnold*

Date:	#	Problem:	
8/15/91	1	Rectal bleeding hemorrhoidectomy 8/6/91.	S— Admitted 6/1/91 with history of rectal bleeding for 2 months. O— Vital signs stable. No bleeding on admission. Following surgery mild discomfort controlled with Talwin. A— Pre-and postoperative course uneventful. Was relieved to learn bleeding due to benign lesion. P— Discharged to home. Instructed by physician to take daily baths. I— Instructed patient about keeping rectal area clean and importance of daily sitz baths. Reinforced necessity of follow-up in physician's office. E— Is able to describe methods she will use to keep rectal area clean. M. Wilson RN

Figure 2-6 Discharge summary.

nurses realize that they are using the nursing process already, in whole or in part, while carrying out their professional responsibilities.

Sometimes the detailed collection of subjective and objective data is neither practical nor possible. The basics of the nursing process can still apply, however, even though the technique must be tailored to fit the situation. The POMR method differs radically from the conventional source-oriented method of record keeping. Although some problems may arise initially with POMR, nurses are able to adapt to this method of record keeping.

Suggested Readings

☐ Alfaro R. Applying nursing diagnosis and nursing process: a step-by-step guide. 2nd ed. Philadelphia: JB Lippincott, 1990. *(Additional coverage of subject matter)*

☐ Bates BA, Hoekelman RA. Guide to physical examination and history taking. 4th ed. Philadelphia: JB Lippincott, 1987. *(In-depth coverage of subject matter)*

☐ Bowers AC, Thompson JM. Clinical manual of health assessment. 2nd ed. St Louis: CV Mosby, 1988. *(In-depth coverage of subject matter)*

☐ Carpenito LJ. Handbook of nursing diagnosis, 1989–1990. Philadelphia: JB Lippincott, 1990. *(In-depth coverage of subject matter)*

☐ Carpenito LJ. Nursing diagnosis: application to clinical practice. 3rd ed. Philadelphia: JB Lippincott, 1989. *(In-depth coverage of subject matter)*

☐ Grimes J, Burns E. Health assessment in nursing practice. Boston: James and Bartlett, 1987. *(In-depth coverage of subject matter)*

☐ Hagopian GA, Hymovich DP, Lynaugh JE. Clinical assessment: a guide for study and practice. Philadelphia: JB Lippincott, 1987. *(In-depth coverage of subject matter)*

☐ Iyer PW, Taptich BJ, Bernocchi-Losey D. Nursing process and nursing diagnosis. Philadelphia: WB Saunders, 1986. *(Additional coverage of subject matter)*

☐ Kim MJ, McFarland GK, McLane Am. Pocket guide to nursing diagnosis. 2nd ed. St Louis: CV Mosby, 1987. *(Additional coverage of subject matter)*

☐ McElroy D, Herbelim K. Writing a better patient care plan. Nursing '88 February 1988;18:50. *(Additional coverage of subject matter)*

☐ Merry JA. Take your assessment all the way down to the toes. RN January 1988;51:60. *(Closely related to subject matter)*

☐ Schamel K. How to assess the patient on long-term care. RN October 1987;50:65. *(Additional coverage of subject matter)*

☐ Seidel HM, Ball JW, Dains JE, Benedict GW. Mosby's guide to physical examination. St Louis: CV Mosby, 1987. *(In-depth coverage of subject matter)*

☐ Tribulski JA. Nursing diagnosis: waste of time or valued tool? RN December 1988;51:30. *(Additional coverage of subject matter)*

☐ Ziegler SM, Vaughn-Wrobel BC, Erien JA. Nursing process, nursing diagnosis, nursing knowledge: avenues to autonomy. Norwalk, CT: Appleton-Century-Crofts, 1986. *(Additional coverage of subject matter)*

Chapter 3
Care of Adults Throughout the Life Cycle

On completion of this chapter the reader will:

■ Identify physical and mental commonalities and differences at various levels of human development

■ Discuss the implications of physical and mental changes for the development of an individual nursing care plan

■ Describe and compare specific physical changes in the aging process and the effects these changes may have on the nursing management of the patient

■ Discuss the physical and emotional effects of the aging process

■ Describe and discuss the special needs and problems relative to young, middle-aged, and elderly people

■ Discuss the problems of the elderly person

DEVELOPMENTAL PROCESS

Growth, decline, change, and development—they are all part of the dynamic thing we call living. Some of the changes that people experience over a lifetime are described as *aging*. Every one does not age at the same rate. Just as the age at which menstruation begins varies, so do the ages at which changes occur later in life vary. One person may be mentally alert, vigorous, and active at age 80, whereas another person may be infirm at age 60. For purposes of discussion, young adulthood is that period when a person is establishing himself or herself, roughly between ages 18 and 35. Middle life, from about age 35 to 65, may be termed the established years. During this time of life, many people advance and secure their positions at their places of employment, become more involved in political, social, or religious organizations, and lead a more consistent life-style. Age 65 has become a common designation for the beginning of old age because pension and retirement plans normally start at this age. In some people, pronounced physiologic and mental aging may begin before age 65.

It is important to understand the developmental pattern of the adult, so that normal changes are not confused with the changes of disease. Some changes are obvious and familiar to all. For example, as a person advances in age, hair gradually turns gray and reflexes become slower. Compare the speed of a 17-year-old on crutches with the movement of an 80-year-old getting out of bed for the first time after surgery. If the nurse knows what to expect from patients on the basis of development and aging, a plan of care may become more effective and patient teaching more realistic.

Developmental Tasks of Adults in Our Culture

The infant has to learn to walk. One of the 6-year-old's tasks is to learn to read, and the adolescent is expected to establish relationships with the opposite sex that are different from those of childhood. In our society, the young adult is responsible for setting up a home and choosing a career. For the middle-aged person there is increasing community responsibility, and the elderly person shares with others the wisdom gathered over a lifetime.

Every stage of development has its own tasks—hurdles to be surmounted, things to be learned, changes to be accomplished. Developmental tasks are achieved most readily at certain ages; failure to accomplish these at the expected time may make their later realization difficult.

There is a progression in the scope of developmental tasks as the person grows from childhood to adulthood. For example, in adjusting to his or her body, it is the young child's task to learn what is part of the physical self and what is not (the toes are, but the toy is not) and to develop skill in walking, holding a spoon, dressing, running, and other activities. It is the adolescent's task to make a socially satisfactory adjustment to the maturing changes that are occurring, and to accept and use these changes. The adult's task is to maintain a healthful physical regimen despite the pressures of life and to learn what new motor skills are needed at work, at home, or in recreational activities. And it is the older adult's task to adapt to living with diminished strength and agility.

Many developmental tasks are *culturally determined.* In some cultures, when adolescents reach young adulthood they become independent of their parents, whereas in other cultures, young adults, even after marriage, continue to live in the parental household and obey their parents' wishes. Although our society places great emphasis on working, making money, and getting ahead, some people place a major value on enjoying each moment of life as it is lived. In planning health care, such differences must be taken into account.

Oversimplification of the concept of developmental tasks should be avoided. Adjustments must be made as each period of life, or each change in the environment, makes new demands. For example, a fear of being alone that is experienced in childhood may seem to subside during middle life because of close relationships with a growing family, only to reappear later in life when family and friends die or move away. Rather than view developmental tasks as achieved or not achieved, it is more accurate to recognize that people of all ages are in the process of realizing these tasks, and that the degree of success with each task may vary markedly at different periods of life.

Some Intangibles

Although the more tangible accomplishments of establishing a home and earning a living are easier to observe, the search for meaning, for identity, and for lasting values involves tasks that determine the quality of the patient's life and relationships. The degree to which one performs these tasks may influence one's response to illness.

Whether a person is successfully dealing with these inner tasks is likely to become evident in times of stress such as illness or bereavement. Some people are aided by a strong religious faith. Illness, aging, and the loss of loved ones raise fundamental questions, such as, "What is the purpose of my life?" or "Now that I am old and cannot work, of what use am I?" Some patients voice these thoughts to the nurse when given an opportunity; many patients do not ask these questions directly, but imply them by their attitudes and reac-

tions. The nurse sees people under circumstances that tend to reveal inner strength, or a lack of it. Just as it is important to accept patients whose values and beliefs are different from one's own, it also is important to accept the patient's progress, as far as the achievement of various life tasks is concerned. A patient who has been primarily concerned with superficial and unimportant events may continue to focus on them during illness. The nurse should respect this attitude and not seek to change it. If a patient wants to discuss some concerns about the meaning of life or about an illness, the nurse can help by listening and by displaying an understanding attitude. Some patients mobilize themselves after illness and misfortune; others do not. The magnitude of a person's inner strength may not be known until it is tested by an ordeal. This inner strength is related to the ability and willingness to withstand the pain and anxiety involved in facing some of the fundamental issues of one's life, and to accept help from others when it is needed. The patients to whom the nurse can be of most genuine and lasting service are those who can accept help and use it to strengthen their own forces in their struggle with illness or disability.

A person's ability to cope with illness depends on (1) how well that person has learned to handle stress, (2) the severity of the condition, and (3) the support given by family and friends. In some instances, the nurse may play a significant role in supporting the ill patient.

THE YOUNG ADULT

The young adult usually is physically more resilient than the older person. Two days after undergoing an appendectomy, the young adult may be able to carry out activities that the middle-aged patient who had the same operation must postpone for a week. Most young people have an emotional resilience that enables them to mobilize energy quickly after a shock or a loss. This does not necessarily mean that the patient has adequately dealt with the experience inwardly.

The young person also is more likely to have intact family relationships than is the elderly person. Many young adults maintain strong ties with their parents, even after they have started families of their own.

Because many young people have other sources of support and assistance, the nurse may fail to notice the ways in which young patients require help. Visits from friends and family may seem to imply that the young adult has many meaningful relationships with others. This is not necessarily so. The relationships may be superficial, leaving the patient very much alone. The nurse must not assume that young patients (or those of any age) who are surrounded by cards, flowers, and candy do not require attention to their physical and emotional needs.

The patient's resilience may be another factor that could deter the nurse from recognizing the need for a supportive listener. It is important to help the patient assimilate painful experiences. Too often family and friends discourage the patient from talking about the experience. They may be eager to forget an event that is painful for them too. Because the nurse listens, patients can be helped to review what has happened and to confront some of their feelings about an illness. Such nursing intervention may or may not help a patient deal with the experience.

The hospital is an environment in which authority and rigid adherence to a routine are much in evidence, and in which patients usually have little voice in making the rules. If young adults are hospitalized for more than a brief period, the rigidity of rules and authority is likely to become especially irritating. They may find various ways to express dissatisfaction, for example, by turning up the volume of the radio or television or disregarding the physician's orders. To whatever extent possible, it is important to include the young patient in the decision-making process, while making a special effort to interpret hospital rules to him or her. Even if rules cannot be changed, they are less likely to cause anxiety or irritation when the patient understands their purpose.

Relationships with physicians and nurses also can reveal to the young person that basic human questions affect people of all ages. Although one's perspectives on these questions differ with age, sharing views can lead each person to deeper understanding. The physician and nurse can provide experience with rational authority. The young patient may have viewed authority as essentially arbitrary and negative—inciting antagonism. Professional people, by the nature of their work, have many opportunities to emphasize the rational aspects of authority. The physician recommends bed rest, not to restrict the patient's freedom, but because the patient's condition necessitates it. The nurse encourages the postoperative patient to walk, not out of a wish to inflict pain, but because walking will speed the patient's recovery. Emphasizing the reasons behind the medical team's actions and decisions and avoiding the arbitrary use of authority may help the young person to appreciate the positive aspects of authority and discipline.

What of the nurse's own reactions to working with young adults? The nurse who is in this age-group may identify with the patient, which may be a problem if the patient has a terminal illness. Caring for a fatally ill young person is a stark reminder of the unpredictability of each person's life span. Working with young adults may make it especially difficult for a young nurse to keep professional and social roles differentiated. The older nurse may carry over to the patient past experiences of conflicts with adolescent children. For nurses of all ages, the challenge in caring for young adults lies in helping them to move forward with the developmental tasks of their age period to the extent that the illness allows, and in providing appropriate care.

Physical Changes

Between ages 18 and 20, after the rapid changes of puberty, a slow and barely perceptible decline in many physical abilities begins. At about age 20, the body and general appearance no longer change quickly.

Visual Accommodation. The ability of the eye to adjust to near and far vision is one of the reliable physiologic indicators of age. Children can see an object clearly when it is held almost at the tips of their noses. Even before puberty, this ability begins to diminish.

Changes in Hearing. Hearing is most acute at about age 14; thereafter it gradually declines. The ability to hear high tones begins to decline in childhood. Many people who are exposed to loud noise over a prolonged period suffer hearing loss. Those who work in areas where loud noise is unavoidable should wear protective devices over their ears. Such devices usually are supplied by the safety divisions of industrial organizations. Those who work in and around the home and are exposed to loud noise also should consider taking steps to prevent hearing loss. Exposure to loud music as well as the use of stereo headphones can cause *permanent and irreversible hearing loss.*

Position Sense and Speed of Reaction. Position sense and reaction time reach their peak between ages 20 and 30. Some youths think that their reaction time is faster than what it is, and attempt feats that are beyond normal capabilities.

Developmental Tasks

A task of young adults in our culture is to work toward independence and self-esteem. One achieves independence by gradually differentiating oneself from one's parents. To be successful in this endeavor, one must develop values and make decisions. An aspect of developing self-esteem is to learn to respect one's own competence. This, in turn, fosters respect for others and their competence; it also furnishes a basis for finding one's place as a productive member of society.

Young adults are expected to become independent

of their parents, to gradually develop a different type of relationship with them, one in which the young adults begin to accept the consequences of their actions. Such development does not take place suddenly; it has its beginnings when children are encouraged to make decisions on their own. Young people whose parents have helped them to gradually assume more independence usually find it easier to make the transition than those whose parents continue to exert strict control through late adolescence.

As a means of achieving independence from their parents, young adults are expected to learn a trade or a profession and to begin to support themselves. Learning a profession usually entails extended schooling and prolongs economic dependence on parents well beyond the point at which physical maturity has been reached.

Young adults are expected to make decisions, stick to them, and take the consequences. They should be able to face reality and differentiate between it and fantasy. Progress in this task, as in others, is achieved gradually throughout childhood and adolescence.

Implications for Nursing

Most people have been taught throughout their childhood to control expressions of strong emotion. Before surgery, children may plainly express fear, giving those who care a chance to offer reassurance and comfort. Young adults may be no less frightened but show their fear in less obvious ways. They, too, require reassurance, but sometimes it is harder to recognize their needs.

Because they are involved in achieving independence from their parents, many young people find it difficult to accept their parents' suggestions, even when the suggestions could prove useful. The nurse can be especially helpful to young adult patients by allowing them to express ideas and ask questions about matters that interest or concern them, and by conveying respect for them as individuals. Counseling in matters of personal health, such as the hygiene of menstruation or skin care for acne, is an example of the kind of help young people may seek from the nurse.

Almost all patients find illness frightening because it represents a threat to body function and body image. Young people who are still developing a concept of their physical self and working through their feelings about sex, illness, or the need for surgery can develop great anxiety. It is helpful to carefully explain necessary procedures and provide privacy when exposure could cause embarrassment. Such measures can convey to young people that the hospital staff is con-

cerned with their welfare, understands their feelings, and respects their right to privacy.

Growth as well as activity have high energy requirements; hence the caloric needs of those who have not attained their full growth are higher than those of older people who engage in the same amount of activity. Young patients may require a diet higher in calories, larger food portions, or between-meal snacks.

At any age, success in coping with a difficult problem can increase a person's confidence in dealing with similar situations in the future. Pain, fear, loneliness, and anger occur many times in the lives of most people. The young patient who is helped to deal with these emotions during an illness is prepared for future encounters with serious problems.

Creating a Positive Environment. Young patients with a chronic disease or a permanent disability are in danger of missing the challenges and learning opportunities appropriate to their age. The nurse might search for ways to change the environment so that they have experiences that are more typical of their culture. Are there courses that the homebound or hospitalized adolescent can take? Can transportation to an activity be provided? When parents, adolescents, and nurses plan and work together and community resources are investigated, ways often can be found to provide the handicapped young person with needed experiences.

Working With Parents. In addition to working with young adults, the nurse has a role in working with their parents. When young adults become ill, their parents can be greatly reassured by the nurse's explanations. Even though they share a home, communication between family members may be inadequate. This is often the case with adolescents and their parents.

Because of the tension and conflicting demands of everyday life, family members may not always be as perceptive of one another's needs or as generous in giving of their time and attention as they believe they should be. When illness occurs, they may express their guilt for such actions in such questions as, "Is this partly my fault?" and "Is there something I should have done to prevent it?" The nurse must allow family members and friends to discuss the matter but should avoid making any comment that implies blame. After the initial shock of the illness has past and the patient has received treatment, the nurse can assist family members to recognize ways in which they can help to prevent or promptly detect similar problems in the future.

It is important to help young adults deal with their illness, whether temporary or permanent, and teach them how to avoid unnecessary threats to their health. They will be better able to meet their individual health needs in the future if they have some understanding of their bodies' reactions in health and in illness. Understanding one's own illness is never purely an intellectual undertaking; it is a combined intellectual and emotional process that includes accepting what has happened and planning what to do about it.

THE ADULT IN MIDDLE LIFE

The middle years usually are characterized by productivity, self-satisfaction, and responsibility toward others. A change from independence and productivity to dependence and curtailment of productivity may constitute a major crisis for this age-group. To become partially or totally dependent on others, even for short periods of time, is often difficult for those accustomed to independence in thinking and actions.

Physical Changes

Strength. Change occurs continuously but so gradually that it often is not noticed. A particular event can suddenly bring the change into sharp focus. The loss of strength that may be revealed in an adult in his or her mid-50s has actually been taking place for two or three decades. This process can go relatively unnoticed until an event demands a physical response that is no longer possessed. Some loss of strength may be attributed to disuse, suggesting that regular exercise over a lifetime contributes to well-being. The middle-aged laborer may note less loss of strength than the middle-aged secretary who has spent much of her life sitting at a desk.

Height and Weight. Height remains constant until old age, when posture and settling of bones cause a slight decline. In contrast, weight continues to increase until about age 60. Usually there is a lessening of exercise and a slowing of metabolism without a corresponding decrease in caloric intake. It is undesirable for a person who has reached optimal weight during young adulthood to continue to gain weight during the middle and late years.

During middle life, there is a gradual slowing of metabolism and reaction time, as well as a gradual decline in visual and auditory perception. Other early signs of aging also begin to appear. These changes can be traumatic for some people, especially in cultures that attach great importance to youth and glamour.

Pace. During the middle years, the pace gradually slows. This modification by no means indicates "sitting back"; these usually are the busiest years of life, but there is a subtle change in the tempo of living. During active adult life, many of the extremes of physi-

cal strength are not required, and their gradual loss is scarcely noticed.

The ill effects of lack of exercise, particularly during middle and later life, have received increased recognition. Failure to exercise regularly may contribute to obesity, lessened efficiency of the circulatory and respiratory systems, and decreased muscle tone and strength. Rather than slipping into a routine that affords too little exercise, people who are in the middle and later years should regularly undertake activities that provide exercise as well as enjoyment, such as brisk walking, swimming, gardening, and bicycling. The middle-aged person who has not been physically active should consult a physician before beginning an exercise program.

Physical examinations in the middle years emphasize the detection of illnesses most commonly found in this age-group, such as heart and blood vessel disease, cancer, and diabetes.

Menopause. This alteration in a woman's reproductive activity normally occurs between ages 45 and 55, but this may vary considerably. Puberty is marked by rapid growth, the maturation of reproductive organs, and the development of secondary sex characteristics in response to the stimulation of sex hormones. Menopause, on the other hand, is characterized by the shrinkage of reproductive organs because of a reduction in the secretion of sex hormones. Ovulation and menstruation gradually cease.

This period of life may be difficult for some women, especially when the symptoms of menopause are severe. There is no physiologic climacteric or "change of life" in men as there is in women, but sexual vigor may decrease. The fact that menopause usually coincides with the growing independence of children causes profound changes in many women's responsibilities and activities, whereas men may continue to be very much absorbed in their careers during middle life. Contrary to popular belief, a marked decrease in sexual response does not necessarily accompany menopause.

Changes in Vision. Loss of visual accommodation, or *presbyopia,* interferes with reading, sewing, and other close work. Presbyopia usually becomes apparent between ages 40 and 50. A person can achieve artificial accommodation by using reading glasses for close work. Gradual decline in visual acuity also occurs, but significant changes usually do not appear until after age 40.

Changes in Hearing. Auditory acuity diminishes with age, and some people, particularly those in the later middle years, find that the decrease is sufficient to interfere with their communicating with others. Loss of hearing that occurs as a result of aging is called *presbycusis.*

By speaking slowly and clearly, the nurse can improve communication with the hearing-impaired patient. Patients fitted with hearing aids may need to be reminded to wear their hearing aids when communicating with others. The nurse should face the patient when speaking so that the patient can see lip movement and facial expression.

Developmental Tasks

Middle life is the period when society makes the greatest demands on people who are not only responsible for themselves, but also for the care of their children and often one or both aging parents. At this time people reach their maximum earning power and acquire most of their material possessions.

Adjusting to the Independence of Children.
It is difficult for many middle-aged parents to accept their children's growing independence. The necessary changes in attitude may be especially hard for the mother who does not work outside the home and whose entire life has been devoted to her children. Women who are employed may view the independence of their children differently from those who have remained at home. For these women, employment may provide involvement and a challenge during their children's transition from dependence to independence, as well as mental and emotional diversion.

Adjusting to Dependence of the Aged.
The increasing dependence of the aged presents strains on people in middle life, not only financially, but also socially and emotionally.

Because more people are living to an advanced age, when the likelihood of physical and mental infirmity increases, the middle-aged adult may become involved in the care of one or more aged parents. When the aged parents are living with one of their children, there may be two or three generations residing under one roof. This living arrangement often results in strains and conflicts between family members. The needs of the aged parents, which become more pressing as time passes, revive the old problem of independence from parents. This time the problem is set in a different context because the child is stronger and the parents are weaker, the child is better off financially and the parents often are less so. A middle-aged person may have difficulty meeting the needs of both growing children and aged parents.

At some point it may become necessary for grown children to place their aged parents in a nursing home. The children often feel guilty about taking this action, even though it is not feasible for them to care for their parents in their own homes. This guilt often leads them to express anger and dissatisfaction toward the nursing home and the care given. Understanding the purposes of various treatments, such as exercises, helps to lessen the grown children's tendency to view the facility and its staff with dissatisfaction. The reluctance that many people have in acknowledging the declining abilities of their parents presents problems in setting realistic rehabilitation goals. Having one's parents cared for in a geriatric setting need not mean the severance of close family ties or the termination of responsibility and participation in the care of one's parents. The nurse can help the family choose a facility that has well-planned menus, a qualified staff, and opportunities for rehabilitation and that is safe.

Observing the changes that occur with advanced age, such as forgetfulness, loss of physical strength, and diminution of vision and hearing, is distressing. For some people the experience of watching their parents age is so painful, particularly if the aging process is complicated by illness or marked impairment of function, that they find ways to withdraw from it. They may avoid visiting the parent or not give assistance that seems within their ability to provide.

The Single Person.
For a variety of reasons, some people never marry. Individual, creative, or religious fulfillment may best be served by remaining single. Many who remain unmarried develop a certain self-reliance that serves them well in later life. They tend to plan ahead and provide for the time when loneliness, diminished physical abilities, and a decrease in income occur.

Satisfactions of Middle Age.
Just as young adulthood has its satisfactions as well as its stresses, so also does middle life have a mixture of the two. At this period the person has a chance to reap the harvest of struggles to establish a home and earn a living.

Those in middle life perceive their own assets and can use them for the good of their families, their communities, and society, as well as for their own self-development. They can harness energies to accomplish goals that are significant and worthwhile. With a channeling and focusing of energies may come additional time for enjoyment.

Middle life makes many people increasingly aware of choices. Some of the choices they have made; others have been made by circumstances. If the direction of one's life is recognized as essentially consistent with one's values, middle life can be richly satisfying.

Implications for Nursing

A major problem that confronts a person who becomes ill during middle life is the change from independence and productivity to dependence and curtailment of productivity. This change creates problems at other age periods as well, but its impact is particularly severe during middle life.

When people become ill during the middle years, it is important to support their remaining independence and ability to make decisions and participate in planning their own care. Because the shift from independence to dependence is already a problem, it is particularly important to use nursing approaches that foster the degree of independence of which the patient is capable. For example, a man who is recovering from a myocardial infarction must rest. He must stay in bed and allow the nurse to bathe him. Such patients commonly express anger at curtailment of their activities and, particularly, at having decisions made for them. Suddenly, with the onset of an illness, the patient is reduced to the helpless physical dependence of an infant. One of the things a nurse can do for these patients is to allow them to make some decisions, such as selecting food from a special diet menu.

Sometimes those who work with the hospitalized patient forget that the patient is part of a family. It is easy for the nurse to sympathize only with the patient, since it is the patient's needs that the nurse sees, and to view the family in a supporting role. It is important that the needs of both patient and family receive fair and equal recognition.

THE OLDER ADULT

Associated with the physiologic changes of aging are increased susceptibility to illness and slowness to recover from it. In our society, many older people join the ranks of the disadvantaged with regard to family ties, income, housing, and opportunities to perform useful and respected work.

Caring for the aged is the responsibility not only of their children, but also of society. The view that families alone are responsible for the care of their aged members has resulted in outcomes that are tragic for people and, in the long run, for society.

It is essential for nurses to understand that responsibility for the care of an aged relative may significantly affect the lives of several family members. Nurses also need to recognize that their role involves helping families make their own decisions in these matters, rather than making the decisions for them or subtly influencing them about what course of action to take. Both the nurse who is quick to recommend a nursing home and the nurse who subtly implies that placing a relative in a nursing home is tantamount to abandonment are imposing their own values on others, rather than helping the elderly person and his or her family consider alternatives and decide for themselves what is best.

Sometimes the assumption is made that later life is synonymous with incapacity. The achievement of an older person often is received with astonishment. Such responses convey the idea that the significant part of life is over once one has passed middle age. They also can undermine the confidence and resilience of many older people who sense that they are not seriously expected to seek new experiences, whether in work or in personal relationships. The aging process generates many doubts and uncertainties about one's ability to support oneself financially and to find companionship and useful work. *Attitudes of younger people, including those in the health care professions, are especially important.* Young health care professionals can convey the idea that there is nothing odd or humorous about an older person's wanting to work or remarry and, particularly, not wanting to be overcome by surprise that important achievements can occur later in life. Instead of asking "Why, at your age?" health care professionals can ask, "Well, why not?"

With aging, people experience many losses—in personal relationships, income, health, agility, and opportunities to learn new things and to continue employment. Such losses should not be viewed in the context of the values and goals of youth and middle life, but *in the context of later life.* Thus, a decrease in physical strength or agility is normal at this time of life, and should be viewed as an expected change, not as a loss. The stark reality of physical decline must be seen from the perspective of the older person, not just in terms of measurement of the loss of youthful vigor and physiologic efficiency.

Physical Changes

Knowledge of normal physiologic changes that occur with aging can help the nurse plan for the care of elderly patients and assist patients and their families in coping with the aging process.

Nutrition. Nutritional deficiency may be a serious problem during old age. Weight loss in older people may be related to lack of dentures, boredom at eating alone, or lack of money. Chronic constipation also may be a problem. Diet planning for elderly patients should aim to limit calories to match lessened energy output but also maintain weight unless the patient is obese. Well-seasoned foods should be included because the sense of taste dulls with age. The older person requires a well-balanced diet that includes fresh fruit and vegetables, milk, eggs, and meat. There should be enough fluid and roughage to encourage normal bowel function. Many older people find that a light supper (perhaps of soup, cereal, bread, or fruit) is sufficient for them at the end of the day, when they are tired. Their heavier meal is eaten at midday. Serving unrecognizable puréed or ground foods insults the taste and the sensibilities of some elderly people; their intake increases when foods are offered in other forms, such as stews. The patient's appetite may increase when he or she is served food that can be eaten with a minimum of assistance. Patients who cannot feed themselves an entire meal may be able to eat a small part of it, provided the meat is cut, containers (milk or juice) are open, and hot beverages have been poured.

Position Sense and Speed of Reaction.
Position sense and reaction time decline gradually until about age 70, when the rate of decline becomes rapid. The deterioration of these two faculties, together with diminished vision, is a common cause of accidents. Many elderly people are injured in falls.

Skin.
Gradual changes in the skin and in the body's ability to adjust to heat and cold occur with age. The skin is drier and prone to wrinkling, and may become thin, flaky, and susceptible to irritation. The hair also becomes drier, thinner, and gray. Nails, particularly toenails, often thicken and become brittle as a result of poor circulation to the extremities.

During later middle life and old age, the body gradually loses some of its ability to adjust to extremes of temperature. It is harder for older people to keep warm in cold weather because their metabolism is slower, and they lack physical vigor for the strenuous exercise that would help them to keep warm. In hot weather, they do not dissipate heat as efficiently as younger people because the blood vessels in their skin may not dilate and their sweating mechanism may not function as effectively as it once did.

Elderly people must be encouraged to dress warmly during the cold months. An elderly patient may require an extra blanket as well as a sweater or other article of clothing around his or her shoulders. When the person is sitting in a chair, care should be taken to adequately cover the legs, shoulders, and feet. He or she should wear slippers and socks, if possible, because the floor may be noticeably cooler than other levels of the room or corridor.

Elderly people may not be able to adequately heat their rooms, apartments, or homes. Prolonged exposure to a cool temperature can quickly cause death because of lowered body temperature (hypothermia). Such deaths are not uncommon among the elderly population. To prevent these occurrences, the elderly person should be checked daily by family, relatives, or friends; loss of adequate heat in the living area requires prompt attention.

Teeth.
Because considerable individual differences exist in the resistance of teeth to decay, some people lose their teeth as they grow old despite good dental care. Others have almost all their own teeth. Older people who need dentures should be encouraged to obtain them, because the dentures will improve their appearance and nutrition. In addition, saliva production decreases, which may cause difficulty in chewing and swallowing some types of food and retard the initial digestion of starches by the salivary enzyme, ptyalin.

Vision and Hearing.
Visual acuity may diminish with age because of macular degeneration or other eye pathologies, such as cataracts.

Most people over age 70 have some degree of cataract formation, but cataracts may be seen in middle-aged people and newborns (congenital cataracts). Children also may develop cataracts as a result of eye trauma.

Hearing loss may begin during the middle years, but it becomes more pronounced during the later years. A person who has difficulty understanding all the words that are spoken to him or her or cannot hear low-volume sounds may need a hearing aid.

Other Physical Changes.
Other important physical changes occur with aging, including a considerable decrease in cardiac output, which in turn affects all organs and structures of the body, and in vital capacity (the amount of air that can be expelled after taking a deep breath). The older person also has a diminished ability to maintain homeostasis during stress and has less reserve energy to deal with exertion, infection, and fatigue.

A person's physiologic response to exercise changes with age. The circulatory system cannot respond as efficiently to the demands of exercise, because the heart and blood vessels cannot supply the muscles' increased demand for blood.

Developmental Tasks

Some people assume that there is only one acceptable pattern of aging. In our society, continued active involvement in work and family affairs is admired. Others adapt successfully by withdrawing somewhat from activities and relationships and investing more time and energy in solitary pursuits, such as gardening, reading, and reflection (Fig. 3-1).

Behavior that is considered maladaptive in one period in life may be an asset in another period. For example, those who were regarded in youth as somewhat distant in their relations may be able to cope particularly well later in life with situations in which they are alone a great deal. Conditions that for some older people might spell intolerable loneliness may

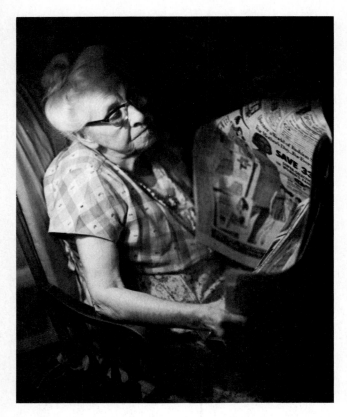

Figure 3–1. Many older adults remain active even into the late years, gardening, reading, and enjoying other hobbies. (Photograph by D. Atkinson).

for others constitute welcome relief from the pressure of maintaining close personal relations.

Coping with Dependence.

Many problems of aging revolve around dependence. People who live long enough become dependent on others, to some extent, for companionship, financial support, and physical care. The change from independent to dependent living usually is gradual unless, for example, a sudden illness renders a previously self-sufficient person dependent. Many older people find dependence on others difficult to accept, even though they may recognize the need for it. Some deny that they need any help, and occasionally jeopardize their safety. Others readily become completely dependent.

Economic Concerns.

One of the tasks of later life involves adjustment to decreased income. Many factors are responsible for the economic plight of the aged. Compulsory retirement has been an important cause. Although legislation has corrected the situation for some, others are forced to retire at age 65 or earlier because of serious illness or a chronic disorder, such as emphysema or heart disease. In addition to their disabilities, they must cope with a reduced income. The fact that more people are reaching old age means that the economic problems of this population are multiplied many times over.

The reluctance of some employers to hire older workers shows that the attitudes of society have played a part in the problem. The liabilities of age have been emphasized and the assets have not been recognized. Studies have shown that this stereotype of old age is not completely accurate and that some elements have been magnified beyond their true proportions. The time needed for recovery from accidents or illness increases with age. On the other hand, older workers tend to be careful, accurate, and dependable, although they also are likely to be slower than younger people, and sometimes have greater difficulty adapting to change. One brighter note is that more employers are beginning to recognize the value of the older person, and statistics show that more retired people are entering the work force.

Older people particularly need money to help them overcome or compensate for some of the infirmities of age. Their medical expenses increase, and they need to employ others to carry out tasks that are physically beyond them.

The enactment of federal legislation (Medicare) providing health benefits to the aged has been an important advance in helping the elderly meet health care costs. Medicare also has eased the burden on the families of elderly people, many of which formerly bore the entire cost of medical care.

Lack of money is not the only problem caused by retirement. Because work has absorbed so large a portion of most people's time and interest and has provided many contacts with other people, idleness, boredom, and loneliness often occur. A person may suffer a loss of self-esteem because the ability to earn has been removed.

Use of Time.

The problem of how to spend time looms large because there often is so much free time. During a person's working life, leisure after a day's work may have been highly prized because it was limited. Too much leisure may lead to feelings of futility and uselessness. The elderly person needs to have opportunities for meaningful, productive work and relationships. The eager response of some older people to opportunities to serve, such as by helping disadvantaged children learn to read, underscores the need for older people to occupy their time usefully and productively. Senior citizen centers and groups have helped some older people engage in meaningful social and recreational activities.

Coping with Loneliness.

The problem of loneliness is acute for many older people. In addition to lack of contact with coworkers on the job, separations occur among family and friends. Inevitably, one spouse dies first. Grown children may live at a considerable distance. Regardless of physical distance, the emotional and social distance between generations may be hard to bridge. Some older people outlive most of their contemporaries, and the physical difficulties associated with travel make it hard for them to see old friends or make new ones. Those who have cultivated an interest in activities that they can enjoy alone are in a better position to cope with the problems of loneliness than are those who have seldom undertaken any project or diversion by themselves. Tolerating and enjoying periods of being alone are assets at any age, but they are particularly important during later life.

An older person who has the capacity and energy to develop new relationships has an advantage in dealing with loneliness. Some older people seek out settings in which they will have more opportunities to meet people and form new friendships, such as retirement villages and senior citizen centers.

Securing Adequate Housing. Finding living accommodations is difficult for many older people from the standpoints of affordability and need for companionship. Lack of money forces many older people to seek less expensive and less desirable accommodations. Usually the new dwelling is smaller, and the reduction in living space makes it necessary for the older person to part with many treasured objects that he or she has accumulated over a lifetime. Older people sustain so many losses that they tend to cling to their possessions, sometimes hoarding objects that appear to others to be of little value.

Objects with which people must part may remind them of past accomplishments and relationships, and therefore are especially comforting to them. It is important that the elderly be permitted to keep as many of their treasured possessions as possible because these possessions provide a link to the past and a comfortable feeling of "belonging here, among these things." Because being surrounded by familiar possessions is so large an environmental support for older people, it is important to increase facilities for home care for the aged and to be as flexible as possible in permitting them to take some possessions with them if it becomes necessary for them to reside in an institution.

Small communities being established for older people combine a chance to live in apartments or small homes with such conveniences as an infirmary, shopping service, and recreational facilities. In all settings, there is a need to allow aging couples to remain together. Not surprisingly, the greatest need exists among those who are least able to pay for ideal retirement living. Some communities have established centers for older people that serve hot meals at noon and provide recreation and companionship.

Implications for Nursing

Attitudes
Nurses have varied reactions to caring for the elderly. For some it can be an unpleasant reminder that they, too, will grow old and die. Working with elderly patients may remind the nurse of troubling aspects of a relationship with aging parents. The physical appearance and limitations of the aged are distasteful to some nurses. These reactions may lead to avoidance of elderly patients.

Other nurses may respect and admire the elderly, perhaps in response to family teachings. The nurse who has idealized the aged, viewing them as benevolent and kindly and as generously sharing their wisdom with the young, also may do an injustice to elderly patients by expecting them to exemplify her or his ideal. Thus, nurses who have very negative or very positive feelings about aging may fail to take into account an individual patient's strengths and weaknesses.

One's views of aging can be made more realistic by remembering that many of the aged are a disadvantaged group in our society. They are disadvantaged in income, employment, housing, health, and companionship. Although such people may become more patient, tolerant, and generous, in many instances, the reverse is true; they may become selfish, resentful, and demanding. The latter characteristics, when observed, may actually reflect deprivation more than chronological age. In addition, some people simply are more pleasant to be with than others—a fact that is true during every period of life.

Teaching the Older Patient
Many older people believe, incorrectly, that at some point in life they lose the ability to learn. Encouraging self-confidence is the first step in helping these people to learn; it also is an important factor when developing a plan for patient teaching.

When teaching older patients, the nurse must convey the idea that they *can* learn. Often it is necessary to proceed more slowly with older patients, and to give them more time to think about and respond to new ideas. The nurse should speak slowly and distinctly to help the patient compensate not only for his or her slower reaction time, but also for any hearing deficit. If visual aids such as graphs, pictures, or printed material are used, the nurse should allow the patient extra time to study them. He or she also should make sure the patient is wearing glasses (if necessary) and that the lighting is good for reading. It is important to use materials that are clear, uncluttered, and large enough to be seen. If the patient's vision is impaired because of cataracts, the patient have need to have printed materials read to him or her.

The first step in teaching the older patient is to find out what he or she already knows by asking questions and listening to his or her replies. New material can then be related to that knowledge. Older people have accumulated a vast store of experience, and helping them to draw on it aids learning.

Physical Care

Older people have to adjust to their increasing physical limitations. Their need for help with self-care grows as their ability to care for themselves diminishes. The nurse must plan for this need and, before the patient is discharged, encourage the patient's family to do the same.

The prevention of physical discomfort is not the only reason for emphasizing the physical care of older people. Another is to help them maintain dignity and self-respect. Contrast the demeanor of the neglected old person with that of one whose snow-white hair is neatly arranged, whose skin is clean and healthy, and whose dress is attractive. One way to augment this concept of self-respect is to call each patient by name. Self-care is always encouraged.

Decreased circulation to the extremities may result in prolonged healing time for injuries or infections. The skin on the legs and feet usually is very dry, and cream or lotion should be applied after bathing. Thickened, brittle toenails, which also may be seen in those with poor circulation to the extremities, should be carefully trimmed, a little at a time. Toenails can be softened by soaking the patient's feet in water. Very thick nails that have been neglected may require the attention of a podiatrist. If the patient's feet are cold, loose socks and extra blankets may help to warm them.

A cream, emollient, or lanolin lotion can be used for back and skin care. Bathing frequently in very warm water dries the skin; instead of daily tub baths, the patient may have a partial bath daily and a tub bath several times a week. All the soap must be rinsed off the skin to prevent irritation. Friction from clothing and bedding should be minimized; the sleeves on the patient's gown can be drawn over the patient's elbows to decrease irritation caused by rubbing against the sheets.

Bath oils may be ordered and added to the water to relieve dry, itching skin. When oil is used in a tub bath, the patient *must* be assisted in getting in and out of the tub.

A stall shower, when available, usually is desirable because it avoids the need to step over the tub and then lower oneself into the tub. For those who are weak and unsteady, a chair may be placed in the shower so that they can be seated while bathing. The shower provides the most thorough rinsing of soap from the skin, thus helping to minimize skin irrita-

tions. Whatever method of bathing is used, particular care must be taken to ensure privacy, since many older people are distressed when they cannot maintain their usual standards of personal modesty.

Dentures require regular cleaning and brushing. If removed, they should be stored in an opaque, covered jar. The patient should be instructed not to roll them in tissues because this way they can easily be lost. When cleaning dentures, they should be placed in a small basin in a sink. Because they can easily be dropped and broken, they should not be held directly over the sink.

Some older patients require a soft diet and foods that are easy to digest. Chewing may be difficult for some patients because of diminished saliva production or improperly fitted dentures; such patients require more time to eat.

Some older women have a vaginal discharge, or incontinence of urine when they cough or sneeze (stress incontinence). The vaginal mucous membrane becomes thin and subject to infection when a woman reaches old age. If the nurse or family member detects this problem, the physician should be consulted; a cleansing douche or oral medication may be ordered. The patient can be kept clean and comfortable by means of good perineal care and the use of disposable pads.

Bowel and urinary elimination may pose problems in the elderly. Frequency of urination is not uncommon and should be reported to the physician. Many older men have enlarged prostates, whereas many older women have relaxation of perineal structures with less efficient emptying of the bladder. Care must be taken to prevent falls when the patient gets up during the night to urinate. Make sure the call button is nearby so that the patient can obtain assistance. For those who are unable to wait for assistance, the bedpan or urinal may be left within easy reach. Some older people are constipated. This problem is more likely to occur in those who cannot get up and move around, who fail to drink sufficient fluids, or whose diet lacks sufficient bulk. Helping the patient to maintain adequate dietary and fluid intake and to have a regular time for evacuation may eliminate chronic constipation. Enemas, mild laxatives, or stool softeners may be ordered by the physician if other methods of relieving constipation are ineffective.

Being confined to bed can have other adverse effects on older people. They expand their chests less fully because of a loss of elasticity of the structures that increase and decrease the size of the thoracic cavity. Confinement to bed accentuates this problem and often leads to the development of hypostatic pneumonia (pneumonia that occurs as a result of prolonged bed rest with failure to cough, move, and breathe deeply).

Decubitus ulcers (bedsores) are common among the aged because of the diminished ability of the skin and subcutaneous tissues to tolerate pressure. Decreased circulation to the brain may cause disorientation. Muscle tone is readily lost during prolonged bed rest; extreme weakness often results and is difficult to overcome. In view of these complications, physicians usually permit elderly patients out of bed as soon as and as often as possible. Patients are encouraged to take a few steps with help and gradually increase their activities.

Older patients are slower in their movements and responses. Attempts to make them hurry often results in confusion, irritation, and accidents. For instance, if the patient eats slowly, his or her tray is served first and collected last. The thoughtful nurse prepares everything patients require for self-care and then lets them proceed at their own pace to complete those aspects of care that they can perform. Explanations of tests and treatments should be made slowly and, if necessary, be repeated.

Even comparatively minor illnesses or injuries can have serious consequences for older people because they can tip the already precarious balance between independence and dependence. Many older people unnecessarily give up some of their usual activities because others are too quick to assume that they will never be able to resume these activities.

Hospital Care

The nurse can make adaptation to the hospital environment easier and less hazardous for elderly patients. Beds that are left in a high position are a potential danger, since older people may misjudge the distance to the floor and fall when getting out of bed. The bed should be left in the low position except when direct nursing care is being administered. A dim light left on during the night may help the patient become oriented to the surroundings and prevent them from falling or tripping over room objects when getting out of bed. The need for raising the side rails during the night should be explained to the patient, and the call button made readily available.

The elderly usually require less sleep, which may present a problem when a hospital room is shared with others. Keeping these patients awake and interested during the day may help them to sleep better at night.

Nighttime confusion and disorientation are common among the elderly, particularly when they are moved from familiar surroundings to a hospital or nursing home. These episodes of confusion, which are likely to occur at night, are disturbing to the patient and to others and are hazardous to the patient's safety. Unfortunately, this problem is commonly mismanaged, and the patient becomes more confused and disturbed.

The initial reaction to these patients may be to control them and lessen the noise they make by taking various measures, such as scolding. Sometimes restraints are quickly applied before other measures are tried; these devices may increase the patient's agitation, anxiety, and confusion. Sedatives and hypnotics, even when administered in low doses, can result in wakefulness, excitement, and confusion.

The nurse should try to determine the cause of the confusion and then attempt to reduce or eliminate it. Elderly patients should be checked frequently during the night, especially when they are noisy or waken many times. Such checking may help to determine what is keeping them awake. Touching and talking to them or adjusting a pillow or blanket might be all that is needed to calm them; on the other hand, being near or touching these people may aggravate their confusion. Some patients remain noisy and confused despite all efforts, but others try to communicate something without being able to state the problem—the need to

Chart 3–1.   Reality Orientation

Beginning

- ☐ The date is prominently displayed on a sheet of paper placed in the patient's line of vision or on a blackboard situated in the solarium or day-room: "Today is Sunday, January 21, 1991."
- ☐ Each time a nurse or nurse assistant enters the room or gives bedside care (bath, medications, linen change), identification is made: "Hello, Mrs. Green, I'm Mrs. Wilson, your nurse." This is repeated until the patient can identify the nurse by name.
- ☐ The time of day is stated: "Mrs. Green, it's 2 o'clock and time for your pill."

Progressive

- ☐ The patient is given portions of current newspapers or magazines, starting with one or two pages or pictures and increasing gradually.
- ☐ A large clock on the wall is used for orientation to time, and a large calendar for day and date (a calendar that shows one page per day is preferred). Personnel should draw the patient's attention to both.
- ☐ Current events are discussed: changes in the weather, major elections, sports events, and other things of interest to a particular patient. Discussions should become more detailed as orientation increases.
- ☐ Happenings in the patient's life are compared from day to day.
- ☐ Television and radio are used to provide news, weather reports, and entertainment. A routine of daily programs provides continuity and encourages recall of recent events.
- ☐ Social interaction with other patients is encouraged, as are hobbies, cards, and group and individual projects.

use a urinal, the discomfort of constipation, being too hot or too cold, fear, or loneliness.

Measures to help elderly patients maintain contact with reality are necessary at any time and, to some extent, prevent episodes of acute confusion. Elderly, confused patients may benefit from *reality orientation* (Chart 3-1).

There is no quicker way for older people to lose their ability to care for themselves than to be treated as though this capacity has been lost. If the nurse performs activities of daily living for these patients, *when they are capable of performing these activities without help*, they may think that they are no longer considered capable of managing such tasks. Giving up these self-care functions, which would help them to maintain some privacy, independence, and contact with reality, leads to an unnecessary dependence on others as well as a loss of self-esteem.

Communication

An important aspect of encouraging communication during hospitalization involves accepting the desire of older people to talk about experiences and events that took place during a more interesting time of their lives. They often have a need to talk about past events, achievements, and losses. Allowing them time to reminisce may encourage further communication between patient, health care personnel, and the family.

Conclusion

When we recognize that older people have something valuable to contribute at home, at work, and in the community, we can be proud to have a part in helping them to maintain their health and continue to make individual and unique contributions as long as possible.

General Nutritional Considerations

Early Years
- ☐ Eating habits may be irregular, and the patient may not be hungry when a meal is served. He or she may desire snacks that may not be available because of dietary restrictions.
- ☐ Food preferences may lean toward "empty" calories rather than a well-balanced diet. The patient may need to be taught good eating habits.
- ☐ Fad dieting may result in various dietary deficiencies.
- ☐ Certain deficiencies, such as a vitamin C (ascorbic acid) deficiency, may interfere with the healing process.
- ☐ Caloric needs are greater; therefore, portions may need to be larger and snacks offered to meet the patient's caloric requirements.
- ☐ Eating habits may be established. The patient may find it difficult to adjust to hospital food or special diets.
- ☐ The patient may need counseling on nutrition from the dietitian or nurse.

Middle Years
- ☐ Food patterns and eating habits are definitely established, making it difficult for some patients to accept special diets or dietary restrictions.
- ☐ The overweight middle-aged adult may have tried fad diets, with uncertain results.

Late Years
- ☐ The eating habits of the elderly may be determined by such factors as limited income, inadequate cooking facilities, and poor dentition.
- ☐ A dietary deficiency may complicate medical or surgical problems.
- ☐ The general physical condition of the patient may affect digestion and absorption of food.
- ☐ Food preferences may be hard to change, making special diets or regulation of food intake difficult.

General Pharmacologic Considerations

- ☐ All patients who take medication after discharge from the hospital should be cautioned on the use of any drug—prescription or nonprescription—unless ordered by the physician. Interactions of various drugs may cause serious adverse effects.

☐ Patients should thoroughly understand drug use: quantity of the drug (number of capsules or tablets, amount of liquid), the time it is to be taken (eg, 10 A.M. and 2 P.M.), and any instruction relating to a specific drug.

☐ Sedatives and hypnotics, even in low doses, can cause wakefulness, excitement, and confusion in *any* patient, particularly in the elderly.

☐ Because drugs are excreted more slowly by the elderly patient, lower doses of many pharmacologic agents, particularly narcotics, sedatives, hypnotics, and other central nervous system depressants, may be necessary. In some instances, toxicity may result when normal doses are administered.

Suggested Readings

☐ Andersen GP. A fresh look at assessing the elderly. RN June 1989;52:28. *(Additional coverage of subject matter)*

☐ Burtis G, Davis J, Martin S. Applied nutrition and diet therapy. Philadelphia: WB Saunders, 1988. *(Additional and in-depth coverage of subject matter)*

☐ Carroll M, Brue IJ. A nurse's guide to caring for elders. New York: Springer Publishing, 1988. *(Additional coverage of subject matter)*

☐ Dudek, SG. Nutrition handbook for nursing practice. Philadelphia: JB Lippincott, 1987. *(Additional and in-depth coverage of subject matter)*

☐ Fuller J, Schaller-Ayers J. Health assessment: a nursing approach. Philadelphia: JB Lippincott, 1990. *(Additional and in-depth coverage of subject matter)*

☐ Hogstel MO (ed). Nursing care of the older adult. New York: John Wiley & Sons, 1989. *(Additional and in-depth coverage of subject matter)*

☐ Kohut S, Kohut J, Fleishman JJ. Reality orientation for the elderly. 3rd ed. Oradell, NJ: Medical Economics, 1987. *(Additional and in-depth coverage of subject matter)*

Chapter 4
Nurse–Patient Relationships

On completion of this chapter the reader will:

- Describe and discuss the essential components of and guidelines for nurse–patient relationships

- Discuss frustration, anxiety, fear, anger, conflict, and grief and how the nurse can work with the patient who is experiencing these emotions

- Understand how to provide emotional support to the patient who is undergoing tests and treatments

- Discuss the implications of sustained nurse–patient relationships

- Understand the problems involved in giving nursing care to the patient who is physically unattractive

- List the essentials of teaching the self-care patient who is undergoing diagnostic tests

- Discuss the problems encountered with the patient who refuses treatment

- Evaluate interventions and relationships of the patient's family in the clinical area

Some basic guidelines for nurse–patient relationships are as follows:

1. The nurse should be sincere. Sick people are perceptive, anxious, and suspicious, even if they do not show it. If they think that the nurse is open and forthright, they are more trusting.

2. Small points of care are important. Reactions to something as personal as illness are not always logical or rational. The fact of recovering from an illness may be lost in the little annoyance of being served cold coffee. If patients recognize interest and concern for their welfare and comfort, they are less likely to become angry.

3. The nurse should evaluate her or his relationships with patients. She or he should not rush in with too many busy activities at once, unless they are of vital importance, and should learn to look at and evaluate the patient. What is the patient's general condition? What is he or she expressing? Is he or she in pain? Does the patient seem to be resigned or apprehensive?

4. Besides giving expert technical care, there are several ways in which the nurse can help patients. One way is to help them gather as many facts as possible about their situation so that they can make reasonable decisions. Another way is to teach them new skills they can use to help them live with or recover from their illness. Of particular importance to patients is the nurse's support as they go through the various stages of illness and recovery.

5. If the patient asks no questions or appears reticent to discuss concerns or feelings, the nurse should not pry. On the other hand, the nurse should never assume that the quiet patient has no problem or understands everything that she or he has been told. It is best not to urge discussion on the unwilling patient.

6. The nurse should avoid trivial statements such as, "Don't worry" and "Everything will be all right" because they may be interpreted as "I don't want to hear about your troubles." If a patient expresses concerns, is worried, or does not feel well, it may open the door to further discussion and an expression of feelings. If the nurse unperceptively pushes aside a remark by saying something like, "Everything will be fine," it may appear that the nurse is avoiding involvement or is not concerned with the patient's problems.

7. The nurse should never talk down to a patient. She or he should avoid using such patronizing expressions as, "How are 'we' feeling today?"

8. The nurse should never give patients the kind of attention that retards their ability to become involved in their own care. Doing too much for patients can be as harmful as doing too little. Patients should be given opportunities to make certain decisions, such as when they would prefer to be out of bed. Encouraging participation in the activities of daily living helps patients move from a state of dependence to one of independence.

9. When patients are angry, the nurse should allow them to express their emotions. It also is important to find out why they are angry, rather than ignore their anger or argue with them over a situation.

A general knowledge of nurse–patient relationships can be adapted to the particular requirements of medical–surgical patients.

1. Each patient is a *unique person,* and therefore is different from all other patients.
2. In most instances, medical–surgical patients have sought care for some physical condition that may or may not be aggravated or caused by emotional stress. Keeping in mind that their attention usually is focused on their physical condition and that they are not primarily concerned with solving personal problems helps to set the tone for the nurse–patient relationship. The nurse's ability to give emotional support is enhanced by the knowledge of why treatment is being sought.
3. In caring for medical–surgical patients, the nurse must consider their physical care as well as their emotional reactions to illness and treatment.
4. *Listening is a important part of nursing care.* What patients say may give clues to their physical and mental condition.
5. The manner in which physical care is administered is important. Touch should be gentle, not rough.
6. Frightening and painful procedures are common on medical–surgical units. Although at first the nurse is a stranger to the patient, the stress of such experiences as undergoing surgery can lead the patient to rely on the nurse for emotional support.
7. There is an enormous variety among medical–surgical patients in terms of such factors as age, diagnosis, and degree of illness. Some patients are helpless; others seem able to care for themselves; some readily express personal feelings; others are reticent.

SOME BASIC CONCEPTS

In the following sections, fear, anxiety, frustration, anger, conflict, and grief are discussed.

Fear

Fear is an emotional and physical reaction to danger. The danger may be real or imagined. People who are afraid usually can identify the cause of their fear. Knees may tremble after a narrow escape from an auto crash; trembling and a pounding heart are normal physiologic reactions to danger. The ill patient may have many fears, some of which are real. Other fears the patient has may be imagined or at times exaggerated.

Fear of the Unknown. This is the most intense, and probably the worst, fear a person can experience. This type of fear may be experienced by a patient who is scheduled for a procedure that has not been explained to him or her and who has not had an opportunity to ask questions. Sometimes the nurse can alleviate a patient's fear of the unknown by reassuring the patient as well as through patient teaching. In other instances, it may be impossible to relieve this type of fear, despite efforts by members of the health care team.

Fear of Disfigurement or Alteration in Body Image. Patients may be concerned with the outcome of a surgical or medical procedure and how it will (or might) change their appearance. They also may have fears concerning their relationships with family, friends, and the general public. For example, a patient with scars and disfigurement caused by severe burns may fear going to public places.

Fear of Pain and Suffering. Patients may experience this type of fear when told of a certain diagnosis or that surgery must be performed. When they express these concerns, reassuring them that pain will be controlled may help to dispel this fear. They should be encouraged to vent their feelings about their surgery or diagnosis, as discussion of the problem may give insight into other fears they may have.

Fear of Abandonment. Patients may express concern about their relationships with family and friends during an illness. Although many family members and friends show concern, there are others who are afraid to deal with an ill family member. Patients may think that they are, or may become, a burden to their spouses or children. They also may fear that their needs will not be met by members of the health care team.

Fear of Death. Fear of death also is a fear of the unknown. It is normal for patients—even those hospitalized for minor surgery—to have a fear of dying.

Fear of Separation. Many patients are greatly concerned about being separated from family and friends because of their hospitalization.

Fear of Being Unable to Make Decisions. A patient may fear being unable, at some time in the future, to make certain decisions regarding recommended treatments or surgery. This fear is more common among young and middle-aged adults, but it also can be experienced by older patients.

Anxiety

Anxiety is an emotional response to a threat to one's self-esteem or well-being. Threats to survival, whether physical survival or survival as an integrated personality, elicit profound anxiety.

Anxiety is somewhat different from fear, but these terms often are used interchangeably. In some people, a specific fear may result in anxiety, and the two emotions may coexist. For example, many patients have a fear of pain, which causes them to feel anxious. In anxiety, the external circumstance may not be clearly identified. People may feel uneasy or have a general sense of impending unpleasantness or disaster for no known reason. Although they may be aware of situations that precipitate their anxiety, they may be unable to identify its cause, which makes them feel helpless and overwhelmed. At other times, they know why they are anxious.

Levels of anxiety vary from mild to panic level. In mild anxiety, a person's ability to observe is heightened; in moderate and severe anxiety, he or she has difficulty focusing on details. In mild anxiety, a person's ability to perceive the relation between events is enhanced; as anxiety increases, this ability progressively diminishes. In panic-level anxiety, a person may describe feelings of "disintegrating" or "being swept away." No matter what the patient's physical condition is, he or she is helpless while in this state and requires assistance to reduce the anxiety to more manageable levels. Staying with the patient is one measure that is useful. Listening is another. At first the patient may describe his or her feelings in a distorted manner. Then, as the nurse listens and as anxiety is reduced, the patient begins to communicate more coherently, thus enabling the nurse to respond.

When patients are anxious, they cannot see all aspects of a problem. They see and magnify only a few details, and sometimes make the wrong connections. Anxious patients often become confused and are unable to follow directions or the explanations given about a treatment.

The nurse should avoid cutting off patients when they begin to talk. Although verbalizing does not in itself relieve anxiety, it can be the beginning of understanding. The problem will never be solved until it is understood. Letting a patient talk opens the way to understanding and dealing with problems.

There also are times when a matter should not be pursued or may need to be postponed. For example, the nurse's skills may not be adequate for the amount of help the patient seems to need. In this instance, another person with more expertise in this area may be required. Other factors, such as the patient's physical condition, may make discussion of anxiety-producing situations unwise.

When a patient has a life-threatening physical need and also is experiencing great fear over a situation, caring for the physical need is the priority; psychological needs can be considered after the emergency is over. Attending to physical needs is one way of communicating support to the patient. Ignoring physical needs—even such simple ones as giving fresh water or lowering the bed to a more comfortable position— sends a message to the patient that no one cares, and this increases his or her anxiety. Words should not be used when action is more appropriate.

Some patients prefer not to discuss their emotional problems with the nurse, and the nurse should respect this preference for privacy. The nurse's need to help should be guided by an understanding of what will bring relief to a particular patient. Some patients find it most helpful when the nurse gives support in nonverbal ways; others are helped when they are encouraged to talk about how they feel.

Dealing With Personal Anxiety.   What are some things a nurse can do when he or she becomes anxious? If possible, the nurse can leave the situation for a moment to think it through. Trying to concentrate on some objective task may give the nurse time to decide what to do next.

When nurses recognize personal anxiety—except in an emergency—they should stop, think the situation through, and seek help; they should not race blindly ahead with what they are doing. Extreme anxiety can keep one from functioning and can cause hazardous behavior; so can physical illness or excessive loss of sleep. Every health care professional has the responsibility to stop work when they are unable to function. None of these "excuses" is legally acceptable if a patient is harmed.

Knowledge and competence are insurance against anxiety. Nurses who are not familiar enough with a certain procedure so that they can perform it almost automatically may become anxious when they are confronted with the necessity to carry out the procedure. On the other hand, nurses should not expect too much of themselves. As knowledge increases, so will competence.

Frustration

Frustration results from the inability to meet a goal. It may consist of anger and a feeling of helplessness. The amount of frustration one feels depends on how important the goal was, what similar past experiences one has had, and how one handled these experiences. A patient who fails to walk well on a newly fitted artificial leg feels frustrated, especially if his or her employment depends on the ability to walk well. We do not always know what goals others have set for themselves, and we cannot assume that a failure that does not frustrate one person will not frustrate another.

Anger

Anger is aggression caused by frustration, anxiety, and a feeling of helplessness. When a person has to hide his or her anger, it becomes subconscious. This type of anger may be harder to handle because the person is unaware of its existence. Feelings and reactions of which one is unaware complicate and obscure the situation, making a rational solution to the problem difficult to achieve.

Patients have many reasons for being angry. Merely being sick creates frustration and a feeling of helplessness. Having to restrict one's activities because of illness or disability is frustrating. Being unable to control the most ordinary daily routines, such as getting a hot cup of coffee or brushing one's teeth, is frustrating. Confinement to a room makes small details seem more important. Some minor causes of patient anger can be remedied (eg, seeing that a patient receives hot coffee if cold coffee is disliked) but unfortunately many major causes cannot.

In addition to giving patients an opportunity to express their anger, the nurse should help them find ways to use up the excess energy generated by anger. Physical activity is especially beneficial. Patients who have their legs in traction can still exercise their arms. These exercises not only prepare them for crutch-walking, but also give them an outlet for their anger.

Conflict

Conflict is a clash between two opposing forces. The medical–surgical patient may have to make some decisions that have far-reaching consequences, and is expected to make these decisions promptly. Such situations set the stage for conflict, with a patient feeling torn between opposing goals. It is not uncommon for a patient to have to choose the lesser of two evils when neither alternative is desirable, and the question revolves around which choice has more assets. Often the situation is complicated by the fact that no one can predict the outcome of a particular treatment or surgery. The nurse can act as a sounding board while the patient expresses the conflict and considers the alternatives.

When patients are in conflict, it is important to supply the information they need to help them make a decision, but not make the decision for them.

Grief

Grief is an intense sadness, an emotional reaction to a severe loss. Appropriate responses are crying, withdrawal, depression, and loss of appetite. Other responses include anger, feelings of emptiness, and despair.

The intensity of grief usually depends on the cause: the greater the loss, the more intense the grief. People grieve for what is important to them and for those they love, regardless of the appropriateness of their reactions. Some physicians and nurses have preconceived

standards that they use to measure the appropriateness of reactions. Such standards alter their perception of what certain experiences mean to patients. Losses have personal and exclusive meanings that may be affected by the magnitude of other serious losses, the recovery from those losses, and the person's personal resources and assets.

SUPPORTING THE PATIENT DURING TESTS AND TREATMENTS

Usually the nurse has primary responsibility for providing emotional support and observing the patient's response during various procedures. However routine such procedures may seem to the professional staff, they usually represent stressful experiences for the patient (Fig. 4-1).

The physician, nurse, and patient are typically the three persons involved during a treatment or test, but additional personnel may be required for some procedures. The primary focus of each is different, and the interaction among them important. The physician concentrates on the procedure, although this does not mean that the the patient is being ignored. The patient's role involves getting through a painful, humiliating, frightening, or sometimes simply tedious experience as best as possible. The nurse must support the patient, both physically and emotionally, as well as assist the physician, obtain necessary equipment, and so on. The patient's confidence is increased if nurse

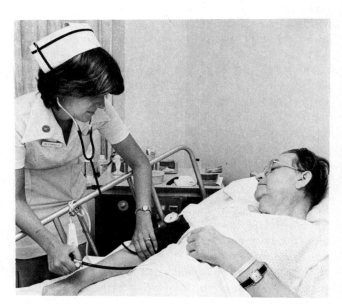

Figure 4-1. Even routine nursing procedures and diagnostic tests can produce stress in the patient. (Photograph by D. Atkinson).

and physician are collaborating and appear to genuinely respect each other.

The nurse should make it a practice to begin a procedure (especially if the nurse has not worked with the physician before) by asking the physician whether anything additional or different is needed. This step helps to prevent tension during the procedure. Particularly if the procedure proves difficult (such as a lumbar puncture in which the spinal fluid is difficult to obtain), a minor problem with equipment can assume major proportions as physician and nurse vent their tension and frustration over the situation.

The nurse's failure to provide emotional support during the stress of diagnostic tests and treatments may anger some patients and make them critical of their care. It is important to observe the patient's reactions and recognize that each patient responds somewhat differently and requires a slightly different approach.

SUSTAINED NURSE–PATIENT RELATIONSHIPS

Working with patients who have long-term illnesses provides many satisfactions but also poses some problems. Some patients improve, but others remain unchanged or become more ill. The nurse is called on to continue working with the patient and the family during extended periods that may be marked by exacerbations as well as remissions of illness.

Long-term patients in a general hospital setting often get lost in the shuffle. The acutely ill surgical patient or the accident victim may claim the staff's time and attention in a way that an elderly patient with chronic congestive heart failure may not. In a general hospital setting or a facility for long-term patients, the nurse should be alert to the special requirements of these patients. There may be activities in which they can participate, such as using the library, playing cards, or sitting in a chair to eat meals in the company of others, if they are able.

Many long-term patients find it hard to adapt to the restrictions imposed by their illness. Listening to these patients and their families and helping them adjust to their situation are important factors in their nursing management.

Necessary care measures must be faithfully performed each day, even though the patient shows little improvement. In some patients, there is no improvement, and one realizes that treatment is serving only to hold ground that might otherwise be lost. The daily routines of care can be discouraging to both nurse and patient. Almost anyone can perceive the drama of bringing a patient out of anaphylactic shock, but not every nurse is attuned to helping a patient with emphysema perform breathing exercises daily, and to experiencing a sense of accomplishment when a patient shows slight improvement.

The relation that the nurse has with the long-term patient is especially important because the patient may have few ties with family and friends. Because other significant relationships often are lacking, the nurse may be the only person who will listen to the patient and be concerned about her or his welfare. The nurse can show interest and support by attending to those daily matters that help long-term patients acquire greater freedom and control over their lives. The nurse also can help these patients use the abilities they have and help them keep in touch with those who are important to them.

Patient Behavior

The facial expression assumed by a patient is not necessarily a true indication of what is happening internally. Cheerfulness can be a mask behind which are hidden fears and anger of a most urgent nature. The need of the quiet person to talk may be great, but the person may find it difficult to express a concern or problem. On the other hand, the patient may attempt to please the staff by not complaining. It should be remembered that any type of patient behavior *may* mask a more serious disease, disorder, or problem.

Other patients, by their behavior, may make it hard for nurses to accept them. For example, an adult patient may act like an uninhibited child, demanding more service than anyone could give. Patients who exhibit what appears to be abnormal behavior may cause anxiety in some nurses because they do not meet the nurses' personal expectations: a patient should be reasonable and cooperative. The nurse should remember that a patient who seems to be willful and obstinate may be trying to maintain integrity and a will to fight. A patient who gives in to every demand may have given up.

Some adults may be ashamed of having to depend on others for their care. These feelings may result in their complaining about every aspect of care. If a patient is embarrassed by a dependence on others, the nurse can point out the temporary nature of the situation. The nurse must help dependent patients *maintain their dignity and self-esteem*.

It is important to assess changes in patients' behavior. Although it is not only useless, but also possibly harmful to demand that patients exercise greater control than they are capable of, a plan of care that enables them to maintain at least a partial degree of control over their environment and activities of daily living needs to be established. For example, a patient with multiple sclerosis has hand tremors. Each time she takes a sip of water, some water spills on the bed. The nurse, noting the difficulty, can place the water glass, half full, on an over-the-bed table close to the patient and put a flexible straw in the glass. The table can then be drawn close to the bed and the patient can sip the water without having to handle the glass.

Cultural Differences

The nurse may avoid some patients for reasons other than personal behavior. They may speak a different language, or their customs may be so different that there seems to be no common ground for communication. It is not unusual for people to avoid the unfamiliar because it usually provokes more anxiety and stress than the familiar. We may be uncertain about what to do or say because we do not know what to expect.

Use of a translator, when possible, may alleviate a language barrier. In some instances, sign language, simple drawings, and demonstrations may be used as methods of communication. It also may be helpful for one to gather information about the background and customs of a person whose cultural patterns and behavior are strikingly different from one's own. Knowledge of the characteristics and behavior patterns of a given group of people is the first step in creating an atmosphere of understanding and mutual respect. This, in turn, may help to reduce the anxiety produced by unfamiliar situations.

GUARDING AGAINST SUICIDE

Depressed patients bear watching, as they may be thinking of committing suicide. Signs of depression include lack of enthusiasm, prolonged insomnia, listlessness, reluctance to speak, neglect of appearance, withdrawal, lack of interest, and feelings of worthlessness. A nonpsychotic patient who attempts suicide may be trying to escape an overwhelming situation. Hostility also may result in suicide. Anger at self and the wish to hurt others usually are influencing factors that are unrecognized by the patient. Suicide may be averted if the patient knows that there is at least one person who cares. That one person can be the nurse. There can be a long, complicated chain of events and feelings leading to suicide. The nurse must recognize depression and then protect the patient by promptly reporting these observations to the physician. Obvious hazards, such as sharp objects, should be removed from the patient's immediate surroundings. Depending on the patient and the physician's orders, other materials such as articles of clothing (belts, ties), glassware, scissors, and pens also may be removed.

A patient who threatens suicide may intend to carry out the threat, and should not be left alone. The physician should be notified immediately, and the pa-

tient's suicidal conversations should be documented in his chart. All nursing personnel must be made aware of threats. Where pain, incurable disease, crippling disability, and impending death are present—as they may be on any general hospital floor—suicide, like fire, is an ever-present possibility.

PATIENTS' COMPLAINTS

Some patients continually complain about pains and aches or the service of the hospital. It is important to determine the reason for the patient's bitterness and continual complaints. Perhaps it is the patient's way of expressing frustration, anger, or hostility, or of getting attention. A patient is cut off from his or her family and friends, work, and home. The usual sources of satisfaction are not available in the hospital. Frequent patient contact as well as listening may help to reduce complaints.

Some nurses may label patients who voice many complaints chronic complainers, those who are never satisfied, or uncooperative people as a way of putting distance between themselves and those who make them anxious. Such labeling reveals a lack of perception and understanding. By stereotyping and labeling a patient, the nurse will, in a sense, absolve guilt feelings that may have occurred because of any lack of attention or care. Stereotyping can be done by a whole group, with disastrous effects on the patient. Once labeled uncooperative, the patient probably will not disappoint anyone and will be uncooperative.

Who are the "good" patients? Many nurses think that submissive patients are good. By bestowing approval on the quiet ones, they force patients to hide their feelings. Some patients do not complain because they are at the mercy of the nurse. Patients lying in bed, sick and in pain, depend on the hospital staff. They are vulnerable, and the danger of being ignored—psychologically and physically—is real.

APPROACH TO THE PATIENT
The Physically Unattractive Patient

Our culture places great emphasis on cleanliness, beauty, pleasant odors, and an attractive appearance. The nurse is bound to be affected by unpleasant sights and odors, but must learn to accept these situations. Odors often can be controlled, but a disfigurement may or may not be able to be corrected by surgery. The nurse must be aware of outward reactions, such as facial expressions, when giving care. What is most important is that *no* negative feelings or emotions be conveyed to the patient. Sometimes nurses are unaware of how facial expressions or gestures come across to others. Another indication of the nurse's approach is the patients' reaction. Patients may show embarrassment or withdraw because of their own reaction to the situation; on the other hand, they may react this way because they perceive that they are not accepted by others.

The Self-Care Patient

Self-care patients present no less of a challenge than the more physically helpless patients in the establishment of the nurse–patient relationship, but the challenges are somewhat different. Patients who are able to attend to their own activities of daily living may be ignored by the nurse, yet their needs may be just as great as the critically ill patient. Many self-care patients are bored and frustrated, and feel helplessness while they wait for surgery, the results of diagnostic tests, or discharge from the hospital.

Nurses can meet the needs of the self-care patient by continuing interpersonal relationships as well as ongoing assessments. Many of these patients want to ask questions, or talk about their diagnosis, their upcoming surgery, or their time at home recovering from surgery. Others require motivation to engage in the self-care activities that play an important part in their rehabilitation.

The Patient Undergoing Diagnostic Tests

Patients who are undergoing diagnostic tests frequently have a good deal of free time and, in some instances, are self-care patients. The experience can be one of constant waiting to go to scheduled appointments or for test results. Such waiting is commonly accompanied by anxiety. Until a diagnosis is made, patients have no concrete enemy to grapple with. Instead, they may have vague fears about what may be wrong and a general feeling of helplessness.

One important aspect of caring for these patients is the explanation of diagnostic tests. Patients should know what will be involved, for example, fasting from food or fluids, having radiologic examinations, having blood drawn, or saving urine samples. They also should be informed of the time of the test, who will perform the test, how long it will take, and where it will be performed. Depending on the type of test, some or all of the information may be given by the nurse. It is the initial responsibility of the physician to provide patients with information about what tests are needed and why, and to interpret the test results to them. The nurse should talk with the physician so the

nurse knows what explanations the patient has received. Within this framework, the nurse reviews and clarifies information with the patient. If a patient is scheduled for a test or procedure about which he or she seems to know nothing, the nurse should bring this to the physician's attention.

Patients need to talk about the results of their tests, the diagnosis, and the treatment that has been prescribed. Often, after the physician has discussed test results with the patient and family, there may be a need to talk about it again—to review what was said and to clarify terms after the first shock of the diagnosis has diminished. Threatening situations may require repeated opportunities for discussion. Some questions may need to be referred to the physician. The patient also may have forgotten or become confused about the information given.

The Unconscious Patient

Some nurses find it difficult to care for a patient who cannot respond; others are relieved not to have to relate verbally to a patient. The nurse must avoid treating these patients as though they were objects, rather than people, and not feel overwhelmed by the seriousness of their condition. When caring for these patients, the nurse should try to think of concrete, individual nursing needs that can be observed, and plan ways to meet these needs. Concentrating on such practical and individualized observations helps to prevent the nurse from being overwhelmed by the gravity of the patient's condition and from thinking of the patient as an object.

Care of unconscious adults, particularly if they are heavy, is best undertaken by two nurses working together. The physical and emotional burdens are made lighter when they are shared. Each can encourage the other and trade information on how best to give mouth care, prevent obstruction of catheters, and so on. It is essential for the nurse not to say anything that the patient should not hear. Even though the patient is unconscious, he or she may still be able to hear.

The Patient Who Refuses Treatment

The patient, on admission to the hospital, is expected to take orders unquestioningly and comply with routines that may be perceived as indignities. No matter how necessary these may be from the standpoint of running the hospital, they can upset patients. The abrupt change from being in charge of their own affairs to following the directions of others is difficult for many. Anxiety over the diagnosis and its implications plays a part in patients' refusal to follow treatment. Patients may refuse treatment for a number of reasons, such as denial that they have a specific illness or disease, fear of the consequences of a treatment or surgery, fear over the pain or disfigurement that may occur, or the cost of treatment.

One crucial consideration, when working with patients who refuse treatment, is recognizing that the patient has the right to do so (except under unusual circumstances that concern legal aspects of nursing). The nurse who understands this can more realistically assess the patient's role, and the role of the nurse in patient care. The nurse must try to help patients make the best possible decision about their own welfare.

THE FAMILY

All patients who are admitted to the hospital have some type of relationship with others. Some patients have no immediate family members, and their "family" may consist of friends and neighbors. Other patients come from large families and also have many relatives and friends. It is not unusual to meet patients who have strong ties to a dog or cat, which may be an important member of the family. Whatever involves the patient also involves the family.

Nurses have specialized knowledge and skills that help patients to recover. But a loved one can make contributions to the peace of mind and comfort of a patient that, because of the closeness of the relationship, have a greater effect than any professional skill. When appropriate, the nurse should involve family members and capitalize on what they can do for the patient.

The family may feel guilty about the patient's illness. Such feelings are often unfounded, but this does not lessen their emotional impact. Being able to participate in the patient's care may help to ease the guilt. The nurse should provide opportunities for the family to talk about the experience.

Several other challenges must be considered when working with the family, particularly when the patient has a long-term illness. It is easy for the nurse to view family members only in their role of helping the patient and to disregard their other responsibilities. In an acute illness, it is common for relatives to discontinue other responsibilities temporarily to help and be with the patient. If illness continues, family members must begin to resume other obligations. In talking with them, the nurse must consider the problems they face. Topics of conversation other than the patient's illness should not be ignored if family members introduce them. As the nurse listens to some of their other concerns, an understanding of and insight into their problems can occur.

Society sets certain standards of responsibility when a family member is ill. Perhaps nowhere are these standards so forcefully upheld as in health care institutions. At morning reports and team conferences, there may be negative comments about patients' families: the family does not take the patient home, they do not visit, and so on. This criticism is understandable; health care personnel rely on families to give emotional and sometimes physical support to the patient. When families do not meet these expectations, not only do patients lack the emotional and physical support that they need, but also the work of physicians and nurses is made more difficult. Not all families can help the patient, for a variety of reasons, many of which may remain unknown. As the nurse works with a family, he or she must be alert to the family's attitudes and abilities to help the patient. This approach enables the nurse to plan for patient and family teaching as well as to determine what federal, state, and local resources may be useful and available to them.

Illness is a powerful force in mobilizing the anxiety of family members, relatives, and friends. They may show their anxiety in various ways—by withdrawing, by becoming too clinical, or by blaming the family's difficulties on the patient's illness. The more nurses recognize the part anxiety plays in such reactions, the better they are able to help the family care for the patient.

The transition from hospital to home can be a stressful experience for both the patient and the family. Often it is possible for patients to reestablish ties with family and friends when they return home. Sometimes it is not, and these patients must recognize that their place in the lives of others, to which they were so eager to return, no longer exists, and they must begin to develop new or different relationships. An appreciation of these factors helps both the patient and the family to assess the situation realistically.

General Gerontologic Considerations

☐ The nurse may need to provide more emotional and physical support to elderly patients because this group of patients often have few family members or friends able to offer support during illness.

☐ Elderly patients are not given the kind of attention that retards their ability to do as much for themselves as they can. Encourage these patients to engage in as much self-care as they are physically able to perform.

☐ Elderly patients are often frustrated because of illness, the inability to participate in activities of daily living, and failure to respond to therapy. Frustration ends in anger and, at times, hostility. The setting of reasonable goals may help to reduce frustration and anger.

☐ Elderly patients require additional support during tests and treatments because they may not understand the treatment being performed or the instructions given by the physician or nurse. Problems with hearing also may be a factor.

Suggested Readings

☐ Barry PD. Mental health and mental illness. 4th ed. Philadelphia: JB Lippincott, 1990. *(In-depth coverage of subject matter)*

☐ Beck CK, Rawlins RP, Williams SR. Mental health–psychiatric nursing: a holistic life-cycle approach. St Louis: CV Mosby, 1988. *(In-depth coverage of subject matter)*

☐ Hogarty SS. How we prepared to prevent suicide RN May 1988;51:21. *(Closely related to subject matter)*

Concepts Related to Health and Illness

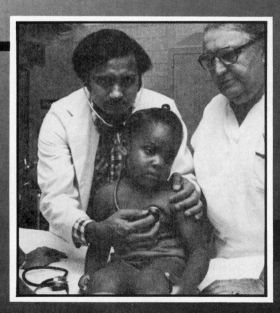

Unit 2

Chapter 5
Interaction of Body and Mind

On completion of this chapter the reader will:

- List the signs and symptoms of psychosomatic illness, hypochondriasis, and conversion disorders

- Discuss the treatment and nursing management of psychosomatic illness, hypochondriasis, and conversion disorders

- Discuss the problems that may be encountered when the patient is a malingerer

- List the signs and symptoms of delirium

- Discuss the treatment and nursing management of the delirious patient

- Discuss the signs and symptoms of chronic brain syndrome

- Discuss the treatment and nursing management of the patient with chronic brain syndrome

PSYCHOSOMATIC DISORDERS

Psycho means mind, and *soma,* body. Psychosomatic illness is the occurrence of bodily symptoms that are psychological or emotional in origin. Mind and body are not separate; one affects and is affected by the other. It is not unusual to experience some manifestation of emotional stress. Experiences such as headache after a quarrel or urinary frequency or diarrhea before an examination are not uncommon and are of a transitory nature for most people. No treatment may be needed, or the person may use simple remedies to relieve discomfort.

Psychosomatic Reactions

Psychosomatic illness is anxiety that results in physical symptoms manifested in an organ or an organ system such as the stomach, bowel, or skin. In other words, a psychological disorder contributes to the occurrence or increase in severity of a physical disorder. In psychosomatic reactions, a physical disorder can be documented by such means as a physical or a radiologic examination. In some people, the occurrence of peptic ulcer, eczema, colitis, and bronchial asthma, as well as other diseases and disorders, *may* be psychosomatic in origin.

Personality profiles have been formulated to describe the characteristics of people who develop psychosomatic reactions. Another point of view is that humans are more complex and varied in their responses than such profiles would indicate, and that factors such as heredity and environment also play a role. Much remains to be learned about the interaction of the body and the mind and about the relation between stress and physical illness.

Hypochondriasis

Patients with hypochondriasis, or *hypochondriacal neurosis,* are preoccupied with the belief that they are physically ill. They have an unrealistic belief that the physical symptoms they experience are caused by a disease. Even when a thorough physical examination does not reveal a disease, they continue to believe that they are physically ill. An example of hypochondriasis is the occurrence of abdominal discomfort that leads the person to believe that cancer must be the cause, even though radiographic and other diagnostic studies reveal nothing more than excessive gas in the bowel. Even though the patient is assured that gas is the cause of the discomfort, the belief that cancer is present continues. Additional bowel complaints may develop, and the patient returns to the same or another physician for further testing.

Note the difference between hypochondriasis and psychosomatic reactions. The person with a psychosomatic reaction has symptoms that *can* be documented by radiography, physical examination, or other diagnostic tests, whereas the hypochondriacal patient has physical symptoms that *cannot* be documented.

Conversion Disorders

The patient with a conversion disorder, or *hysterical neurosis,* attempts to reduce anxiety by developing a disturbance or alteration of a function that suggests a physical illness. The symptoms of this somewhat uncommon personality disorder are not under the patient's voluntary control. An example of a conversion disorder is the development of blindness when there is no organic disorder or disease to cause the blindness. Other symptoms seen in conversion disorders include hearing loss, paralysis of an extremity, and speech impairment. The reason the person particularly develops blindness or paralysis usually is deep-seated and not easy to determine.

Treatment

The first step in helping patients with psychosomatic disorders is to accept and acknowledge their illness. If possible, the cause of the disorder must be found, and measures taken to eliminate it and prevent a recurrence of symptoms. Thorough physical and psychological examinations are essential. Although the physician may suspect that the illness is due to emotional rather than physical causes, a physical disease must be ruled out. An illness that at first is considered to be emotional in origin may later be diagnosed as physical.

A thorough search for physical causes of symptoms is necessary, because it helps these patients to gain confidence and realize that their condition and welfare are being taken seriously. If no organic basis for the symptoms is found, they may find the news easier to accept if they have had a thorough physical examination.

Patients with a psychosomatic reaction (eg, anxiety that results in physical symptoms) may require drug therapy. In some instances, such as with a bleeding peptic ulcer, surgery may be necessary. Hypochondriacal patients often are difficult to treat. Because there is no physical illness, drug therapy or surgery is not necessary. Sometimes, by talking with these patients, the physician or nurse may learn about the emotional difficulties they are experiencing and can help them see the possible relation between their symptoms and emotional stress. Until these patients begin to see this relation, the relief of symptoms is transitory and random. When they understand the cause-and-effect relation, they may find other ways of handling their emotional problems. Patients with a conversion disorder also are difficult to treat, and may respond poorly to therapy. Psychotherapy may help these patients find a way to cope with their problem.

Each situation has many diverse and subtle aspects. Sometimes the patient's physician recommends the services of a psychiatrist. The two physicians may work together, one concentrating primarily on the emotional causes and the other concentrating primarily on the relief of physical symptoms.

Nursing Management

Nursing management of patients with a psychosomatic reaction requires tact, insight, and judgment. These patients need someone to listen to them, to be concerned about their symptoms, and to respect them. Prying or attempting to force on them an acceptance of the relation between their symptoms and their emotional problems can make them more anxious. Such efforts may intensify their physical symptoms and their resistance to any later suggestion that they receive psychotherapy.

When talking to these patients, the nurse may make observations that point to a relation between their physical symptoms and other events in their lives. Do the symptoms come and go, leaving the patient free of discomfort for part of the day, or do they persist most of the day and night? What relieves the symptoms? Medication? Diversion? Such observations can help to identify the anxiety-producing aspects of a person's life.

The nurse should develop a relationship with those who have psychosomatic illnesses. Listening is an important part of the nurse–patient interaction. Often there may be opportunities to help these patient see the connection between their symptoms and their reactions to daily experiences. Ultimately they may understand the relation between the bodily symptoms they experience and the emotion they are describing.

Patients with a psychosomatic illness are likely to be neglected. It is not uncommon for the same staff members who give excellent care to other patients to ignore them because they have no physical illness. Condemnation of those with a psychosomatic illness can persist despite intellectual understanding of theories about its causes. These patients can immediately sense whether those who care for them are trying to help. It is important to understand two points:

1. The patient with psychosomatic illness can no more "snap out of it" at will than can the patient with a disease like pneumonia, whose need for care is readily acknowledged.
2. The patient with psychosomatic illness develops symptoms as a manifestation of largely unconscious psychic conflicts. These symptoms are real.

MALINGERING

A malingerer is one who deliberately fakes illness to achieve some secondary gain, such as financial compensation, obtaining drugs, or excuse from work or school. Malingering may be seen in all age-groups. It is not unusual for children to occasionally complain of a headache, nausea, or some other illness so that they will not have to attend school. Adults also use excuses such as these to stay home from work or school or to avoid other obligations. People who fake an illness to obtain financial compensation (eg, insurance claims and malpractice suits) may go to great lengths to prove that they are ill or have been physically injured.

Chronic malingering is an unhealthy and unsatisfactory solution to a problem. It can have serious consequences, such as loss of employment and failure in school. Often it adds to the person's difficulties because she or he makes elaborate attempts to avoid detection. Malingering must be resolved by the person or the employer, or by some other method.

Nursing Management

A person with psychosomatic illness may be confused with a malingerer. The essential difference is that the malingerer fakes symptoms of a disease or disorder; it is a conscious process, and the person is aware that he or she is pretending to be sick. The person with a psychosomatic disorder experiences real symptoms.

Sometimes it is difficult to detect malingering; at other times it is obvious. The nurse must record all symptoms presented by the patient, followed by an assessment of the areas of complaint. Prejudging a person as a malingerer may be in error, since the person may indeed be ill.

One problem associated with malingering is misdiagnosis. Because the person offers a series of fake complaints, unnecessary tests may be ordered and drugs prescribed for an illness that does not exist. The far-reaching consequences of these diagnostic tests and prescriptions include harm to the patient and unwarranted costs to an insurance carrier. In addition, absence from work may place an extra burden on others.

The physician must decide if the patient's complaints are real (and this may be difficult), or if the patient is a malingerer. Some chronic malingerers can be helped to cope with their difficulties in other ways, but many who are in the habit of faking an illness find that this way of handling problems surpasses other methods. Unless detected and punished (eg, fired from work or expelled from school), the successful malingerer usually persists.

DELIRIUM

Delirium is an acute, reversible state of disorientation caused by interference with metabolic processes of the brain. Causes include fever, the immediate postoperative phase of cardiac surgery, drug overdose, acute alcoholism, and the terminal phases of some illnesses, such as renal or hepatic failure.

Symptoms

Delirious patients are disoriented with respect to time and place and may have illusions and hallucinations. An *illusion* is an inaccurate interpretation of stimuli within the environment. For example, the patient may believe that his wife is calling him, when actually it is the nurse. *Hallucinations* are subjective sensory experiences that occur without stimulation from the environment. For example, the patient may hear a voice when no one is calling.

Delirious patients are restless and confused, and show defects in memory and judgment. They may behave impulsively and act on incorrect interpretations of their environment, which could result in physical harm to themselves or others.

Treatment

Delirium often develops suddenly and can subside quickly. The main goal of treatment is to remove the cause. The patient may require sedation with tranquilizers.

Nursing Management

Delirious patients need to be protected from harming themselves and others and helped to minimize their disorientation. Care measures include the following:

1. Keep sensory stimuli to a minimum. The room should be quiet, and unnecessary noise avoided. Conversation should be specific and repetitive. For example, repetition of the phrase, "You're in the hospital, and I am your nurse," can help these patients orient themselves to their environment. Explanations should be brief and simple. The nurse should try not to reflect the patient's restlessness and agitation. Feelings can be contagious. Speaking quietly and slowly may help to lessen the patient's apprehension.
2. Keep the room softly lit during the night to prevent the increased disorientation that usually occurs when the patient is left in a darkened room.
3. Protect the patient from harm. A physician's order is required before restraints can be used. If restraints are ordered, the nurse should be sure that the restraints *do not impair circulation* and that they give the patient as much movement as is compatible with safety. Many people, delirious or not, react to physical restraints with

anger. The delirious patient may be made more excited when restraints are applied. Restraints must be removed at least every 2 hours, and the patient supervised during the entire time the restraints are removed. The area beneath the restraint should be inspected for redness, bruising, abrasions, and cuts. The family should be informed of the necessity for restraining measures.

4. Delirious patients usually are incapable of feeding themselves. Feed them slowly and give them time to chew their food. An adequate fluid intake is encouraged, unless there is an order to limit fluids.
5. Side rails help to keep patients in bed. Explain their purpose, so that they are not considered a confining cage from which the patient must escape. A patient who is physically strong can climb over side rails.
6. Observe delirious patients at frequent intervals. This contact may assure them that they are being cared for, can lessen their agitation, and may prevent them from hurting themselves. A family member can be asked to stay with the patient.
7. Keep objects that are capable of causing harm away from the patient. For instance, cigarettes and matches should not be left within reach.
8. Because these patients cannot control their behavior, scolding is both inappropriate and ineffective.

Delirious patients require a great deal of nursing care. Their unpredictable behavior often interferes with the goals of those caring for them. As far as possible, the environment and the plan of care should be modified to help prevent incidents that can upset the patient and those around him.

CHRONIC BRAIN SYNDROME

Chronic brain syndrome is a general term used to describe symptoms found in specific mental disorders that are organic in origin. This disorder results from irreversible and diffuse damage to the brain. Causes include advanced arteriosclerosis of cerebral vessels, cerebrovascular accident, Alzheimer's disease, heavy metal (lead, mercury) poisoning, cerebral tumors, syphilis, and metabolic disorders such as severe, untreated hypothyroidism. In some instances, the cause may be unknown.

Symptoms

The onset of chronic brain syndrome usually is slow and insidious. This disorder is most common in those over age 70, but it also may be observed in younger people. Early in the disorder, the patient demonstrates poor judgment and has frequent memory lapses. There also may be impairment in abstract thinking, a decline in personal hygiene, shallow emotional responses (emotional lability), apathy, and periods of disorientation. She or he may become depressed or irritable, or develop anxiety over these symptoms. As the disorder progresses, hallucinations (especially at night), restlessness, insomnia, incoherent speech, and manic behavior may occur. The patient may wander away from home, become difficult to manage, and exhibit bizarre behavior.

Treatment

Treatment varies, depending on the severity of the disorder. In some instances, tranquilizers may be used to control behavior and make the patient more manageable. In most cases, treatment is supportive.

Nursing Management

Nursing management is directed toward helping patients with chronic brain syndrome live their lives to the fullest. The following guidelines can be used for providing such care:

1. Treat these patients with respect and kindness and help them maintain their dignity.
2. Identify the patient's needs and then develop realistic short- and long-term goals to meet these needs and the nursing interventions necessary to attain the stated goals.
3. Periodically evaluate each patient to determine if the stated goals are being met. Determine which nursing interventions require alteration because of changes in the patient's condition or failure to attain the stated goals.
4. Treat these patients like adults, even though their behavior is childlike. Do not scold them for their behavior or talk to them as if they were children.
5. Encourage interaction with others by providing daily recreational activities.
6. Avoid the use of restraints unless they are absolutely necessary. Restraints may only add to the patients' confusion as well as result in frustration and anger.
7. Encourage independence by allowing patients to engage in the various activities of daily living as much as possible.
8. Provide reality orientation (see Chart 3-1) to decrease confusion.
9. Make any changes in routine slowly. To help reduce confusion, explain any change and be with the patient when the change is made.

General Nutritional Considerations

☐ Patients who are under stress may lose their appetite; it is important to provide them with simple, attractive, nutritious foods and liquids.

☐ If a patient is placed on a psychotropic drug, the nurse should read the package insert accompanying the medication, check drug information in text references, or check with the hospital pharmacist for any dietary considerations that affect the specific drug. For example, some psychotropic medications should *not* be given with a diet that includes cheese, chocolate, alcohol, or caffeine.

General Pharmacologic Considerations

☐ A complete current medication history should be obtained for each patient. Many people who experience stress take over-the-counter drugs, stimulants, and tranquilizers that they may not mention unless asked.

☐ Some patients under stress increase their consumption of alcohol.

☐ Disorientation may be an adverse effect of medications; appropriate action to withdraw the drug or reduce the dosage must be taken promptly.

General Gerontologic Considerations

☐ Some elderly patients are prone to periods of disorientation and memory impairment.

☐ When patients with chronic brain syndrome are no longer able to assume responsibility for their activities, they may require a supervised environment, such as a nursing home or living with those who can assume responsibility for their care.

☐ Patients' families often require help, understanding, and emotional support while making the decision to move a parent from an independent to a supervised environment.

Suggested Readings

☐ Barry PD. Mental health and mental illness. 4th ed. Philadelphia: JB Lippincott, 1990. *(In-depth coverage of subject matter)*

☐ Barry PD. Psychosocial nursing assessment and interventions of the physically ill person. 2nd ed. Philadelphia: JB Lippincott, 1988. *(In-depth coverage of subject matter)*

☐ Beck CK, Rawlins RP, Williams SR. Mental health–psychiatric nursing: a holistic life-cycle approach. St Louis: CV Mosby, 1988. *(In-depth coverage of subject matter)*

☐ Birckhead LM. Psychiatric mental health nursing: the therapeutic use of self. Philadelphia: JB Lippincott, 1989. *(In-depth coverage of subject matter)*

☐ Johnson BS. Psychiatric mental health nursing: adaption and growth. 2nd ed. Philadelphia: JB Lippincott, 1989. *(Additional coverage of subject matter)*

☐ Pedersen LM, Fingerote E, Powell C, Edmund L. Avoiding restraints: why it can mean good practice. Nursing '89 December 1989;19:66. *(Additional coverage of subject matter)*

☐ Shives LR. Basic concepts of psychiatric/mental health nursing. 2nd ed. Philadelphia: JB Lippincott, 1989. *(In-depth coverage of subject matter)*

☐ Stuart GW, Sundeen SJ. Principles and practice of psychiatric nursing. 3rd ed. St Louis: CV Mosby, 1987. *(In-depth coverage of subject matter)*

Chapter 6
Fundamental Processes of Health and Illness

On completion of this chapter the reader will:

- Define and use correctly the disease terminology in this chapter

- Discuss homeostasis and the basic concepts of stress in relation to illness and health

- Discuss the methods that may be used to modify stress

- Discuss the role of the nurse in dealing with stress and the clinical situations that produce stress

- Discuss the basic principles of the major internal and external body defenses

Nursing, as a health profession, helps people to reach and maintain optimal health or wellness. It also is concerned with preventing disease and caring for those who are ill.

Wellness and illness are relative states that are constantly changing. A state of wellness or illness depends on the body's ability to meet biologic, physiologic, and sociologic needs and make suitable adaptations to internal and external stresses as they arise.

TERMINOLOGY

A standard terminology is used in describing disease conditions and patient problems. It is important to have a clear understanding of the following terms and concepts.

Acute, Chronic. The word *acute* can be misleading to patients and their families. It does not necessarily refer to the seriousness of a disease or disorder, but describes the rapid nature of its onset and progress. In contrast, the term *chronic* describes the lengthy, sometimes endless persistence of a condition without much change for the better. Examples of the use of these two terms are *acute* appendicitis and *chronic* osteoarthritis.

Severe, Moderate, Mild. Severe, moderate, and mild are used to describe or grade the seriousness of a problem. For example, pain may be described as severe, moderate, or mild, or the joint deformity of rheumatoid arthritis can be graded as severe, moderate, or mild. These terms may be either general and individualized (eg, the patient's description of his pain) or accurate (eg, the physician's grading of the degree of deformity in an arthritic joint).

Early, Late, Terminal. A stage of a disease or disorder may be described as early, late, or terminal. These terms are more general than exact. *Early* refers to a stage of a disease when symptoms and the effects on body organs or structures are less widespread or serious. For example, in an early stage of cancer, no symptoms may be present and the tumor confined to one area with no evidence of metastasis (spread). *Late* refers to more serious or severe symptoms with a decided effect on one or more organs or structures of the body. *Terminal* means the stage preceding death.

Primary, Secondary. A disease also may be described as *primary* or *secondary*. A *primary* condition is assumed to have developed independently of any other condition; it is the original illness. A subsequent disorder that develops as a result of an original illness is called *secondary*. To illustrate, a patient sustained multiple injuries in an automobile accident, one of which was a compound fracture of the femur. Because

51

part of the femur punctured the skin, causing the wound to become contaminated with bacteria, an infection of the bone (osteomyelitis) developed. The fracture is the primary condition; the osteomyelitis is a result of the injury and, therefore, a secondary condition.

Morbidity, Mortality.

Morbidity means sickness. It usually is expressed as a rate in relation to population. If 39 out of 1,000 persons are ill, the morbidity rate is 39 per 1,000. *Mortality* means death. If 25 out of 1,000 persons die, the mortality rate is 25 per 1,000.

Hereditary Diseases and Disorders.

A *hereditary disease* or *disorder* is inherited from one or both parents. From the moment of conception, the destiny of thousands of traits is decided. Some inherited diseases and disorders can impair body function to a major or minor degree, whereas others are potentially fatal. Hemophilia and color blindness are examples of disorders that are transmitted by the genes from parent to child. Hemophilia, which often requires intensive, lifelong treatment, is potentially fatal, whereas color blindness has little or no effect on a person's health. Some hereditary diseases are carried in the genes as recessive traits, and are not manifested in every generation.

Congenital Defects and Disorders.

A *congenital defect* or *disorder* is present at the time of birth. It may have been caused by some unfavorable event or unfortunate environmental condition experienced by the fetus during pregnancy, or its cause may be unknown.

The development of the fetus can be affected by maternal factors such as diet, cigarette smoking, exposure to radiation, and ingestion of certain drugs. Other, as yet unknown factors or events also may have a harmful effect on the developing fetus. An illness of the mother during pregnancy can impair normal fetal development. An example of such an illness is German measles, which can result in a congenital disorder related to sight or hearing or both.

A congenital defect can be a serious threat to life, as when an infant is born with part or all of a vital organ or structure missing; it may be disfiguring, as in polydactylism (more than the usual number of fingers or toes); or it may be so slight as to escape notice.

Trauma.

Trauma means injury, and applies to both physical wounds, such as those suffered in an automobile accident, and psychic wounds, such as those experienced after the loss of a loved one.

Hypoxia, Anoxia.

Hypoxia means a deficiency of oxygen reaching the body tissues. Examples of medical disorders that can cause hypoxia are emphysema, shock, anemia, neuromuscular disease, and edema. A person also can become hypoxic by being trapped in a fire, which consumes much of the available oxygen in the immediate vicinity. The effects of hypoxia are dramatic because all body cells require an adequate and uninterrupted supply of oxygen.

Anoxia means a total lack of oxygen. It may occur in such conditions as respiratory obstruction, lack of circulation of blood to body tissues, and profound shock. The cerebral cortex of the brain is sensitive to an inadequate supply of oxygen. Irreversible damage occurs if the cortex is deprived of oxygen for more than 3 to 7 minutes, with the amount of time dependent on the person's age and adequacy of cerebral circulation as well as other factors.

Ischemia.

A reduction in the blood supply to a local area is called *ischemia*. It is possible for specific areas of the body to be deprived of oxygen while other areas receive a sufficient supply. Thus, if a patient has a narrowing of the coronary arteries, a reduced amount of blood flows through these arteries, and the myocardium (heart muscle) becomes ischemic.

Ischemia may damage nerves irreparably; it also may harm less sensitive tissue, like muscle. If the ischemia is relieved and has not been too severe or prolonged, the injury may be reversed. Serious and continued ischemia can cause necrosis (death) of the involved tissues. When an area of tissue is deprived of its blood supply long enough to become necrotic, it is described as an area of *infarction*.

Neoplasms.

A *neoplasm* is the new formation of abnormal tissue. Neoplasms also are called *tumors*. A *benign* neoplasm usually is covered by a capsule of fibrous tissue and is similar to the tissue in which it originates. It may have little activity except local growth, or it may carry on the processes characteristic of the tissue from which it started. Benign tumors of endocrine glands can produce the hormone of the gland; for example, a certain type of benign tumor of the pancreas is capable of secreting insulin. Benign tumors typically stay within their capsules and do not spread to other sites.

Although considered less dangerous than a malignant tumor (cancer), a benign tumor may be a cause for concern for several reasons. In certain locations, it is disfiguring, as, for example, a fatty tumor (lipoma) of the face. In other cases, it grows to occupy too much space and crowds the normal structures so that they cannot function correctly. A benign tumor growing in an inoperable area in the brain or the spinal cord can be fatal. A benign, hormone-producing tumor (eg, a thyroid adenoma) may function outside of the organized body commands, secreting the hormone in excess or at inappropriate times.

Once located, benign tumors usually can be surgically removed. The surgical trauma involved in removal of tumors in some areas or structures, such as the brain, can result in permanent damage to surrounding tissues.

Malignant neoplasms (collectively called *cancers*) grow and act in total disregard of body order (Fig. 6-1). Their cells may differ considerably from those of the tissue of their origin, and they tend to spread (metastasize) to other parts of the body. A malignant tumor can invade, crowd, and weaken normal structures. Some malignant tumors that arise from endocrine glands may secrete hormones. (For further discussion of cancer, see Chapter 19. The characteristics of benign and malignant tumors are compared in Table 19-2.)

Infection. An *infection* is the invasion of the body by a microorganism that is capable of causing harm. Such a microorganism is called a *pathogenic microorganism*, or a *pathogen*.

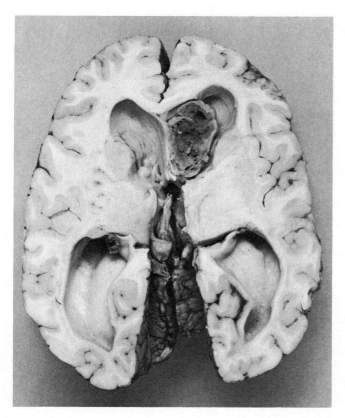

Figure 6–1. Tumor (ependymoma) of the lateral ventricle of the brain. (Courtesy of K. L. Terplan, MD. Photograph by D. Atkinson).

Microorganisms are classified as protozoa, yeasts, molds, bacteria, rickettsiae, and viruses. They harm human cells by growing within them or by producing toxins. Microorganisms must live in an environment or a specific tissue site that is suited to their needs. For example, the microorganism of tetanus cannot survive in oxygen but must multiply and produce the toxins it needs to live deep in a wound.

Because we do not live in a sterile environment, we come in contact with many types of pathogenic and nonpathogenic microorganisms, but we are not always sick. The development of an infection depends on several factors: (1) the type and number of invading microorganisms, (2) the virulence of the microorganisms, and (3) the resistance of the host. (See Chapter 7 for a more thorough discussion of infectious disease concepts.)

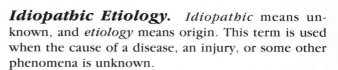

Idiopathic Etiology. *Idiopathic* means unknown, and *etiology* means origin. This term is used when the cause of a disease, an injury, or some other phenomena is unknown.

HOMEOSTASIS

Homeostasis is a relatively stable state of equilibrium (balance). To maintain homeostasis, the body must constantly balance the components (eg, hormones, water, electrolytes, proteins, vitamins, minerals, and oxygen) of its internal environment; it must obtain the substances it needs and convert or eliminate what it does not need. An imbalance can arise from deprivation, such as a vitamin deficiency, or from excess, such as too many sodium ions.

CONCEPT OF STRESS

Stress, according to Engel (1953), can be "any influence, whether it arises from the internal environment or from the external environment, that interferes with the satisfaction of basic needs or that disturbs or threatens to disturb the stable equilibrium."

In Selye's theory (1956), stress is a specific physiologic condition manifested by a general adaptation syndrome. Whether stressors (events that cause stress) are biologic (eg, surgical trauma or bacterial toxins), psychological (eg, worry, fear, or rage), or sociologic (eg, a new job or increased family responsibilities), the same nonspecific general adaptation syndrome results if the stress is excessive, ill-timed, or too sudden in onset.

The general adaptation syndrome consists of three stages: alarm reaction, resistance, and exhaustion or death. Most stressors evoke the first two stages of response. A person goes through these defensive stages many times. They are purposeful and necessary homeostatic reactions.

The general response to a stressor is accomplished through the coordinated efforts of the endocrine, musculoskeletal, immune, and autonomic nervous systems. When stress occurs, nerve endings in the autonomic nervous system produce the neurohormones norepinephrine and epinephrine. Through the endocrine system, stressors stimulate the pituitary to secrete adrenocorticotropic hormone, which in turn acts on the adrenal cortex to produce the predominantly antiinflammatory glucocorticoids cortisone and cortisol. Glucocorticoids tend to be inhibitory and catabolic. The adrenal gland also produces the mineralocorticoids aldosterone and desoxycorticosterone. Mineralocorticoids tend to be stimulative and anabolic. The musculoskeletal response includes increased muscle tone (or tension) because of increased activity of the reticular formation. Prolonged muscle tension can result in such complaints as stiff neck, sore muscles, headache, and backache. Suppression of the immune system may occur in those who are subject to stress. The exact mechanism of immune system suppression is unknown, but it is thought to be related to a feedback mechanism between the hypothalamic-pituitary-adrenal system and the immune system.

Stress is not an entirely negative concept. Inherent in each person's growth and development are markedly stressful situations that, if mastered, give zest and fullness to life. In the oyster, a pearl is produced in response to a stressor, a foreign body such as a grain of sand. Each stage of development has its stressful tasks to be learned and mastered that ready one for the next stage of development.

The person who subjects herself to the stress of attaining the physical conditioning required for a daily 2-mile run gradually increases the efficiency of her cardiovascular system. This is beneficial stress, which is denied to the person who limits his exercise to brief periods of physical activity. Trying something for the first time, whether it be a new job, a new skill, or a new role in life, often is a stressful experience. But as one perseveres and as ability and confidence increase, apprehension diminishes and life is enriched because of the continuing effort to learn and grow.

Biologically, a person's method of adaptive responses is limited by genetic endowment as well as by morphologic characteristics and physiochemical structure. Psychological adaptation also depends on genetic endowment plus one's relations with significant others and one's beliefs. Although people have greater latitude sociologically for new adaptive modes, inertia and cultural tradition may impede the

development of new coping mechanisms, particularly if they contradict old values.

Sometimes the body, despite its marvelous capacity for coping with stressors of various types and intensities, reaches a point where excessive stress cannot be compensated for, and symptoms result. These symptoms may represent damage caused by excessive stress. Although symptoms have classically been categorized as mental or physical, each disease process involves all tissues of the body, directly or indirectly, in varying degrees.

Although symptoms may reflect an organic disturbance, they may not have been initiated by cellular pathology. Disease usually is the result of multiple factors. A female diabetic patient who is well controlled with diet and insulin may be considered as being in a state of equilibrium. But the social and psychological stressors associated with her husband's sudden death may be sufficient to provoke acute symptomatic illness. Organic disorders are concomitants in the complex of biologic, psychological, and social patterns of adaptation, and illness should be looked on as a breakdown in total living. Good treatment, then, emphasizes the function of the person in all of her or his dimensions.

Modification of Patient Stress

Each patient reacts differently to stress-producing situations. One person may show little concern if served food that is cold, whereas another may become angry and refuse to eat. This difference in people also applies to stress caused by an illness or surgery. Two patients who are the same age may have the same illness. One recovers quickly, whereas the other takes longer than usual to recover. One of the reasons for the prolonged recovery time may be the person's inability to respond to the stress caused by an illness.

The mechanism of response to stress is complex and sometimes not well understood. The following points should be considered to reduce or modify the patient's physical and emotional stress.

Preventing, Modifying, Reducing, or Eliminating Stressors.
Nurses can anticipate the adaptive tasks faced by patients through knowledge of the specific developmental needs and tasks for each stage in the life cycle. The prevention of illness at crisis points in life is enhanced when people are prepared for new adaptive tasks. Nurses can assist in the maintenance of homeostasis by effective patient teaching and participation in health education programs at the family and community levels.

Hospitalized patients are almost constantly subjected to stress. Nurses often can eliminate patient stress by explaining a procedure before it is performed, staying with a patient while a test is carried out, and allowing the patient to verbalize fears and concerns. A well person can successfully deal with most annoying events at home or work (eg, the noise of a television set, an uncomfortably cool room, or a cup of cold coffee), but for a hospitalized person, these events can become stressful situations.

Although the stress of illness cannot be eliminated, it can be modified by good nursing care. For example, the development of a decubitus ulcer, which is a stressor, can be prevented by good skin care, adequate nutrition, and frequent position changes. Administering medications on time, reporting changes in the patient's condition, and monitoring the patient's response to treatment are other examples of how the nurse can reduce the stress of illness.

Patient Support. The adaptive processes used by patients in their attempt to establish a new state of equilibrium must be supported. During illness, the nurse can accomplish this by managing the patient's internal environment through such measures as controlling pain with analgesics, accurately administering fluids and electrolytes, and encouraging the patient to eat.

Understanding the mental mechanisms that patients use to cope with threats to their integrity enables the nurse to be supportive. Listening nonjudgmentally as patients confront their weaknesses, identify their strengths, and attempt to reassess the direction of their lives relieves them of the burden of carrying this load internally.

Management of the patient's external environment often is necessary to promote rest, a major treatment for many illnesses. Two examples of nursing measures that promote rest are arranging for a comfortable room temperature and spacing care activities for the benefit of the patient rather than for the convenience of hospital departments.

Stress Acceptance. A certain amount of stress is beneficial, and the application of stressors is a necessary part of the treatment process. Optimal stress tolerance levels need to be accurately assessed so that patients are guided to use their adaptation energy at a rate and in a direction appropriate to the capacity of their minds and bodies.

The nurse who encourages a patient who has had a cholecystectomy to cough up secretions introduces another stressor but minimizes its effect by splinting the incisional area when the patient coughs and deep-breathes. Stress during the postoperative period can be minimized by teaching the patient how to cough correctly during the preoperative period, when he is probably more comfortable. Introducing minimal stress through the performance of coughing and deep-breathing exercises prevents a major stress factor that would occur with atelectasis and hypostatic pneumonia. Administering an analgesic (if one is ordered) about 30 minutes before the patient performs his exercises and supporting the incision as the patient coughs and deep-breathes reduce the stress resulting from the pain that accompanies these maneuvers. Judgment arising from knowledge and experience enables the nurse to determine how much stress is appropriate for the individual patient, when to apply it, and when and how to lessen or eliminate it.

BODY DEFENSES
Sources of Body Protection

The body maintains many reserves. When a blood vessel fails, the body may be able to replace its function by developing other vessels that go to the stricken part (collateral circulation). The body has a supply of minerals, some vitamins, food, and fluid beyond its immediate requirements. Many vital functions of the body also have a reserve capacity. For example, there is more lung tissue than normally is required; there are two kidneys (although one could provide satisfactory renal function); there is reserve liver function; and there are dual organs of sight and hearing.

Hyperplasia and Hypertrophy. In certain tissues, in time of increased demand, extra growth occurs. For example, the removal of one kidney often results in an enlargement of the remaining kidney, increasing the amount of available kidney function. The extra growth (proliferation) of normal tissue is called *hyperplasia.* An increase in the size of an organ or structure without an increase in the number of cells is called *hypertrophy.*

Hyperplasia also can occur when no apparent need for it exists, as, for example, the development of hyperplasia of the thyroid gland, with an excess production of thyroid hormone.

Autonomic Nervous System. In response to the ever-changing environment, the autonomic nervous system makes many adjustments in the body that are beyond voluntary control. For example, it regulates body temperature, alters the size of the pupils, and increases or decreases the heart rate.

External Defenses. The skin, with its superficial layer of dead cells, is a relatively impermeable covering. As long as it remains intact, it is the body's major external protection against invasion by microorganisms. The outer layer of skin also prevents liquids, gases, and chemical irritants from coming in contact with living cells below the skin surface. The skull shields the delicate tissues of the brain. The rib cage provides protection for the heart, lungs, and large blood vessels.

Openings into the body also have their protection. Hydrochloric acid in the stomach creates an environment in which most microorganisms cannot survive. The lungs are protected from infection by producing mucus that washes away particles of dust and microorganisms and by tiny cilia that help to move foreign matter out of the respiratory tract. The reflexes of blinking and tear production protect the eyes. Body openings have a rich blood supply and abundant lymphatic tissue to protect the cells of the area if they are invaded by microorganisms.

Internal Defenses.

Internal defenses are highly organized reactions that occur when the body is threatened. For example, in times of sudden, urgent distress, certain sensations, such as dry mouth and a rapid heartbeat, are experienced. These sensations are the result of the release of the neurohormones epinephrine and norepinephrine. The alert state produced by these hormones has been described as preparation for fight or flight.

A second hormonal reaction can occur when the pituitary orders the adrenal cortex to discharge its adrenal cortical steroid. Hydrocortisone constitutes a major part of this substance. Blood pressure, fluid and electrolyte regulation, the membranes covering cells, and the metabolism of glucose are some of the structures and mechanisms affected. Particularly during periods of prolonged stress, the hormonal activity of the adrenal cortex provides a key to the widespread reaction that defends the body. Other hormones also regulate processes to maintain a normal cellular environment. Hormones help to prevent the harm that could follow those occasions when excessive fluid, sugar, or salt ingestion would otherwise radically upset normal cell environment.

Inflammatory Response

Inflammation is the body's response to cell damage. Regardless of the cause, whether a cut, a burn, or a bruise, the reaction is similar. The signal that starts the reaction appears to be the release of histamine, plasma proteases, prostaglandins, and other substances. These substances have a profound effect on the capillaries. The capillaries dilate widely, bringing greatly increased amounts of blood to the area. If the action takes place in the skin or in tissues just below the skin surface, the redness produced by this flushing is visible. The site is warm because it has a greater supply of blood than the tissue around it.

Not only do the capillaries dilate, but the mesh of their walls is opened. Capillaries normally are permeable to the passage of fluid and electrolytes; in this situation, however, they permit extra fluid and some plasma protein to escape. This extra fluid in the tissue spaces results in swelling, accompanied by discomfort and throbbing. Often the swelling is sufficient to stimulate the pain receptors. The blood vessel changes are responsible for the cardinal symptoms of inflammation: swelling, pain, redness, and heat.

Among the substances released by the injured cells is one that attracts white blood cells (leukocytes), which pass through the capillary walls into the damaged tissues. When there is extensive tissue damage, a large amount of this substance is released. It may be absorbed and circulate in the blood. It appears to stimulate the production of more leukocytes. A blood count taken at this time reveals an increase in the number of leukocytes (leukocytosis).

Fever may accompany inflammation. How inflammation influences the temperature-regulating center is not clear. A substance absorbed from the injured cells may be the signal that stimulates this response.

The effects of inflammation might prove to be beneficial. The protein that escapes into the damaged tissue tends to gel and impede the movement of materials within the site. Swelling and pain encourage the person to keep the injured part at rest, which prevents activity from dispersing the contents of the injured area. Bacteria or an offensive substance, such as a foreign chemical, could create additional harm if distributed beyond the local tissue.

Inflammation attracts attention. The patient feels its effects, and the physician relies on its features to help locate and identify the injury. By watching the sequence of symptoms, it is possible to determine whether the body is overcoming the problem or is in need of additional therapy.

At times it is desirable to combat inflammation by countering the vascular dilatation. For example, cold compresses may be prescribed for a sprained ankle because there is no apparent benefit from the painful swelling and no microorganism needs to be isolated. The removal of necrotic tissue still occurs, but at a slower pace because of the vasoconstriction induced by the cold. Sometimes the physician prescribes cold compresses for the first 24 hours to impede swelling, and then warmth to increase blood supply and hasten the removal of waste.

Inflammation and other mechanical and physiologic defense mechanisms against infection are discussed in Chapter 7.

General Nutritional Considerations

☐ Stress necessitates an increase in caloric and protein requirements.

☐ Stress may cause a decrease in appetite, and food intake may be reduced. Diet modifications, such as small, frequent feedings or a diet high in protein and calories, may be necessary.

☐ A balanced diet is necessary for restoring and maintaining health in both the ill and the well person.

General Pharmacologic Considerations

☐ The administration of certain drugs may reduce or modify stress when they alter the disease process.

☐ Pain is a common stressor in the hospitalized patient. When ordered, analgesics are best given before the patient experiences intense pain.

General Gerontologic Considerations

☐ The elderly are less able to adapt to stress and may have deficient protective mechanisms.

☐ The mechanisms of homeostasis become less effective with aging; thus, stress may reduce the reserve power of the body and make the patient more vulnerable to disease.

Suggested Readings

☐ Burton GRW. Microbiology for the health sciences. 3rd ed. Philadelphia: JB Lippincott, 1988. *(Additional coverage of subject matter)*

☐ Memmler RL, Wood DL. The human body in health and disease. 6th ed. Philadelphia: JB Lippincott, 1987. *(Additional coverage of subject matter)*

☐ Porth CM. Pathophysiology: concepts of altered health states. 2nd ed. Philadelphia: JB Lippincott, 1986. *(In-depth, high-level coverage of subject matter)*

☐ Taylor MC, Lillis C, LeMone P. Fundamentals of nursing: the art and science of nursing care. Philadelphia: JB Lippincott, 1989. *(Additional coverage of subject matter)*

Chapter 7

Infectious Diseases: Concepts

On completion of this chapter the reader will:

- List the agents of infection

- List the factors involved in the spread of an infectious disease

- List the types of microorganisms responsible for infectious diseases

- List and describe the mechanical and physiologic defense mechanisms used by the body to defend itself against agents that cause disease

- Define active and passive immunity

- Define the three types of immunity

- List the signs and symptoms of generalized and localized infections

- List and describe the methods used in the diagnosis of an infectious disease

- Describe the causes of decreased resistance to infection

Infectious diseases are a major health problem in both the community and hospital environment. By definition, an *infectious disease* is the invasion and establishment of a pathogenic (disease-causing) microorganism on or within the body. Although many microorganisms are present in the environment as well as on or within the body, not all are capable of producing an infectious process in any one person. An example is the bacterium *Staphylococcus aureus,* which is present in the nose and throat of many people. In a susceptible host, such as a seriously ill or debilitated person, this microorganism can cause an infectious disease.

Once a pathogen enters the body, one of three events occurs: (1) the body's defense mechanisms eliminate the pathogen, (2) the pathogen resides in the body without causing disease, or (3) the pathogen causes an infectious disease.

A *communicable* disease is an infectious disease that is transmissible to other people. Examples of communicable diseases are measles, streptococcal sore throat, sexually transmitted diseases, and tuberculosis.

INFECTIOUS PROCESS

Several important factors are involved in producing an infectious disease. The development of an infection depends on factors such as the following:

- Nature of the infectious agent, its invasiveness, the number present, and the duration of exposure
- Source of the agent and the mode of transmission
- Virulence of the microorganism
- Susceptibility of the host

Like the links in a chain, these factors are interdependent (Fig. 7-1). It is possible to control an infection by removing one or more of the links and breaking the chain.

Agents of Infection

Many varieties of microorganisms are present in the environment. Some varieties are harmful, or *pathogenic,* and can produce disease in a susceptible person, or *host.* Under certain circumstances, microorganisms can reside in or on the body without causing disease, for example, the normal microbial flora (bacteria) that are present in the intestine, some of which are responsible for the synthesis of the B vitamins, vitamin K, and folic acid. Microorganisms that live in the host and do not cause disease when they remain in that area are called *commensals.* If commensals invade or are released into other areas of the body, such as the genitourinary tract or the abdominal cavity, they can become pathogenic microorganisms.

The agent's ability to cause infection depends on a number of factors. The microorganism must be able to

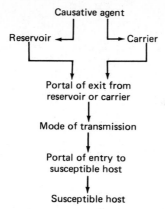

Figure 7–1. Factors involved in the spread of an infectious disease.

survive outside the body until it enters the host, and it must overcome the body's mechanical and physiologic defense mechanisms. Some infectious agents can enter the host only by a specific portal of entry; others are not restricted in this way. The number of microorganisms present and the length of time during which the host is exposed to them are also important factors in the development of an infectious disease. Some microorganisms have greater invasive power and virulence than others. They may have special structures that protect them against the host's defensive mechanisms, or they may produce toxic substances, or *toxins*.

Infectious agents include bacteria, viruses, fungi (yeasts and molds), rickettsiae, protozoans, and mycoplasmas, all of which are microorganisms, and helminths, which are parasitic worms.

Bacteria. Bacteria are single-celled microorganisms. They may be either round (cocci), rod-shaped (bacilli), or spiral (spirochetes). Bacteria also may be *aerobic* or *anaerobic*. Aerobic bacteria require oxygen for growth and multiplication, whereas anaerobic bacteria grow and multiply only in an atmosphere that lacks oxygen.

Viruses. A virus, the smallest agent known to cause disease, is a submicroscopic, filterable (ie, passes through a bacterial filter) microorganism. Viruses can be divided into two types, depending on whether their nucleic acid composition consists of DNA (deoxyribonucleic acid) or RNA (ribonucleic acid). They invade living cells because they must use the metabolic and reproductive materials of living cells or tissues to multiply.

Some viral infections, such as the common cold, are minor and self-limiting. Others, such as rabies, poliomyelitis, and viral hepatitis, are more serious and may be fatal. On occasion, a virus may exist in a living host and from time to time cause a recurrent infection. An example of this phenomenon is the herpes simplex virus, which causes cold sores (fever blisters).

Fungi. Fungi are living organisms of the plant kingdom. They are divided into two basic groups, *yeasts* and *molds*. Only a small number of fungi are known to produce disease in humans.

Fungus (mycotic) infections may be divided into the following three types:

- Superficial mycotic infections, or dermatophytoses, that affect the skin and hair
- Intermediate mycotic infections that chiefly affect subcutaneous tissues
- Deep (or systemic) mycotic infections that affect deep tissues and organs

Rickettsiae. Rickettsiae are microorganisms that resemble, but are different from, bacteria. Like viruses, these microorganisms invade living cells and cannot exist outside of a living organism or host. Rickettsial diseases are transmitted by arthropods (invertebrate animals with a segmented body, an external skeleton, and jointed, paired appendages), such as the flea, tick, louse, or mite.

Protozoans. Protozoans are single-celled animals that are classified according to their motility (ability to move). Some protozoans move like the ameba, which also is a protozoan. Others move by means of cilia (hairlike projections) or flagella (whiplike appendages). Still others have little or no movement.

Mycoplasmas. Mycoplasmas are single-celled microorganisms that lack a cell wall and, therefore, are pleomorphic (ie, assume many shapes). They are similar, but not related, to bacteria. Mycoplasmas primarily infect the surface linings of the respiratory, genitourinary, and gastrointestinal tracts.

Helminths. Helminths (worms) are intestinal parasites. They are divided into three major groups: (1) the nematodes, or roundworms; (2) the cestodes, or tapeworms; and (3) the trematodes, or flukes.

The life cycle of helminths is complex. Briefly stated, some types enter the human body in the egg stage, whereas other forms spend the larval stage in an intermediate host or reservoir and then enter the human host. The organisms mate and reproduce in the definitive host and then are excreted, and the cycle begins again.

Transmission of Infection

The transmission of infection involves the transfer of the infectious agent from the place where it lives and multiplies (reservoir) to the host.

Reservoir. The reservoir is the environment in which the infectious agent is able to survive and reproduce. The reservoir may be human, animal, or nonliving. Some common inanimate (nonliving) reservoirs (*fomites*) are contaminated food and water, eating utensils, books, and clothing.

The term *carrier* refers to a human or animal that harbors (or is the reservoir of) an infectious organism but does not show active evidence of the infectious disease. The carrier is thus a potential source of infection. Human carriers who show no evidence of the infectious disease are called healthy carriers; carriers who are recovering from the infectious disease and have no symptoms, although they continue to harbor the infectious agent, are convalescent carriers; and carriers who are in the incubation period, the time between contact with the infectious agent and the appearance of the first symptoms of the infectious disease, are incubatory carriers.

Portal of Exit. The route by which the infectious agent escapes from the reservoir or the infected host is its portal of exit. The infectious organism may leave the body through the respiratory, gastrointestinal, or genitourinary tract, and through the skin and mucous membranes when the continuity of these structures has been interrupted by an open lesion. Some causative agents leave the reservoir by way of an insect bite (malaria) or by some mechanical means, such as an infected hypodermic needle (type B hepatitis and acquired immunodeficiency syndrome). The term *vector* is commonly used to designate the insect or animal that transfers an infectious agent from one host to another; for example, the *Anopheles* mosquito is the vector that transmits malaria.

Portal of Entry. To cause disease, the infectious agent must gain entrance by an appropriate portal of entry. Most infectious agents are restricted to only one portal of entry, but some agents may use several routes. Staphylococci, for example, can cause disease by entering through the respiratory tract (pneumonia), the skin (boils), the blood (internal abscesses), or the gastrointestinal tract (food poisoning).

Mode of Transmission. Infectious agents may be transmitted to the host by direct or indirect contact or by vectors. *Direct contact* refers to body contact with infected secretions, excreta, or drainage. Gonorrhea, for example, is spread by direct contact. Transfer by *indirect contact* can occur in several ways. It involves contact with an object or substance that has been contaminated by an infected person or a carrier. Contaminated eating utensils, hypodermic needles, food, and water are common reservoirs of infection. When an infected person coughs or sneezes, the air may be contaminated by infected droplets. Insect vec-

tors, such as mosquitoes, flies, mites, and ticks, are responsible for transmitting many infectious diseases.

Susceptibility of the Host

Increased susceptibility to infection may arise from a number of factors, such as the host's age and nutritional status and the presence of other diseases or conditions that alter the state of physical and mental wellness and the host's immune system.

MECHANICAL AND PHYSIOLOGIC DEFENSE MECHANISMS

The body defends itself in many ways against agents that cause disease. These methods are called *defense mechanisms.*

Skin and Mucous Membranes

The first line of defense against invading microorganisms is provided by unbroken and healthy skin and mucous membranes that mechanically separate underlying body tissues from microorganisms present in the environment. The normal flora (eg, microorganisms) found on the skin and mucous membranes compete with pathogenic microorganisms for nutrients, thereby retarding the growth of pathogens in these areas. In addition, the skin, which is acidic (because of the acetic acid in perspiration), creates an undesirable medium for the multiplication of pathogenic microorganisms.

Mucous membrane secretions of the vagina favor the growth of nonpathogenic acid-producing bacteria, such as Döderlein's bacillus. The normal vaginal flora help to maintain an acid pH environment that is unfavorable for the multiplication of pathogenic bacteria and fungi. A change in vaginal pH or destruction of the normal flora can favor the development of a vaginal infection.

Cilia

Hairlike projections called *cilia* arise from the mucous membrane lining the upper respiratory tract (nasal cavities, trachea, and bronchi) and mechanically trap microorganisms, dust, and other foreign particles suspended in inspired air. Microorganisms and foreign particles also may be trapped by mucus secreted by the lining of the respiratory tract and moved upward toward the pharynx by wavelike motions of the cilia. They are then either swallowed or expectorated.

Mucus also is believed to be antibacterial, thus adding to the protective defense mechanism of the upper respiratory tract.

Lysozyme and Gastric Juices

Lysozyme (muramidase), an enzyme capable of splitting (lysing) the cell wall of some gram-positive bacteria, is present in tears, saliva, mucus, skin secretions, and some internal body fluids. This enzyme is bactericidal (destroys bacteria), and thus acts as a defensive barrier to some pathogenic bacteria.

Gastric juices, which are strongly acidic, destroy many of the microorganisms that enter the body by way of the mouth.

Interferon

Interferon is a protein substance produced by white blood cells and probably other body cells in response to viral infections as well as other factors. When a cell is invaded by a virus, it produces and releases interferon, which appears to trigger a cell to manufacture an antiviral protein. Because interferon also appears to inhibit cell reproduction, it is used in the treatment of some types of cancers. Although the use of interferon in cancer treatment remains experimental and at times disappointing, there have been some positive results. Its use in the treatment of viral disorders also has been the subject of investigation.

Reticuloendothelial System

Two major defense mechanisms are provided by the reticuloendothelial system: phagocytosis and the immune response.

Phagocytosis. The reticuloendothelial system is a group of specialized cells that line many vascular and lymphatic channels. Some of these cells are capable of *phagocytosis,* which is the ingestion and digestion of foreign agents, such as bacteria, viruses, and protozoans, and other matter, such as red blood cells that become fragmented at the end of their (about) 120-day life span. These specialized cells are called *phagocytes.* The larger phagocytes are called *macrophages* and the smaller ones, *microphages.* Phagocytes may be stationary, or fixed, such as those located in the alveoli of the lungs, the liver, the spleen, or bone marrow. Others may move about, and are called *wandering phagocytes.* Neutrophils and monocytes, which are two types of white blood cells (leukocytes), are wandering phagocytes.

The invasion of microorganisms or other foreign debris triggers a phagocytic response by various cells of the reticuloendothelial system. These cells mobilize to destroy the invading microorganisms, and thereby prevent infection. Sometimes the number of invading microorganisms is so great that despite phagocytic activity, an infection occurs. Some diseases, such as leukemia and aplastic anemia, may reduce the number of wandering phagocytes, and thereby increase susceptibility to infection.

Immune Response. The stem cells of bone marrow are capable of producing different types of blood cells: monocytes, lymphocytes, neutrophils, basophils, eosinophils, red blood cells (erythrocytes), and platelets. During fetal life, some of the lymphocytes are influenced to become T cells and others are influenced to become B cells (Fig. 7-2).

Any foreign substance (eg, a microorganism) that enters the body and is capable of stimulating the formation of antibodies is called an *antigen* (or immunogen). When an antigen enters the body, one of three responses may occur: (1) a response negotiated by B cells, (2) a response negotiated by T cells, or (3) a response negotiated by both B cells and T cells.

When the response is negotiated by B cells, it is called *humoral immunity,* and antibodies, or *immunoglobulins,* are formed. These immunoglobulins (Ig) are subdivided into groups—IgA, IgD, IgE, IgG,

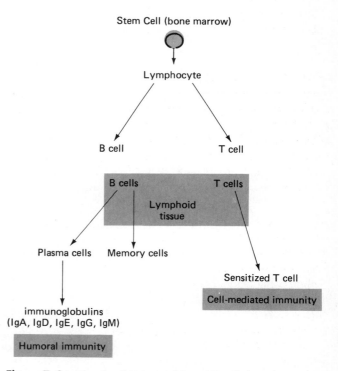

Figure 7–2. The development of B and T cells from bone marrow stem cells.

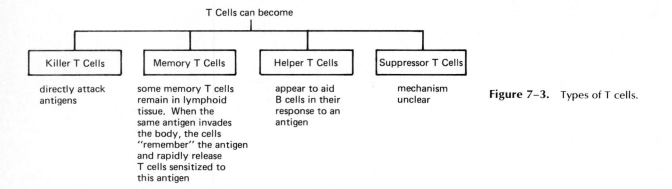

Figure 7–3. Types of T cells.

and IgM—and are part of the body's serum (plasma) proteins called *gamma globulins.* Immunoglobulins (antibodies) are capable of destroying invading microorganisms (antigens). B cells also may produce memory cells (see Fig. 7-2) that "remember" the invading antigen. If the same antigen invades the body again, these memory cells can produce a more rapid and intense response to the antigen invasion.

When the response is negotiated by T cells, it is called *cell-mediated immunity.* This type of immunity involves the release of several types of sensitized T cells (see Fig. 7-2). Some T cells become memory cells (Fig. 7-3). Like the memory B cells, they react rapidly to a later invasion by the same antigen. Some become killer T cells that directly attack the invading antigen. Killer T-cell response also is seen in organ transplantation; in this case, the donor organ, such as a kidney, liver, or heart, is the antigen. This response causes the body to reject the transplanted organ. Rejection of a transplanted organ can be prevented by the use of drugs as well as other modes of therapy.

There are three types of immunity: naturally acquired active immunity, artificially acquired active immunity, and passive immunity (Fig. 7-4).

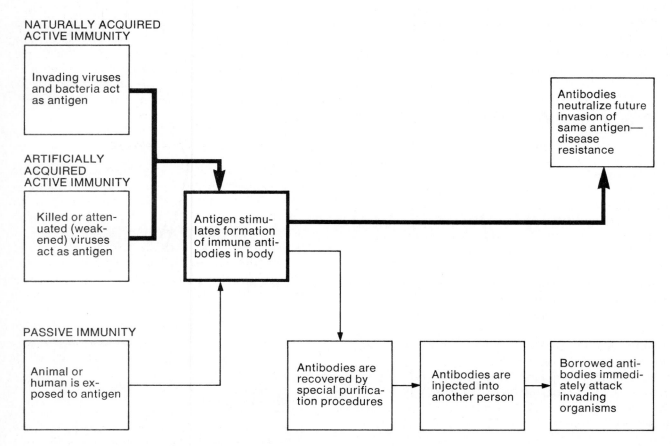

Figure 7–4. Active and passive immunity.

Naturally Acquired Active Immunity. Immunity to a specific microorganism as a result of a previous invasion by the microorganism is known as naturally acquired active immunity, or actively acquired immunity. An example of this type of immunity is a lifelong immunity to measles that is acquired after having the disease. Not all invading microorganisms produce an antibody response that gives lifelong immunity. At times immunity may be short-lived or even nonexistent (eg, the immunity that results from the invasion of viruses that cause the common cold).

The initial invasion by a microorganism (antigen) produces both humoral and cell-mediated immunity. *Humoral immunity* involves the B cells that manufacture immunoglobulins (antibodies) that are capable of destroying the invading antigen. The person develops signs and symptoms of the infection because the body requires a period of time to produce a sufficient number of antibodies. There is recovery from the infection because of antibody production. Exposure to the same antigen at a later time normally provides a sufficient number of antibodies to destroy the invading antigen. Lifelong immunity to certain disease-producing antigens occurs because some antibodies from the original infection are still present, and the memory cells are able to "remember" the specific antigen. If the body were unable to produce antibodies, the infection would not only continue, but also become severer as the microorganisms continued to multiply. Death from an overwhelming infection could be the result.

Cell-mediated immunity involves the production of T cells, some of which are killer T cells. The killer T cells migrate to and directly attack the invading antigen.

Artificially Acquired Active Immunity. Artificially acquired immunity is similar to actively acquired immunity in the sense that a microorganism invades the body and elicits a response from the immune system. The difference between actively acquired and artificially acquired immunity is that the latter results from the administration of a killed or attenuated (weakened) microorganism (antigen) or toxoid (an attenuated toxin) followed by manufacture of antibodies against the disease. The body's defense mechanisms cannot distinguish between a killed or attenuated antigen and a virulent (live) antigen, and manufactures antibodies in the presence of antigens in any of these forms. The killed or attenuated antigen does not cause disease symptoms that are as severe as the symptoms produced by a live antigen; however, some minor symptoms of the infection may be noted. The B cells manufacture antibodies, and the B and T memory cells "remember" the killed or attenuated antigen and recognize it if a future invasion occurs.

Passive Immunity. Passive immunity uses antibodies produced by another organism, either animal or human. These antibodies are injected to provide immediate, short-lived immunity and protection from the invading antigen. No memory cells are produced, and the level of the injected antibodies diminishes over a period of several weeks to a few months. Passive immunity may involve the injection of an *antitoxin,* a substance formed after exposure to a toxin. A *toxin* is a substance produced by some bacteria (eg, the bacterium that causes tetanus). The body's defense mechanisms respond to a toxin by producing an antitoxin, in the same way that they produce antibodies against an antigen. Antitoxins for passive immunity are obtained from animal or human sources, and are available for the treatment of botulism, diphtheria, gas gangrene, and tetanus. Snake antivenin, a form of passive immunity, contains protective substances obtained from the gamma globulin of horses. The antivenin is administered after a bite by some species of poisonous snakes.

Human immune serum may be used for passive immunization against measles, pertussis (whooping cough), hepatitis B, chickenpox, and tetanus. Immune serum globulin, also called *gamma globulin,* is recovered from *human pooled plasma.* Because there is more than one plasma donor, the serum is likely to contain a variety of specific antibodies. Newborn infants also receive passive immunity to some diseases from their mothers because the maternal circulating antibodies cross the placental barrier. As with other forms of passive immunity, the newborn infant is immune, for a few months after birth, to those diseases for which the mother has manufactured antibodies.

Inflammatory Response

Although the inflammatory response is a general defense mechanism, it usually is greater when tissue injury is caused by microorganisms than when physical trauma has occurred (Fig. 7-5). Inflammation is marked by heat, redness, swelling, and pain.

The inflammatory response serves to bring nutrients necessary for the repair of tissues (healing), destroy microorganisms, and remove debris; it thus contains or localizes the infection. Despite the body's protective mechanisms or, in some instances, because of the lack of an effective protective mechanism, not all infections can be contained and controlled; microorganisms may move to adjacent structures such as the lymph nodes or bloodstream.

The inflammatory response has three stages:

1. *Vascular response.* Shortly after tissue injury (physical or invasion by microorganisms), there is localized vasoconstriction immediately followed by vasodilatation. This vasodilatation, caused by the release of histamine

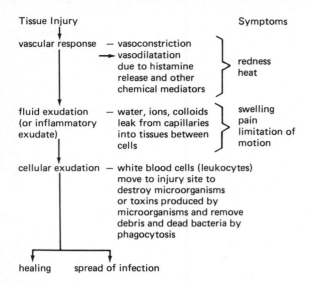

Tissue Injury   Symptoms

vascular response — vasoconstriction
                → vasodilatation   ⎫ redness
                  due to histamine   ⎬ heat
                  release and other   ⎭
                  chemical mediators

fluid exudation   — water, ions, colloids ⎫ swelling
(or inflammatory   leak from capillaries ⎬ pain
exudate)   into tissues between ⎭ limitation of
                     cells   motion

cellular exudation — white blood cells (leukocytes)
                     move to injury site to
                     destroy microorganisms
                     or toxins produced by
                     microorganisms and remove
                     debris and dead bacteria by
                     phagocytosis

healing   spread of infection

Figure 7–5. Mechanisms of the inflammatory response.

and probably other chemical substances at the site of injury, results in increased blood flow to the injured part. Two early signs of inflammation—heat and redness—are now apparent.

2. *Fluid exudation.* At the time of vasodilatation, capillary walls become more permeable, allowing the passage of molecules of water and colloids as well as ions into the tissues between the cells of the injured area. This also is called the *inflammatory exudate.* The collection of fluid between the cells accounts for the swelling and pain or tenderness at the site of injury. Limitation of motion also may occur because of the pain and swelling.

3. *Cellular exudation.* White blood cells move to the injury site to destroy microorganisms or the toxins produced by the microorganisms and to remove debris and dead bacteria produced by phagocytosis.

LOCALIZED INFECTIONS

An infection that has not spread is said to be *localized.* The initial reaction to an invading microorganism is a vascular response, which produces redness and heat (see Fig. 7-4). This is followed by leakage of fluid, colloids, and ions from the capillaries into the tissues between the cells, producing swelling, pain, and, at times, limitation of motion. Lymphocytes move to the injury site to destroy the pathogens or the toxins produced by the pathogens and to remove debris from the area. To prevent the spread of pathogenic microorganisms to adjacent tissues, a fibrin barrier is formed around the injured area. The exact mechanism of the formation of this barrier is unclear. Inside the barrier, a thick, white exudate (pus) accumulates. This collection of pus is called an *abscess.* The abscess may break through the skin and drain, or it may have to be opened and drained by a physician. Internal abscesses,

such as on the lung or liver, require surgery for incision and drainage of the abscess.

Some microorganisms localize more readily, whereas others spread once they have become established. The streptococcus, for example, can produce a substance that breaks down the wall of fibrin, enabling the bacterium to spread to adjacent tissues and invade lymphatic channels. If any microorganism invades the lymph nodes, the resulting inflammation is called *lymphadenitis.* The swelling in the lymph nodes produces a tender, firm lump, a signal that the microorganisms have reached this area (Fig. 7-6). If the microorganisms are sufficiently numerous and virulent, this defense mechanism may be unable to contain the infection, and the microorganisms begin to travel from node to node. Because the lymphatic system drains into the venous system, the microorganisms may eventually reach the bloodstream. When the microorganisms circulate in the blood, the condition is called *septicemia.*

Localized infections may produce generalized symptoms. An example is an abscess of a body organ or structure such as the liver, lung, brain, or anorectal area. Symptoms include fever, chills, fatigue, headache, and anorexia (loss of appetite). Leukocytosis (an increase in the number of white blood cells) and an increase in the erythrocyte sedimentation rate may occur. Depending on the type of infection, other laboratory tests also may show changes. Other signs and

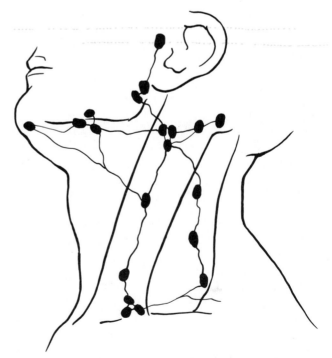

Figure 7–6. Lymph nodes of the neck help to prevent the spread of infection from a primary site in the head or neck to the rest of the body.

symptoms may be present, depending on the location of the abscess. For example, a person with a lung abscess also may experience shortness of breath, coughing, and hemoptysis (expectoration of blood). The sputum may be dark brown, and contain old red blood cells and pus.

GENERALIZED INFECTIONS

Generalized infections are those that are widespread or involve a large area or one or more organs. The signs and symptoms of a generalized infection are variable. During the early stages, some patients have few symptoms and do not appear acutely ill, whereas others experience many symptoms. Fever usually is present, and body temperature may rise as the infection worsens. A sudden high fever is not uncommon. Chills, which may occur before there is a rise in body temperature, signal that the body is responding to the infection. They also may be an indication that the microorganisms have entered the bloodstream. During chills, the patient feels cold because superficial blood vessels constrict to prevent loss of heat from the blood. Sweating also stops, and circulation is diverted away from superficial blood vessels to blood vessels deep within the body. Muscles begin to contract in uncontrollable shivering, and heat is produced by this increased muscle activity. The pulse and respiratory rates usually are elevated.

Some patients may experience a drop in blood pressure. Hypotension occasionally becomes severe, and shock ensues. This type of shock, referred to as *septic shock, bacteremic shock,* or *toxic shock,* more commonly occurs in the person with an infection caused by gram-negative microorganisms. Severe infections caused by *S. aureus* and streptococcal microorganisms, which are gram-positive, also may cause septic shock. Other signs and symptoms of a generalized infection include headache, muscle aches and pains, rash, joint pain, anorexia, weakness, and fatigue. The symptoms of an infection caused by a specific pathogen depend on the toxigenicity or virulence of the pathogen and the response of the individual host. To illustrate, an invasion by a pathogen that normally is considered nonvirulent or of low toxigenicity produces a different response in a person with a decreased resistance to infection than it does in a person with adequate resistance to infection.

The signs and symptoms of some communicable diseases may be fairly uniform and predictable. The complaints related by the patient and physical signs noted during examination are often diagnostically significant. Children with rubella (German measles) have a typical diffuse macular and punctate rash, and lymph node enlargement is common. The rash and other signs and symptoms of rubella are different from the rash of measles (rubeola). Patients with rubeola also have upper respiratory tract symptoms (bronchitis and nasal secretions) and the characteristic Koplik spots on the buccal mucosa. Fever and a particular type of cough are typical signs of pertussis (whooping cough), and swelling of the parotid and other salivary glands is a sign of mumps.

Signs and symptoms of other communicable diseases, such as helminth infestations (eg, hookworm and roundworm), may be vague, and specific diagnostic tests may be required.

DIAGNOSIS OF AN INFECTIOUS DISEASE

A physical examination and thorough patient history are essential for the diagnosis of an infectious disease. Sometimes they are all that is required for diagnosis. The diagnosis of some infectious diseases, however, requires additional studies or a laboratory examination of body fluids to identify the microorganism.

The type and number of tests or studies required for diagnosis depends on several factors. An extremely ill patient may require not only those tests pertinent to the infectious disease but also other tests to determine any additional problems that may be caused by the infection. Various tests and diagnostic studies also may be required at certain intervals to monitor the patient's response to treatment. For example, a patient with a bacterial pneumonia confirmed by sputum culture and a chest radiograph (also called x-ray) may have these tests repeated one or more times to monitor the effectiveness of antibiotic therapy.

Bacteriologic Studies

To identify the pathogen causing an infection, bacteriologic studies are performed. The source of the specimen may be body fluids or wastes, such as blood, sputum, urine, or feces, or the purulent exudate. For direct examination, the specimen is smeared on a slide and examined microscopically. Because bacteria are colorless, it is often necessary to stain or dye the specimen to examine it in this manner. One stain that may be applied is the Gram stain. Those bacteria that absorb the dye (or color) are classified as *gram-positive,* such as *S. aureus.* Those that do not absorb the dye are *gram-negative,* such as *Neisseria gonorrheae.*

The bacterium *S. aureus,* the causative microorganism of some *nosocomial* (hospital-acquired) infections, may be tested for pathogenicity or virulence (its power to produce disease) by the coagulase test. When a culture of *S. aureus* is reported as coagulase-positive, it is more virulent than a culture of the same microorganism that produces a negative (coagulase-negative) response to this test.

Often specimens are cultured. This involves placing a small amount of the specimen on the surface of or in a special growth medium, such as broth or blood agar. The plates or tubes are then incubated for a specific period of time, removed, and examined visually and microscopically.

Sensitivity studies also may be done to determine which antibiotic will inhibit the growth of a microorganism and be effective in treating the infection. To determine bacterial sensitivity to chemotherapeutic agents, disks impregnated with different antibiotics are placed on a culture plate that has been smeared with the specimen to be tested. After a specified time, each disk is inspected for growth, or the lack of growth, of bacterial colonies. Lack of growth indicates bacterial sensitivity; therefore, the drug should be effective in treating the infection. Bacterial growth around the disk indicates bacterial resistance and probable ineffectiveness of the drug. Sensitivity tests may be ordered along with a culture.

Skin Tests

Skin testing may be done for some infectious diseases to determine the presence of a specific active or inactive infection. Diseases for which skin testing may be done include histoplasmosis, mumps, tuberculosis, diphtheria, and coccidioidomycosis.

The material for skin testing is injected intradermally, preferably on the inner (volar) aspect of the forearm. The reaction is read after a specified period of time—usually 48 to 72 hours. The time interval between injection of the testing material and the reading of the reaction is important; therefore, the manufacturer's recommendations (as stated in the package insert accompanying the testing material) for each test must be followed.

Immunologic Tests

The following immunologic tests may be used to determine the presence of antigen–antibody reactions:

1. *Agglutination* (or *clumping*) *tests*. Examples include the cold agglutinins test, which may reveal the presence of high titers in such diseases as cirrhosis, lymphatic leukemia, peripheral vascular disease, and atypical pneumonia, and the hemagglutination inhibition test, to determine immunity to rubella.
2. *Precipitation tests*. Examples include C-reactive protein, which can be used to determine the severity of some inflammatory diseases, and the fungal antibody test for coccidioidomycosis.
3. *Complement-fixation test*. This test is used to diagnose histoplasmosis, blastomycosis, and rickettsial diseases.
4. *Immunofluorescence tests*. These tests identify immunoglobulins, which are antibodies formed by the immune system. Two examples are the fluorescent treponemal antibody absorption test for syphilis and the indirect fluorescent antibody test for the Epstein-Barr virus and antinuclear antibodies. The indirect fluorescent antibody test also may be used to diagnose toxoplasmosis.

Tissue Biopsy

Small samples of tissue obtained during major or minor surgical procedures may be examined microscopically and cultured for microorganisms.

Other Tests

Depending on the infectious disease, other methods of diagnostic testing may be used. Radiography (plain films or contrast studies), computed tomography scanning, and magnetic resonance imaging may be used to locate abscesses, identify displacement of organs or structures that may indicate abscess formation, and detect changes in tissues in areas such as the bones or the lung. Laboratory tests such as a complete blood count, erythrocyte sedimentation rate, and white cell count and differential may be ordered, since changes in these results also may indicate the presence of an infectious process.

CAUSES OF DECREASED RESISTANCE TO INFECTION

Physiologic and mechanical defense mechanisms are major lines of defense against invasion by pathogenic microorganisms. If one or more of these defense mechanisms is weakened or lacking, an atmosphere conducive to infection may be created. For example, the mucous membranes lining the vagina favor the existence of nonpathogenic microorganisms that help to maintain an acidic environment that is unfavorable for the establishment of pathogenic microorganisms. A change in the vaginal pH or destruction of the normal flora can occur with frequent douching or the use of some types of antibiotics, such as the tetracyclines. Either of these activities can create a favorable environment for the growth of pathogenic microorganisms such as the fungus *Candida albicans*.

The use of some brands of vaginal tampons for the absorption of the menstrual flow has been linked to the development of toxic shock syndrome. Whether the use of a highly absorbable type of tampon that requires frequent changing favors the multiplication of pathogens or interferes with vaginal defense mechanisms is not known. Toxic shock syndrome also has occurred in nonmenstruating women and men, but the incidence is lower in these groups. The pathogen responsible for the syndrome is believed to be a penicillin-resistant strain of *S. aureus*.

Conditions That Affect the Reticuloendothelial System

Two major defense mechanisms of the body—phagocytosis and the immune response—are provided by the reticuloendothelial system. Certain diseases or conditions can alter the ability of one or more of the components of the reticuloendothelial system to respond to invading pathogens. One example is the hematologic disorder agranulocytosis, a decrease in the production of white blood cells by the bone marrow, including those cells capable of phagocytosis. People with some forms of leukemia also are highly susceptible to infection because their bone marrow produces many immature white blood cells that are incapable of dealing with invading pathogens.

Drugs

Any drug that possesses the ability to depress bone marrow activity decreases the body's resistance to infection by altering this normal physiologic defense mechanism. Corticosteroid preparations, when given in high doses or for prolonged periods, can suppress the immune response. Some drugs—for example, the antibiotic chloramphenicol (Chloromycetin), the antithyroid preparation propylthiouracil, and the antirheumatic agents indomethacin (Indocin) and phenylbutazone (Butazolidin)—are capable of causing varying degrees of bone marrow depression, resulting in a decrease in the production of blood cells, including white blood cells. Patients who receive these and other drugs that are capable of affecting the bone marrow are closely observed for signs and symptoms of bone marrow depression (eg, unusual bleeding or bruising, fever, chills, sore throat, and malaise). Frequent laboratory studies usually are necessary to detect severe bone marrow depression.

The immunosuppressive agent azathioprine (Imuran) is given to prevent rejection of a transplanted kidney. The ability of this drug to suppress the immune system is a desirable action of the drug, since the body rejects transplanted organs, which are recognized by the immune system as foreign proteins (antigens). The recognition of other antigens, such as

pathogenic microorganisms, also is suppressed. A patient who receives this drug becomes highly susceptible to invading pathogens, even those that are normally present in the environment.

Alterations in Mechanical Barriers

The unbroken skin serves as a protective barrier by separating the underlying tissues from the surrounding environment, including pathogenic microorganisms. Any break in the continuity of the skin, such as would be caused by cuts, abrasions, puncture wounds, and surgery, allows both pathogenic and nonpathogenic microorganisms to invade underlying tissues. Some interruptions in the skin's continuity are minor, and the healthy person's physiologic defense mechanisms are able to control the invasion. Even a major interruption, such as a surgical incision or a large wound or puncture, frequently is controlled by the healthy person's defense mechanisms. Antibiotics are administered to aid the person's defense mechanisms in controlling invading pathogens.

Some people (eg, those with leukemia) may develop severe infections after a small break in the skin's continuity because the reticuloendothelial system is producing immature cells that are incapable of attacking invading microorganisms. Local and systemic infections are common complications of severe and extensive burns because the skin's protective abilities have been destroyed. Microorganisms in the environment also are a source of infection despite strict aseptic techniques, correct isolation procedures, and intensive antibiotic therapy.

Skin disorders, such as exfoliative dermatitis and herpes zoster (shingles), and lesions, such as superficial carcinomas (arising particularly from carcinoma of the breast), may lead to secondary infections. For example, exfoliative dermatitis involves widespread loss of the superficial layers of the skin, thus permitting the invasion of pathogens. Skin breaks caused by scratching (itching may be severe in the healing phase of shingles) also contribute to the introduction of pathogens. A superficial carcinoma leads to necrosis of tissues over the neoplasm, thus destroying the protection afforded by unbroken skin.

The action of the cilia lining the upper respiratory tract may be impaired by smoking or prolonged exposure to heavy concentrations of industrial pollutants. Damage to these structures lessens their ability to effectively clear the respiratory tract of mucus that has trapped inhaled foreign particles, including microorganisms contained in inspired air. This decreased effectiveness of the cilia may lead to infections of the respiratory tract.

Systemic Diseases

Some systemic diseases interfere with one or more physiologic defense mechanisms, and thus decrease resistance to invading pathogens. Diseases such as multiple myeloma, Hodgkin's disease, and some forms of leukemia directly affect structures that are responsible for antibody formation. Others may indirectly affect the body's defense mechanisms. An example of this is peripheral vascular disease, which involves constriction of the peripheral arterial system, resulting in decreased arterial blood flow. As a result, tissues of the extremities fail to receive an adequate supply of oxygen and nutrients as well as circulating antibodies and protective lymphocytes. The decreased blood supply ultimately may lead to ulcerations and gangrene of the affected areas, and the protective skin barrier is lost.

Congenital Deficiencies

X-linked infantile agammaglobulinemia is a deficiency in the development of B cells (see Fig. 7-2) with resultant lack of antibody formation (humoral immunity). T-cell development (cell-mediated immunity) is normal. This sex-linked disorder occurs only in males, and may be treated with gamma globulin concentrations and antibiotics.

In DiGeorge's syndrome, infants are born without a thymus gland, and therefore lack or have a deficiency of T-cell formation (cell-mediated immunity). Patients with this disorder have been treated with thymus obtained from a human fetus.

Severe combined immunodeficiency is a genetic disorder in which both B and T cells are deficient or absent. Many of these patients succumb at an early age despite intensive therapies. Bone marrow transplantation has been successful in some cases. Others have survived by being placed in highly specialized germ-free environments.

Other Factors

Malnutrition, age, a serious debilitating illness, and possibly other factors may directly or indirectly cause decreased resistance to infection. Often there is a combination of several complex factors rather than an isolated simple one. It is important for nurses to realize that many factors play a role in any one person's ability or inability to resist infection. Hospitalized patients are especially prone to infection because of their enhanced susceptibility to infection and the potential for direct transmission of pathogenic microorganisms from the hospital environment and personnel.

Suggested Readings

☐ Burton GRW. Microbiology for the health sciences. 3rd ed. Philadelphia: JB Lippincott, 1988. *(Additional coverage of subject matter)*

☐ Fischbach FT. A manual of laboratory diagnostic tests. 3rd ed. Philadelphia: JB Lippincott, 1988. *(Additional coverage of subject matter)*

☐ Halpern SR. Quick reference to clinical nutrition. 2nd ed. Philadelphia: JB Lippincott, 1987. *(Additional coverage of subject matter)*

☐ Kirkis EJ, Grier M. Nurse's guide to infection control practice. Philadelphia: WB Saunders, 1988. *(In-depth coverage of subject matter)*

☐ Lewis LW, Timby, BK. Fundamental skills and concepts in patient care. 4th ed. Philadelphia: JB Lippincott, 1988. *(Additional coverage of subject matter)*

☐ Wallach JB. Interpretation of diagnostic tests: a handbook synopsis of laboratory medicine. Boston: Little, Brown & Co, 1986. *(In-depth, high-level coverage of subject matter)*

☐ West KH. Infectious disease handbook for emergency care personnel. Philadelphia: JB Lippincott, 1987. *(In-depth coverage of subject matter)*

Chapter 8

Community-Acquired and Nosocomial Infections

On completion of this chapter the reader will:

■ Differentiate between nosocomial and community-acquired infectious diseases

■ List and discuss the methods of preventing and controlling community-acquired infections

■ List and discuss the methods of preventing and controlling nosocomial infections

■ Describe the various types of isolation techniques

■ Use the nursing process in the management of the patient with an infectious disease

Infectious diseases may be divided into two types: community-acquired infections and nosocomial (hospital-acquired) infections.

COMMUNITY-ACQUIRED INFECTIONS

Many communicable diseases have been either contained or eliminated because of advances in the prevention and treatment of infectious diseases and in general health measures aimed at controlling the spread of such diseases. These advances include the discovery of antibiotics, the development of immunizing agents, guidelines for the proper disposal of human wastes, legislation controlling the preparation and sale of foods, immunization programs, and public education. Some of the community-acquired infections seen in the United States are listed in Table 8-1.

Despite these intensive efforts, new problems arise. The discovery of antibiotics greatly reduced the number of deaths attributed to some infections (eg, pneumonia). Although a wide variety of antiinfective drugs are available, some microorganisms are resistant to these agents. Consequently drug resistance has made some infectious diseases increasingly difficult to treat. Apathy toward immunization programs also poses a potential health problem. Parents who have never seen or known a person with diphtheria or poliomyelitis may not recognize or believe that there is a need for early and effective immunization against these communicable diseases. Some communities require all children who are entering or currently enrolled in school to be properly immunized; other areas have few or no immunization requirements. In addition, all preschool children are entirely dependent on their parents for obtaining immunizations during early childhood.

An effective immunization program can solve some of the problems associated with childhood communicable diseases. Active immunization against mumps, measles (rubeola), diphtheria, tetanus, pertussis (whooping cough), poliomyelitis, and rubella (German measles) is recommended by the U.S. Public Health Service. Free immunization offered by local public health departments reduce or eliminate the financial burden for those who cannot pay for these services. Legislation requiring adequate immunization before entering school as well as during the school years has been passed by some states and local communities. Although these requirements are objectionable to some people on legal or moral grounds, they appear to be justified.

Several sound reasons exist for the adequate immunization of all children against some communicable diseases. The immunization of children protects *all* people—adults as well as children. For example, older boys and men who have not had mumps or been

Continued on page 74

Table 8–1. Community-Acquired Infections

Infectious Disease	Causative Microorganism	Reservoir	Mode of Transmission	Methods of Treatment and Control
Amebiasis	Entamoeba histolytica	Human carriers (healthy, chronic)	Infected water, raw vegetables; insect vectors	*Treatment:* amebicide drugs *Intestinal form:* paromomycin, (Humatin), iodoquinol, metronidazole (Flagyl), carbarsone, emetine HCl, tetracyclines (in conjunction with amebicides), erythromycin. Extraintestinal form: metronidazole, emetine HCl, chloroquine *Control:* sanitary disposal of human wastes, fly control, routine examination of food handlers, chlorination *and* filtration of drinking water
Ancyclostomiasis (hookworm)	Nector americanus, Ancyclostoma duodenale	Infected person	Eggs in feces deposited on ground, larvae penetrate bare skin (usually of foot)	*Treatment:* thiabendazole (Mintezol), mebendazole (Vermox), pyrantel pamoate (Antiminth) *Control:* sanitary disposal of human wastes
Encephalitis; eastern and western, St Louis	Specific virus for each type	Mosquito + ? birds, rodents, etc	Bite of infected mosquito	*Treatment:* supportive *Control:* elimination of mosquito breeding places, avoid contact with mosquito
Candidiasis	Candida albicans	Humans	Direct contact with those infected or with carriers	*Treatment:* deep-seated/systemic–amphotericin B (Fungizone), nystatin (intestinal), flucytosine (Ancobon), miconazole (Monistat); superficial—topical application of gentian violet, miconazole, clotrimazole (Lotrimin), nystatin, amphotericin B *Control:* treat infections, avoid contact, in newborn nurseries isolate those with oral candidiasis
Chancroid	Haemophilus ducreyi (Ducrey bacillus)	Humans	Direct sexual contact	*Treatment:* sulfonamides, tetracyclines, streptomycin *Control:* avoid sexual contacts, identify and report known cases, treat contacts
Chicken pox (varicella)	Varicella-zoster virus	Infected person	Direct contact, airborne, fomites	*Treatment:* supportive, immune serum globulins for high-risk patients *Control:* disinfect articles soiled by discharges (nose, throat, lesions)
Dermatophytosis (ringworm), tinea capitis (scalp); tinea corporis (body); tinea pedis (foot)	Various species of Microsporum and Trichophyton	Humans, animals	Direct or indirect contact	*Treatment:* griseofulvin (t. capitis); tolnaftate (Tinactin), undecylenic acid (Desenex), miconazole (Micatin), clotrimazole (Lotrimin); triacetin (Enzactin), iodochlorhydroxyquin (Vioform) *Control:* disinfect/launder clothing, towels, socks; general cleanliness; disinfect floors and benches if contact is public facility, keep feet dry

Continued

Table 8–1. Community-Acquired Infections *Continued*

Infectious Disease	Causative Microorganism	Reservoir	Mode of Transmission	Methods of Treatment and Control
Diphtheria	*Corynebacterium diphtheriae* (Klebs-Loeffler bacillus)	Humans	Contact with patient or carrier, fomites	*Treatment:* active disease, diphtheria antitoxin + supportive therapy with antibiotics *Control:* immunization with diphtheria toxoid
Giardiasis	*Giardia lamblia*	Humans	Probably fecal contamination of water	*Treatment:* quinacrine, furazolidone (Furoxone) *Control:* Improve water sanitation facilities; improve water purification methods, identify and treat contacts
Gonorrhea	*Neisseria gonorrhoeae*	Humans	Direct contact (usually sexual)	*Treatment:* penicillin preceded by probenecid, erythromycin, spectinomycin (Trobicin), tetracycline *Control:* avoid sexual contacts, investigation and treatment of infected people and their contacts
Hepatitis type A (infectious hepatitis)	Hepatitis A virus	Humans	Direct contact	*Treatment:* supportive; ISG may offer protection against clinical manifestations if given early *Control:* enteric and blood precautions; ISG for contacts
Hepatitis type B	Hepatitis B virus	Humans	Parenteral administration of human blood and blood products (eg, serum, packed cells, fibrinogen) from infected person; contaminated needles and syringes, intravenous equipment	*Treatment:* supportive *Control:* enteric and blood precautions; careful screening of blood donors
Infectious mononucleosis	Epstein-Barr virus	Humans	Probably direct contact	*Treatment:* supportive *Control:* properly dispose of articles soiled with nose and throat secretions
Influenza A, B, C; subtypes of A	Virus type A, B, C	Humans	Direct contact	*Treatment:* supportive, amantidine HCl (for type A virus influenza) *Control:* active immunization with specific virus vaccine, especially high-risk people
Legionnaires' disease	*Legionella pneumophila*	? Environment	Probably airborne droplets from contaminated water and other sources	*Treatment:* erythromycin *Control:* locate source of infection
Lymphogranuloma venereum	*Chlamydia trachomatis*	Humans	Sexual contact, contact with articles contaminated by discharges	*Treatment:* tetracyclines *Control:* identify and treat sexual contacts

Continued

Table 8–1.   Community-Acquired Infections *Continued*

Infectious Disease	*Causative Microorganism*	*Reservoir*	*Mode of Transmission*	*Methods of Treatment and Control*
Malaria	Plasmodium (P. vivax, P. falciparum, P. malariae, P. ovale)	Humans	Bite of infectious *Anopheles* mosquito, transfusion of blood from infected people	*Treatment:* antimalarial drugs specific to type of malaria being treated
				Control: eradication of mosquito breeding areas, prophylactic administration of antimalarial drugs, blood donor screening
Measles (rubeola)	Virus of measles	Humans	Direct contact, droplet spread	*Treatment:* supportive
				Control: active immunization with measles vaccine, live, attenuated
Meningococcal meningitis	Neisseria meningitides	Humans	Direct contact	*Treatment:* sulfonamides, extended-spectrum penicillins (eg, ampicillin, hetacillin), tetracycline (IV), chloramphenicol (Chloromycetin)
				Control: prophylactic treatment of contacts with sulfonamides, treatment of known carriers with rifampin (Rifadin); meningococcal polysaccharide vaccine to high-risk people in endemic areas
Mumps	Virus of mumps	Humans	Direct contact, droplet spread	*Treatment:* supportive
				Control: active immunization with live mumps virus vaccine; proper disposal of articles soiled with secretions from nose, throat
Mycoplasmal pneumonia (eaton agent, PPLO)	Mycoplasma pneumoniae	Humans	Direct contact, droplet spread	*Treatment:* tetracyclines, erythromycin
				Control: proper disposal of articles soiled with secretions from nose, throat
Paratyphoid fever	Salmonella paratyphi, S. schottmuelleri, S. hirschfeldii	Humans	Direct contact; contact with feces, urine of carrier and contaminated food and water	*Treatment:* ampicillin, chloramphenicol (Chloromycetin)
				Control: periodic bacteriologic examination of food handlers, proper disposal of human wastes, identification and treatment of carriers
Poliomyelitis	Poliovirus types 1, 2, 3	Humans	Direct contact	*Treatment:* supportive
				Control: active immunization with oral (Sabin) or parenteral (Salk) vaccine
Rabies	Virus of rabies	Wild and domesticated animals: dog, fox, bat, raccoon, skunk, cat, rat	Virus-laden saliva of infected animal introduced by bite	*Treatment* (prophylactic): Rabies vaccine (duck embryo) dried killed virus plus rabies immune globulin (human) or rabies vaccine human diploid cell cultures (HDCV)
				Control: destruction of rabid animals; vaccination of pets; preexposure immunization of high-risk people with rabies vaccine (duck embryo) or HDCV

Continued

Table 8–1. Community-Acquired Infections *Continued*

Infectious Disease	Causative Microorganism	Reservoir	Mode of Transmission	Methods of Treatment and Control
Rocky Mountain spotted fever	*Rickettsia rickettsii*	Infected wild rodents, other animals	Bite by infected tick	*Treatment:* tetracyclines, chloramphenicol (Chloromycetin) *Control:* avoid tick-infected areas; remove ticks promptly without crushing
Rubella (German measles)	Virus of rubella	Humans	Direct contact, nasopharyngeal secretions	*Treatment:* supportive *Control:* active immunization with rubella virus vaccine, live; gamma globulin, ISG to contacts
Salmonellosis (acute gastroenteritis)	*Salmonella enteriditis* plus subtypes	Domestic and wild animals, humans	Ingestion of pathogens in food, meat, poultry; direct contact	*Treatment:* supportive; at times antibiotics may be necessary *Control:* periodic examination of food handlers; thorough washing of foods: meat and poultry inspection
Syphilis	*Treponema pallidum*	Humans	Sexual contact	*Treatment:* penicillin, erythromycin, tetracycline *Control:* investigation and treatment of contacts
Tetanus	*Clostridium tetani*	Animals (especially horses), humans	By injury such as puncture wound contaminated with spores	*Treatment:* wound débridement, tetanus immune globulin (passive immunization); if immune globulin not available give tetanus antitoxin *Control:* active immunization with tetanus toxoid
Trichinosis (intestinal roundworm)	*Trichinella spiralis*	Pigs and some wild animals	Eating raw or insufficiently cooked meat from infected animal	*Treatment:* thiabendazole (Mintezol), mebendazole (Vermox) *Control:* adequate processing, preparation, and cooking of pork, pork products
Trichuriasis (whipworm)	*Trichuris trichiura*	Humans	Fecal-oral route (ingestion of eggs passed in feces and found in soil)	*Treatment:* thiabendazole (Mintezol), mebendazole (Vermox) *Control:* adequate disposal of human wastes, sanitary habits in using restroom facilities and preparing food
Tuberculosis	*Mycobacterium tuberculosis*	Humans; cows (in some countries)	Direct contact, airborne	*Treatment:* antitubercular agents *Control:* early case finding by skin testing. Chest radiographic examination recommended only for those with abnormal skin test results
Typhoid fever	*Salmonella typhii*	Humans	Contaminated food, water	*Treatment:* chloramphenicol (Chloromycetin) *Control:* adequate water purification, sanitary disposal of human wastes, milk pasteurization, proper processing and handling of foods, identification of carriers

Continued

Table 8–1. Community-Acquired Infections *Continued*

Infectious Disease	*Causative Microorganism*	*Reservoir*	*Mode of Transmission*	*Methods of Treatment and Control*
Whooping cough (pertussis)	*Bordetella pertussis*	Humans	Direct contact with discharges from laryngeal/bronchial membranes	*Treatment:* supportive; erythromycin for severe cases *Control:* active immunization with pertussis vaccine; pertussis immune globulin for contacts

ISG, immune serum globulin.

immunized against this disease may become sterile if they become infected with the mumps virus. Another example is the birth defects caused by the rubella virus. An insufficient rubella antibody titer (eg, the person has few circulating rubella antibodies) in a pregnant woman can, on exposure to a person with rubella, result in one or more birth defects, such as blindness, deafness, and mental retardation. Any woman of childbearing age who wants to become pregnant should have a hemagglutination inhibition test to determine her susceptibility to rubella. If her rubella antibody titer is too low, she should receive the rubella virus vaccine, live, for active immunization against this disease. Before the vaccine can be given, the woman must be tested for pregnancy and the results must be negative. She also must not become pregnant for 3 months after she receives the vaccine.

Prevention and Control

As stated earlier, an effective immunization program is one method of controlling some of the communicable diseases of childhood. Table 8-2 lists the recommended childhood immunization schedules. Other methods of controlling community-acquired infections are those activities that interrupt the chain of factors (see Chapter 7) necessary for the spread of an infectious disease. These factors are as follows:

- Causative agent
- Reservoir or the carrier
- Portal of exit from the reservoir or carrier
- Mode of transmission
- Portal of entry to a susceptible host
- Susceptible host

Table 8–2. Recommended Immunization Schedules

	2 mo	*4 mo*	*6 mo*	*15 mo*	*18 mo*	*4–6 yr*
Diphtheria toxoid*†	✓	✓	✓		✓	✓
Tetanus toxoid*†	✓	✓	✓		✓	✓
Pertussis vaccine*	✓	✓	✓		✓	✓
Trivalent oral polio vaccine	✓	✓	✓		✓	✓
Measles vaccine‡				✓		
Rubella vaccine‡				✓		
Mumps vaccine‡				✓		

* Usually given as diphtheria and tetanus toxoids combined with pertussis vaccine (DPT).
† Tetanus and diphtheria toxoid boosters. Give at 10-year intervals to maintain immunity.
‡ May be given as combined measles, mumps, and rubella (MMR) vaccines in a single dose.
(Adapted from the American Academy of Pediatrics, Committee on Infectious Diseases, 1982 and MMWR 1983 January 14;32:1–17. Refer to these sources for recommended immunization schedules of infants and children [up to the 7th birthday] and people over 7 years old, not immunized according to the above schedule.)

Many federal, state, and local laws are concerned with the food we eat. Inspection of poultry and live-stock farms, slaughterhouses, food-processing plants, restaurants, retail food markets, and other facilities involved in the preparation, storage, and sale of food has reduced the risk of transmitting some infectious diseases. The periodic health examinations required of food handlers also reduce the risk of disease transmission.

Improved water purification methods and proper sewage and garbage disposal eliminate some reservoirs of infection. Inspection and bacteriologic testing of water wells in rural areas and more stringent laws governing septic tank systems have done much to eliminate diseases that are transmitted through fecal contamination of drinking water.

Local, state, and federal health agencies and the World Health Organization cooperate in the detection and control of communicable diseases. Because of their combined efforts, the incidence of many infectious diseases has been reduced and some (eg, smallpox) have been virtually eliminated. Local agencies responsible for insect and rodent control help to reduce the incidence of diseases transmitted by animals and insect vectors.

Strict housing and building codes, when passed and enacted, have done much to eliminate overcrowding, which in turn reduces the number of infections transmitted by close contact. Inspection of facilities concerned with all aspects of health care and maintenance has decreased the incidence of diseases once prominent in the institutional setting.

School lunch programs and meals served to the elderly at senior citizens' centers or by volunteer agencies have helped to improve the nutritional intake of these segments of the population. Maintaining good nutrition is one way of reducing susceptibility to infectious diseases.

Another method of preventing and controlling infectious diseases is education of the public. Ideally, education about general health measures should begin early in life. Parents should instruct their children in proper hand washing and in personal cleanliness and grooming. School health education programs should begin in the early grades because they help to reinforce what has been taught in the home. For some children, the school may be the only source of health education because their parents have neglected this part of their education.

NOSOCOMIAL INFECTIONS

A nosocomial infection is one that is acquired during hospitalization and that was not present, as either an active, incubatory, or chronic infection, at the time of admission.

The microorganisms most commonly responsible for nosocomial infections are *Staphylococcus aureus, Escherichia coli, Proteus, Pseudomonas aeruginosa, Klebsiella,* and the *Enterobacter* species. Other pathogens also may be seen.

Hospitalized patients are more susceptible to infections than are well people. Among those most susceptible to infections are newborn infants, debilitated patients, patients who are receiving corticosteroid or immunosuppressive therapy, patients with extensive burns, patients with certain metabolic disorders, and patients who have undergone major surgery.

Some nosocomial infections are caused by microorganisms that are present in the hospital environment (floors, utensils, other patients, visitors, and hospital personnel). These are referred to as *exogenous* (arising or coming from outside the organism) infections. Other nosocomial infections are caused by the patient's own normal bacterial flora. These are referred to as *endogenous* (arising or coming from within) infections.

Patients are constantly exposed to pathogenic microorganisms by virtue of the hospital's environment. Hospital personnel are in frequent and direct contact with many patients throughout the day, thus providing an excellent mode of transmission for pathogens. These pathogens usually pose no problem for the healthy person, but they may be the source of infection for those whose resistance is low. Visitors from diverse areas of the community also may introduce additional pathogens into the hospital environment.

Some patients are admitted to the hospital with infections (eg, a draining abscess, pneumonia, or hepatitis). Even though special precautions—isolation for instance—are taken, some of the microorganisms enter the general hospital environment.

Another way nosocomial infections are transmitted is by patient-to-patient use of equipment such as ventilators, intermittent positive-pressure breathing apparatus, physical therapy aids, wheelchairs, and carts. Although some items are thoroughly cleaned after each direct use by a patient, they still may harbor a small number of pathogens. Areas of the hospital frequented by other patients (eg, shared bathrooms, shower and tub facilities, pay telephones, and lounges) also may be sources of infection.

Prevention and Control

Most hospitals include an infection control committee in their organizational systems. This committee is composed of representatives from various areas and departments of the hospital, such as medical staff, nursing service, clinical laboratories, pathology, operating room, housekeeping, and dietary service. The responsibilities of the infection control committee are surveillance, education of hospital personnel, provision of guidelines for the prevention of infectious diseases, and investigation and follow-up of outbreaks of nosocomial infections.

Surveillance. Surveillance is the detection, reporting, and recording of nosocomial infections. Detection may be accomplished in several ways; the procedures or policies to be followed are developed by the committee.

One method of detection is the collection of periodic bacteriologic cultures from various hospital departments, such as the newborn nursery, the laundry, food preparation areas, and the operating room. Some types of hospital equipment, such as humidifiers, respirators, air conditioning systems, and sterilizers, are included in these surveys. Samples may be collected from the air or from surfaces. Because airborne transmission of pathogens appears to be an important factor in nosocomial infections, air samples are taken in various areas of the hospital. The frequency of sampling usually is determined by the infection control committee. Surface sampling uses various techniques to obtain cultures from floors, shelves, counters, walls, and so on. This procedure also can be used to determine the effectiveness of cleaning procedures performed by the housekeeping department.

The reporting of infections to the infection control committee by physicians, nurses, and other hospital personnel helps to identify possible sources of infection.

To detect pathogenic microorganisms in hospital personnel, the preemployment physical examination may include a chest radiograph, a tuberculin skin test, nose and throat cultures, and a stool examination for ova and parasites. After employment, all or some of these tests may be repeated at periodic intervals. Some hospitals may require postemployment testing only of food handlers and those who work in areas concerned with patient care.

Education. Several ways exist in which the infection control committee may inform all hospital personnel of the accepted methods of reducing nosocomial infections. One method involves inservice programs for each hospital department. Another entails the meeting of department heads and supervisory personnel to discuss the findings of recent surveillance procedures and, when necessary, to recommend possible solutions to the identified problems.

Provision of Guidelines. The infection control committee helps to establish guidelines for the prevention of infections by setting criteria for some hospital activities. These criteria may be concerned with preemployment and postemployment health ex-

aminations, sterilization procedures and methods, disposal of garbage and infectious materials, isolation techniques, cleaning techniques for housekeeping, and so on. Surveillance also may point out a need for reevaluation of criteria. The infection control committee may be responsible for adding to or changing hospital policies and procedures concerned with the prevention of nosocomial infections. The committee also designates the isolation procedure and precautions to be followed for a specific infection, and defines the procedures to be followed in labeling and disposing of contaminated bed linen or other articles that have come into contact with the patient.

Investigation and Follow-Up. If an outbreak of a nosocomial infection occurs, the infection control committee plays a major role in identifying the source or cause of the infection. If the source or cause can be identified, the committee recommends additional policies, criteria, or guidelines, when necessary, to prevent future outbreaks.

Good Housekeeping Techniques. Proper cleaning of floors, walls, bathrooms, and patient equipment such as beds, chairs, and stands is essential because the recommended cleaning methods for these areas and items do have a positive effect on the bacterial content of the air. The techniques for handling and laundering bed linens used in the hospital differ from those used in the home because laundered bed linens that are contaminated with even a small number of pathogens are sources of infection.

Disposal of Contaminated Materials. Most hospitals have written policies detailing the techniques to be used for handling and disposing of articles contaminated with infectious matter (eg, syringes, dressings, and bed linens). Such techniques effectively reduce the number of pathogens that can harm patients in the hospital as well as people in the community.

Contaminated articles should be placed in a nonpenetrable bag. The bag should be sealed and its contents clearly marked on the outside. Double-bagging may be used when the outside of the original bag becomes contaminated. Used disposable needles should not be broken before they are placed in a container, to avoid accidental puncture of the hands or fingers. Because acquired immunodeficiency syndrome and hepatitis can be spread by accidental contact with infected blood, the proper disposal of needles is extremely important.

Hand Washing. Hand washing is the single most important measure for preventing the spread of infection. The following four elements are necessary to reduce the number of microorganisms on the hands: (1) a cleansing agent, (2) friction, (3) running water, and (4) time. The hands must be washed with a cleansing agent such as soap. Friction and the lather from the cleansing agent lift the microorganisms from the skin's surface. Running water removes the cleansing agent and many of the microorganisms. Time is essential because a brief rinsing of the hands is ineffective. From 30 to 60 seconds of washing is recommended for hands not grossly contaminated with blood, secretions, purulent exudate, and the like.

The hands should be washed routinely between every patient contact, no matter how brief, and after handling contaminated articles. Hands also should be washed before leaving the hospital unit as well as on returning to it. They should be dried with paper towels, and the towels disposed of in proper containers. *Hand washing is especially important when coming in contact with those patients on isolation precautions.*

Personal Grooming.
Hospital personnel should change their clothing or uniforms daily. Hair should be clean and kept short or at least close to the head. The fingernails should be kept short and clean; long fingernails, as well as rings and other jewelry, can scratch the patient's skin during direct patient care as well as harbor microorganisms. As stated earlier, one method of invasion by pathogens is through broken skin.

Isolation and Precautions.
Methods for controlling the spread of pathogens are recommended by the Centers for Disease Control. Category-specific isolation and precaution procedures include those detailed in the following sections.

Strict Isolation.
This form of isolation prevents the spread of highly contagious and virulent infections. A private room is necessary, and masks, gowns, caps, and gloves are worn by everyone who enters the patient's room. Articles that have come in contact with the patient or that have been soiled with infected material are disposed of according to hospital policy. Infected articles are placed in specially marked or colored bags or containers.

Contact Isolation.
This form of isolation is similar to strict isolation, except that another patient with the *same* contagious disease may be placed in the room. Gowns and masks are worn if there is close patient contact or handling of infected materials. Contaminated articles are handled in the same manner as for strict isolation.

Respiratory Isolation.
This type of isolation (which includes tuberculosis isolation for pulmonary tuberculosis) is instituted when the patient has a contagious disease that is spread by way of the respiratory tract. A private room is used, but another patient with the same infection may be placed in the room. Masks are worn by those in contact with the patient, but gowns and gloves usually are not necessary. Contaminated articles are handled in the same manner as for strict isolation.

Enteric Precautions.
Enteric precautions are initiated to prevent the spread of gastrointestinal infections caused by infectious organisms transmitted through the feces. Gowns, masks, and gloves are not necessary, but gowns and gloves are worn when handling articles contaminated with feces. Contaminated articles are handled in the same manner as for strict isolation.

Drainage and Secretion Precautions.
These precautions protect patients and hospital personnel from infected secretions or drainage. Gowns and gloves are worn when handling secretion-contaminated articles. Such articles are handled in the same manner as for strict isolation.

Blood and Body Fluid Precautions.
These precautions help to prevent transmission of infection by infected blood or body fluids. They are similar to drainage and secretion precautions. Gowns and gloves are worn when handling contaminated articles. Particular care is taken to avoid needlestick injury. Contaminated articles are handled in the same manner as for strict isolation, and particular care is exercised in disposing of needles.

Protective Isolation.
Protective, or reverse, isolation protects patients with impaired resistance to infection against contact with pathogenic microorganisms. A private room is necessary. Everyone who enters the patient's room must wear gowns, masks, and gloves. Some hospitals require that head coverings be worn as well.

Effective Sterilization of Reusable Articles.
Some articles used for patient care must be sterilized after each use. These include operating room instruments, linens, and articles used in the diagnosis and treatment of diseases and disorders, such as radiograph catheters and some types of tracheostomy tubes. Methods of sterilization include dry heat, pressurized steam, gas (ethylene oxide), and chemical disinfectants. When chemical disinfectants are used, the article must be thoroughly washed to remove secretions before it is immersed in the disinfectant. To

obtain the desired results, the time limit for immersion must be satisfied.

Disposable Equipment and Supplies.
Because they are used for only one patient, disposable articles such as needles, syringes, drainage pads, and catheterization trays have helped to reduce the number of nosocomial infections.

NURSING PROCESS —THE PATIENT WHO HAS AN INFECTIOUS DISEASE

Assessment
A thorough patient history and physical examination are of equal importance when assessing a patient with any type of infection. The general areas of history and physical assessment of those with community-acquired or nosocomial infections are shown in Charts 8-1 and 8-2. The history of a patient with a community-acquired infection may identify the source of infection, which in turn may indicate public health measures that may be necessary to prevent the spread of the disease. The history of a patient with a nosocomial infection may be obtained from the patient's chart as well as from the patient. The hospital's infection control committee may find it necessary to investigate the patient's contact with visitors and hospital personnel as well as review recent bacteriologic studies from areas of the hospital.

Nursing Diagnosis
The following nursing diagnoses may apply to a patient with an infectious disease:

- Pain related to an infectious process
- Hyperthermia related to infectious process
- Impaired skin integrity; altered oral mucous membrane related to fever, drug therapy, dry mouth, other factors (specify)
- Diarrhea related to infection of gastrointestinal tract, antibiotic therapy
- Constipation related to drug therapy (narcotics), failure to drink an adequate amount of fluids
- Bathing and hygiene, dressing and grooming, and feeding self-care deficits related to fever, fatigue, malaise, severity of illness
- Fluid volume deficit related to fever, diarrhea, diaphoresis, failure to drink fluids
- Altered nutrition: less than body requirements related to anorexia, impairment of oral mucous membranes, other factors (specify)
- Potential for infection transmission related to failure of medical personnel to observe proper techniques (eg, hand washing, isolation procedures)
- Social isolation related to restriction of visitors, decreased interaction with health care personnel

- Self-esteem disturbance related to odors, prolonged hospitalization, discouragement, other factors (specify)
- Knowledge deficit of the transmission and prevention of infection, hospital procedures used to control infection

Planning and Implementation
The major goals of the patient include increased fluid and food intake, normal bowel elimination, an absence of infection, an absence of pain or discomfort, and an understanding of the methods of preventing a (future) infection.

The major goals of nursing management include the prevention of the transmission of the infection to others, the relief of the symptoms of the infection, and satisfaction of the patient's immediate and long-term needs. The nursing diagnoses made during the initial and ongoing assessments determine the goals to be attained. For example, if the patient has a decreased food and fluid intake because of ulcerations of the oral cavity, a soft, bland diet high in calories and protein and frequent offering of fluids may enable the patient to meet nutritional and fluid needs.

A positive and empathetic attitude should be a major component of the patient care plan. The patient and the family need emotional support and understanding. Physical discomfort may be a serious problem, and the hospital stay prolonged. Visits by family and friends, which are important to most patients, may be restricted. Odors may permeate the room and be difficult to control. Depression may occur, and the patient and the family frequently may become discouraged.

Altered Comfort.
Pain, itching, soreness, burning, and other symptoms may accompany an infection. Assessments for pain or discomfort are made periodically, and medications administered as prescribed. When a topical drug is used, the skin must be gently cleansed of any previous application before the drug is applied again. Any break in the continuity of the skin may spread the infection or introduce additional pathogenic microorganisms.

Hyperthermia.
Fever, with or without chills, is common, but the body temperature of some patients is normal or slightly above normal. Vital signs are monitored every 4 hours or as ordered. If the patient's temperature fails to respond to therapeutic measures, such as the administration of an antipyretic, the physician should be notified. If the patient is perspiring, the gown is changed as needed and the bed linen kept clean and dry.

Skin and Mucous Membrane Integrity.
The skin or mucous membranes may be broken either directly

Chart 8–1. Assessment of the Patient Who Has a Community-Acquired Infection

I. Patient History
A. Symptoms: type, onset, severity, order, and progression of symptoms
B. Questions relative to symptoms and possible diagnosis
1. Direct contacts
    a. Human: People with a known infection of any type; people who appeared ill; large crowds; sexual (if a sexually transmitted disease is suspected)
    b. Animal: Domesticated animals (eg, cats, dogs, birds); farm animals; wild animals (eg, rabbits, deer, raccoons). Types of contact: handling, eating of animal, bite by animal, scratch or wound from handling animal, skin break or injury before handling animal
    c. Insect: Travel to areas of heavy insect population; known or suspected bite by insects
2. Indirect contacts
    a. Environmental: Puncture wounds, cuts, abrasions, or other injury causing break in the skin, including the place and circumstances of the injury (eg, farm, fields, desert)
    b. Food and water consumption: History of recent food and water intake, including place of consumption, eating of home canned food, drinking of water from city water system, well water, bottled water
    c. History pertinent to diseases transmitted by blood and blood products: Recent blood transfusions, dental procedures, parenteral injections, donation of blood
    d. Contact with contaminated objects used by a person with an infection
C. Other
1. History of drug use: Prescription, nonprescription, and illegal drugs and the method of administration
2. History of travel: Foreign countries, continental United States; mode of travel (eg, bus, airplane, automobile, ship); all areas visited on way to and from destination, including hotels, restaurants, cities, towns
3. Immunization history: All active and passive immunizations, including those required for foreign travel
4. History of past and current diseases (medical, surgical), including childhood diseases

II. Physical Assessment
A. Head and neck
1. Evidence of discharge from nose, eyes, ears
2. Redness or swelling in or around eyes, nose, lips
3. Palpation of parotid glands, lymph glands of neck
4. Visual inspection of the nose, mouth (including buccal areas), tongue, throat
5. Evidence of rash or other skin lesions or changes
B. Trunk
1. Evidence of rash or other skin lesions or changes
2. Evidence of puncture wounds, scratches, abrasions, insect bites, or other breaks in the skin
3. Palpation of axillary and femoral areas for lymph node enlargement
4. Auscultation of lungs
5. Palpation of abdomen
C. Extremities
1. Evidence of rash or other skin lesions or changes
2. Evidence of muscle weakness, muscle fasciculations, tetany
3. Evidence of puncture wounds, scratches, abrasions, insect bites, or other breaks in the skin. Look for needle marks on known or suspected drug users
4. Evidence of a localized infection in soft tissues and around nail beds
D. Other
1. Sputum: Color, amount, general appearance
2. Stool: Consistency, color, number, visual inspection for helminths
3. Urine: Evidence of blood, general appearance
4. Vomitus: Amount, color
5. Exudate: Color, amount, peculiar odor (describe)

by the infection or as a result of drug therapy, dry mouth, or other factors. Any break in the skin or mucous membrane is documented during the initial assessment and in subsequent periodic assessments of the area. Any increase or decrease in the integrity of these areas also is recorded. A topical anesthetic may be ordered to relieve pain and discomfort.

Diarrhea or Constipation. Some infectious diseases are accompanied by diarrhea. The source of this problem as well as a description of the number, consistency, and color of the stools may be determined during the patient history. The physician may order the collection of one or more stool specimens to determine the causative agent. Each bowel move-

---

Chart 8–2. Assessment of the Patient With a Nosocomial Infection

I. *Patient History*

A. Review of onset of symptoms (may be taken from chart) as well as the patient's own description of symptoms

B. Investigation of patient contacts: Visitors, hospital personnel

C. List of all areas occupied by or visited by patient: X-ray, operating room, physical therapy, lounges, telephone booths, shower and tub rooms

D. Food history: Type of hospital diet, eating of food brought in by visitors

II. *Physical Assessment (pertains largely to the type of infection)*

A. Wound: Type, color, and amount of drainage or exudate (also note characteristic odor, if present), signs of inflammation around the wound

B. Vital signs: Present vital signs as well as review of recent vital signs and changes in same

C. Assess for general signs and symptoms that may be associated with a specific infection

1. Pulmonary: Cough, type, color, and amount of sputum, respiratory difficulty, auscultation of chest

2. Gastrointestinal (upper): Nausea, vomiting, color and amount of vomitus, anorexia, epigastric pain or distress

3. Gastrointestinal (lower): Abdominal cramping, tenderness, or pain; diarrhea; character and frequency of stools

4. Genitourinary: Appearance of urine, daily output, evidence of discharge around urethral meatus

5. Skin: Presence of rash or other skin lesions or changes, type and amount of drainage from wounds, incisions, abscesses

6. Neurologic: Evidence of central nervous system irritability or other changes (eg, tetany, change in the level of consciousness)

7. Hematologic: Evidence of generalized septicemia (abrupt onset of high fever, shaking chills, nausea, vomiting, hypotension or shock)

---

ment is inspected for amount, color, and consistency; if blood is noted, this also is recorded and the physician notified. Enteric precautions are necessary if diarrhea is caused by an infectious microorganism such as a bacterium, protozoa, or ameba.

The patient is instructed to clean the perineal area after each bowel movement, and the perineal area is inspected daily for excoriation. If this problem occurs, ointments or creams may be ordered to relieve discomfort and aid in the healing of the area.

Causes of constipation include the administration of a narcotic for pain and inadequate fluid or food intake. When a narcotic analgesic is being administered for pain, the patient is observed for constipation. Laxatives or enemas may be needed to relieve constipation.

Self-Care. The patient is assessed for the ability to carry out activities of daily living, and assisted as needed.

Fluid Volume Deficit. Fever and sweating increase the body's need for fluids. Dehydration and electrolyte loss may occur as a result of fever, decreased intake of food or fluids, or diarrhea. Fluids are offered frequently (unless the physician orders otherwise), and vital signs monitored every 2 to 4 hours. The intake and output are monitored, and the physician notified if urine output falls below 500 mL/day. Oral or intravenous replacement of fluids and electrolytes may be necessary. Laboratory monitoring of electrolytes may be ordered, and the patient observed for signs of potassium, sodium, or chloride deficiency.

Nutrition. Food and fluid intake may be decreased because of the anorexia (loss of appetite) and malaise (a feeling of discomfort or uneasiness) that often accompanies an infection. Infections that involve the mouth may impair swallowing. Prolonged illness and a decreased food intake can result in a state of catabolism, which uses protein as a source for energy.

The patient may require a well-balanced diet high in protein and calories. Food intake is monitored and recorded. The dietitian should be notified if the patient is eating poorly; a diet suited to the patient's condition and food preferences may be necessary to maintain an adequate food intake. If anorexia persists, the patient should be weighed once or twice a week, and significant weight loss reported to the physician.

Potential for Infection Transmission. When isolation is necessary, the techniques of the procedure are followed in accordance with hospital policy. The type of isolation depends on the type of infection. *Hand washing is an important element in preventing the spread of infection.*

Preventing the transmission of a nosocomial infection to other patients is extremely important. Many of the pathogens responsible for these types of infections have developed an increased resistance to antibiotic therapy. This problem, coupled with many patients with decreased resistance to infection, adds to the dangers associated with nosocomial infections.

Social Isolation. Visits by family and friends, which are important to most patients, may be restricted. In addition, family members may be reluctant, for any number of reasons, to visit the patient. The family should be encouraged to visit as often as possible. Frequent interaction with health care personnel also reduces the effects of isolation and shows the patient that needs are being identified and met.

Self-Esteem Disturbance. The patient and family need emotional support and understanding. In addition to the illness that required hospitalization, new problems have arisen. Physical discomfort is increased, and the hospital stay may be prolonged. Odors may permeate the room and be difficult to control. Depression is common, and the patient and the family frequently become discouraged. In addition to meeting the patient's physical needs, a positive and empathetic attitude should be a major component of the patient care plan.

Knowledge Deficit. Examples of community-acquired infections that may require explanation of preventive measures include helminthic infections, staphylococcal food poisoning, and salmonellal infections. The patient and the family may require instruction regarding the prevention of future infections (as may be seen in cases of staphylococcal food poisoning) or the spread of the infection to others. For example, to prevent spreading the infection to others in the household, the family may be advised to use separate dishes, bed linens, towels, and so on for the person with an infection.

The hospitalized patient as well as visitors require an explanation of isolation techniques and why they are necessary. They also need to be given an explanation of all treatments necessary to control the infection. If the patient is placed in isolation, the wearing of the required coverings (mask, gown, gloves, and cap) by visitors and medical personnel tend to isolate the patient emotionally from human contact. Isolation techniques also can give the impression that the patient's condition is critical. Although the prognosis may be poor, most patients are expected to recover. The nurse must take the time to explain the purpose of the procedure to the patient as well as to the family. When the patient is ready for discharge from the hospital, education about the prevention of future infection may be necessary.

Evaluation

- Comfort is maintained as much as possible
- Attains normal body temperature
- Attains integrity of skin and mucous membranes
- Attains normal defecation pattern
- Maintains adequate fluid intake
- Attains and maintains normal food intake
- No evidence of spread of infection to self or others
- Acquires understanding of illness and preventive measures
- Understands and accepts change in social interactions
- Demonstrates improvement in self-concept

General Nutritional Considerations

- Fruit juices and gelatin desserts can be offered to increase the fluid intake of the person with an infectious disease.
- A well-balanced diet prepared in small amounts and offered four times a day may be necessary if the patient has anorexia.
- A referral to the dietitian may be necessary if anorexia is present or the patient has difficulty eating his diet.
- Meals for the patient in isolation are served on disposable dinnerware. The tray should be made as attractive as possible to encourage eating and minimize the manner in which the food is served. Uneaten food and the dinnerware are disposed of in plastic containers before removal from the room.
- If the infection is prolonged and severe, meals high in calories and protein may be necessary.

General Pharmacologic Considerations

- Antipyretic drugs (eg, aspirin and acetaminophen) usually are ordered if the patient has a fever. If the patient is unable to take or tolerate the drug orally, the physician should be consulted about a different route of administration.
- When an antipyretic drug is administered rectally, the suppository is inserted high in the rectum. The patient is checked in 30 minutes to ensure that the suppository has not been expelled from the rectum.

☐ Antibiotics must be given *on time* to maintain the therapeutic blood levels necessary to control the infection.

☐ When antibiotics are administered, the patient should be observed for adverse drug effects. Nausea, vomiting, anorexia, diarrhea, and rash are adverse effects of some antibiotics, but also are symptoms associated with some infectious diseases. An accurate patient history and physical examination at the time of admission, plus ongoing documentation of the patient's symptoms, may help to distinguish between those symptoms related to the infectious disease and those possibly caused by antibiotic therapy.

General Gerontologic Considerations

☐ The elderly patient may be more prone to nosocomial infections because of the effects of aging on the immune system, which in turn decreases the ability to fight infection.

☐ Infection in the elderly patient may be more serious because homeostatic mechanisms and the ability to fight infection are less efficient.

☐ When isolation technique is necessary, the elderly patient may become confused because of the decrease in contact with other people and the lack of environmental stimulation from television, radio, windows facing the outside, reading materials, and so on.

☐ Some infectious diseases are accompanied by such symptoms as severe vomiting and diarrhea, high fever, and shock. These symptoms can lead to such problems as electrolyte imbalances, dehydration, and decreased vital organ perfusion. The elderly patient usually has a decreased physical reserve, and thus may be unable to withstand the problems associated with an infection.

Suggested Readings

☐ Abrams AC. Clinical drug therapy: rationales for nursing practice. 2nd ed. Philadelphia: JB Lippincott, 1987. *(Additional and in-depth coverage of subject matter)*

☐ Burton GRW. Microbiology for the health sciences. 3rd ed. Philadelphia: JB Lippincott, 1988. *(Additional coverage of subject matter)*

☐ Coleman D. The when and how of isolation. RN October 1987;50:50. *(Additional coverage of subject matter)*

☐ Cornell C. Tuberculosis in hospital employees. Am J Nurs April 1988;88:484. *(Additional coverage of subject matter)*

☐ Gurevich I. How to make every culture count. RN August 1988;51:49. *(Additional coverage of subject matter)*

☐ Johnson GE, Hannah KJ. Pharmacology and the nursing process. Philadelphia: WB Saunders, 1987. *(In-depth coverage of subject matter)*

☐ Mooney BR, Armington LC. Infection control: how to prevent nosocomial infections. RN September 1987;50:20. *(Additional coverage of subject matter)*

☐ Pagana KD, Pagana TJ. Diagnostic testing and nursing implications: a case study approach. St Louis: CV Mosby, 1986. *(Additional coverage of subject matter)*

☐ Pritchard V. Preventing and treating geriatric infections. RN March 1988;51:36. *(Additional coverage of subject matter)*

☐ Whiteman KF. Why bother with flu shorts? Am J Nurs November 1987;87:1408. *(Additional coverage of subject matter)*

Chapter 9
Sexually Transmitted Diseases

On completion of the chapter the reader will:

- Discuss the incidence of STDs
- Discuss the factors contributing to the spread of STDs
- Discuss methods of preventing and controlling the spread of STDs
- Discuss the symptoms, diagnosis, and treatment of the more common STDs
- Use the nursing process in the management of a patient with an STD

Sexually transmitted diseases (STDs) are a diverse group of infections acquired through sexual activity with an infected person (Table 9-1). Included in the STDs are the venereal diseases syphilis, gonorrhea, chancroid, and granuloma inguinale as well as such diseases as human papillomavirus, herpes simplex virus, chlamydial infections, acquired immunodeficiency syndrome (AIDS), and trichomonal vaginitis.

INCIDENCE

The incidence of STDs has been on the increase. Many factors contribute to this increase, including a change in sexual attitudes and a decrease in the use of the condom along with an increase in other methods of birth control such as contraceptives, tubal ligation, and vasectomy. Not all STDs must be reported to public health authorities, making accurate recording of the incidence of some STDs unreliable. Some physicians also fail, for any number of reasons, to report all or some of the STDs treated in private practice. The law requires that venereal diseases such as gonorrhea and syphilis be reported. Chlamydial infections usually are not reported, but are common.

FACTORS THAT CONTRIBUTE TO THE SPREAD OF STDS

Certain elements and behaviors contribute to the transmission of STDs. These factors include the following:

- Unknown carrier of the disease. Some STDs have few or no outward symptoms. The person has no indication that an infection is present, and the sexual partner has no observable warning that an STD infection may occur.
- Casual sex between heterosexual, bisexual, or homosexual partners
- Sharing of needles to administer drugs, especially needles used for administration by the intravenous route
- Absence of laws that require the reporting of *all* STDs. Acquired immunodeficiency syndrome or human immunodeficiency virus (HIV)-positive antibody titers are not required to be reported to health authorities. In addition, screening for AIDS remains a controversial issue, thereby possibly exposing health care workers as well as all people to AIDS.
- Unfaithful sexual partner
- Length of time between exposure to an STD and the appearance of symptoms or positive antibody tests. The infected person does not know that he or she has an STD and, therefore, unknowingly infects others. If the infected person frequently engages in casual sex, many people may be infected with the disease before symptoms appear in the infected person.
- Failure to recognize the signs and symptoms of an STD followed by failure to seek early treatment as well as to refrain from sexual activity until treatment is complete
- Lack of proper knowledge regarding STDs and their prevention

Table 9-1. Sexually Transmitted Diseases

Microorganism	*Disease or Syndrome*
Bacteria	
Calymmatobacterium granulomatis	Granuloma inguinale (donovanosis)
Campylobacter species	Enteritis (homosexual men)
Chlamydia trachomatis	Nongonococcal urethritis, epididymitis, proctitis, cervicitis, salpingitis, conjunctivitis, pneumonia, lymphogranuloma venereum, Reiter's syndrome
Gardnerella vaginalis	Vaginitis
Haemophilus ducreyi	Chancroid
Mycoplasma hominis	Pelvic inflammatory disease, postpartum fever
Nisseria gonorrhoeae (gonorrhea)	Urethritis, epididymitis, proctitis, bartholinitis, endometritis, salpingitis, conjunctivitis, arthritis, dermatitis, amniotic infection
Shigella species	Enteritis (homosexual men)
Treponema pallidum	Syphilis
Ureaplasma urealyticum	Nongonococcal urethritis
Fungi	
Candida albicans	Vulvovaginitis, balanitis
Parasites	
Phthirus (pubis)	Lice (pubic)
Sarcoptes scabiei	Scabies
Protozoans	
Entamoeba histolytica	Amebiasis, enteritis (homosexual men)
Giardia lamblia	Enteritis (homosexual men)
Trichomonas vaginalis	Vaginitis
Viruses	
Cytomegalovirus	Infant mortality, birth defects
Hepatitis A virus	Hepatitis (homosexual men)
Hepatitis B virus	Hepatitis (especially in homosexual men)
Herpes simplex virus	Genital herpes, meningitis, disseminated infection in newborns
Human immunodeficiency virus (human T-lymphocytic virus)	AIDS
Human papillomavirus	Condyloma acuminata, cancer of the cervix
Molluscum contagiosum virus	Molluscum contagiosum of the genitals

- Exposure of health personnel to blood and body fluids from a person infected with an STD who has not been diagnosed
- Administration of blood and blood products that are contaminated with the AIDS virus. Although transmission of AIDS by this means has decreased because of screening tests done on donated blood, there still remains the possibility that the donated blood will test negative if the donor has recently become infected with AIDS yet has not manufactured antibodies against the virus.
- Failure of the sexually active person to heed the warnings about STDs or adhere to methods of prevention

PREVENTION

A multifaceted approach is necessary to prevent the spread of STDs. Education of the public remains one of the most important methods of controlling the spread of these infections. In 1988, the U.S. Department of Health and Human Services mailed a pamphlet titled "Understanding AIDS" to all households in the United States. School systems have instituted programs that explain AIDS as well as other STDs to students. Television and the printed media present advertisements for condoms as well as recommendations for preventing the spread of STDs.

The person with an STD must refrain from sexual activity until the infection has been eradicated. Physicians and nurses must emphasize the importance of completing a course of therapy to control the infection as well as the consequences of sexual activity while the infection is still active.

Another important aspect of prevention is locating and treating sexual contacts. The person with an STD must be willing to name the people with whom he or she has had sexual contact so that these people also may be tested and treated. Unfortunately, the identification of sexual contacts often proves to be inaccurate or incomplete.

Many STDs can be cured with antimicrobial drugs; some of the microorganisms that cause STDs have mutated or changed, however, and are resistant to certain drugs. Continued research on the part of pharmaceutical companies as well as independent and government research laboratories is necessary to develop new methods of treatment. Facilities to diagnose and treat STDs must be available in all areas as well as to all segments of the population.

To prevent the spread of AIDS, health professionals as well as others who may be exposed to blood or body fluids (eg, policemen, firemen, ambulance personnel, boxing referees) must wear gloves when contact with these products may occur. Blood banks must screen all donated blood for HIV antibodies. This test is called the enzyme-linked immunosorbent assay (ELISA).

TYPES OF SEXUALLY TRANSMITTED DISEASES
Chlamydial Infections

The causative organism of chlamydial infections is *Chlamydia trachomatis*. These infections may coexist with other STDs, primarily gonorrhea.

Symptoms
Urethritis and epididymitis in men and cervicitis along with a mucopurulent discharge in women are the most common symptoms, although some patients are asymptomatic. Chlamydial infections also may be transmitted from mother to infant at birth. Additional problems associated with a chlamydial infection include pelvic inflammatory disease, ectopic pregnancy, sterility, and systemic infections.

Diagnosis
Diagnosis is made by direct microscopic examination and culture of secretions or tissue scrapings.

Treatment
Antimicrobial drugs, such as the tetracyclines, erythromycin, and the sulfonamides, are used for treatment. The length of treatment is 7 to 21 days, during which time the person should refrain from sexual activity. Treatment failure usually is due to either reinfection or patient noncompliance (failure of the patient to finish a course of therapy or take the antimicrobial agent as directed by the physician).

Gonorrhea

The causative organism of gonorrhea is *Neisseria gonorrhoeae*. Gonorrhea and chlamydial infections, probably the most common STDs, often coexist.

Symptoms
Symptoms usually appear 2 to 6 days after infection. Urethritis with a purulent discharge and pain on urination are the most common symptoms in men. The infection may spread to the prostate, seminal vesicles, and epididymis. Sometimes there are no symptoms of infection in men. In homosexual men, there may be gonococcal infection of the pharynx and the rectum. About half of the women with gonorrhea experience no symptoms. When symptoms are present, they include a vaginal discharge, abnormal menstrual bleeding, and painful urination. If untreated, the infection may progress upward to the cervix, endometrium, and fallopian tubes.

Diagnosis
Diagnosis is made by microscopic examination using the Gram's stain method as well as by culture. When a culture is obtained, the specimen must immediately be placed on the culture plate and taken to the laboratory. In men, a specimen of the urethral discharge is obtained. Anal and pharyngeal smears may be obtained if the person has practiced oral or anal sex. Cultures also may be done at this time. In women, specimens for examination are obtained by direct visualization of the cervix. Lubricants are not used on the speculum because these products may destroy the gonococci. Cultures of the cervix as well as microscopic examination of cervical smears are performed.

Treatment
Because some men and about half of the women infected with gonorrhea experience no symptoms, these people seldom seek medical care. This increases the risk of the infection being spread to others. Those who are diagnosed are treated with antibiotics such as ampicillin, cefoxitin, tetracycline, spectinomycin, and penicillin. Some strains of gonorrhea are resistant to some antibiotics; therefore, repeat therapy with a dif-

ferent antibiotic may be necessary. The person must refrain from sexual activity until follow-up smears are negative.

Syphilis

The spirochete *Treponema pallidum* is the causative organism of syphilis. If untreated, syphilis can progress through the secondary and tertiary stages. Only during the primary and secondary stages can it be transmitted to others.

Symptoms

The time between infection and the first occurrence of symptoms is about 21 days. In the primary (early) stage, a chancre (painless ulcer) may appear on the genitals, anus, cervix, or other parts of the body (Fig. 9-1). At first it resembles a small papule, but it later appears ulcerated. If untreated, the chancre heals in several weeks, and the patient progresses to the secondary stage of syphilis. The symptoms of this stage include fever, malaise, rash, headache, sore throat, and lymph node enlargement. Late, or tertiary, syphilis is noninfectious because the microorganism has invaded the central nervous system as well as other organs of the body. Symptoms of tertiary syphilis include tabes dorsalis (a degenerative condition of the central nervous system that results in loss of peripheral reflexes and of vibratory and position senses, and ataxia), joint changes (Charcot's joints), incontinence, and impotence. There also may be cardiovascular symptoms, including aortic aneurysm and aortic valve insufficiency.

Diagnosis

Diagnosis is made by microscopic (darkfield) examination of scrapings from the chancre. Laboratory tests include the VDRL (Venereal Disease Research Laboratory) flocculation test, the rapid plasma reagin card test, the fluorescent treponemal antibody absorption test, and the microhemagglutination assay.

Treatment

Penicillin G benzathine, penicillin G aqueous benzyl, and penicillin G procaine are used for treating early (primary and secondary) syphilis. Patients who are allergic to the penicillins may be given tetracycline or erythromycin. Follow-up examinations and laboratory tests are recommended 3, 6, and 12 months after initial treatment. Those with tertiary syphilis require larger doses of penicillin. The response is poor in those with cardiovascular syphilis.

Acquired Immunodeficiency Syndrome

The acquired immunodeficiency syndrome is caused by the retrovirus HIV, also called human T-cell lymphotrophic virus type III (HTLV-III). Human retroviruses are divided into two groups: HTLV-I and HTLV-II are leukemia viruses, and HTLV-III, the AIDS virus. In the United States, AIDS was first detected in homosexual men about 1981. Shortly thereafter, it was found in intravenous drug abusers who shared needles. The Haitian population also had a high incidence of AIDS. Studies since then have shown that the virus infects heterosexuals as well as those who receive the virus by means of infected blood. The exact origin of the disease or how it developed is still not clearly understood, but it has been theorized that the retrovirus (HTLV-I) infecting certain species of African monkeys may have undergone a genetic change and become the HTLV-III virus.

Since the early 1980s, AIDS has become a primary health issue. Because the virus was being transmitted to those receiving blood transfusions infected with the AIDS virus, there was major concern over the effect AIDS would have on the general population. In 1984, a screening test for donated blood became available, and the danger of transmitting AIDS by means of a blood transfusion was greatly reduced.

The acquired immunodeficiency syndrome affects the body's immune system by destroying T-cell lymphocytes, which are concerned with antibody formation. The virus also uses T-cell lymphocytes for producing more HTLV-III viruses. When the body's natural production of T-cell lymphocytes is impaired, the person becomes susceptible to infection by other microorganisms.

AIDS-Related Complex. AIDS-related complex (ARC) describes those with HIV antibodies who have

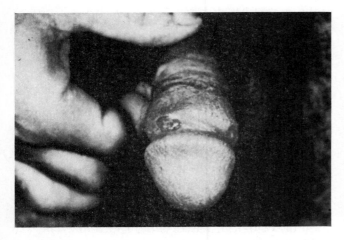

Figure 9-1. Chancre, the primary lesion of syphillis. (Medichrome, Clay-Adams, Inc, New York, NY).

at least two signs of immunodeficiency as shown by laboratory tests, such as a decrease in the number of T-cell lymphocytes, leukopenia, elevated serum globulin levels, and anemia. The person may or may not show clinical signs and symptoms such as fever, weight loss, and lymph node enlargement. It is not known what percentage of those with ARC ultimately develop AIDS.

Mode of Transmission. The AIDS virus is transmitted by contact with blood, blood products, and body fluids such as semen and vaginal secretions. Contact with these fluids may occur through anal or vaginal intercourse, intravenous administration of AIDS-contaminated blood or blood products, the sharing of contaminated intravenous needles, in utero transmission from mother to child, and accidental contact with contaminated blood or blood products. Accidental contact refers to needlesticks or direct contact by way of open skin lesions or breaks in the skin. Although the virus has been found in urine, tears, saliva, and cerebrospinal fluid, there is no evidence that the virus can be transmitted through these body fluids.

An important aspect in controlling the spread of AIDS is identification of those who have the disease and those who test positive for AIDS antibodies but do not have symptoms of the disease. Anyone who has had multiple sexual partners of either sex, sex with one or more prostitutes, or sex with homosexual or bisexual men or who has used intravenous drugs should consider being tested. Health care personnel who work with AIDS patients or those who are exposed to blood or blood products also should consider being tested. This is especially important for those who work in areas where the incidence or chance of exposure is high.

Symptoms

Initial symptoms, which may appear weeks or months (and perhaps years) after the original infection, include fever, malaise, sweating, arthralgia, sore throat, anorexia (which may be severe), nausea, vomiting, and a rash. Diarrhea, stiff neck, and abdominal cramps also may be present. Lymph node enlargement, anemia, and a decreased platelet count are common. Some patients are asymptomatic. As the disease progresses, pulmonary, gastrointestinal, and neurologic symptoms may occur. Some of these symptoms are due to infections with microorganisms that can no longer be handled by the body's immune system. These include *Pneumocystis carinii* pneumonia, infectious diarrhea, oral fungal infections (candidiasis), cytomegalovirus infections, and viral infections such as herpes simplex. These are called opportunistic infections, since they result from a failure of the immune system. Kaposi's sarcoma, a malignant neoplasm of the endo-

thelial layer of blood and lymphatic vessels, frequently is seen. Neurologic manifestations such as subacute encephalitis also may occur.

Diagnosis

Diagnosis of AIDS is based on the symptoms as well as laboratory tests. Often the development of *P. carinii* pneumonia causes the patient to seek medical help. Laboratory diagnosis for AIDS (or HIV) antibodies includes immunofluorescent assays, the Western blot, and the ELISA. It may take from 2 weeks to 12 months or longer for the HIV antibodies to appear in the blood. If HIV antibodies are found, the person is said to be seropositive. Additional diagnostic tests, although not specific for HIV antibodies, include routine laboratory tests such as a complete blood count, platelet count, serum globulin levels, and cultures (when an opportunistic infection is apparent).

Treatment

There is no way of knowing whether a seropositive person will progress to having AIDS. Currently there is no cure for AIDS, and treatment is mainly supportive. Antimicrobial therapy may be used to control opportunistic infections associated with AIDS. Zidovudine (Retrovir), also known as AZT (azidothymidine), is given to those with AIDS as well as ARC, but drug therapy specifically aimed at the AIDS virus is currently experimental. Zidovudine has helped some patients, and, although not a cure, it may prolong life. The focus is on prevention until such time as drug therapy or a vaccine will prove effective. Most patients die of overwhelming opportunistic infections as well as Kaposi's sarcoma.

People who are seropositive should immediately stop having unprotected sex. This protects the uninfected partner and avoids the risk of again being exposed to the AIDS virus. It is thought that repeated exposure to the AIDS virus increases the chance of the disease progressing more rapidly. It also is believed that some strains of the virus are more virulent than others.

Herpes Simplex Virus

The herpes simplex virus type 1 (HSV-1) and herpes simplex virus type 2 (HSV-2) are responsible for cold sores of the lips (HSV-1) and genital and perineal lesions (HSV-1 and HSV-2). HSV-2 also is known as genital herpes. Transmission of *either* of these viruses is by direct contact with oral or genital secretions. Either virus may be introduced into the eye, the mouth, the genital area, or a skin site. HSV-2 can be transmitted from mother to infant during vaginal birth.

HSV infections often occur in those with AIDS as well as those who are undergoing cancer chemotherapy or organ transplantation or who are immunocompromised (eg, have an ineffective immune system).

Symptoms

Those infected with the HSV-1 virus may exhibit no symptoms, or may have oral lesions along with a low-grade fever, malaise, and enlargement of the lymph nodes in the neck. The oral lesions may be seen in the mouth or on the lips, and appear as yellowish vesicles. Other symptoms include pharyngitis, keratoconjunctivitis (inflammation of the cornea and conjunctiva), chills, muscle soreness, and difficulty swallowing. HSV-1 infections recur, since after the first infection, the virus remains dormant in the ganglia of the nerves that supply the area.

The symptoms of HSV-2 include vesicular lesions on the buttocks, penis, perineum, vulva, cervix, and vagina. If anal intercourse is the method of transmission, lesions may appear in the rectum and perianal area. The lesions are painful, and may persist for several weeks. Malaise, fever, chills, and headache may be seen. As with HSV-1, HSV-2 recurs because it lies dormant in the ganglia of the nerves that supply the area. Some patients note that stress, emotional situations, exposure to sunlight, menstruation, and fever trigger the recurrence of the lesions.

Diagnosis

Diagnosis of HSV-1 and HSV-2 is made by examination of the lesions. If HSV-2 is suspected, the lesions may be cultured. The specimen is immediately transferred to a culture plate and taken to a laboratory.

Treatment

HSV-1 may not require treatment, since the infection often is self-limiting. HSV-2 may be treated with oral, topical, or intravenous acyclovir (Zovirax). Intravenous acyclovir is used if the patient has a severe initial episode of HSV-2, or if the patient is immunodeficient. If the infection is in the eye, vidarabine, idoxuridine, or trifluridine ophthalmic ointment may be prescribed. Topical acyclovir is ineffective in controlling recurrent appearances of the lesions. Some people may require analgesics for pain or discomfort.

Those with HSV-2 infections are instructed to refrain from sexual intercourse or use a condom. If there is a periodic recurrence of the lesions, it is recommended that they use a condom at all times.

Human Papillomavirus

A human papillomavirus infection causes a condition known as genital warts. The incidence of this STD is rising. There appears to be an increased risk of cancer of the vulva, vagina, and cervix in women with genital warts. The incubation period normally is about 1 to 2 months, but it may be longer.

Symptoms

Genital warts usually are painless, and appear as soft, fleshy wartlike growths on the genitalia or cervix or in the vagina. Anyone may become infected with genital warts after having sexual relations with an infected person. People with AIDS as well as others with an immunodeficiency are prone to this infection.

Diagnosis

Diagnosis is made by visual examination of the area.

Treatment

There is no available cure for genital warts. They may be treated with a topical solution of podophyllin, which is left on for 4 to 6 hours and then washed off. The use of a condom is recommended during treatment and until the warts disappear.

Candidiasis

Candidiasis, or infection with one of the *Candida* fungi, is most commonly caused by *Candida albicans*. A candidal infection may occur in many types of situations, such as during antibiotic therapy and after skin or mucous membrane trauma. It is not a true STD but is included with the STDs because the infection can be transmitted between sexual partners. The incidence of a candidal infection is high in those with other STDs.

Symptoms

Symptoms depend on the area affected. Oral candidiasis is manifested by the appearance of a gray membrane-type covering of the area. If the vulvovaginal area is affected, itching and a vaginal discharge are noted.

Diagnosis

Diagnosis is made by microscopic examination of scrapings from the affected area.

Treatment

Topical application of an antifungal agent such as clotrimazole or miconazole is used for vulvovaginal infections. Topical nystatin may be used to treat oral candidiasis. Candidiasis infections recur in some people, despite therapy.

Mycoplasmas

Two mycoplasmal infections, caused by *Mycoplasma hominis* and *Ureaplasma urealyticum*, affect the genitourinary tract. Infection may result in nongonococcal urethritis and inflammation of the prostate, cervix, vagina, upper urinary tract, and female pelvic organs.

Symptoms

Symptoms depend on the area affected. Those with nongonococcal urethritis have symptoms that are similar to those of gonorrhea. Inflammation of other areas of the genitourinary tract may give rise to a variety of symptoms, such as dysuria and abdominal pain or discomfort.

Diagnosis

Diagnosis is made by history as well as cultures.

Treatment

The erythromycins or tetracyclines are prescribed for mycoplasmal infections.

Trichomoniasis

Infection with the protozoan *Trichomonas vaginalis* may occur alone or along with one or more other sexually transmitted infections.

Symptoms

Most men and some women with this infection are asymptomatic. Women may experience a yellow, creamy vaginal discharge that produces itching and burning.

Diagnosis

Diagnosis is made by microscopic identification of the microorganism.

Treatment

Trichomoniasis is treated with metronidazole.

Other STDs

Granuloma inguinale, or donovanosis, is caused by *Calymmatobacterium granulomatis*, and is relatively uncommon in the United States. The infection is characterized by lesions in the genital, inguinal, and anal areas, and is treated with antimicrobials, usually tetracycline or sulfisoxazole.

Chancroid is caused by the *Haemophilus ducreyi* bacillus. The infection is characterized by the appearance of a macule, followed by vesicle-pustule formation and, finally, a painful ulcer. It is treated with erythromycin or tetracycline.

Lymphogranuloma venereum, caused by a strain of *Chlamydia trachomatis*, is characterized by a small erosion or papule and enlargement of adjacent lymph nodes. The affected lymph nodes can become necrotic. The usual site of infection is the genital area. The infection may be treated with tetracyline or a sulfonamide.

Molluscum contagiosum is a viral infection of skin cells that results in dome-shaped papules that appear on the trunk, genitals, and face. Treatment involves removal of the warts with cantharidin or podophyllin.

Pubic lice and scabies are parasitic infestations that can be transmitted between sexual partners when one of the partners is infected. Although not true STDs, both infestations may be seen alone or along with one or more other STDs.

Hepatitis, *Shigella* infections, enteritis caused by the *Campylobacter* species and *Giardia lamblia*, cytomegalovirus infection, vaginal infections caused by *Gardnerella vaginalis*, and amebiasis are not STDs, but may be sexually transmitted.

NURSING PROCESS —THE PATIENT WHO HAS A SEXUALLY TRANSMITTED DISEASE

Assessment

A thorough patient history is important when the patient has an STD. The patient is questioned about recent sexual contacts, the date of exposure, and any past history of an STD. For some STDs, all recent sexual contacts must be reported to public health authorities, but laws concerning which diseases are reportable vary from state to state. It is important to obtain the names of all people with whom the infected person has had sexual contact. These people are then contacted and advised to seek examination by a physician, even if they are not experiencing any symptoms of an infection. Unfortunately, some patients refuse to name any or all sexual contacts, thus contributing to the spread of STDs.

Physical assessment depends on the patient's complaints. A patient who complains of a rash, urethral discharge, or perianal itching requires a visual examination of the area. In addition to examining the area of the primary complaint, the entire body surface is examined for rash, sores, signs of infection or inflammation, signs of burrows (which may indicate scabies), scratches or other open areas, and trauma. The pubic area is inspected for lice. The genital and rectal areas are examined for redness, swelling, discharge, warts, drainage, and lesions. *Gloves must be worn by the person performing the physical assessment and disposed of as potentially infected materials.*

The nurse must assume a nonjudgmental attitude during history taking and physical assessment of a patient with an STD. Unfortunately, some patients refuse to follow a treatment regimen or take precautions to prevent the spread of the infection because of the attitude of health care professionals. Confidentiality is important, and privacy must be maintained when the history is taken and a physical assessment performed. By assuming a professional yet understanding attitude, the nurse can help the patient deal with the fears and anxieties associated with this type of infection.

Nursing Diagnosis

The following nursing diagnoses may apply to a patient with an STD:

- Pain related to the infectious process
- Hyperthermia related to the infectious process
- Anxiety related to the diagnosis, treatment
- Diarrhea related to infection of the gastrointestinal tract, drug therapy
- Ineffective individual coping related to inability to accept diagnosis, inability to place blame on the appropriate person
- Altered family processes related to family member infected with an STD, other factors (specify)
- Fear related to diagnosis, consequences of an STD
- Potential for infection transmission related to presence of infectious agent
- Altered sexuality patterns related to presence of infectious agent
- Social isolation related to diagnosis, embarrassment, other factors (specify)
- Noncompliance (potential or actual) related to knowledge, indifference, other factors (specify)
- Knowledge deficit of modes of transmission, treatment, prevention

Planning and Implementation

The major goals of the patient include control of the infection, relief of symptoms, prevention of transmission, and avoidance of another infection.

The major goals of nursing management include eradication of the infection (when possible), prevention of transmission, relief of symptoms, education, and alleviation of the anxiety and fears associated with the infection. Many STDs can be cured, but eradication of the infection depends on patient compliance to a course of treatment. This is why information regarding the importance of completing a course of therapy as well as methods of preventing a future infection assumes a major role in planning.

Some STDs, for example gonorrhea and nongonorrheal urethritis, invade the genitourinary tract, and cause dysuria and difficulty in urinating. These symptoms usually disappear a few days after treatment begins. If gonorrhea goes untreated, urethral strictures may develop, requiring periodic dilatation of the urethra or, possibly, reconstructive surgery of the urethra.

Some STDs can only be controlled (eg, HSV infections). AIDS, however, cannot be cured and is fatal. When the patient is faced with this diagnosis, emotional support as well as planning to meet the patient's physical, social, and financial needs are important aspects of nursing management.

Pain. The patient is reassured that the pain or discomfort associated with some STDs is relieved when the infection is eradicated. Severe discomfort or pain is reported to the physician, since an analgesic may be necessary.

Hyperthermia. Fever may be associated with some STDs and may persist until the infection is brought under control. Any temperature elevation at the time of the physical assessment as well as a history of a fever is reported to the physician, who may order an antipyretic.

Anxiety. Most patients with an STD experience varying degrees of anxiety. Those who have been successfully treated for previous STDs may have less anxiety than patients who have multiple problems associated with the infection. Some patients openly express their feelings, whereas others give no indication of a problem. Often a health care worker with an understanding and empathetic attitude can encourage these patients talk about their problems. These patients also may express anger and frustration.

Diarrhea. Diarrhea may be a symptom of some STDs (eg, enteritis caused by a protozoan infection). It also can occur as an adverse effect of some antimicrobial agents, especially when the drug is taken orally over an extended period. Until the infection is controlled, these patients are instructed to increase their fluid intake as well as attain a normal food intake. If diarrhea is severe, they are informed of the signs of electrolyte imbalance and instructed to notify the physician if any one of these occurs.

Ineffective Individual Coping. People express various emotions when they discover that they have an STD. They may be unable to accept the diagnosis, and express inappropriate reasons for the infection, inappropriately place the blame for the infection on one or more persons, or blame society in general for their problem. Some of the ineffective coping mechanisms may remain firm in the patient's mind, but others may be directed toward positive attitudes by means of education about and prevention of STDs.

Altered Family Processes. A married patient may have difficulty explaining the infection to his or her spouse as well as asking the spouse to seek medical attention. An STD indicates that one spouse has had sexual activity outside the marriage, which creates various emotional responses. The infected person may not want to communicate with the spouse for any number of reasons.

These patients must be allowed to express the fears, anxieties, and emotions that accompany this type of problem, and the nurse must show understanding of the problems associated with informing the spouse. The nurse also must explain the consequences of silence on the part of the infected spouse, and recommend that the couple seek marriage counseling.

Fear. A patient diagnosed as having AIDS probably knows that there is no cure and that the infection is fatal. Some patients with gonorrhea fear the consequences that the infection may have on their marriage, and teenagers may be concerned about how the infection will affect their sexual partners and their reputation with their peers. Other patients, through lack of knowledge, fear that the infection may not be cured, when indeed many STDs do respond well to treatment.

The nurse must try to identify any fears the patient may have as well as attempt to dispel those fears by means of explanation, education, and, possibly, referral to a social agency, such as a marriage counseling service or a group that deals with teens who have an STD.

Potential for Infection Transmission. All patients with STDs are capable of transmitting the infection until it is cured. Patients are advised to return for laboratory tests to be sure they are no longer contagious. The exceptions are those with AIDS or active herpes simplex virus infections. Patients with AIDS remain capable of spreading the disease if they continue to engage in unprotected sexual activity. Those with herpes simplex virus are infectious when the disease is initially active or recurs at a later time.

Altered Sexuality Patterns. A person with an STD needs to refrain from sexual activity until the infection is cured. When the STD cannot be cured, as, for example, with AIDS or herpes simplex virus infection, instructions are given regarding the use of condoms (eg, practice safe sex). This alteration in sexual activity may not be accepted by all patients. Health care personnel must emphasize the importance of the patient's changing his or her pattern of sexual activity. An atmosphere of mutual trust between the nurse and the patient must be established, and the patient given time to ask questions.

Social Isolation. A person may be embarrassed by his or her situation, and therefore avoid social as well as sexual contact with others. The person with AIDS is especially prone to social isolation because of the information—and sometimes misinformation—about the disease that has been given to the public. Nurses can help AIDS patients, as well as those with other STDs, understand and accept the actions of others by being good listeners and allowing patients to talk through their emotions. The physician may find it necessary to refer the patient to a psychiatrist, a psychologist, or group therapy.

Noncompliance. Despite the information they receive, some patients with STDs fail either to seek treatment or to complete a course of therapy. Others fail to use protective measures or change their sexual activities to prevent a recurrence of the infection or the acquisition of a different STD. Still others do not care, and believe that (some) STDs can be cured with an injection or a few pills. Health care professionals must inform the patient of all the risks and dangers of certain sexual practices or activities and repeated STD infections. Information given in a positive manner may help the patient to understand the importance of seeking treatment, completing a course of therapy, preventing the transmission of the infection to others, and using methods of avoiding infection in the future.

Knowledge Deficit. Many people have wrong or no information about STDs. Some people disregard the information they do receive. People diagnosed as having an STD should be given information regarding the importance of treatment, the prevention of spread to others, and methods that may be used to avoid future infections. The nurse must first determine what these patients know and then add to their knowledge or correct facts that are wrong. Some cities have hot lines that adolescents and young adults with STDs can call for answers to their questions and that can help people with an STD get in touch with a support group. A nationwide hot line (1-800-227-8922) provides information about and referral services for STDs.

Evaluation

■ Pain controlled as much as possible
■ Attains normal body temperature
■ Anxiety and fear reduced or eliminated

- Diarrhea controlled
- Demonstrated a more positive attitude and ability to cope with the infection
- Expresses a desire to discuss the infection with the noninfected spouse
- Understands the reactions of others to an STD

- Identifies past sexual partners so that examination and treatment of these people can be instituted
- Acquires knowledge and demonstrates understanding of STDs, their signs and symptoms, the importance of treatment, methods of prevention, and the risks involved with certain types of sexual activity

General Nutritional Considerations

☐ A patient with AIDS must be encouraged to eat a well-balanced diet. Because severe anorexia often accompanies this disease, it may be necessary to offer high-calorie liquids between meals.

☐ Intravenous supplementation of fluids and calories may be necessary if an AIDS patient fails to eat or drink an adequate amount.

General Pharmacologic Considerations

☐ Antipyretic drugs (aspirin and acetaminophen) usually are ordered if the patient has a fever.

☐ A *complete* course of the recommended antimicrobial therapy is necessary to cure (most) STDs.

☐ Drugs currently used in the treatment of AIDS are expensive. Some patients are able to obtain their drugs through various social agencies or groups that pay for the cost of therapy.

☐ Free clinics for the detection and treatment of STDs are available in most areas.

☐ An allergy history is obtained before administration of any antimicrobial agent (eg, penicillin, sulfonamides, and tetracycline). The physician is informed of an allergy to any antimicrobial agent, so that a different drug can be ordered.

☐ The prescribed drug regimen is explained to the patient. Information should include the number of capsules or tablets per dose, the time of day the drug is to be taken, food restrictions (if any), and possible adverse effects. Emphasis is placed on the importance of completing a course of therapy.

General Gerontologic Considerations

☐ The elderly patient may be sexually active, and therefore develop an STD.

☐ Some older patients may have limited knowledge about STDs, and therefore not recognize some of the symptoms or seek treatment.

Suggested Readings

☐ Baril MT, Jaser SK. Living with AIDS. RN March 1988;51:81. *(Additional coverage of subject matter)*

☐ Barrick B. Caring for AIDS patients: a challenge you can meet. Nursing '88 November 1988;18:50. *(Additional coverage of subject matter)*

☐ Brennan L, Editors of Nursing '88. The battle against AIDS: A report from the nursing front. Nursing '88 April 1988;18:60. *(Additional coverage of subject matter)*

☐ Corless IB. AIDS: principles, practices, and politics. New York: Hemisphere Publishing, 1987. *(Additional coverage of subject matter)*

☐ Flaskerud JH. Aids/HIV infection: a reference guide for nursing professionals. Philadelphia: WB Saunders, 1989. *(Additional and in-depth coverage of subject matter)*

☐ Frumkin LR, Leonard JM. Questions and answers on AIDS. Oradell, NJ: Medical Economics, 1987. *(Additional coverage of subject matter)*

☐ Grabbe LL, Brown LB. Identifying neurologic complications of AIDS. Nursing '89 May 1989;19:66. *(Additional coverage of subject matter)*

☐ Gurevich I. Counseling the patient with herpes. RN February 1990;53:22. *(Additional coverage of subject matter)*

☐ Hamilton D. For AIDS patients, little things can mean a lot. Nursing '88 May 1988;18:61. *(Additional coverage of subject matter)*

☐ Kennedy M. AIDS: coping with the fear. Nursing '87 April 1987;17:45. *(Additional coverage of subject matter)*

☐ Loucks A. Chlamydia: an unheralded epidemic. Am J Nurs July 1987;87:920. *(Additional coverage of subject matter)*

☐ McElhose P. The "other" STDs: as dangerous as ever. RN June 1988;51:52. *(Additional coverage of subject matter)*

☐ Nettina SM. When patients with genital herpes turn to you for answers. Nursing '89 August 1989;19:61. *(Additional coverage and illustrations that reinforce subject matter)*

☐ Perdew S. Facts about AIDS: a guide for health care providers. Philadelphia: JB Lippincott, 1989. *(Additional coverage of subject matter)*

☐ Plank CS. Aerosolized pentamidine: A new weapon against PCP Nursing '89 February 1989;19:48. *(Additional coverage of subject matter)*

☐ Scherer P. How AIDS attacks the brain. Am J Nurs January 1990;90:44. *(Additional coverage of subject matter)*

☐ Schmitz D. When IV drug abuse complicates AIDS. RN January 1990;53:60. *(Additional coverage of subject matter)*

☐ Shilts R. And the band played on: politics and the AIDS epidemic. New York: St Martin's Press, 1987. *(Additional coverage of subject matter)*

☐ Sipes C. Should hospital patients be screened for AIDS? Nursing '88 February 1988;18:49. *(Additional coverage of subject matter)*

☐ Tribulski JA. The true odds of getting AIDS from a patient. RN May 1988;51:64. *(Additional coverage of subject matter)*

☐ Ungvarski P. Coping with infections that AIDS patients develop. RN November 1988;51:53. *(Additional and in-depth coverage of subject matter)*

☐ Wallach JB. Interpretation of diagnostic tests: a handbook synopsis of laboratory medicine. Boston: Little, Brown & Co, 1986. *(In-depth coverage of subject matter)*

Chapter 10
Allergic Disorders

On completion of this chapter the reader will:

- List and discuss the types of allergic disorders
- List the substances that commonly cause allergy
- Discuss the methods of diagnosing an allergy
- Describe the methods used in the treatment of allergies
- Use the nursing process in the management of the patient with an allergic disorder

Allergy refers to a state of *altered* immunologic reactivity whereby the body is injured in the course of its immune response against a substance that is recognized as something foreign to the body. An allergic reaction may affect various organs and structures such as the skin, nasal mucosa, and gastrointestinal tract.

An *antigen* is a substance that evokes the production of *antibodies*. If tissue injury results, the antigen is then called an *allergen*, that is, a substance capable of causing an allergic response in tissues (tissue injury). When an antigen produces an immune response, as may be seen with the production of antibodies against an invading microorganism, the microorganism is called an *immunogen*, that is, a substance capable of producing an antibody response that produces immunity (see Chapter 7).

Allergy can occur at any age, and the pattern of allergic response may vary in the same person over the years. People may suddenly show an allergic reaction to a substance with which they have had contact for years. On the other hand, allergic responses to one agent may gradually disappear, to be replaced by sensitivity to another substance. Why these changes occur is not clear.

SUBSTANCES THAT COMMONLY CAUSE ALLERGY

Allergens may be inhaled or ingested, or they may come in contact with the skin. Drug allergy is common and can be caused by almost any drug. Certain drugs, such as penicillin, are especially likely to cause allergic reactions.

Substances that are present in the environment may produce an allergic response in sensitive people. Dust, pollen, animal hairs and dander, molds, grasses, and trees are examples of such substances. These substances are airborne and therefore are inhaled.

Some people are sensitive to substances that come in contact with the skin, thus producing a skin reaction (allergic dermatoses). Examples of substances that may produce an allergic skin reaction are soap, drugs, deodorant, hair spray, and cosmetics.

DIAGNOSIS

Diagnosis of an allergy may be simple and clear-cut, or it may require multiple tests and a thorough patient history. Some people develop typical symptoms of allergic rhinitis only when ragweed is producing pollen, leading the physician to suspect that ragweed is the offender and to perform a skin test to confirm the diagnosis. Other patients have symptoms throughout the year without any apparent relation to the substances they eat or come in contact with in the environment. Skillful interviewing and careful observation may uncover clues that indicate an allergy to a specific substance or group of substances. Diagnosis is complicated by the fact that the patient may be allergic to more than one substance, and the tendency to develop symptoms may vary with fatigue or emotional stress and with the presence of infection.

Skin Tests

There are two methods of skin testing, the intradermal injection and the scratch test. Extracts of various substances (antigens) such as pollens, animal danders, food, and dust may be used for testing. In the intradermal test, a dilute solution of an antigen is injected intradermally. A positive reaction, marked by the appearance of a raised wheal or localized erythema (redness), indicates sensitivity (allergy) to the injected antigen. The scratch test involves making a scratch on the skin and applying the test antigen to the scratch. If a raised wheal or localized erythema appears, a positive reaction to the antigen has occurred.

TREATMENT

The type of treatment used to relieve the symptoms of allergy depend on the type of allergy present. Once the diagnosis has been confirmed and the offending allergens identified, the physician selects the most appropriate treatment. One or more of the following methods may be used in the treatment of an allergy.

Antihistamines. Available as prescription or nonprescription agents, antihistamines are a large group of drugs that relieve the symptoms of allergy. They may be given by the oral, intravenous, intramuscular, or topical route.

Nasal Decongestants. Used to relieve nasal congestion, nasal decongestants are available as topical drops or sprays.

Avoidance of the Allergen. Sometimes the allergen can be removed from the environment. For example, a person who is allergic to feathers must avoid the use of feather pillows.

Modification of the Environment. Environmental changes such as air conditioning and electrostatic air cleaners may help some people who are allergic to airborne allergens such as dust and pollen.

Immunotherapy. The injection of extracts, which are dilute amounts of the offending allergens, appears to stimulate antibody formation against the injected allergens. The injections are given on a regular basis, such as every 3 to 6 weeks. When the person is allergic to substances that are present year-round, the extracts are given during the entire year. Those who are allergic to seasonal substances, such as grasses and trees, require immunotherapy for only part of the year.

Immunotherapy is begun with very dilute extracts of the offending allergens. Weekly injections are required until the maximum dose is achieved. The patient then receives subsequent booster injections every 4 to 6 weeks.

Corticosteroids. Because of their antiinflammatory activity, corticosteroids are of value in treating the inflammatory responses seen with allergies.

Epinephrine. Epinephrine is a sympathomimetic agent used for emergency treatment of serious allergic reactions, such as an reaction to bee stings or anaphylactic shock. Epinephrine or related sympathomimetic agents also may be included in topical nasal decongestants.

TYPES OF ALLERGIES
Allergic Rhinitis

Allergic rhinitis, also called hay fever or pollinosis, is the most common form of allergy. It is caused by environmental airborne allergens such as pollens and molds. If untreated, chronic allergic rhinitis can result in asthma, chronic bronchitis, asthmatic bronchitis, nasal polyps, and otitis media.

Symptoms

Sneezing, itching of the nose, nasal congestion, thin, watery nasal discharge, and itching and redness of the eyes are symptoms of allergic rhinitis. Headache, earache (caused by otitis media), malaise, and fatigue also may occur. The intensity of symptoms may vary.

Diagnosis

Diagnosis is based on symptoms and a thorough patient history. The physician may perform skin tests to determine the offending allergens.

Treatment

Antihistamines, nasal decongestants, corticosteroids, immunotherapy, avoidance of the offending allergens, and modification of the environment may reduce or eliminate symptoms. Eye drops that contain antihistamine may be prescribed for eye symptoms.

Contact Dermatitis

Contact dermatitis is a skin reaction that results from contact with a substance to which the person is sensitive or allergic. It also may occur when a person comes in contact with an irritating substance. This latter skin response is not a true allergic reaction, and may occur in those who do not have allergies.

Symptoms

Itching, burning, redness, and rash are seen. The size of the lesions may vary from small to large. The rash may appear as raised, fluid-filled lesions (vesicles). Infection may occur.

Diagnosis

Diagnosis is based on physical examination of the affected areas and a thorough patient history.

Treatment

Avoidance of the allergen or irritating substance is necessary. Changing the brand of the offending substance may alleviate the problem. If the substance cannot be avoided, providing protection for the exposed skin may be of value. Topical or oral antihistamines and topical or oral corticosteroids may be prescribed. Skin infections are treated with antibiotics.

Dermatitis Medicamentosa

Dermatitis medicamentosa occurs when the person is allergic to a drug. Many drugs list rash as a possible adverse effect. The appearance of a rash may indicate the development of a more serious reaction (eg, anaphylaxis) with repeated administration of the drug.

Symptoms

The rash appears suddenly. It usually is generalized but may appear in one area, such as on the arms or trunk. The rash may be bright red, and itching may occur.

Diagnosis

Diagnosis is made by examination of the affected area and a thorough patient history of recent drug therapy.

Treatment

The drug is stopped *immediately*. The rash usually disappears in a few hours. Antihistamines may be prescribed. The patient is closely observed for more serious symptoms (see later discussion of drug allergy).

Food Allergy

Food allergies most commonly occur in children but may be seen in adults.

Symptoms

Nausea, vomiting, diarrhea, abdominal cramps, malaise, itching, rash, and respiratory symptoms (wheezing, cough) may occur.

Diagnosis

Diagnosis is based on a thorough patient history. Often it is difficult to identify the foods to which the person is allergic. In some instances, skin testing is negative. To determine which foods are the source of allergy, the physician may have the patient fast for 1 or 2 days and drink distilled water. One food at a time is then added to the diet, starting with foods that are known to be hypoallergenic, such as rice and tapioca.

Treatment

Avoidance of the food causing the allergic reaction is the only treatment. In some instances, the person is not allergic to particular food groups but is allergic to the chemicals (eg, fertilizers, dyes, and preservatives) contained in the food. To reduce or eliminate symptoms, the patient may have to eat only food that is organically grown and contains no preservatives or dyes.

Drug Allergy

Other symptoms besides dermatitis medicamentosa may occur if the person is allergic to a drug. Reactions may be immediate or delayed for several hours or days. Although an allergic reaction may occur with the first dose of a drug, it is more commonly seen at the time of the second or subsequent doses. A variety of allergic responses may occur, ranging from mild to serious and even life-threatening.

Drug allergy probably results from the drug or its metabolite combining with a protein to form a complex that stimulates the immune response. The occurrence of adverse drug effects after administration of a drug is not a true drug allergy. These effects are probably an exaggerated response to the pharmacologic effects of the drug or its metabolites.

Symptoms

The most serious drug allergy reaction is anaphylaxis. Drug-induced lupus syndromes, dermatitis medicamentosa, drug fever, pulmonary reactions, lymph node enlargement, and hepatic syndromes are examples of responses caused by drug allergy.

Diagnosis

Diagnosis is based on symptoms and the patient's drug history.

Treatment

The offending drug is stopped immediately. Additional treatment is aimed at controlling or eliminating the symptoms until the drug is eliminated from the body or the damaged organ or structure recovers.

Urticaria and Angioedema

Urticaria and angioedema (also called *angioneurotic edema*) may occur as a response to an allergen. The allergen may be a drug or an environmental substance, or result from exposure to cold, food, blood (as a transfusion), or chemicals.

Symptoms

Urticaria, or hives, involves the superficial layers of the skin and is marked by itching, swelling, redness, and the development of wheals. When the edema extends deeper into tissues of the skin or mucous membranes, it is termed *angioedema*. Urticaria and angioedema may occur together. Angioedema usually involves the head and neck areas. When the mucous membranes of the mouth, pharynx, larynx, and bronchi are affected, the consequences can be serious. The causes of angioedema include certain drugs, heredity, and exposure to cold. In many cases, the cause is unknown. Angioedema can result in respiratory arrest because the swelling may obstruct the respiratory passages.

Diagnosis

Diagnosis is made by examination of the affected areas.

Treatment

Topical or oral antihistamines and corticosteroids may be prescribed for urticaria. Angioedema of the larynx and epiglottis may cause severe respiratory distress. The status of the cardiac and respiratory rate is determined. It is important that an adequate airway be established. Endotracheal intubation or an emergency tracheostomy may be required. Bronchospasm may be treated with intravenous administration of epinephrine or aminophylline.

Anaphylaxis

Anaphylaxis is a sudden reaction that occurs after exposure to an allergen to which the person is extremely sensitive.

Symptoms

Symptoms appear suddenly. In the beginning, the patient may have a sensation of warmth. Urticaria, angioedema, and itching may occur. Swelling may be present in the nose, mouth, throat, and bronchi, resulting in moderate to severe upper airway obstruction, which can be life-threatening. Bronchoconstriction also may be seen. The most serious manifestation of anaphylaxis is hypotensive or anaphylactic shock (see Chapter 18).

Diagnosis

Diagnosis, which must be made immediately, is based on symptoms.

Treatment

To begin immediate treatment, early recognition is necessary. If the offending allergen (eg, a drug or insect venom) was injected into an extremity, a tourniquet is placed above the area. Subcutaneous injection of 0.2 to 0.5 mL of epinephrine 1:1,000 is given immediately in the upper arm. If necessary, the dose may be repeated two more times at 20- to 30-minute intervals and the patient closely observed. Antihistamines and corticosteroids may be given to prevent additional skin manifestations. Patients with a known hypersensitivity to insect venom may be prescribed an emergency treatment kit. Products available contain premeasured doses of epinephrine in a disposable syringe. The kit also may contain a tourniquet.

Anaphylactic shock requires immediate and intensive treatment. An intravenous line with normal saline solution is established immediately. Epinephrine is administered intravenously. Other vasopressors, such as dopamine, may be given to treat hypotension. Supportive treatment, such as oxygen and mechanical ventilation, also may be used. If cardiac or respiratory arrest occurs, cardiopulmonary resuscitation is begun immediately. Drugs and equipment (eg, intravenous equipment and epinephrine) usually used to treat anaphylaxis are brought to the bedside by another member of the medical team. Measures to treat hypoxia and shock are instituted (see Chapters 18 and 21).

NURSING PROCESS —THE PATIENT WHO HAS AN ALLERGIC DISORDER

Assessment

With the exception of the occurrence of anaphylaxis, a thorough patient history is important when the patient has an allergic disorder. Areas covered include a complete medical and surgical history, a food history (with particular attention to those foods that cause any type of problem), and a family allergy history. The patient's symptoms are recorded in detail, and those factors that appear to increase or decrease symptoms (eg, exposure and time of year) are explored. All drugs, both prescription and nonprescription, taken in the past are recorded, with special attention to those agents that may have caused a problem. If there are skin manifestations, the affected areas are examined and the lesions described in detail.

Nursing Diagnosis

Depending on the type and symptoms of allergy, one or more of the following nursing diagnoses may apply to a person with an allergic disorder:

- Impaired home maintenance management related to inability to work in an environment that produces moderate to severe symptoms
- Noncompliance related to indifference, lack of knowledge, other factors
- Impaired skin integrity caused by dermatitis, pruritus
- Potential for infection related to impaired tissue integrity, scratching
- Ineffective airway clearance caused by angioedema
- Ineffective breathing pattern caused by angioedema
- Impaired gas exchange caused by angioedema of the upper airway
- Altered oral mucous membrane related to angioedema of oral cavity
- Knowledge deficit of treatment modalities

Planning and Implementation

The major goals of the patient include relief of symptoms and a thorough understanding of the prescribed treatment modalities.

The major goals of nursing management are to reduce or eliminate the symptoms associated with the allergic disorder, reduce anxiety, and supply information regarding the patient's specific treatment regimen.

The major goal of nursing management of a patient with anaphylaxis is immediate recognition and reversal of symptoms.

Once the offending allergens are identified, suggestions are made regarding treatment and avoidance of the allergens. In some cases, a printed list of required tasks is given by the physician. These tasks and possible alternatives can be discussed by the nurse.

The nurse can minimize the possibility of allergies developing because of contact with drugs by working neatly, avoiding spills, and washing the hands before as well as after preparing a drug for administration.

Prevention.   To eliminate possible allergic drug reactions, a *thorough* drug history is taken at the time of the initial assessment as well as before any new drug is added to the patient's therapeutic regimen. Any patient with a history of drug allergy is *closely observed each time a new drug is added to the therapeutic regimen.* If anaphylaxis should occur, emergency equipment is brought to the bedside and help is summoned immediately.

Those with known sensitivity to an allergen that results in anaphylaxis should carry identification, such as a Medic Alert tag, to inform medical personnel of their allergies. Those sensitive to insect venom (eg, bees, wasps, and hornets) should carry an emergency kit containing epinephrine.

Avoidance of environmental substances to which the person is allergic can decrease or eliminate some symptoms.

Impaired Home Maintenance Management.   The patient is encouraged to explore possibilities and their alternatives regarding avoidance of the offending allergen. In some instances, the nurse must ask questions and offer solutions until the problem is resolved. Examples of solutions that may be proposed for various types of allergies include discontinuing the use of feather pillows, using air conditioning and special furnace filters, using hypoallergenic products, and wearing gloves (rubber or plastic) when coming in contact with an offending allergen or irritable substance.

Noncompliance.   Treatment may extend over many years. Some patients, for any number of reasons, fail to comply with the recommended treatment modalities. For others, changes in the environment may not be financially or physically possible. The nurse must listen to the patient, identify possible areas of noncompliance, and work with the patient to solve immediate and long-range problems.

Impaired Skin Integrity; Potential for Infection.   Scratching of lesions may result in breaks in the skin, which allow pathogenic microorganisms to enter and cause infection. Topical agents may be prescribed or recommended to control itching. The patient should be advised to keep the nails clean and short and, if necessary, to wear cotton gloves at night to prevent scratching while sleeping. Any signs of infection or a spread of skin lesions requires examination by a physician as soon as possible.

Ineffective Airway Clearance and Breathing Pattern; Impaired Gas Exchange; Altered Oral Mucous Membrane.   A patient with a known allergy to one or more drugs or a history of angioedema is closely observed each time a new drug is ordered. The respiratory rate and character are assessed at frequent intervals, and the oral cavity inspected for changes in the appearance of the mucous membranes.

Immediate recognition of this disorder is necessary, as edema of the upper airway can result in severe respiratory distress and become a life-threatening situation.

Knowledge Deficit. Once the diagnosis of allergy is made and the offending allergens tentatively or positively identified, treatment modalities are explained to the patient in detail. A thorough teaching program helps the patient to understand what can and must be done to relieve symptoms. Once the patient is made aware of what must be done and what results might be expected, he or she may be more willing to follow recommendations for modification of his or her environment and for treatment.

If environmental modifications are recommended, the nurse should go over each recommendation in detail. Time must be allowed for the patient to read printed material (when used) and ask questions. The patient may be unable to eliminate certain environmental factors, and the nurse must take time to explore alternatives.

The medical regimen prescribed by the physician is thoroughly explained, and the patient encouraged to adhere to the prescribed methods of treatment. The patient is cautioned against the overuse of nose drops or sprays and advised to use only prescribed or recommended drugs and only in the dosage suggested by the physician. Overuse of products containing sympathomimetic amines, such as epinephrine, can result in rebound congestion, a period of nasal congestion that may be worse than before the drug was used.

If immunotherapy is recommended, the patient is told that it will be necessary to keep all appointments during the initiation of therapy as well as for follow-up booster injections. If initial or booster injections are missed, the series of injections must be restarted, using the lowest dose. The grace period for missing injections varies. Missing a weekly injection by 5 to 7 days during the initial series or missing a booster injection by more than 2 or 3 weeks usually requires starting therapy from the beginning.

If a food allergy is suspected and a hypoallergenic diet ordered to determine the offending food or chemical allergens, the diet and the method of adding new foods must be thoroughly explained. The patient is told to keep a record of the symptoms, or lack of symptoms, experienced each time a new food is added.

If epinephrine is prescribed for the treatment of anaphylaxis, the symptoms that necessitate its administration are explained in detail. Instruction in the application of a tourniquet and self-administration of the drug is given. The patient is told that there is an expiration date for the epinephrine, and that the prescription must be refilled on or before the date stamped on the carton.

Evaluation

- Verbalizes awareness of what must be done and what results might be expected once treatment is begun
- Verbalizes understanding of changes necessary to reduce symptoms and participates in solving problems related to home maintenance management
- Verbalizes willingness to participate in a treatment program
- No evidence of anaphylaxis
- Verbalizes understanding of the treatment modalities necessary to reduce or eliminate symptoms
- Verbalizes understanding of hypoallergenic diet
- Demonstrates understanding of the symptoms of anaphylaxis and ability to administer emergency epinephrine

General Nutritional Considerations

☐ Special diets prescribed for those with food allergies require an explanation of the initial foods as well as when and how each new food is added to the diet.

General Pharmacologic Considerations

☐ Most antihistamines cause drowsiness. The patient is told to avoid driving a car, operating machinery, or performing any tasks that require alertness.

☐ The physician is consulted before nonprescription products that contain antihistamines are used.

☐ The use of nonprescription eye preparations to reduce redness should be avoided. Itching and redness of the eyes should be evaluated and treated by a physician.

Suggested Readings

☐ Berkow R, Fletcher AJ, eds. Merck manual of diagnosis and therapy. 15th ed. Rahway, NJ: Merck & Co, 1987. *(In-depth coverage of subject matter)*

☐ Dong FM. All about food allergy. Philadelphia: JB Lippincott, 1984. *(Additional and in-depth coverage of subject matter)*

☐ Karb VB, Queener SF, Freeman JB. Handbook of drugs for nursing practice. St Louis: CV Mosby, 1988. *(Additional coverage of subject matter)*

Chapter 11
Substance Abuse

On completion of this chapter the reader will:

- Define the terms used when discussing substance abuse

- Discuss the dangers associated with substance abuse

- List and discuss the drugs and substances subject to abuse

- Discuss the immediate treatment of the toxic effects related to substance abuse

- Describe some of the methods of treating substance withdrawal and dependence

- Use the nursing process in the management of the patient with a substance abuse problem

Substance (or drug) abuse has become one of the leading problems worldwide. The terms *drug* and *substance* often are used interchangeably. Substance (or drug) abuse is the use of a natural or synthetic substance to alter mood or behavior in a manner that differs from its generally accepted use. For example, morphine may be prescribed by a physician for severe pain; this is an acceptable use of the drug. When morphine is used to produce euphoria or prevent symptoms of narcotic withdrawal, it is an unacceptable use of the drug.

Every patient seen in the home, clinic, or hospital setting must be considered a *potential* candidate for substance abuse and withdrawal symptoms.

Terminology

The following terms may be used when discussing substance abuse.

Habituation. Habituation is a pattern of repeated use. The user exhibits little or no tendency to increase the dose, and withdrawal symptoms usually do not occur if the substance is withdrawn. The abuser may have some degree of psychological dependence on the effect of the substance.

Dependence. Dependence is a strong need to continue taking or using a substance and an ambivalence toward it. Withdrawal symptoms occur when the substance is withheld. There are two types of dependence: psychological and physical. *Psychological dependence* is a compulsion to use a substance to obtain a pleasurable experience. The need for use ranges from mild to severe. Continued use may lead to physical dependence. *Physical dependence* is a compulsive need to use a substance repeatedly to avoid mild to severe withdrawal symptoms. The time required for development of either type of dependence varies with the person and the type and amount (dose, frequency) of the substance used.

Addiction. Addiction is a state of periodic or chronic intoxication produced by the repeated consumption of a natural or synthetic substance. Characteristics include an overpowering desire or need to continue taking the drug and to obtain it by any means, a tendency to increase the dose, a psychological and, usually, a physical dependence on the effects of the drug, and a detrimental effect on both the addict and society. Addiction may be used interchangeably with physical dependence or severe habituation.

Tolerance. Tolerance is a need to increase the dose or the frequency of use to obtain the original or desired effect.

Withdrawal Symptoms. Withdrawal symptoms are psychological and physical symptoms that occur when the abused substance is abruptly discontinued. These symptoms vary and depend on the substance used.

Problems Associated With Substance Abuse

Substance abuse and dependence can cause major health and economic problems. Some of these problems are as follows:

1. Because he or she may not be able to properly perform his or her job, the substance abuser may endanger the health, safety, or welfare of the general public.
2. The care of substance abuse patients in both general and mental hospitals as well as in correctional institutions is costly to the community.
3. Substance abuse is expensive. Many addicts soon find themselves without funds and turn to theft, prostitution, and other illegal activities to support their drug dependence.
4. Major health problems, such as cirrhosis, and the transmission of diseases, such as hepatitis and acquired immunodeficiency syndrome, may be associated with substance abuse.
5. Injury or death to self and others may occur if the substance abuser loses control.
6. Loss of time from and inefficiency at work or school may increase employer expenses, reduce employee income, or result in dropping out of school.
7. The family structure and integrity may be altered when one or more members abuse drugs.

ALCOHOL ABUSE

Alcohol (ethanol) is a central nervous system (CNS) depressant. The effects of alcohol on the CNS are related to the levels of alcohol in brain tissue and blood. They include changes in judgment, behavior, motor coordination, and consciousness.

Alcohol abuse is found in all occupations and at all socioeconomic levels; it may be a single abuse or coexist with the use of other abused substances, such as tranquilizers, cocaine, and narcotics. Despite the many problems associated with alcoholism, many alcoholics have an amazing ability to maintain themselves in the community. They continue to work and may conceal their substance abuse. The condition may persist, with varying degrees of severity, for a large part of a person's life. Today, more teenagers, and even young children, are becoming alcoholics.

Alcoholics who are admitted to the hospital for reasons other than alcoholism may try to hide their drinking problem. Some bring a supply of alcohol with them. Others, such as acute surgical patients, are, of necessity, deprived of oral fluids, including alcohol.

Such patients usually develop signs of alcohol withdrawal syndrome (also called delirium tremens or DTs) in a few hours to 3 days or more.

Symptoms of Acute Alcohol Intoxication

Symptoms of acute alcohol intoxication include drowsiness to stupor, slurred speech, ataxia, and behavioral changes such as euphoria and aggressive or belligerent behavior. The alcoholic may develop alcohol withdrawal syndrome, a condition that results from sudden withdrawal from alcohol or a prolonged heavy intake of alcohol.

Early signs of alcohol withdrawal syndrome include nausea, vomiting, anorexia, disorientation, agitation, hallucinations, and diaphoresis. Seizures also may be seen. As the condition progresses, restless, violent, unceasing activity occurs, and may be so great that it leads to death from heart failure or exhaustion. Tremors, anxiety, insomnia, and visual, auditory, and tactile hallucinations usually intensify. Perspiration may be profuse, and dehydration and electrolyte imbalance may occur. Respiratory and pulse rates, blood pressure, and often temperature are elevated. If alcohol withdrawal syndrome occurs when the body is under an added strain, such as an illness, the body's resistance to alcohol poisoning is decreased.

Treatment and Rehabilitation

After assessment, the most serious effects of alcohol toxicity are given priority. It is important to determine whether the patient has taken one or more other drugs immediately before, during, or after the time he or she has consumed alcohol. The use of CNS depressants (such as barbiturates or tranquilizers) with alcohol can potentiate the effects of the depressant, possibly resulting in respiratory depression and coma. Death has occurred when even small amounts of alcohol have been combined with a CNS depressant.

The patient must be protected from injury. Physical restraints are avoided whenever possible because they often aggravate the patient's condition. The presence of a nurse or a nursing assistant who is calm, firm, and watchful helps to protect the patient from injury as well as to lessen extreme agitation.

Drug therapy for withdrawal symptoms is symptomatic, and includes the following:

- Vitamins, especially the vitamin B group. Alcoholics usually suffer from vitamin deficiency; vitamin B deficiency may be so severe that the patient develops pellagra.
- Paraldehyde, which may be used as a sedative during periods of acute agitation
- Tranquilizers, which may be used to lessen the patient's restlessness and agitation and to control withdrawal symptoms

■ Anticonvulsants, to prevent convulsions that may occur with alcohol withdrawal syndrome or acute alcohol intoxication

Intravenous fluids and electrolytes may be given until anorexia, nausea, and vomiting are sufficiently controlled to permit an adequate intake of oral fluids. A nutritious diet is essential as soon as the patient can tolerate oral fluids and food.

After the acute phase has passed, the patient requires long-term treatment. Sometimes disulfiram (Antabuse) is used as an adjunct to other kinds of therapy for chronic alcoholism. This drug causes no apparent effects when given alone, but the ingestion of even small amounts of alcohol causes severe nausea, vomiting, and diarrhea. Hypotension, which may become severe, also may be seen. Patients must give their informed consent before they are given disulfiram and must be fully aware of the symptoms that will occur if they take a drink. Continued use of other drugs such as tranquilizers and sedatives presents hazards because alcoholics are likely to transfer their dependence on alcohol to other substances.

Individual or group psychotherapy may help the patient to gain greater insight into the emotional problems that have led to alcohol dependence. Family support also is essential. Alcoholics Anonymous, an organization composed of and run by alcoholics, has been beneficial for many people; it is noted for its success in helping those who have not been helped by other means. The philosophy of Alcoholics Anonymous is expressed in a prayer its members use: "God, grant me the serenity to accept the things I cannot change, courage to change the things I can, and the wisdom to know the difference." Families may be helped by referral to such groups as Al-Anon, for families of alcoholics, and Alateen, for teenagers with parents who are alcoholics.

COCAINE

Cocaine use is the number one substance abuse problem in the United States. Cocaine, which is obtained from the leaves of the coca plant, is a CNS stimulant. A highly addicting substance, it has caused death, even when used in small doses.

The powder form of cocaine is snorted (inhaled through the nose) or dissolved and injected intravenously. Crack, a purified form of cocaine with a crystalline or rocklike appearance, is smoked either by placing it in a pipe or by sprinkling it onto or mixing it with tobacco. Cocaine may be freebased, which reduces it to its purest form. It is then smoked by sprinkling it onto a cigarette or inhaling it through a pipe. This method of using crack or free base produces a more immediate rush than when the substance is used by nasal inhalation.

Symptoms of Acute and Chronic Toxicity

Signs and symptoms of acute toxicity include agitation, psychotic behavior, violent behavior, hyperthermia, seizures, dysrhythmias, hypertension, respiratory failure, and dilated pupils. Signs and symptoms of chronic toxicity include dysrhythmias, hypertension, memory impairment, personality and behavioral changes, ulceration of the nasal mucosa and perforation of the nasal septum (in those who inhale cocaine), needle marks along the pathways of veins (in those who use cocaine intravenously), anorexia, weight loss, psychosis, and hallucinations.

Cocaine use results in physical dependence. In some people, dependence occurs rapidly—sometimes after one or two uses. Withdrawal usually is characterized by depression, psychosis, lethargy, restlessness, an intense craving for the drug, inability to concentrate, and irritability.

Treatment and Rehabilitation

Immediate treatment of cocaine toxicity depends on the patient's symptoms. Aggravated behavior may be treated with sedatives or tranquilizers. Dysrhythmias may be treated with antiarrhythmic drugs. Respiratory and circulatory problems may require oxygen, mechanical ventilation, and an intravenous line to administer drugs and fluid. Seizures require administration of an anticonvulsant, and extreme hyperthermia, use of a hypothermia blanket.

Children of cocaine-addicted mothers may be born with birth defects as well as an addiction to cocaine.

Addiction often is difficult to treat. The chronic cocaine user must be encouraged to enter a rehabilitative program that focuses on detoxification as well as counseling and peer group support. Referral to groups such as Cocaine Anonymous has helped some people continue abstinence from the drug.

HEROIN AND OTHER NARCOTICS

Heroin (diacetylmorphine), a potent and illegal narcotic, produces an intense high, or a state of euphoria. Other narcotics that are abused include codeine, morphine, meperidine (Demerol), methadone, hydromorphone (Dilaudid), oxycodone, and opium (often as paregoric). Tolerance and physical dependence can occur rapidly, and often depend on the dose and frequency of use. Eventually, the abuser uses the drug to prevent withdrawal symptoms, rather than to obtain a high.

Intravenous administration of heroin, as well as other abused substances, can lead to acquired immunodeficiency syndrome, hepatitis, and septicemia. Heroin and other narcotics cross the placental barrier. A child born to a mother who is addicted to one or more of these substances also is addicted to the drug. Addiction in the newborn is extremely serious, and the mortality rate is high, despite early recognition and treatment.

Symptoms of Acute and Chronic Toxicity

Signs and symptoms of acute toxicity include respiratory depression (which may be severe), stupor to coma, hypotension, bradycardia, and cold, clammy skin. Pinpoint pupils may be seen when an opiate has been used. Chronic toxicity is evidenced by anorexia, weight loss, constipation, malnutrition, needle marks and scarring (tracks) along the path of arteries and veins, and, possibly, unkempt appearance.

Withdrawal symptoms usually begin 8 to 12 hours after the last dose and reach a maximum in 2 or 3 days. Symptoms of mild withdrawal include tearing eyes, runny nose, sneezing, yawning, gooseflesh, and sweating. As withdrawal continues, extreme agitation, nausea, vomiting, anxiety, irritability, restless activity, chills, fever, generalized body aches, tremors, muscle spasms, and elevated blood pressure and pulse rate occur.

Treatment and Rehabilitation

Withdrawal symptoms may be halted by the administration of methadone, which also is a narcotic. If methadone is not used, withdrawal symptoms—which are not life-threatening—are treated symptomatically.

Rehabilitation methods vary. One method is the administration of methadone over a prolonged period. After a variable time, the dose of methadone is slowly reduced until the patient no longer needs the drug. The symptoms experienced during slow withdrawal from methadone usually are less severe than those that occur with withdrawal from an opiate.

Patients who take methadone in doses that reduce or eliminate the craving for an opiate are able to carry on activities that require mental alertness and motor coordination. Lassitude, nausea, vomiting, dizziness, sweating, anorexia, and insomnia still may occur and last for weeks, but the most acute symptoms of withdrawal usually are avoided. Another drug used for opiate addiction is naltrexone (Trexan), which is a long-acting narcotic *antagonist*. This drug is not addicting. If patients return to opiate abuse while receiving naltrexone, they do not experience the desired effects. A patient must be opiate-free for at least 7 days before starting naltrexone therapy.

Psychotherapy is an important aspect of rehabilitation. It involves not only breaking the pattern of addiction to a narcotic, but also—even more difficult— treating the underlying personality disorder and dealing with the complex web of social problems that accompany the addiction.

PSYCHOTOMIMETIC (HALLUCINOGENIC) DRUGS

A psychotomimetic drug produces an acute change in the perception of reality. Included in this group are mescaline, LSD (lysergic acid diethylamide), DOM (2,5-dimethoxy-4-methylamphetamine; also called STP), psilocybin, phencyclidine (PCP, angel dust) and DMT (dimethyltryptamine).

Use of these agents causes visual hallucinations and mood changes. The results are inconsistent and differ from person to person—and even within the same person—when the drug is taken under varying circumstances. Psychotic episodes may occur during and after use, and may progress to periodic occurrences even when the drug is not being used. These events take place more frequently in those who have underlying emotional problems. Another problem that may occur for many years after use has been discontinued is flashbacks, which are more common with LSD use. Flashbacks are brief episodes of the original sensations experienced during use of the substance. The frequency of flashbacks is variable.

Although physical dependence on these drugs does not occur, a user can develop a psychological dependence. No physical withdrawal symptoms if abuse of the drug is discontinued.

Symptoms of Use

Symptoms of use vary widely and depend on the purity and amount used, the individual person, and the atmosphere in which the drug was taken. The desired effects are euphoria and vivid images, colors, and sounds. Sometimes undesirable sensations, such as panic, terror, severe depression, and frightening images and sounds, may be experienced. This effect is referred to as a *bad trip*. Phencyclidine use may result in a severe psychotic disorder (which may be permanent) as well as violent behavior.

Treatment and Rehabilitation

Treatment involves placing the patient in a quiet atmosphere and talking to him or her in a calm, reassuring manner (talking down). A mild sedative may be ordered if the patient is experiencing severe panic or is extremely restless and unmanageable.

Rehabilitation is aimed at redirecting the patient's thinking regarding the use of these substances. Psychotherapy may be necessary for some people, especially those who experience repeated psychotic episodes or flashbacks.

AMPHETAMINES

Amphetamines (or speed) are CNS stimulants. They increase a person's sense of alertness and wakefulness and alter mood. Misuse of amphetamines ranges from brief and relatively infrequent use of moderate amounts to postpone fatigue, to abuse by "speed freaks," who take massive doses, seeking extended periods of euphoria and wakefulness until they crash, that is, come down off a high. After using amphetamines to produce an unnatural wakefulness and alertness, a person often experiences a let-down characterized by physical and mental exhaustion.

Symptoms of Use and Toxicity

Amphetamine use is characterized by an increase in the pulse rate and blood pressure, wakefulness, nervousness or excitation, anorexia, dilatation of the pupils, and hyperactive reflexes. Large doses may produce extreme agitation, aggressiveness, severe hypertension, hostility, erratic behavior, convulsions, toxic psychosis (which may resemble paranoid schizophrenia), and death. Use by people with or without a history of hypertension could result in a cerebrovascular accident (stroke) or other serious consequences.

Authorities believe that amphetamine use results in physical dependence. Psychological dependence also can occur. Symptoms of withdrawal include lethargy, fatigue, depression, and muscle discomfort or pain. A toxic psychosis also may be present during the withdrawal period.

Treatment and Rehabilitation

Treatment depends on the seriousness of the symptoms. Respiratory and cardiovascular support may be necessary. Diazepam (Valium) may be given intravenously for sedation. An antihypertensive agent may be ordered for hypertension.

Rehabilitation of the physically dependent abuser usually involves individual or group psychotherapy and rapid or slow withdrawal of the drug. Although a person may have abused only amphetamines, it also is possible that other substances have been abused and that dependence on these substances has occurred.

MARIJUANA

Marijuana is derived from the *Cannabis sativa* plant, which grows in many areas of the world. The main active substance that gives the user various pleasurable effects is delta-9-tetrahydrocannabinol, which is concentrated in the leaves and flowering tops of the plant.

The leaves and flowering tops are dried and then loosely rolled in cigarette paper. The resin extracted from the plant's flowers is called *hashish*. It may be smoked in a pipe, eaten, or added to drinks or food and is 5 to 10 times as potent as marijuana smoked as a cigarette.

Two cannabinoids are used to treat nausea and vomiting associated with cancer chemotherapy when the patient has not responded to other forms of treatment. They are dronabinol (Marinol), the principle psychoactive substance of the *Cannabis sativa*, and nabilone, a synthetic cannabinoid. Marijuana also is being used on a limited basis in the treatment of glaucoma that does not respond to other approved methods of treatment.

Symptoms of Use

The effects of smoking marijuana are variable and usually described as pleasurable changes in mood, perception, and consciousness. Light-headedness, drowsiness, and a pleasant feeling, which may be accompanied by a heightened sensitivity to sounds, colors, and other elements in the environment, may be experienced. Impairment of coordination and motor reflexes may occur. People who use marijuana or hashish before or during the performance of tasks that require motor coordination and mental concentration (eg, driving a car or operating heavy machinery) increase the risk of accidental injury to themselves as well as others. Higher concentrations of tetrahydrocannabinol (the main active ingredient in marijuana) also may produce hallucinations and mind-altering effects similar to, although not as intense as, those experienced during the use of the hallucinogens. Other physical effects include tachycardia, decreased intraocular pressure, increased appetite, and reddening of the eyes.

Treatment and Rehabilitation

Treatment after use seldom is necessary unless some type of physical injury has occurred. Those who experience more intense effects, such as vivid images or personality changes, may need to be placed in a quiet room until the effects wear off. Rehabilitation must focus on the dangers of substance abuse.

BARBITURATES

Barbiturates such as pentobarbital (Nembutal), secobarbital (Seconal), and amobarbital (Amytal) are used most often to produce euphoria. At times, they are used along with, before, or after other abused substances such as alcohol, tranquilizers, or opiates, which increase the depressant effect of the barbiturate. Barbiturate use can result in both physical and psychological dependence.

Symptoms of Toxicity

The symptoms and degree of toxicity depend on the amount ingested and whether one or more other CNS depressants were taken with the barbiturate. Overdose (toxicity) can produce slurred speech, disorientation, and confusion. Large doses or use with another CNS depressant may result in respiratory depression, cyanosis, dilated pupils, rapid and weak pulse, hypotension, ataxia, change in the level of consciousness (sleepiness to comatose), and death. Withdrawal symptoms include weakness, insomnia, anxiety, mental confusion, tremors, nausea, vomiting, malaise, headache, and, possibly, hallucinations, delirium, and seizures.

Treatment and Rehabilitation

Treatment depends on the severity of the toxicity. Vital signs are monitored every 5 to 30 minutes. Mechanical ventilation or a tracheostomy may be necessary if respiratory depression is severe. An intravenous line is inserted immediately, since drugs to support the blood pressure or prevent seizures may be required. Mild toxicity may only necessitate observation of the patient and measures to prevent self-harm during periods of confusion or disorientation.

Many people who are dependent on barbiturates require psychiatric counseling. Withdrawal from the drug may be treated by substituting phenobarbital (also a barbiturate) for the original abused substance to decrease the severity of withdrawal symptoms. The dose is slowly tapered over a period of several weeks, and then the drug is discontinued. This treatment is best conducted in an inpatient setting where the administration of the drug can be controlled.

NONBARBITURATE SEDATIVES AND TRANQUILIZERS

Diazepam (Valium), chlordiazepoxide (Librium), ethchlorvynol (Placidyl), and glutethimide (Doriden) are examples of nonbarbiturate drugs that can be abused. These drugs can produce physical and psychological dependence.

Although a person may abuse only one of the drugs in this group, she or he may use the agent before, in conjunction with, or after another substance subject to abuse. Methaqualone, which has been withdrawn from the market, remains available as a popular underground drug, because only a basic knowledge of chemistry is needed to manufacture it.

Some people become dependent on these drugs when they are repeatedly prescribed for the treatment of anxiety or insomnia. Dependency can occur in as little as 2 months of daily use. Withdrawal symptoms resemble those of barbiturate withdrawal and can be severe. Withdrawal from diazepam can be especially severe.

Symptoms of Toxicity

Symptoms of overdose vary, according to the drug, the dose, and the length of use. Drowsiness to coma, confusion, slurred speech, memory impairment, ataxia, hypothermia, respiratory depression, dysrhythmias, convulsions, and hypotension may be seen.

Treatment and Rehabilitation

The immediate and serious symptoms, such as respiratory depression, dysrhythmias, convulsions, and severe hypotension, are treated first. Mechanical ventilation may be necessary if respiratory depression is severe. Anticonvulsant and antiarrhythmic drugs, and agents to support the blood pressure may be necessary.

For those with physical dependence, rehabilitation involves withdrawal from the drug. The dose may be tapered over time; this is best done in an inpatient setting, wherein administration of the drug can be controlled.

VOLATILE HYDROCARBONS

Benzene, acetone, carbon tetrachloride, trichlorethane, and toluene are examples of volatile hydrocarbons that can be found in many household products, such as nail polish remover, cleaning fluids, glue, and some types of paint. Because they are inexpensive and legal, these substances are more commonly abused by young people. To obtain the desired effects, the substance usually is placed in a handkerchief or plastic bag and inhaled, or it is inhaled directly from the container. The effects include excitation, light-headedness, exhilaration, and, occasionally, hallucinations. These effects are short-lived (about 30 minutes or less), which may prompt the user to repeat its use in a short period of time. Although physical dependence apparently does not occur, psychological dependence may be seen with repeated use.

Symptoms of Toxicity

Overdose can produce dysrhythmias, hypotension, delirium to coma, and respiratory depression. Prolonged use can damage the lungs, heart, and liver.

Treatment and Rehabilitation

Treatment may require respiratory support by means of mechanical ventilation and drug therapy for dysrhythmias and hypotension. Rehabilitation must focus on the serious consequences associated with the use of these substances.

NICOTINE

Nicotine is an alkaloid found in the tobacco of cigarettes and cigars and in loose tobacco for chewing and pipe-smoking. The undesirable effects of smoking constitute a real health hazard to a large segment of the population who are heavy smokers and to those non-smokers who passively inhale tobacco smoke. Consequently, the problem of tobacco habituation and dependence is a rightful concern for all health care professionals.

An increased risk of developing lung cancer is related to the number of cigarettes smoked per day and the duration of smoking. Pipe and cigar smokers, who usually do not inhale, develop cancer of the lung more frequently than do nonsmokers, but less frequently than do cigarette smokers. Pipe smokers are especially prone to oral cancer, as are those who chew tobacco.

Nicotine causes breathlessness, both at rest and on exertion, decreased pulmonary function, and a chronic productive cough. Paralysis of the cilia caused by smoking prevents the clearing away of foreign particles, such as those found in tobacco smoke, which are then deposited on the epithelium. In addition, the abnormality seen in chronic bronchitis can be caused by smoking. Smoking has been identified as a cause of emphysema, and the death rate from emphysema, like that from bronchitis, is higher in the smoker than in the nonsmoker. The symptoms of bronchitis and emphysema tend to be progressive, especially in smokers, and may result in respiratory crippling to the extent that these people are unable to work or even walk because they cannot breathe adequately.

When these smokers stop smoking, they may experience such symptoms as constipation, irritability, slowing of the pulse, hunger, weight gain, and a craving for tobacco. The craving may disappear after a few days or months, or it may persist for years.

The nurse may be asked to give suggestions on how to stop smoking. No method helps all people, but anti-smoking clinics and hypnosis have helped some. Others find serious reasons for stopping and do so themselves by either quitting suddenly or slowly decreasing the number of cigarettes smoked per day.

NURSING PROCESS —THE SUBSTANCE ABUSE PATIENT

Assessment

The substance abuse patient may be seen in the emergency department or the general hospital setting. Chart 11-1 lists areas that may be covered dur-

---

Chart 11–1.   Assessment of the Patient Suspected of or Diagnosed as a Substance Abuser

General Appearance
- ☐ Clean, neat, dirty, disheveled

Speech Pattern
- ☐ Normal, rapid, slurred, incoherent

Neuromuscular
- ☐ No symptoms, tremors, depressed tendon reflexes, motor incoordination

Eyes
- ☐ *Pupils:* Normal, dilated, pinpoint, reaction to light (normal, slow, fixed)
- ☐ *Nystagmus:* Absent, present
- ☐ *Vision:* Normal, blurred

Nose
- ☐ Normal, evidence of ulceration of nasal membranes, perforation of nasal septum, excessive secretions

Skin
- ☐ *Integrity:* Normal, evidence of bruising, cuts, abrasions, needle marks, scars, sores, signs of infection
- ☐ *Color:* Normal, pale, cyanotic, flushed
- ☐ *Appearance:* Normal, dry, moist, perspiring (heavy, mild)

Respirations
- ☐ Normal, rapid, shallow, depressed

Pulse
- ☐ Rate, rhythm (describe abnormalities)

Blood Pressure
- ☐ Within normal limits, hypotensive, hypertensive

Temperature
- ☐ Normal, elevated, below normal

Sensorium
- ☐ Clear, clouded, disoriented, apparent hallucinations (if possible, describe as visual, auditory, or both)

Memory
- ☐ Evidence of memory loss

General Behavior
- ☐ Passive, aggressive, agitated, hyperactive, euphoric, combative, uncooperative

Level of Consciousness
- ☐ Awake, stuporous, semicomatose, comatose

Breath
- ☐ Odor (describe)

---

ing a physical assessment. In addition, a history is taken that includes all the symptoms the patient has experienced or that have been observed by others. When possible, a history of substance use (type, frequency, and amount) is obtained. Laboratory studies may be performed to validate the type of substance used and to detect the presence of other medical problems, such as dehydration and electrolyte imbalance.

Nursing Diagnosis
Depending on such factors as the substance that is being abused and the patient's symptoms, one or more of the following may apply:

- Ineffective airway clearance related to the inability to cough
- Anxiety related to loss of control
- Sensory/perceptual alterations related to confusion, memory impairment, withdrawal, impaired judgment
- Altered nutrition: less than body requirements related to anorexia
- Potential for injury to self or others related to disorientation, impaired judgment, tremors
- Fluid volume deficit related to nausea, vomiting, diarrhea, anorexia, mental impairment
- Potential for violence related to disorientation, hallucinations, impaired judgment, impulsive behavior
- Sleep pattern disturbance related to anxiety, insomnia, irritability
- Self-esteem disturbance related to guilt, mistrust
- Ineffective individual coping related to substance dependence, loss of family support
- Knowledge deficit of the dangers of substance abuse, treatment and rehabilitation programs, other factors (specify)

Planning and Implementation
The major goals of the patient include a relief of symptoms associated with drug use or withdrawal and a desire to enter a rehabilitation program.

The major goals of nursing management depend on the assessment and nursing diagnoses as well as the treatments prescribed by the physician. Some nursing goals may be unrealistic because not all patients can be cured of substance dependence. The reasons for abuse may be many, and some may never be detected, despite intensive therapy.

After assessment, the most serious symptoms, such as respiratory depression, hypotension, and dysrhythmias, are treated first. Laboratory studies may be ordered to detect the substance (or substances) taken by the patient, but not all abused substances can be detected by these methods.

Less serious problems are attended to after the patient is stabilized and vital signs are normal. Intake and output and vital signs are closely monitored until the effects of the abused substance are diminished. The patient history may reveal the substance abused, the amount, and the frequency of use.

If a decision is made to institute detoxification, the patient and his or her family must be informed of the necessary steps to be taken and where they will be accomplished. Some patients may be admitted to special hospitals or other facilities that specialize in detoxification. When withdrawal occurs, the patient is treated symptomatically, but sedatives or other types of drug therapy and treatment modalities may be prescribed.

Ineffective Airway Clearance. Blood pressure and pulse rate are monitored at the prescribed intervals, and the respiratory status is evaluated frequently, especially if the abused substance depresses the CNS. Any change in the vital signs is reported to the physician immediately.

Anxiety, Disturbance in Self-Esteem, Ineffective Individual Coping. Anxiety and panic may be seen as a effect of the abused substance, but they also may be seen in patients who are oriented to their surroundings, but fear they have lost control of their lives.

Depending on their mental and physical condition, these patients need to talk about their drug problem. Some feel guilty, whereas others find it difficult to trust family members or medical personnel. Some patients have trouble coping with their drug problem or loss of family support.

Group therapy often helps to relieve tension and provides an opportunity for members to ventilate their feelings. This type of therapy also may help the abusers to share their problems with others and to gain insight into why they have developed a substance abuse problem.

Sensory/Perceptual Alterations, Potential for Injury and Violence. These patients require frequent assessment of their mental status. If they are disoriented, exhibit erratic behavior, or appear to be in danger of harming themselves or others, steps need to be taken to protect the patient as well as those caring for him.

Altered Nutrition, Fluid Volume Deficit. Many patients with a long history of substance abuse suffer from various stages of malnourishment. Patients are encouraged to eat and often are allowed to select a diet that includes their food preferences. These patients should be weighed weekly. Failure to gain or maintain their weight is brought to the attention of the physician.

If nausea, vomiting, diarrhea, or anorexia occurs, the patient may develop a fluid volume deficit. Intake and output is measured, and the patient is encouraged to drink extra fluids.

Sleep Pattern Disturbance. Many substance abuse patients find it difficult to sleep. A tranquilizer may be ordered if the patient is extremely irritable or has not slept for several days.

Knowledge Deficit. Rehabilitation is aimed at getting the patient to acknowledge his dependence and accept treatment.

There are many types of rehabilitation programs. The method chosen depends on the individual patient and the substance abused.

Although patients may be aware of the dangers associated with substance abuse, these facts should be repeated during the recovery phase. Allowing these patients time to discuss all matters related to their substance abuse problem and helping them through recovery offer them the opportunity to learn about themselves and possibly stay free of drugs.

Evaluation

- Vital signs are stable
- Symptoms of toxicity are controlled
- Respiratory function is adequate
- Fluid volume deficit (if present) is corrected
- Harm to self and others is prevented or controlled
- Patient is mentally clear
- Patient demonstrates a beginning ability and desire to cope with problems associated with or caused by substance abuse
- Patient understands potential or actual mental, physical, and social problems that accompany substance abuse
- Patient accepts fact of substance dependence and shows willingness to obtain treatment
- Patient refrains from substance abuse

General Nutritional Considerations

☐ The substance abuse patient may have a vitamin and nutritional deficiency. A well-balanced diet usually is ordered.

☐ The nurse should encourage the patient to eat. Small, frequent feedings may be better tolerated than three regular meals.

☐ Patients who are going through medically supervised drug withdrawal may require dietary supplements and between-meal feedings.

☐ The meal trays of alcoholic or drug-dependent patients should be checked after each meal, as these patients tend to eat poorly. Any evidence of reduced dietary intake should be reported to the physician.

General Pharmacologic Considerations

☐ It is essential that alcoholic patients receive vitamin therapy.

☐ Paraldehyde, which may be used as sedation during periods of acute alcohol withdrawal, may be given orally (undiluted or diluted in juice) or by the intramuscular route.

☐ Because of postural hypotension, alcoholics who are receiving phenothiazine-type drugs (eg, chlorpromazine [Thorazine]) should be warned against rising rapidly from a lying or sitting position.

☐ Disulfiram (Antabuse) may be given to alcoholics as part of their rehabilitation program. These patients should be fully informed of the symptoms (eg, severe nausea, vomiting, and diarrhea) they will experience if they drink alcohol while taking the drug.

☐ Phenothiazine-type tranquilizers must be administered cautiously because they potentiate the depressant and hypotensive effects of alcohol.

☐ Patients who are receiving tranquilizers or barbiturates should be warned against using alcohol while taking these drugs. The combination of alcohol and tranquilizers or barbiturates can be hazardous and could lead to coma and death.

☐ Patients who are receiving methadone as part of a rehabilitation program should have this noted on the front of their charts and on the patient Kardex. Because it is a narcotic, methadone can potentiate the action of certain drugs, most notably narcotics, tranquilizers, barbiturates, and anesthetics.

☐ Patients who are receiving methadone usually require lower doses of such drugs as tranquilizers and barbiturates when it is necessary to administer these agents.

☐ Naltrexone is a narcotic antagonist used for maintenance of an opioid-free state in those formerly dependent on opioids. Hospitalized patients who are receiving this drug must not be given opioids for analgesia.

General Gerontologic Considerations

☐ Drug abuse and drug dependence are not restricted to young and middle-aged people; it also can be found in the elderly.

☐ Some drugs that are used to sedate or make elderly patients more manageable in the home, hospital, or nursing home setting may cause drug dependence.

☐ In older patients, self-administration of narcotics, tranquilizers, and barbiturates may not be reliable because they may fail to read or understand the directions for taking the medication or the substances to avoid while taking these drugs.

Suggested Readings

☐ Acee AM, Smith D. Crack. Am J Nurs May 1987;87:614. *(Additional coverage of subject matter)*

☐ Adams FE. Drug dependency in hospital patients. Am J Nurs April 1988;88:477. *(Additional coverage of subject matter)*

☐ Barry PD. Mental health and mental illness. 4th ed. Philadelphia: JB Lippincott, 1990. *(In-depth coverage of subject matter)*

☐ Birckhead LM. Psychiatric mental health nursing: the therapeutic use of self. Philadelphia: JB Lippincott, 1989. *(In-depth coverage of subject matter)*

☐ Cooper KL. Drug overdose. Am J Nurs September 1989;89:1146. *(Additional coverage of subject matter)*

☐ Estes NJ, Heineman ME. Alcoholism: development, consequences and interventions. 3rd ed. St Louis: CV Mosby, 1986. *(Additional coverage of subject matter)*

☐ Goodman L. Would your assessment spot a hidden alcoholic? RN August 1988;51:56. *(Additional coverage of subject matter)*

☐ Johnson BS. Psychiatric mental health nursing: adaption and growth. 2nd ed. Philadelphia: JB Lippincott, 1989. *(Additional coverage of subject matter)*

☐ McCaffery M. When your patient is a drug abuser. Nursing '88 November 1988;18:49. *(Additional coverage of subject matter)*

☐ Powell AH, Minick MP. Alcohol withdrawal syndrome. Am J Nurs March 1988;88:312. *(Additional coverage of subject matter)*

☐ Rich J. Action stat! Acute alcohol intoxication. Nursing '89 September 1989;19:33. *(Additional coverage of subject matter)*

☐ Vandegaer F. Cocaine: the deadliest addition. Nursing '89 February 1989;19:72. *(Additional coverage of subject matter)*

Chapter 12

Water, Acid–Base, and Electrolyte Imbalances

On completion of this chapter the reader will:

- Describe the basic principles of water and electrolyte regulation

- List and discuss the causes of fluid volume deficit and excess

- Describe the diagnosis and treatment of fluid volume deficit and excess

- Use the nursing process in the management of the patient with a fluid volume deficit or excess

- List the four types of acid–base imbalances and give some of the causes of each imbalance

- Describe the diagnosis and treatment of each type of acid–base imbalance

- Use the nursing process in the management of the patient with an acid–base imbalance

- List and discuss the principal roles of sodium, potassium, calcium, and magnesium

- List the symptoms of electrolyte deficit and excess

- Describe the diagnosis and treatment of electrolyte deficit and excess

- Use the nursing process in the management of those with an electrolyte imbalance

About 60% of the adult human body is water; of an adult who weighs 125 lb, about 75 lb is water. Body water is kept within cells (*cellular* or *intracellular*), between cells (*interstitial*), and in the bloodstream (*intravascular*). The interstitial and intravascular spaces are called, somewhat misleadingly, the *extracellular* (outside the cells) *compartment*.

Each of the countless number of cells that make up skin, muscle, or tissue is a tiny pond of fluid held together by the cellular membrane. Around these cells is the bath of interstitial fluid. Within each cell, there is constant chemical activity, as well as constant interchange with the interstitial fluid.

Fluid Volume Imbalances

Most cell membranes are permeable to water, and the total exchange is enormous. The net exchange of water is governed by changes in osmotic pressure. *Osmotic pressure* (power to draw water) is exerted by concentrated solutions on one side of a semipermeable membrane that draw water from dilute solutions on the other side. Osmosis takes place whenever a concentration gradient exists across a semipermeable membrane. If the concentration is higher within the cell, water is drawn through the membrane into the cell from the interstitial space until the concentration of particles in the fluid is the same on both sides of the membrane. If the concentration is higher in the interstitial space, water is pulled from the cell. By means of osmosis, the system tends to achieve a situation of uniform osmotic pressure (Fig. 12-1).

A healthy person normally consumes more water and electrolytes than are needed. Water is in everything that is eaten, and is formed within the body during metabolic processes. Fluid requirements vary, depending on the size, activity, and conditions in the external environment that affect fluid loss (eg, temperature). Normal daily fluid requirements for an adult range from 1.5 to 3 L.

Water and electrolytes normally leave the body by way of the skin, lungs, kidneys, and bowel. *Insensible fluid loss* is that which is lost through the skin and the lungs; it can be measured only with special equipment. Perspiring is the primary cause of insensible loss, but water also is exhaled from the lungs as vapor. The largest amount of fluid is excreted by the kidneys, and a relatively small amount is lost in feces. The tubules of the kidneys select and return to the general circulation electrolytes needed by the body. Those ions not needed by the body are excreted in the urine.

The kidneys remove about 180 L of fluid from the bloodstream each day. All but about 1 to 1.5 L is reabsorbed into the blood and passes into the renal pelvis

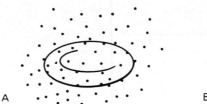
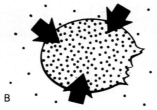
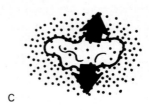

Figure 12–1. Concentration of particles in cells in relation to surrounding fluid. (*A*) Isosmotic: the number of particles within the cell and in the fluid surrounding the cell are about equal. Water passes across the cell wall in both directions. (*B*) Hypo-osmotic: the number of particles in the fluid outside the cell is less than the number inside the cell. Water flows into the cell until the concentration is equal on both sides of the wall, or until the cell bursts. (*C*) Hyperosmotic: the number of particles in the fluid outside the cell is greater than the number inside the cell. The cell becomes dehydrated as the water leaves it.

[handwritten annotation: urine ^very concentrated = ↑HIGH Specific Gravity]
[handwritten annotation: urine not concentrated = Low Specific Gravity]
[handwritten annotation: ↑spec. grav.]
[handwritten annotation: ↑Hct]

in the form of urine. The kidney also makes a continuous adjustment in ion selection according to the needs of cells. Thus, if salt intake increases and there is an excess of sodium and chloride ions in the body, the healthy kidney adjusts by excreting these excess ions.

The urine output for a healthy adult is less than 2 L/day, and total fluid output ranges from 1.85 to 3.6 L/day. To keep the body in good condition, the amount of fluid lost each day should be balanced by the amount taken in.

The normal functioning of the body depends on the maintenance of constant conditions within the body's internal environment. Body fluids carry nutrients and oxygen to and remove waste products from the cells. If an imbalance occurs, severe symptoms, damage to tissues, and even death may result.

Fluid Volume Deficit *= hypovolemia*

A deficit or decrease in the body's fluid volume is called *fluid volume deficit* (FVD), or *hypovolemia.* Some of the causes of FVD are decreased intake of water and electrolytes; a loss of water and electrolytes, as may be seen in severe diarrhea and vomiting, brisk and rapid diuresis without adequate replacement of water and electrolytes, and prolonged gastrointestinal suction; bowel obstruction; severe burns; and crush injuries.

[handwritten: FVD and causes]

Symptoms

Symptoms vary according to the severity of the deficit and include dry mucous membranes, slow filling of hand veins, decreased urine output, concentrated urine, weak and rapid pulse, orthostatic hypotension, decreased body temperature, central venous pressure below 4 cm of H_2O, and cool to cold extremities. In the later stages of FVD, stupor or coma, hypotension, and marked oliguria are common.

[handwritten: know some]

Diagnosis

Diagnosis is made by the patient's symptoms as well as by results of laboratory tests such as hematocrit, blood urea nitrogen level, serum creatinine and electrolyte levels, and urinalysis. The hematocrit usually is increased, and the blood urea nitrogen level may be elevated out of proportion to the serum creatinine level. The urine may have a high specific gravity and appear concentrated. Serum electrolyte levels may be increased or decreased. An increased serum sodium level often accompanies FVD.

Treatment

[handwritten: if mild - oral fluids]

Treatment of FVD depends on the severity of the disorder. In mild FVD, oral fluids that provide water and electrolytes may be given. In severe cases, intravenous administration of an isotonic electrolyte solution, such as lactated Ringer's solution or isotonic saline solution, may be ordered.

[handwritten: if severe - IV fluids]

NURSING PROCESS —THE PATIENT WHO HAS A FLUID VOLUME DEFICIT

Assessment

[handwritten: assess pt.]

A history (eg, prolonged episodes of diarrhea or prolonged gastrointestinal suction) may determine the cause of the FVD. Complete medical, drug, and allergy histories should be obtained.

Skin turgor and elasticity is tested by gently pinching and then releasing the skin over the back of the hand, sternum, forehead, or inner thigh. The skin normally returns quickly to its previous position, but in the patient with FVD, the skin returns more slowly. Because elasticity of the skin decreases with age, this test may not be reliable in the elderly. The oral

[handwritten: Test turgor, oral membranes, capillary refill, P. P. other pulses]

membranes should be inspected for evidence of dryness.

Nursing Diagnosis

Depending on the degree of FVD, one or more of the following nursing diagnoses may apply:

- Fluid volume deficit. If the cause is known, it may be stated as part of the diagnosis (eg, fluid volume deficit related to blood loss).
- Altered thought processes related to fluid volume deficit and possibly electrolyte imbalances

Planning and Implementation

The major goals of the patient are to attain and maintain a normal fluid volume.

The major goals of nursing management are to correct the FVD, closely monitor the patient for changes (improvement or deterioration), and protect the patient from injury if she or he should become confused and restless.

Fluid Volume Deficit. Oral fluids should be given if the FVD is mild to moderate and the patient is able to swallow. Oral fluids that contain electrolytes also may be ordered. Severe FVD usually requires intravenous fluid replacement. If the oral membranes are dry and cracked, frequent oral care is necessary.

Vital signs should be monitored every 2 to 4 hours, and the patient observed for a rise in pulse rate, an increase or a decrease in body temperature, and signs of postural hypotension. The patient should be weighed daily, or as ordered, and continually observed for a decline in the symptoms associated with FVD. Skin turgor and oral mucous membranes should be assessed two or three times a day.

Intake and output should be closely monitored (Chart 12-1), and the physician notified if the patient is unable to consume an adequate amount of fluid or if urine output decreases despite increased oral intake or infusion of intravenous fluids. The specific gravity of the urine should be checked every 4 hours. Concentrated urine may have a specific gravity of 1.025 or above.

Altered Thought Processes. Because severe FVD may result in mental changes, the patient should be observed for confusion and restlessness. If intravenous solutions are being administered, the insertion site should be checked at frequent intervals to make sure the needle has not been displaced. Needle displacement may cause extravasation (escape of fluid from a blood vessel into surrounding tissues while the needle or catheter is in the vein) or infiltration (collection of fluid in tissues—usually subcutaneous

tissue—when the needle or catheter is out of the vein).

Evaluation

- Fluid volume deficit is corrected
- Urine output is increased, and urine is of normal amount, color, and specific gravity
- Vital signs are normal
- Symptoms of FVD are absent; skin turgor returns to normal; oral mucous membranes assume a normal appearance
- Is alert and oriented
- Normal fluid intake is resumed
- Able to perform activities of daily living

Fluid Volume Excess

An excess or increase in the body's fluid volume is called fluid volume excess (FVE), or *hypervolemia*. Some of the causes of FVE are renal failure, congestive heart failure, excessive intake of salt (sodium chloride), corticosteroid therapy (usually in high doses), Cushing's syndrome, cirrhosis, excessive oral intake or parenteral administration of large amounts of water over a short period of time, and rapid administration of parenteral fluids that contain sodium. FVE also may be seen in those with normal or increased fluid intake and decreased renal function.

Symptoms

Symptoms include peripheral edema, rapid weight gain, full bounding pulse, central venous pressure above 11 cmH2O, distended neck veins, moist crackles in the lungs, polyuria and dilute urine (if renal func-

Chart 12–1. Intake and Output: Important Points to Remember

- Intake includes all fluids plus those foods that are liquid at room temperature (gelatin, ice cream, ice chips).
- Output includes urine as well as vomitus, diarrhea, drainage, and blood.
- A physician's order is not needed for measurement of intake and output.
- Remind the ambulatory patient that all urine must be measured; therefore, a urinal or bedpan must be used, and the urine is not to be discarded until it is measured.
- The intake and output record should include the amount and the time of day fluid is taken in or excreted.
- The intake and output record is checked and totaled at the end of each shift.

tion is normal), and slow emptying of the hand veins. In severe FVE, ascites and pulmonary edema may occur.

Diagnosis

Diagnosis is made by the patient's history and symptoms as well as by the results of laboratory tests, which may include measurement of serum electrolyte levels, and urinalysis. Serum electrolyte levels may be abnormal. The specific gravity of the urine may be decreased (if renal and cardiac function are normal) and the color pale to almost colorless. Other laboratory or diagnostic tests relating to the possible cause of FVE (eg, cirrhosis or congestive heart failure) may be ordered.

Treatment

Treatment depends on the severity of the disorder. In mild FVE, fluid intake (oral or parenteral) should be limited until the condition is corrected. Diuretics also may be administered for moderate to severe FVE. If pulmonary edema occurs, additional treatment modalities (eg, cardiac glycosides, oxygen, and diuretics) are required.

NURSING PROCESS —THE PATIENT WHO HAS A FLUID VOLUME EXCESS

Assessment

A history may determine the cause of FVE. Complete medical, drug, and allergy histories should be obtained. The extremities should be examined for edema. In patients who are confined to bed rest, the sacral area also should be examined for edema. The neck veins, which normally are not prominent when the patient is in a sitting position, should be observed for distention. The lungs should be auscultated for crackles, and the general appearance of the skin noted.

Nursing Diagnosis

Depending on the degree of FVE, one or more of the following nursing diagnoses may apply:

- Fluid volume excess. If the cause is known, it may be stated as part of the diagnosis (eg, fluid volume excess related to overhydration).
- Impaired tissue integrity related to edema
- Ineffective breathing pattern related to hyperventilation secondary to pulmonary crackles or pulmonary edema (specify)

Planning and Implementation

The major goal of the patient is to cooperate with the treatment regimen necessary to correct FVE.

The major goals of nursing management are to correct the FVE and closely monitor the patient for changes (improvement or deterioration). Depending on the cause and severity of FVE and other coexisting pathologic conditions, treatment may include sodium restriction, diuretics, administration of oxygen and elevation of the head of the bed if breathing becomes labored, and elevation of the extremities when the patient is out of bed, to reduce edema. Vital signs should be monitored every 1 to 4 hours, depending on the severity of the FVE.

Fluid Volume Excess. If oral fluids are restricted, they should be offered at evenly spaced intervals throughout the waking hours. The patient should be weighed daily or as ordered. The physician should be notified of any significant increase in weight.

Intake and output should be *closely* monitored (see Chart 12-1), and the physician notified if there is a significant change in urine output.

Impaired Tissue Integrity. The patient's position should be changed every 2 hours, and pressure points checked for signs of skin breakdown, as edematous tissue is fragile and subject to decubitus formation.

Ineffective Breathing Pattern. Respiratory rate and pattern should be monitored, and the lungs auscultated for crackles. If dyspnea or orthopnea occurs or is originally present and worsens, or if cyanosis is noted, the physician should be notified immediately.

Evaluation

- Fluid volume excess is corrected
- Urine output is normal
- Vital signs are normal
- Edema is corrected and skin turgor returns to normal
- Breath sounds are normal, and there is no evidence of dyspnea, orthopnea, cyanosis, or distended neck veins

Acid–Base Imbalances

The normal composition of body fluids depends on the concentration of acids, alkalies, and electrolytes. A ratio of 20 parts bicarbonate to 1 part carbonic acid is necessary to maintain a normal plasma pH of 7.34 to 7.45, or a slightly alkaline state. The symbol pH refers to the amount of hydrogen ions in a solution. The more hydrogen ions in a solution, the more acid it is. The body adjusts the hydrogen ion concentration by two mechanisms: one is a chemical mechanism and the other, an organ mechanism.

The *chemical mechanism* involves the use of chemical buffers that either add or subtract hydrogen ions. Because the pH depends on the amount of hydrogen ions in a solution, adding hydrogen ions makes a solution more acid and removing hydrogen ions makes a solution more alkaline. The major chemical buffers of the body are carbonic acid (H_2CO_3) and bicarbonate (HCO_3). These substances constitute the bicarbonate–carbonic buffer system.

The *organ mechanism* primarily consists of the lungs and kidneys. The lungs, by releasing carbon dioxide (which, when dissolved in water, becomes carbonic acid) in expired air, affect the carbonic acid concentration in extracellular fluid. Rapid respirations increase the amount of carbon dioxide released in expired air over a given period and, therefore, decrease the amount of carbonic acid in extracellular fluid. A decrease in the respiratory rate or volume, or both, reduces the amount of carbon dioxide released in expired air over a given period and, therefore, increases carbonic acid concentration in extracellular fluid. The kidneys, by retaining or excreting hydrogen and bicarbonate ions, help to restore balance when acidosis or alkalosis occurs.

There are four types of acid–base imbalance: *metabolic acidosis, metabolic alkalosis, respiratory acidosis,* and *respiratory alkalosis.*

Metabolic Acidosis *loss bicarbonate or gain in acid (not carbonic)*

Metabolic acidosis is a bicarbonate deficit that may occur when there is a loss of bicarbonate or a gain in an acid other than carbonic acid. Conditions that may result in metabolic acidosis include diarrhea, lactic acidosis, uremia (uremic acidosis), insulin deficiency resulting in diabetic ketoacidosis, shock, and starvation. The anion gap (or R factor) is a laboratory test used to determine the type of metabolic acidosis. The normal anion gap is ±12 mEq/L, and is a determination of the difference between sodium and potassium ion concentrations and the sum of chloride and bicarbonate anions, with the difference reflecting the concentration of anions in extracellular fluid.

Metabolic acidosis may be classified as either *normal anion gap acidosis* or *high* (increased) *anion gap acidosis.*

1. *Normal anion gap acidosis* results from a loss of bicarbonate, such as may be seen in severe diarrhea, ileostomy, intestinal or biliary fistula, ureterosigmoidostomy, renal tubular acidosis, intestinal suction, and increased chloride levels.

2. *High anion gap acidosis* results from excessive production of metabolic acids (other than carbonic acid), such as lactic acid or ketones, or from a decreased loss of metabolic acids. Causes of high anion gap acidosis owing to excessive production of metabolic acids include salicylate poisoning, lactic acidosis, diabetic ketoacidosis, alcoholism (alcoholic ketoacidosis), and fasting or starvation states. High anion gap acidosis owing to a decreased loss of metabolic acids may be seen in renal failure.

Symptoms

Symptoms include anorexia, nausea, vomiting, headache, confusion, flushing, lethargy, malaise, drowsiness, abdominal pain or discomfort, and weakness. Severe metabolic acidosis may result in stupor, coma, and death because of the depression of vital functions.

Diagnosis

Diagnosis is made by measuring arterial blood gases, which show a decrease in pH, plasma bicarbonate, and $Paco_2$. Diagnosis also is based on the patient's symptoms.

Treatment

Treatment includes elimination of the cause and replacement of fluids and electrolytes that may have been lost. Bicarbonate also may be administered.

Metabolic Alkalosis   *↑ in base bicarbonate*

Metabolic alkalosis is an increase in base bicarbonate. Base bicarbonate may be increased when there is an excessive oral or parenteral use of bicarbonate-containing drugs or other alkaline salts, or a rapid decrease in extracellular fluid volume (eg, in diuretic therapy). Base bicarbonate also may be increased when there is a loss of hydrogen and chloride ions (eg, in vomiting, prolonged gastric suctioning, hypokalemia, or hyperaldosteronism). The loss of hydrogen and chloride ions results in retention of sodium bicarbonate and an increase in base bicarbonate.

Symptoms

Symptoms include anorexia, nausea, vomiting, circumoral paresthesias, confusion, carpopedal spasm, hypertonic reflexes, tetany, and a decreased respiratory rate.

Diagnosis

Diagnosis is made by laboratory test results. Arterial blood gas studies show an increase in pH, plasma bicarbonate, and $Paco_2$. Serum bicarbonate levels and, possibly, urine pH are increased. Serum potassium and, possibly, serum chloride levels are decreased. Diagnosis also is based on the patient's symptoms.

Treatment

Treatment includes elimination of the cause. Potassium (as a potassium salt) may be given if hypokalemia (potassium deficiency) is present. Sodium chloride may be given to correct volume depletion when there has been a rapid decrease in extracellular fluid volume.

NURSING PROCESS —THE PATIENT WHO HAS METABOLIC ACIDOSIS OR ALKALOSIS

Assessment

Once the diagnosis of metabolic acidosis or alkalosis has been confirmed, the nurse must carefully document all presenting symptoms to provide accurate baseline data. Evaluation of the patient's mental status as well as documentation of any neurologic symptoms (metabolic alkalosis) also is necessary. If gastrointestinal symptoms (nausea and vomiting) are present, the amount of fluid loss must be determined. The patient with an acid–base imbalance also may have an electrolyte imbalance, and this must be considered during assessment.

Complete medical, drug, and allergy histories are obtained. Vital signs are taken, and the patient is weighed.

Nursing Diagnosis

Depending on the degree of metabolic acid–base imbalance, one or more of the following nursing diagnoses may apply:

- Anxiety related to discomfort, respiratory distress, nausea, vomiting
- Fluid volume deficit related to nausea and vomiting
- Altered nutrition: less than body requirements owing to nausea, confusion, or other symptoms of the imbalance
- Sensory/perceptual alterations related to metabolic acid–base imbalance

Planning and Implementation

The major goals of the patient are to attain and maintain normal metabolic acid–base balance.

The major goal of nursing management is the correction of metabolic acidosis or alkalosis. It is accomplished by accurate observation of the patient's symptoms and response to therapy, as well as administration of prescribed treatments.

Bicarbonate may be administered to a patient with metabolic acidosis. Sodium chloride may be ordered for the patient with metabolic alkalosis to aid in the restoration of fluid volume as well as to enhance the excretion of the excess bicarbonate. Vital signs are monitored every 4 hours or as ordered. The physician may order daily to weekly weight measurement.

Anxiety. Anxiety and confusion may be reduced by frequent patient contact and reassurance.

Fluid Volume Deficit, Altered Nutrition. Intake and output and vital signs should be closely monitored, and significant changes reported to the physician. If the patient has been vomiting, oral fluids should be offered at frequent intervals. Interval feedings of soft, bland foods also may be necessary.

Sensory/Perceptual Alterations. If confusion occurs, the patient must be observed at frequent intervals. In some instances, restraints are necessary. If the patient is acutely ill, is confused, or has neurologic symptoms, she or he requires assistance with activities of daily living.

Evaluation

- acid–base imbalance is corrected
- Anxiety is reduced as much as possible
- Normal fluid balance is attained and maintained
- Nutritional deficits are corrected
- Vital signs remain stable

Respiratory Acidosis

Respiratory acidosis, which may be either acute or chronic, is caused by carbonic acid excess. Acute respiratory acidosis may be caused by pneumothorax or hemothorax, pulmonary edema, acute bronchial asthma, atelectasis, hyaline membrane disease or other forms of respiratory distress in the newborn, pneumonia, and some drug overdoses or head injuries when there is a decrease in the respiratory rate and volume. Chronic respiratory acidosis may be caused by chronic respiratory disorders such as emphysema, bronchiectasis, bronchial asthma, and cystic fibrosis.

Symptoms

Symptoms of acute respiratory acidosis include behavioral changes (mental cloudiness, confusion, disorientation, hallucinations), tremors, muscle twitching, flushed skin, headache, weakness, paralysis, stupor, and coma. Symptoms of chronic respiratory acidosis are less prominent, and include a dull headache and weakness.

Diagnosis

Arterial blood gas analysis shows a decrease in pH and an increase in the $Paco_2$ in acute respiratory acidosis, and a low normal or slightly below normal pH and an increase in the $Paco_2$ in chronic respiratory acidosis.

Treatment

Treatment is individualized, depending on the cause of the respiratory acidosis and whether the condition is acute or chronic. Measures include the administration of pharmacologic agents such as bronchodilators to patients with bronchial asthma or chronic emphysema, the administration of oxygen and antibiotics to those with pneumonia (the fluid intake is increased for those with chronic respiratory disorders to aid in the thinning and raising of secretions), and the use of mechanical ventilation. The administration of high concentrations of oxygen to patients with chronic respiratory disorders is contraindicated. These patients have adapted to increased levels of carbon dioxide (and thus carbonic acid), and high levels of oxygen further decrease the respiratory rate, which increases the respiratory acidosis.

Respiratory Alkalosis

Respiratory alkalosis is due to a carbonic acid deficit that occurs because excessive carbonic acid is blown off in expired air. The primary cause is hyperventilation. Some causes of hyperventilation are anxiety, high fever, thyrotoxicosis, early salicylate intoxication, hypoxemia, and mechanical ventilation.

Symptoms
Symptoms include light-headedness, numbness and tingling of the fingers and toes, circumoral paresthesias, sweating, panic, dry mouth, short periods of apnea, and, in severe cases, convulsions.

Diagnosis
Laboratory test results show a pH above 7.45; $Paco_2$ is below 35 mmHg, and the serum bicarbonate level usually is below 24 mEq/L.

Treatment
Treatment aims to correct the cause of hyperventilation. Sedation may be required if hyperventilation is caused by extreme anxiety. Having the patient rebreathe expired air from a paper bag that is held over the nose and mouth also may be useful.

NURSING PROCESS —THE PATIENT WHO HAS RESPIRATORY ACIDOSIS OR ALKALOSIS

Assessment
Once the diagnosis has been confirmed, the nurse must carefully document all presenting symptoms to provide accurate baseline data. Evaluation of the patient's status and documentation of any symptoms are necessary. The patient with an acid–base imbalance also may have an electrolyte imbalance, and this must be considered during assessment.

Complete medical, drug, and allergy histories should be obtained. Vital signs should be taken, and the patient weighed.

Nursing Diagnosis
Depending on the degree of respiratory acidosis or alkalosis, one or more of the following diagnoses may apply:

- Ineffective breathing pattern related to respiratory alkalosis
- Anxiety related to difficulty breathing
- Feeding and bathing/hygiene self-care deficit related to fatigue, behavioral changes, and other symptoms caused by the acid–base imbalance

Planning and Implementation
The major goals of the patient are to attain and maintain normal a normal acid–base balance.

The major goal of nursing management is correction of respiratory acidosis or alkalosis.

Planning is directed toward correcting the underlying cause, restoring a normal acid–base balance, and managing, when possible, the symptoms of the imbalance. This may be accomplished by improving ventilation (respiratory acidosis) or decreasing or eliminating episodes of hyperventilation (respiratory alkalosis). Planning includes administering prescribed treatments or drugs and closely monitoring vital signs and laboratory studies.

Intake and output, and vital signs should be closely monitored, especially if the acid–base imbalance is severe.

Anxiety. The patient with respiratory alkalosis caused by episodes of hyperventilation should be told about the effects of this breathing pattern. He or she should be instructed to concentrate on breathing and to take deep breaths. In some instances, a rebreathing device, such as a paper bag, is helpful.

Ineffective Breathing Pattern. The patient with respiratory acidosis may be placed in a high semi-Fowler's position to aid breathing. The airway must be kept patent. In some instances, tracheal suctioning is necessary. The patient must be frequently assessed for respiratory distress. Other treatment modalities depend on the cause of the imbalance, and include drugs such as bronchodilators and antibiotics.

Feeding and Bathing/Hygiene Self-Care Deficit. Patients who are acutely may require assistance with their activities of daily living. Between these activities, rest periods are provided to reduce demands on the respiratory system.

Evaluation

- Acid–base imbalance is corrected
- Normal breathing pattern is established
- Anxiety is reduced, and patient with respiratory alkalosis understands that anxiety may provoke episodes of hyperventilation
- Able to resume activities of daily living
- Vital signs remain stable

Electrolyte Imbalances

Electrolytes are in the water of both cellular and extracellular spaces. They include ions such as potassium, magnesium, sodium, phosphate, sulfate, calcium, chloride, bicarbonate, and protein, and organic acids such as carbonic acid and the amino acids. A striking difference exists between extracellular and cellular fluids in terms of the concentration of ions. The sodium, calcium, and chloride ion concentrations are many times higher in extracellular fluid than in cellular fluid. In contrast, potassium, magnesium, and phosphate concentrations are many times higher within the cell than outside the cell. These differences are responsible for electrical potentials that develop across the cell membrane and perhaps also for the degree of permeability of the membrane. An incorrect concentration of these ions on both sides of a membrane affects the transmission of impulses across nerve fibers. Deficits or excesses of sodium, calcium, and potassium are of particular concern.

SODIUM

The sodium cation (Na^+), the chief electrolyte found in extracellular fluid, is essential for the maintenance of normal nerve and muscle activity, the regulation of osmotic pressure in body cells, and the maintenance of acid–base balance. The principal role of sodium is the regulation and distribution of fluid volume in the body. Normal sodium concentration ranges from 135 to 145 mEq/L.

Sodium Deficit

Sodium deficit, or *hyponatremia,* may occur when there is profuse diaphoresis along with the ingestion of plain water, excessive administration of nonelectrolyte intravenous fluids, profuse diuresis, loss of gastrointestinal secretions (eg, in prolonged gastrointestinal suction or draining fistulas), or Addison's disease.

Symptoms

Symptoms include confusion, weakness, restlessness, elevated body temperature, tachycardia, muscle twitching, and abdominal cramping. If the deficit is severe, convulsions or coma may be seen.

Diagnosis

Diagnosis is based on the patient's symptoms and laboratory test results, primarily the serum sodium level that is less than 135 mEq/L. Other laboratory tests also may be done, as the patient may have more than one imbalance.

Treatment

Treatment includes administration of sodium by the oral route (foods high in sodium content, salt water, and salt tablets) if the deficit is mild, or by the intravenous route (using isotonic [0.9%] sodium chloride or lactated Ringer's solution) when the deficit is severe.

Sodium Excess

Sodium excess, or *hypernatremia,* may occur when there is an excessive intake of salt without ingestion of water or when excessive water is lost without an accompanying loss of sodium. Some of the causes of hypernatremia are profuse watery diarrhea, high fever, decreased water intake (eg, in elderly, debilitated, unconscious, or retarded patients), excessive administration of parenteral solutions that contain sodium, use of hypertonic saline solution to induce abortion, and severe burns.

Symptoms

Symptoms include thirst; dry, sticky mucous membranes; decreased urine output; fever; a rough, dry tongue; and lethargy, which may progress to coma if the excess is severe.

Diagnosis

Diagnosis is based on the patient's symptoms and laboratory test results, especially the serum sodium level, which is more than 145 mEq/L. Other laboratory tests also may be done, as the patient may have more than one imbalance.

Treatment

Treatment depends on the cause of the imbalance, and includes the administration of plain water orally or a hypotonic sodium solution (usually 0.3% sodium chloride). In mild cases of hypernatremia, restriction of sodium intake may be instituted until laboratory test results are normal.

NURSING PROCESS —THE PATIENT WHO HAS A SODIUM IMBALANCE

Assessment

Sodium deficit or excess must be detected early, as serious consequences may result if the imbalance becomes severe. Patients at risk for developing a sodium imbalance should be closely monitored. If an imbalance occurs, the patient's mental status as well as other symptoms are noted and recorded.

Medical, drug, and allergy histories should be obtained, and the patient weighed.

Nursing Diagnosis

Nursing diagnoses are based on the patient's symptoms and the severity and possible cause of the deficit or excess. They may include one or more of the following:

■ Activity intolerance related to lethargy, confusion, fever, other symptoms (specify)
■ Hyperthermia related to sodium imbalance
■ Pain related to muscle twitching, abdominal cramping secondary to hyponatremia
■ Altered oral mucous membrane related to dry mouth secondary to hypernatremia
■ Knowledge deficit of methods of preventing of sodium imbalance

Planning and Implementation

The major goals of the patient are to attain and maintain normal sodium balance.

The major goals of nursing management are early detection of sodium imbalance, especially in those at risk to develop this imbalance, and correction of the imbalance.

Intake and output should be measured, and vital signs should be monitored every 1 to 4 hours, depending on the severity of the deficit or excess. The patient's symptoms should be evaluated and compared with the baseline data obtained during assessment.

HYPONATREMIA. If intravenous administration of normal saline solution is ordered, the rate of infusion should be closely monitored. If sodium replacement by dietary means is ordered, the feedings should be evenly spaced throughout waking hours. The patient should be frequently assessed for an increase or decrease of symptoms associated with this deficit, and the physician notified if symptoms become worse or laboratory values show a significant change.

HYPERNATREMIA. Fluids should be offered at regular intervals, and the physician notified if the urine output remains low or the patient has difficulty taking oral fluids. If oral intake is inadequate, parenteral fluids or tube feedings may be necessary. When tube feedings are administered, sufficient water must be added to the feeding as well as water given by way of the tube between feedings. The patient should be assessed frequently for an increase or a decrease of symptoms, and the physician should be notified if symptoms become worse or laboratory values show a significant change.

Activity Intolerance. Assistance with activities of daily living may be necessary in those with a moderate to severe sodium deficit or excess. To reduce or eliminate fatigue, the patient should be encouraged to rest between activities.

Hyperthermia. The patient's temperature should be monitored every 4 hours, and the physician should be notified of any significant elevation, since an antipyretic drug may be necessary to correct hyperthermia.

Pain or Discomfort. The patient with muscle twitching and abdominal cramping should be told that these symptoms will subside when the deficit is corrected. When pain or discomfort is severe, the physician may order an analgesic or a tranquilizer with muscle-relaxing effects.

Altered Oral Mucous Membrane. Dryness of the mucous membranes may be relieved by frequent sips of water. Glyceride or another type of protective ointment may be applied to the lips and oral care given as needed. The oral cavity should be inspected daily for signs of inflammation, cracking, or other abnormalities.

Knowledge Deficit. Patients with a sodium imbalance should be informed of its symptoms and instructed to notify their physicians if symptoms should occur.

Patients with hyponatremia caused by profuse diaphoresis should be instructed to follow the recommendations of the physician when this event develops. Those with hypernatremia caused by an excessive sodium intake should be advised to avoid foods with a high sodium content. A list of these foods should be given to and reviewed with the patient.

Evaluation

■ Serum sodium returns to normal or near normal level
■ Patient is mentally clear and oriented to time and place
■ Urine output is normal

- Signs and symptoms of hyponatremia or hypernatremia are absent
- Oral mucous membranes are intact and show no evidence of injury
- Vital signs are stable
- Patient takes an adequate amount of fluid daily
- Patient demonstrates understanding of symptoms of hyponatremia and hypernatremia and the methods that may be used to avoid a sodium imbalance

POTASSIUM

The potassium cation (K^+) is the chief electrolyte found in intracellular fluid. It is essential in the maintenance of normal nerve and muscle activity, the regulation of osmotic pressure of body cells, and the maintenance of acid–base balance. Potassium has the same functions intracellularly as sodium has extracellularly. Normal potassium concentration ranges from 3.5 to 5.5 mEq/L.

Potassium Deficit

A potassium deficit, or *hypokalemia,* may occur in conjunction with the following: use of potassium-wasting diuretics (eg, furosemide, ethacrynic acid, and the thiazides); loss of fluid from the gastrointestinal tract (eg, in severe vomiting or diarrhea, draining intestinal fistulas, or prolonged gastrointestinal suction); taking large doses of corticosteroids; intravenous administration of insulin and glucose; and prolonged administration of nonelectrolyte parenteral fluids.

Symptoms
Symptoms include fatigue, weakness, anorexia, nausea, vomiting, dysrhythmias (abnormal heart rate or rhythm, especially in people receiving cardiac glycosides), leg cramps, muscle weakness, and paresthesias. Severe hypokalemia may result in hypotension, flaccid paralysis, and death caused by cardiac or respiratory arrest.

Diagnosis
Diagnosis is based on the patient's symptoms and laboratory test results, particularly serum potassium. Other laboratory tests also may be ordered, as the patient may have more than one imbalance.

Treatment
Treatment includes (when possible) elimination of the cause. Mild hypokalemia may be treated by increasing potassium intake by eating potassium-rich foods or using an oral potassium salt. Severe hypokalemia usually is treated with the intravenous administration of a potassium salt such as potassium chloride.

Potassium Excess

A potassium excess, or *hyperkalemia,* may develop in conjunction with the following: severe renal failure when the kidneys are unable to excrete potassium; severe burns; the administration of potassium-sparing diuretics; overuse of potassium supplements, salt substitutes (which contain potassium instead of sodium), or potassium-rich foods; crush injuries; Addison's disease; and rapid administration of parenteral potassium salts.

Symptoms
Symptoms include diarrhea, nausea, muscle weakness, paresthesias, and dysrhythmias. If severe hyperkalemia is not corrected, death can result from cardiac or respiratory arrest.

Diagnosis
Diagnosis is based on the patient's symptoms and laboratory test results, particularly serum potassium. Other laboratory tests also may be ordered, as the patient may have more than one imbalance.

Treatment
Treatment depends on the cause and severity of the excess. Mild hyperkalemia may be treated by decreasing the intake of potassium-rich foods or discontinuing oral potassium supplements until laboratory values are normal. Severe hyperkalemia may be treated with the administration of a cation-exchange resin such as Kayexalate, a regular insulin and glucose mixture, or sodium bicarbonate; peritoneal dialysis; or hemodialysis.

NURSING PROCESS —THE PATIENT WHO HAS A POTASSIUM IMBALANCE

Assessment
The patient's symptoms can be identified by a patient history and physical examination. Vital signs should be taken, paying particular attention to cardiac rate and rhythm. The possible cause may be identified during the patient history, for example the patient taking diuretics without potassium replacement therapy (hypokalemia) or the patient overusing a salt supplement that contains potassium (hyperkalemia).

Nursing Diagnosis
Nursing diagnoses are based on the patient's symptoms and the severity and possible cause of the deficit or excess. One or more of the following may apply:

- Activity intolerance related to fatigue, weakness secondary to potassium imbalance
- Fluid volume deficit related to vomiting secondary to hypokalemia
- Pain related to leg cramps secondary to hypokalemia
- Feeding and bathing/hygiene self-care deficit related to muscle weakness and paresthesia secondary to potassium imbalance
- Knowledge deficit of methods of preventing a potassium imbalance

Planning and Implementation

The major goals of the patient are to attain and maintain a normal potassium balance.

The major goals of nursing management are to prevent and correct the potassium imbalance and to closely monitor the patient so that a deficit does not recur.

HYPOKALEMIA. If the deficit is mild, potassium-rich foods may be eaten or oral potassium salts ordered. A severe deficit may require the intravenous administration of potassium. When potassium is given intravenously, *it is diluted in an intravenous solution* and *administered at a rate not to exceed 10 mEq/h.* In critical situations, such as the development of a dysrhythmia, the physician may order the potassium given at a more rapid rate. The rate of administration should be closely monitored, as patient movement may speed up or slow down the infusion. Vital signs should be monitored, paying special attention to heart rate and rhythm. The physician should be notified immediately if there is a significant change in heart rate or rhythm because emergency treatment may be necessary.

HYPERKALEMIA. Persons with mild hyperkalemia caused by excess ingestion of potassium should be advised to follow a diet low in potassium.

Severe hyperkalemia requires more intensive treatment, such as peritoneal dialysis or the administration of a cation-exchange resin. Vital signs should be closely monitored, and any change in heart rate or rhythm reported to the physician, as high serum potassium levels can lead to cardiac arrest.

Activity Intolerance, Feeding and Bathing/Hygiene Self-Care Deficit.

Persons with severe imbalances require partial or complete assistance with their activities of daily living. These tasks should be spaced so that the patient has time to rest between activities.

Fluid Volume Deficit.

Intake and output should be monitored. The physician should be informed if the patient with hypokalemia has repeated episodes of emesis, because intravenous fluid replacement may be necessary.

Pain and Discomfort.

Patients with hypokalemia may develop moderate to severe muscle cramps. The physician should be notified of this problem, as a tranquilizer with muscle-relaxing effects may be ordered.

Knowledge Deficit.

Patients with hyperkalemia should be advised to avoid foods or preparations that are high in potassium. A list of potassium-rich foods is given to and reviewed with the patient. The patient also should be instructed to read food labels carefully. Those who require additional potassium in their diet also should be given a list of potassium-rich foods.

The symptoms of hypokalemia or hyperkalemia should be reviewed with these patients, and they should be instructed to notify their physicians immediately if one or more of these symptoms should occur.

Evaluation

- Serum potassium returns to normal or near normal level
- Symptoms of potassium imbalance are absent
- Heart rate and rhythm are normal
- Patient with hypokalemia eats potassium-rich foods to balance potassium loss
- Patient demonstrates understanding of symptoms of hypokalemia and hyperkalemia and methods that may be used to avoid a potassium imbalance

CALCIUM

Most of the body's calcium (Ca^{2+}) is found in the bones and teeth. A small percentage (about 1% of total body calcium) is found in the blood. The level of calcium in the blood is regulated by the parathyroid glands. Calcium is necessary for the clotting of blood; smooth, skeletal, and cardiac muscle function; the transmission of nerve impulses; and the absorption and utilization of vitamin B_{12}. Vitamin D is necessary for the absorption of calcium in the intestine. Normal calcium concentration ranges from 9 to 11 mg/dL.

Calcium Deficit

A calcium deficit, or *hypocalcemia,* may be seen in people whose calcium intake is insufficient; in those with vitamin D deficiency (vitamin D is necessary for the absorption of calcium), hypoparathyroidism, burns, acute pancreatitis, or intestinal malabsorption disorders; and in those whose parathyroid glands have been surgically removed accidentally.

Symptoms

Symptoms include tingling in the extremities and the area around the mouth (circumoral paresthesias), muscle and abdominal cramping, carpopedal spasms, mental changes, positive Chvostek's sign (spasms of the facial muscles when the facial nerve is tapped), laryngeal spasms with airway obstruction, tetany (hypocalcemic), convulsions, bleeding, and dysrhythmias.

Diagnosis

Diagnosis is based on the patient's symptoms and laboratory test results. The serum calcium level is decreased, but other abnormal values, such as a decrease in the serum albumin level, also may be seen.

Treatment

Treatment includes administration of oral calcium and vitamin D for mild deficits, and intravenous administration of a calcium salt, such as calcium gluconate, for severe hypocalcemia.

Calcium Excess

An excess of calcium, or *hypercalcemia,* may be seen in conjunction with tumors of the parathyroid glands, multiple fractures, Paget's disease, hyperparathyroidism, excessive doses of vitamin D, prolonged immobilization, some chemotherapeutic agents (estrogens, androgens, progestins, and antiestrogens) used in the treatment of neoplastic disease, and malignant diseases such as multiple myeloma, tumors with or without bony metastasis, acute leukemia, and lymphomas.

Symptoms

Symptoms include deep bone pain, constipation, anorexia, nausea, vomiting, polyuria, thirst, pathologic fractures, and mental changes (usually decreased memory and attention span). Chronic hypercalcemia can result in the formation of kidney stones.

Diagnosis

Diagnosis is based on serum calcium levels and the patient's symptoms.

Treatment

Treatment includes determining and correcting the cause, when possible. Mild hypercalcemia may be treated by forcing fluids and limiting the oral calcium intake until the results of laboratory studies are normal. Acute hypercalcemia may be treated by the administration of one or more of the following: intravenous sodium chloride (0.45% or 0.9%), to increase calcium excretion in the urine; the diuretic furosemide, to promote calcium excretion; oral phosphates,

or calcitonin. Hypercalcemia associated with cancer or the chemotherapeutic regimen for cancer is treated on an individual basis. A decrease in drug dosage or the discontinuation of therapy may be necessary. Corticosteroids or plicamycin (an antineoplastic agent also used to treat the hypercalcemia of malignant diseases that do not respond to other forms of therapy) also may be used.

NURSING PROCESS —THE PATIENT WHO HAS A CALCIUM IMBALANCE

Assessment

A general assessment identifies such symptoms as carpopedal spasm, tetany, and deep bone pain. The history may identify the cause of the calcium imbalance, for example the administration of hormones as a cancer treatment (hypercalcemia).

Nursing Diagnosis

Nursing diagnoses are based on the patient's symptoms and the severity and possible cause of the imbalance. One or more of the following may apply:

- Pain related to muscle cramping and tetany secondary to hypocalcemia, or bone pain secondary to hypercalcemia
- Potential for injury related to pathologic fractures associated with hypercalcemia
- Knowledge deficit of methods of preventing a calcium imbalance

Planning and Implementation

The major goals of the patient are to attain and maintain a normal calcium balance.

The major goal of nursing management is correction of the calcium imbalance.

HYPOCALCEMIA.   The patient should be closely monitored for neurologic manifestations (tetany, convulsions, amd spasms), dysrhythmias, and airway obstruction, as emergency interventions may be necessary. If the deficit is severe, seizure precautions should be taken.

A mild calcium deficit may be treated with oral calcium supplements and a calcium-rich diet. A severe deficit is treated with intravenous administration of calcium salts. Because calcium aids in clotting, the patient should be routinely checked for signs of bruising or bleeding.

HYPERCALCEMIA.   Mild hypercalcemia may be corrected with the administration of oral fluids and a low-calcium diet. Severe cases require more intensive therapy. Fluids should be offered at frequent intervals, and the patient encouraged to ambulate.

Pain and Discomfort. The patient's position should be changed every 2 hours, and an effort made to keep the patient as comfortable as possible by supporting the extremities with pillows or pads. The pain associated with muscle cramping and tetany usually subsides once the hypocalcemia is corrected. The physician should be informed if the patient continues to experience pain, as an analgesic or a tranquilizer with muscle-relaxing effects may be ordered.

Potential for Injury. Patients with chronic hypercalcemia and the potential for pathologic fractures should be protected from injury. They should be assisted when ambulating and should wear shoes rather than loose slippers when they are out of bed.

Knowledge Deficit. Persons with hypercalcemia or hypocalcemia may require diets that are low or high in calcium, respectively. A high- or low-calcium diet is given to and reviewed with the patient. The drug regimen for those with hypocalcemia is reviewed with the patient.

Evaluation

- Serum calcium returns to normal or near normal level
- Symptoms of calcium imbalance are absent
- Patient eats diet high in calcium (hypocalcemia) or adheres to diet low in calcium (hypercalcemia)
- Patient takes oral fluids and ambulates at frequent intervals (hypercalcemia)
- Patient demonstrates understanding of dietary and drug regimens

MAGNESIUM

Magnesium (Mg^{2+}) is found in bone cells and in specialized cells of the heart, liver, and skeletal muscles. Only a small percentage of the total magnesium found in the body is present in the extracellular fluid compartment. Magnesium is involved in the transmission of nerve impulses and plays a role in muscle excitability. It also is an activator for a number of enzyme systems, including the functioning of B vitamins and the utilization of potassium and calcium. Normal magnesium concentration is 1.5 to 2.5 mEq/L.

Magnesium Deficit

A magnesium deficit, or *hypomagnesemia,* may be seen in chronic alcoholism, diabetes mellitus, severe renal disease, a high intake of calcium, severe malnu-

trition, toxemia of pregnancy, intestinal malabsorption syndromes, excessive diuresis (drug-induced), hyperaldosteronism, and prolonged gastric suction.

Symptoms

Symptoms include tachycardia and other dysrhythmias, neuromuscular irritability, paresthesias of the extremities, leg and foot cramps, hypertension, mental changes, positive Chvostek's sign (see section on calcium deficit) and positive Trousseau's sign (muscle spasm of the arm and hand produced by application of pressure to nerves and vessels of the upper arm), dysphagia, and convulsions.

Diagnosis

Diagnosis is based on serum magnesium levels and the patient's symptoms.

Treatment

Treatment includes administration of oral magnesium salts or the addition of magnesium-rich foods to the diet. A severe magnesium deficit may be treated with intravenous administration of magnesium sulfate.

Magnesium Excess

A magnesium excess, or *hypermagnesemia,* may be seen in conjunction with renal failure, Addison's disease, the excessive use of antacids or laxatives that contain magnesium, and hyperparathyroidism.

Symptoms

Symptoms include flushing and a feeling of warmth, hypotension, lethargy, drowsiness, bradycardia, muscle weakness, depressed respirations, and coma.

Diagnosis

Diagnosis is based on serum magnesium levels and the patient's symptoms.

Treatment

Treatment includes decreasing oral magnesium intake. In severe hypermagnesemia, hemodialysis may be necessary. If respiratory failure occurs, mechanical ventilation is necessary.

NURSING PROCESS —THE PATIENT WHO HAS A MAGNESIUM IMBALANCE

Assessment

A general assessment identifies symptoms. A patient history may identify the cause of the imbalance, for example a history of prolonged gastric suction (hypomagnesemia), or hyperparathyroidism (hypermagnesemia).

Nursing Diagnosis

Nursing diagnoses are based on the patient's symptoms and may include one or more of the following:

- Pain related to neuromuscular irritability secondary to hypomagnesemia
- Potential for injury related to drowsiness, lethargy, muscle weakness secondary to hypermagnesemia
- Knowledge deficit of methods of preventing magnesium imbalance

Planning and Implementation

The major goals of the patient are to attain and maintain a normal magnesium balance.

The major goals of nursing management are correction of the magnesium imbalance and the prevention of recurrences.

Vital signs should be taken at frequent intervals, and the physician informed of any changes in blood pressure or the development of a dysrhythmia.

HYPOMAGNESEMIA.   The patient should be closely observed for dysrhythmias and early signs of neuromuscular irritability, which should be reported to the physician immediately. If intravenous magnesium sulfate is administered, the patient should be closely monitored for a sharp drop in blood pressure. If dysphagia is noted, care should be taken in the administration of fluids and food. Patients who are receiving a digitalis preparation should be closely monitored for digitalis toxicity, which can be precipitated by a magnesium deficit. A diet high in magnesium may be prescribed for a mild deficit.

HYPERMAGNESEMIA.   If magnesium excess is due to excessive use of antacids or laxatives, the patient should be instructed to avoid these preparations. Severe magnesium excess may require hemodialysis.

Vital signs should be monitored, and the patient observed for episodes of hypotension and bradycardia or other dysrhythmias.

Pain and Discomfort.   The patient should be assured that pain and discomfort will subside once treatment is instituted. If muscle pain persists because of prolonged neuromuscular irritability, the physician may order an analgesic or a tranquilizer with muscle-relaxing effects.

Potential for Injury.   Patients with magnesium deficits should be assisted when getting out of bed until all neuromuscular symptoms related to the disorder are relieved.

Respiratory Function.   When the magnesium excess is moderate to severe, the patient's respiratory rate should be closely monitored, and the physician contacted immediately if there is any change in the respiratory rate, rhythm, or depth.

Knowledge Deficit.   Persons with magnesium deficits may be placed on a diet high in magnesium. A list of foods high in magnesium should be given to and reviewed with the patient. If drug therapy is prescribed, the drug regimen should be reviewed with the patient.

Patients with magnesium excesses caused by excessive use of laxatives or antacids that contain magnesium should be warned to check with the physician before using these products. If use is allowed, the patient should be warned to follow the physician's recommendations regarding the frequency of their use.

Evaluation

- Serum magnesium returns to normal or near normal level
- Symptoms of magnesium imbalance are absent
- Vital signs are stable
- Patient understands dangers of laxative and antacid overuse (hypermagnesemia)
- Patient demonstrates understanding of the treatment regimen and methods to prevent a magnesium imbalance

General Nutritional Considerations

- ☐ Some of the foods high in sodium are bacon, bread, green olives, sweet pickles, some salad dressings, regular butter and margarine, catsup, corn flakes, cheddar and Parmesan cheese, peanut butter, and food to which salt is routinely added, such as potato chips, peanuts, and pretzels.
- ☐ Some of the foods high in potassium are bananas, tomatoes, orange and prune juice, dates, potatoes, milk and some milk products, apricots, avocados, raisins, soybeans, salt substitutes, lima beans, and honeydew melon.
- ☐ Some of the foods high in calcium are cheese, cream, milk, ice cream, yogurt, broccoli, spinach, farina, collards, kale, mustard greens, and turnip greens.

☐ Some of the foods high in magnesium are bananas, chocolate, almonds, tofu, bran, peanut butter, raw beet greens, dried apricots, and graham crackers.

General Pharmacologic Considerations

☐ Electrolytes may be given as drugs for replacement of lost electrolytes.

☐ The dosage of electrolytes must be carefully measured and given only as directed by the physician because these agents are potentially dangerous.

General Gerontologic Considerations

☐ The elderly patient has a tendency to drink less water, and therefore may incur chronic FVD as well as other electrolyte imbalances.

☐ A poor appetite, erratic meal patterns, the inability to prepare nutritious meals, or financial circumstances may influence nutritional status, resulting in electrolyte imbalance.

☐ The aging process often is accompanied by chronic disorders such as cardiac and renal disease, which may be treated by drug therapy. The effect of certain drugs (eg, digitalis preparations) may be modified in the presence of some electrolyte imbalances.

☐ Poor respiratory exchange caused by chronic lung disease, inactivity, or thoracic skeletal changes may lead to chronic respiratory acidosis.

☐ Overuse of sodium bicarbonate (baking soda), an inexpensive substitute for commercial antacids, may lead to metabolic alkalosis.

Suggested Readings

☐ Barta M. Correcting electrolyte imbalances. RN February 1987;50:30. *(Additional coverage of subject matter)*

☐ Calloway C. When the problem involves magnesium, calcium or phosphate. RN May 1987;50:30. *(Additional coverage of subject matter)*

☐ Fischbach FT. A manual of laboratory and diagnostic tests. 3rd ed. Philadelphia: JB Lippincott, 1988. *(Additional coverage of subject matter)*

☐ Horne MM, Swearingen PL. Pocket guide to fluids and electrolytes. St Louis: CV Mosby, 1988. *(Additional coverage of subject matter)*

☐ McAdams R, McClure K. Hypovolemia: when to suspect it. RN December 1986;49:34. *(Additional coverage of subject matter)*

☐ Metheny NM. Fluid and electrolyte balance: nursing considerations. Philadelphia: JB Lippincott, 1987. *(Additional and in-depth coverage of subject matter)*

☐ Rinard G. Water intoxication. Am J Nurs December 1989;89:1635. *(Additional coverage of subject matter)*

☐ Schwartz MW. Potassium imbalances. Am J Nurs October 1987;87:1292. *(Additional coverage of subject matter)*

☐ Sommers M. Rapid fluid resuscitation: how to correct dangerous deficits. Nursing '90 1990;20:52. *(Additional and in-depth coverage of subject matter)*

☐ Toto KH. When the patient has hyperkalemia. RN April 1987;50:34. *(Additional coverage of subject matter)*

☐ Toto KH. When the patient has hypokalemia. RN March 1987;50:38. *(Additional coverage of subject matter)*

☐ Weldy NJ. Body fluids and electrolytes: a programmed instruction. 5th ed. St Louis: CV Mosby, 1988. *(Additional coverage of subject matter)*

☐ Young Me, Flynn KT. Third-spacing: when the body conceals fluid loss. RN August 1988;51:46. *(Additional coverage of subject matter)*

Medical–Surgical Nursing Interventions

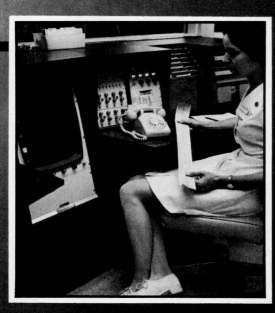

Unit 3

Chapter 13
Intravenous Therapy

On completion of this chapter the reader will:

■ State the rationale for intravenous administration

■ List the various types of solutions (infusates) used for intravenous therapy and give the rationale for the use of each

■ Discuss the techniques used in parenteral administration by a peripheral vein

■ Discuss the techniques used in parenteral administration by a central vein

■ Discuss patient preparation for intravenous therapy

■ Calculate the flow rate of a given amount of intravenous solution

■ List the factors that influence intravenous flow rates

■ List and discuss the complications of intravenous therapy

■ Use the nursing process in the management of the patient who is receiving intravenous therapy

Intravenous (IV) therapy demands skillful administration technique, close observation of the patient, and a number of special nursing considerations. Drugs, solutions (eg, dextrose, plasma expanders, and amino acids), and whole blood and blood components may be given by the IV route in specific situations.

RATIONALES FOR INTRAVENOUS ADMINISTRATION
Administration of Pharmacologic Agents

The IV route is used when the following conditions apply:

■ The drug can be given only by the IV route
■ A rapid drug effect is desired
■ The patient cannot be given the drug orally (eg, during the immediate postoperative period or when the patient is not permitted to receive anything by mouth)
■ Severe vomiting or diarrhea will not allow sufficient time for drug absorption
■ A continuous therapeutic blood level of a drug is desired

Administration of Solutions

Solutions may be given by the IV route when it is necessary to perform any of the following therapies:

■ Replace or supplement fluid, electrolytes, amino acids, lipids, or vitamins
■ Supply carbohydrates, as a source of calories, in a readily usable form
■ Administer a temporary substitute for whole blood
■ Keep a vein open for the emergency administration of drugs or solutions

Types of Solutions

Dextrose (D-glucose) in water is available in various concentrations, and supplies carbohydrates in a readily usable form. The 2.5%, 5%, and 10% solutions are used for peripheral vein infusion. The 20% solution is used to supply adequate calories in a minimal amount of solution. The 25% and 50% solutions are used for treatment of acute hypoglycemia. The 10%, 20%, 30%, 38.5%, 40%, 50%, 60%, and 70% solutions are used for central venous infusions. The calorie content of each of these solutions is shown in Table 13-1.

Dextrose in sodium chloride (saline) is available in various concentrations, and supplies carbohydrates in a readily usable form along with sodium chloride. Concentrations include dextrose 2.5% in 0.45% sodium chloride; dextrose 5% in 0.2%, 0.33%, 0.45%, and 0.9% sodium chloride; and dextrose 10% in 0.45% and 0.9% sodium chloride.

Alcohol in dextrose solutions are available as 5% alcohol and 5% dextrose in water, which supplies 450

Table 13–1. Calorie Contents of Dextrose in Water Solutions

Concentration (%)	Cal/L
2.5	85
5	170
10	340
20	680
25	850
30	1,020
38.5	1,310
40	1,360
50	1,700
60	2,040
70	2,380

cal/L, and 10% alcohol and 5% dextrose in water, which supplies 720 cal/L. Alcohol in dextrose solutions are used for increasing the calorie intake and for fluid replacement.

Solutions of 10% *fructose (levulose) in water* and 10% *invert sugar in water* are used for calorie and fluid replacement. Each supplies 375 cal/L.

Combined electrolyte solutions contain many of the electrolytes found in the cellular and intracellular spaces, along with various concentrations of dextrose or fructose. Examples of these solutions are Plasma-Lyte 56 and 5% dextrose, dextrose 5% in lactated Ringer's solution, Isolyte G with 10% dextrose, and Normosol-M 900 Cal.

Sodium chloride solutions are available in concentrations of 0.45%, 0.9%, 3%, and 5%. The 0.45% solution is used to provide fluid replacement when fluid losses exceed electrolyte depletion. The 0.9% solution, also called normal saline solution, is used to supply fluid and sodium chloride. The 3% and 5% solutions are used to provide sodium and chloride in hyponatremia and hypochloremia (decrease of chloride in the blood) caused by electrolyte losses, drastic dilution of body water after excessive water intake, and emergency treatment of severe salt depletion.

Intravenous fat emulsion is used for the prevention and treatment of essential fatty acid deficiency. It provides nonprotein calories for those whose calorie needs cannot be met with glucose.

Amino acid solutions promote protein synthesis, reduce the rate of protein breakdown, and promote wound healing. They are primarily used in debilitated patients as well as in those who are receiving long-term parenteral nutrition. Examples of these solutions

include Aminosyn, 3.5%, 5%, 7%, 8.5%, and 10%; Travenol, 5.5%, 8.5%, and 10%; and FreAmine III, 8.5% and 10%. Amino acid solutions for renal failure include Aminosyn-RF, NephrAmine 5.4%, and RenAmin.

Plasma expanders can be used as substitutes for whole blood and plasma to maintain the volume of circulating blood and treat shock. Plasma expanders include hetastarch, low-molecular-weight dextran (Dextran 40), and high-molecular-weight dextran (Dextran 70 and Dextran 75).

Whole blood supplies blood cells and plasma. Packed red cells contain a minimal amount of plasma and are used when red blood cell administration is required but a minimal amount of fluid replacement is needed.

Platelets in platelet-rich plasma (eg, platelets suspended in a small amount of plasma) may be administered to those with hemorrhagic disorders.

Plasma can be used to replace coagulation factors that are found to be deficient in bleeding disorders.

Serum albumin is a protein fraction of blood. It can be used in the treatment of shock, burns, hypoproteinemia (a decrease in the amount of protein in the blood), acute liver failure, and acute nephrosis. It is available as 5% and 25% normal (human) serum albumin.

Administration of Whole Blood and Blood Components

Whole blood and blood components are administered IV in the following circumstances:

- It is necessary to replace blood loss or blood cell destruction with whole blood, packed red blood cells (red blood cells separated from whole blood), frozen red cells, or platelets (platelet-rich plasma)
- Plasma protein fraction and human albumin (normal serum albumin 5%, 25%) are necessary for the treatment of hypovolemic shock, hypoproteinemia, severe burns, acute nephrosis, acute liver failure, peritonitis, pancreatitis, exchange transfusions, and cardiopulmonary bypass surgery.

ADMINISTRATION BY A PERIPHERAL VEIN

Peripheral parenteral administration is the administration of a drug, solution, whole blood, plasma expanders, or blood components by way of a peripheral vein. Preparation for the IV administration of fluids includes the following:

- Selection of the necessary equipment for administration
- Preparation of the patient
- Selection of the site
- Performance of the venipuncture

Equipment

Equipment includes the IV solution, the prescribed medication to be added to the solution, and the following administration equipment: IV tubing, skin antiseptic, tourniquet, needle, IV pole, dressings for the venipuncture site, tape to anchor the needle and dressings, antibiotic for the venipuncture site (as prescribed by the physician or hospital policy), splints or restraints to immobilize the extremity used for administration, and, when necessary, an electronic pump or controller or a pressure infusion sleeve. A fluid warmer also may be used to raise the temperature of parenteral solutions as well as blood because administration of solutions that are below body temperature causes a loss of body heat.

Intravenous electronic controllers regulate the gravity flow of an IV solution and may be volumetric or nonvolumetric. Volumetric controllers are set to deliver a specific volume (amount) at a specific rate (drops per minute). Nonvolumetric controllers are set to deliver the IV solution at a specific rate. *Intravenous electronic pumps* exert positive pressure, which is greater than arterial or venous pressure, to deliver IV solutions. Pumps also may be volumetric or nonvolumetric. A *pressure infusion sleeve* is a cuff that holds the plastic IV solution container. Inflation of the cuff exerts a squeezing action on the plastic container, thus permitting a more rapid infusion of the solution.

One or more drugs may be prescribed for addition to the solution, and may be added by the nurse or the pharmacist, depending on hospital policy or the type of drug being added to the solution. Because many drugs are incompatible, and therefore cannot be added together to an IV solution, the nurse must check with the pharmacist before adding two or more drugs to a parenteral solution.

Whole blood and some blood components are obtained from the hospital blood bank. Whole blood (fresh, frozen, or packed red cells) must be typed and cross-matched before administration to a patient.

IV lines (or tubing) come in various types, such as a single (primary) line or Y-tubing (which provides two lines), shown in Figure 13-1. The tubing may have a simple drip chamber or a volume-control drip chamber. It also may have a piggyback port for the intermittent administration of solutions or drugs. The clamp supplied with the IV line is used to regulate the IV flow or rate of administration. An in-line filter may be used to decrease the risk of bacterial contamination.

The type and size of the needle used depend on several factors, for example the planned total time of administration (hours versus days), the viscosity of the fluid (blood versus dextrose in water), the site selected for administration, the condition of the veins,

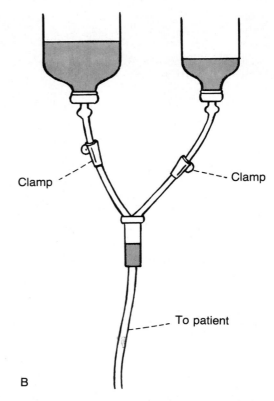

Figure 13–1. Bottles connected in parallel (Y-type) setup. (Metheny NM, Snively WD Jr. Nurses' handbook of fluid balance. 4th ed. Philadelphia: JB Lippincott, 1983)

and patient cooperation (alert and cooperative versus semiconscious and restless).

The types of needles include the straight needle, the winged-tip or butterfly needle, the over-the-needle catheter, the inside-the-needle catheter, and the winged-tip needle units used for intermittent administration of drugs (heparin lock). The straight needle is used for short-term administration of an IV solution or for administration of whole blood or blood components. The winged-tip needle is used for infants and children, when the dorsum of the hand is selected as the venipuncture site, for elderly or debilitated patients, and for patients who are receiving short-term therapy. The over-the-needle catheter is used for long-term IV therapy as well as for administration of viscous fluids such as blood. The inside-the-needle catheter is used for long-term therapy, the administration of viscous fluids, central venous pressure monitoring, and central parenteral administration of drugs and nutrients.

Needle sizes are given in gauge, which is the outside diameter of the needle. The larger the gauge number, the smaller the needle. Thus, a 26-gauge needle is smaller than a 19-gauge needle. Most routine venipunctures on adults require the use of a 20- to 22- or

23-gauge needle. Administration of whole blood, serum albumin, and other viscous solutions usually requires the use of a 19-gauge needle.

Needles also are available in various lengths. Straight needles vary in length from 0.75 to about 2 inches. Wing-tipped needles are short, and over-the-needle and inside-the-needle catheters are available in a range of lengths.

An IV prep tray is kept in the hospital unit. It usually contains tourniquets, tape, sterile gauze pads, skin antiseptic, a variety of needles, immobilization devices, and an antimicrobial ointment for application to the venipuncture site. Various types of skin antiseptics, such as alcohol or povidone-iodine, may be used to prepare the venipuncture site. The use of nonallergenic tape is preferable, especially when IV therapy continues for an extended period. An antimicrobial ointment may be applied to the venipuncture site after insertion and stabilization of the needle or catheter.

Patient Preparation

The patient is given an explanation of the purpose of the procedure at his or her level of understanding. This is best done *before* the equipment is brought to the patient's room. Every effort should be made to make the explanation clear, concise, and informative without causing the patient undue anxiety. Time should be allowed to answer the patient's questions. The following points may be included in the explanation:

- Why IV therapy is needed
- About how long the procedure will take
- The site to be used
- The amount of discomfort that normally accompanies insertion of the needle or catheter
- Instructions regarding limitation of activities

Site Selection

Sites for the administration of IV drugs or solutions include the superficial veins of the arm and hand (antecubital fossa, or inner elbow; dorsum, or back, of the hand; and forearm veins) and of the scalp, which are primarily used in infants. The superficial veins of the hand and forearm are shown in Figure 13-2. Selection of a vein depends on several factors, such as the patient's age, the condition of the veins, the duration of IV therapy, the IV solution ordered, needle or catheter size, and patient cooperation. Veins that have been used frequently for IV administration may be in poor condition, and therefore not desirable for further use. The use of veins that are difficult to palpate after the application of a tourniquet also may be contraindicated because insertion of the needle may be a problem.

Venipuncture

The procedure for venipuncture is as follows:

1. Apply a tourniquet above the selected venipuncture site. Wait for the veins in the area to dilate, and select the best vein (if more than one is available) according to the position of the vein, and thus the final position of the needle or catheter.

2. Prepare the site with a skin antiseptic. Apply the antiseptic in a circular motion, starting over the selected site and moving outward. Hospital policy or physician preference may determine the type of skin antiseptic used. If iodine is used, allow the area to dry, and wipe the area with an alcohol sponge. If the patient is allergic to iodine, use alcohol as a skin antiseptic.

3. Use a finger or the thumb to pull the skin taut over the vein. Insert the needle (with the bevel up and at a 20- to 30-degree angle) below the point where you plan to penetrate the vein wall. Once the skin is pierced, decrease the angle of the needle to enter the vein. If the needle is in the vein, a backflow of blood is visible in the plastic area above the needle hub. Slowly and carefully advance the needle until about three quarters of the needle length is below the skin. Remove the tourniquet, and open the flow clamp on the tubing to allow the solution to flow into the vein. Adjust the flow rate according to the desired infusion rate.

4. For insertion of an over-the-needle catheter, follow the same procedure as in step 3. Once the catheter is in the vein and blood backflow occurs, hold the needle hub with the thumb and forefinger and advance the catheter (or cannula) into the vein. Open the flow clamp on the tubing, and adjust the flow rate.

5. For insertion of an inside-the-needle catheter, follow the procedure described in step 3. Once the catheter is in the vein and blood backflow occurs, push the flow control plug into the adapter to prevent blood from leaking out of the catheter. Next, advance the catheter into the vein. Then remove the tourniquet and open the flow clamp on the tubing. *Note:* The nurse should achieve proficiency in the insertion of over-the-needle and inside-the-needle catheters before attempting to use these types of needle for IV administration.

6. Secure the needle or catheter with tape, taking care to leave the venipuncture site uncovered. Then apply antimicrobial ointment to the venipuncture site, cover the site with a sterile gauze pad, and tape the pad in place. Use additional tape to further secure the needle and tubing. Print the date and time of insertion on a small piece of tape and place it on top of the dressing.

7. Immobilize the extremity with an arm board, splint, or other device that may have to be tailored to the patient's activity.

ADMINISTRATION BY A CENTRAL VEIN

Central venous lines are used for administering total parenteral nutrition (TPN), monitoring central venous

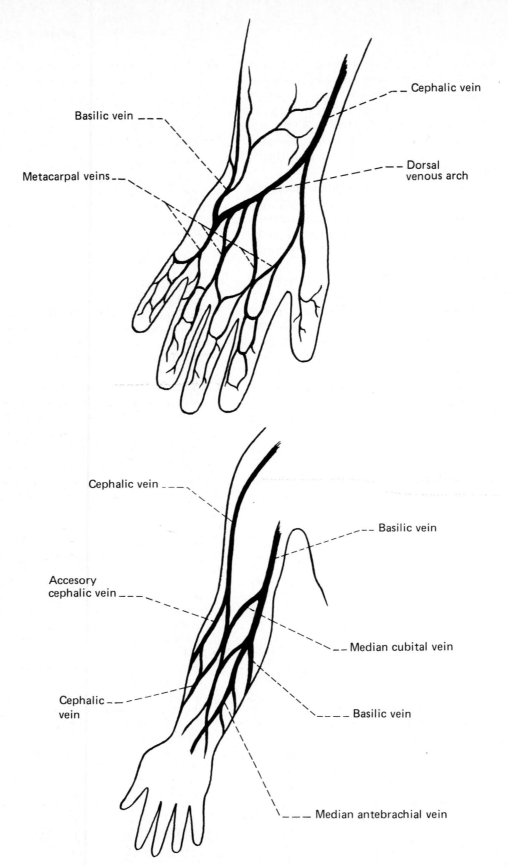

Figure 13–2. Venipuncture sites. (*Top*) Superficial veins of the hand. (*Bottom*) Superficial veins of the forearm. (Metheny NM, Snively WD Jr. Nurses' handbook of fluid balance. 4th ed. Philadelphia: JB Lippincott, 1983)

pressure, and administering IV solutions when peripheral veins have collapsed, or when long-term IV therapy or thrombophlebitis has reduced the availability of peripheral veins. A central venous catheter is inserted by a physician. Catheter placement is shown in Figure 13-3.

Equipment

The physician orders the size and type of catheter to be inserted. The size may range from 14- to 18-gauge. The following equipment also is needed: sterile gloves, skin antiseptic, sterile drapes and masks, local anesthetic, sterile scissors and hemostat, syringes and needles, suture, tape, sterile gauze pads, antimicrobial ointment, a priming solution (usually dextrose 5% in water), and the solution to be administered. Some hospitals prepare trays for the insertion of central venous or arterial lines. Physician preference also may dictate the equipment necessary for catheter insertion.

Insertion of a Hickman, Broviac, or Groshong catheter requires general or local anesthesia, and is guided by fluoroscopy. These catheters provide long-term access to the venous system (eg, for parenteral nutrition administration and the collection of venous blood samples).

Patient Preparation

The patient is given an explanation of the procedure at his or her level of understanding. This is best done *before* the equipment is brought to the room. Every effort should be made to make the explanation clear, concise, and informative without causing the patient undue anxiety. Time should be allowed to answer the patient's questions about the procedure. The following points may be included in the explanation:

- Why this type of therapy is needed
- About how long the procedure will take
- The site to be used
- The positions that will be used for catheter insertion
- Equipment attached to the central lines (infusion or controller pumps, IV solution containers) and the dressing and filter changes that will be performed on a regular basis

Site Selection

The physician selects the site to be used. The three sites that may be used are the jugular vein, the subclavian vein, and a peripheral vein with the catheter threaded into the superior vena cava.

Catheter Insertion

If the patient is a male, the selected insertion site is checked for hair and shaved as needed. Before insertion of the catheter, the patient is placed in the Trendelenburg position to dilate the veins and reduce the risk of air embolism. When the subclavian vein is selected, a rolled blanket or towel is placed under the shoulder that is on the side of the insertion site. For

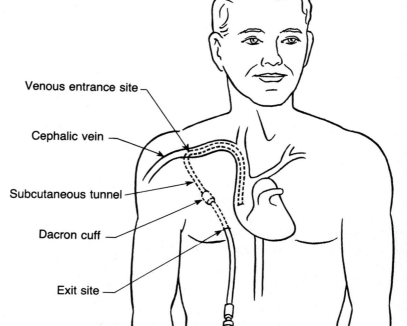

Figure 13–3. Indwelling central venous catheter for prolonged TPN or chemotherapy. (Metheny NM, Snively WD Jr. Nurses' handbook of fluid balance. 4th ed. Philadelphia: JB Lippincott, 1983)

Venous entrance site

Cephalic vein

Subcutaneous tunnel

Dacron cuff

Exit site

jugular insertion, a rolled blanket or towel is placed under the shoulder opposite the insertion site. The patient's head is turned away from the site to minimize contamination by airborne pathogens and to make the site more accessible. The physician may alter these positions, depending on the patient as well as personal preferences.

The physician inserts the catheter using strict aseptic technique. After insertion of the catheter, a chest radiograph may be ordered to confirm catheter placement.

FLOW (INFUSION) RATE CALCULATION

When calculating IV flow rates, the following three factors must be known:

1. Amount of solution ordered (eg, 500 mL, 1,000 mL)
2. Total time of infusion (eg, infuse the prescribed amount in 8 hours)
3. Number of drops per milliliter in the macrodrip or microdrip system

The first step is to take the amount of solution ordered and divide it by the total time of the infusion to determine the number of milliliters to be given each hour.

$$\frac{1,000 \text{ mL}}{8 \text{ hr}} \times 125 \text{ mL/hr}$$

Next, check the manufacturer's labeling on the drip system to determine the number of drops required to deliver 1 mL. Macrodrip systems may deliver 10, 15, or 20 drops/mL, whereas microdrip systems usually deliver 50 or 60 drops/mL. To determine the number of drops per minute to infuse the solution, either of the following formulas may be used:

$$\frac{\text{volume of fluid (mL)}}{\text{time of infusion (in min)}} \times$$

$$\text{drops/mL of system used} = \qquad (1)$$

$$\text{flow rate in drops/min}$$

$$\frac{\text{drops/mL}}{60 \text{ sec}} \times \text{volume of fluid/hr} \qquad (2)$$

To illustrate, using 1,000 mL of fluid to be administered in 8 hours and using a macrodrip system that delivers 15 drops/mL.

$$\frac{1,000 \text{ mL}}{480 \text{ min}} \times 15 = 31 \text{ drops/min} \qquad (1)$$

$$\frac{15 \text{ drops/mL}}{60 \text{ sec}} \times 125 \text{ mL} = 31 \text{ drops/min} \qquad (2)$$

Factors That Influence Flow Rates

The following factors may affect the rate of flow:

- The viscosity (thickness) of the solution. The more viscous the solution, the slower the flow rate.
- The size of the needle or catheter. Large needles and catheters allow delivery of greater amounts of fluid through the lumen.
- The height of the infusion container. The higher the container, the faster the infusion rate.
- The amount of fluid in the container. Solution flows faster from a full container than from one that is partially empty.
- Loose clamp on tubing
- Obstructed tubing. The flow may either stop or slow if the patient is lying on the tubing, the tubing is pinched or kinked, or a clot forms in the needle or catheter.
- Alteration of needle or catheter position in the vein. If the bevel of the needle or catheter lies against the vein wall, the outflow of solution is affected. The patient's movements can cause the bevel to lie against the vein wall.
- Kinking or bending of a plastic catheter within the vein. This reduces or may stop the flow of solution, and may occur when the catheter is located over a joint such as the elbow and the patient bends his arm.
- Obstruction of the air vent or outlet of the IV solution container. Improper venting or obstruction of the air vent or outlet creates a partial vacuum in the container, thus slowing and finally stopping the flow of solution.
- Use of certain filters
- Tampering with the IV line clamp by the patient or visitors

COMPLICATIONS
Intravenous Therapy Complications

A number of complications are associated with IV therapy. One or more of these complications may occur during peripheral IV therapy or TPN. The nurse should be aware of potential problems and know how to manage them appropriately. The following are some of the major complications of IV therapy.

Extravasation and Infiltration. Although they often are used synonymously, extravasation and infiltration have different meanings. *Extravasation* refers to the escape of fluid from a blood vessel into surrounding tissues while the needle or catheter is in the vein. *Infiltration* is the collection of fluid into tissues (usually subcutaneous tissue) when the needle or catheter is out of the vein. Both events necessitate discontinuation of the infusion and insertion of an IV line in another vein. Some drugs are capable of causing severe tissue damage if extravasation or infiltration occurs.

Phlebitis, Thrombophlebitis, and Thrombosis. Phlebitis, thrombophlebitis, and thrombosis are believed to be caused by localized irritation of the vein wall. Irritation may be caused by the needle or catheter, chemical irritation (eg, drugs added to the IV solution or the IV solution itself), or infection.

Fluid (or Circulatory) Overload. Fluid overload refers to an excessive amount of fluid in the body, which accumulates faster than it can be excreted by the kidneys. The amount of solution required to produce fluid overload varies, depending on the patient's size, age, and cardiac and renal status. Fluid overload can cause congestive heart failure and pulmonary edema, and may result after rapid infusion of a large volume of fluid. Rapid infusion of IV solutions that contain one or more drugs also can produce toxic reactions because rapid delivery of the solution produces a high concentration of the drug in the blood.

Clot Formation. A clot may form in the needle or catheter when the flow of the solution is stopped. The needle or catheter must be removed and a new IV line inserted in another vein.

Infection. Whenever pathogenic organisms are introduced into the bloodstream, infection may occur. Causes include contamination of the IV solution at the time of manufacture or during preparation for administration; contamination of any part of the delivery system (eg, needle, catheter, or IV tubing), and contamination of drugs added to the IV solution.

Embolism. Embolism may result from air entering the IV system (air embolism) or from the breaking away of all or part of a thrombus that has formed on the vein wall (thromboembolism). Rarely, pieces of IV catheter that were broken off during insertion or removal have entered the bloodstream.

Transfusion Complications

The following complications can result from the transfusion of blood or blood products:

Allergic Reaction. The symptoms of an allergic reaction include urticaria, pruritus, and bronchial wheezing. Rarely, anaphylaxis may occur. This reaction is thought to be caused by allergens in the donor blood reacting with antibodies in the recipient's blood.

Hemolytic Reaction. A hemolytic reaction occurs because the donor's blood is incompatible with the recipient's blood. Causes include incorrect typing and cross-matching and administration of the wrong type of blood.

Febrile Reaction. A febrile reaction may be caused by bacterial contamination of the blood, but also may occur with a hemolytic reaction.

Disease Transmission. Hepatitis (some types), acquired immunodeficiency syndrome, and malaria can be transmitted in the blood of the donor. Although donor blood is screened for hepatitis C (formerly type non-A, non-B), hepatitis B, and acquired immunodeficiency syndrome, a small chance still remains that these infections may be transmitted.

NURSING PROCESS —THE PATIENT UNDERGOING INTRAVENOUS THERAPY

Assessment
The patient's admission history and most recent laboratory values are reviewed before the physical assessment. The patient is assessed with regard to hydration (see section on fluid volume deficit in Chapter 12). Recent conditions or situations that may have decreased the patient's oral fluid intake (eg, nausea, anorexia, or unconsciousness), or increased the excretion of fluid (eg, diarrhea or vomiting) or urine output (eg, administration of diuretics) without adequate oral fluid intake are considered at this time.

The veins of the hand, forearm, and antecubital fossa are inspected for adequate filling when a tourniquet or blood pressure cuff is applied. Previously used venipuncture sites are examined for redness and swelling and palpated for soreness. The presence of these symptoms may contraindicate the use of these areas. The approximate diameter of the vein and the gauge of the needle are compared, as the vein must be large enough to accommodate the needle. The patient's preference for an IV site also is considered.

Nursing Diagnosis
Depending on the degree of fluid volume deficit and the type of solution administered, one or more of the following diagnosis may apply:

- Anxiety related to need for IV therapy or preconceived discomfort related to this treatment
- Fluid volume excess related to excessive IV fluid intake
- Fluid volume deficit related to condition warranting IV therapy, incorrect infusion rate, failure to meet the patient's fluid needs
- Diarrhea related to effects of TPN solution

- Constipation related to effects of TPN solution
- Impaired physical mobility related to IV therapy
- Feeding and bathing/hygiene self-care deficits related to use of an extremity for peripheral IV therapy
- Potential for infection related to break in aseptic technique or contamination of IV line, skin site, IV solution
- Hyperthermia related to infection

Planning and Implementation

The major goals of the patient are to attain and maintain an adequate fluid or nutritional intake.

The major goals of nursing management are to administer the IV solution (eg, fluids, blood, or TPN) as prescribed, observe the patient for potential complications, and observe and record the patient's response to therapy.

Hospital policy may dictate that certain members of the health care team be responsible for starting various types of infusions. In some institutions, a team of specially trained personnel are assigned to initiate IV therapy.

The intake and output of all patients who receive IV therapy should be monitored. If the intake-output ratio shows a decided change, the physician should be notified.

The patient should be observed for signs of complications, such as systemic or local infection, fluid overload, blood transfusion reactions, and phlebitis.

If the patient is receiving TPN, the urine should be checked for glucose and ketone bodies every 4 to 6 hours, because the patient may or may not be producing a sufficient amount of endogenous insulin. The physician should be notified if the urine tests positive for glucose or ketones. Serum electrolyte and albumin determinations usually are ordered and the TPN formula adjusted by the physician.

Some drugs (eg, water-soluble vitamins and potassium chloride) are added directly to an IV solution before administration because they *must* be given in dilute form. Unless there is a specific written order to the contrary, solutions that contain potassium should not be infused at a rate faster than 40 mEq every 4 to 6 hours. A rapid rise in the serum potassium level, which can result from a too-rapid infusion rate, may produce dysrhythmias, which can be fatal. In an emergency, the maximum rate of infusion is 40 mEq every 2 hours, and a written order stating the time limit of the infusion must be obtained.

Some drugs are administered at specified intervals and need not be diluted by a full container of an IV solution. Additive sets, such as a volume-control set or an IV piggyback set, are used for intermittent IV drug administration. When a volume-control set is used, the medication is administered over a 15- to 30-minute period. Drugs administered by IV piggyback are given over a time period ordered by the

physician or recommended by the drug manufacturer. When drugs are added to an IV solution, the container should be labeled with the name and dose of the drug added and the date and time the drug was added to the solution.

For a summary of the principles that apply to IV therapy, see Chart 13-1.

Anxiety. The patient should be given an explanation of the procedure, and be informed of the potential for momentary discomfort when the needle or catheter is inserted.

Administration. Maintenance of the correct infusion rate is important to prevent fluid (circulatory) overload. The infusion rate should be monitored every 15 minutes (more frequently if the patient is restless), and adjusted as needed. At the time the infusion rate is checked, the area around the needle should be examined for signs of extravasation or infiltration, such as swelling and blanching of the skin. If extravasation or infiltration occurs, the infusion must be discontinued and a new line inserted in another vein. Some IV drugs (eg, levarterenol [Levophed]) can cause *severe* tissue damage if extravasation or infiltration occurs, and the physician must be notified immediately because treatment of the area usually is required.

The rate of administration usually is expressed as number of drops per minute. The usual flow rate is 30 to 60 drops/min, depending on the number of drops per milliliter delivered by a specific type of IV administration set. Unless a pump or controller is used to control the rate of infusion (or the number of drops per minute), the nurse is responsible for making sure that the volume and flow rate are correct. IV pumps and controllers must still be checked at peri-

---

Chart 13–1. Intravenous Therapy: Important Points to Remember

- ☐ Use aseptic technique to prevent the introduction of microorganisms into the bloodstream.
- ☐ Clearly label all intravenous solution bottles or bags when drugs are added.
- ☐ Maintain correct flow (infusion) rate.
- ☐ Observe patient for signs of complications of intravenous therapy.
- ☐ Observe site of infusion (point where needle enters the skin and the surrounding area) for extravasation of solution into surrounding tissues.
- ☐ Discontinue infusion before bottle (or bag) and tubing are empty.

odic intervals, since equipment failure or other problems may occur. The visual and audio alarm systems must be turned on whenever the unit is in use. The physician may order more rapid administration in patients who are severely dehydrated, or slower administration in elderly patients or those with cardiovascular disease, or when the solution contains a potent drug.

If a large volume of any IV solution has infused at a rapid rate, the patient is closely observed for signs of fluid overload. Signs and symptoms include headache, weakness, blurred vision, behavioral changes (confusion, stupor, disorientation, delirium, drowsiness), weight gain, incoordination, isolated muscle twitching, a rise in intracranial pressure accompanied by a rise in blood pressure and a decrease in pulse rate, and hyponatremia. Cardiopulmonary signs and symptoms include dyspnea; orthopnea; pulmonary rales; wheezing; coughing; increase or decrease in blood pressure; distended neck veins; elevated central venous pressure; dizziness; fatigue; weight gain; peripheral edema; oliguria; severe anxiety; extreme restlessness; confusion; weak, rapid pulse rate; cold, cyanotic, or mottled extremities; and copious amounts of frothy, blood-tinged sputum.

An infusion should be discontinued (or more solution added as ordered) before the bag or bottle and tubing are empty. This prevents air from entering the vein from the container. In addition, allowing the container to completely empty can cause a blood clot to form in the needle. As a result, the needle must be reinserted, causing the patient unnecessary discomfort.

If a needle is used and it enters an arm vein over a joint or in the back of the hand, the arm or hand should be supported with a splint, a special metal holder, or other supportive device. If the arm does not have excessive hair, it can be loosely fastened to the board with adhesive tape or Velcro straps at both ends and near the needle. If the patient's arm has an abundance of hair, the site can be shaved before the infusion is started. The support should be snug enough to hold, but not so tight that it compresses the blood vessels.

Before administering whole blood or packed red blood cells, the nurse should make sure that the patient's name, blood type, and Rh type on the blood bag label matches the information on the patient's chart. There also should be documentation on the container that a type and cross-match were performed. Vital signs should be taken before the infusion is started. During and after administration, the patient should be observed for signs and symptoms of a transfusion reaction, which include chills, fever, dyspnea, cyanosis, sudden sharp pain in the lumbar region, headache, nausea, tightness in the chest, urticaria, pruritus, and wheezing. If one or more of these occur, hospital policy regarding transfusion reactions should be followed. In most institutions, the transfusion is discontinued, normal saline solution is infused at a keep-vein-open rate, and the physician is notified immediately. If it is been determined that a transfusion reaction has occurred, the blood container and IV tubing should be sent to the blood bank. Hemoglobinuria (blood in the urine) may occur after a hemolytic transfusion reaction. Specimens from three or four consecutive voidings or urine collected from an indwelling catheter for a total of 6 to 8 hours (depending on hospital policy) is sent to the laboratory for examination for hemoglobinuria.

An allergic transfusion reaction is treated with antihistamines. Treatment of a hemolytic reaction is directed toward prevention of renal damage that may follow hemoglobinuria. Mannitol (an osmotic diuretic) may be administered to increase urine output. Intake and output should be monitored and the physician notified immediately of any decrease in urine output.

Diarrhea or Constipation. Patients who are receiving TPN may develop diarrhea or constipation because of the formula or other factors. Bowel function should be monitored, and alterations (constipation, diarrhea) brought to the attention of the physician, as a change in formula may be necessary.

Feeding and Bathing/Hygiene Self-Care Deficits, Impaired Physical Mobility. The administration of an IV infusion must not interfere with nursing care. The patient should be assisted with the activities of daily living as needed. In some instances, complete care is required.

The arm used for IV therapy should be firmly supported and the tubing kept loose when the patient is turned or repositioned, to avoid dislodging the needle or catheter.

Potential for Infection. The dressings over the venipuncture site should be changed every 48 to 72 hours, or according to hospital policy. The site should be inspected daily for inflammation, redness, and streaking. If these symptoms occur, the physician should be notified.

Aseptic technique should be followed when IV therapy is started, when additional IV solution is added, when medications are administered by the IV route, and when dressings are changed over the TPN infusion site. Failure to adhere to the principles of aseptic technique can result in the introduction of pathogenic organisms into the bloodstream. Hospital protocol for dating and changing the IV tubing and filter should be followed.

Hyperthermia. Vital signs should be monitored every 4 hours. If the patient's temperature is elevated or the patient has chills, the physician should be notified *immediately*.

Evaluation

■ Fluid volume deficit is corrected
■ Anxiety caused by institution of IV therapy is reduced or eliminated
■ Fluid volume deficit or excess does not occur during administration
■ Diarrhea is detected early and reported to the physician
■ Altered nutrition (less or more than body requirements) does not occur during administration
■ Patient performs activities of daily living within limits of immobility related to IV therapy
■ No signs of systemic or local infection are present
■ Body temperature remains normal
■ Complications related to IV therapy are absent
■ Hospital protocol regarding administration and observation of IV solutions is followed

General Nutritional Considerations

☐ Patients who are receiving IV therapy may not be permitted food or fluids by mouth. Such patients, however, may be permitted to have ice chips.

☐ TPN formulas are tailored and adjusted to meet individual patients' requirements. The glucose content provides calories, and essential amino acids, electrolytes, vitamins, and minerals are added during preparation by the hospital pharmacist.

☐ Patients who are receiving TPN require administration of IV lipid solutions, usually twice per week.

General Gerontologic Considerations

☐ IV solutions usually are given at a slower rate because most elderly patients have cardiac or renal disorders.

☐ The elderly patient's skin may be traumatized by the application of a tourniquet. Placing a hand towel, a washcloth, or the sleeve of the patient gown over the area may reduce skin trauma.

☐ Because the veins of elderly people tend to be rigid, difficulty may be encountered during a venipuncture procedure. Poor skin turgor also may make it difficult to keep the skin taut over the vein (which stabilizes the vein while the needle or catheter is being inserted).

☐ Confused or disoriented patients must be observed at frequent intervals because excessive movement or pulling on the IV line may dislodge the needle.

☐ Elderly patients are more prone to fluid (circulatory) overload and should be closely observed for signs and symptoms of this complication, even when the solution is infusing at a slower rate.

Suggested Readings

☐ Barrus D, Danel G. Should you irrigate an occluded IV line? Nursing '87 March 1987;17:63. *(Additional coverage of subject matter)*

☐ Channell SR. Manual of IV therapy procedures. 2nd ed. Oradell, NJ: Medical Economics, 1985. *(Additional coverage of subject matter)*

☐ Delaney CW, Lauer ML. Intravenous therapy: a guide to quality care. Philadelphia: JB Lippincott, 1988. *(Additional and in-depth coverage of subject matter)*

☐ Delaney CW, Lauer ML. Intravenous therapy: guide for quality practice. Philadelphia: JB Lippincott, 1988. *(Additional coverage of subject matter)*

☐ Dunn D, Lenihan S. The case for saline flush. Am J Nurs June 1987;87:798. *(Additional coverage of subject matter)*

☐ Gahart BL. Intravenous medications: a handbook for nurses and other allied health personnel. 5th ed. St Louis: CV Mosby, 1988. *(Additional coverage of subject matter)*

☐ Gasparis L, Murray EB, Ursomanno P. IV solutions: which one's right for your patient? Nursing '89 April 1989;19:62. *(Additional coverage of subject matter)*

☐ Klass K. Troubleshooting central line complications. Nursing '87 November 1987;17:58. *(In-depth coverage of subject matter)*

☐ LaRocca JC, Otto SE. A pocket guide to intravenous therapy. St Louis: CV Mosby, 1988. *(Additional coverage of subject matter)*

☐ Magdziak BJ. There's just no excuse for IV complications. RN February 1988;51:30. *(Additional coverage of subject matter)*

☐ Millam DA. Managing complications of IV therapy. Nursing '88 March 1988;18:34. *(Additional coverage of subject matter)*

☐ Millam DA. Tips for improving your venipuncture techniques. Nursing '87 June 1987;17:46. *(Additional coverage of subject matter)*

☐ Morris LL. Critical care's most versatile tool RN May 1988;51:42. *(Additional coverage of subject matter)*

☐ Northridge JA. Calculating IV medications with confidence. Nursing '87 September 1987;17:55. *(Additional coverage of subject matter)*

☐ Peck NL. Action stat! Blood transfusion reactions. Nursing '87 January 1987;17:33. *(Additional coverage of subject matter)*

☐ Sherman JE, Sherman RH. IV therapy that clicks. Nursing '89 May 1989;19:50. *(Additional coverage and illustrations that reinforce subject matter)*

☐ Viall CD. Your complete guide to central venous catheters. Nursing '90 February 1990;20:34. *(Additional coverage and illustrations that reinforce subject matter)*

Chapter 14
The Patient in Pain

On completion of this chapter the reader will:

- Discuss the physiologic and neurologic mechanisms of pain

- List the factors that can influence response to pain

- Discuss the effects of pain

- Discuss the noninvasive and invasive methods of relieving pain

- Use the nursing process in the management of the patient experiencing pain

Pain is a complex phenomena that is not fully understood. Various theories have been expounded for the manner in which pain is received by higher centers of the brain.

Pain is a disagreeable sensation caused by a potentially harmful stimulus. What may be mild pain for one person can be moderate or even severe pain for another. There is no way a nurse can determine the amount of pain experienced by a patient. The only information the nurse has is what comes from the patient—an expression, a statement, an emotional reaction. When patients say they have pain—*they have pain!* The exceptions are the malingerer, and the narcotic addict who is faking pain to obtain an opioid and prevent withdrawal symptoms.

Not everyone reacts to pain in the same manner; nor does everyone experience it in a like way. The patient who cries when in pain is *no different* from the patient who bears severe pain in silence. For each, pain is a real and private sensation.

PHYSIOLOGIC AND NEUROLOGIC MECHANISMS OF PAIN

The theories of pain include the specificity theory, the pattern theory, and the gate control theory. Two substances produced endogenously, endorphins and enkephalins, also appear to mediate pain perception.

Specificity Theory. The specificity theory states that pain occurs because specific pain receptors, when stimulated, transmit the sensation of pain to higher centers of the brain.

Pattern Theory. The pattern theory involves the sharing of pain receptors with other sensory modalities, and the same nerve (or neuron) can transmit both painful and nonpainful stimuli.

Gate Control Theory. A modification of the specificity theory, the gate control theory states that "gates" in the spinal cord control the transmission of pain sensations to higher levels of the brain. The simultaneous firing of large nerve fibers carrying stimuli evoked by touch and of smaller fibers that carry pain information creates a gate effect that blocks the transmission of pain impulses going to the brain. This theory may explain why the use of transcutaneous electrical nerve stimulation (TENS) has helped some people with chronic pain.

Endorphins and Enkephalins. Endorphins and enkephalins are produced by the central nervous system. These substances mimic the actions of morphine, and thus bind to opioid receptor sites in the brain. By binding to these receptor sites, they provide analgesia by raising the threshold to pain, and thus can produce varying degrees of pain relief.

FACTORS THAT INFLUENCE PAIN RESPONSE

Many factors influence a person's interpretation of and response to pain. Physical activity may increase the amount of pain a person feels, or it may make him or her temporarily forget about it. Anticipation can heighten the response to pain; for example, the patient who watches the nurse prepare an injection may anticipate pain. Response to pain also may be learned, as is the case with children who imitate their parents' reactions to pain. On the other hand, parents may suggest to their children what they believe is the correct response to pain. A son may be reminded that "men don't cry if they have pain," or a daughter may be encouraged to miss school when she has only mild menstrual discomfort.

Pain experienced in the past may influence a person's current or future response to pain. This is an important point to remember during preoperative preparation of the patient who has had previous surgery. The pain or discomfort experienced at that time may influence a response to pain during the postoperative period.

Response to pain or discomfort may be culturally influenced. In one culture or ethnic group, pain may evoke a highly charged emotional response in either or both sexes; in another group, pain is expected to be borne with stoic silence. Emotional reactions to pain are by no means consistent for all members of any particular group, and the nurse must avoid stereotyped opinions when evaluating the patient who is in pain.

Pain may be acute or chronic. *Acute pain* describes a painful stimulus that lasts for a short time, usually less than 6 months. *Chronic pain* lasts for more than 6 months. These terms usually are used to describe the duration of pain rather than its severity.

EFFECTS OF PAIN

Sudden, severe pain can cause shock; if the patient is already in shock, it can deepen the disorder. Severe pain must be relieved as soon as possible. Severe pain also can increase restlessness, which may be undesirable in patients with severe injuries or cardiac problems. Another consequence of pain is anorexia, which can be serious if food intake is decreased over a long period. A nutritious, well-balanced diet often is an important part of medical treatment. It may be necessary for the nurse or the dietitian to discuss this problem with the patient, choosing favorite foods while staying within the range of a well-balanced diet suited to meet the patient's nutritional requirements. Small, frequent meals may be needed to supply an adequate and nutritious diet.

Pain affects the mind as well as the body. Constant pain wears down a person's ability to tolerate any pain or discomfort. People who experience chronic pain may be subject to a variety of physical and emotional problems, such as depression, ulcers, increased blood pressure, and difficulty sleeping. Some patients' need for analgesics may increase, or they may become exhausted, severely depressed, or suicidal.

NONINVASIVE PAIN RELIEF MEASURES

Analgesics. Narcotic and nonnarcotic analgesics are used to relieve pain. Narcotic analgesics, such as meperidine, morphine sulfate, and hydromorphone, are used to control moderate to severe pain. Other narcotic analgesics, such as propoxyphene and codeine sulfate, are indicated for mild to moderate pain. Nonnarcotic analgesics, such as acetaminophen, aspirin, ibuprofen, and salicylate derivatives, are used for mild to moderate pain. Nonsteroidal antiinflammatory agents, such as naproxen and piroxicam, are used for certain arthritic disorders. Other drugs used specifically in the treatment of conditions such as gout, rheumatoid arthritis, and migraine headaches are not classed as analgesics, but do relieve the pain associated with these disorders.

There are two concerns associated with the long-term use of narcotic analgesics. One is the development of addiction; the second is drug tolerance, which in turn requires an increased dose of the drug to produce the desired result. Neither of these concerns applies to the terminally ill patient, who must be kept as comfortable as possible without fear of addiction or drug tolerance, but they must be considered in the treatment of chronic pain.

Some nonnarcotic analgesics, when used daily over an extended period, can cause undesirable side effects, such as gastrointestinal bleeding and hemorrhagic disorders. Because some of these drugs are available over the counter, they may be overused, and their adverse effects may go undetected by the patient.

Patient-Controlled Analgesia. Patient-controlled analgesia allows patients to administer their own analgesic by means of an intravenous pump system. The dose and the time interval permitted between doses is programmed into the device to prevent accidental overdosage.

Intraspinal Analgesia.

In intraspinal analgesia, a narcotic or local anesthetic is infused into the subarachnoid or epidural space of the spinal cord by means of a catheter inserted by the physician. The analgesic is administered as ordered, usually several times per day or as a continuous low-dose infusion. This method of analgesia relieves pain with minimal systemic drug effects. When used in terminally ill patients or those who require long-term analgesia, there is less chance that the subcutaneous tissues will be affected by repeated injections or fail to provide analgesia because of poor drug absorption.

Transcutaneous Electrical Nerve Stimulation.

Transcutaneous electrical nerve stimulation is used to treat some forms of acute and chronic pain. It is safe and does not produce systemic side effects. This procedure involves the use of a battery-operated unit with electrodes that are placed on the skin at appropriate sites, for example directly over the affected area or structure, at areas along a nerve pathway, or at points distal to the painful area. Placement sites may be changed by the physician or dentist if the patient's pain is not relieved.

The electrodes deliver an electrical impulse (or stimulus) at a prescribed amplitude (the amount of current delivered), pulse width (or duration of the impulse as measured in microseconds), and pulse frequency (the number of impulses per second). In some instances, the patient is instructed to change the amplitude and pulse width of the electrical stimulus when using TENS on an outpatient basis.

The electrodes usually are covered and secured with a karaya pad. They must be removed once a day, the skin cleansed and allowed to dry, and the site checked for redness. Persistent redness of the area may necessitate a change in electrode placement.

Outpatients who use TENS should be examined periodically for effectiveness of the unit. Some patients may receive only minimal relief from these units or find that the units become less effective after a period of time, whereas others experience long-term full or partial pain relief.

Heat and Cold.

Application of heat, by means of a heating pad or moist hot packs, may provide relief of minor pain such as that caused by arthritis, muscle strain or sprain, and soft-tissue injury. In addition to controlling bleeding and swelling resulting from minor injuries, cold may be used for pain. Neither heat nor cold applications are effective in controlling deep-seated, severe pain. Some forms of chronic pain respond to the application of heat or cold.

H-Wave Dental Anesthesia.

The H-wave device uses an electronic signal delivered to gum tissue. This signal intercepts the pain messages going to and being perceived by the brain. The patient can increase or decrease the signal by means of a control box.

This type of anesthesia is started at a low amplitude, at which time the patient feels a tingling sensation. The amplitude is slowly increased until it reaches a level where anesthesia occurs. The time required to reach anesthesia varies, but the average appears to be 10 to 20 minutes. During the time of painful manipulations or procedures, the patient can increase the amplitude for a brief period. H-wave anesthesia is being tested for other uses, such as relieving pain caused by sports injuries.

Acupuncture.

Although not accepted by all medical personnel, acupuncture has provided pain relief for some patients. Needles are inserted at selected sites and twirled or vibrated by means of an electric current or by the fingers. Relief of pain, especially the chronic type, is not permanent, and repeated treatments are almost always necessary.

Other Noninvasive Techniques.

Other noninvasive techniques used in pain management include distraction, relaxation, guided imagery, biofeedback, and hypnosis. The effectiveness of any of these techniques is not predictable. Some patients may benefit greatly from any one of these techniques, whereas others do not.

INVASIVE PAIN RELIEF MEASURES

Sometimes pain cannot be controlled by analgesic medications, other noninvasive measures, and appropriate nursing management. This type of pain is termed *intractable pain,* and the physician may decide to perform a neurosurgical procedure to provide relief. A laminectomy must first be performed on the patient who has a rhizotomy or cordotomy, to expose the operative area. Care during the postoperative period is the same as for any laminectomy procedure.

Posterior Rhizotomy.

Posterior rhizotomy involves the sectioning of the posterior nerve root just before it enters the spinal cord. Posterior spinal nerves are sensory, thus sectioning prevents sensory impulses from entering the spinal cord and going to the brain. This results in a *permanent* loss of sensation in the area supplied by the sectioned nerve. More than one nerve may need to be sectioned to produce the desired results. Some patients, especially those who are terminally ill, may be unable to tolerate this surgery. A chemical rhizotomy (using chemicals such as alcohol or phenol to destroy the nerve) is an alternative, and

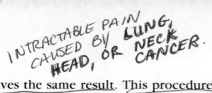
INTRACTABLE PAIN CAUSED BY LUNG, HEAD, OR NECK CANCER.

often gives the same result. This procedure usually is reserved for those with intractable pain caused by lung cancer and head or neck cancer.

Cordotomy.
Cordotomy is an interruption of pain pathways in the spinal cord. Like a rhizotomy, this is a major surgical procedure. Sensory nerve tracts in the vertebral column are destroyed, thus preventing sensory nerve impulses from going to the brain. Loss of sensation is permanent.

Percutaneous Cervical Cordotomy.
Percutaneous cervical cordotomy is basically the same procedure as a cordotomy, but it carries less surgical risk and usually is better tolerated by terminally ill patients. Guided by fluoroscopy, the surgeon inserts a needle through the skin (percutaneous) in the area of the neck (cervical) near the mastoid process. Pain pathways are interrupted by movement of the needle. This procedure is performed under local anesthesia.

NURSING PROCESS —THE PATIENT EXPERIENCING PAIN

Assessment
Any patient who has pain deserves *immediate* attention. Before nursing measures are instituted, the patient must be quickly and accurately evaluated (Chart 14-1). The exact location of the pain is important. The patient who has had abdominal surgery but complains of pain in the incision *and* leg requires additional assessment of the leg pain plus examination by a physician. Pain in the incision is to be expected, but leg pain may be a complication of surgery. If the patient is not asked *where* the pain is, a potentially serious condition may go unnoticed.

A description of pain is patient-oriented; in other words, it gives the patient's view. An exact description may aid in diagnosis. Pain that changes from dull to sharp, pain that begins in the chest and radiates down the arm, intermittent pain that becomes a steady pain—all may indicate a specific disease, problem, or change in the patient's condition. In turn, such a change may prompt the physician to institute a different medical or surgical treatment, order diagnostic studies, or prescribe additional medication. Noting whether a specific situation or activity brings on the pain may clarify the diagnosis or indicate a need for additional therapeutic measures.

It also is important to note what, if anything, relieves the pain. For example, the patient who has abdominal pain may notice that the pain is relieved after she eats, or the patient who experiences chest pain while walking may observe that the pain disappears when he is resting. *VERY IMP!*

Nursing Diagnosis
The nursing diagnoses are based on such factors as the type of pain, the patient's response to pain, the type of analgesic administered, and the patient's response to the analgesic. The following diagnoses may apply:

- Anxiety related to anticipation of pain or to nonrelief of pain by means of conventional methods
- Fear related to pain or the illness causing pain
- Self-care deficits (partial to total) related to the central nervous system (CNS) depressant effects of a narcotic analgesic
- Activity intolerance related to the effects of the administered analgesic
- Constipation related to the effects of the narcotic analgesic on the gastrointestinal tract
- Potential for injury related to the CNS depressant effects of a narcotic analgesic
- Fluid volume deficit related to failure to take oral fluids secondary to the CNS depressant effects of an analgesic
- Altered nutrition: less than body requirements secondary to the CNS depressant effects of an analgesic
- Impaired gas exchange related to the respiratory depressant effect of a narcotic analgesic
- Sleep pattern disturbance related to sleeping at intervals throughout the day secondary to the periodic CNS depressant effect of a narcotic analgesic, presence of unrelieved pain
- Ineffective individual coping related to chronic pain
- Knowledge deficit of precautions taken after an invasive procedure to relieve pain, precautions taken after administration of a narcotic analgesic, postdischarge therapy with narcotics

---

Chart 14–1. Assessment of Pain

Initial Assessment
- Location
- Description of the pain: Sharp, dull, stabbing, throbbing, squeezing, radiating, intermittent, steady, severe, mild, bearable, superficial
- Relation to circumstance: What (if anything) brings on the pain? Does anything relieve the pain (eg, change of position, walking)?
- Onset: Sudden, gradual

Evaluation of Nursing Management
- Was the pain relieved by an analgesic?
- Were nursing measures used? Were they successful?

Planning and Implementation

The major goals of the patient are to attain and maintain a pain-free state.

The major goal of nursing management is to relieve pain by using prescribed therapy (eg, administering analgesics or applying warm soaks) or nursing interventions (eg, changing the patient's position).

Analgesics should be administered *promptly* (Fig. 14-1). Sometimes nurses become hardened to demands for analgesics, and the patient may be labeled a clock-watcher or accused of being a "baby about pain." Making a patient wait creates anxiety, and anxiety may increase pain. If an analgesic is not administered promptly and pain is allowed to reach maximum intensity, the drug will not be as effective as when it is given before the pain becomes intense.

After administering an analgesic, it is important to determine the effect of the drug. Many analgesics relieve most or all of the pain in about 30 to 45 minutes, at which time the patient should be questioned about the effect of the analgesic. If the pain has not been relieved, the patient should be reassessed and the physician notified.

In addition to administering an analgesic, the nurse can institute the care measures listed in Chart

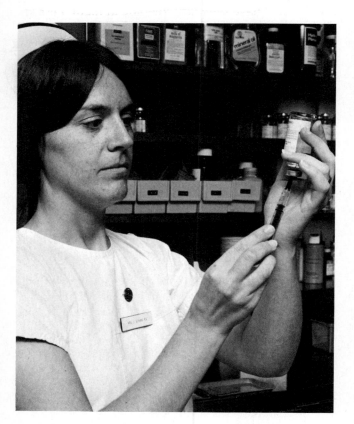

Figure 14–1. When the patient has pain, analgesics should be prepared and administered promptly. (Photograph by D. Atkinson)

Chart 14–2. Nursing Management of the Patient With Pain

- Administer analgesics promptly. Note whether the medication relieves pain.
- Create a position of comfort for the patient.
- Provide distraction or diversion: television, radio, the companionship of other patients.
- If the pain is caused by pressure on one or more parts of the body, attempt to relieve the pressure. Change the patient's position frequently.
- Reduce or eliminate noise and disturbances.
- Be gentle in giving care.
- Reduce as much as possible excessive and unnecessary activities during morning care—turning, feeding, changing bed linen, and so on.
- Ice (chips, collar, packs) can relieve certain types of pain. A physician's order for them usually is needed.
- Moist heat may relieve muscle pain and stiffness. It usually requires a physician's order.
- Surgical patients need support for the incision when they are coughing, turning, and doing deep-breathing exercises.

14-2 to relieve pain or discomfort. These measures may not be effective for all patients.

Pain can be intensified by *additional* discomforts. An example is the patient with pain in a surgical incision *and* back pain from lying in one position for an extended period. Noise also may decrease the patient's ability to tolerate pain; it may even exacerbate the pain. The nurse should speak softly when talking to a patient and perform activities quietly.

Although narcotic and nonnarcotic analgesics reduce pain during the postoperative period, nursing measures may be used to further reduce discomfort. Before surgery, the patient should be taught how to support the incision while coughing and breathing deeply, to take the strain off the incision and reduce the pulling or tearing sensation often felt during these movements. Chest tubes, urethral catheters, and suprapubic tubes may cause discomfort or pain, and should be checked for excessive tension. Uncomfortable positions, rigid restraint of the arms during administration of intravenous fluids, wrinkles or lumps in the bedding, and drafts can add to the patient's discomfort. Extra effort and ingenuity go a long way toward relieving these problems.

Initially, patients who have undergone invasive procedures to relieve pain are likely to complain of pain in the operative site; they also may state that there is no relief from the pain for which the surgery was performed. They should be reassured that it takes several days before relief is noted. In reality, the patient has no pain in the areas supplied by the sectioned spinal nerves or spinal tracts. Possibly the brain has "learned" that this is a painful area, and the pain may remain for several days or longer, even though no sensory impulses are reaching the brain. Other patients may notice relief almost immediately.

Postoperative assessments include checking for sensory and motor integrity. The physician may order sensory evaluation of the area by use of a (sterile) pin. The area is pricked with the pin, and the patient is then asked if anything is felt. The nurse's fingertip should be used several times, instead of the pin, to confirm the validity of the patient's response. The patient should be asked to move all four extremities (motor loss is abnormal) as a check for motor ability. Any change in motor ability must be reported at once. The bed usually is kept flat and the patient logrolled every 2 hours.

Anxiety and Fear. Some patients express or show anxiety or fear regarding the pain they are experiencing, or the pain they anticipate experiencing, as well as concern over the effect of drugs to relieve pain. Anxiety and fear also may be caused by the seriousness of the patient's disease. These patients must be reassured that all members of the health care team are working toward relieving their pain.

Feeding and Bathing/Hygiene Self-Care Deficits. Patients who are receiving narcotics or other drugs capable of causing CNS depression may be unable to carry out activities of daily living. Assistance should be given as needed, and these activities scheduled so that the patient can participate in self-care as much as possible. The timing of the activities depends on the patient's reaction to the analgesic.

Constipation. Some analgesics, especially the narcotics, cause constipation. Bowel movements should be recorded, and the physician notified if the patient goes longer than 2 days without a bowel movement; a laxative or stool softener may be ordered.

Potential for Injury. Patients who are receiving analgesics that affect the CNS may be lethargic, confused, and drowsy, and may suffer injury when getting out of bed or performing activities of daily living. The call button should be placed within easy reach, and the patient instructed to ask for help when getting out of bed. Side rails should be raised, but the use of restraints should be avoided unless this becomes absolutely necessary. A restrained patient can become confused and extremely restless.

Food and Fluid Intake. Patients who are receiving narcotic analgesics may lose their appetite as well as decrease their fluid intake. Fluids should be offered at intervals throughout the waking hours. Anorexia may necessitate offering the patient small meals four or more times per day and encouraging him or her to eat or be fed, if necessary. The dietitian should be consulted regarding between-meal feedings as well as the selection of food.

Impaired Gas Exchange. Some narcotics have a depressant effect on the respiratory system. Before a narcotic is administered, the patient's respiratory rate should be checked. If it is 10 or fewer breaths/min, the drug should be withheld. Because the potential for respiratory depression exists for 1 or more hours after the drug is administered, the patient is encouraged to deep-breathe and cough every 1 or 2 hours during the time when the respiratory rate is decreased. The respiratory rate also is monitored after the narcotic is administered, and the physician notified if the rate falls below 10 breaths/min. A narcotic antagonist, which will reverse the effects of the narcotic, may be required.

Sleep Pattern Disturbance. Some patients who are receiving narcotic analgesics experience a sleep pattern disturbance. They sleep for short periods during the day and have difficulty sleeping at night. Disruption in the sleep pattern may result in restless, confusion, and personality changes. The physician should be consulted when the patient appears to have difficulty sleeping during the night or exhibits signs that may indicate a sleep pattern disturbance. Depending on circumstances, such as the patient's need for and response to an analgesic, the physician may prescribe a change in the dose or time interval or a change in the type of analgesic.

Ineffective Individual Coping. Some patients with chronic pain become depressed, withdrawn, or demanding. They may cope poorly with problems and have frequent emotional outbursts. They also may believe that no one is concerned about their pain or is interested in helping them find relief. Patients with chronic pain may need to talk about their pain. Just talking may help to ease the emotional impact of the experience. Sometimes nurses think that unless they are actively doing something, they are not helping their patients. This is not so. Listening is an art, and being an attentive and interested listener may be as valuable as administering medications and treatment. No one task stands alone as the accepted method in the management of pain.

Knowledge Deficit. When a surgical procedure has been performed for pain relief, the patient and the family must be cautioned against exposure of these areas to excessive heat or cold. This includes the application of ice or heating pads and prolonged exposure to the sun. The affected area should be inspected daily for signs of injury, since the patient cannot feel the pain of injury if it should occur. If there is a break in the skin, it also is inspected daily for signs of inflammation or infection. Any severe injury, any injury that does not heal within a reasonable amount of time, or any inflammation or infection that occurs should be reported to the physician immediately.

If an analgesic is ordered for pain relief after discharge from the hospital, the patient should be instructed to take the medication exactly as prescribed and not to increase the dose if the pain worsens. Instead, the patient should contact the physician.

Because CNS depression (eg, sleepiness and slowed reflexes) may occur, the patient is warned not to performed tasks that require alertness, such as driving.

Evaluation

- Pain and discomfort is reduced or eliminated
- Patient obtains full effect of the analgesic
- Anxiety and fear are reduced or eliminated
- Activities of daily living are carried on alone or with assistance
- Patient is able to tolerate activities because of planning and management
- Bowel function is normal
- Injuries are avoided
- Food and fluid intake meets the patient's daily requirements
- Patient takes deep breaths during time of narcotic analgesic effect
- Patient sleeps during the night and stays relatively awake during daytime hours
- Patient exhibits ability to cope with pain and understands concern of medical personnel in relieving pain
- Patients demonstrates an understanding of postoperative care of the area involved after an invasive procedure for relieving pain
- Patient demonstrates an understanding of postdischarge analgesic use

General Nutritional Considerations

☐ An effort should be made to determine which foods the patient particularly likes and can tolerate.

☐ Painful procedures should be timed so that the patient is at maximum comfort at mealtime.

☐ Small portions and between-meal feedings may be particularly helpful if the patient develops drug- or pain-related anorexia.

General Pharmacologic Considerations

☐ If an analgesic is administered before pain reaches maximum intensity, it is more effective.

☐ Administration of pain-relieving medication should be timed to permit maximum patient cooperation in care, such as turning, walking, and coughing.

☐ The patient should be observed for untoward side effects, especially depressed respirations, when narcotic analgesics are administered.

General Gerontologic Considerations

☐ Pain perception may be diminished in the elderly patient.

☐ Confused, senile, or disorientated patients may not be able to communicate that they have pain or describe the type, location, and intensity of their pain.

☐ Elderly patients usually require a smaller dose of a narcotic analgesic.

☐ Aging may result in chronic diseases such as arthritis, which in turn may produce varying degrees of chronic pain.

☐ Pain perception may be so diminished that the acute pain of disorders such as cholelithiasis, myocardial infarction, and bowel obstruction may not be perceived, and thus not reported to medical personnel.

Suggested Readings

☐ Baquie ML. What matters most in chronic pain management. RN March 1989;52:46. *(Additional coverage of subject matter)*

☐ Fitzgerald J, Shamy P. Let your patient control his analgesia. Nursing '87 July 1987;17:48. *(Additional coverage of subject matter)*

☐ Height K. What you should know about epidural analgesia. Nursing '87 September 1987;17:58. *(In-depth coverage of subject matter)*

☐ Malseed R, Girton SE. Pharmacology: drug therapy and nursing considerations. 3rd ed. Philadelphia: JB Lippincott, 1990. *(Additional and in-depth coverage of subject matter)*

☐ McCaffery M, Beebe A. Pain: clinical manual for nursing practice. St Louis: CV Mosby, 1989. *(Additional and in-depth coverage of subject matter)*

☐ McCaffrey M. Patient-controlled analgesia: more than a nightmare. Nursing '87 November 1987;17:63. *(In-depth coverage of subject matter)*

☐ Owen AS. Nurses plunged me into the pain cycle; nurses pulled me out. RN August 1988;51:22. *(Additional coverage of subject matter)*

☐ Thiederman S. Stoic or shouter, the pain is real. RN June 1989;52:49. *(Additional coverage of subject matter)*

☐ Watt-Watson J. What do we need to know about pain? Am J Nurs September 1987;87:1217. *(Additional coverage of subject matter)*

Chapter 15
Care of the Dying Patient

On completion of this chapter the reader will:

■ Recognize some of the problems of the dying patient

■ Describe the important aspects of nursing care of the dying patient

■ Discuss the needs of the family of the dying patient

■ Begin to formulate personal ideas about death and the dying process

■ Use the nursing process for the management of the dying patient

Our society gives many indications that death is a taboo subject. Euphemisms such as *passed away* are widely used in place of the word *death,* and a great deal of effort and money often go into preparing and showing the body of the deceased in a way that makes it appear that death has not occurred.

Most people have little contact with death because it usually occurs in hospitals, nursing homes, and skilled nursing facilities or as a result of an accident. More often people die surrounded by awesome equipment and busy physicians and nurses dedicated to saving lives. To these health care professionals, the death of a patient may signify their failure as healers. Seldom in the hospital environment is death viewed and discussed as a natural and universal experience. The role of health care workers in supporting these patients and their loved ones during this experience often is neglected because emphasis is placed on the details of therapy that, although necessary and important, do not in themselves convey human caring. Nurses have the opportunity to be involved with patients and families at the time of death—an opportunity that can enable them to help others during one of life's crucial experiences, as well as to grow personally in their understanding and acceptance of death as part of life.

There is growing recognition that attitudes of falseness and denial interfere with providing supportive care for the patient and the family. Patients whose illness is terminal still encounter evasion and a false and superficial cheerfulness that they usually are quick to detect. Family members who realize that the death of a loved one is near frequently have little opportunity to discuss their feelings with nurses and physicians. Avoidance of the dying patient and the family is common, and serves to protect staff members from confronting their own anxieties about death and their own feelings when one of their patients has a terminal illness. Although death can occur in any clinical setting, it is most common on medical–surgical units and in geriatric services.

INSIGHTS AND ATTITUDES

Recent studies of death and dying have provided new insights into the needs of dying patients, their families, and those who care for them in a hospital setting.

Personal Attitudes

Of primary concern are one's personal view of death and the recognition that many patients and their families come to this experience quite unprepared to deal with it. The person whose only experience with death has been a visit to a funeral home is not well prepared for the reality of the change that occurs with the cessation of breathing and sudden stillness, as the patient crosses the threshold from life to death.

The development of one's philosophy and religious beliefs concerning death and of one's ability to accept the reality of death are lifelong tasks to be dealt with again and again as life makes new demands and presents new challenges. People who thought that they understood their views on death may find that they have hardly begun this process when confronted by a sudden death. For the nurse, as well as all people, understanding and facing the idea of death is part of the growth process. Those in the health professions have the opportunity, by their care of patients and their families at the time of death, to enhance their personal growth. The nurse's ability to help patients and families at the time of death is based on understanding and inner growth. It is through understanding, humility, and the recognition and acceptance of death as part of life that the nurse ministers to dying patients and their families. The emphasis is on recognizing what this experience means to these patients and to those who are close to them, helping them to express their thoughts and feelings, and supporting them as they go through the stages of the experience.

Stages of Emotional Reaction

Elisabeth Kübler-Ross defines the five stages before death as denial, anger, bargaining, depression, and acceptance. These stages apply to those who are aware that they have a terminal illness; they may be summarized as follows.

Denial. Patients first deny that their illness is terminal or may have serious consequences, if untreated. They may believe that radiographs are in error, that the diagnosis is incorrect, or that their laboratory tests were mixed up with those of another patient. Some patients go through elaborate mental gymnastics to prove to themselves that this illness is not happening. They may be experiencing symptoms of a potentially fatal illness, yet do not seek medical help because they are denying the fact that they have an illness.

Anger. The second stage is anger: "Why me?" The anger may be directed toward others: physicians, nurses, family, or other patients. Anger also may be expressed in other ways. Patients may complain about care, blame the medical profession for their illness or failure to get better, or make statements such as "If John had a heart attack and went back to work in 8 weeks, why am I so sick?"

Bargaining. The third stage is an attempt to postpone death by bargaining. Usually these bargains are secretly made with God or some other abstract being, with the patient promising to do something if death is postponed.

Depression. The fourth stage is marked by depression as patients realize the truth of the situation. During this stage, they may have a sense of great loss that is multifaceted. They may mourn the loss of money, a change in body image, the loss of employment, or what their illness and, finally, death are doing to the family.

Acceptance. In the fifth stage, patients appear detached, are tired and weak, and may sleep often. They may want to be left alone.

All patients do not follow these stages in an orderly progression, and some may even be in several stages at once (eg, a patient who is angry as well as depressed). It may be difficult to recognize all of these stages, especially if the patient is going through more than one at the same time, and has mixed symptoms or characteristics.

One consideration that is particularly important in working with dying patients is their right to know the seriousness of their condition. Informing patients of the nature and gravity of their illness is the physician's responsibility. It is important that those who care for the patient be made aware of what the patient has been told. Lack of this knowledge greatly interferes with the nurse's relationship with dying patients. For example, the nurse may avoid all but the most superficial subjects of conversation, out of uncertainty about how to respond if the patient should ask, "Am I going to die?"

Most of these patients gradually recognize clues in the behavior of others that indicate that their illness is terminal. Thus, the view of the patient as being thoroughly unaware and seeking a disclosure from the nurse often is incorrect. When patients are given the opportunity, they often bring up awareness of their approaching death by a remark about plans for providing for their children, leaving gifts for their families, and so on. Such comments, when they reflect the patient's realistic assessment of the situation, should be accepted, rather than refuted by such replies as, "You shouldn't talk like that." Sometimes no verbal reply is necessary because the feeling of acceptance of what has been said is expressed nonverbally in the way the nurse conveys caring.

NURSING PROCESS —THE DYING PATIENT

Assessment

Some dying patients are only kept comfortable, whereas others are surrounded by highly technical equipment such as ventilators, intravenous lines, and other methods of treatment or life support. The patient may be resting quietly in bed, sitting in a chair, or lying in a bed in an intensive care unit. Assessment, then, is first based on the patient's *basic* physical problems and needs, such as relief from pain and the need for food and fluids. This is followed by an assessment of the problems and needs that arise from the patient's medical or surgical disorder, such as inadequate ventilation (respiratory) or circulation (cardiac). Finally, assessment is focused on the patient and the family and on their attitudes and approach to the fact that the patient is dying.

Nursing Diagnosis
The following nursing diagnoses are related to the family and the patient's terminal condition. The relation to the nursing diagnosis is highly variable, and can be stated as either directly related to the disorder or related to the fact that the patient is in a terminal stage of illness.

Each may or may not be present, depending on the disease that is the cause of the terminal illness and the patient's condition and individual needs or problems at the time of assessment. Some of these diagnoses (eg, hypothermia) may be seen as the patient nears death; others may be seen days or weeks preceding death. Additional diagnoses may be added if the patient is receiving drugs, such as a narcotic analgesic for pain, or when various forms of medical and surgical interventions are instituted to prolong or support life.

- Activity intolerance
- Impaired adjustment
- Ineffective airway clearance
- Potential for aspiration
- Hypothermia
- Hyperthermia
- Ineffective breathing pattern
- Ineffective family coping: compromised
- Altered family processes
- Fear
- Fluid volume deficit (actual or potential)
- Fluid volume excess (actual or potential)
- Anticipatory grieving
- Hopelessness
- Impaired physical mobility
- Altered nutrition; less than body requirements
- Powerlessness
- Impaired skin and tissue integrity (actual or potential)
- Impaired swallowing
- Sleep pattern disturbance
- Total incontinence
- Altered oral mucous membrane
- Social isolation
- Spiritual distress
- Altered thought processes

Planning and Implementation
The major goal of the patient is to die with dignity.

Four important goals of the nursing management of dying patients are (1) to provide physical care and comfort; (2) to support them as they begin to consider their approaching death; (3) to foster communication with them so that they do not face this experience in increasing isolation from others; and (4) to openly discuss problems with the family.

Physical Care. Primarily, dying patients need consideration as human beings. They require thoughtful attention to physical comfort: position change, mouth care, sips of fluids if they are able to tolerate them, and, when possible, a quiet, restful environment. A disturbance in the sleep pattern may occur because of anxiety, fear, the use of narcotic analgesics, or the presence of bright overhead lights. Bright lights usually are used in intensive care areas, where patients are being extensively monitored and life-support equipment is present. When possible, bright lights should be turned off or dimmed, especially when patients appear to be sleeping.

Because many physical activities cannot be tolerated, these patients need assistance with all or most of their activities of daily living. They should be protected from routine, impersonal care, typified by large numbers of health care workers arriving to take their temperature, provide water pitchers, or check on the liter flow of oxygen. Time should be allowed for talking during physical care and treatments. The patient may bring up concerns or problems at these times, and should not be rushed.

Difficulty in swallowing may create a potential for aspiration of fluids as well as a decrease in food intake. If the patient is able to take oral fluids or food, these should be offered in small amounts. Intake and output should be measured, as intravenous fluid supplementation may be necessary. Providing fluids, calories, electrolytes, and vitamins by either or both of these methods makes the patient more comfortable but does not always prolong life. Because cardiac output may be decreased, the patient who is receiving intravenous fluids should be watched for signs of fluid overload.

These patients may have difficulty breathing, and oxygen therapy or mechanical ventilation may be necessary. They may be unable to cough and raise secretions, and gentle suctioning may be required. If the patient has pulmonary edema, suctioning will *not* clear the lungs or make breathing easier.

A drop in blood pressure or advanced heart failure may result in poor tissue and organ perfusion. The skin must be protected from injury, and the patient's position changed every 2 hours or as needed. Drugs for blood pressure support or cardiac improvement may be administered intravenously. Intramuscular administration of drugs to those with poor tissue perfusion usually produces inadequate drug absorption and, therefore, minimal drug effectiveness.

Incontinence of the bowel or bladder or both may be seen, either because of the patient's disease process or because the patient is in the terminal stages of life. An indwelling catheter may be necessary when bladder control is lost. Bowel incontinence should be recognized immediately, and the anal and perineal areas cleaned and bedding or incontinence pads changed as needed.

Hypothermia may occur as death nears, and the patient may complain of feeling cold. Light blankets may be applied, but they may not make the patient feel warmer. Some patients have an overwhelming infection, and therefore the body temperature may be elevated. Measures such as the administration of an antipyretic drug or the use of a hypothermia blanket may be necessary.

Emotional Support. Because dying patients tend to become isolated from others (Fig. 15-1), it is particularly important to provide additional time when the primary objective of nursing management is to listen and support the patient as death nears.

The family and the patient may go through actual or anticipatory grieving. The *actual grieving* is experienced during the time the patient is dying as well as after death. *Anticipatory grieving* occurs when the family or patient realizes that death is inevitable. Grieving is a normal emotion that is evidenced in many ways. Some may remain quiet, whereas others openly weep or have emotional outbursts. The family as well as the patient should be allowed to go

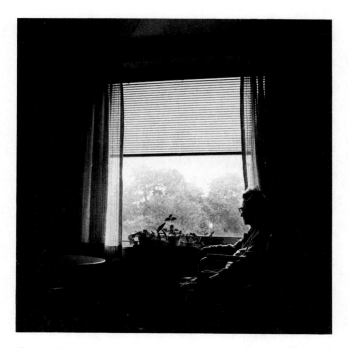

Figure 15–1. The dying patient tends to become isolated from others. (Photograph by D. Atkinson)

through the grieving process without restraint or misunderstanding, and the nurse should be available to be with the family and offer emotional support as needed.

It is important to be sensitive to the patient's spiritual concerns and to help obtain the desired religious counseling and rites. When patients are too ill to express their wishes, the family should be consulted about spiritual care.

Some patients have difficulty adjusting to a terminal illness. They may fear death, the medical treatments that may be necessary, pain, and separation from those they love. A feeling of hopelessness and powerlessness may be present, since they cannot assume responsibility for their decisions. As death nears, or as a result of the disease process or an altered sleep pattern, they may not be aware of their surroundings or recognize family and friends.

Some patients grow and mature as they approach death. Their philosophical and religious views deepen; they develop a broader view of their life and death as natural events in the ebb and flow of life. They may experience a tenderness and closeness toward family and friends they did not feel before. Other patients become progressively disengaged from others as death approaches. In such cases, the family needs to be helped to understand this change. Often patients have a particular need for familiar, treasured possessions. It is especially important to keep the possessions they value nearby.

Fostering Communication. Families of dying patients particularly need the support a nurse can give. Their own process of grieving often begins when they learn that the patient's illness is terminal. Some family members begin to withdraw emotionally from the patient at this time because they find the experience too painful. Others draw closer, realizing that they have only a short time left to be with their loved one. The family's feelings do not necessarily conform to others' idealized views of what these feelings should be.

The more family members can express their feelings to an understanding listener, the better. Sharing helps them to recognize and deal with their innermost emotions and feelings, and allows them to ventilate and share their grief with another. The possible harm that can result from direct expression of feelings between relatives and the dying person is overestimated. Family members may be so cautioned against showing any but cheerful feelings that they assume an air of false cheerfulness when visiting the patient. The patient senses the "mask" and feels isolated from those they turn to for closeness. When family members can no longer keep up the pretense, and show grief, both the relative and the patient often experience relief at the honest communication between them. This does not mean that it is helpful for family members to burden the patient with their grief. One big problem among family members of dying patients in our culture seems to lie in the inability to communicate frankly with the dying person—to express feelings and accept expressions of feelings. Failure to show their tenderness for the dying family member is a source of poignant regret for grieving relatives. The nurse who can accept direct, straightforward communication from families can help them to be more direct with the patient, thereby assisting them to have this enriching experience.

Supporting Family Members.   It is important for the family to have a room where they can have privacy to talk with other relatives, to cry, and to rest. In some hospitals or health care centers, facilities are extremely limited in this regard, and often family members must stand for long periods in the corridor while one or two relatives remain with the patient. Every effort should be made to find a place where the family can have some privacy and be seated comfortably. Frequent visits can be made if they show they want this contact. Just sitting with the family for a short time, expressing concern for their comfort and welfare and listening to some of their concerns, can provide strong emotional support. The family frequently worries about how much the patient is suffering. It is helpful to explain that as life ebbs, so usually does awareness of pain and discomfort. Thus, as death draws near, these patients may seem detached and unaware of those around them. Often they slip into unconsciousness before death. It is then that the family's suffering is likely to be acute, although the patient's is lessened.

Nurses should listen to statements or ideas expressed by dying patients and their families. Some terminally ill patients fear that their lives will be prolonged by mechanical equipment and sophisticated technologies, which only adds physical and emotional pain and suffering to the act of dying. Out of this dilemma have arisen the Living Will, which is not legally binding in all states, and other documents such as the Christian Affirmation of Life. The Living Will requests that physicians allow patients to die if their condition is irreversible; the Christian Affirmation of Life requests that extraordinary means not be used to prolong life. Both documents are capable of creating legal as well as moral and ethical problems because the terms *irreversible* and *extraordinary means* may be difficult, at times, to interpret or define. Ultimately, the determination to prolong life must rest with the physician, who must use legal,

medical, and ethical guidelines as well as discussion with the family to reach a decision.

Helping the family to express their emotions and, as much as possible, to understand what is occurring can help them recover from grief after the patient's death. The nurse has many opportunities to assist the family to deal with the reality of death. After the patient dies, most families leave the hospital at once. Some may want to remain for a time with the body of the deceased, and they should be allowed a period of privacy before postmortem care is given. If family members or relatives seem unusually distraught, it is wise to telephone another family member to come and be with them or call the hospital chaplain.

The nurse who cares for a dying patient also experiences grief and needs support from colleagues and supervisors.

Evaluation

The use of some of the following evaluations depends on the stage of the terminal illness, the physical condition of the patient, and the type and length of the terminal illness. Some occurrences cannot be improved or eliminated, and may need to be omitted or restated.

- Activities of daily living are carried out by the patient (with assistance and as tolerated) or by nursing personnel
- Patient adjusts emotionally to terminal illness
- Airway is kept as clear as possible
- Aspiration of fluids or food is avoided
- Body temperature is normal
- Breathing pattern is normal, or breathing is assisted with oxygen therapy or mechanical ventilation
- Drugs are administered as ordered for improvement of cardiac output
- Family members appear able to cope with the patient's terminal illness
- Family members show support and offer comfort to the patient
- Patient appears less fearful and feelings of hopelessness are diminished
- Patient's fatigue is lessened because of assistance by nursing personnel
- Fluid volume excess or deficit is corrected
- Family and patient exhibit signs of grieving
- Bowel and bladder incontinence is recognized and incontinent care is given
- Patient's nutritional needs are met (orally or intravenously)
- Patient's skin remains intact with no signs of breakdown
- Impaired swallowing is corrected (when possible) by means of frequent oral care
- Sleep pattern is normal
- Patient visited often by family, nursing personnel
- Patient's spiritual needs are met

General Nutritional Considerations

☐ Dietary considerations vary, depending on the cause and nature of the patient's illness.

☐ Patients who have abandoned hope may have little or no appetite. Providing a selection of their favorite foods, mealtime companions, and attractive preparation may encourage them to eat.

☐ Sound nutrition should be encouraged as an aid to helping patients feel as well and as strong as possible, for as long as possible (see Chapter 14).

General Pharmacologic Considerations

☐ Control of pain often is a great challenge (see Chapter 14).

☐ Fears of the patient and staff regarding the possibility of the patient's developing a tolerance to pain-relief medications should be discussed.

☐ Drugs for raising the blood pressure, improving tissue and organ perfusion, and correcting cardiac or circulatory problems may be ordered.

General Gerontologic Considerations

☐ Elderly patients may die alone, without the support of family members, relatives, and close friends. The nurse may be the only person to give close emotional support during the final hours of living.

☐ Nurses may administer less emotional support to dying patients who are elderly. Even though these patients, by reason of age, have reached the termination of life, they still require as much emotional support before death as do young and middle-aged patients.

Suggested Readings

☐ Amenta MO, Bohnet NL. Nursing care of the terminally ill. Boston: Little, Brown & Co, 1986. *(Additional and in-depth coverage of subject matter)*

☐ Anderson D. Death and dying: ethics at the end of life. RN October 1988;51:42. *(Additional coverage of subject matter)*

☐ Clough J. Making life and death decisions you can live with. RN May 1988;51:28. *(Additional coverage of subject matter)*

☐ Cohen CB. Casebook on the termination of life-sustaining treatment and the care of the dying. Bloomington: Indiana University Press, 1987. *(Additional and in-depth coverage of subject matter)*

☐ Davis AJ, Aroskar MA. Ethical dilemmas and nursing practice. Norwalk, CT: Appleton-Century-Crofts, 1983. *(Additional and in-depth coverage of subject matter)*

☐ Ellis K. The slow code dilemma. RN June 1987;50:28. *(Additional coverage of subject matter)*

☐ Ferszt GG, Taylor PB. When your patient needs spiritual comfort. Nursing '88 April 1988;18:48. *(Additional coverage of subject matter)*

☐ Fowler M, Levine-Ariff J. Ethics at the bedside: a source book for the critical care nurse. Philadelphia: JB Lippincott, 1987. *(Additional and in-depth coverage of subject matter)*

☐ Kübler-Ross E. Death: the final stage of growth. Englewood Cliffs, NJ: Prentice-Hall, 1975. *(Closely related to subject matter)*

☐ Kübler-Ross E: On death and dying. New York: Macmillan, 1969. *(Closely related to subject matter)*

☐ Kübler-Ross E: Questions and answers on death and dying. New York: Macmillan, 1974. *(Closely related to subject matter)*

☐ Martin NF. How nursing takes over when medicine gives up. RN March 1988;51:30. *(Closely related to subject matter)*

Chapter 16

Management of the Surgical Patient

On completion of this chapter the reader will:

- Discuss and list routine preparations of the patient going to surgery
- Use the nursing process in the management of the patient during the preoperative period
- Discuss nursing responsibilities during the intraoperative period
- Use the nursing process in the management of the patient during the intraoperative period
- Discuss nursing responsibilities during the postanesthesia period
- Use the nursing process in the management of the patient during the postanesthesia period
- Discuss nursing responsibilities during the recovery period
- Recognize, list, and discuss the major complications that may occur during the postoperative period
- Use the nursing process in the management of the patient during the recovery period

The performance of a surgical procedure is a common event. Many operations are emergencies because they are performed to correct conditions that are life-threatening (eg, bowel obstruction and dissecting aortic aneurysm). Other surgical procedures are less urgent, and may be performed days after the need for surgery is recognized. Some operations are elective procedures, that is, they are scheduled at the convenience of the physician and patient.

A surgical procedure may be performed for one or more of the following reasons:

- Removal of a diseased organ or structure (eg, appendectomy)
- Biopsy or diagnosis (eg, biopsy of a breast lesion)
- Repair or restoration of an organ or structure (eg, colostomy for a bowel obstruction)
- Cosmetic improvement (eg, rhinoplasty)
- Relief of pain (eg, rhizotomy)

TISSUE REPAIR

Any wound or injury results in repair, a mechanism by which the body repairs damage to the skin and underlying structures. As damaged tissue is being cleared of debris, the signal for repair is given. The three types of wound repair are shown in Figure 16-1.

Healing by *first intention* is the ideal method of wound healing. An example of healing by first intention is a surgical scar. The incision edges are approximated and sutured. The suture holds the tissues firmly in this position. Healing occurs, using normal cells and some scar tissue to fill in the defect.

The edges of some wounds may be so far apart that they cannot be pulled together satisfactorily. Infection also may cause a separation of tissue surfaces and prevent wound approximation. The wound defect is left open, and granulation tissue, followed by scar tissue, is allowed to form. Epithelium ultimately grows over the scar tissue. This is healing by *second intention*.

In *third-intention* healing, the wound is first allowed to heal by second intention and then closed surgically when there is no evidence of infection (Fig. 16-2). This type of healing may occur when a deep wound has not been sutured or when a wound breaks down and then is resutured after granulation tissue has formed.

Granulation tissue is delicate and vascular. Great care should be used when changing dressings to avoid damaging newly forming tissues, as well as to spare the patient any unnecessary discomfort. Before removing packing or gauze that has adhered to the tissues, the area should be moistened with sterile saline solution or other solution ordered by the physician.

When the union of tissues is satisfactory, a signal stops further work by the fibroblasts (cells from which connective tissue develops). In the weeks that follow, fibrils (small fibers) harden and contract. The drawing tight of the network of tough fibrils can cause defor-

First Intention

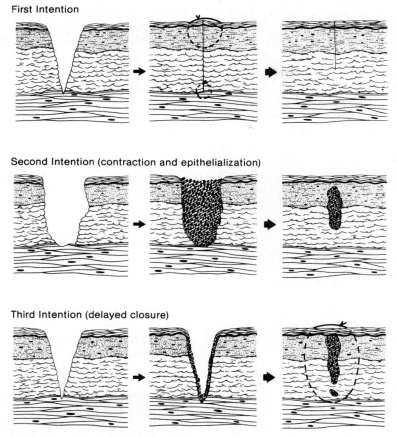

Second Intention (contraction and epithelialization)

Third Intention (delayed closure)

Figure 16–1. Classification of wound healing. *First intention:* A clean incision is made with primary closure; there is minimal scarring. *Second intention* (contraction and epithelialization): The wound is left open to allow formation of granulation tissue with resultant large scab and abnormal dermal–epidermal junction. *Third intention* (delayed closure): The wound is left open and closed secondarily when no evidence of infection is present. (Hardy JD. Hardy's textbook of surgery. Philadelphia, JB Lippincott, 1983:109)

mity. The pull of a contracted scar is strong enough to tilt the head or keep an entire limb in a contorted position. This problem is one reason for attempting care that allows healing with minimum scar formation.

The scar is as strong at 3 weeks as it will ever be, but it continues to change for a long time. With contraction, the scar squeezes out the capillaries that once richly infiltrated its network. It begins to blanch, and over months and years becomes colorless.

Adequate blood flow is the key to healing. Healing is delayed when the blood supply to the wound site is poor. The anterior portion of the lower leg is such a site, and injuries to this area heal more slowly than those to other areas of the leg. Adipose (fat) tissue also has poor vascularity, and heals slowly. Extra care and time are required for healing in an obese person because pads of fat have been joined together within the wound. Circulation should never be impaired. When the patient has a wound on the leg, she should be encouraged to avoid assuming an unfavorable posi-

tion, such as crossing the legs. Excessive tension or pulling on wound edges can delay healing. The nurse should be alert for any signs or symptoms of impaired circulation, such as swelling, coldness, absence of pulse, pallor, or mottling, and should report them immediately. In applying a dressing, particularly to an extremity, the nurse should make certain that it does not impair circulation.

WOUND DISRUPTION

Dehiscence means the separation of wound edges without the protrusion of organs. *Evisceration* means the separation of wound edges with the protrusion of organs. These complications are most likely to occur between the 6th and 8th postoperative days. Predisposing factors include those that interfere with normal healing, such as malnutrition (particularly insufficient protein and vitamin C), defective suturing, and un-

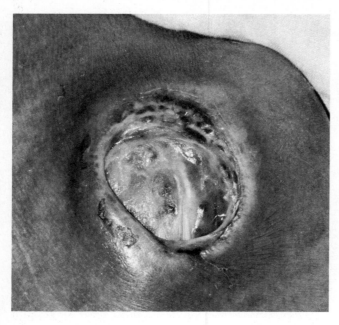

Figure 16–2. Decubitus ulcer showing third-intention healing with the wound filled with granulation tissue. (Photograph by D. Atkinson)

usual strain on the wound from severe coughing, sneezing, retching, or hiccuping. Extreme obesity, an enlarged abdomen, and an abdomen weakened by prior surgeries also may contribute to the occurrence of wound dehiscence and evisceration.

The patient may complain of a sensation of something "giving way." Pinkish drainage may suddenly appear on the dressing. If wound disruption is suspected or has occurred, the patient should be placed at complete rest in a position that puts the least strain on the operative area. If evisceration has occurred, sterile dressings moistened with sterile normal saline solution should be placed over the protruding organs or tissues. The physician should be notified immediately if wound dehiscence or evisceration occurs. Emotional support and reassurance are necessary.

Surgical Procedure

PREOPERATIVE PERIOD

The immediate preoperative preparation of the patient may take place on the nursing unit. Some patients who are scheduled to undergo elective operations are admitted to the hospital on the morning of surgery, arriving at the hospital at least 2 hours before surgery is to take place. Some operations, such as cataract surgery, can be performed on an outpatient basis, with the patient assigned to a special ambulatory unit for preoperative as well as postoperative care.

The preoperative preparation of the patient varies

according to hospital policy, the physician's preoperative orders, the condition of the patient, the type of surgery to be performed, and the time when the patient is admitted to the hospital. A preoperative checklist is used to ensure completion of observations and nursing tasks. Examples of these tasks include taking vital signs and making sure that the operative consent has been signed and that the patient has voided. When these and other details have been carried out with careful attention and due consideration for the patient and the family, the patient is helped onto the stretcher for safe transport to the surgical suite.

Patients who consent to have surgery—particularly operations that require general anesthetics—depend completely on the knowledge, skill, and integrity of health care personnel (Fig. 16-3). In accepting this trust, members of the surgical team have an obligation to make the patient's welfare their first consideration.

Ambulatory Surgery

Some surgical procedures that once required hospitalization are now performed on an outpatient basis. An

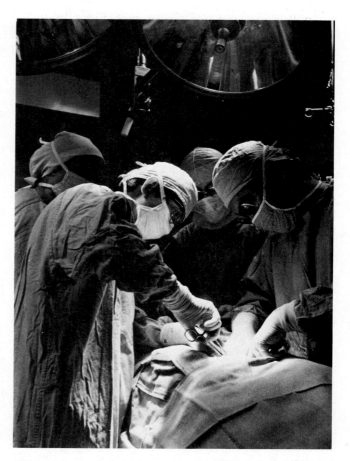

Figure 16–3. The patient who consents to surgery is completely dependent on the abilities of the surgical team. (Photograph by D. Atkinson)

example of an outpatient operation is the removal of a cataract. A special unit may be used for admitting the patient, receiving the patient for recovery from anesthesia, and discharging the patient. Most of these operations are performed under local anesthesia, but an intravenous sedative or relaxant may be administered immediately before as well as during the procedure. An anesthesiologist often is assigned to be with the patient in case administration of a general anesthetic is necessary.

Patients who undergo ambulatory surgery receive the same preoperative and postoperative care as hospitalized patients. Because an intravenous sedative may be administered or a general anesthetic required, these patients are advised to withhold food and fluids beginning at midnight the night before the procedure. During a preoperative visit to the surgeon's office, oral and written instructions are given to the patient. On admission to the unit, a review of the surgeon's preoperative instructions is conducted to be sure the patient has followed instructions. Medications and skin preparation, such as shaving and scrubbing around the surgical area, may have been ordered to be performed by the patient at home. If the patient has neglected one or more of the preoperative instructions, the surgeon is notified immediately.

NURSING PROCESS —PATIENT MANAGEMENT DURING THE PREOPERATIVE PERIOD

Assessment

Surgery may be an emergency, and certain tasks may need to be omitted because of the patient's condition or the urgency for rapid preparation for surgery. In this situation, there may be no time for a thorough assessment, written nursing diagnoses, and thorough evaluation of nursing management. The patient may have conditions or disease states present, such as a fluid volume deficit or altered comfort (pain), that may alter the extent of the assessment and nursing diagnosis.

Some patients are admitted to the hospital during the early morning hours before surgery. In these instances, time for preoperative assessment, nursing diagnoses, and evaluation of nursing management also may be limited. Recognition of the patient's immediate preoperative needs is important, however, and the preparation for surgery still can include the use of the nursing process.

Nursing Diagnosis

The type of surgery to be performed, as well as other factors, may influence the number and extent of the nursing diagnosis. The following diagnoses may apply:

- Anxiety or fear related to surgical procedure and outcome of surgery
- Spiritual distress related to the outcome of the surgical procedure or potential serious consequences of surgery
- Ineffective individual coping related to the results of surgery
- Anticipatory grieving related to the results of surgery
- Altered family processes related to the outcome of the surgical procedure
- Knowledge deficit of the surgical procedure, preparations required before surgery, postoperative tasks performed by the nurse and patient, other factors (specify)

Planning and Implementation

The major goals of the patient are to understand the preparations for surgery, understand and practice those tasks required after surgery, and effectively participate in preparations for surgery.

The major goal of nursing management is to physically, emotionally, and spiritually prepare the patient for surgery.

Anxiety or Fear. Patients who are extremely frightened respond poorly to surgery; they seem to be particularly prone to such complications as cardiac arrest and irreversible shock. Unless the operation is an emergency, many surgeons delay surgery if the patient is very frightened. Patients who are extremely fearful before surgery may show unusual behavior afterward, perhaps not recognizing changes in their bodies that have resulted from surgery, or they may withdraw from others and show signs of depression. The nurse must be on the alert for any unusual emotional reactions exhibited by the patient during the preoperative period, and report them promptly. A tranquilizer may be ordered to relieve the patient's preoperative anxiety.

Preoperative fear and anxiety may be resolved by careful preoperative teaching. Many patients experience these emotions because they know little or nothing about what will happen before, during, and after surgery. Often a simple, brief explanation of some of the tasks performed by nursing personnel or of what will occur in the recovery room helps to allay apprehension. In some hospitals, nurses from the recovery room, postsurgical unit, or intensive care unit visit the patient the evening before surgery. They explain routine postoperative procedures and allow the patient time to ask questions.

PREOPERATIVE TEACHING.   A clear, careful explanation by the surgeon is most important because the patient must understand the reason for surgery and know what results to expect. When the nurse knows what information the physician has given to the patient, she or he is in a better position to help the patient understand any points that are not clear, or to dispel any misconceptions the patient or the family may have.

Before surgery, patients usually are alert and may be free of pain. During the immediate postoperative period, they are drowsy from medication and anesthesia and often have pain. Pain and sleepiness interfere with learning. Thus, it is preferable to teach patients during the preoperative period. Repetition and review may be necessary postoperatively, but patients are better able to participate in their recovery because they know what to expect. The patient is probably anxious, and *anxiety can interfere with learning*. For this reason, the nurse must learn to recognize defenses, such as denial or forgetting, and plan explanations in accordance with the patient's readiness and ability to receive information. Simple, factual explanations, adjusted to the patient's ability and need, are an essential part of a teaching plan. Patients who understand what they can do to help themselves are prepared to cooperate with all members of the health care team.

The information included in the preoperative teaching plan varies with the type of surgery that is to be performed. The following are examples of explanations and demonstrations that may be given to the patient:

- Preoperative medication—when it will be given, what it will do
- Postoperative control of pain
- Explanation and description of the recovery room or specialized postsurgical area
- Why blood pressure and pulse and respiratory rates are monitored frequently during the immediate postoperative period
- How to perform deep-breathing and coughing exercises, and why it is necessary to perform these exercises at regular intervals
- How to splint the incision when deep-breathing and coughing
- How to move the legs and feet and change position, and why it is necessary to change position at regular intervals
- How to use the incentive spirometer

Depending on the type of surgery performed, the nurse also may inform the patient about the possible need to administer intravenous fluids or blood transfusions and to insert an indwelling catheter, a nasogastric tube, or other types of drainage tubes. The patient should be given the opportunity to practice, under supervision, deep-breathing and coughing exercises, foot and leg exercises, splinting of the incision, and position changes.

Many patients fear pain and severe discomfort after surgery. The nurse should explain that medication will be ordered for the relief of pain and discomfort, and that every effort will be made to relieve any postoperative pain.

Patients who are admitted to the hospital for emergency surgery must be prepared as quickly as possible. There is no time for detailed explanations of preoperative preparations and the postoperative period. Even though explanations must be brief, they should be given if the patient is alert enough to understand them. When the patient recovers from surgery, extra thought and attention should be given to helping the patient understand the illness or accident that has occurred.

Spiritual Distress. Religious faith is a source of strength and courage for many patients. Opportunities for them to have contact with their clergymen are especially important as they prepare for surgery. Every effort should be made to help patients maintain their religious ties, either through the services of their own clergymen or through the hospital chaplain.

Ineffective Individual Coping, Anticipatory Grieving. The surgery may result in the loss of a body part or in some other type of change in body function (eg, amputation of a limb or a colostomy). Some people accept the changes that will result from surgery; others have great difficulty doing so. Grieving over the future loss of a part or a function also may begin at this time. The nurse should be aware of patients' verbalizations regarding their surgery, and thus be attuned to their needs. For some, a referral to a support group (eg, the United Ostomy Association) for a preoperative visit may be an advantage, but referrals are made only with physician approval. Despite a great deal of emotional support, some patients cope poorly and are unable to adjust to changes.

Altered Family Processes. Family members need to understand what measures are necessary to prepare a patient for surgery, so that they can participate in the preoperative and postoperative care and provide further explanation and encouragement. Some patients can better accept the necessity for surgery if it is explained by a relative. Family members want to be near patients and help in any way they can during the preoperative period. Their presence helps the patient to feel less alone and conveys the family's concern and interest.

The patient who is admitted for emergency surgery is prepared as quickly as possible. These preparations often are distressing to family members because they are concerned about their relative's welfare. As soon as emergency measures have been carried out, the nurse should spend time talking with the family and help them to understand what has happened.

Patients who have no family members may have friends present before surgery. Friends should receive the same considerations as family members.

Some types of surgery affect not only the patient, but also the family. Family members may be unable to accept the physical changes or losses that result from surgery. Sudden changes in their life-style and the family structure may prompt emotional reactions such as depression, hopelessness, and grief. The nurse should be aware of any family problems that become evident during the preoperative period. If the patient is to be seen by members of a support group before surgery, it may be helpful for the family to be present during the meeting. It may be necessary to allow the family members time to ask questions and talk about their problems. If they appear unable to accept the situation, the nurse should relay this information to the physician.

Knowledge Deficit. Preoperative preparation may extend over a period of several days, and may include many tests, radiographic studies, and laboratory procedures, as well as education of the patient and the family. The nurse plays an important part in explaining the necessity for preoperative tests and in carrying out the preparation for these tests. A summary of preoperative preparations is given in Chart 16-1.

A medical history is taken and a physical examination performed before surgery. In addition, laboratory tests such as urinalysis, complete blood count, hemoglobin, and hematocrit usually are ordered. These studies are performed to discover any preexisting disease that might alter the patient's response to or recovery from surgery. In many hospitals, a routine chest radiograph is taken to make certain that the patient has no unsuspected pulmonary disease. In some hospitals, an electrocardiogram is ordered for all patients over age 40. If unsuspected pulmonary or cardiac disease is discovered, the surgery may be delayed while measures to treat or control the condition are instituted. Those who are scheduled for elective surgery may have these tests performed as an outpatient, usually within 1 week of surgery.

Often surgery must be undertaken despite the presence of other illnesses such as heart disease or chronic obstructive pulmonary disease. The presence of coexisting diseases or disorders frequently

Chart 16–1. Checklist for Preoperative Care

General Goals
- ☐ Emotional support
- ☐ Explanation and instruction
- ☐ Spiritual needs; visit from clergyman
- ☐ Planning with family; teaching family

Afternoon/Evening Before Surgery
- ☐ Check preoperative orders carefully; note orders for enemas, catheterization, medications, any other preoperative procedures.
- ☐ Check surgical consent form for patient's signature and proper wording of operative procedure.
- ☐ Prepare skin of operative area.
- ☐ Safeguard patient's valuables.
- ☐ Give hypnotic, if prescribed, to promote sleep.
- ☐ Withhold food and fluids as instructed (usually after midnight).
- ☐ Make certain that all specimens requested have been collected (eg, urine, blood)

Morning of Surgery
- ☐ Take and record temperature and blood pressure.
- ☐ Assist patient with personal hygiene as necessary.
- ☐ Help patient to dress for operating room.
- ☐ Remove prostheses (including dentures, if it is hospital policy to do so).
- ☐ Have patient void.
- ☐ Administer preanesthetic medication.
- ☐ Leave patient resting in bed, with call button handy.
- ☐ *Note:* These measures cannot and should not always be carried out in this order. *The needs of the individual patient are more important than any routine.*

affects nursing management during the postoperative period.

Immediate Preoperative Preparation

Immediate preparation for surgery usually starts the afternoon or early evening before surgery. If the patient is admitted the morning of surgery, these preparations are begun shortly after admission to the unit.

SKIN PREPARATION.   Although the procedure for skin preparation varies, cleanliness of the skin and the removal of hair from its surface without injury or irritation are fundamental. The skin cannot be made completely sterile, but the number of microorganisms on it can be substantially reduced. Shaving is necessary to prevent contamination of the surgical area because microorganisms are present on the hair. Shaving also prevents hair from entering the wound, where it acts as a foreign body that interferes with healing. Sometimes plain soap and water are used for cleansing the skin. Topical antiseptics, such as povidone-iodine, which are effective in decreasing the number of microorganisms on the skin, also may be used. Most hospitals formulate guidelines describing the areas of the skin to be shaved. Figure 16-4 shows areas of the body customarily prepared for common types of surgery. If there is any question about the area to be prepared, the surgeon should be contacted. It is important to have the skin preparation complete before surgery.

Before starting the procedure, the nurse should briefly explain to the patient what will be done and why. The patient should be draped and screened to prevent unnecessary exposure. Preparation for orthopedic surgery must be done with great care because infections of the bone are difficult to manage, even with intensive antibiotic therapy.

ELIMINATION. Distention of the bladder makes lower abdominal surgery more difficult and increases the risk of injury to the bladder during surgery. For this reason, some surgeons request that the patient be catheterized and a catheter be left in place. Patients who are not catheterized should be instructed to void immediately before or after the preoperative medication is given.

Enemas may be ordered before surgery to clean out the lower bowel. The act of straining to have a bowel movement is painful after any abdominal operation. If fecal matter is left in the bowel before surgery, it may harden and even become impacted before the patient is able to bear down painlessly enough to evacuate it. An enema or series of enemas is particularly important when surgery is performed on the bowel. Sometimes enemas are ordered when surgery involves areas other than the intestines, thus eliminating the need to strain to have a bowel movement during the immediate postoperative period. In addition, general anesthetics relax the muscles; having the bowel empty prevents the occurrence of an involuntary bowel movement during or immediately after surgery.

FOOD AND FLUIDS. The physician gives specific directions about the length of time food and fluids are to be withheld before surgery. Midnight preceding surgery usually is specified as the time for terminating fluid intake, and the supper hour the last time the patient takes solid food. Before these times, the patient is encouraged to eat and drink to maintain fluid and electrolyte balance and to meet the body's increased need for nutrients during the healing process. Protein and ascorbic acid (vitamin C) are especially important in promoting wound healing. Except in emergencies, surgery on a patient whose nutrition is poor usually is postponed until deficiencies of food, fluids, or electrolytes can be corrected. If the patient is unable to take a sufficient amount of oral fluids, preoperative administration of intravenous fluids may be necessary.

CARE OF VALUABLES. Attention should be given to the care of valuables on admission. Sometimes, despite these measures, the nurse finds that a patient has valuable jewelry or documents in his or her possession on the morning of surgery. It is the policy in most hospitals that valuables be placed in the hospital safe before the patient goes to surgery. It is important to chart what has been done with valuables, such as giving them to relatives or depositing them in the hospital safe.

Rings should be removed and given to a family member or placed in the hospital safe. If the patient is reluctant to remove a wedding band, gauze may be slipped under the ring and then looped around the finger and wrist. Care should be taken to avoid tying the gauze tightly, as it could impair circulation to the finger or hand. Adhesive tape also can be applied over a plain wedding band and may be preferable to gauze.

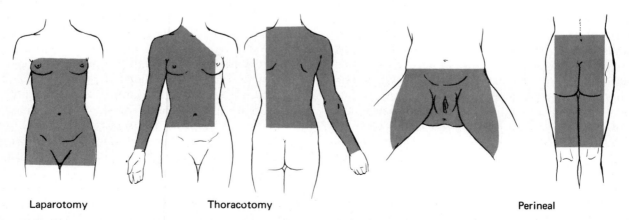

Laparotomy   Thoracotomy   Perineal

Figure 16–4. These diagrams indicate areas of skin prepared before laparotomy, thoracotomy, and surgery in the perineal area. Skin preparation is extensive in each of these examples. The procedure of each hospital varies somewhat in the designation of the areas to be prepared.

ATTIRE. The patient should be given a clean hospital gown; personal clothing should not be worn in the operating room.

PROSTHESES. In most hospitals, patients are asked to remove full or partial dentures so that these objects will not become dislodged and cause respiratory obstruction during the administration of a general anesthetic. Some anesthesiologists, however, prefer that well-fitting dentures be left in to preserve the contours of the face. If dentures are to be removed, patients should be tactfully asked if they have any. If they do, they should be given an opaque denture jar; then, unless they need help, they should be left alone for a few minutes while they remove and clean their dentures and place them in the container. In most hospitals, the container for dentures is left at the patient's bedside until he returns to his room. Other prostheses, such as artificial limbs, also should be removed before surgery.

MOUTH CARE. All patients should have thorough mouth care before surgery; a clean mouth makes them more comfortable and prevents the aspiration of particles of food that may be left in the mouth.

MAKEUP AND GROOMING. During surgery, the anesthesiologist periodically inspects the face, lips, and nail beds for evidence of cyanosis. Patients should be asked to remove any makeup and nail polish. Details of personal grooming, such as trimming the nails and shaving, should be completed before surgery. Women should be asked to remove any metal or plastic objects in the hair because these might cause injury if the patients become restless during or immediately after surgery. A special cap that covers the hair is placed on the patient's head either in the operating room or just before the patient leaves the room.

SURGICAL CONSENT. Before surgery can be performed, a surgical consent form, or operative permit, must be signed by the patient. If the adult patient is not mentally competent or is unconscious or semiconscious, the consent may be signed by a family member or guardian. If the patient is a minor (ie, under age 18), the consent form is signed by a parent or legal guardian. In some instances, a person under age 18 who is living away from home and is self-supporting is considered an emancipated minor, and she or he may sign the form. The nurse should be familiar with laws governing the age of consent as well as the legal implications when a person other than the patient signs the consent form.

Because consent must be informed and voluntary, the physician gives the patient a full explanation of the surgery and its possible adverse effects. The patient or family member also must understand that a signed consent form grants permission to health care personnel to perform the surgery. If the patient needs more information, the nurse notifies the physician. The consent form must be signed before sedative medications are administered, so that the patient is mentally alert when signing. The patient's or family member's signature must be witnessed by an adult, usually a member of the medical team or personnel in the admissions department. The signed consent form should be inserted in the patient's chart.

PREOPERATIVE MEDICATION. Tranquilizers, such as chlordiazepoxide, or sedatives, such as phenobarbital, may be given several days before surgery to relieve severe anxiety. The evening before surgery a hypnotic drug, such as flurazepam (Dalmane), may be given. About 30 to 60 minutes before the patient is taken to the operating room, a preoperative medication may be administered. This medication may consist of one, two, or three drugs: a narcotic or sedative, an antiemetic, and a drug to decrease secretions of the respiratory tract. Examples of these drugs are meperidine (Demerol), a narcotic used to sedate the patient; perphenazine (Trilafon), an antiemetic that also has sedative properties, especially when administered with a narcotic; and atropine, a cholinergic blocking agent that decreases secretions of the nose, mouth, throat, and bronchi. The preoperative medication usually is ordered by the anesthesiologist; the choice of drugs is based on the patient, the surgery, and the type of anesthetic that will be used. Older patients, semiconscious or unconscious patients, and those with certain diseases or disorders may not be given a preoperative medication, since one or more of these drugs may be contraindicated. If there is any question regarding the preoperative medication or the absence of an order for a medication, the anesthesiologist should be notified.

Before the immediate preoperative medication is administered, the blood pressure and pulse and respiratory rates should be obtained (Fig. 16-5). The patient should be given an explanation of the effects that will be experienced after the preoperative medication is administered. If a narcotic or antiemetic is administered, the patient should be told that drowsiness will occur in about 20 minutes; administration of a cholinergic blocking agent will result in extreme dryness of the mouth. The patient should be instructed to remain in bed. The side rails should be raised and the call button placed within easy reach. The patient should be cautioned not to smoke after the preoperative medication has been given.

TRANSPORTATION OF THE PATIENT TO THE OPERATING ROOM. Patients normally are transported to the operating room on a cart. They should be covered with cotton blankets and a restraint fastened to prevent them from falling off the cart. All necessary information should be recorded on the chart before

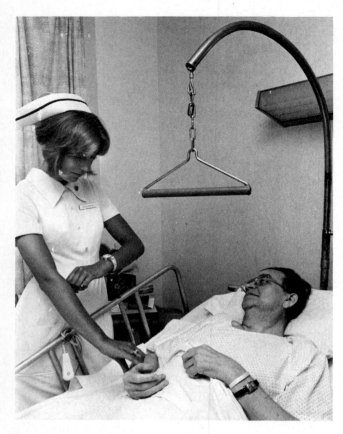

Figure 16–5. The blood pressure and pulse rate of the surgical patient are taken before the administration of narcotics. (Photograph by D. Atkinson)

the patient leaves the room: vital signs, weight, preoperative medications, voiding, preoperative procedures such as enemas, disposition of valuables and dentures, and pertinent observations on the patient's condition. The consent form should be checked to be sure it is correctly signed and witnessed. The patient's identification bracelet should be checked before leaving the room to be sure the right patient is being taken to surgery.

Evaluation

- Preoperative anxiety is reduced or eliminated
- Patient's spiritual needs are met
- Patient demonstrates ability to cope with the potential results of surgery
- Family demonstrates evidence of coping with the potential results of surgery
- All surgical preparations for surgery are carried out
- Patient demonstrates an understanding of type and purpose of surgical procedure, preoperative preparations, postoperative tasks performed by self and nursing personnel.

INTRAOPERATIVE PERIOD

The intraoperative period is the time when the patient is in the operating room. The nurse may assume one or more duties relevant to patient care. Basically, the scrub nurse assists the surgeon and wears a sterile gown and gloves. Responsibilities during surgery include handing instruments to the surgeon and assistant surgeon, preparing sutures, receiving specimens for laboratory examination, and counting sponges and needles. The circulating nurse wears operating room attire but does not wear a sterile gown and gloves. Responsibilities include obtaining and opening wrapped sterile equipment and supplies before and during the surgery, keeping records, adjusting lights, receiving specimens for laboratory examination, and coordinating the activities of other personnel, such as the pathologist and the radiology technician.

NURSING PROCESS —PATIENT MANAGEMENT DURING THE INTRAOPERATIVE PERIOD

Assessment
Assessment of the patient in the operating room is largely based on the type or extent of surgery performed, the age of the patient, and any preexisting disease. Depending on circumstances, assessment may include the following:

- Blood pressure, pulse and respiratory rates, and level of consciousness
- Evaluation of the patient's general physical condition
- Examination for the presence of catheters and tubes (eg, nasogastric, chest)
- Review of the patient's chart, including a signed surgical consent, administration of preoperative medications (time, dose, and patient response), voiding, skin preparation, carrying out of other preoperative orders, and laboratory and diagnostic tests

Nursing Diagnosis
The nursing diagnosis is based on the assessment of the patient, and may include one or more of the following:

- Potential for infection related to entrance of microorganisms into the surgical wound, lack of strict aseptic technique
- Fluid volume excess or deficit related to inaccurate administration of intravenous fluids, blood, or blood products

Planning and Implementation
Planning and implementation of nursing management depends on routine tasks performed by nurs-

ing personnel in surgery as well as variables such as the surgery performed, the type of anesthesia used (general, local, or spinal), the age and condition of the patient, and the occurrence of complications during surgery.

Potential for Infection.   Strict aseptic technique must be followed before and during surgery. If any break in technique is noted, it should be immediately brought to the attention of the surgeon and other operating room personnel.

Fluid Volume Excess or Deficit.   The anesthesiologist and the circulating nurse usually are responsible for adding fluids to the intravenous lines. The circulating nurse may be responsible for recording and keeping a running total of intravenous fluids. During the procedure, the surgeon may periodically ask how much intravenous fluid has been administered. If the patient has an indwelling catheter, urine output may be measured during surgery.

Observations   Although the patient is covered by sterile surgical drapes, it usually is possible to observe the face and possibly the hands for evidence of cyanosis. The administration rate of some intravenous fluids and the amount of urine output also may be the responsibility of the circulating nurse. Adverse situations, such as malfunctioning equipment, is brought to the attention of the surgeon or anesthesiologist.

Other Duties   The recording of pertinent observations usually is the duty of the circulating nurse. Once surgery is completed and the patient transferred to the recovery area, the scrub or circulating nurse may communicate information regarding the surgery to recovery room personnel. If biopsies or samples are taken during surgery, the circulating nurse is responsible for labeling and sending tissue and fluids to the appropriate laboratory.

All drugs or fluids (blood, plasma, and intravenous solutions) given to the scrub nurse or anesthesiologist are identified both visually and verbally. The label on the solution or drug container is shown to the person receiving the material at the same time the name and, in certain instances, the dose, such as 50 mg/mL, are stated. This is especially important during emergency situations. Communication with other hospital departments, such as the blood bank or pathology, may be the responsibility of the circulating nurse.

Evaluation

■ Aseptic technique is observed before and during the surgical procedure

■ Accurate recording of data is carried out
■ All tissue and fluid samples are accurately labeled and sent to the appropriate departments
■ Information is related to recovery room personnel

POSTANESTHESIA AND RECOVERY PERIODS

The *postanesthesia period* designates the time the patient spends recovering from the effects of anesthesia. The *recovery period* designates the time from the end of the postanesthesia period until the patient can resume most activities, such as returning to work or managing a household.

Postanesthesia Period

Factors such as the patient's age and nutritional status, preexisting diseases, and the type of surgery performed may affect the duration of the postanesthesia period and the type of nursing management. Immediately after completion of the surgical procedure, the patient is transported to the recovery room (or postanesthesia recovery room). The recovery room normally has accommodations for a group of patients who are under the continuous surveillance of highly skilled personnel (Fig. 16-6). Equipment is available for immediate use if necessary. Vital signs are recorded at frequent intervals, and the progress of recovery from anesthesia is entered in the patient's record.

NURSING PROCESS —PATIENT MANAGEMENT DURING THE POSTANESTHESIA PERIOD

Assessment
When the patient arrives in the recovery room or postanesthesia recovery room, pertinent information regarding the surgery and any complications that arose during surgery is given to nursing personnel by the anesthesiologist or circulating nurse. Further assessment may include the following:

■ Rapid assessment of the patient's general condition (color, respiratory rate, airway patency, and level of consciousness) while connecting the airway, tubes, or drains to the proper equipment, such as suction (Fig. 16-7), mechanical ventilator, or wall oxygen
■ Measurement and recording of vital signs
■ Inspection of the surgical dressing as well as tubes, drains, and intravenous lines

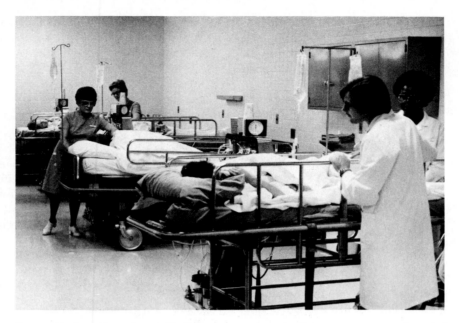

Figure 16–6. The patient in the recovery room is under the continuous surveillance of highly skilled personnel. (Photograph by D. Atkinson)

Nursing Diagnosis

One or more of the following nursing diagnoses may apply to the patient during the immediate postanesthesia recovery period:

- Ineffective airway clearance related to the effects of anesthesia and drugs administered before and during surgery

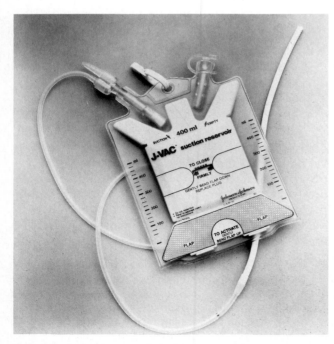

Figure 16–7. The J-VAC closed wound drainage system suction reservoir may be used to drain fluid from a surgical area. (Courtesy of Johnson & Johnson Patient Care, Inc, New Brunswick, NJ)

- Ineffective breathing pattern related to the effects of anesthesia or airway obstruction
- Anxiety related to the results of surgery or biopsy during surgery
- Pain related to the surgical procedure
- Fluid volume deficit related to loss of blood and fluids during surgery
- Potential for injury related to excitement, restlessness, or pain while recovering from anesthesia

Planning and Implementation

The major responsibilities of the nurse during the patient's postoperative recovery room stay are to ensure a patent airway, help to maintain adequate circulation, prevent or treat shock, and attend to the proper positioning and function of drains, tubes, and intravenous infusions.

Ineffective Airway Clearance, Ineffective Breathing Pattern. If a general anesthetic has been administered, the patient will arrive in the recovery room with an endotracheal tube or an oropharyngeal airway in place (Fig. 16-8). Either of these devices helps to maintain a patent airway. The endotracheal tube may be connected to a mechanical ventilator. Although it usually is removed by the anesthesiologist, it also may be removed by the nurse. After removal, an oropharyngeal airway is inserted to prevent the tongue from obstructing the passage of air during this phase of recovery from anesthesia. The airway is left in position until the patient begins to regain consciousness, giving evidence of the return of the swallowing and cough reflexes. The patient should be positioned so that vomitus or secretions will not

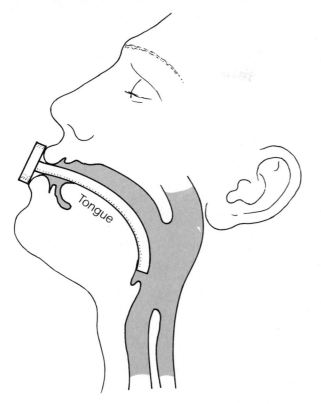

Figure 16-8. An oropharyngeal airway in place. The airway prevents the tongue of the unconscious patient from blocking the air passages. As long as the airway is unobstructed and in place, air has a free route between the pharynx and the outside.

be aspirated into the tracheobronchial passages. To prevent aspiration, vomitus or secretions should be removed promplty by suction.

Maintaining Circulation. Positioning the patient is an important measure in preventing interference with circulation; normal body alignment should be maintained. Precautions should be taken to prevent displacement of the intravenous needle because maintenance of the infusion is important to adequate circulatory function. Blood pressure and pulse rate should be monitored every 5 to 15 minutes and compared with the patient's preoperative and intraoperative vital signs.

Fluid Volume Deficit. Postoperative shock caused by blood loss, fluid shifts, and neurogenic factors usually is mild and amenable to therapy. Intravenous fluids should be regulated to prevent overhydration, but specified in amount and rate of flow to treat dehydration. The kind and specific amount of intake for fluids and blood depend on the patient's requirements and the kind of surgery performed. The rate of flow should be carefully determined at the start and checked frequently.

Pain. Medication for pain relief or sedation is ordered by the surgeon. The recovery room nurse exercises judgment in administering the first postoperative medication. Judgments in this matter are based on knowledge of the drugs used for anesthesia, their effect on the action of the prescribed analgesic, the patient's condition, and the vital signs.

Anxiety, Potential for Injury. Anxiety related to the effects of anesthesia, pain, and the outcome of surgery may be seen as the patient recovers from anesthesia. The final outcome of some surgical procedures may not be known until the pathologist has examined tissue or the internal organs or structures. Although patients may have been told preoperatively what surgery will be performed, they may begin to show concern about the surgical procedure when recovering from anesthesia. Although still sedated, anxiety, and in turn restlessness, may be noted. At this time, the patient must be protected from injury as well as causing displacement of drains, tubes, or dressings.

Family. It is important to keep family members informed of the patient's condition. Some hospitals provide a visitors' lounge near the area of the operating and recovery rooms. Opportunities for contact with the staff are fostered by such an arrangement because of its convenience to all concerned. If the surgeons and nurses know that family members are nearby, they can more easily stop to speak to them.

Drains, Tubes, and Intravenous Lines. The number and kind of drains and tubes vary with the surgical procedure. When drains are not functioning properly, measures should be instituted to correct the malfunction. To prevent further complications and delayed healing, indwelling drains must be kept in proper position and perfect working order. Catheters and tubes must be checked to prevent kinking or clogging that interferes with adequate drainage of urine or bile.

Intravenous fluids usually are administered throughout surgery and into the recovery phase until the patient's blood pressure is stabilized. This routine precaution is desirable in the event of shock. Maintenance of adequate circulation is essential for prompt treatment of vascular collapse, even in a mild form. If the surgical procedure is a major one, fluids are needed to maintain nutritional status until the patient is able to resume oral nourishment.

Discharge from the Recovery Room. Although the length of time varies, the average duration of the postanesthesia period ranges from 30 minutes to 2 or more hours. When patients have fully recovered from anesthesia and there is no evidence of complications, they are prepared to return to the unit. A summary of the recovery from anesthesia and all vital information, such as fluid intake and output and the color and amount of drainage, should be recorded on the chart. A summary of recovery from anesthesia should be given orally to nursing personnel when the patient is returned to the unit. If the type of surgery requires intensive nursing care, the patient may be transferred to an intensive care unit where special equipment is available to help detect and prevent serious complications.

Evaluation

- Airway remains open and breathing pattern is normal
- Vital signs are stable
- Pain is controlled or lessened
- Fluid intake meets requirements; hypovolemia (if present) is corrected
- Nutritional needs are met (intravenous fluids, calories)
- Patient does not injure self or disturb dressings; drains, intravenous lines, and catheters remain intact and functioning
- Patient's anxiety is reduced or eliminated

RECOVERY PERIOD

The recovery period begins when the patient arrives in the hospital room or a postsurgical unit and extends until after discharge from the hospital and full activity is resumed. Some patients have a smooth, uncomplicated recovery from surgery, and are discharged from the hospital in a few days. Others experience a prolonged mental and physical recovery that may include complications arising from surgery.

NURSING PROCESS —PATIENT MANAGEMENT DURING THE RECOVERY PERIOD

Assessment

Immediate assessment of the patient returning from the postanesthesia recovery area or postsurgical unit includes the same tasks as those performed in the recovery room. They are as follows:

- Rapid assessment of the patient's general condition (color, respiratory rate, and level of consciousness) while connecting the airway, tubes, or drains to the proper equipment, such as suction machines, mechanical ventilator, or wall oxygen
- Measurement and recording of vital signs
- Inspection of the surgical dressing as well as the airway, tubes, drains, and intravenous lines

- Review of the patient's surgical procedure and recovery from anesthesia

Assessment is continuous throughout the patient's hospitalization and may alter, delete, or add to the nursing diagnoses.

Nursing Diagnosis

Nursing diagnosis depends on many factors, such as the type of surgery performed, the patient's age and general physical condition, preexisting diseases or disorders, and the presence of internal or external devices, such as a pacemaker, indwelling catheter, chest tubes, and intravenous lines. For example, a patient with an ileostomy may develop an impairment of skin integrity around the stoma, whereas a young patient recovering from an appendectomy will probably not develop a problem with skin integrity. Some nursing diagnoses may apply to a particular patient or situation, and can be added to the following:

- Activity intolerance (immediate or long-range) related to surgery
- Anxiety related to the results of surgery, recovery from surgery, other situations (specify, if known)
- Potential for aspiration related to impaired swallowing, surgery to the head or neck, gastrointestinal tubes, other (specify)
- Hypothermia related to the effects of anesthesia, drugs administered during surgery
- Hyperthermia related to infection or other factors (specify)
- Diarrhea related to antibiotic therapy, diet, or surgery
- Constipation related to analgesics, diet, or surgery
- Pain related to surgical procedure, postoperative activities
- Ineffective individual coping related to the surgical procedure
- Fluid volume deficit related to surgery, inappropriate administration of intravenous fluids, excessive drainage, other factors (specify)
- Fluid volume excess related to cardiovascular disorder, incorrect administration of intravenous fluids
- Impaired physical mobility related to surgery
- Potential for infection related to surgery, break in aseptic technique after surgery
- Impaired skin integrity related to surgery, lack of mobility, infection, nutritional status, wound separation, other factors (specify)
- Feeding, bathing/hygiene, dressing/grooming, and toileting self-care deficits related to surgery
- Body image disturbance related to the results of surgery
- Impaired social interaction related to the results of surgery
- Social isolation related to the results of surgery
- Ineffective breathing pattern related to failure to cough and deep-breathe

- Ineffective airway clearance related to immobility, failure to deep-breathe and cough
- Knowledge deficit of management after discharge from the hospital

Planning and Implementation

Depending on the patient's condition, long-term planning and management may be instituted shortly after the patient's arrival on the unit, or they may be delayed.

The major goals of the patient include relief of pain and discomfort, adequate tissue perfusion, optimum respiratory function, avoidance of complications, return of normal bowel and bladder function, avoidance of infection, normal food and fluid intake, acceptance of the results of surgery, reduction in anxiety, maintenance of skin integrity, and return to normal activities.

The major goals of nursing management are prevention and detection of complications, protection of the patient from injury during this period of helplessness, relief discomfort and pain, helping the patient regain independence, and teaching and informing the patient.

Immediate Postoperative Complications. During the first 24 hours after surgery, each member of the nursing team must watch for the signs of four important complications that may occur during this period: hemorrhage, shock, hypoxia, and vomiting.

HEMORRHAGE.   Hemorrhage can be internal or external. If a large amount of blood has been lost, there will be signs and symptoms of shock (fall in blood pressure, weak and rapid pulse, pallor, increased respiratory rate, restlessness, and cool moist skin). The amount of blood lost need not be great enough to cause serious complications. For example, after thyroidectomy, a small amount of blood seeping from a capillary may be sufficient to compress the trachea, resulting in respiratory difficulty.

Dressings should be inspected regularly for any sign of bleeding. The bedding and the dressing under the patient also should be inspected because blood may pool under the patient's body and be more evident under the patient than on the dressing. If the patient is bleeding internally, it may be necessary to return him or her to surgery for ligation of bleeding vessels. Blood transfusions may be ordered to replace the blood lost.

When reporting bleeding, the color of the blood is noted. Bright red blood signifies fresh bleeding. Dark, brownish blood indicates that the bleeding is not fresh. When the patient is transferred from one unit or area to another, it is important to find out whether drains have been inserted and what type of drainage is expected. Dressings that become soiled may be reinforced, but usually are not changed except at the direction of the surgeon. If drainage is to be expected, the patient should be told that the drainage is a normal consequence of the surgery and does not indicate any complications.

The color and amount of any drainage are described accurately on the patient's chart.

SHOCK.   The loss of fluids and electrolytes, trauma (both physical and psychological), anesthetics, and preoperative medications may all play a part in causing shock. Signs and symptoms include pallor, fall in blood pressure, weak and rapid pulse, restlessness, and cold, moist skin. Narcotics should never be administered to a patient who is in shock or to one in whom shock seems imminent until the patient has been evaluated by a physician. Narcotics given to a patient who is in shock may not be absorbed because of the decreased volume of circulating blood. As the patient recovers from shock and circulation improves, several doses of the narcotic may be absorbed at once, resulting in an overdose. Narcotics may precipitate shock in patients in whom this complication is imminent.

The patient who is in shock should be kept lying flat unless the physician orders otherwise. Some physicians advocate elevation of the legs to enhance the flow of venous blood to the heart. Patients who have had brain surgery or spinal anesthesia should be kept lying flat unless the physician orders otherwise.

Shock must be detected early and treated promptly. Prolonged, severe shock can result in irreversible damage to vital organs such as the brain, kidneys, and heart. The treatment of shock varies, and often depends on the cause, if known. Whole blood, plasma expanders, parenteral fluids, oxygen, and drugs such as adrenergic agents may be used.

HYPOXIA.   Hypoxia may complicate postoperative recovery. Anesthetics and preoperative medications may depress respirations, thus interfering with oxygenation of the blood. Because mucus may block tracheal or bronchial passages and interfere with breathing, the amount of oxygen entering the lungs may be decreased. Oxygen and suction equipment should be ready for emergency use and the patient watched carefully for cyanosis and dyspnea. If breathing is obstructed because the tongue has fallen back and obstructed the nasopharynx, the lower jaw should be pulled forward and an oropharyngeal airway inserted. This type of obstruction also can be relieved by turning the patient on her side.

Other factors, such a residual drug effect or a drug overdose, pain, poor positioning that causes pressure, a pooling of secretions in the lungs, or an obstructed airway, also predispose to hypoxia.

Restlessness, crowing or grunting respirations, diaphoresis, bounding pulse, and rising blood pressure should arouse suspicion of respiratory obstruction.

When indicated, positive-pressure ventilation should be applied by the use of a mechanical ventilator. Any one of several types may be used. Many hospitals have the advantage of inhalation therapy services. Personnel in these services are specially trained to take care of the equipment and to assist with this important aspect of care.

VOMITING. Vomiting after surgery can be due to the anesthetics used, to drugs administered before, during, or immediately after surgery, or to the surgery itself. Some patients experience nausea and vomiting when taking fluids for the first time after surgery. Other patients vomit in the immediate postanesthesia period, before they have even attempted to take oral fluids.

During the early postoperative period, an emesis basin should be kept within easy reach of the patient. If vomiting is severe or prolonged, oral feedings should be temporarily discontinued, intravenous fluids administered, and, in some instances, a nasogastric tube inserted and connected to suction. The patient should be observed for signs and symptoms of dehydration and electrolyte imbalance. The physician may prescribe an antiemetic agent if nausea and vomiting persist.

Spinal Anesthesia. Nursing care and observation are important after spinal anesthesia. The fact that the patient is conscious simplifies some aspects of postoperative care; however, it is important to remember that the patient usually has been given medication that makes him sleepy. Side rails should be raised and the call button handy.

At first, the patient experiences numbness and a feeling of heaviness in the lower extremities. Even though the patient has been advised beforehand that these effects would occur, it is important for the nurse to repeat the explanation that numbness is usual and will subside in a short time. Many patients become apprehensive because of this symptom, and fear that the anesthetic has paralyzed their legs.

Patients usually are kept lying flat in bed for 6 to 12 hours after surgery, and unless ordered otherwise, they may be turned from side to side. As the spinal anesthesia wears off, they begin to have a sensation in the anesthetized parts that is described as "pins and needles." They also begin to experience pain in the operated area. Patients who develop a headache after spinal anesthesia may have to remain lying flat for a longer period. There has been much discussion about "spinal headache," and some patients think that it is an inevitable sequel to spinal anesthesia. The nurse should not contribute to this impression by the power of suggestion. A statement such as "I'll keep the bed flat so you can rest" is preferable to "I'll keep the bed flat so you won't get a headache."

Activity. Immediately after surgery, patients are totally dependent on nursing personnel for their activities of daily living. Many patients are ambulated shortly after surgery; some, however, may be unable to get out of bed for days or even weeks after surgery because of the seriousness of the surgery, complications, or other factors.

The ability to ambulate as well as to perform activities of daily living are based on many factors, such as the type of surgery and the patient's physical condition before and after surgery. An assessment reveals the patient's needs, and the meeting of these needs are planned according to such factors as pain tolerance, response to analgesics, general physical condition, and the desire to participate in activities. Some patients need to be encouraged to be active after surgery, and the importance of increasing activities must be stressed. Some patients experience moderate to severe fatigue after surgery. Nursing management should be planned so that activities such as ambulation and personal care are spaced throughout the day.

The term *early ambulation* is widely used to describe one aspect of postoperative treatment. Patients are helped to walk early in the postoperative period. The patient is helped to a sitting position at the side of the bed. If dizziness occurs and is *more than* momentary, the patient should be returned to a supine position.

Exercise and erect posture help the patient to breathe more deeply, and the change of position helps to prevent congestion of the lungs with fluid. Walking stimulates circulation in the lower extremities, thus lessening the problem of venous stasis. Erect posture and exercise also help to overcome the problems of urine retention, constipation, and abdominal distention caused by gas. Early ambulation helps patients to regain their appetite, and greater activity during the day helps them to sleep better at night. The following are some important points that pertain to ambulation:

1. Early ambulation is a therapeutic measure. Its primary purpose is to prevent complications.
2. Ambulation means walking, not sitting. Prolonged sitting puts pressure on the legs, resulting in thrombophlebitis. The patient should sit for short periods and take frequent, short walks.
3. Walking soon after surgery often causes pain and apprehension. The purpose of walking is explained, and its importance emphasized.
4. Early ambulation helps the patient to feel less helpless. One of the dangers of early ambulation is overconfi-

dence. Because patients feel more self-sufficient, they may be misled into taking on too much activity too soon.

5. Special equipment, like catheters and intravenous equipment, need not restrict the patient to bed. Its management does require some ingenuity, however, so that the treatment may be continued safely and effectively while the patient is out of bed.

Hiccups. Hiccups (singultus) result from intermittent spasms of the diaphragm, and may occur after surgery, especially surgery of the abdomen. They may be mild, and last for only a few minutes. Prolonged periods of hiccups are not only unpleasant, but also may cause pain or discomfort in the incision. Hiccups also may result in wound dehiscence or evisceration, inability to eat, nausea and vomiting, exhaustion, and fluid and electrolyte and acid–base imbalances. The physician should be contacted if hiccups persist for more than a few minutes or if symptoms of wound disruption are apparent.

Anxiety and Fear. Many patients exhibit anxiety and fear before surgery as well as after. Some worry about their recovery; others worry about the results of surgery and possibly the changes that will take place in their lifestyles. For example, patients who have had coronary bypass surgery may show concern over the necessity to alter their eating habits, and patients with colostomies may exhibit a great deal of anxiety over performing stoma care. The nurse should listen to the patient as many times as these anxieties and fears are mentioned in conversation with nursing personnel. Being aware of postoperative anxiety and fear may prompt a discussion of the problem with the physician and referral of the patient to such sources of information as a support group, a social worker, and a dietitian.

Potential for Aspiration. A danger of aspiration exists until the patient is fully awake and able to swallow without difficulty. Vomiting after surgery also may result in aspiration. Most patients can begin to take fluids within 8 to 24 hours after surgery, unless the surgical procedure has involved the gastrointestinal tract.

Hypothermia and Hyperthermia. Hypothermia that occurs shortly after surgery may result from the administration of intravenous fluids that are cooler than body temperature, open cavities (abdominal, chest) during surgery, advanced age, muscle inactivity, drugs administered during surgery, and cool temperatures in the operating and recovery rooms. The body temperature usually returns to normal shortly after surgery. Administering warmed intrave-

nous fluids, using light blankets in cool rooms, and encouraging the patient to move all extremities aid the body temperature to return to normal.

A mild increase in body temperature is not unusual after surgery; a significant rise, however, may indicate infection or some other process, such as the development of a thrombus, and requires immediate attention. The patient's temperature should be monitored every 4 hours after surgery. A significant increase in temperature should be reported to the physician. Measures to reduce body temperature include the administration of antipyretic drugs, such as aspirin and acetaminophen, and the application of hypothermia blankets. Infection is treated with antibiotics.

Constipation, Diarrhea. Constipation may occur after the patient begins to take solid food, and may be caused by inactivity, diet, or narcotic analgesics. On the other hand, the patient may experience diarrhea, which may be caused by diet, drugs such as antibiotics, or the surgical procedure. A record of the patient's bowel movements should be kept and the physician notified if either of these two problems occur. Because diarrhea may be caused by antibiotic therapy, the physician should be notified of this problem before the next dose of the drug is due.

Abdominal distention results from the accumulation of gas (flatus) in the intestines. It is caused by a failure of the intestines to propel gas through the intestinal tract by peristalsis, and is aggravated by the tendency of some patients to swallow large quantities of air, especially when they are frightened or in pain. Manipulation of the intestines during abdominal surgery may cause postoperative distention because handling temporarily inhibits normal peristalsis. Contributing factors are inactivity after surgery, interruption of a normal food and fluid intake necessitated by surgery, and anesthetics and drugs given during or after surgery.

If the symptoms are mild, they can be relieved by nursing measures. When patients are permitted out of bed, they should be encouraged (and assisted) to ambulate. Sometimes walking, plus some privacy in the bathroom, helps to expel the gas. Patients should be encouraged to change their position frequently and to eat as normally as possible within the limits specified by the physician. If discomfort is severe, or if it is not relieved promptly by nursing measures, the physician should be notified. The physician may order the insertion of a rectal tube to dilate the anal sphincter and release the gas that may have accumulated in the rectum. The tube is inserted in the same manner as when giving an enema. The best results are achieved by leaving the rectal tube in place for 20 minutes, removing and cleaning it, and then reinserting it every 2 to 3 hours until abdominal distention is relieved. Continuous use can render it ineffective as well as cause unnecessary discomfort.

Sometimes a serious condition called *paralytic ileus* occurs. The patient has paralysis of the intestines, and thus absence of peristalsis. There is an absence of bowel sounds as well as abdominal distention and pain. Vomiting also may occur. A nasogastric tube usually is inserted and food and fluids withheld until bowel sounds return.

Acute gastric dilatation, a condition in which the stomach becomes distended with fluids that do not normally pass through the gastrointestinal tract, is another complication similar to paralytic ileus. The patient may regurgitate small amounts of liquid, the abdomen appears distended, and, as the condition progresses, symptoms of shock may develop. Acute gastric dilatation is treated by passing a nasogastric tube to the patient's stomach, applying suction, and removing the gas and fluid. Some surgeons routinely use suction of the gastrointestinal tract to prevent paralytic ileus and acute gastric dilatation.

Pain. Because a certain amount of pain is expected after surgery, analgesics are included in the postoperative orders. The severest pain occurs during the first 48 hours after surgery. Pain arouses varying degrees of anxiety and emotional responses. Some patients take it in stride; others greatly fear it. Anxiety, accompanied by tenseness and fear, increases pain. *Intense pain also can cause shock.* Thus, it is most important that pain and discomfort be relieved during the postoperative period.

The nurse is responsible for evaluating the patient's need for a narcotic. Usually an analgesic such as morphine or meperidine can be repeated at 3- to 4-hour intervals. What at first appears to be a simple procedure (the patient has pain; the nurse gives the analgesic) is really a complex one. One should consider the following factors before administering a narcotic:

1. Narcotics are not without adverse effects. Morphine as well as other narcotics may depress respirations; meperidine can cause hypotension.
2. The timing of the administration of narcotics should be considered in relation to getting patients out of bed. Some patients require medication for the relief of pain before they can tolerate the additional discomfort entailed in getting up. In such instances, it usually is advisable to allow patients to rest in bed for about an hour after administering an analgesic, to permit relaxation, and then, when helping them out of bed, to have the assistance of a second person in case the patient becomes faint or dizzy.
3. If narcotics are continued for *prolonged* periods, the danger of addiction arises. Administration during the

early postoperative period usually does not pose a danger of addiction.
4. Nursing measures also should be used to relieve pain or discomfort. Sometimes pain at the operative site is intensified because the patient has minor physical discomforts. Along with the administration of a narcotic, the nurse should try simple comfort measures such as changing the patient's position, using a small pillow for supporting the back or shoulders, and gently massaging areas subject to pressure, such as the elbows and hips. These nursing actions also may enhance the effect of the narcotic. A comfortable patient can rest and receive the full benefit of the analgesic without being disturbed for nursing tasks.
5. A narcotic should never be given to a patient whose blood pressure is low and unstable unless the physician is consulted first. If shock is imminent, administration of a narcotic can precipitate it.
6. It usually is advisable to wait until patients have fully recovered from anesthesia before giving them a narcotic. Although they may mumble about pain, they often are not fully aware of it until they open their eyes and become oriented to their surroundings. A patient's condition and recovery from anesthesia can be evaluated more accurately if the analgesic is withheld until the patient is at least partially awake.
7. The purpose of the medication is to relieve pain, not to render the patient stuporous. Oversedation makes it impossible for the patient to practice such preventive measures as deep-breathing and coughing.
8. Morphine depresses respirations. If the patient's respirations are fewer than 10 to 12 breaths per minute, it should be withheld and the physician consulted.
9. Narcotics and sedatives should be given cautiously to older people because they tend to become restless and disoriented as a result of the drug.
10. When giving medicine for the relief of pain, the nurse should capitalize on its psychological as well as physiologic effect by informing the patient that the injection being given is for pain.
11. Analgesics should be administered promptly when they are required. Minutes seem like hours to the patient who is in severe pain.
12. The nurse should try to determine whether the pain is incisional pain, for which the analgesic is ordered, or whether it stems from another source. If abdominal surgery was performed and the patient complains of pain in the chest, for example, the narcotic should not be given and the physician contacted immediately so that the cause of the pain can be determined and measures taken to control it.
13. Most patients do not require frequent administration of narcotic analgesics after the third postoperative day. At this time, the physician may either decrease the dose of the drug or increase the time interval between injections (eg, from every 4 hours to every 6 hours). Another alternative is to order a less potent analgesic. There is no set time limit on how long after surgery narcotic analgesics are needed because much depends on the type and extent of surgery and on the patient. If the patient continues to complain of

pain after the dose, the drug, or the time interval has been changed, the physician should be notified, as a complication such as wound infection or thrombus formation may be developing. Another possible cause of continued requests for an analgesic is the patient's growing dependence on the drug to relieve worry and anxiety rather than pain. This tendency should be noted early because it can lead to addiction.

Ineffective Individual Coping, Body Image Disturbance, Impaired Social Interaction.

Some surgeries (eg, an amputation or a colostomy) change the patient's life-style. Although the surgery was necessary, and the patient may have understood this fact, it is still difficult for the patient to cope with a change in body image. The nurse should constantly be aware of the clues that may indicate ineffective coping mechanisms and, if apparent, these should be discussed with the physician. A referral to appropriate people or agencies may be necessary.

Inability to cope with the results of surgery also can affect the patient's ability to socially interact with his or her spouse, family members, friends, medical personnel, and other patients. The patient may prefer to be alone, appear depressed and withdrawn, communicate poorly, and appear reluctant to participate in activities of daily living. Some surgical procedures (eg, a colostomy) make it necessary to teach the patient about personal hygiene and how to care for the part affected by surgery. The effectiveness of a teaching plan may be influenced by the patient's inability to cope with the results of surgery.

It usually is necessary to assist the patient in coping with a change in body image *before* a teaching plan can be instituted. Being an understanding listener, identifying the areas of concern, and working with other medical personnel may help the patient to work through this problem and become receptive to a teaching plan. Often the patient's family can offer support for the patient. Family members are less worried when they are kept informed of the patient's condition, given opportunities to express their interest and concern, and allowed to learn about and participate in long-range planning and management for care.

Family Coping.

Seeing the patient, if only for a few moments, often does a great deal to assure the family and lessen their apprehension and anxiety. Careful explanation of what to expect (eg, that the patient is drowsy or confused, or that intravenous fluids are being given) is essential in lessening apprehension. A brief visit from the family shortly after returning from the recovery room also assures the patient that the family is there and that they are concerned.

Sometimes it is possible and desirable to allow a responsible member of the family to sit quietly beside the patient during the early postoperative period. Having a member of the family near is especially helpful if the patient is aged or extremely apprehensive, or if the patient is unable to speak English.

Fluid Volume Excess or Deficit.

Intravenous fluids usually are administered after surgery. The length of administration depends on the type of surgery performed and the ability of the patient to take oral fluids after surgery. The flow rate of intravenous fluids should be closely monitored and adjusted as needed. If an electronic infusion device is used (see Chapter 13), the device should still be monitored for accuracy and to make sure that is working properly. The patient also should be observed for signs of fluid excess or deficit (see Chapter 12).

Regardless of how much intravenous fluid the patient is receiving, nothing soothes a parched, dry mouth and throat like cool liquids that the patient can and is allowed to swallow. Patients usually ask for water almost as soon as they begin to complain of pain in the incision. The following points should be considered before the patient is given fluids by mouth:

1. Check to make sure that the physician's orders allow fluids to be given. The instructions may specify food and fluid as tolerated; on the other hand, they may state "Ice chips" or "Nothing by mouth."
2. If the patient is not allowed oral fluids, use mouth rinses and place a cool, wet cloth or some ice chips against the patient's lips to help relieve dryness.
3. Make certain that the patient has recovered sufficiently from anesthesia to be able to swallow. Ask the patient to try swallowing without drinking anything. If this can be done, give the patient a small sip of water.
4. Give only a few sips of water at a time. Fluids should be introduced slowly and given in small amounts; otherwise, vomiting may occur. Give fluids through a straw rather than directly from the glass, so that the patient does not have to sit up. If the patient vomits, assure him that he will soon be able to retain fluids. Offer mouthwash to help get rid of the taste of anesthetics and of vomitus. Change the patient's gown and bedding as needed.

Altered Patterns of Urination.

Most patients who have had abdominal surgery, particularly of the lower abdominal and pelvic regions, have difficulty voiding after surgery. Operative trauma in the region near the bladder may temporarily decrease the patient's sensation of needing to void. The fear of pain also causes tenseness and difficulty in voiding. Position is important. Many women cannot void while lying down, but they can if they are allowed to sit up.

Most men also have difficulty voiding while recumbent, but they can void normally if they are permitted to use the urinal while standing at the bedside.

Patients who have had major surgery on or near the bladder almost always have an indwelling (retention) catheter inserted. If a catheter was not inserted, any surgery—major or minor—on any area of the body can cause difficulty in voiding. Catheterization entails the risk of bladder infection and is avoided when simple nursing measures, plus a little patience, can result in adequate voiding.

The time and amount of each voiding should be recorded for 1 or 2 days after surgery. The length of time that this part of the record should be kept depends on how quickly normal function is resumed. A written order is not required for the measurement of intake and output. The physician also may write specific orders regarding the measurement of intake and output (eg, measuring the urine output every hour).

For the patient who is unable to void, 8 to 12 hours is the usual time that is allowed postoperatively before catheterization is considered. Overdistention of the bladder should be avoided because it makes the patient restless and uncomfortable, and, in the case of abdominal surgery, puts extra pressure on the operative site. Signs and symptoms that indicate a distended bladder include the following:

- Restlessness
- Distention of the area just above the symphysis pubis. Careful palpation of this area causes discomfort, and the patient may feel the need to void.
- Large intake of oral or parenteral fluid with no unusual loss of fluid (eg, from prolonged vomiting or profuse sweating)

Potential for Infection. The postoperative patient must be carefully observed for signs and symptoms of wound infection. In normal recovery, pain in the incision decreases over a period of days. If an infection in or below the incision is occurring, increased pain often is noted. Other signs and symptoms of infection include localized heat, redness, swelling, fever, and purulent exudate. Signs and symptoms of a systemic infection include fever, chills, headache, and anorexia.

If there is drainage from the incision, culture and sensitivity studies may be ordered. It may be necessary to place the patient in isolation to prevent the spread of the infection to other patients. The treatment of infection includes administration of antibiotics, measures to drain purulent material (when applicable), and maintenance of the patient's resistance through rest and nutritious diet.

Ineffective Breathing Pattern, Ineffective Airway Clearance. Patients with chronic respiratory diseases such as bronchitis and elderly patients whose breathing has become more shallow are especially susceptible to postoperative respiratory complications. Pneumonia may result from failure to sufficiently expand the lungs; accumulation of fluid in the lungs is exacerbated by failure to change position and to deep-breathe and cough. This type of pneumonia is called *hypostatic*, or *postoperative, pneumonia*. It occurs because the condition of the patient's lungs favors infection (any fluid that stagnates in the body becomes a culture medium for bacteria) rather than because the patient has been exposed to virulent organisms, such as those that can cause pneumonia in healthy people. Because conditions in the patient's own respiratory system offer little resistance, organisms harbored in the mouth and throat that usually are not harmful are able to cause infection. The signs and symptoms of pneumonia include fever, cough, expectoration of purulent or blood-streaked sputum, dyspnea, and malaise. Treatment involves the use of antibiotics.

Obstruction of a large or small bronchial passageway results in failure of a part of the lung to expand. This is called *atelectasis*. In postoperative patients, the most common cause of obstruction is a mucous plug. Because unconsciousness, immobility, and failure to cough and deep-breathe are predisposing factors, this and other pulmonary complications also can develop in nonsurgical patients.

To avoid respiratory complications, the nurse should help the postoperative patient maintain conditions that help to prevent pneumonia and atelectasis. Specific nursing interventions include the following:

- Suctioning mucus from the nose and mouth while the patient is unconscious
- Instructing the patient to cough and deep-breathe
- Changing the patient's position every 2 hours
- Encouraging and supervising the use of an incentive spirometer, if one has been ordered

The performance of coughing and deep-breathing exercises helps to remove secretions from the lungs and bronchi. Usually ordered every 1 to 2 hours, these exercises are essential if postoperative respiratory complications are to be prevented. Coughing usually places a strain on an incision, especially if surgery was in the chest or abdomen. Using a pillow or hand to support the incision may eliminate some of the discomfort experienced when the patient is coughing. Also of value is the administration of a narcotic followed in 45 minutes to 1 hour by deep-breathing and coughing exercises. The nurse can time these exercises during the early postoperative period, as shown in Table 16-1.

The physician may order intermittent positive-

Table 16–1. Schedule for Postoperative Exercises

Time	Nursing Action
12 noon	Narcotic analgesic administered
12:45 1:45 2:45	Deep-breathing and coughing exercises*
4:30	Narcotic analgesic administered
5:30 6:30 7:15	Deep-breathing and coughing exercises*
8:45	Narcotic analgesic administered

* The deep-breathing and coughing exercises were performed six times during the 8-hour period and were planned according to the analgesic effects of the narcotic.

pressure breathing to be performed two or more times per day. This procedure delivers air or oxygen into the lungs and removes carbon dioxide. It also may be used to administer medications, by the aerosol method, into the lungs. Intermittent positive-pressure breathing is particularly effective for those who cannot or will not attempt deep-breathing after surgery. Pain associated with coughing that usually follows the procedure may cause a patient to be uncooperative and refuse the treatment. It then becomes essential that the nurse *stress* the importance of the procedure and try to gain the patient's cooperation.

An incentive spirometer may be used to encourage deep-breathing and thus prevent atelectasis. The several types of spirometers provide visual or auditory recognition of the results of its use. Some units can be set at a certain level for inhalation. An incentive spirometer usually is used for about 5 days after surgery. Patients with chronic pulmonary disorders may use the unit for a longer time.

Altered Tissue Perfusion. When patients lie still for long periods without moving their legs, venous circulation may be impaired. Blood may flow sluggishly through the veins (venous stasis). This condition predisposes a patient to the development of inflammation, with consequent formation of clots within the veins, a condition called *thrombophlebitis*. Another condition in which clots form but in which inflammation is minimal or absent is called *phlebothrombosis*. These conditions occur most frequently in the legs. Clots that do not adhere to the wall of the vein, but travel in the bloodstream are called *emboli*. By lodging in a distant blood vessel, emboli may obstruct circulation to a vital organ (eg, a lung) and cause severe symptoms and even death.

The nurse may help to prevent thrombophlebitis by making sure that prolonged pressure that might impair circulation is not applied to the patient's legs and by encouraging the patient to perform leg exercises. Unless specifically ordered by the surgeon, the use of pillows under the knees or calves should be avoided. The use of elastic stockings or elastic bandages can help to prevent thrombophlebitis and phlebothrombosis. If elastic bandages are used, they are removed and reapplied *every 6 to 8 hours*. Elastic stockings are removed and reapplied once or twice a day.

Leg exercises usually are ordered in an effort to prevent the formation of a thrombus. Unless the physician leaves orders to the contrary, postoperative patients should begin to move their legs as soon as consciousness returns. These exercises are not complicated; they can be taught readily during the preoperative period and then reviewed with the patient postoperatively. Patients should be instructed to move their toes and feet, alternately flexing and extending them. Next, they should flex and extend their legs by bending the knees and then straightening their legs. These exercises should be repeated at regular intervals.

Knowledge Deficit. Before discharge from the hospital, the patient needs to receive instruction on the correct way to carry out treatment at home. The following points may be included in a patient teaching plan:

1. Keep the incision clean and dry.
2. Follow the physician's recommendations regarding cleaning the incision, applying a dressing, showering or bathing, diet, and activity.
3. Contact the physician if any of the following occurs: chills or fever; drainage from the incision (some drainage may be expected in certain cases); foul odor or pus coming from the incision; redness, streaking, pain, or tenderness around the incision; any other symptoms not present when discharged from the hospital (eg, vomiting, diarrhea, cough, chest pain, and pain in the legs).

Evaluation

- Needs caused by activity intolerance are met
- Anxiety and fear are reduced or absent
- Body temperature is normal
- Bowel elimination is normal
- Pain is controlled with analgesics
- Patient is able to cope with the results of surgery
- Planned nursing activities diminish fatigue
- Intake and output is normal
- Signs of fluid volume excess or deficit are absent

- Electrolyte studies are normal
- Physical mobility progressively improves
- Patient socializes with family, relatives, friends, medical personnel
- Patient's skin remains intact with no signs of impairment of tissue integrity
- No evidence of wound infection is seen
- Breathing pattern is normal; patient performs deep-breathing exercises

- Normal blood gas studies are maintained because of normal breathing pattern
- Complications related to surgery are absent or identified and corrected immediately
- Patient demonstrates understanding of incision care, treatment modalities, problems that require contacting the physician

General Nutritional Considerations

☐ Food and fluid requirements may be provided by the intravenous route until the patient is able to take oral feedings.

☐ Anesthesia decreases peristalsis; therefore, food and fluids are not given orally until peristalsis returns.

☐ Depending on the surgery, the physician usually orders a progressive diet: clear liquid diet, full liquid diet, soft diet, regular or house diet. Some patients may progress from a liquid to a house diet.

☐ Vitamins B and C may be added to intravenous fluids because these vitamins aid wound healing; they are given daily because they are water-soluble vitamins and are not stored in the body.

☐ Before discharge from the hospital, some surgical patients may require special instructions on dietary intake and limitations.

☐ Proteins are necessary for the maintenance and repair of body tissues. Damaged tissue, such as skin ulcerations and surgical incisions, may require additional dietary protein to encourage proper healing.

General Pharmacologic Considerations

☐ Some patients experience acute anxiety before surgery, and the physician may prescribe a tranquilizer or sedative during the preoperative period. The nurse should notify the physician if the medication does not appear to be effective.

☐ The evening before surgery a hypnotic drug may be ordered to ensure rest. The results of the medication should be documented on the patient's chart.

☐ Explanations to patients on the effects of the preoperative medication depend on the drug administered; these explanations usually include (1) the drowsiness and the extreme dryness of the mouth, nose, and throat that will occur; and (2) the importance of remaining in bed after the injection has been given.

☐ Narcotic analgesics should be administered as ordered and as needed. The patient should not be made to wait for relief of pain, provided the established interval between doses has passed.

☐ Narcotic analgesics should *not* be administered to a patient who is in shock or if shock appears imminent without first checking with the physician.

☐ Morphine and other opiates depress respirations; therefore, the respiratory rate is counted *before* these drugs are administered, and the medication is withheld if the respiratory rate is 10 to 12 breaths per minute or below.

General Gerontologic Considerations

☐ Sometimes the risk of surgery is greater in the elderly because they may have disorders (eg, cardiac or renal disease) that interfere with recovery.

☐ A detailed history of drugs taken before admission is important because some drugs persist in the body for a period of time, and may interfere with the administration of anesthetic agents or drugs given before, during, or after surgery.

☐ A diminished ability to hear, see, and understand may interfere with preoperative and postoperative teaching. Explanations and demonstrations of the material presented may need to be repeated.

☐ Detailed assessments and tests of various body systems usually are required during the preoperative period.

☐ Elderly patients usually receive smaller doses of preoperative, intraoperative, and postoperative drugs, especially those that affect the central nervous, cardiovascular, or renal system.

☐ Elderly patients are prone to postoperative complications such as shock, atelectasis, pneumonia, paralytic ileus, gastric dilatation, and venous stasis.

☐ Postoperative ambulatory activities are essential, but planned carefully according to the patient's tolerance, which usually is less than that of the younger person.

☐ The postoperative convalescence period usually is longer. The patient may require positive reinforcement during his progress through the postoperative period, as well as extensive discharge planning.

☐ If the elderly patient lives alone, or with a spouse who is about the same age or who is ill or infirm, additional consideration should be given to discharge planning. It may be necessary to use the services of relatives or friends, a public health nurse, a visiting nurse, or home health care personnel during the convalescent period. In some instances, it is necessary to admit the patient to a skilled nursing facility for convalescent care.

☐ A loss of subcutaneous tissue and thinning of the skin accompanies the aging process. This, in turn, may lead to stress-producing situations such as poor wound healing, tissue breakdown owing to excessive pressure on a part, or inadequate development of granulation tissue in healing wounds.

Suggested Readings

☐ Alfaro R. Applying nursing diagnosis and nursing process: a step-by-step guide. 2nd ed. Philadelphia: JB Lippincott, 1990. *(Additional coverage of subject matter)*

☐ Burden N. Post-anesthesia: while the patient is unconscious. RN April 1988;51:34. *(Additional coverage of subject matter)*

☐ Burden N. Regional anesthesia: What patients—and nurses—need to know. RN May 1988;51:56. *(Additional coverage of subject matter)*

☐ Chitwood LB. Unveiling the mysteries of anesthesia. Nursing '87 February 1987;17:53. *(Additional coverage of subject matter)*

☐ Cuzzell JZ. Wound care forum: the new RYB color code. Am J Nurs October 1988;88:1342. *(Additional and in-depth coverage of subject matter)*

☐ Demling RH, Wilson MD. Decision making in surgical intensive care. St Louis: CV Mosby, 1988. *(In-depth coverage of subject matter)*

☐ Fraulini KE, Borchardt AC. Guide to solving post-anesthesia problems. Nursing '88 May 1988;16:66. *(Additional coverage of subject matter)*

☐ Frost E, ed. Recovery room practice. St Louis: CV Mosby, 1985. *(In-depth coverage of subject matter)*

☐ Gruendemann BJ, Meeker MH. Alexander's care of the patient in surgery. 8th ed. St Louis: CV Mosby, 1987. *(In-depth coverage of subject matter)*

☐ Kneedler EA, Dodge GH. Perioperative patient care. 2nd ed. St Louis: CV Mosby, 1987. *(In-depth coverage of subject matter)*

☐ McConnell EA. Clinical considerations in perioperative nursing: preventive aspects of care. Philadelphia: JB Lippincott, 1987. *(In-depth coverage of subject matter)*

☐ Moriarty MB. How color can clarify wound care. RN September 1988;51:49. *(Additional coverage of subject matter)*

☐ Sarasny Sl. Are you ready for this bedside emergency? RN December 1987;50:32. *(Additional coverage of subject matter)*

☐ Schulteis AH. When and how to extubate in the recovery room. Am J Nurs August 1989;89:1040. *(Additional coverage and illustrations that reinforce subject matter)*

☐ Stotts NA. Seeing the red and yellow and black: the three-color concept of wound care. Nursing '90 February 1990;20:59. *(Additional coverage and illustrations that reinforce subject matter)*

☐ Weinberger B. The sooner, the better. Nursing '89 February 1989;19:75. *(Additional coverage of subject matter)*

☐ Wells MM. Decision making in perioperative nursing. St Louis: CV Mosby, 1987. *(In-depth coverage of subject matter)*

Chapter 17
Nursing in Emergencies

On completion of this chapter the reader will:

- Discuss principles of emergency nursing in the hospital setting

- List and discuss general principles of first aid

- Describe and demonstrate the Heimlich maneuver

- Describe and discuss the emergency treatment of respiratory obstruction

- Describe and discuss the management of respiratory arrest

- List the symptoms and initial management of shock

- Describe and discuss the treatment of animal bites

- List the more common causes of food poisoning

- Describe and discuss the treatment and prevention of food poisoning

- Describe and discuss the treatment of drug, chemical, and gas poisoning

- Describe and discuss the treatment of psychiatric emergencies

- Describe the treatment of wounds

- Describe and discuss the treatment of heatstroke, frostbite, and sunburn

- Describe and discuss the treatment of bites and stings

EMERGENCY NURSING

Emergency nursing requires judgment, timing, alertness, and knowledge. An emergency department's primary purpose is to treat the serious, often life-threatening events that require immediate attention. Major emergencies that call for prompt action include hemorrhage, cessation of respiration or cardiac function, shock, electric shock, serious wounds (eg, fractures, puncture wounds, burns, gunshot wounds), animal or poisonous snake bites, poisoning (due to contaminated food, toxic substances, drugs, or gas), psychiatric emergencies, substance abuse, and exposure to extremes of temperature (eg, heatstroke, frostbite).

Many patients seen in an emergency department do not have life-threatening emergencies but still require treatment. Some individuals seeking treatment may have minor injuries or ailments that could be treated in a physician's office, but for various reasons the individual seeks treatment at a hospital. General principles for emergency nursing include the following:

1. Evaluate each patient to assess the seriousness and extent of the illness or injury and to prioritize the patient's needs. Then schedule an examination by a physician or nurse. Patients with serious illnesses or injuries are given priority over those with less serious or minor problems.

2. Recognize an emergency. Learn enough about each patient's condition to recognize when an illness is or has become serious.

3. Apply the principles of first aid. Because nurses are often the first to see patients in an emergency, they must be able to establish priorities of care. Severe hemorrhage, acute respiratory difficulty, shock, severe chest pain, multiple injuries, high fever, and coma are examples of conditions that have the highest priorities.

4. Adjust pace to rapidly changing situations. The nurse must move fast to aid respiration, stop bleeding, and attend to other major emergencies. The report given to the physician, however, must be as accurate as it is prompt.

5. The nurse is often the first person to see the patient and the family. An appropriate word can help assure them that the physician will treat the patient as soon as possible.

6. Meeting physical and emotional needs, supporting the family or relatives, and attending to spiritual needs are all part of emergency nursing.

7. The extent of the patient's injuries should be explained clearly by the physician, but the nurse must be prepared to repeat explanations to the patient or family.

8. The nurse must be especially observant for symptoms that seem in excess of the injury, or for denial of the injury.

9. Supplies must always be available and ready for use. It is the responsibility of all personnel to know where the emergency supplies and equipment are located and how to use them.

10. If the patient is discharged from the emergency department, clear and complete instructions regarding home

care of the injury or illness are given to the patient and the family. Patients tend to be anxious, and instructions are easily confused or forgotten. When possible, instructions should be written as well as given verbally.

11. Many emergency nursing procedures have legal ramifications; therefore, all emergency department personnel must be familiar with local, county, and state laws. Basic precautionary actions include the following:

— All incidents and observations are carefully and accurately documented.

— When a patient is seriously injured, valuables are removed and sent home with the family or deposited in the hospital safe. The disposition of the valuables is entered in the patient's record.

— It may be necessary to work with the police to help establish the identity of an unaccompanied, helpless person or to document the results of criminal acts, such as rape, assault, and child abuse.

— All clothing is handled with care, even if it is bloody or dirty. If clothing must be cut, it is cut along a seam whenever possible.

— If an adult patient is unable to sign a consent for surgery, the family must be located.

GENERAL PRINCIPLES OF FIRST AID

First aid may be defined as the tasks designed to keep a person with an injury or serious illness alive and to prevent further damage or complications until medical treatment can be initiated. Usually applicable to incidents that occur outside of the hospital, first aid also can be used in the emergency department when a patient must wait to be seen by a physician. Important general principles of first aid, adaptable to particular situations, include the following:

1. Establish an airway and adequate respiration.
2. Stop any bleeding.
3. Obtain vital signs.
4. Assess for injuries systematically and as soon as possible. Assessment is made after bleeding is stopped and respiration is established. It begins at the head and continues to the toes. A wound that is small or hidden by clothing may still present a serious problem.
5. Consider underlying anatomy and physiology. For example, a chest wound that sucks in air with every breath is a sign that the wound probably extends into the pleural cavity. When the rib cage expands, air is pulled into the pleural space through the wound, collapsing the lung. Immediate action in this instance would be to place a pressure dressing over the area to prevent more air from entering the chest through the puncture wound.
6. Prevent chilling. Almost all emergency conditions entail a degree of shock; both chilling and excessive heat may further increase shock and must be avoided.
7. Do not give the patient anything to eat or drink until

the full extent of the injuries has been determined by a physician.

8. Stay with seriously ill or injured people until they are examined by a physician.
9. Report symptoms that were noted and the initial emergency treatment, if any, that was given.
10. Communicate calmness. Fear and confusion can be minimized by a calm but firm manner.

Emergency Situations

HEMORRHAGE

It is important to look for bleeding and to stop it quickly. Most people can tolerate the loss of a pint of blood, but losing a quart or more leads to shock. A patient can die of hemorrhage in less than 1 minute if a large artery is severed. Most bleeding, however, can be stopped by pressure on and around the area and elevation of the affected extremity. Emergency management of hemorrhage is as follows:

1. If the hemorrhage is external, remove or cut away clothing over and around the injured area. Apply direct continuous pressure to the wound or on a major artery leading to the wound. Press the artery against the bone (Figs. 17-1 and 17-2). When able, apply a firm pressure dressing. If an extremity is involved, it should be immobilized.
2. If the hemorrhage is external, elevate the injured part. If bleeding of an extremity cannot be controlled by the application of pressure and elevation of the part, the physician may order a tourniquet. An extremity that is mangled, crushed, or amputated requires a tourniquet to stop bleeding. Periodic release of the tourniquet depends on the severity of the injury. A tourniquet of the inflatable (pneumatic) type is preferable. A blood pressure cuff can be used as a tourniquet; the cuff is inflated to a level above the patient's systolic blood pressure. If the blood pressure is not obtainable, the cuff is inflated until bleeding stops. An inflatable tourniquet should not be removed except by a physician.
3. If the hemorrhage is internal and in the lower part of the body, a medical antishock trouser (MAST) may be ordered. This device applies counter pressure around the legs and abdomen. When available, a MAST may be applied by emergency personnel before transporting the victim to the hospital.
4. Insert an intravenous line to provide a method to replace lost fluid and to obtain blood samples for the laboratory. Add dextrose in saline to the intravenous line until the physician orders other replacement solutions (eg, whole blood or plasma). The rate of infusion of any intravenous fluid is dependent on several factors, including the amount and type of fluid lost and the patient's cardiac status.
5. Every 3 to 15 minutes, monitor vital signs, the appearance of the area of hemorrhage, and the effectiveness of treatment.

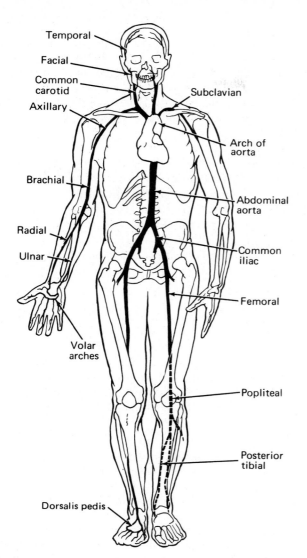

Figure 17–1. Arteries that may be palpated (except the aorta and the common iliac) and compressed. The line on the left leg indicates that the arteries travel along the back of the leg.

6. Keep the patient in a supine position.
7. If emergency surgery is indicated to control internal or external bleeding, prepare the patient according to the physician's orders. The family, if present, are informed of the decision to take the patient to surgery.

RESPIRATORY EMERGENCIES
Respiratory Obstruction

Obstruction of the respiratory tract may be partial or complete. Most often it is due to a foreign body lodged in the upper respiratory tract. Complete airway obstruction results in respiratory arrest. In adults, one of the most common causes of partial or complete respiratory obstruction is food lodged in the airway. In children, toys small enough to fit in the mouth as well

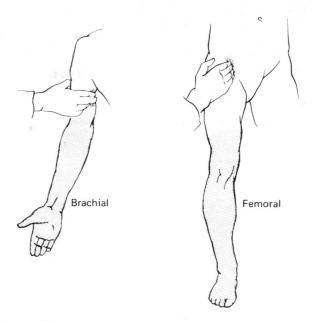

Figure 17–2. Methods of occluding the brachial and femoral arteries to control bleeding from injuries in the shaded areas. Pressure is applied to the artery and to the bone behind it.

as food are the most common causes of respiratory obstruction.

Management

If a foreign body has obstructed the air passages, the Heimlich maneuver is attempted and is performed by standing behind the patient. One fist is clenched, with the fingers of the clenched hand placed against the patient's abdomen about midway between the navel and the xiphoid process. The other hand is placed over the clenched fist. The fist is pressed into the abdomen using a quick upward thrust and repeated until the foreign body is expelled and the patient is able to breathe. If the patient is unconscious and lying on his or her back, the nurse should kneel and face the patient's head. The heel of the hand is placed in the same position as the clenched fist when the patient is standing. The other hand is placed on top. The hands are pressed into the abdomen with a quick upward thrust and repeated as needed.

Respiratory Arrest

Respiratory arrest is the complete cessation of breathing. The causes of respiratory arrest include drowning, electric shock, carbon monoxide or other gaseous poisoning, drugs, certain central nervous system and thoracic diseases and injuries, and complete obstruction of the respiratory tract. Respiratory arrest must be treated immediately because brain death occurs in minutes, depending on the age of the patient. Infants and young children may tolerate 8 minutes without oxygen, whereas the elderly person may only tolerate 3 to 4 minutes. It is most important to determine the possible or probable cause of respiratory arrest.

Management

The steps for emergency management of respiratory arrest are as follows:

1. Place the patient on a firm, flat surface. Clear the airway of any mucous, dirt, or other particles by wiping the inside of the patient's mouth with the index and middle fingers. Look for a possible cause of obstruction, such as an object in the back of the mouth. Do not attempt to remove an object in this area; an effort to do so may push the object further down and thus make removal difficult or impossible. Instead, use the Heimlich maneuver (see earlier discussion of respiratory obstruction).
2. Use either of the following maneuvers to open the airway.
    — Head-tilt–chin-lift maneuver: Place the palm of one hand on the victim's forehead and use firm backward pressure to tilt the head back. Place the fingers of the other hand under the lower jaw (mandible) near the center and lift. This action brings the chin forward and clenches the teeth.
    — Jaw-thrust maneuver: Use the fingers of both hands (one on each side of the jaw) to grasp the victim's lower jaw near the angle of the jaw and lift forward while simultaneously tilting the head backward.
3. Insert an oropharyngeal airway and begin cardiopulmonary resuscitation to bring oxygen to the brain and other vital organs until further treatment, such as the insertion of an endotracheal tube, mechanical ventilation, and drug therapy, can be instituted.

SHOCK

The loss of blood or any type of injury is capable of causing shock. In shock, the patient's skin is cold and moist; the lips and fingers are pale or cyanotic. A detailed discussion of the types, symptoms, and treatment of shock is found in Chapter 18. The following measures are carried out until the cause of shock is determined and medical treatment is instituted:

1. Insert an intravenous line immediately, if one is present, and run at a rate to keep the vein open (KVO) until the patient is seen by a physician.
2. Keep the patient lying flat with the feet 8 to 12 inches higher than the head (unless dyspnea occurs in this position).
3. Keep the patient as still and as quiet as possible.
4. Keep the patient warm, but avoid overheating. Excessive heat results in vasodilatation, which can increase shock.
5. Do not give anything by mouth.

WOUNDS

A wound is a break in the continuity of the skin. Wounds seen in the emergency department range from small lacerations to serious, widespread injuries, such as gunshot and stab wounds. The victim incurring multiple injuries may have many types of wounds.

History

Assessment reveals the seriousness of the victim's condition. If multiple injuries have occurred, the most serious problems, such as hemorrhage or shock, are treated first. The patient is also assessed for other problems, such pneumothorax and internal bleeding, which may not be readily apparent but which also require immediate attention. After the patient's condition has been stabilized and other potentially life-threatening problems treated, attention may be given to the wounds.

If the wound is minor in nature, it is important to determine when and how the wound occurred. In some instances, part of the treatment may depend on the cause of the wound. For example, a wound caused by an instrument contaminated with soil may require administration of tetanus prophylaxis, whereas a wound caused by a kitchen knife may not.

Treatment

When applicable, clothing covering the wound is carefully removed. If the clothing has stuck to the wound, it is necessary to soak the clothing with saline or hydrogen peroxide before removal. Hair around the wound is clipped or shaved, and the area around the wound cleansed with an antiseptic agent. If suturing is necessary, a local anesthetic is injected. The physician then cleans and debrides the wound, removing any foreign particles or objects before suturing the wound edges. If suturing is not necessary, the physician approximates the edges and applies a dressing that keeps the edges together until the area has healed. A sterile dressing is applied. When an extremity is involved, the part may be immobilized.

Depending on the extent and cause of the injury, antibiotics (topical or systemic) may be prescribed. If the patient is discharged from the emergency department, instructions are given regarding care of the area and the time to return for removal of the sutures.

ANIMAL BITES
Snake Bites

People bitten by snakes native to the United States usually recover, but a snake bite can be fatal. In all likelihood, the victim is extremely apprehensive. It is most important to identify the snake because treatment may include the administration of snake antivenin. If the person saw the snake, it is important to obtain its description, mainly its color and the shape of its head.

Treatment is directed toward keeping the snake venom from entering the bloodstream, thus, spreading to other areas of the body. The patient is kept quiet, and the affected part is immobilized. The physician may order the application of a tourniquet above and below the area of the bite and, possibly, the application of a cold compress. If available, antivenin is administered.

Warm-Blooded Animal Bites

Bites from any warm-blooded animal must be regarded as potential transmitters of rabies. The wound is washed and debrided if necessary by a physician. Tetanus immunization is given. If a person is bitten by an animal that may have rabies, the rabies vaccine is given if (1) the animal is found and appears rabid or develops rabies after it has been impounded, or (2) the animal cannot be found, but the type of animal is known to carry rabies (eg, bats, skunks, raccoons, or dogs).

INSECT BITES AND STINGS

Ticks

The tick may be killed with a few drops of turpentine, or a hot needle may be used to make it release its hold. Tweezers may be used to gently remove the tick from the skin. Crushing the tick could transmit virulent pathogenic microorganisms that are carried by some ticks. Excessive force in trying to remove a tick must be avoided. The area should be scrubbed with soap and water afterward.

Lyme Disease
Lyme disease is caused by a spirochete carried by the ticks of some wild animals such as deer, mice, and some domesticated animals, such as dogs. Early symptoms include a red macule or papule at the site of the tick bite, which may be followed by headache, neck stiffness and pain, and fatigue. Symptoms that may occur weeks or months later include arthritic joint swelling and pain, fatigue, cardiac involvement (heart block), and neurologic abnormalities (eg, facial palsy, meningitis, encephalitis). Treatment is with tetracycline, phenoxymethyl penicillin, or erythromycin. Intravenous penicillin G may be given for meningitis or encephalitis.

Bees, Wasps, Hornets

The stinger should be removed with a sterile needle or tweezers (only honey bees shed their stinger). An ice bag or a paste made of baking soda reduces swelling and itching. Antihistamines may also be used to control itching. If the person is allergic to the venom of the insect, anaphylactic shock may occur (see Chapter 18). For those with a known allergy to a particular stinging insect venom, the physician may prescribe a kit containing epinephrine in a sterile syringe. The drug is self-injected after a bite by the offending insect.

Poisonous Spiders, Tarantulas, and Scorpions

Death of a healthy adult from spider bite or scorpion sting is rare, but the symptoms can be extremely painful. Deaths have occurred in children and in adults with weakened conditions. The best known toxic spider is the black widow, which secretes a neurotoxin. This spider has a shiny black color with a red to orange hourglass shape on its ventral surface. The less well-known brown recluse spider is at least as dangerous. It is somewhat smaller than the black widow and ranges from light tan to dark brown in color, with a banjo-shaped spot on its abdomen. The brown recluse is shy and usually hidden from view. It appears to bite when it is threatened. Unfortunately, it sometimes lives in old clothing or shoes kept in a garage or basement. When a person tries to put these garments on, the spider, presumably in self-defense, bites. The initial bite is seldom painful and often is unnoticed. The toxin, however, contains an extremely potent digestive enzyme, and, after a few hours, it destroys a large amount of tissue, leaving an open wound that may not heal for many months.

Secondary infections can follow spider bites. For this reason, a report of a spider bite must be taken seriously, even if no pain or toxicity is initially evident. If possible, the spider should be identified. If identification cannot be made, any person bitten by a spider of unknown species should be seen by a physician for immediate observation and definitive management. For temporary relief, cold applications to the bitten area are helpful, but freezing of tissues must be avoided. Specific medical treatments for black widow spider bites include the intravenous injection of calcium gluconate and the use of an antivenin. No antivenin is available for brown recluse spider venom.

POISONING

The forms of poisoning most frequently encountered are food poisoning, drug or chemical poisoning, and poisoning by gas inhalation.

Food Poisoning

Food poisoning results when food is contaminated with microorganisms such as *Clostridium botulinum, Staphylococcus aureus,* and *Salmonella enteritidis.* Food poisoning may be of nonmicrobial origin, as for example, poisoning caused by contamination of food by insecticides. Naturally toxic plants, such as various strains of mushrooms, berries, and wild plants, may be ingested through accident or ignorance.

Botulism

Botulism is caused by *Clostridium botulinum,* an anaerobe which produces a neurotoxin. This microorganism is found most often in foods that have been improperly canned at home. The neurotoxin is destroyed by heat just below the boiling point. The spores, which are produced by the microorganism, are killed by temperatures over the boiling point, about 120°C. Any can that is swollen or seems to contain gas should be discarded unopened. Symptoms of botulism include nausea and vomiting, headache, lassitude, double vision, muscular incoordination, and inability to talk, swallow, or breathe.

Treatment includes administration of botulinal antitoxin, mechanical ventilation, and intravenous therapy. Early treatment is important. Death is often due to respiratory failure.

Other Types of Food Poisoning

Microorganisms that cause food poisoning grow in food, especially those products that have not been refrigerated before or after eating. Symptoms of food poisoning may include weakness, diarrhea, nausea, vomiting, and abdominal cramps developing a few hours after ingesting the contaminated food. They may last for 1 or 2 days. Death is rare but has occurred. Poisoning due to certain varieties of mushrooms, wild berries, and other naturally toxic substances can be more serious.

Food poisoning may not be recognized until the food is absorbed and the patient begins to experience symptoms. When a patient is admitted to the emergency department with possible food poisoning, the following steps are vital:

1. Identification of the contaminated food. The family is instructed to bring the possibly contaminated food to the hospital as soon as possible for examination and laboratory tests (cultures). If the food was eaten at a restaurant, information about the name and address of the facility, the time the food was served, and the foods that were eaten must be obtained.
2. History. The patient or a family member is questioned about the type of symptoms, when symptoms began in relation to the time the suspected food was eaten, and the number of times the victim vomited or had a bowel movement.

3. Treatment. Parenteral fluids may be ordered to correct fluid loss. An antiemetic may be prescribed to control nausea and vomiting. Vital signs are monitored, with the frequency depending on the condition of the patient. Samples of vomitus and feces are saved for possible laboratory examination.
4. Teaching. To prevent future episodes of food poisoning, a teaching plan includes the following instructions:
   — Hands are washed before as well as during food preparation. When handling fresh poultry, the hands are washed before preparing other foods. Uncooked poultry may contain *Salmonella* organisms, which can be transferred to other foods, such as fresh vegetables.
   — Foods, including fresh fruits and vegetables, are thoroughly washed before cooking or eating.
   — Food should be cooked for adequate times and at recommended temperatures. Although raw foods such as fish can be eaten safely, improper preparation and refrigeration can contaminate this type of food.
   — Immediately refrigerate leftover food. Do not allow food to stand in the kitchen or dining area. Refrigerate foods prepared for picnics and buffet meals until they are ready to be served.
   — Avoid the use of wooden cutting boards. The surface and grain of the wood cannot be cleaned adequately and tends to harbor pathogenic microorganisms. Use cutting boards with smooth, nonporous surfaces.

Drug and Chemical Poisoning

Poisoning from drugs and chemicals is a common problem. Small children (Fig. 17-3) are prone to ingesting common household substances; these may be relatively harmless, or they may be capable of causing permanent disability or death. Adults may ingest drugs or chemicals by accident or on purpose. Accidental ingestion may occur in the elderly, who may not be able to read a label or who may not remember that a prescribed dose of a medication has already been taken. Accidental overdose of a drug may occur with substance abuse. Poisoning by ingestion of a drug or chemical may occur in suicide attempts.

History

After ingestion of a drug or chemical, it is extremely important to determine the following factors:

- Substances involved
- Amount or dose ingested
- Route (oral, parenteral)
- Approximate time of ingestion
- What treatment, if any, was given before admission to the emergency department
- Patient's general condition

Treatment

Correct treatment or administration of an antidote depends on substance identification. If the substance is unknown, a thorough assessment of the patient's physing vital signs, administration of oxygen, mechanical ventilation, suctioning, insertion of a nasogastric tube, and monitoring urinary output.

Teaching

Prevention is the goal of any teaching plan associated with drug and chemical poisoning. The public must be made aware of the dangers associated with certain types of chemicals and the hazards of substance abuse.

1. The public should know about local poison information centers with 24-hour telephone answering services. If a child or adult has ingested a drug or chemical, the poison center can provide information about emergency treatment and antidotes.
2. All cases of accidental or intentional drug or chemical ingestion must receive prompt medical attention. The victim should be transported to the hospital as quickly as possible. Delay in seeking medical attention or inappropriate treatment by family members can result in permanent damage or death.
3. All prescription and nonprescription drugs and household chemicals (eg, soaps, insecticides, cleaning solutions, drain cleaners, bleach, paint and paint thinners, ammonia) are kept in a safe place and out of the reach of small children. In some instances, these substances should be kept in locked cupboards.
4. If the container of the drug or chemical ingested by the person is found, it must be saved; if the container is not found, a specimen of the person's vomitus or urine should be saved and brought to the emergency department.
5. Ipecac syrup, a drug that causes vomiting, does not require a prescription and should be in all households with small children. This drug should not be given, however, until the family member has contacted a poison information center, physician, or hospital emergency department.

Poisoning by Gas

Carbon Monoxide

Carbon monoxide, an odorless, colorless gas, is the most common gas involved in poisoning. Inhalation of carbon monoxide may result from industrial or household accidents and suicide attempts. The running of a gas engine (eg, a car engine) in an unventilated area results in a rapid buildup of carbon monoxide. A defective furnace or other heating device may also emit carbon monoxide. Improper ventilation with the use of kerosene heaters, charcoal burning, and furnaces may also result in carbon monoxide poisoning.

Symptoms of carbon monoxide poisoning include headache, muscle weakness, slurred speech, dizziness, difficulty walking, and mental confusion. Skin color may change from pale or cyanotic to pink or cherry red.

When carbon monoxide poisoning is suspected, the

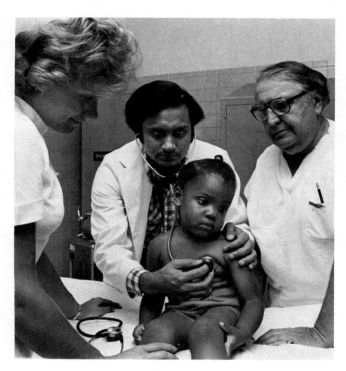

Figure 17–3. Children frequently ingest drugs and chemicals found in and around the home and should be treated as soon as possible. (Photograph by D. Atkinson)

ical and mental status may provide important information. Burns on the mouth suggest that a corrosive acid or alkali has been swallowed; drowsiness, stupor, or coma may indicate ingestion of a substance affecting the central nervous system. Laboratory tests may also be used to identify some substances as well as determine blood levels.

The goals of treatment are (1) to remove or inactivate the substance as soon as possible, (2) to treat the symptoms, and (3) to administer an antidote if the substance is known and an antidote is available.

After ingestion of a drug or chemical, the following steps may be taken:

1. If the container is not found immediately, the poison may be diluted by giving the patient (if conscious) as much water as possible. Rapid action is important.
2. Vomiting is induced or a nasogastric or gastric lavage tube is passed to empty stomach contents. Do not induce vomiting if: the substance is ammonia or a strong acid or alkali (which would reburn the tissues of the mouth and esophagus when brought up), or any petroleum product, such as gasoline, lighter fluid, or kerosene; the patient is already comatose or convulsing, or the patient complains of severe pain or a burning sensation in the mouth and throat.
3. Supportive care is given and depends on the symptoms as well as the substance ingested. Supportive care may include maintaining an airway, starting an intravenous line for the administration of fluids and drugs, monitor-

patient must be removed from the area. If the patient is not breathing, mouth-to-mouth resuscitation is started. The patient is hospitalized as rapidly as possible.

If carbon monoxide poisoning has occurred, oxygen (100%) is administered by mask and blood is drawn to determine carboxyhemoglobin levels. An intravenous line is inserted to support blood pressure and administer drugs.

Radon

Radon, a colorless, odorless gas, is the radioactive by-product of the decay of the radioactive element radium. It is found in soil in many areas of the country and can enter the home through cracks and other openings in the floor and walls of the basement. Inhalation of radon gas over a prolonged period of time is thought to increase the risk of lung cancer and other types of cancer.

Test kits are available for detecting high levels of radon gas. If a home area is found to have levels higher than those recommended, several changes to the basement can be made. Vents and fans installed to move air from the basement to the outside appear to lower the concentration of radon. No treatment for prolonged inhalation of radon gas has been found.

EXPOSURE TO TEMPERATURE EXTREMES
Heatstroke

In this potentially serious disorder, the body's normal responses to increasing atmospheric temperature do not function properly. Symptoms of heatstroke include confusion, dizziness, and weakness. The skin is red, hot, and dry to the touch and little or no perspiration is seen. The body temperature can be 105°F (40.6°C) or higher. Elderly or debilitated people and those taking certain drugs (eg, diuretics, major tranquilizers) are especially prone to heatstroke during hot, humid weather. People who engage in heavy physical activities during hot, humid weather also can suffer from heatstroke.

Treatment

The victim should be taken to a hospital as soon as possible. The most important goal of treatment is to bring down the body temperature. Clothes are removed. The entire body is covered with wet, cold towels, or the patient is immersed in a tepid or cool bath. Other methods of lowering body temperature include application of ice packs to the forehead, axillae, body and legs, or a hypothermia blanket. If conscious and able to swallow, small amounts of a cool drink may be given. A temperature probe is placed in the rectum, and vital signs are monitored frequently.

An intravenous line is inserted to administer fluids. The intake and output is monitored because renal failure may occur after severe heatstroke. Cooling is continued until body temperature is about 101°F. Sustained high fever may result in brain, liver, kidney, and central nervous system damage.

Teaching

People who are more susceptible to heatstroke or who have had heatstroke are warned of its dangers and informed of the methods to avoid it. Emphasis is placed on the importance of maintaining an adequate fluid intake, reducing activities, avoiding prolonged exposure to the sun, and wearing loose clothing during hot, humid weather. Air conditioning also is recommended but may not always be feasible or affordable.

Frostbite

Severe cold causes injury to tissues. Extreme vasoconstriction and thrombosis and direct injury to the walls of the blood vessels and the cells occur. Exudate escapes from the damaged vessel walls, resulting in edema. Ischemia of the tissues is found, and the skin blanches. The frostbitten part becomes numb and stiff. As it warms, it turns a bright pink and blisters.

Treatment

Clothing around the affected area is carefully removed, and the extremity immersed in a warm solution, with the temperature about 100°F. Slow warming of a frostbitten part causes more tissue damage than rapid warming. The extremity is immersed for about 30 to 45 minutes, or until the part appears to regain some of its normal color. Moving the extremity in the warm bath or using a whirlpool type bath is necessary to keep the water warm. Warm water is added to the solution as needed. As the part warms, pain may be experienced and analgesics may be needed.

After bathing, the skin is blotted dry, and a dry sterile dressing applied, using sterile gauze or cotton to separate skin surfaces such as those between the fingers or toes. The affected part requires elevation to prevent swelling. If legs or feet are involved, the patient should not walk.

Debridement and skin grafting may be necessary if blistering has occurred. Because deep circulation is affected less than superficial circulation, this surgical treatment usually is effective.

The degree of injury varies in severity. In mild cases, recovery is complete. In severe cases, amputation may be necessary. Patients who have been severely frostbitten may, for years afterward, experience numbness and tinging when the affected area is exposed to cold.

These patients are advised to protect this area in the future from injury or exposure to cold.

Teaching

Measures for the prevention of frostbite include the following:

1. Wear adequate clothing, such as thermal undergarments and windproof outer clothing, when exposed to low temperatures.
2. Keep normally exposed areas (face, ears, neck, hands) adequately protected from cold air and wind.
3. Be aware that even moderate cold accompanied by wind (wind chill factor) can produce frostbite.
4. Avoid constrictive clothing, such as shoes and socks that are too tight. Keep the entire body as warm and dry as possible when exposed to extreme cold.
5. Exercise legs, feet, arms, and fingers if they are in a situation that is likely to cause frostbite.
6. Observe the skin for the development of yellow-white patches and heed such sensations as pricking or pain, which may be early signs of frostbite.
7. Snow or cold water is never applied to the frostbitten areas.

Sunburn

A first-degree burn may be soothed by cool compresses. To avoid further trauma to the skin, the patient must be handled gently. Blisters should be dressed with sterile gauze. If the sunburn is extensive, intravenous fluids, analgesics, and the topical application of an antibiotic ointment may be necessary.

PSYCHIATRIC EMERGENCIES

In a psychiatric emergency, the individual may be brought to the emergency department by the family, neighbors, or the police. In this type of emergency, the person exhibits a disturbance in behavior, thought, or affect which may coexist with physical injuries that have been self-inflicted or inflicted by others.

History

Whenever possible, it is important to determine the events that led to the behavioral changes. The people accompanying the patient to the emergency department are questioned. A medical history is obtained, because various diseases or disorders, such as diabetes mellitus with hypoglycemia or alcohol or drug withdrawal, may cause behavioral changes.

Treatment

Treatment depends on the patient's mental condition and behavior. This type of emergency requires the emergency department personnel to consider the patient's safety and their own safety, while maintaining a calm and confident manner.

Violent or aggressive patients usually require immediate and rapid sedation with a tranquilizer. They must be protected from harming themselves and others and must not be left alone. Restraints may be necessary if behavior cannot be controlled by medication or if the patient refuses to accept the medication.

The individual who appears out of contact with reality but who is not physically aggressive or aggravated may also require a small dose of a sedative or a tranquilizer. They also must be under observation at all times.

The depressed patient may be quiet and communicate poorly or may show some evidence of agitation. Some depressed patients are suicidal and, therefore, require constant observation and, possibly, administration of an antidepressant drug.

Depending on the diagnosis and the degree of illness, the patient may be admitted to a psychiatric unit for further treatment, referred to another hospital with a psychiatric unit, or referred to a private physician.

OTHER EMERGENCIES

Other situations seen in the emergency department are covered in appropriate chapters. Shock is covered in Chapter 18, substance abuse in Chapter 11, fractures in Chapter 55, and thermal injuries in Chapter 56.

General Pharmacologic Considerations

☐ Emergency department nurses must be familiar with the use, action, and adverse effects of drugs used in emergency situations.

☐ Accidental chemical ingestion is a relatively common occurrence, especially among children. Patient discharge teaching should include instructions regarding safekeeping of drugs and household products.

☐ It is important to locate the drug or chemical container in accidental or intentional cases of poisoning or overdose to identify the material and possibly the amount ingested.

☐ Ipecac syrup, a drug that induces vomiting, should be kept in all households with small children. This drug is available in a 1-oz size and directions for use are printed on the label. For children older than 1 year, give half of the container (15 mL). Parents are advised to contact the local poison center, their physician, or a hospital emergency department before giving this drug.

General Gerontologic Considerations

☐ The elderly are prone to injuries that require emergency attention. Such injuries may include falls, hypothermia, burns, accidental drug overdose, and heatstroke.

☐ The injured elderly patient may become confused and frightened after an injury. Continual assurance is necessary during transportation to the hospital and during the time of treatment in the emergency department.

☐ After an accident or injury, the elderly patient may not be able to communicate accurate information regarding circumstances surrounding the injury or accident and the location of family members.

Suggested Readings

☐ Beyea SC. What people expect you to know about poison ivy. RN August 1989;52:23. *(Additional coverage of subject matter)*

☐ Cardonna VD, Hurn PD, Mason PJ, Scanlon-Schilpp AM, Veise-Berry SW. Trauma nursing: from resuscitation through rehabilitation. Philadelphia: WB Saunders, 1988. *(Additional and in-depth coverage of subject matter)*

☐ Cerrato PL. Food poisoning makes a dangerous comeback. RN October 1989;73. *(Additional coverage of subject matter)*

☐ Kitt S, Kaiser J. Emergency nursing: a physiologic and clinical perspective. Philadelphia: WB Saunders, 1989. *(Additional and in-depth coverage of subject matter)*

☐ Mancini ME. Decision making in emergency nursing. St Louis: CV Mosby, 1987. *(Additional and in-depth coverage of subject matter)*

☐ Redheffer GM. Treating wounds on the scene: part 1. Nursing '89 July 1989;19:51. *(Additional coverage and illustrations that reinforce subject matter)*

☐ Redheffer GM, Baily M. Assessing and splinting fractures. Nursing '89 June 1989; 19:51. *(Additional coverage and illustrations that reinforce subject matter)*

☐ Rich J. Action stat! Snakebite. Nursing '87 June 1987;17:33. *(Additional coverage of subject matter)*

☐ Sheehy SB. Mosby's manual of emergency care. 3rd ed. St Louis: CV Mosby, 1989. *(Additional and in-depth coverage of subject matter)*

☐ Sheehy SB, Marvin JA, Jimmerson CL. Manual of clinical trauma care: the first hour. St Louis: CV Mosby, 1988. *(Additional and in-depth coverage of subject matter)*

☐ Smith GA, Savinski-Bozinko G. Giving emergency care for burns. Nursing '89 December 1989;19:55. *(Additional and in-depth coverage of subject matter)*

☐ Talley MA, Luterman A. . . . About burns. Nursing '89 January 1989;19:21. *(Additional coverage of subject matter)*

Chapter 18
The Patient in Shock

On completion of this chapter the reader will:

- Define shock
- List the types of shock
- Describe and discuss the physiologic changes that occur with each type of shock
- List and discuss the symptoms of shock
- Discuss measures that may be used to prevent shock
- Discuss the prognosis and complications of shock
- List and briefly describe the assessment of a patient in shock
- Use the nursing process in the management of a patient in shock

A serious disorder, *shock* occurs when inadequate peripheral blood flow decreases the amount of oxygen that reaches vital tissues and organs and reduces the removal of the waste products of metabolism.

The faster the shock state can be reversed, the greater the chance of uncomplicated recovery. Regardless of the cause, prolonged shock is incompatible with life. In few instances is the careful attention to nursing practices and principles more important to a patient's recovery than it is in the management of a patient in impending or actual shock.

TYPES OF SHOCK
Hypovolemic Shock

In hypovolemic shock, the volume of fluid is reduced because of a loss of blood, plasma, or body fluids. Hypovolemic shock can be caused by, for example, severe burns, in which a large amount of plasma seeps from the circulatory system into the injured area, the loss of large amounts of fluid, as with protracted vomiting and diarrhea, and hemorrhage.

Cardiogenic Shock

In cardiogenic shock, a decrease in the contraction ability of the heart or an interference with the normal function of the heart occurs. When the contraction (or contractile) ability of the myocardium is diminished, the cardiac output, which is the amount of blood leaving the heart with each ventricular contraction, decreases. A reduction in cardiac output results in a decreased blood supply and, therefore, a decreased delivery of oxygen to body tissues and organs. Interference with the normal function of the heart, as might be seen with some cardiac dysrhythmias or cardiac tamponade, also reduces cardiac output.

Vasogenic Shock

In vasogenic shock, diffuse vasodilatation results in an increase in the size of the vascular bed. When blood becomes trapped in small vessels and in the viscera, it is lost temporarily to the mainstream of circulating fluid. The skeletal muscles and the viscera may become engorged with blood. Vasogenic shock is normovolemic because the amount of fluid in the circulatory system is not reduced; however, the fluid is not circulating in a way that permits effective perfusion of the tissues. Anaphylactic shock is an example of vasogenic shock.

Neurogenic Shock

Neurogenic shock results from an insult to the nervous system, which leads to decreased arterial resistance.

Intracranial damage and certain drugs can cause neurogenic shock. Vasodilatation, a prominent feature, is due to the loss of sympathetic nervous system control over the size of the arterioles.

Bacteremic (Septic) Shock

Bacteremic shock can be seen with an overwhelming bacterial infection, usually in a patient who is succumbing to the infection. Bacteremic shock is more common in patients with bacteremia caused by gramnegative organisms. Endotoxins released by these organisms are probably a major cause.

SYMPTOMS OF SHOCK

The nurse must watch for signs that the body is being forced to call on major defenses to maintain blood pressure. Although deep shock can develop in minutes, there may also be a warning period.

Arterial Blood Pressure.   In shock, the systolic and diastolic blood pressure falls. Blood pressure is a valuable but not an infallible index of shock. Organ blood flow and tissue perfusion, not blood pressure, are the critical determinants.

Blood pressure falls because cardiac output decreases or the size of the vascular bed increases. For the adult, the average, normal systolic blood pressure is 100 to 130 mmHg. A systolic blood pressure of 90 to 100 mmHg may indicate impending shock, whereas 80 mmHg or below would indicate shock. These figures generally apply to normotensive (normal blood pressure) individuals. For example, a blood pressure of 120/82 is considered normal; if an individual with untreated hypertension and an original blood pressure of 190/112 develops a blood pressure of 120/82, however, shock may be present.

To determine if shock is present, the patient's previous blood pressure must be known. Regardless of the numeric figure, a progressive fall in blood pressure with a rapid, thready pulse is a serious sign. In the early stages of shock, the blood pressure may not fall because the body attempts to compensate by, for example, decreasing the size of the vascular bed (vasoconstriction) or shifting fluids from around and inside body cells to the vascular compartment (inside blood vessels). A rapid pulse, apprehension, or air hunger may be the only indications of impending shock. The physician is made aware of any fall in systolic blood pressure below 100 mmHg or any fall of 20 mmHg or more below the patient's usual systolic blood pressure.

In some instances, measurements of blood pressure may be difficult or even impossible to obtain or may be falsely low, particularly in patients with peripheral arteriosclerosis compounded by the effects of vasopressor drugs. When peripheral arterioles are constricted in shock, diastolic pressure rises initially because an increased pressure is necessary for the blood to flow through the constricted vessels. Intraarterial blood pressure monitoring is more accurate than the usual, indirect auscultatory method of a blood pressure cuff.

The systolic blood pressure may be quickly determined by palpation, using a sphygmomanometer with the fingertips on the radial pulse. After the cuff has been inflated sufficiently to obliterate the pulse, air is let out of the cuff slowly to allow blood to begin flowing through the radial artery. The systolic blood pressure is recorded when the radial pulse is palpable.

Skin.   Peripheral blood vessels constrict to direct blood from the skin to more vital organs, such as the kidney and brain. Ischemia renders the skin pale and cold. The skin is clammy due to activation of the sweat glands. Cyanosis, especially of the nail beds, lips, and earlobes, indicates a deficiency of oxygen. Lack of cyanosis, however, does not prove the absence of hypoxia (decrease of oxygen in inspired air). Recognition of cyanosis may be obscured by deep skin pigmentation, anemia, and poor lighting conditions.

Pulse Rate and Rhythm.   Cardiac output is decreased in shock. A compensatory tachycardia occurs in an attempt to increase cardiac output. The minimum essential myocardial perfusion pressure needed to maintain coronary artery blood flow is considered to correspond to a systolic pressure of about 80 mmHg. Below this level, the myocardium becomes increasingly hypoxic. The force of myocardial contraction decreases, and the potential for dangerous cardiac dysrhythmias, including ventricular fibrillation, increases.

Pulse Pressure.   Pulse pressure is the numerical difference between the systolic and diastolic blood pressures. If a patient has a blood pressure of 120/80, the pulse pressure is 40. In shock, a fall in systolic blood pressure with a rise in diastolic blood pressure results in a narrowed pulse pressure. The small spurts of blood passing in the artery feel more like a quiver than the thump of a full pulse. This pulse is often described as a rapid, thready pulse. In the later stages of shock, the pulse may be imperceptible.

Respirations.   In shock, the tissues receive less oxygen. In response, the patient tries to obtain more oxygen by breathing faster (tachypnea). Rapid respirations help move blood in the large veins toward the heart. The respirations are shallow, and grunting may be heard. In earlier stages, the patient is hungry for air; but in profound shock the respiratory rate decreases. To treat hypoxia, humidified oxygen is given.

Temperature. Heat-regulating mechanisms are depressed in shock, and heat loss is increased by added diaphoresis. With the possible exception of bacteremic shock, subnormal temperature is characteristic.

Restlessness and Pain. Restlessness in shock is caused more often by hypoxia than by pain and may be relieved by oxygen administration. Pain, which can cause or enhance shock, lessens a patient's adaptive response.

Narcotics cause further respiratory and circulatory depression. When symptoms of shock are present, the nurse should call the physician and, in the meantime, withhold all previously ordered drugs. Narcotics should be given judiciously to a postoperative patient whose blood pressure is falling or a patient who shows other symptoms that shock may be approaching. The physician may give the drug in such situations intravenously in a diluted bolus dose, administered slowly and titrated to the patient's response.

Kidneys. A decreased cardiac output diminishes renal blood flow. Vasoconstriction, the body's physiologic response to shock, also contributes to a marked reduction in renal blood flow. In many instances, the rate of urine formation is the most important indicator of the status of a patient in shock. A patient in shock or impending shock needs an indwelling urethral catheter and hourly measurement of urine output. The physician should be notified of urinary output below 30 mL/hr so that therapy may be initiated promptly to promote adequate renal perfusion.

With rapid reversal of the shock, urine output usually returns to normal. Continued oliguria indicates renal damage, which is thought to have been caused by the reduced blood flow to the kidney.

Brain. Alteration in cerebral function often is the first sign of inadequate oxygen delivery to the tissues. Mild anxiety, increasing restlessness, agitation, or other change in behavior can be clues in advance of the more obvious signs of shock. As the condition deteriorates, the patient becomes listless and stuporous and ultimately loses conscious.

pH and Arterial Blood Gases. The measurement of hydrogen ion concentration (pH), oxygen tension (PaO_2), and carbon dioxide tension ($PaCO_2$) in arterial blood is an effective way to evaluate lung function, lung adequacy, and tissue perfusion. In shock, the PaO_2 is below 60 mmHg and the $PaCO_2$ may be normal or decreased.

Arterial blood gas specimens are drawn from a direct arterial puncture and may be serially or continuously monitored with an indwelling arterial catheter.

Central Venous Pressure. Central venous pressure (CVP) is the pressure of the blood in the right atrium or the venae cavae. It serves to distinguish relationships among the hemodynamic variables in shock: the venous return, the quality of the function of the right ventricle, and the vascular tone. Its measurement is a critical guide in the management of a patient in shock. Normal CVP is 4 to 10 cm of water.

An isolated CVP reading is of little value unless it is unusually high or low. To evaluate CVP readings, obtain a baseline value first, and then take frequent readings to measure a patient's response to drug therapy or to blood volume increase or decrease. To be accurate, the zero level on the manometer must also be at the same height in relation to the patient's right atrium.

Pulmonary Artery Pressure. Although right ventricular failure can be measured by CVP, left ventricular failure cannot. When left ventricular failure is anticipated, suspected, or known, a pulmonary artery (PA) pressure or pulmonary wedge capillary (PWC) pressure is obtained. A Swan-Ganz catheter with two, three, or four lumens is inserted into the vena cava and advanced through the right atrium to the right ventricle. The catheter is then advanced to the pulmonary artery. This procedure obtains a reading for the PA pressure. Further advancement of the catheter, with the balloon inflated, into a wedged position gives a reading for the PWC pressure. Normal PA pressures range from 20 to 30 mmHg systolic and 8 to 12 mmHg diastolic. Normal PCW pressures range from 4 to 12 mmHg. References may vary on these figures.

The Swan-Ganz catheter may be used in patients with myocardial infarction, congestive heart failure, and pulmonary embolus, and in any critically ill patient who requires monitoring of cardiac and pulmonary status.

PREVENTION

Though not in all cases, shock can sometimes be prevented. The key to preventing shock lies in the recognition of conditions that may lead to shock (eg, identifying situations that cause severe hypovolemia, which may eventually lead to hypovolemic shock). Recognition of the early signs of shock is equally important. If shock is recognized early and treatment instituted immediately, the condition may be reversed and the patient may recover with no ill effects.

To maintain an appraisal of the circulatory state, the patient's vital signs are monitored until the occurrence of shock is no longer considered probable. All postoperative patients belong in this category. Even if the surgical procedure involves almost no blood loss, the stress of going to surgery, the anesthetic, and the necessary trauma of the surgical incision can all lead to shock.

PROGNOSIS AND COMPLICATIONS

If shock has progressed too far before treatment is started, if a patient fails to respond despite prompt treatment, or if an underlying condition, such as a massive myocardial infarction, cannot be effectively treated, death follows.

Failure of the kidneys to resume work after the blood pressure improves may be a serious complication. Other complications may not be immediately observable or may not occur until the patient has recovered from shock. Even in uncomplicated recovery, a patient requires a period of convalescence, during which the effects of the body's defensive response to shock can subside.

When shock is treated adequately and promptly, the patient usually recovers. As vital signs return to normal, therapeutic measures can be gradually withdrawn.

NURSING PROCESS —THE PATIENT IN SHOCK

Assessment
Recognition of the early signs of shock followed by immediate medical intervention may improve the situation while the body's defenses are still in control. The early signs of shock can be identified by means of continuous assessment of those with conditions, diseases, or disorders that may produce shock.

If shock is suspected, the following signs are checked: condition of the skin, pulse rate and rhythm, blood pressure, rate and quality of the respirations, body temperature, urinary output, and a general evaluation of the level of consciousness. The physician is notified immediately.

Nursing Diagnosis
The number and extent of the nursing diagnoses often depend on the cause, type, and degree (severity) of shock.

- Anxiety related to a change in physical status (early stages of shock)
- Fear related to a change in physical status (early stages of shock)
- Hypothermia related to shock

- Hyperthermia related to bacteremic shock
- Pain related to initial disorder (specify), procedures necessary for the treatment of shock
- Altered family processes related to the seriousness of the patient's condition
- Potential for infection related to the use of invasive devices necessary for hemodynamic monitoring
- Spiritual distress (family, patient) related to seriousness of patient's condition and possible prognosis
- Knowledge deficit (family) of information about the patient's condition

Planning and Implementation
The major goals of the patient include attaining and maintaining normal blood pressure.

The major goals of nursing management include reversal of the condition as rapidly as possible, reduction or elimination of any excessive demands placed on the heart, and observation of the patient for complications associated with this disorder.

The treatment of shock depends on the cause of shock (when known) and the seriousness of the disorder. Treatment of hypoxia, pain, and cardiac dysrhythmias proceeds concurrently with the treatment of shock.

If a patient has no intravenous line, one should be started for drug therapy and fluid replacement. Obvious causes of shock, such as external hemorrhage, are controlled.

Drug Therapy. The pharmacologic treatment of shock depends on the type of shock present as well as the intensity of the shock and the presence of concurrent medical diseases (if any). Vasopressors, drugs which constrict blood vessels, are sympathomimetic agents (ie, they mimic the activity of the sympathetic nervous system) and, therefore, are given frequently for the treatment of some types of shock because the body's own sympathetic nervous system fails to compensate for the prolonged or severe drop in blood pressure. Vasopressors decrease the size of the vascular bed, causing in turn an increase in blood pressure.

In some instances, more than one drug may be administered in the treatment of shock. For example, a patient in cardiogenic shock due to a cardiac dysrhythmia may be given a vasopressor and an antiarrhythmic agent. The pharmacologic treatment of shock may also change, depending on the patient's response to treatment.

Anxiety and Fear. In the early stages of shock, patients may exhibit varying degrees of anxiety or fear. These feelings may be due to various factors, such as sensing a change in their condition or realizing the increased activity of nursing tasks (eg, frequent blood pressure readings). Calmly performing the tasks necessary to monitor the patient's condition as well as reassuring the patient and family may reduce anxiety. The procedures that must be performed (eg, the insertion of a CVP line, the use of local anesthetics) are explained briefly to the patient in a quiet and calm manner.

Hypothermia or Hyperthermia. In most types of shock, the body temperature decreases; in bacteremic shock, the body temperature often increases. Because a specific temperature range is necessary for cellular function and enzyme activity, a patient with hypothermia is kept comfortably warm through control of environmental temperature and light blankets. Direct heat to the skin is not used because heat causes vasodilatation, further increasing heat loss and the size of the vascular bed, which, in turn, may reduce blood flow to vital organs. Heat also raises the metabolic rate, increasing tissue requirement for oxygen.

If the body temperature is elevated, the physician may order an antipyretic drug, such as aspirin. A hypothermia blanket may also be necessary if the temperature elevation does not respond to antipyretic agents.

Cardiac Output and Tissue Perfusion. Shock decreases cardiac output. The patient's activity, therefore, is kept to a minimum without introducing hazards of immobility. Physical and emotional activity increase cellular needs for oxygen and nutrients and increase the formation of metabolites, all of which place further demands on the heart and other organs of the body. Nursing tasks, such as bathing and linen changes, are reduced or eliminated. Positioning, lifting, and turning are done gently. Certain necessary tasks are spaced at intervals to allow the patient time to rest and should disturb the patient as little as possible. Reducing anxiety also reduces cardiac demands.

A decrease in cardiac output results in a decrease in the blood supply to all tissues and organs of the body. Decreasing the workload of the heart, administering oxygen, correcting a fluid volume deficit, correcting the cause of shock, and administering drug therapy to increase the blood pressure combine to improve cardiac output and help increase tissue and organ perfusion.

Pain. Pain may be caused by the original disorder, such as a myocardial infarction, or may be related to procedures necessary for the treatment of shock. Because acute pain can intensify shock, narcotics are given as ordered. Because narcotics also may lower blood pressure, the nurse must use judgment and consult with the physician before administering a narcotic analgesic.

Opiates administered subcutaneously or intramuscularly to patients already in shock may not be absorbed effectively from the tissues because of diminished circulation. If several injections of narcotics or any drug are given during shock, the multiple doses may be absorbed when the patient's circulation improves, causing serious toxic effects.

Altered Family Processes. The seriousness of the patient's condition may result in certain changes within the family, who may be unable to accept the seriousness of the situation or unable to communicate their feelings with other family members. The nurse must take time to listen to the family's problems, even if only for a few moments. If the family does not appear to accept the seriousness of the patient's condition or prognosis, the nurse must relay this information to the physician.

Fluids. Hypovolemic shock is best treated with the type of fluid that is being lost. In hemorrhage, this is whole blood; in burn shock, plasma; in extreme vomiting and diarrhea, fluids containing electrolytes. When blood is given, the physician usually orders rapid infusion while the blood pressure is low and a slower rate of administration when the blood pressure rises. To keep pace with blood loss, several simultaneous transfusions may be given. A pressure sleeve may be used to force the blood into circulation more rapidly than could be accomplished by gravity. When whole blood is desired but not available, the intravenous infusion may be started with plasma, concentrated albumin, low molecular weight dextran, or saline until whole blood can be obtained.

A CVP line may be inserted to monitor a patient's response to fluid replacement. Infusing measured increments of fluid while observing CVP response serves to establish a true CVP value (initial low or normal levels are meaningless unless the response to an additional fluid load is observed) and, as a therapeutic measure, serves to increase the effective circulating blood volume and increase cardiac output.

When the CVP is initially elevated or rapidly rises to high levels with volume increments of fluid, the administration of intravenous fluids is deferred or slowed. Drug therapy is then used to improve the pumping effectiveness of the heart.

Although intravenous fluids are necessary in the treatment of shock, a decrease in cardiac output and decreased renal perfusion inhibit the normal excretion of excess fluid. Since a potential or actual fluid volume excess may occur, the urinary output is monitored at frequent intervals (usually hourly). A decrease in urinary output despite adequate administration of intravenous fluids may indicate a fluid volume excess.

Fluid volume excess also may occur if intravenous fluids are administered too rapidly. Intravenous infusion rates are checked frequently to ensure proper hourly administration of fluids. If an intravenous pump or controller is being used, it is checked for accuracy and possible malfunction.

The CVP readings are also monitored. A rise in the CVP above 15 cm of water indicates the inability of the right heart to accept a further fluid load (eg, intravenous fluids). If more fluid arrives at the heart than the left side of the heart can hold and move forward, pulmonary pressure rises. A rise in pressure in the pulmonary vessels squeezes some fluid from the vessels into the alveoli. This condition is called *pulmonary edema*, which is serious and only adds to the patient's critical condition.

Potential for Infection.   Many times the treatment of shock includes insertion of intravenous and CVP lines as well as other devices, such as an intraaortic balloon pump which may be used for cardiogenic shock due to a massive myocardial infarction. Local or systemic infection may result from the use of these devices. Intravenous lines and indwelling urethral catheters are changed according to hospital policy. The dressings covering CVP lines and other invasive devices are changed as per hospital or unit policy, and an antibiotic ointment is applied to the insertion site as per hospital or unit policy. The patient's temperature is monitored at least every 4 hours and elevations reported to the physician. Increased redness or the appearance of purulent drainage around insertion sites is also brought to the attention of the physician.

Positioning.   Unless ordered otherwise, the patient in shock is kept supine with the legs elevated 20 to 30 degrees. A small pillow may be placed beneath the head; a large pillow flexes the head forward and interferes with breathing. Keeping the patient flat increases blood flow to the brain. Patients in cardiogenic shock may benefit from a low Fowler's position. Slight elevation of the head of the bed prevents the abdominal organs from pushing up against the diaphragm and, thus, decreasing lung expansion and resulting in shallow respirations and impaired gas exchange.

Oxygen.   Humidified oxygen usually is ordered for the patient in shock because of impaired gas exchange. The patient is observed for evidence of cyanosis and increased respiratory rate. Blood gas studies may be performed to monitor the patient's response to therapy.

Urinary Output.   Urinary output often is decreased because of the decrease in renal blood flow. Urine output is measured hourly and the physician notified if it falls below 30 mL/hr. Correction of shock may result in the return of a normal urinary output.

Spiritual Distress.   In the early stages of shock, patients may be aware of the seriousness of their disorder, and they may be disturbed because of their religious beliefs. Although the nurse's primary focus is the treatment and intervention necessary to correct shock, it is still important to listen to the patient. A request for clergy should be attended to as soon as possible, even if it is necessary to ask another nurse or other unit personnel to make the contact. The patient is also reassured that a member of the clergy has been contacted.

The family may also experience spiritual distress due to the gravity of the situation. Again, nursing personnel must listen to statements made by family members and honor requests for a visit by a member of the clergy.

Knowledge Deficit.   Shock is a serious disorder that requires intense and sophisticated medical intervention. Medical personnel often only have time to discuss the situation with the family briefly and quickly. Although the time with the family may be limited, medical personnel should attempt to keep the family informed of the patient's progress as often as possible. If the family appears to have many questions regarding treatment and prognosis, the physician is notified.

Evaluation

- Anxiety or fear is reduced
- Body temperature is normal or near normal
- Cardiac output is improved
- Pain and discomfort are reduced or eliminated
- Family appears to accept seriousness of patient's condition and understands necessity for certain treatment modalities
- Fluid volume deficit or excess is corrected
- No apparent evidence of localized or systemic infection
- Demonstrates improved gas exchange
- Demonstrates improved tissue perfusion
- Urinary output normal
- Spiritual needs (patient, family) are met
- Family is aware of patient's condition, necessary treatment modalities, prognosis
- Shock is corrected; vital signs are normal

General Pharmacologic Considerations

☐ Shock demands intensive treatment. Drugs used in the treatment of shock include adrenergic drugs that have profound vasopressor action; examples are epinephrine, levarterenol, metaraminol (Aramine), phenylephrine (Neo-Synephrine), and the norepinephrine precursor, dopamine (Intropin). Other agents that may be used include whole blood, blood products (eg, plasma, albumin), and plasma expanders (eg, dextran 40).

☐ Other drugs relevant to a patient's physical problems and the underlying conditions that may be the cause of shock are often concurrently administered. Drugs in this category might include cardiac preparations (eg, digoxin, lidocaine, procainamide), diuretics, and corticosteroids.

☐ Administration of powerful vasopressors demands constant nursing supervision. The patient's blood pressure must be monitored every 2 to 5 minutes if the patient is receiving levarterenol and every 3 to 8 minutes for other vasopressors (circumstances may change these intervals). The rate of administration by intravenous infusion is adjusted according to the patient's blood pressure. The site of intravenous infusion and surrounding areas are frequently inspected for signs of extravasation or infiltration.

☐ If extravasation or infiltration should occur, the infusion has to be discontinued, especially if levarterenol is being administered. (This drug causes severe tissue necrosis.) It is important to start an identical infusion in another extremity before the original infusion is discontinued. Failure to keep the intravenous solution infusing (even though extravasation into tissue is occurring) may result in circulatory collapse. If the intravenous needle is totally displaced from the vein, the infusion can be discontinued as or before another is started. In the latter case, speed in restarting the infusion is of the utmost importance.

☐ The patient in shock is observed for signs of fluid overload. If this condition occurs while a vasopressor is still required, a more concentrated form of the drug, which uses less fluid as a vehicle for the administration, may be given.

Suggested Readings

☐ Abrams AC. Clinical drug therapy: rationales for nursing practice. 2nd ed. Philadelphia: JB Lippincott, 1987. *(Additional and in-depth coverage of subject matter)*

☐ Blake P. Precision moves that counter cardiogenic shock. RN May 1989;52:52. *(Additional coverage of subject matter)*

☐ Briening EP. Septic shock: tough cases that teach the most. RN September 1988;51:36. *(Additional coverage and illustrations that reinforce subject matter)*

☐ Gawlinski A. Saving the cardiogenic shock patient. Nursing '89 December 1989;19:34. *(Additional coverage of subject matter)*

☐ McConnell EA. Clinical considerations in perioperative nursing: preventive aspects of care. Philadelphia: JB Lippincott, 1987. *(Additional and in-depth coverage of subject matter)*

☐ McConnell EA. Is it hypovolemic or septic shock? Nursing '88 October 1988;18:88. *(Additional coverage of subject matter)*

☐ Sarsany SL. Massive bleeding. RN February 1988;51:36. *(Additional coverage of subject matter)*

☐ Sumner S. Action stat! Septic Shock. Nursing '87 February 1987;17:33. *(Additional coverage of subject matter)*

☐ Wahl SC. Septic shock: how to detect it early. Nursing '89 January 1989;19:52. *(Additional and in-depth coverage of subject matter)*

Oncologic Nursing

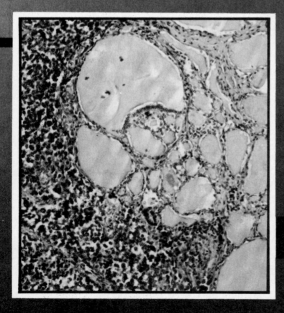

Unit 4

Chapter 19

Care of the Patient Who Has Cancer

On completion of this chapter the reader will:

■ Discuss the pathology and etiology of cancer

■ List and discuss the symptoms of cancer

■ Name the seven warning signs of cancer

■ Discuss the prevention of cancer

■ Discuss factors or situations that may predispose an individual to cancer

■ Differentiate and describe malignant and benign tumors

■ Discuss the various methods of diagnosis and treatment of cancer

■ Discuss the emotional impact associated with the diagnosis of cancer

■ Use the nursing process in the management of a patient with cancer

PATHOLOGY

Body cells can undergo changes in structure and appearance, begin to multiply, and eventually form a colony of cancer cells (Fig. 19-1). These cells can form in any part of the body at any time and from any cell. They usually multiply rapidly, invading and destroying surrounding normal tissues by causing pressure and competing with normal cells for nutrients and oxygen. Though cancer cells change in appearance, they usually retain enough resemblance to the tissues from which they were formed to be recognized if found in other parts of the body. For example, if a tumor from the neck shows malignant cells formed from breast tissue, it is known to have spread from the breast. Sometimes the secondary tumor is found before the primary tumor has been discovered.

Although all forms of malignant growth may be referred to as cancer, more specific terms are used to describe particular types of cells that have undergone malignant transformation. Malignant tumors may arise from any or all three embryonal tissues.

Embryonal tissues are described as follows:

Ectoderm   outer layer of the embryo; produces the skin and the nervous system
Mesoderm   middle layer of the embryo; produces bones, cartilage, muscle, fat, blood, and all other connective tissues
Endoderm   inner layer of the embryo; produces the linings of the gastrointestinal (GI) tract, respiratory system, spleen, liver, and so forth

Usually, tumors are named after the types of tissues from which they are formed. When a tumor contains all three embryonal components, it is referred to as a *Teratoma*. Examples of names of tumors that relate to types of tissue are given in Table 19-1.

Table 19-2 describes how malignant tumors differ from benign tumors. Benign tumors usually are encapsulated, whereas malignant tumors tend to infiltrate surrounding tissue and may metastasize (spread). Cancer is known to spread to the lymph nodes that drain the tumor area. For this reason, a lymph node dissection may be performed in addition to wide excision of the tumor (Fig. 19-2).

Cancer can spread in the following ways:

■ Direct extension to adjacent tissues
■ Extension from lymph vessels into the tissues that lie alongside lymphatic vessels
■ Transportation by the lymph or vascular system, often to distant sites
■ Diffusion within a body cavity

The area in which malignant cells first form is called the *primary site*. The regions of the body to which cancer cells spread are termed *secondary* or *metastatic sites*. Metastasis is one of the most discouraging characteristics of cancer because even one malignant cell can start a metastatic lesion in a distant part of the body. Metastatic tumors are treated aggressively when-

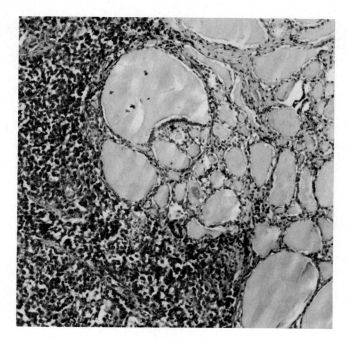

Figure 19–1. A microscopic section of thyroid tissue showing normal thyroid cells (*right*) and malignant anaplastic metastatic melanoma (*left*). (Courtesy of P. S. Milley, MD. Photograph by D. Atkinson)

ever possible. Because of this treatment, more patients are long-term survivors. The patient and family are told of the importance of good follow-up care with periodic evaluations and examinations.

Benign tumors remain at the original site of their development. They may grow large, but their rate of growth is slower than that of malignant tumors. Benign tumors usually do not cause death unless their location impairs the function of a vital organ, such as the brain. On the other hand, malignant tumors grow rapidly, and, unless completely removed before metastasis has occurred, they are likely to spread.

ETIOLOGY

Certain factors appear to be related to the development of cancer, at least in some individuals. Environmental and social factors strongly influence the incidence of some types of cancer. Skin cancers may be caused by prolonged exposure to sunlight. Fortunately, these cancers are easy to detect and are highly curable. Physical agents such as x-rays and gamma rays are well-established causes of squamous cell carcinomas and bone sarcomas. Chemicals have been known to produce skin cancers in industrial workers. Prolonged exposure to such substances as coal dust or asbestos has also been implicated in the cause of cancer. The inhalation of cigarette smoke over a period of years has been a major cause of lung, pharyngeal, oral, and laryngeal cancers.

Some factors are thought to predispose the individual to cancer. Leukoplakia of the mouth or genitals, for instance, may remain benign or may undergo malignant change. Leukoplakia are removed when feasible.

SYMPTOMS

Cancer is an insidious disease that may have few or no early symptoms. In some instances, early signs are

Table 19–1.   Classification of Tumor Cells

oma = tumor

Origin	Malignant (cancer)	Benign (non) cancerous
Skin	Squamous cell carcinoma	Papilloma
	Malignant melanoma *Killer*	Nevus (mole)
Epithelium	Adenocarcinoma	Adenoma
Muscle	Myosarcoma	Myoma
Connective tissue		
Fibrous tissue	Fibrosarcoma	Fibroma
Adipose (fatty) tissue	Liposarcoma	Lipoma
Cartilage	Chondrosarcoma	Chondroma
Bone	Osteosarcoma	Osteoma
Nerve tissue	Neurogenic sarcoma	Neuroma
	Neuroblastoma	Ganglioneuroma
	Glioblastoma	Glioma
Bone marrow	Multiple myeloma	
	Leukemia	

Table 19–2.   Characteristics of Malignant and Benign Tumors

Malignant	Benign
Grow rapidly	Grow slowly
Rarely enclosed in a capsule	Almost always enclosed in a capsule (encapsulated)
Infiltrate surrounding tissues	Do not infiltrate surrounding tissues
Spread from original site by metastasis	Remain localized
May recur after being removed	Usually no recurrence after removal
Harmful to host	Usually not harmful to host
Prognosis dependent on the type and location of the tumor, speed of diagnosis, presence or absence of metastasis	Prognosis almost always good*

* The exception may be the presence of a benign tumor causing compression of a vital organ (eg, a benign brain tumor).

vague and offer no real indication of the presence of a malignant tumor. Every effort must be made to discover cancer in its earliest stage. The seven warning signals of cancer listed by the American Cancer Society should be familiar to all:

C   Change in bowel or bladder habits
A   A sore that does not heal
U   Unusual bleeding or discharge
T   Thickening or lump in breast or elsewhere
I   Indigestion or difficulty in swallowing
O   Obvious change in wart or mole
N   Nagging cough or hoarseness — 3 wks. or longer

PREVENTION

In people fearful of cancer, every symptom, however minor or transient, can cause near panic. These reactions indicate the need for better information on the ways by which cancer can be controlled and cured. Education, through the media and in schools, has developed an awareness of the warning signals of cancer as well as those factors that may influence the development of cancer.

Public education must stress the importance of periodic physical examinations and cancer screening programs. Self-examination of the breasts, testicles, and all skin surfaces is valuable and should be taught. The avoidance of factors that predispose an individual to cancer and early detection of cancer increase the chances of curing the disease.

DIAGNOSIS

The diagnosis of cancer begins with the recognition that the disease may assume many forms and guises.

Sometimes the symptoms are so obvious that patients know they probably have cancer. At other times, the physician's suspicion is aroused by an apparently minor condition, such as a chronic cough or nausea, that does not respond to therapy.

Complete, periodic physical examinations are important for discovering cancer in its early stages. Every clinic, physician's, and dentist's office should be a cancer detection center. Another way to detect cancer in its early stages is for the individual to recognize the physical changes revealed through self-examination of the breasts (see Chapter 50), inspection of the skin for any changes or new growths, and palpation of the testicles (especially in young men). In addition, the seven warning signs of cancer also should alert the individual to seek medical advice if other physical changes occur.

Cancer is diagnosed by using a careful patient history, a physical examination, and diagnostic studies. A careful history defines the patient's complaints and, on occasion, reveal information that raises the suspicion of a malignant process. The physical examination may reveal a suspicious growth, a change in the size of a body organ or structure, enlarged lymph nodes, or other abnormalities that may indicate a malignancy. At times, the physical examination may be unrevealing, but the patient's history raises questions.

Many diagnostic tests and studies can be used to establish a diagnosis of cancer. The physician, using information obtained during the physical examination and patient history, selects the tests or studies that help establish a diagnosis.

Laboratory Tests.   Results from laboratory tests may be indicative of certain types of malignancies. Tests which may be useful include the serum alkaline

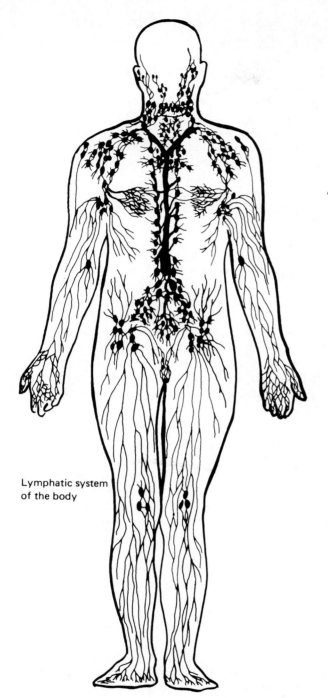

Lymphatic system
of the body

Figure 19–2. One route by which malignant cells can spread to other areas of the body is the lymphatic system. Cancer cells also can be carried by the blood.

and acid phosphatase tests, the carcinoembryonic antigen (CEA) test, and serum and urine calcium determinations. While these tests are not specific for cancer, abnormal results may indicate a malignant process. For example, a markedly elevated acid phosphatase may be seen in metastatic carcinoma of the prostate, and moderately elevated values may be seen in

other malignancies, such as multiple myeloma and bone cancer.

Other laboratory tests may be useful in establishing a diagnosis, and, although abnormal values do not directly indicate a malignant process, they may help in formulating a total clinical picture. For example, anemia present in an individual with a possible cancer of the large intestine may be revealed by means of a complete blood cell (CBC) count.

Radiographs. Radiographs are frequently employed in the diagnosis of a malignancy. They can be used as plain film or with contrast media or specialized equipment. Plain films are radiographic films used alone. A contrast medium is a substance that is injected, inserted, or swallowed to highlight, outline, or provide detail that is not visible with plain film. Examples of studies performed with contrast media are upper GI series, barium enemas, and intravenous pyelograms (IVPs).

Radiographic procedures that require special machines or additional equipment are tomography, xeroradiography, and computed tomographic (CT) scan. Tomography uses a series of radiographic films taken at calibrated levels (or planes) of a specific area, organ, or structure. These films provide more detail of an area than can be obtained with plain films. Xeroradiography differs from regular radiography in the type of material used to record the image. Traditional radiography uses special photographic film, whereas xeroradiography employs special copy paper that gives greater detail to the recorded image.

CT Scan. The CT scan uses radiography and a computerized scanning system (Fig. 19-3). Multiple x-ray beams are passed through the body at various angles and levels. The computerized scanning system sorts and records the varying degrees of x-ray penetration and produces an image on a television screen. The image may be recorded for further study. Machines capable of scanning the brain or the entire body may be used to identify malignant lesions as well as nonmalignant disorders, such as cerebral hematomas, cirrhosis of the liver, and aortic aneurysms.

Radioisotopes. Radioisotope studies use radioactive materials in the diagnosis of various malignancies. The radioactive substance is injected intravenously or taken orally, depending on the type of study and the radioisotope used. A scanner is then used to identify areas of increased, decreased, or normal distribution of the radioactive material. The use of radioisotopes and a scanning device is called a *scintillation scan.*

Emission Computer Tomography. Positron emission tomography (PET) and single photon emis-

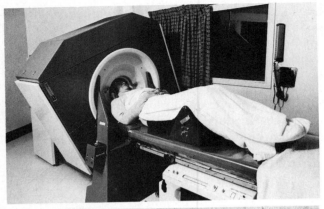

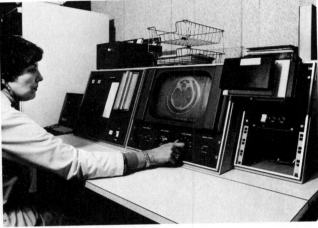

Figure 19–3. CT scan uses x-rays (*top*) and a computerized scanning system (*bottom*). (Photographs by D. Atkinson; courtesy of W. Kinkel, MD, Dent Neurological Institute, Buffalo, NY)

sion computerized tomography (SPECT) may be used for the diagnosis of a malignancy. Both studies require the use of radionuclides to determine the function of an organ. These studies differ from a CT scan, which depicts the structure or anatomy of an organ.

Cytology. Microscopic examination of cells obtained from various areas of the body may be used to diagnose malignant and premalignant disorders. One example of a cytologic examination is the Papanicolaou (Pap) smear used in diagnosing malignant and premalignant changes of the endometrium, cervix, and vagina. Cells obtained from the bronchi or GI tract by washings, body fluids such as urine or cerebral spinal fluid, and accumulated fluids in body cavities may also be examined microscopically for cell changes.

Biopsy. Samples of tissue taken from the body can be examined microscopically for changes that may indicate a malignant or premalignant process. Tissue samples may be obtained at the time of surgery, by insertion of a special biopsy needle using local anesthesia, and during special procedures such as endo-

scopic examination of the esophagus, stomach, bladder and rectum.

Endoscopic Examinations. Fiberoptic instruments are flexible tubes containing optic fibers that enable light to travel in a straight line or at various angles. When a flexible tube is bent or twisted, light continues to travel along the optic fiber to illuminate the area being observed. Endoscopic examinations, for example, gastroscopy, bronchoscopy, and sigmoidoscopy, may be performed to directly visualize specific areas. When malignancy is suspected, tissue biopsies may be taken. Endoscopic examinations may also be performed for nonmalignant disorders.

Ultrasound. This type of study uses high-frequency sound waves to detect internal abnormal variations of a body organ or structure. The reflection of sound waves is projected on a screen and may also be recorded on photographic film or videotape. This technique, also called an *echogram,* is employed in the diagnosis of malignant as well as nonmalignant disorders. Examples of ultrasound procedures in the diagnosis of malignancies include echograms of the male and female pelvis, kidney, pancreas, brain, lymph nodes, and liver.

TREATMENT

Three basic methods are employed in the treatment of cancer: (1) surgery, (2) radiation therapy, and (3) chemotherapy. These methods may be used alone or in combination; one is not superior to the others, nor does one or more methods produce better results. It must be remembered that the patient rather than the cancer is being treated; therefore, many factors may enter into a decision as to which methods to use.

Surgery

Surgery may range from excision of the tumor alone to extensive surgical excision, which includes removal of the tumor and adjacent structures, such as bone, muscle, and lymph nodes. What and how much is removed depends on facts the surgeon learns, including the pathologist's initial findings at the time of surgery, the age and physical condition of the patient, and the results that can be expected. An extensive operation may be followed by reconstructive or plastic surgery to functionally or cosmetically correct defects caused by the original surgery. Not all patients are candidates for reconstructive surgery, especially if tumor growth was not halted or their physical condition is poor and they are unable to tolerate additional surgery.

Some surgeries are necessarily disfiguring and some

so profound that the patient has great difficulty in adjusting to body changes and disfigurement. Although plastic and reconstructive surgery may restore most of the function or appearance of an area, at times it cannot, and the areas remain drastically changed, especially as in radical surgery involving the head and neck.

Radiation Therapy

Radiation is the emission of energy that is able to travel through space or matter, as, for example, the heat given off by the sun. _Ionizing radiation_ is radiation that uses alpha, beta, or gamma rays to directly or indirectly cause injury or death to cells. Both normal and malignant cells are affected by ionizing radiation. X-rays and radioisotopes, such as radium and cesium, produce ionizing radiation of the type used in the treatment of cancer. _Radioactivity_ is the ability of a substance to emit alpha, beta, and gamma rays. A _radioisotope_ (or radioactive isotope) is a chemical element with radioactivity. Hydrogen is an element that has no radioactive properties. Radium is an element that emits alpha, beta, and gamma rays and is, therefore, classified as a radioisotope. Radioisotopes are used for both diagnostic and therapeutic procedures.

Radiation therapy is the treatment of cancer using x-rays or radioisotopes. The aim of radiation therapy is to orderly destroy malignant, rapidly dividing cells, while leaving the rest of the body well or able to recover and eliminate the dead cancer cells. Rapidly dividing cells are more sensitive to radiation (termed _radiosensitivity_) than those that divide slowly. Radiation therapy may be applied externally or internally. When a malignancy is far advanced, radiation therapy is used palliatively to cause a remission of symptoms so that the patient is more comfortable. Like surgery, radiation therapy can result in painful and unpleasant side effects.

**External Radiation Therapy.** External radiation therapy may be selected for the treatment of some cancers and may be used before or after surgery or for palliative measures. External radiation therapy uses machines capable of delivering x-rays, gamma rays, protons, neutrons, and alpha and beta particles or electrons, all of which are capable of producing ionizing radiation.

This type of therapy is normally delivered over a period of several weeks and may be given on an outpatient basis if the patient is well enough to remain at home. In some instances, external radiation therapy may precede or follow internal radiation therapy. For example, the patient with cancer of the cervix may not have surgery but may be given external radiation therapy followed by internal radiation therapy.

**Internal Radiation Therapy.** In certain instances, it is more advantageous to insert a radioactive substance into the tumor (interstitial), rather than use a distant source (external radiation therapy). This method has the advantage of delivering the highest dose within the tumor. Radioisotopes may also be administered orally or intravenously for a systemic effect, placed in solid tumors inside the body or into body cavities for a local effect, or applied topically to skin lesions using various kinds of applicators.

An applicator may be used to hold the radioactive source within the body. The radioactive substance may be inserted along with the applicator, or it may be introduced after the applicator has been put in place (the afterloading technique).

The patient's chart lists specific orders for treatment and the precautions that are to be taken during treatment. A notation is made regarding the type and dosage of radioactive substance, the time and area of insertion, the type of applicator used, and the time the material is to be removed. The chart may also give the name of the individual to be notified if an emergency occurs, such as the dislodging of a radium applicator inserted into the vagina. If any orders are unclear, the nurse should contact the radiologist.

In preparing the private room before treatment, the nurse must check to see that essential items are available: paper tissues and bags, water glass, straws, and so on. Furnishing these items before treatment reduces exposure of nursing personnel once treatment has begun. The patient should have adequate reading material or other forms of diversion, because these items will not become radioactive unless directly contaminated with radioactive material. Some hospitals use a special room that accommodates more than one patient. The beds are kept a specific distance apart for the safety of other patients in the room.

All personnel and workers in the area should be made aware of internal radiation therapy, even though a radiation sign is posted on the wall (Fig. 19-4). Cleaning and maintenance personnel who may not be aware of the signs especially should be informed. Visitors for other patients may inquire about the radiation

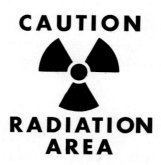

CAUTION

RADIATION AREA

Figure 19–4.   International radiation symbol.

signs and should be assured that neither they nor the patients are in danger.

Everyone involved in the care of patients who receive internal radiation therapy must recognize the necessity for limitations to radiation exposure. The degree of possible hazard depends on the type and amount of radioactive material used for treatment. Generally, no special precautions are required when patients receive small amounts of a radioactive substance for diagnostic studies. If necessary, precautions are specified by the radiologist.

When radioisotopes are used in the treatment of cancer, three safety principles must always be kept in mind: time, distance, and shielding (where applicable).

Time.   Time refers to the length of exposure. The less time spent in the vicinity of a radioactive substance, the less radiation received. Nurses should plan carefully so that less time actually is spent at the bedside. The nurse must learn to work quickly and efficiently. Careful psychological preparation helps the patient to accept the limited amount of nursing time.

Distance.   Distance refers to the distance from the radioactive source. The patient's bed assignment and degree of isolation are determined by the radiation safety officer after monitoring the patient. The inverse square law applies to radiation exposure. The rate of exposure varies inversely to the square of the distance from the source (patient). Nurses standing 4 feet away from the source of radiation receive 25% of the radiation they would receive if they were standing 2 feet away from the source (Fig. 19-5).

Shielding.   Shielding is the use of any type of material to lessen the amount of radiation that reaches an area. The material usually used is lead (eg, lead-lined gloves and lead aprons). Other materials, such as concrete walls, have the capability of shielding.

Because radiation produces no immediate symptoms, one can receive radiation injury without being aware of it. The National Committee on Radiation Protection publishes guides for radiation safety. The effects of long and short exposures must be taken into account. The latent period between the exposure and the accumulated biologic effect is often long, and great care is taken to protect occupationally exposed workers from radiation injury that can accumulate over the years. Pregnant women (whether staff members or visitors) should avoid exposure to radioactive substances.

Chemotherapy

Chemotherapy uses drugs as a method of treating cancer (Table 19-3). Generally, antineoplastic drugs

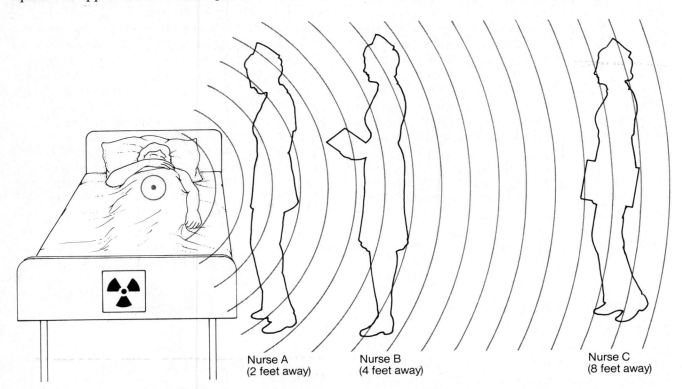

Nurse A
(2 feet away)

Nurse B
(4 feet away)

Nurse C
(8 feet away)

Figure 19–5.   Examples of distance. Nurse B receives about 25% of the radiation received by Nurse A, and Nurse C receives about 25% of the radiation received by Nurse B.

can be divided into the following categories: (1) alkylating agents, (2) antimetabolites, (3) miscellaneous agents, (4) antibiotics, (5) mitotic inhibitors, and (6) hormones. Antineoplastic drugs may be given by the following routes: topical, oral, intramuscular, subcutaneous, intravenous, arterial, intraarterial, intravesicle, intratumor, intrathecal, or intracavity. Many of these drugs affect cells that divide at a rapid rate, such as tumor cells but also normal body cells, such as bone marrow, lymph tissue, and the epithelial cells that line the GI tract. Most antineoplastic agents can cause mild to severe adverse effects. Appropriate references should be consulted about the adverse effects of each agent.

In chemotherapy, nursing management of the patient varies with the drug, the dose administered, and the route used. Some patients experience little discomfort, while others have a wide range of symptoms.

Adverse effects that may be encountered during chemotherapy include fatigue, stomatitis, alopecia, leukopenia, easy bruising, nausea, vomiting, and diarrhea. Many of these drugs depress the bone marrow, thus inhibiting the manufacture of red and white blood cells and platelets. In some instances, a profound decrease in these blood components may occur, resulting in anemia, a tendency toward bleeding, and a low white blood cell count. The anemia and bleeding tendencies may be treated with blood transfusions (whole blood, packed cells, or platelets). A decrease in white blood cells decreases resistance to infection; in some cases, the white blood cell count can drop so low that even a minor infection could result in death. Patients with a low white blood cell count may be placed in reverse isolation. Some hospitals use special isolation rooms (eg, germ-free units, laminal air-flow rooms) for those undergoing intensive chemotherapy, whole body radiation therapy, or those who develop seriously low white blood cell counts.

Corticosteroids may be used in the treatment of some forms of acute and chronic leukemia and lymphomas. These drugs also can depress the bone marrow, especially the manufacture of white blood cells. By a mechanism not fully understood, they provide symptomatic relief, and, for a time, the patient looks and feels better. Corticosteroids also reduce elevated serum calcium levels seen in cancers that have metastasized to the bone.

Supportive Therapies

In addition to chemotherapy, surgery, and radiation therapy, the treatment of cancer includes supportive therapies, such as special diets, the fitting of prosthesis, and occupational and diversional therapies. Drugs, such as analgesics, electrolytes, vitamins, and intravenous fluids, may also be needed. Emotional support may be given by special support groups, such as Reach for Recovery for mastectomy patients or a local ostomy group for those with a colostomy. Members of the clergy, relatives, and friends also are essential components of physical and emotional support.

PATIENT REACTION TO DIAGNOSIS

Once a diagnosis of cancer has been confirmed, the question arises: should patients be told? Patients have a right to know their diagnoses, the treatment that will best cure or control their malignancies, and their prognoses. Exceptions do exist, however. Some patients cannot emotionally accept the diagnosis, at least early in the disease, and others may be too ill to understand. A family may ask the physician not to discuss the diagnosis of cancer with the patient, or ask the physician to delay telling the patient. The family should understand that it is often difficult to keep the diagnosis from these patients for an indefinite period of time. If radiation treatments or chemotherapy are the chosen methods of treatment, either in conjunction with or instead of surgery, these patients ultimately will realize they have cancer. Nurses must respect the decision of the family or physician to withhold information, regardless of their own feelings in the matter. Such a decision has usually required much thought and consideration. A notation on the Kardex states exactly what the patient has been told about the diagnosis and the terms used by the physician. If the patient has not been told of the diagnosis, the alternative terms used (tumor, growth, cyst, and so on) can be noted on the Kardex.

Even though progress has been made in the treatment of cancer, the word *cancer* still has a tremendous emotional impact. When the diagnosis is first known, most patients respond with shock, disbelief, fear, anguish, denial, and worry. These feelings may last indefinitely. Eventually, many patients decide to face the problem, do all they can to recover, and try to live a normal life. Others may never recover emotionally; this emotional problem has been known to affect their physical progress. Sometimes acceptance of the diagnosis and a positive outlook can be fostered by the family, the physician, and the nurse. How the patient is told is important. The physician and nurse who show sincere interest and concern may help the patient through this traumatic period.

THE TERMINALLY ILL PATIENT

Management of the terminally ill patient can be both physically and emotionally difficult. Not only must the patient be considered, but the family, who must face

Table 19–3. Antineoplastic Agents

Generic Name	Trade Name	Use
Alkylating Agents		*inhibit cell division* *induce mutation*
Busulfan	Myleran	Palliative treatment of chronic myelogenous leukemia
Carmustine (BCNU)	BiCNU	Brain tumors, multiple myeloma, Hodgkin's disease, non-Hodgkin's lymphomas
Chlorambucil	Leukeran	Chronic lymphocytic leukemia, malignant lymphomas, giant follicular lymphoma, Hodgkin's disease
Cisplatin	Platinol	Metastatic testicular and ovarian tumors, advanced bladder cancer
Cyclophosphamide	Cytoxan Neosar	Malignant lymphomas, multiple myeloma, leukemias, neuroblastoma, ovarian adenocarcinoma, retinoblastoma, carcinoma of the breast
Lomustine (CCNU)	CeeNu	Brain tumors, Hodgkin's disease
Mechlorethamine HCl	Mustargen	Hodgkin's disease, lymphosarcoma, chronic myelocytic or lymphocytic leukemia, polycythemia vera, bronchogenic carcinoma
Melphalan	Alkeran	Multiple myeloma, nonresectable epithelial ovarian carcinoma
Pipobroman	Vercyte	Chronic granulocytic leukemia, polycythemia vera
Streptozocin	Zanosar	Metastatic islet cell carcinoma of the pancreas
Triethylenethiophosphora-mide	Thiotepa	Adenocarcinoma of the breast and ovary, control of intracavity effusions secondary to diffuse or localized neoplastic disease, lymphomas
Uracil mustard	—	Chronic lymphocytic leukemia, non-Hodgkin's lymphomas, chronic myelogenous leukemia, early stages of polycythemia vera
Antimetabolites		
Cytarabine	Cytosar-U	Acute myelocytic and lymphocytic leukemia in adults and children
Floxuridine	FUDR	Intra-arterial infusions in the palliative management of GI adenocarcinoma metastatic to the liver
Fluorouracil	Adrucil	Palliative management of carcinoma of breast, colon, rectum, stomach, pancreas not amenable to surgery or radiation
Mercaptopurine	Purinethol	Acute leukemia, chronic myelogenous leukemia
Methotrexate	Folex, Mexate	Gestational choriocarcinoma, chorioadenoma destruens, palliation of acute lymphocytic leukemia, breast cancer, epidermoid cancers of the head and neck, lung cancers, advanced lymphosarcoma
Thioguanine	—	Acute lymphatic leukemia, acute myelogenous leukemia
Antibiotic Agents		
Bleomycin sulfate	Blenoxane	Squamous cell carcinoma of the head and neck, lymphomas, testicular carcinoma
Dactinomycin	Cosmegen	Wilms' tumor, rhabdomyosarcoma, choriocarcinoma, nonseminomatous testicular carcinoma, Ewing's sarcoma, sarcoma botryoides
Daunorubicin HCl	Cerubidine	Acute nonlymphocytic leukemia of adults, acute lymphocytic leukemia in children, adults
Doxorubicin HCl	Adriamycin	Acute lymphoblastic and myeloblastic leukemia, Wilms' tumor, neuroblastoma, soft tissue and bone sarcomas, breast and ovarian carcinomas, transitional cell bladder carcinoma, thyroid carcinoma, Hodgkin's and non-Hodgkin's lymphomas, bronchiogenic carcinoma
Mitomycin	Mutamycin	Disseminated adenocarcinoma of the stomach or pancreas
Plicamycin	Mithracin	Malignant testicular tumors
Mitotic Inhibitors		
Etoposide	VePesid	Refractory testicular tumors
Vinblastine sulfate	Velban	Hodgkin's disease, lymphocytic and histiocytic lymphoma, advanced testicular carcinoma, Kaposi's sarcoma, choriocarcinoma, breast cancer
Vincristine sulfate	Oncovin	Acute leukemia, Hodgkin's disease, lymphosarcoma, reticulum cell sarcoma, rhabdomyosarcoma, neuroblastoma, Wilms' tumor

Continued

Table 19–3. Antineoplastic Agents *Continued*

Generic Name	Trade Name	Use
Hormones Androgens		
Testolactone	Teslac	Advanced or inoperable breast carcinoma in postmenopausal women
Estrogens		
Diethylstilbestrol diphosphate	Stilphostrol	Prostatic cancer
Polyestradiol phosphate	Estradurin	Prostatic cancer
Estrogen/Nitrogen Mustard		
Estramustine phosphate sodium	Emcyt	Prostatic cancer
Antiestrogen		
Tamoxifen	Nolvadex	Breast cancer in postmenopausal women
Progestins		
Medroxyprogesterone acetate	Depo-Provera	Endometrial or renal carcinoma
Megestrol acetate	Megace Pallace	Advanced carcinoma of the breast or endometrium
Miscellaneous Agents		
Asparaginase	Elspar	Acute lymphocytic leukemia
Dacarbazine	DTIC-Dome	Metastatic malignant melanoma
Hydroxyurea	Hydrea	Melanoma, chronic myelocytic leukemia ovarian carcinoma
Interferon alfa 2a	Roferon-A	Hairy cell leukemia plus clinical trials for treatment of other neoplastic diseases
Interferon alfa 2b	Intron A	Same as interferon alfa 2a
Mitotane	Lysodren	Adrenal cortical carcinoma
Procarbazine HCl	Matulane	Hodgkin's disease

separation from a loved one in the near future, must be considered as well.

Good nursing management is essential to keep the patient as comfortable as possible. Each nursing task must be carried out in a gentle manner to reduce the possibility of pain and discomfort. Attention is given to providing an adequate fluid and nutrition intake, keeping the patient warm and dry, and controlling odors (when present). Pain is managed by the administration of analgesics. An important part of nursing management is to help the patient maintain dignity, despite an illness that often requires almost complete dependence on others for all activities of daily living (ADLs).

In the past, terminally ill patients were often hospitalized because family members were unable to care for them. The organization of hospice units now allows many terminally ill patients to be at home with their families or to be placed in a specially designated hospice unit in a hospital. The hospice unit in a hospital differs from a standard hospital room in that it has a warm, homelike atmosphere. The hospice team includes physicians and nurses, as well as other personnel such as social workers, clergymen, and dietitians. When established in the home, the needs and desires of the patient and family form a focal point for patient management. Equipment and supplies, such as a hospital bed, ambulatory devices, dressings, bed linen, and drugs, are obtained. The family may require instruction in the handling of special equipment and the administration of drugs or solutions used for total parenteral nutrition. The patient and family are usually visited daily by a nurse or other member of the hospice team. Problems that arise are dealt with on an individual basis, with each member of the hospice team used as needed. When the patient dies, members of the hospice team continue to offer emotional support, as needed, to family members.

NURSING PROCESS —THE PATIENT WHO HAS CANCER

Assessment
Meeting the needs of patients with cancer are varied and complex and depend on their reactions to the diagnosis, the location of the cancer, impairment of body functions that may result from the disease or its

treatment, the stage of the disease, and the prognosis. Assessment must include a complete evaluation of these patients, including their physical and emotional states. Assessment includes the following:

- A review of the patient's chart for biopsy reports, laboratory tests, and other diagnostic studies, previous treatments or surgeries for cancer (if any), the stage of the disease (eg, early, late, terminal, in remission, metastatic), present or planned treatment modalities (if any), and physician's comments
- A history of past and present symptoms
- A head to toe appraisal of the patient's physical status
- An assessment of the patient's nutritional status
- An appraisal of the patient's ability to carry out daily living activities
- An evaluation of the patient's emotional response to the diagnosis
- An assessment of what the patient knows about the diagnosis, treatment, and prognosis
- An evaluation of the family's response to the patient's illness and their ability to act as a support group during therapy

A review of the patient's chart usually gives a total picture of the patient's past and present status. It is important to know the type and location of the malignancy and if evidence of metastasis exists. Before starting treatment, the tumor is staged and graded. *Staging* determines the size of the tumor and evidence of metastasis, as noted by the presence or absence of lymph node involvement and other factors. *Grading* determines the classification of the tumor cells and seeks to determine the origin of the tumor. For example, a tumor of the lung may be graded as well differentiated, which means that the cells of the tumor resemble the cells of the lung tissue where the tumor originated. If a tumor is graded as poorly differentiated, the tumor cells do not resemble the cells of the tissues in which they are found.

Abnormal laboratory tests, which should be carefully noted, may influence the nursing diagnosis and planning and implementation by identifying potential or real problems, such as bleeding tendencies or risk of infection. For example, bleeding tendencies, as noted by a decrease in the platelet count, would alert the nurse to the dangers associated with any break in skin integrity or trauma to the skin.

A careful and thorough head to toe physical assessment is most important. Plans are made, using proper nursing management, to correct or alleviate the problems that are found, such as early decubitus formation, gingivitis, and bleeding tendencies. Other problems, such as bladder or bowel incontinence, ulcerations of the oral mucous membranes, changes in alertness or mental acuity, dry fragile skin, and

muscle weakness, may also influence patient management.

It is especially important to assess patients with metastatic cancer for complications. Bleeding or even serious hemorrhage may occur if a blood vessel is eroded by malignant tissue. Infection, manifested by such symptoms as fever and chills, may occur because the tissues undergoing malignant change are vulnerable to infection. Pathologic fractures may result if the patient has metastasis to bone. In addition, complications (eg, thrombophlebitis or pneumonia) may occur as a result of physical inactivity.

The nutritional status of the patient must be determined. Many patients with cancer have episodes of decreased food intake or absorption as a result of the disease or of chemotherapy or radiation therapy. It is important to identify the patient's present weight, the amount of weight lost (if any), and the presence of anorexia, nausea, vomiting, or diarrhea. Patients in poor nutritional states often have difficulty with cancer treatments and may require supplemental feedings, either orally or parenterally, before therapy can be instituted.

With cancer, the threat to the body's wholeness is severe. The disease and the treatment are often destructive of tissue and can be disfiguring. Hair loss, weakness, loss of a body part or function, weight loss, and skin changes are effects that may be experienced. Some patients fear the pain or disfigurement or any other specific aspect of the illness less than they fear the possible overall loss of self-control and dignity during the final stages of the illness.

The reactions of family members to the diagnosis and to the knowledge of the changes in the relationship that may result between patients and their family members are also considered during assessment. Loss of income and change in lifestyle are two examples of problems facing the family. The demands placed on the family during and after treatment may make coping with the changes in their own lives difficult.

During assessment, actual or potential threats to the patient's self-image and the emotional responses of the patient and family must be identified.

Nursing Diagnosis

The extent and number of nursing diagnoses depend on many factors, such as the stage of the patient's disease, the prognosis, and the patient's age. Patients may remain relatively stable for a period of time, or they may experience frequent changes in their physical and emotional states. Consequently, the nursing diagnosis and nursing management may need to be updated frequently.

■ Activity intolerance related to chemotherapy, radiation therapy, stage of the disease

■ Anxiety related to surgery, diagnostic procedures, treatments, prognosis

■ Constipation related to the effects of narcotic analgesics

■ Diarrhea related to the effects of chemotherapy or radiation therapy, dietary intake

■ Pain related to the progress of the disease, ineffectiveness of analgesics to control pain

■ Impaired verbal communication related to the effects of surgery (specific surgical procedure such as laryngectomy, radical oral surgery)

■ Ineffective individual coping related to inability to accept diagnosis, depression, other factors (specify)

■ Altered family processes related to ill family member

■ Fear related to the diagnosis, disfigurement, necessary treatments, prognosis (specify)

■ Fluid volume deficit related to decreased oral intake or abnormal fluid loss (specify)

■ Dysfunctional grieving related to alteration in body image or loss of a body part or function

■ Hopelessness related to diagnosis, prognosis, drastic change in lifestyle

■ Potential for infection related to effects of chemotherapy, radiation therapy on bone marrow

■ Altered nutrition: less than body requirements related to disease process, chemotherapy, radiation therapy

■ Feeding, bathing and hygiene, and dressing and grooming self-care deficits related to the effects of illness or treatments

■ Self-esteem disturbance related to changes in body image and role functions

■ Altered sexuality patterns related to the effects of illness or surgery, chemotherapy, or radiation therapy

■ Impaired social interaction related to changes in body image or function

■ Impaired tissue integrity related to the effects of disease or treatments

■ Potential for injury related to a bleeding disorder

■ Knowledge deficit of diagnosis, treatments, prognosis, home care, other (specify)

Planning and Implementation

The major goals of the patient include the attainment of comfort, prevention of infection, prevention of injury, attainment of an optimal nutritional status, maintenance of tissue integrity, and the preservation of self-respect and dignity.

The major goals of nursing management include the relief of pain and discomfort, the emotional support of the patient and the family, the reduction of anxiety, and the performance of tasks that help patients maintain a state of wellness within their capabilities.

The process of physical care is often demanding: tubes to keep patent, skin care, and many other tasks can tax the resources of the nursing staff. Every effort should be directed toward helping patients maintain their dignity; for example, use care in draping during treatments, pay strict attention to cleanliness, and allow patients to participate in planning and participating in their care when they can.

Activity Intolerance. Patients may vary in their ability to participate in their ADLs. Some require assistance in getting out of bed, walking, or taking care of their personal needs, whereas others do not. Patients are encouraged to be active within the limits of their ability. Activities, such as ambulating or bathing, are planned and spaced so that patients do not tire easily. Letting them do small tasks, such as brushing their teeth or washing their face, even when fatigued, fosters independence.

Anxiety. One of the most prominent emotions experienced by patients with cancer is anxiety. Although unable to identify the cause of their anxiety, it is ultimately rooted in their disease and the effects it will have on themselves, their family, and friends. Symptoms that may be noted are nervousness, uneasiness, irritability, crying, angry outbursts, and withdrawal. The nurse may alleviate some anxiety by allowing patients time to talk through their problems, by understanding and accepting their emotional reactions, and by using kindness and gentleness when carrying out those tasks necessary for treatment and basic patient management. Explaining procedures and the adverse effects associated with treatments may also help reduce anticipatory anxiety.

Patients must be given basic information during radiation therapy. Silence or vague answers often increase anxiety more than the truth does. Most patients tolerate therapy and bear some discomfort if given simple explanations. Lay terminology should be used because technical terms may increase anxiety. It is important, however, not only to explain the treatment but also to listen to their views, doubts, and concerns. Discussion of the side effects of therapy should be minimized until they are imminent or actually occur.

When patients are faced with surgery, they may have many questions about how the surgery will affect their bodies, what it will do for their illness, and whether the cancer will be cured or controlled. While some questions are answered originally by the physician, the nurse can restate the information. Because of the anxiety about surgery, many patients hear and understand only part of what they have been told originally. Later they realize that they still have many questions.

The use of chemotherapy in the treatment of

cancer also creates a variety of emotional responses. Often, patients have heard about the effects of antineoplastic drugs on the skin, hair, and GI tract. The physician must explain the reason for therapy, length of therapy, what adverse drug effects may occur, how these effects will be treated, and the expected outcomes. The nurse, however, may find it necessary to reemphasize or reexplain instructions and information given by the physician. Once patients know what to expect, their level of anxiety may be reduced.

Constipation.   The administration of narcotic analgesics often causes constipation. Patients are checked daily for bowel movements. Lack of a bowel movement for several days is brought to the attention of the physician; a laxative, enema, or stool softener may be prescribed.

Diarrhea.   Diarrhea may occur during chemotherapy and radiation therapy. Some antineoplastic drugs and internal or external radiation therapy to the abdomen have a profound effect on the GI tract, resulting in severe and prolonged diarrhea. When diarrhea occurs, the number, frequency, approximate amount, and color of the stools are recorded and the patient observed for signs of a fluid volume deficit. The physician is kept informed of the number of bowel movements because intravenous fluids or parenteral nutrition may be necessary. If the patient is able to take oral food and fluids, these are encouraged at regular intervals during waking hours. If diarrhea becomes severe and cannot be controlled by other methods, therapy may need to be postponed until the GI tract recovers.

Pain.   Many patients fear pain more than any other aspect of cancer. Pain must be controlled as much as possible by administration of analgesics. If the prescribed analgesic cannot control the pain, the physician must be notified. Nursing measures, such as repositioning the patient every 2 hours, finding positions of comfort, and good oral care, often lessen pain and discomfort.

Brompton's mixture, a mixture of drugs such as morphine or methadone, a phenothiazine, and an aromatic elixir, is an oral preparation used for the control of severe pain. This mixture is given every 3 or 4 hours around the clock. The addition of a phenothiazine enhances the effect of the narcotics and the alcohol of the aromatic elixir and prevents the nausea that may occur during the administration of an opiate.

Patients who express fear that the pain may later become unbearable can consider the medications available to relieve pain and the fact that all members of the medical team will help them remain as comfortable as possible.

It has been observed repeatedly that patients who receive emotional support from the nursing staff and who are in an atmosphere that fosters dignity, self-care to the extent possible, recreation, and companionship experience less pain.

Impaired Verbal Communication.   Difficulty in or absence of the ability to speak creates anxiety, frustration, anger, and feelings of abandonment. A patient with radical head or neck surgery may have lost the power of speech (total or partial). Those with severe stomatitis or other oral problems may have the power of speech but are unable to speak clearly because of changes in the oral mucosa or other structures in the mouth.

If patients are unable to communicate, a pad and pen or pencil can be provided. If they cannot communicate in this manner, the nurse must take the time to question them and instruct them to nod their head for yes or no. Asking patients to point to where it hurts or to print letters on their hand or in the air to spell out words provides a way to answer more specific questions. It is most important to remember that patience is required when trying to communicate with those who have totally or partially lost the power of speech.

Impaired communication can also mean a breakdown in relationships between patients, their family, and those involved in their care. When communication is impaired, the patient suffers the most.

Ineffective Individual Coping.   Many patients are unable to cope with their diagnoses, the changes in their bodies as a result of surgery, or the effects of radiation therapy and chemotherapy. Cancer patients often have many frustrating moments. During chemotherapy or radiation therapy, they may be acutely ill on some days; or, the prognosis may be good, but months later a recurrence of the disease is discovered. The effects of the disease on a patient's body and life, as well as the far reaching effects on members of the family, often cause many obstacles. While some patients are able to overcome obstacles, others experience many difficulties or are unable to accept each problem as it occurs.

Helping patients cope with their emotional and physical problems is not an easy task. Most of these patients are extremely sensitive to the attitudes and abilities of those involved in their care. By accepting their emotional state, nursing personnel can help the patients accept therapy and come to terms with their illness. By being a good listener, a nurse can sometimes help these patients work through their problems. At other times, a nurse may identify problems that need referral to another professional, such as a physician, social service worker, psychologist, dietitian, or occupational therapist.

Families are usually devastated when a member has been diagnosed as having cancer. Lifestyles are disrupted, financial security threatened, and the possibility of death confronted. While medical personnel attempt to help the family as well as the patient, problems that occur within the family structure may go unrecognized. Both family members and patients may give clues about the problems that are occurring. By listening carefully, the nurse may be able to identify problems and offer suggestions or referrals to appropriate people or agencies.

Altered Family Processes.   When a member of the family is ill, disruption in normal everyday routine occurs. Problems include a breakdown in communication between family members (including the patient), poor adaption to crisis, failure of one or more family member to share in burdens arising from the crisis, and failure of one or more family member to meet the physical and emotional needs of other family members.

The nurse may note overt changes in the relationship between family members or the patient and one or more family member. The patient and family may openly express emotions, such as hostility and anger, or concerns about a particular situation or problem.

Since the family is important to these patients and plays a vital role in their mental and physical support during illness, it is vital that breakdown in the family support structure be recognized. Whenever possible, patients and families must be supported and the family unit restored to a healthy, functioning one. The type of problems and the manner in which the patient and family respond to support from nursing personnel affect the way the problems can be addressed.

Nurses must help patients and their families realize that a diagnosis of cancer is not synonymous with death; they must help them make use of available treatment and establish a regimen that encourages as full a return to normal activities as possible. The patient who is physically able to continue working is encouraged to do so, as well as encouraged to continue normal home life and recreation. Professional staff can help families realize that patients benefit (as do those in close association with them) from encouragement to live as full a life as possible.

Patients who have cancer and who continue most of their usual activities have many concerns. The nurse can help by listening, clarifying, and assisting patients and families in finding their own solutions. When family members are able to express their own misgivings and questions to the staff, they are then better able to assist and support the patient. The patient or family is referred to the social worker for assistance with matters such as housing, transportation, and family problems.

Fear.   Cancer patients and their families may have many fears related to the diagnosis, prognosis, disfigurement, treatments, and pain of the disease. Although some fears are unfounded, they nonetheless exist. Others fears are real. While difficult to dispel, fear often can be reduced by explaining treatments and surgeries in understandable terms, showing concern, listening, and using gentleness when administering treatments that are painful or that cause discomfort.

It is important to listen to the patients, to assist them in expressing their fears, and to discuss their fears with them. In so doing, the vague and threatening fears may be lessened and made more manageable. It may help patients to speak of their fear of death, of separation from loved ones, of loss of control, and of disfigurement.

Fluid Volume Deficit.   A fluid volume deficit may occur when patients are receiving chemotherapy, radiation therapy, or as part of the clinical picture of cancer. It is not unusual for these patients to have marked anorexia along with a decrease in oral fluid intake.

Radiation sickness is sometimes experienced by patients undergoing radiation therapy. The amount of radiation sickness depends on the site, dose, and size of area treated. Symptoms may include weakness, nausea, vomiting, diaphoresis, and sometimes chills. Vomiting may be severe and prolonged, resulting in a fluid volume deficit. This and other symptoms are handled prophylactically and symptomatically. If radiation reactions become severe, the physician may halt treatments to give the body a chance to recover. The reason for stopping treatment should be explained to the patient and family to avoid misunderstandings, feelings of discouragement, and notions of a setback. It should be explained that deviations from the original plan of therapy are not unusual.

Destruction of the tumor is facilitated by the large amounts of water and oxygen present in the tissues. Because large amounts of tumor are being affected during therapy, it is important to avoid uric acid crystalluria (crystals in the urine) and possible kidney shutdown. Good hydration and maintenance of dilute urine are measures used to prevent this complication. The patient should take up to 3 L of fluid daily. If the fluid intake is inadequate, the physician may order intravenous fluids to make up the deficit. Accurate intake and output records are essential.

The maintenance of good hydration for those receiving radiation therapy is an important nursing responsibility.

Chemotherapy often involves the administration of two or more antineoplastic drugs. Some antineoplastic drugs cause severe nausea, vomiting, or diarrhea. The intake of oral fluids and food and the absorption of food and fluid from the GI tract may be decreased. If symptoms become severe, therapy may need to be temporarily or permanently discontinued or other antineoplastic agents prescribed.

Terminally ill patients often poorly consume oral food and fluids. To keep the patient comfortable, parenteral fluids may be necessary. To prevent a fluid volume deficit, the nurse must offer these patients frequent sips of water and other liquids throughout waking hours, even if they are receiving parenteral fluids.

Dysfunctional Grieving. Although many patients are cured of cancer, initial responses to the diagnosis and possible prognosis include thoughts of death, loss of a body part or function, and pain and suffering. Many decisions must be made about the treatment and the changes in the family structure that may occur during treatment. Although all decisions are ultimately the responsibility of the patient and family, the medical team can help them make decisions by explaining the proposed treatment (surgery, chemotherapy, radiation therapy) as well as alternatives, discussing anticipated outcomes, and allowing them time to ask questions.

During the various stages of treatment, grieving can occur with changes in physical appearance. A patient who was once healthy may now experience, for example, hair loss, skin pigmentation, weakness, or weight loss. Surgery may have resulted in body changes greater than what had been anticipated. Treatment may require equipment whose appearance is frightening.

As the patient and family progress through the grieving process, they may react with various emotions, such as anger, frustration, hostility, and depression. Any change in the patient's status or the prognosis may further complicate existing problems. Additional responsibilities placed on family members and long hours at the patient's bedside often stretch emotional resiliency, and the family begins to find it more and more difficult to cope with each new problem as it arises.

The nurse must take the time to listen and encourage the patient and family to verbalize their feelings. The nurse may be able to offer suggestions or make referrals to a professional or agency that could provide physical and emotional assistance.

Hopelessness. Many emotional feelings are associated with the diagnosis of cancer. Feelings of hopelessness are often present, even though they may not be openly expressed. Allowing time to ask questions and discuss feelings may identify areas where the nurse can offer support and encouragement. Although this problem can be treated in many ways, support groups whose members also have had the same type of cancer can help dispel the idea that every diagnosis of cancer is associated with prolonged suffering and death.

Potential for Infection. Infection may be associated with various types of invasive procedures, such as intravenous or intraarterial lines, surgery, breakdown in skin integrity, immobility, and decreased intake of food and fluids. Certain forms of cancer, such as leukemia, can affect the ability of bone marrow cells to manufacture the white blood cells necessary to fight infection. Patients who receive radiation therapy or chemotherapy may develop varying degrees of bone marrow depression.

Periodic complete blood cell counts, weekly or more often, are ordered to monitor the patient's response to therapy and to detect early indications of an infectious process or bone marrow depression. In addition to laboratory tests, the temperature is monitored every 4 hours and the patient frequently assessed for other signs of infection, such as inflammation, malaise, sore throat, chills, nausea, vomiting, or sudden appearance of or change in the type of drainage. Any slow or rapid rise in body temperature or the appearance of other signs of infection is reported to the physician immediately.

Treatment of infection usually includes the administration of one or more antibiotics. Whole blood, packed cells, or platelet transfusions may be necessary if the patient has a decrease in the red or white cell count or shows signs of bone marrow depression. If the reduction in white blood cells (leukopenia) is severe, the physician may temporarily halt treatment and place the patient in isolation. The type of isolation used depends on the severity and cause of leukopenia or bone marrow depression. Visitors and hospital personnel with colds or other infections should not be in close contact with these patients.

Despite the many types of antibiotics available, the use of strict aseptic technique, and the technological advances in medicine, cancer patients can die from overwhelming infections.

Altered Nutrition: Less Than Body Requirements. Anorexia, along with weight loss, nausea, vomiting, and diarrhea, may be seen in the cancer patient. Nutritional problems may be due to the treatment being given; for example, nausea and vomiting are associated with the administration of antineoplastic agents or radiation therapy. Inadequate ingestion, digestion, and absorption of food also may be associated with the illness.

Poor response to radiation therapy is evident more often among the cachectic than the well-nourished patients. On entering tissues, radiation produces ionization (the breaking up of molecules into their constituent ions) and chemical alteration of tissue proteins. To avoid nausea and vomiting after radiation therapy, the nurse and dietitian should plan the patient's meals so that no food is served for at least 1 hour before and after therapy.

Patients receiving chemotherapy often experience anorexia, nausea, and vomiting at some point during the course of therapy. GI symptoms can occur shortly after the first dose or after several doses. Symptoms may persist for only a few hours or may last for days. Some patients respond to the administration of an antiemetic and may be able to take oral food and fluids within 24 hours. Those having severe and prolonged vomiting or diarrhea may require intravenous fluids or total parenteral nutrition.

Some patients are helped by the administration of an antiemetic before administration of antineoplastic drugs. The physician may prescribe an antiemetic a half hour before each radiation or chemotherapy treatment and also an antiemetic for 12 or more hours after treatment. If the patient continues to have severe nausea and vomiting and the oral intake of food or fluid is low, the physician is notified.

All patients are weighed regularly (eg, daily to weekly), depending on the type of treatment being given and the status of the patient. Each meal tray is checked for the amount of food consumed, and intake and output records are kept. Significant or steady weight loss and failure to consume an adequate amount of food are brought to the attention of the physician.

Terminally ill patients require adequate amounts of food and fluid to keep them comfortable and to improve the quality of life.

Self-Care Deficits.

A patient's ability to take care of daily living activities is monitored throughout the hospitalization. When patients are no longer able to perform these tasks, they must be assumed by nursing personnel. Many patients prefer to do as much as possible for themselves until they are no longer able to do so. Allowing patients to participate in their self-care often helps them maintain dignity and independence.

When possible, activities such as bathing, oral care, and grooming should be spaced so that the patient does not become exhausted. These activities are also planned to be carried out before rather than after certain treatments, such as the administration of an antineoplastic drug that results in prolonged episodes of nausea and vomiting.

Self-Esteem Disturbance.

Surgery performed for the treatment of cancer can result in radical changes to the patient's appearance or body function. Also, prolonged illness or treatment modalities may result in changes such as marked weight gain or loss, changes in skin pigmentation, scarring, hair loss, or decreased or absent sexual drive. A patient's role in the family structure may be changed. Often, a positive approach by members of the health team, as well as by support groups and the family, helps to restore self-esteem.

Patients must be encouraged and motivated to become independent. Encouraging participation in ADLs and decision-making may help establish a more positive self-image. Allowing patients time to express concerns about the changes made in their lives is also necessary.

Altered Sexuality Patterns.

Certain treatments or surgeries may temporarily or permanently alter the patient's sexual function or image. Patients who experience a change in sexual pattern are encouraged to discuss this problem with the physician as well as their sexual partner. In some instances, counseling by a qualified sexual therapist is necessary.

Impaired Social Interaction.

Some patients find it difficult to face family members, relatives, and friends during and after therapies used in the treatment of cancer. Some are ashamed of their diagnosis, whereas others are concerned about their appearance or an odor. Patients may exhibit various emotional reactions, such as depression or anxiety. They may refuse to see visitors or communicate poorly with their family and members of the health team.

Many times, impaired social interactions occur because of a change in body image. The nurse must be alert to a patient's difficulty in communicating with others. Listening to their fears and concerns, a nurse may help them begin to work through this difficult time in their lives. In addition, a support group may help them verbalize their fears and feel comfortable with others. Continued difficulty in social interactions is discussed with the physician; it may be necessary to refer a patient to a therapist skilled in dealing with the emotional problems encountered by the patient with cancer.

Impaired Tissue Integrity. Chemotherapy, radiation therapy, long periods of immobilization, primary or metastatic malignant tumors of the skin, and weight loss may affect the skin and mucous membranes.

SKIN. Maintenance of skin integrity is important in the management of a patient with cancer. A break in the continuity of the skin is a potentially serious problem. Entrance of microorganisms found in the environment may result in an overwhelming superficial or systemic infection, especially in those with bone marrow depression and decrease in the white blood cell count. The skin must be inspected daily for changes in appearance, signs of infection, decubitus formation, and evidence of any break in or injury to the skin. Immobile patients are turned and repositioned every 2 hours, day and night. The skin must be kept clean and dry, especially if the patient is incontinent. The skin around a stoma (colostomy, ureterostomy) is watched carefully for redness and irritation, indicating early skin breakdown.

During radiation therapy, a patient may have skin reactions, which can vary from mild to severe. The skin over the treated area is kept clean and dry and checked daily for signs of redness, ulceration, and infection. The patient should be advised to report any discomforts experienced during radiation therapy to the nurse and the radiologist. The patient is told that the skin in the treated area may become reddened and that this is a normal reaction to therapy.

The outpatient is instructed to avoid the use of unprescribed ointments or creams and to avoid extremes of heat or cold. Heating pads, ultraviolet light, diathermy, whirlpool, sauna or steam baths, and direct sunlight are avoided. Careful bathing is advised, and soap and friction over the treated skin must be avoided. The skin markings must *not* be washed off because they are used as guides by the radiologist and technicians. These marks are necessary for the setting and adjusting of the x-ray machine over the area to be radiated. Loose clothing is advised to avoid irritation of the irradiated areas.

Intense itching may be experienced. A type of steroid cream or aerosol spray can be prescribed for relief. Cornstarch may be used over radiated areas where two skin surfaces are in contact, for example, axillary and groin areas, and areas under the breasts, provided the skin has not broken down. If the scalp is being irradiated, shampoo, tinting, and permanent waving are avoided. On completion of therapy, the physician may recommend a mild baby shampoo.

Temporary or permanent changes in skin pigmentation may be due to radiation therapy or chemotherapy or may be part of the illness. When therapy involves exposed skin surfaces of the head and neck, patients can be advised to use makeup on the face or scarves and high collars around the neck to cover the affected areas after a full course of therapy is completed and the skin has healed.

ALOPECIA. Hair loss or thinning (alopecia) may be seen as a result of radiation therapy, chemotherapy, or poor nutritional intake. The amount of hair lost often depends on the dose of the drug and duration of administration. Alopecia, while not life-threatening, poses a major threat to the patient's self-image and esteem.

Patients who receive therapy that will probably result in hair loss must be told of this effect before therapy is instituted. The patient is also told that hair loss may be gradual or may occur over a short period of time. The nurse may recommend the purchase of a wig, cap, or scarf before therapy begins. These devices can then be used before hair loss becomes prominent. Regrowth of the hair usually occurs within 4 to 6 months after therapy is finished. The new growth of hair may be a slightly different color and texture.

STOMATITIS. Inflammation of the mucous membranes of the mouth (stomatitis) may occur during chemotherapy and radiation therapy. The degree of stomatitis may range from mild redness and discomfort to large, painful ulcerated areas. Speech, chewing food, and swallowing may present problems.

The mouth is inspected daily, using a lightly padded tongue blade and flashlight. The lips are inspected, especially at the corners, for cracks or open sores. Any changes in the mouth or lips are reported to the physician. If pain occurs, the physician may order a local anesthetic gel, such as benzocaine or tetracaine, to be held in the mouth for several minutes at prescribed intervals throughout the day. A soft bland diet and frequent, small feedings of high caloric foods are usually ordered. If the patient is still unable to eat, total parenteral nutrition may be necessary.

Good oral care is essential for those with or predisposed to developing stomatitis. Frequent mouth rinses with warm water and application of glycerin and lemon to dry lips may make the patient more comfortable. Dental care may be difficult, but a soft tooth brush or the use of toothpaste on a cotton swab may help remove accumulated debris from the teeth. Severe stomatitis may require a dental consultation if the teeth appear to be affected by the disorder.

Bleeding Tendency. Bleeding in the cancer patient is usually due to a decrease in the number of platelets (thrombocytopenia). Tumors invading the bone marrow and chemotherapy and radiation therapy can result in thrombocytopenia.

The patient is assessed daily for evidence of easy bruising, blood oozing from small cuts or abrasions, bleeding gums, or the appearance of blood in the stool or urine.

Some episodes of bleeding and bruising can be prevented or lessened by the following measures:

- Using a soft toothbrush or cotton-tipped swabs for oral care
- Gentleness in moving, lifting, and assisting the patient
- Placing prolonged pressure or a pressure dressing on intravenous, intramuscular, and subcutaneous injection sites after withdrawal of the needle
- Using an electric rather than a safety razor
- Taking oral rather than rectal temperatures
- Taking special precautions to prevent falls as well as other types of injuries, such as bumping into or furniture or parts of the bed (eg, side rails, over-the-bed stands)

Knowledge Deficit.   A lack of knowledge can alter a patient's ability to cooperate with members of the medical team. Cancer patients and their families often have many questions. Because of fear and anxiety, patients and families may not fully comprehend all they have been told, and explanations and instructions need to be repeated. A patient and family have the right to know the following:

- The diagnosis and prognosis
- What further diagnostic studies will be necessary
- The adverse effects associated with treatment
- What type of treatment will be necessary
- What alternative to treatment is possible
- What changes (if any) in body image or function will occur
- How lifestyle will or must change
- What special care or treatment will be required after discharge from the hospital

In addition to the above general areas, more detailed and specific information is usually necessary and often based on the treatment given and the questions raised by the patient or family. Examples of areas that may be covered in more detail include the frequency of laboratory tests, the length of hospital stay, home care, chemotherapy or radiation therapy appointments, how to care for a colostomy, when hair will grow back, and when the individual may return to work. Patients who have had surgery require information regarding the care of their incision (see Chapter 16). If the patient is discharged on a special diet, the dietitian should review the diet with the patient. Patients who must take drugs at home require a complete explanation of the drug regimen as well as information regarding adverse drug effects and the effects that require contacting the physician.

All members of the health care team must be aware of any explanations or information given the patient and family. This awareness includes discussions by professionals, such as the physician, other nurses, dietitian, or the therapist or specialist assigned to instruct a patient in a specific area, such as colostomy care. The nurse can help by listening and allowing patients to express their feelings and by identifying areas or facts that are not completely understood. Once these areas are recognized, an appropriate member of the health team can supply additional information.

Evaluation

- Activity tolerance is improved
- Able to perform ADL within limits of ability
- Anxiety and fear is reduced
- Attains normal defecation pattern
- Pain and discomfort are reduced or eliminated
- Communicates effectively with family, relatives, visitors, hospital personnel
- Shows a more positive attitude and ability to cope with present situation
- Family shows evidence of coping with patient's diagnosis, prognosis, condition, treatments
- Problems relating to alterations in family processes identified and resolved
- Normal fluid balance is attained and maintained
- Shows evidence of progressing through a normal grieving process
- No evidence of local or systemic infection
- Acquires understanding of illness, treatment modalities
- Attains normal food intake; nutritional deficits are corrected; weight remains stable
- Demonstrates improvement in self-concept
- Understands and is able to accept altered sexual patterns
- Socializes with family, relatives, friends, medical personnel
- Attains and maintains skin and oral mucous membrane integrity
- Family members are aware of patient's diagnosis, necessary treatment modalities, prognosis
- Patient and family demonstrate understanding of treatment regimen after discharge from the hospital

General Nutritional Considerations

☐ Many patients develop anorexia due to radiation therapy, chemotherapy, or the course of their disease. A well-balanced diet is important during cancer treatment; intake of food and fluids is encouraged. Some patients may require frequent small feedings rather than three standard meals.

☐ Adequate fluid intake is necessary to prevent dehydration and electrolyte imbalance, especially in those who have frequent episodes of vomiting.

☐ Patients with stomatitis can be given a soft, bland diet. Patients who develop diarrhea due to radiation therapy or chemotherapy may require a bland or low-residue diet.

☐ To avoid nausea during treatment, no meals should be served 1 hour before or after a treatment has been given.

☐ Patients who experience nausea during the days or weeks required for external radiation therapy may find food more palatable and acceptable when served in small amounts.

General Pharmacologic Considerations

☐ Antineoplastic drugs used in the treatment of cancer are potentially toxic agents. Nurses should be thoroughly familiar with adverse effects and toxicity of these agents. The dose or length of treatment depends in some cases on the patient's response to therapy.

☐ Combination chemotherapy, rather than the use of a single agent, may be employed in the treatment of neoplastic diseases.

☐ Many antineoplastic drugs have a profound effect on the bone marrow. Patients should be observed for signs of bone marrow depression, namely, fever, sore throat, and chills for infection; and for bleeding, oozing from venipuncture or parenteral drug injection sites, bleeding from the gums, or signs of blood in the urine or stools.

☐ Intravenous or intraarterial administration of antineoplastic agents may lead to thrombophlebitis. Sites should be inspected daily for tenderness, pain, swelling, or induration above or below site of use.

☐ Nausea, vomiting, and diarrhea may be observed during administration of many antineoplastic agents. These adverse effects must be reported immediately because dehydration and electrolyte imbalance often occur rapidly. Antiemetic or antidiarrheal drugs or intravenous fluid and electrolyte replacement may be needed.

☐ Allopurinol is sometimes prescribed when the uric acid level rises during chemotherapy.

☐ Patients referred to outpatient clinics for further drug therapy must be encouraged to keep clinic appointments and to report all unusual symptoms or effects experienced between treatments.

☐ Nausea is a common adverse effect of radiation therapy; an antiemetic may be needed.

☐ Drugs may be ordered for other adverse effects that may occur during radiation therapy: aspirin for fever, antibiotics for infection, various ointments and creams for the skin over the radiated area. When creams or ointments are ordered, these products are to be applied exactly as ordered (eg, sparingly or liberally).

General Gerontologic Considerations

☐ An elderly patient with a terminal neoplastic disease may pose additional problems with nutrition, adequate fluid intake, skin care, and prevention of the complications related to inactivity.

☐ An elderly patient often has decreased resistance to infection, which may pose additional problems if the patient receives antineoplastic agents that have a depressant effect on the bone marrow.

☐ Because of concurrent disease, as well as the effect of the aging process on the body's tissues and organs, an elderly patient may not receive the same surgical or chemotherapeutic treatment for a neoplastic disease that a younger patient does.

☐ An elderly patient, faced with the long and sometimes rigorous treatment of a neoplastic disorder, may refuse treatment.

☐ An elder patient who has undergone extensive surgery for treatment of a neoplastic disease requires detailed home care planning before discharge from the hospital.

☐ Arthritis, as well as general muscular stiffness, may make lying supine on an x-ray table difficult for the time required for radiation treatment. It may be necessary to pad bony prominences and provide support to the back or legs during a radiation treatment.

☐ The skin of the elderly patient is often dry. Intense itching and dryness may be experienced during and after radiation therapy. Additional treatment of skin problems arising from radiation therapy may be necessary. The skin should be inspected frequently for signs of breakdown, evidence of excessive scratching, and infection.

☐ Elderly patients are often more prone to electrolyte imbalance than younger patients. Excessive vomiting during or after a course of radiation treatments may result in a serious electrolyte imbalance.

☐ An elderly patient who receives internal radiation therapy with an applicator inserted into a body cavity may experience difficulty in lying still until the end of the treatment. These patients should be checked more frequently for displacement of the applicator.

Suggested Readings

☐ Andersen AR. Are your IV chemo skills up-to-date? RN January 1989;52:40. *(Additional coverage of subject matter)*

☐ Baird SB. Decision making in oncologic nursing. St Louis: CV Mosby, 1987. *(Additional coverage of subject matter)*

☐ Beers L. "I want to live until I die": Working to control a cancer patient's pain. Nursing '88 October 1988; 18:70. *(Additional coverage of subject matter)*

☐ Beyers M, Durburg S, Werner J. Complete guide to cancer nursing. Oradell, NJ: Medical Economics, 1984. *(In-depth coverage of subject matter)*

☐ Birdsall C, Neliboff A. How do you manage chemotherapy extravasation? Am J Nurs February 1988;88:228. *(additional coverage of subject matter)*

☐ Bruera E, MacDonald N. Overwhelming fatigue in advanced cancer. Am J Nurs January 1988;88:99. *(Additional coverage of subject matter)*

☐ Cerrato PL. Meeting your CA patient's nutritional needs. RN February 1988;51:63. *(Additional coverage of subject matter)*

☐ D'Agostino NS. Managing nutrition problems in advanced cancer. Am J Nurs January 1989;89:50. *(Additional and in-depth coverage of subject matter)*

☐ Gullatte MM. Managing an implanted infusion device. RN January 1989;52:44. *(Additional coverage and illustrations that reinforce subject matter)*

☐ Holman SR. Essentials of nutrition for the health professions. Philadelphia: JB Lippincott, 1987. *(Additional and in-depth coverage of subject matter)*

☐ Johnson BL, Gross J, eds. Handbook of oncology nursing. New York: John Wiley & Sons, 1985. *(In-depth coverage of subject matter)*

☐ Lenehan JK. Cancer with metastasis to family life. RN June 1988;51:31. *(Additional coverage of subject matter)*

☐ Luckmann J, Sorensen K. Medical–surgical nursing: a psychophysioloigic approach. 3rd ed. Philadelphia: WB Saunders, 1987. *(Additional and in-depth coverage of subject matter)*

☐ Masoorli ST, Miller KH. Putting some comfort in chemotherapy. RN August 1988;51:73. *(Additional coverage of subject matter)*

☐ McGowan KL. Radiation therapy: saving your patient's skin. RN June 1989;52:24. *(Additional and in-depth coverage of subject matter)*

☐ Rudolph B. The heart and soul of hospice nursing. RN March 1988;51:33. *(Additional coverage of subject matter)*

☐ Schlesselman SM. Helping your cancer patient cope with alopecia. Nursing '88 December 1988;18:43. *(Additional coverage of subject matter)*

☐ Tenenbaum L. Cancer chemotherapy: a reference guide. Philadelphia: WB Saunders, 1989. *(In-depth coverage of subject matter)*

☐ Valente SM, Saunders JM. Serious depression in cancer patients. Nursing '89 February 1989;19:44. *(Additional coverage of subject matter)*

☐ Walters P. Chemo: the nurse's guide to action, administration, and side effects. RN February 1990;53:52. *(Additional coverage of subject matter)*

The Respiratory System

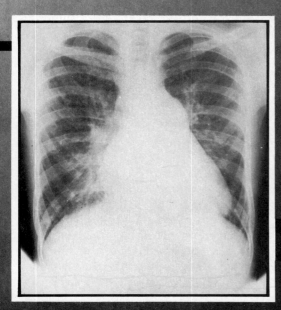

Unit 5

Chapter 20

Introduction to Respiratory Nursing

On completion of this chapter the reader will:

- Be familiar with the anatomy and physiology of the upper and lower respiratory airway

- List and discuss the tests and studies used in the diagnosis of disorders of the upper and lower respiratory airway

- Perform a basic assessment of a patient with an upper or lower respiratory airway disorder

- Use the nursing process in the management of a patient who undergoes diagnostic evaluation of the upper or lower respiratory airway

UPPER RESPIRATORY AIRWAY
Anatomy and Physiology

The upper respiratory tract, or airway, consists of the nose, sinuses, pharynx, tonsils and adenoids, larynx, and the bones and cartilaginous structures surrounding or supporting these structures (Fig. 20-1).

Nose

The internal nose is divided into two passages and separated by the *nasal septum*. The supporting structures of the septum and walls of the nasal cavity are made up of bone and cartilage. The lateral walls of the nasal cavity are formed by three bony protuberances on either side–the superior, the middle, and the inferior–called *conchae* or *turbinates*, which increase the surface of the nasal passages. Between the conchae are grooves that contain openings through which the sinuses drain. Three pairs of openings—superior, middle, and inferior—lie beneath each respective concha. The entire nasal cavity is lined with a highly vascular mucous membrane, the surface of which is composed of ciliated columnar epithelial cells. Interspersed with the columnar cells are numerous goblet cells that secrete mucus which is carried back to the nasopharynx by the movement of the cilia. Air passing through the nose is warmed by the blood vessels that line the air passages. The mucous secreted by the goblet cells traps small particles, such as dust and pollen, in the inspired air.

Paranasal Sinuses

The *paranasal sinuses* are extensions of the nasal cavity and are located in the surrounding facial bones (see Fig. 20-1). The lining of these sinuses is continuous with the mucous membrane lining of the nasal cavity. These sinuses are located in the frontal, ethmoid, sphenoid, and maxillary bones. They function to lighten the weight of the skull and give resonance to the voice.

The two frontal sinuses lie within the frontal bone that extends above the orbital cavities. The ethmoid bone, located between the eyes, contains a honeycomb of small spaces known as the *ethmoid sinuses*. The sphenoid sinuses lie behind the nasal cavity. The maxillary sinuses (antrum of Highmore) are located on either side of the nose in the maxillary bones. The largest of the sinuses, they are the most accessible to treatment.

The olfactory area lies at the roof of the nose; directly above is the cribriform plate that forms a portion of the roof of the nose and the floor of the anterior cranial fossa. Trauma or surgery in this area carries risk of injury to or infection of the brain.

Pharynx

The *pharynx*, or throat, is divided into three continuous areas, the *nasopharynx*, the *oropharynx*, and the

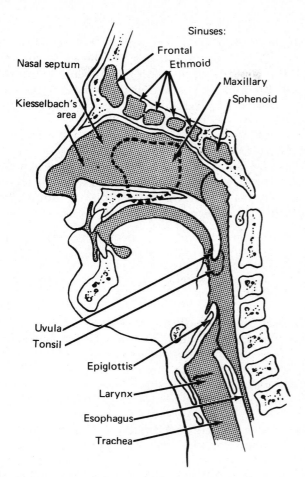

Figure 20-1. Some important structures of the nose and the throat.

laryngeal pharynx. The nasopharynx is the area behind the nasal cavity; the oropharynx is the area behind the oral cavity; and the laryngeal pharynx extends from the end of the oropharynx to the larynx. The pharynx carries air into the bronchi and lungs, and food and liquids into the esophagus.

Tonsils and Adenoids

The *tonsils* are two pairs of elliptically shaped bodies of lymphoid tissue located on either side of the upper section of the oropharynx. They can be viewed by looking into the oral cavity. Tonsils, which consist of lymphoid tissue, protect the body against invasion by microorganisms. People who are subject to chronic throat infections may have had their tonsils removed.

The *adenoids*, also lymphoid tissue, are located in the nasopharynx. They usually are not visible when looking into the oral cavity. The adenoids may have been removed along with the tonsils, or they may have shrunk and become nonfunctional.

Larynx

The *larynx*, or voice box, is located between the pharynx and the trachea and consists of a somewhat rigid framework of cartilages held together by ligaments. Except for the vocal cords, the interior of the larynx is lined by ciliated mucous membrane that is continuous with the mucous membrane of the pharynx and the trachea. The cartilaginous framework of the larynx consists of the *thyroid,* the *arytenoid,* and the *cricoid* cartilages.

On each lateral wall of the laryngeal cavity are two horizontally placed folds of mucous membrane—the ventricular folds, or false vocal cords, and the vocal folds, or true vocal cords. The latter are the lower of the two. The larynx forms a part of the air passages, which constitute an air column that produces sounds of varying pitch. The larynx, however, cannot produce words. The sounds made by the vibrating vocal cords are molded into speech by the pharynx, palate, tongue, teeth, and lips.

The *glottis* is the opening between the vocal chords. The *epiglottis*, situated above the glottis, opens and closes to direct air or food and liquids into the appropriate passages. The epiglottis is closed over the larynx during swallowing and is open during the passage of air from the upper respiratory tract to the bronchi and lungs (Fig. 20-2).

Assessment of the Upper Respiratory Airway

Patient History. The history should include a medical, drug, and allergy history, a full description of the symptoms, the length of time they have been present, what, if anything, caused or relieved the symptoms, and what drugs (prescription, nonprescription) were used to treat the symptoms. If trauma to these structures has occurred, a full description of the injury is obtained.

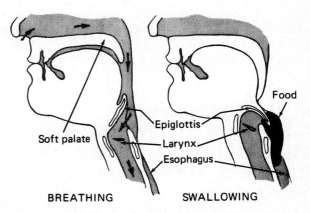

Figure 20-2. During swallowing, the soft palate is elevated to close off air from the nose. Breathing is interrupted momentarily. The larynx rises, and its opening is shut off by the epiglottis until the food has passed down into the esophagus.

Nose and Sinuses. The external part of the nose is inspected for signs of injury, inflammation, symmetry, and lesions. The internal structures of the anterior nasal passages are best seen by use of a light and nasal speculum and inspected for signs of frank bleeding, oozing, drainage or exudate, and deviation of, injury to, or perforation of the nasal septum. The nasal membranes are inspected for color and evidence of swelling, injury, or inflammation. The sinuses cannot be seen but may be transilluminated with a penlight placed in the patients mouth. The area over the sinuses is palpated for tenderness.

Pharynx and Tonsils. A tongue blade and light are used to examine the posterior pharynx and tonsils. These areas are inspected for evidence of inflammation and swelling as well as for changes in the color of the mucous membranes.

Larynx. The physician performs an indirect laryngoscopy (visualization of the larynx) by using a light and laryngeal mirror. To perform a direct laryngoscopy, the physician passes a laryngoscope (a hollow instrument with a light at its distal end) to the larynx after the patient's throat has been anesthetized. A local anesthetic is used to depress the gag reflex and reduce discomfort.

Laboratory Tests

Many general laboratory tests can be performed on the patient with an upper respiratory disorder. Although not specifically intended for the respiratory system, these tests may be used along with other tests for diagnosis. Examples of these tests are culture and sensitivity studies and the white blood cell count and differential.

Diagnostic Tests

Diagnostic tests that may be performed on the upper respiratory tract include biopsy, transillumination of the sinus cavities, radiograph of the sinuses, and direct visualization of upper respiratory structures (eg, laryngoscopy).

NURSING PROCESS —THE PATIENT UNDERGOING DIAGNOSTIC EVALUATION OF THE UPPER RESPIRATORY AIRWAY

Assessment

A thorough patient history includes a description of symptoms and the length of time they have been present, factors that may influence the symptoms (if any), and any drugs (prescription, nonprescription) used previously for treatment or relief of symptoms.

If the problem appears to be associated with the larynx, the patient is asked about symptoms such as weight loss, prolonged hoarseness, or difficulty in swallowing.

Nursing Diagnosis

Depending on the patient's diagnosis, the following may apply to the patient who has a diagnostic test of the upper airway. For some patients, additional nursing diagnoses may be necessary.

- Knowledge deficit of the diagnostic procedure
- Anxiety related to the scheduled procedure
- Pain related to the diagnostic procedure (specify)
- Impaired swallowing related to the diagnostic procedure (specify)

Planning and Implementation

The major goal of the patient may be to understand and perform the tasks necessary for accurate completion of a laboratory study or diagnostic test.

The major goal of nursing management is to prepare the patient properly for diagnostic testing.

Knowledge Deficit and Anxiety. The patient and family require an explanation of the diagnostic procedure. The physician usually explains the procedure and its purpose. When necessary, the nurse may repeat or clarify the physician's initial explanation. A basic explanation of the procedure and information about when it will be done and what patient participation will be required (if any) can reduce anxiety associated with the diagnostic tests.

Fasting may be required for a test. The patient is instructed and later reminded not to eat or drink until the test is completed.

Pain and Impaired Swallowing. Pain and difficulty swallowing may occur after a diagnostic procedure, such as a laryngoscopy. The physician may order the use of ice chips and an ice collar for several hours after the procedure, until the patient can swallow normally and has less discomfort. Continued discomfort or signs of bleeding are reported to the physician.

Evaluation

- Anxiety is reduced
- The patient and family understand the purpose and procedure of the diagnostic test and know when it will be performed and what participation is required by the patient
- Discomfort is relieved
- Swallowing and gag reflexes return

LOWER RESPIRATORY AIRWAY
Anatomy and Physiology

The lower respiratory airway, or tract, consists of the trachea, bronchi, bronchioles, and lungs (Fig. 20-3). Accessory structures are the diaphragm, rib cage, sternum, spine, muscles, and blood vessels.

Trachea

The *trachea* is a hollow tube that extends from the lower edge of the larynx. The end of the trachea bifurcates (divides) to form the left and right *bronchi.* The supporting structure of the trachea is made of up C-shaped cartilages that help keep the trachea open. The solid part of the C faces the anterior chest. The trachea transports air from the laryngeal pharynx to the bronchi and lungs.

Bronchi and Lungs

The *tracheobronchial tree* consists of the trachea and the left and right bronchi. The right bronchus slopes somewhat more acutely downward than the left. The entrance of the bronchus into the lung is called the *hilus* of the lung. The *carina* is a ridge at the lower end of the trachea at the point where the trachea separates into the left and right bronchi. When the carina is stimulated, coughing and bronchospasm usually occur.

The right and left bronchi divide into *secondary bronchi.* Three secondary bronchi are on the right and two on the left. The secondary bronchi supply air to each of the lobes of the lung. The bronchi continue to branch, forming smaller bronchi and finally *terminal bronchioles* (smaller subdivisions of the bronchus). At the end of the terminal bronchioles are the *alveoli,* which are small, clustered sacs. Each alveolus consists of a single layer of squamous epithelium cells. The thin-walled alveoli are surrounded by capillaries. It is at this point that oxygen and carbon dioxide are exchanged. The blood vessels of the lungs are the pulmonary arteries and veins.

The lungs are located in the chest or *thoracic* cavity. The right lung has three lobes and the left has two. The lungs are covered by a serous membrane called the *visceral pleura.* The chest wall is covered by the *parietal pleura.* Serous fluid separates and lubricates the visceral and parietal pleurae. The *diaphragm* separates the thoracic cavity from the abdominal cavity. On inspiration, the respiratory muscles contract and the diaphragm contracts and moves downward, thus enlarging and creating negative pressure in the thoracic cavity. On expiration, the respiratory muscles relax and the diaphragm returns to its normal position, creating positive pressure in the thoracic cavity. The *mediastinum* is between the lungs and contains the heart, esophagus, trachea, lymph nodes, and the left and right pulmonary artery and vein.

Pressure in the thoracic cavity (or thorax) changes during the respiratory cycle. The following pressures are considered:

Atmospheric pressure—the pressure in the surrounding air, which at sea level is 760 mmHg
Intrapulmonary pressure—the pressure inside the airways (trachea, bronchi) and alveoli
Intrapleural pressure—the pressure in the pleural cavity or the pressure between the visceral and parietal pleura; intrapleural pressure is always less than intrapulmonary and atmospheric pressures
Intrathoracic pressure—the pressure in the thoracic cavity; it is equal to the intrapleural pressure.

On inspiration, the intrapulmonary, intrapleural, and intrathoracic pressures are *negative* or less than atmospheric pressure. On expiration, these pressures are *positive* or greater than atmospheric pressure. Under normal conditions, a gas (including air) moves from an area of higher pressure to an area of lower pressure. For example, this type of air movement occurs in the opening of a vacuum-packed can. The sound heard on breaking the vacuum seal is the rush of atmospheric air moving to the area of lower pressure inside the can.

The creation of negative pressure on inspiration allows air to flow into the lungs. On expiration, when intrathoracic pressure becomes positive, air moves out of the lungs.

The main function of the respiratory system is to exchange oxygen and carbon dioxide between atmospheric air and the blood. Usually, the respiratory system has sufficient reserves to maintain the normal partial pressures or tension of these gases in the blood during times of stress. Respiratory insufficiency develops if too much interference with the following aspects of lung function occurs:

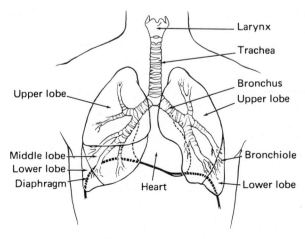

Figure 20-3. The respiratory tract.

Ventilation—the movement of air in and out of the lungs in volumes sufficient to maintain normal arterial oxygen and carbon dioxide tensions

Perfusion—the filling of the pulmonary capillaries with venous blood returning from the systemic circulation by way of the right ventricle

Diffusion—the exchange of oxygen and carbon dioxide across the alveolar–capillary membrane

Distribution—the delivery of (atmospheric) air to the separate gas exchange units in the lung

Abnormalities in ventilation, perfusion, diffusion, or distribution lead to the following conditions:

Hypoxia—decreased oxygen in inspired air
Hypoxemia—decreased oxygen in the blood
Hypercapnia—increased carbon dioxide in the blood
Hypocapnia—decreased carbon dioxide in the blood

Alveolar ventilation determines the amount of carbon dioxide in the body. An increase in carbon dioxide, which is present in body fluids primarily as carbonic acid, decreases the hydrogen ion concentration (pH) below the normal 7.4; a decrease in carbon dioxide increases the pH above 7.4. The pH affects the rate of alveolar ventilation by a direct action of hydrogen ions on the respiratory center in the medulla oblongata. Contributing to the normal pH, the kidneys maintain serum bicarbonate within a normal range by excreting excess hydrogen ions. The lung and the kidneys combine to maintain the ratio of carbonic acid to bicarbonate at 1:20, fixing the pH at about 7.4.

In a critically ill patient, various homeostatic mechanisms operate to compensate for altered physiology. Buffer ratios shift, the lung can blow off carbonic acid as carbon dioxide, or the kidneys can excrete more bicarbonate in an attempt to maintain normal pH. Compensatory mechanisms, however, can become overstressed and fail, causing dangerous clinical conditions. In an intensive care patient, these conditions are generally superimposed on an already serious underlying condition. The patient's condition is said to be compensated as long as the ratio of carbonic acid to bicarbonate remains 1:20.

Disturbances in pH that involve the lung and carbonic acid levels and that result from dissolved carbon dioxide are termed *respiratory;* the other disturbances are termed *metabolic.* At times, metabolic and respiratory derangements coexist. Blood gas studies of an arterial blood sample enable the physician to assess the acid–base balance dependably and rapidly. The blood may be withdrawn by single arterial puncture, or repeated samples may be drawn from an indwelling arterial catheter, such as a Swan-Ganz catheter. A heparinized syringe is used and is carefully filled to avoid bubbles. If delay in analysis is anticipated, the syringe is immediately immersed in ice. This action decreases the metabolic activity of the blood cells and prevents oxygen consumption in the syringe.

Assessment of the Lower Respiratory Airway

Patient History. The history should include a medical, drug, and allergy history, as well as a full description of symptoms, including the length of time they have been present, what, if anything, caused or relieved the symptoms, and what drugs (prescription, nonprescription) were used to treat the symptoms. In addition to symptoms, the patient is asked about smoking (including exposure to others who smoke if the patient is a nonsmoker), a family history of lung disease or allergies, and exposure to pollutants (industrial, environmental).

Trachea. The trachea and its adjacent area are gently palpated and visually inspected for placement and deviation from the midline. The presence of lymph node enlargement is noted.

Bronchi and Lungs. Assessment of the bronchi and lungs uses inspection, percussion, auscultation, and palpation. *Inspection* includes looking at the anterior, posterior, and lateral chest walls for lesions, symmetry, deformities, color of the skin, and evidence of muscle weakness or weight loss. The breathing pattern (eg, rate, rhythm, depth) is observed. Movement of the rib cage, including the intercostal muscles, during inspiration and expiration, as well as any use of abdominal or neck muscles for breathing is observed. The anterior and posterior external chest wall is inspected for evidence of trauma.

Percussion of the chest wall may be performed by the experienced examiner, who can hear the normal and abnormal sounds produced by this maneuver. With the patient in a sitting position, the middle finger is placed on the chest wall and tapped with the middle finger of the opposite hand. Percussion is begun on the posterior chest wall, starting at the top of the shoulder and progressing down in about 5-cm (2-inch) intervals. Percussion of the anterior chest wall follows.

Auscultation of the chest is performed with a stethoscope. A knowledge of normal and abnormal breath sounds is required. The stethoscope is placed at various intervals over the chest wall while the patient deeply inhales and exhales. Because lightheadedness may occur because of hyperventilation, the patient is asked to rest and breathe normally two or three times after taking five or six deep breaths.

Palpation by the experienced examiner is performed to detect tenderness, masses, swelling, and other abnormalities of the chest wall. Vocal fremitus (the feeling of sound through the fingers and palm of the hand placed on the chest wall) may be performed to detect emphysema or pneumonia.

Mental Status. The patient is observed for confusion, delirium, severe anxiety, restlessness, and disorientation.

Laboratory Tests

General Tests. A complete blood cell count, white blood cell count and differential, and serum electrolytes are examples of general laboratory tests that may be ordered when the patient has a known or suspected lower respiratory airway disorder. Other tests include culture and sensitivity studies of fluids (eg, fluid from the pleural space).

Sputum. Samples of sputum may be collected and sent to the laboratory. Microscopic examination of appropriately stained smears may reveal casts, cancer cells, or pathogenic microorganisms. Culture and sensitivity tests may also be ordered. Sputum samples may be collected over a 24-hour period, may be a single specimen raised by the patient by means of suction, or may be secretions removed during a bronchoscopy.

Gastric Contents. Because pathogenic organisms that cause lung disease frequently are swallowed, the fasting contents of the stomach may be examined. This diagnostic procedure may be used when tuberculosis is suspected.

Blood Gasses. Severe disease of the respiratory passages can interfere with oxygen supply. Blood gas studies may be performed on patients with respiratory disorders as well as on any patient that is acutely ill. These studies are the measurement of oxygen, carbon dioxide, and hydrogen (as pH) in either venous or arterial blood. Most blood gas studies are performed on arterial blood (arterial blood gases). Two of these studies—the PaO_2 and the $PaCO_2$—measure the partial pressure or tension of oxygen and carbon dioxide in arterial blood. The normal PaO_2 is 80 mmHg or greater; the normal $PaCO_2$ is 35 to 45 mmHg. The normal arterial blood pH is 7.35 to 7.45.

1. An elevated PaO_2 may be seen with hyperventilation during arterial blood sampling.
2. A decreased PaO_2 may be seen with hypoventilation due to neuromuscular disease, chronic obstructive pulmonary disease, and insufficient oxygen in the atmosphere.
3. An elevated $PaCO_2$ indicates *respiratory acidosis*. This

disorder is seen in those with chronic obstructive pulmonary disease, inadequate ventilation with a mechanical ventilator, or in any patient who has a decreased respiratory rate.
4. A decreased $PaCO_2$ indicates *respiratory alkalosis*. This disorder is seen in those who are nervous or anxious or who have any condition that causes hyperventilation or a rapid respiratory rate.

Oxygen is present in the blood as a gas dissolved in plasma and combined with the hemoglobin of red blood cells. The greatest amount of oxygen in the blood is contained in the hemoglobin. If the PaO_2 is decreased, body tissues do not receive sufficient oxygen. Oxygenation of body tissues depends on the amount of oxygen in arterial blood and the ability of the heart to pump oxygenated blood to all parts of the body. Patients with respiratory disorders can neither get oxygen into the blood nor rid the blood of carbon dioxide, a waste product of cellular metabolism. In addition, patients with cardiac disorders cannot adequately pump oxygenated blood to all areas of the body because of the inefficiency of the pumping action of the heart.

Diagnostic Tests

Radiographic Studies. Radiographic examination of the chest is secondary only to the physician's stethoscope in the diagnosis of acute respiratory disorders. Often, when the physical examination of the patient fails to reveal a respiratory disorder, small lesions may be noted on a chest radiograph. Fluoroscopy enables the physician to view the thoracic cavity with all its contents in motion. A computed tomographic scan or magnetic resonance imaging may be used to produce axial views of the lungs to detect tumors and other lung disorders during early stages of the disease.

Bronchoscopy. The physician may perform a bronchoscopy for direct visual examination of the trachea, the two major bronchi, and multiple smaller bronchi in both the diagnosis and the therapy of acute respiratory disorders. The bronchoscope is a hollow instrument that can be passed into the trachea under local or general anesthesia. Through the lumen of the bronchoscope, the physician may pass suction catheters to obtain secretions for culture and Papanicolaou smears or to remove aspirated foreign bodies.

Bronchography. For this procedure, after the pharynx and larynx have been anesthetized, the physician introduces a catheter into the trachea by either the nasal or oral route and positions it above the bifurcation. Radiopaque dye is injected into the trachea through the tube, and the patient is tilted in various positions so that the dye flows throughout the bronchial tree. Radiographs (bronchograms) are taken to reveal the radiopaque outlines of the bronchi and bronchioles. If tracheobronchial secretions are profuse, postural drainage may be necessary before the examination to clear mucus and to permit better visualization of smaller bronchi. The patient should be informed of the discomfort that may be experienced during the procedure and is advised not to cough during instillation of the contrast material because coughing could drive the dye into the alveoli. Sedation may be ordered before the procedure.

Thoracentesis.   Normally, a small amount of fluid lies between the visceral and parietal pleura. When an excess of fluid occurs, the physician inserts a needle into the chest wall under local anesthesia. This procedure, called a *thoracotomy*, also may be used to obtain a sample of pleural fluid or a biopsy specimen from the pleural wall for diagnostic purposes, such as a culture and sensitivity or microscopic examination.

Mediastinoscopy.   With the patient under local anesthesia, the physician inserts an endoscope above the sternum into the mediastinal space to visualize and obtain a biopsy specimen of the mediastinal lymph nodes.

Pulmonary Function Studies.   Pulmonary function studies are performed to identify abnormalities in respiratory function and to periodically evaluate the status of a patient with a respiratory disease. Examples of these studies include the following:

Vital capacity (VC)—the maximum volume of air that can be exhaled after maximum inhalation (normal, 4,000–4,800 mL)

Forced vital capacity (FVC)—the maximum volume of air that can be exhaled with a forced expiratory effort (normal, 3,000–5,000 mL)

Forced expiratory volume, timed (FEV$_t$)—the time (expressed as t) required, in seconds, to expire a percentage of air (normal, 81%–83% in 1 second; 90%–94% in 2 seconds; and 95%–97% in 3 seconds)

Radioisotope Studies.   The injection or inhalation of a radioisotope (eg, Technetium) may be used to evaluate pulmonary blood flow and diagnose and locate pulmonary emboli. Technetium is injected in a peripheral vein, and the area is scanned with a device such as a scintillation detector. Inhalation of the radioisotopes krypton, technetium, or xenon may be used in a ventilation lung scan, which assesses the movement or lack of movement of air in the lungs.

NURSING PROCESS —THE PATIENT UNDERGOING DIAGNOSTIC EVALUATION OF THE LOWER RESPIRATORY AIRWAY

Assessment
The patient with a respiratory disorder may find it difficult to talk; prolonged questioning may have to be delayed, or a family member may have to be asked about the patient's problems. A complete medical, drug, and allergy history and a history of symptoms are obtained. Vital signs are taken and the patient is weighed.

Nursing Diagnosis
The nursing diagnoses selected for an individual patient depends on the tentative or actual medical diagnosis, the diagnostic procedure performed, and the patient's response to the procedure.

- Anxiety related to the scheduled procedure
- Ineffective airway clearance related to inability to raise secretions, pain, fatigue, other factors (specify)
- Knowledge deficit of diagnostic study

Planning and Implementation
The major goal of the patient may be to understand and perform the tasks necessary for accurate completion of a laboratory study or diagnostic test.

The major goal of nursing management is to prepare the patient properly for diagnostic testing.

A single or 24-hour sample of sputum for laboratory examination may be ordered. Because negative smears do not always indicate the absence of disease, repeated examinations may be ordered on successive days. When collecting sputum, the patient is taught how to handle the container. The inside of the receptacle must be kept sterile. The cup or bottle is covered to keep airborne microorganisms and odor inside and to prevent the contents from being easily viewed. The specimen is refrigerated when a delay in sending it to the laboratory occurs. Sputum specimens should be raised from deep in the bronchi; the sputum first expectorated in the morning, for example, is usually adequate. The patient is instructed to perform good oral care immediately before raising sputum so that no saliva or old food particles are expectorated into the container. Color, consistency, odor, and quantity of sputum are noted and charted. The appearance of blood is reported to the physician.

If an invasive procedure, such as a thoracentesis, is

planned, the nurse must reassure the patient that a local anesthetic will be given. All equipment and supplies for the procedure are brought to the patient's room and left covered until the physician is ready to perform the procedure. The nurse stays with the patient and assists the physician as needed. After the procedure, a pressure dressing may be applied. The dressing is inspected every 2 hours for drainage, and the patient is assessed for difficulty in breathing, tightness in the chest, prolonged episodes of coughing, lightheadedness, tachycardia, and severe chest pain. Vital signs are monitored at frequent intervals. The color and amount of sputum raised (if any) is recorded.

Ineffective Airway Clearance. Before a bronchoscopy or bronchography, the patient should have mouth care, and dentures are removed. The patient is usually given nothing to eat or drink 8 to 12 hours before the procedure to avoid vomiting and aspiration during the procedure. After the procedure, the patient may have an increase in secretions because of irritation caused by the insertion of the bronchoscope. Because the gag reflex was temporarily abolished with a local anesthetic, the patient is given nothing by mouth for several hours after the procedure and observed for signs of respiratory difficulty. Supplied with tissues and a sputum cup or emesis basin, the patient is encouraged to expectorate as often as necessary. After the procedure, the throat

may feel irritated for several days, and the patient is advised to talk as little as possible. Bloody mucus usually is expectorated after the test.

Complications of bronchoscopy include laryngeal edema, which may be so severe that the patient requires a tracheostomy, and bleeding, if a biopsy has been performed. Red streaks of blood may be expected after biopsy, but frank bleeding requires the immediate attention of the physician.

Anxiety and Knowledge Deficit. Although a test may have been explained by the physician or nurse, it may be necessary to repeat, clarify, or simplify the explanation. Often, an explanation of the procedure and information about when it will be done and the tasks the patient is to perform during the procedure (eg, take deep breaths, lie still on the table) help reduce the anxiety associated with diagnostic tests.

Patients scheduled for radioisotope studies are made aware of the fact that no danger of radiation exposure after the procedure exists.

Evaluation

- The patient and family understand the purpose and procedure of the diagnostic test, when it will be performed, and what participation will be required of the patient
- Anxiety is reduced
- Airway is effectively cleared of secretions

General Nutritional Considerations

☐ The patient undergoing bronchoscopy usually is given nothing by mouth for 8 to 12 hours before the test to avoid the danger of vomiting and aspiration. The patient should be informed that fasting from food and fluids is necessary.

☐ Drinking extra fluids may help thin bronchial secretions.

General Pharmacologic Considerations

☐ Patients who have diagnostic tests that involve the use of a contrast media that contains iodine are questioned about allergies, especially allergies to seafood (which contains iodine) and iodine. If the patient appears to have an iodine allergy, the physician must be notified *before* the test. An allergic reaction to iodine can be serious and sometimes fatal.

General Gerontologic Considerations

☐ Older patients may have difficulty understanding explanations or directions given by the physician or nurse. It may be necessary to repeat or restate information or directions given before or during diagnostic testing.

☐ Older patients may be especially fearful of diagnostic tests because of mental confusion or lack of understanding.

Suggested Readings

- [ ] Alfaro R. Applying nursing diagnosis and nursing process: a step-by-step guide. 2nd ed. Philadelphia: JB Lippincott, 1990. *(Additional coverage of subject matter)*
- [ ] Bates BA, Hoekelman RA. Guide to physical examination and history taking. 4th ed. Philadelphia: JB Lippincott, 1987. *(In-depth coverage of subject matter)*
- [ ] Fuller J, Schaller-Ayers J. Health assessment: a nursing approach. Philadelphia: JB Lippincott, 1990. *(Additional coverage of subject matter)*
- [ ] Kozier B, Erb G. Techniques in clinical nursing: a nursing process approach. 2nd ed. Menlo Park, CA: Addison-Wesley, 1987. *(Additional coverage of subject matter)*
- [ ] Memmler RL, Wood DL. Structure and function of the human body. 4th ed. Philadelphia: JB Lippincott, 1987. *(Additional coverage of subject matter)*
- [ ] Memmler RL, Wood DL. The human body in health and disease. 6th ed. Philadelphia: JB Lippincott, 1987. *(Additional coverage of subject matter)*
- [ ] Rifas E. How to listen in on breath sounds. RN March 1984;47:30. *(Additional and in-depth coverage of subject matter)*
- [ ] Shapiro B. Clinical applications of respiratory care. 3rd ed. Chicago: Year Book Medical Publishers, 1985. *(Additional and in-depth coverage of subject matter)*
- [ ] Stevens SA, Becker KL. How to perform picture-perfect respiratory assessment. Nursing '88 January 1988;18:57. *(Additional and in-depth coverage of subject matter)*
- [ ] Taylor DL. Assessing breath sounds. Nursing '85 March 1985;15:60. *(Additional and in-depth coverage of subject matter)*
- [ ] Wilkins RL, Hodgkin JE, Lopez B. Lung sounds: a practical guide. St Louis: CV Mosby, 1988. *(In-depth, high-level coverage of subject matter)*
- [ ] Wilkins RL, Sheldon RL, Krider SJ. Clinical assessment in respiratory care. 2nd ed. St Louis: CV Mosby, 1989. *(In-depth, high-level coverage of subject matter)*

Chapter 21

Disorders of the Upper Respiratory Airway

On completion of this chapter the reader will:

■ List the symptoms, diagnosis, and treatment of infectious and allergic disorders of the upper respiratory airway

■ Use the nursing process in the management of a patient with an infectious or allergic disorder of the upper respiratory airway

■ List the symptoms, diagnosis, and treatment of trauma to or obstruction of the upper respiratory airway

■ Use the nursing process in the management of the patient with trauma to or obstruction of the upper respiratory airway

■ List clinical situations that may require a tracheostomy

■ List clinical situations that may require endotracheal intubation

■ Use the nursing process in the management of a patient with a tracheostomy

■ Use the nursing process in the management of a patient with endotracheal intubation

■ Describe the early symptoms of cancer of the larynx

■ Discuss the emotional impact of radical surgery that may be used for treatment of cancer of the larynx

■ Use the nursing process in the management of a patient with a laryngectomy

INFECTIOUS AND ALLERGIC DISORDERS OF THE UPPER RESPIRATORY AIRWAY

Sinusitis

Sinusitis is an inflammation of the sinuses. The maxillary sinus is affected most often. Sinusitis is caused principally by the spread of an infection from the nasal passages to the sinuses and by the blockage of normal sinus drainage (Fig. 21-1). Lowered resistance to infection is an important predisposing factor. Emotional strain, fatigue, and poor nutrition increase one's susceptibility to sinusitis. Sinusitis that accompanies or follows the common cold illustrates the role played by infection and obstruction. Because the mucous membrane lining of the nasal passages and the sinuses is continuous, infection spreads readily from the nose to the sinuses.

Interference with the drainage of the sinuses predisposes to sinusitis because trapped secretions readily become infected. Allergy frequently causes edema of the conchae, which may also lead to sinusitis. Nasal polyps and deviated septum are other common causes of faulty sinus drainage.

Sinusitis can lead to serious complications, such as spread of the infection to the middle ear or the brain. Bronchiectasis may also follow chronic, longstanding sinusitis.

Symptoms

Symptoms of sinusitis may depend on which sinus is infected and include one or more of the following: headache, fever, pain over the area of the affected sinus, nasal congestion and discharge, pain around the eyes, and malaise.

Diagnosis

Diagnosis is based on the patient's history of symptoms. Culture and sensitivity tests, radiograph of the skull, and transillumination of the sinuses may also be used.

Treatment

Acute sinusitis frequently responds to conservative treatment designed to help the patient overcome the infection. Bed rest, ample fluid intake, humidification, local heat application, and analgesics often are effective. Antibiotic therapy may be necessary if the infection is severe. Vasoconstrictors, such as phenylephrine nose drops, may be used to relieve nasal congestion and aid in drainage of the sinuses. Many nasal preparations can be purchased without a prescription, but people may have a tendency to overmedicate. When nose drops are used too frequently or over a long period, they provide shorter and shorter periods of relief, rebound nasal congestion often occurs, and the nasal congestion becomes worse.

227

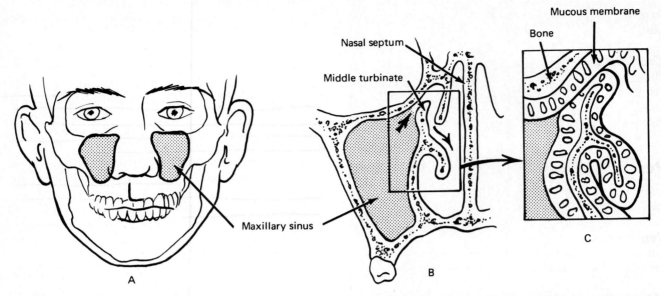

Figure 21–1. Edema can cause obstruction of sinus drainage. (*A*) Location of maxillary sinuses. (*B*) The maxillary sinuses normally drain through the openings that lie under the middle turbinates. The opening for the drainage is near the upper portion of the sinus. (*C*) Edema, such as that which commonly accompanies upper respiratory infections, can obstruct the opening and prevent normal sinus drainage.

Many cold tablets contain antihistamines that thicken nasal secretions. Although this action may temporarily decrease the discomfort of profuse nasal secretions, thickened secretions can block the drainage openings of the sinus cavity and lead to failure of the sinuses to drain adequately. Trapped secretions may become a focus for continuing infection.

To remove the accumulated exudate and promote drainage, the physician may irrigate the maxillary sinus with a catheter inserted through the normal opening under the middle concha. Surgery may be indicated in treatment of chronic sinusitis. An operation, called an *antrotomy* or antrum window operation, makes an opening in the inferior meatus to provide sinus drainage. A more radical procedure, the *Caldwell-Luc operation* occasionally is performed through the mouth, above the upper teeth. The diseased mucous membrane lining of the sinus is removed, and a new opening is made into the inferior meatus of the nose so that adequate drainage can occur.

Nasal Polyps

Nasal polyps are grapelike swellings that are believed to result from chronic irritation, such as that caused by infection or allergy. When polyps grow in the nose, they obstruct nasal breathing and sinus drainage.

Symptoms

Difficulty breathing through one or both sides of the nose is the most common symptom.

Diagnosis

Diagnosis is made by visual examination of the nose.

Treatment

When nasal obstruction becomes severe, the polyps may be removed under local anesthesia. Unfortunately, polyps tend to recur, and the patient often must undergo surgery more than once for the same condition. The excised tissue is examined microscopically to determine whether it is benign or malignant. Most nasal polyps are benign.

Tonsillitis and Adenoiditis

The tonsils and adenoids are lymphatic tissues and, therefore, common sites of infection. Although these disorders are more common in children, they also may be seen in adults.

Symptoms

Symptoms of tonsillitis include sore throat, difficulty or pain on swallowing, fever, and malaise. Enlargement of the adenoids may produce nasal obstruction, noisy breathing, snoring, and a nasal quality to the voice. Chronic infection of the adenoids may result in an acute or chronic infection in the middle ear (otitis media).

Diagnosis

Diagnosis is confirmed by a history of the patient's symptoms as well as visual examination of the tonsils and adenoids. A culture and sensitivity test of the area may be made to determine the causative microorganism.

Treatment

After the results of a culture and sensitivity test, appropriate antibiotic therapy may be ordered. Chronic tonsillitis and adenoiditis may require removal of these structures (*tonsillectomy* and *adenoidectomy*).

Peritonsillar Abscess

A severe tonsillar infection may result in a *peritonsillar abscess*.

Symptoms

Symptoms include difficulty in and pain when swallowing, fever, malaise, and difficulty talking.

Diagnosis

A history and visual examination of the tonsillar area often establish the diagnosis.

Treatment

Culture and sensitivity tests may be ordered, but the physician often prescribes administration of penicillin or another antibiotic to be started immediately after a culture is obtained. Surgical drainage of the abscess may be required if the abscess partially blocks the oropharynx. A local anesthetic is sprayed or painted on the surface of the abscess, and the contents are evacuated. Repeated episodes may require a tonsillectomy.

Acute Pharyngitis

An inflammatory disorder, acute pharyngitis is caused by a virus or bacteria.

Symptoms

Symptoms include fever, malaise, inflammation of the pharyngeal area, enlargement of the cervical lymph nodes, and enlargement of the tonsils (if present).

Diagnosis

A throat culture with sensitivity studies is recommended, especially if a bacterial infection is suspected. If the causative microorganism is a group A streptococcus, all family members should have throat cultures, and those testing positive should be treated with a course of penicillin therapy.

Treatment

When caused by more virulent bacteria, such as *Staphylococcus aureus* or the group A streptococcal organisms (strep throat), prompt treatment is necessary. Untreated acute pharyngitis caused by these microorganisms may result in otitis media, mastoiditis, rheumatic fever, and nephritis. Penicillin is the drug of choice if the infection is caused by group A streptococci. Erythromycin, one of the cephalosporins, tetracycline, or another antibiotic found effective by means of sensitivity tests is used if the patient is allergic to penicillin.

Bed rest, an increased fluid intake, an analgesic and antipyretic for discomfort and fever, and a soft diet are additional treatment measures. The patient should be seen by a physician after completing a course of therapy, and a repeat throat culture should be performed. If the culture is positive, additional antibiotic therapy is usually necessary.

Chronic Pharyngitis

Causes of chronic pharyngitis include prolonged exposure to environmental dust particles, using the voice excessively, and smoking.

Symptoms

Symptoms include difficulty swallowing, irritation of the throat, and mucus production.

Diagnosis

Diagnosis is made by the patient's history as well as visual examination of the pharynx.

Treatment

Treatment includes avoiding the cause of the condition, for example, resting the voice or giving up smoking. Those exposed to environmental dust are encouraged to wear masks during time of exposure.

The Common Cold

The *common cold* is a general term used to describe a respiratory infection that involves the nasal passages and throat. Viral in origin, it is the most common disorder that affects humans.

Symptoms

Sneezing and nasal congestion and discharge accompany the common cold. Other symptoms, which may vary from person to person, include chills, fever, headache, sore throat, cough, and aching muscles. Symptoms usually last for 5 or more days.

Diagnosis

Diagnosis is normally based on a patient's symptoms as well as examination of the throat and nasal passages.

Treatment

No drug cures the common cold. The usual recommended treatment is bed rest, increased fluid intake, and aspirin (adults only) or acetaminophen for fever and muscle aching. Nonprescription nasal deconges-tants and antihistamines may be used to relieve some of the symptoms, but these agents do not shorten the length of time the infection persists. Various nonpre-scription preparations may be used for a sore throat, but salt water gargles can be just as effective. For coughing, many nonprescription antitussive prepara-tions are available; however, some physicians feel that their use should be limited because coughing clears the respiratory tract of secretions.

The common cold can be serious in people, such as elderly or debilitated patients, with chronic respira-tory disorders and those on antineoplastic or pro-longed corticosteroid therapy. In these patients, more intensive therapy may be necessary.

Laryngitis

Laryngitis is an inflammation and swelling of the mucous membrane lining of the larynx. Laryngitis often accompanies upper respiratory infections and is due to the spread of the infection to the larynx. Laryn-gitis also can be caused by excessive or improper use of the voice or by smoking.

Symptoms

Hoarseness or, sometimes, the inability to speak above a whisper are the usual symptoms. A cough and a feel-ing of throat irritation may also be seen.

Diagnosis

The diagnosis may be made by the patient on the basis of the symptoms alone. If the condition persists, the person should seek the advice of a physician. Most physicians believe hoarseness lasting more than 2 weeks warrants an examination of the larynx (laryn-goscopy). Prompt investigation of the cause of persis-tent hoarseness is essential because this symptom may be due to cancer of the larynx.

Treatment

Treatment of laryngitis involves voice rest and the treatment or the removal of the cause. Antibiotics may be prescribed if laryngitis is caused by a bacterial in-fection. Cool steam inhalation therapy by means of a cold vaporizer may also be used.

NURSING PROCESS —THE PATIENT WHO HAS AN INFECTIOUS OR ALLERGIC DISORDER OF THE UPPER RESPIRATORY AIRWAY

Assessment

Assessment involves a thorough patient history, in-cluding the length of time the symptoms have per-sisted and drug therapy to relieve symptoms (if any). The upper respiratory airway passages are examined using a flashlight and nasal speculum or tongue blade. The appearance of the mucous membranes, the presence of swelling or enlargement, and the presence of drainage is noted.

Nursing Diagnosis

One or more of the following may apply to the pa-tient with an infectious or allergic disorder of the upper airway and depend on the symptoms, the pa-tient history, and the physical assessment:

- Hyperthermia related to infection
- Chronic pain related to sinusitis, tonsillitis
- Ineffective airway clearance related to excessive se-cretions, swelling of the oropharynx
- Fluid volume deficit related to hyperthermia or inabil-ity to swallow liquids
- Potential for infection transmission related to pharyn-gitis due to *Streptococcus aureus* or group A strepto-cocci
- Altered health maintenance related to smoking

Planning and Implementation

The major goals of the patient include the relief of symptoms, control of the inflammation or infection, and the prevention of complications.

The major goals of nursing management are to relieve symptoms, to control and eradicate the in-fection or inflammation, to prevent further compli-cations, and to inform the patient of ways to prevent a recurrence of the disorder.

Hyperthermia and Chronic Pain.   Fever may be re-duced by use of an antipyretic drug, such as aspirin or acetaminophen. General discomfort and pain may also respond to these drugs. Local anesthetics sprayed into or held in the mouth may temporarily relieve pain. Antibiotic therapy may also be pre-scribed.

Ineffective Airway Clearance.   Humidification of surrounding air may loosen secretions and make the patient feel more comfortable. Greater fluid intake and mouth washes may also help loosen secretions. Nasal congestion may be relieved by nose drops, such as those containing phenylephrine. When the condition is due to an allergic reaction, antihista-mines may be of value.

Fluid Volume Deficit.   If the patient has difficulty in swallowing because of pain, ice chips or ice water may be offered and the patient encouraged to take small amounts of fluids at frequent intervals.

Potential for Infection Transmission.   The impor-tance of completing a full course of antibiotic therapy to control the infection, prevent complications, and prevent the spread of infection to others is explained to the patient. Contact with others should be avoided until the infection is eliminated.

Altered Health Maintenance. When a condition is due to an upper respiratory infection or to brief overuse of the voice, *voice rest*, that is, writing to communicate rather than speaking, is often the only specific treatment required. The patient must be explained this term and taught that whispering is as harmful as talking. Voice rest facilitates the healing of inflamed mucous membranes.

If smoking is the cause of the disorder, patients are encouraged to stop smoking. If quitting proves to be difficult, the physician should be consulted. Those exposed to environmental hazards, such as dust and other pollutants, are advised to wear a mask to remove suspended air particles during times of exposure.

Evaluation

- Body temperature is normal
- Pain or discomfort is relieved
- Airway is effectively cleared of secretions
- Fluid volume deficit is corrected
- Infection is controlled and not transmitted to others
- Understands the importance of correct health habits to control or eliminate the disorder

TRAUMA TO OR OBSTRUCTION OF THE UPPER RESPIRATORY AIRWAY

Epistaxis (Nosebleed)

Most nosebleeds occur in Kiesselbach's area, a plexus of capillaries located on the anterior part of the nasal septum. Epistaxis may result from local trauma, such as any kind of blow. It may also result from disease, such as rheumatic fever, hypertension, and blood dyscrasias, and from cocaine abuse. Epistaxis that results from hypertension or blood dyscrasias is likely to be especially severe and difficult to control.

Symptoms

Bleeding may be slight or heavy. Blood may trickle or gush out of the nose as well as drip down the back of the throat.

Diagnosis

Diagnosis is made by visual inspection of the nares. The physician may use a tongue blade to examine the back of the throat and a laryngeal mirror to examine the area above and behind the uvula.

Treatment

The physician may apply aqueous epinephrine 1:1000 (on a cotton pledget or as a spray) topically to the bleeding area. Epinephrine causes vasoconstriction and, therefore, should stop the bleeding. Pressure may then be applied to the nares. The physician may also cauterize the bleeding and may need to insert an anterior or posterior nasal packing.

An anesthetic and decongestant to constrict superficial blood vessels is first sprayed into the nose or applied topically with a swab or pledget. An anterior pack is inserted into the anterior nares and left in place. A posterior nasal pack requires insertion with a catheter or forceps. This type of pack has a piece of suture attached to the end that is inserted first. The pack is anchored by drawing the suture through the mouth and taping it to the cheek.

Additional treatment includes eliminating the cause (when possible).

Deviated Septum

The nasal cavity is divided into two passages by a septum consisting of bone and cartilage. Few people have an absolutely straight nasal septum, and some have a markedly crooked one. The crookedness may be congenital; often it is caused by trauma. When the septum is crooked (deviated), one nostril may be much larger than the other. Marked deviation can result in complete obstruction of one nostril and interference with sinus drainage.

Diagnosis

Diagnosis is made by visual inspection of the nose.

Treatment

Surgical correction may be necessary to restore normal breathing and to permit adequate sinus drainage. A septal deviation due to injury may require surgery to correct the deformity and to avoid chronic sinusitis.

The operation performed to correct a deviated septum is called a *submucous resection* (SMR). After a local anesthetic has been administered, the surgeon makes an incision through the mucous membrane and removes the portions of the septum that cause obstruction.

Obstruction of the Larynx

Obstruction of the larynx is an extremely serious and often life-threatening condition. Causes of laryngeal obstruction include edema of the larynx due to an allergic reaction, severe inflammation and edema of the throat, and the aspiration of foreign bodies, such as food. Total obstruction prevents the passage of air from the upper to the lower respiratory airway; partial obstruction results in difficulty breathing. Unless total obstruction is relieved *immediately*, the patient dies of respiratory arrest.

Symptoms
Symptoms include difficulty breathing (partial obstruction), respiratory arrest (total obstruction), and, as the condition progresses, cyanosis.

Diagnosis
Diagnosis must be immediate and is made by viewing the patient's respiratory distress.

Treatment
If a foreign body was aspirated, the Heimlich maneuver is used (see Chapter 17) to try and force the object out of the respiratory passages. Allergic reactions or severe inflammation and edema may be treated with administration of epinephrine or a corticosteroid or with a tracheostomy.

NURSING PROCESS —THE PATIENT WHO HAS TRAUMA TO OR OBSTRUCTION OF THE UPPER AIRWAY

Assessment
Trauma to the upper airway due to violent force, such as a blow to the face, requires visual inspection of the involved areas. The surrounding structures, such as the jaw, neck, forehead, cheeks, and eyes are also inspected, as blunt force can cause multiple injuries. The presence of bleeding, edema, bruising, and lacerations is carefully recorded.

Bleeding in the absence of injury requires inspection of the involved areas and a patient history, which may indicate the cause of bleeding. The blood pressure and pulse are taken, and the ability of the patient to breathe through the nose and mouth is noted.

Laryngeal obstruction is an emergency. Initially, assessment only requires immediate evaluation of the patient's ability to breathe and the possible determination of the cause, such as aspiration of food.

Nursing Diagnosis
Trauma with or without bleeding may elicit the following diagnoses:

- Pain related to injury, surgery
- Anxiety related to pain, injury or bleeding, anticipation of medical or surgical treatment

- Ineffective breathing pattern related to bleeding or edema secondary to obstruction of the upper airway

Planning and Implementation
The major goals of the patient with trauma of the upper respiratory airway include relief of pain or discomfort, relief of anxiety, and improved breathing. The major goal of the patient with an obstruction of the larynx is restoration of normal respiratory function.

The major goals of nursing management include relief of pain, improvement of respiratory function, and control of symptoms associated with trauma.

Pain. Trauma to the nose and surgery for a deviated septum can result in mild to severe pain. The physician may order an analgesic for pain, preferably acetaminophen or another mild analgesic. Aspirin is avoided because this drug can affect the ability of the blood to clot and, thus, may increase bleeding.

Anxiety. Bleeding of or injury to the upper airway can cause moderate to extreme anxiety. Blood oozing from the nose may frighten the patient, and lightheadedness or fainting may occur. Anxiety over the treatment of a nosebleed (eg, the insertion of nasal packing or swabs, inspection of the area) and fear that the bleeding can't be controlled may be seen. Patients are protected from falling or injury if they appear lightheaded. Instruments and materials are kept out of the patient's sight. The patient is assured that the problem can be corrected, and that the nasal pack is slightly uncomfortable but will be removed in 1 or 2 days. The patient is encouraged to breathe through the mouth and spit out any blood.

Bleeding. A nosebleed is a common occurrence and is usually not serious, but it is often frightening for both those who experience it and those who witness it. First aid for a mild nosebleed requires the application of pressure by holding the soft parts of the nose firmly between thumb and forefinger for several minutes. This action often effectively controls bleeding. Patients are shown how to apply pressure; often they can control the bleeding if it occurs when they are alone. They are instructed to breathe through the mouth, while applying firm pressure to the nares. Patients should sit with their heads tilted slightly forward to prevent the blood from running down the throat. Elevation of the head lessens the flow of blood. Because fainting may occur, the patient must be protected from falling. If bleeding is severe, a basin must be provided to catch the blood. The patient should be instructed not to swallow blood that may run into the mouth and throat, but to spit it out. If the bleeding is slight, tissues or a handkerchief may be sufficient to prevent soiling of the clothing.

If bleeding cannot be controlled by simple measures, anterior and posterior nasal packing may be inserted by the physician. The nasal packing usually is kept in place for about 48 hours. The patient's vital signs are monitored, and the anterior nose packing is inspected for continued evidence of heavy bleeding. The patient is encouraged to spit out any blood that may still ooze from the area. Any difficulty in breathing or displacement of the nasal pack is reported to the physician immediately.

Submucous Resection.   When surgery is completed, both sides of the nasal cavity are packed with gauze, which usually is left in place for 24 to 48 hours. A moustache dressing (a folded piece of gauze applied under the nostrils and held in place with tape) is applied to absorb bloody drainage. The patient is assessed at frequent intervals for signs of airway obstruction.

Obstruction of the Larynx.   Aspiration of food or another foreign object that completely obstructs the larynx requires immediate treatment. If the object has lodged in the pharynx and can be seen, removal with a finger is attempted. When the object is in the larynx or trachea, the Heimlich maneuver is used and repeated until the patient coughs up the material and is able to breathe. If this maneuver fails to dislodge the object after three or four tries, the physician may perform an emergency tracheostomy.

When obstruction is due to an allergic reaction that results in edema, and drug therapy is instituted, the patient is closely monitored for relief of airway obstruction. If drug therapy does not reduce edema and improve breathing, or if the obstruction worsens, an emergency tracheotomy may be necessary.

Evaluation

■ Pain related to injury or surgery is reduced or eliminated
■ Anxiety is reduced or eliminated
■ Breathing pattern is normal
■ Foreign object is removed from the larynx or trachea, breathing pattern is normal, airway is clear

MALIGNANT DISORDERS OF THE UPPER RESPIRATORY AIRWAY
Cancer of the Larynx

Cancer of the larynx is most common among people older than 45. Men are affected more frequently than women. Although the cause is unknown, it is believed that chronic laryngitis, irritants such as alcohol, cigarette smoke, and industrial pollutants, habitual overuse of the voice, and heredity may predispose to the condition.

Symptoms

Persistent hoarseness usually is the earliest symptom. Often this condition is slight at first and is ignored. A sensation of swelling or a lump in the throat may be noticed, followed by dysphagia and pain when talking. If the malignant tissue is not removed promptly, the patient develops symptoms of advancing carcinoma, such as weakness, weight loss, and anemia. The importance of consulting a physician about persistent hoarseness or difficulty in swallowing cannot be overemphasized.

Diagnosis

The diagnosis is established by patient history. The physician also visually examines the larynx, called *laryngoscopy*, and may obtain a biopsy specimen for microscopic examination of the lesion and confirmation of the diagnosis. A complete physical examination also is performed.

Treatment

Surgical removal of the tumor, and often the entire larynx, is necessary. Radiation therapy and chemotherapy also may be employed. If the tumor is discovered promptly and has not metastasized, it sometimes can be removed without removing the entire larynx; this less radical procedure is called a *laryngofissure*. Because a laryngofissure does not involve removal of the entire larynx, a patient does not lose his or her voice, but the voice becomes husky.

In more advanced cases, total laryngectomy is necessary. If the disease has extended beyond the larynx, a radical neck dissection (removal of the lymph nodes, muscles, and adjacent tissues) is performed. A patient with a total laryngectomy has a permanent tracheal stoma (opening) because after surgery the trachea is no longer connected to the nasopharynx. The larynx is severed from the trachea and removed completely. The only respiratory organs in use thereafter are the trachea, the bronchi, and lungs. Air enters and leaves through the tracheostomy; the patient no longer feels air entering the nose (Fig. 21-2). Because the anterior wall of the esophagus connects with the posterior wall of the larynx, it must be reconstructed. Tube feeding facilitates healing by preventing muscle activity and irritation of the esophagus.

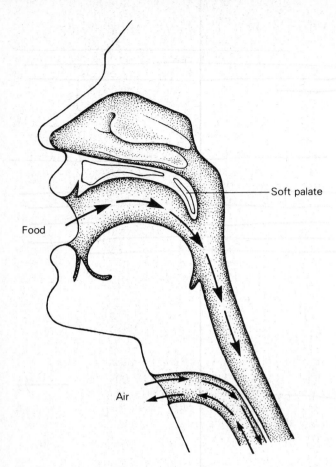

Figure 21–2. Air enters and leaves through a permanent tracheal stoma.

NURSING PROCESS —THE PATIENT UNDERGOING A LARYNGECTOMY

Preoperative Period

Assessment
A complete medical, drug, and allergy history is obtained. A smoking and alcohol intake history is included in the history. Vital signs are taken and the patient is weighed.

The patient's response to the diagnosis and understanding of what the surgery entails are carefully assessed; emotional support before and after surgery depends on the patient's ability to cope with the changes in body image.

Nursing Diagnosis
Depending on the patient, one or more of the following nursing diagnoses may apply:

■ Anxiety related to diagnosis, surgery, loss of voice after surgery

■ Ineffective individual coping related to diagnosis, loss of body part (larynx)
■ Knowledge deficit related to surgery

Planning and Implementation
The major goals of the patient include a reduction in anxiety and understanding of the diagnosis, the reason for surgery, and the results of surgery.

The major goal of nursing management is to prepare the patient physically and emotionally for surgery.

Anxiety and Ineffective Individual Coping. Patients faced with a diagnosis of cancer and voice loss usually experience a great deal of anxiety as well as difficulty in coping with the diagnosis and surgery. During the preoperative period, the nurse should allow these patients time to verbalize their fears and concerns, and questions should be answered by the physician or nurse.

Knowledge Deficit. The physician explains the need for and the expected extent of the surgery. The amount that patients are told during the preoperative period depends on the surgeon. If a total laryngectomy is scheduled, the patient must be informed that the loss of a natural speaking voice is *permanent.* Although most physicians give a careful, detailed explanation before surgery, patients may claim to the nurse that they did not know the voice loss would be permanent. Many times the patient was depressed or refused to accept the diagnosis of cancer and the need for radical surgery when the physician explained the surgery. It may be necessary to repeat information given by the physician. Knowing what to expect after surgery reduces a patient's anxiety associated with surgery and fosters better patient cooperation after the operation.

A detailed explanation of the ways to communicate with others is explained. Patients should know that they can write messages immediately after surgery and that the call light will be answered promptly. Patients are told by the physician that they will have a permanent tracheostomy, or opening in the neck, and that they will be taught how to care for this opening before they are discharged from the hospital. The patient should understand that food will be given through a nasogastric tube during the postoperative period.

Additional preoperative teaching includes a demonstration of deep breathing and leg exercises.

Evaluation

■ Anxiety is reduced
■ Demonstrates ability to cope with diagnosis and surgery
■ Demonstrates understanding of the results of surgery

Postoperative Period

Assessment

On return from the recovery room, the chart is reviewed for the type and extent of surgery, the patient's present condition, and the types of drains used or dressings applied. Vital signs are taken and the patient's general condition evaluated to establish baseline data.

Nursing Diagnosis

Depending on the type and extent of surgery and the individual patient, one or more of the following may apply:

- Anxiety related to change in body image, difficulty in communicating needs, suctioning procedures, other factors (specify)
- Pain related to surgery
- Impaired verbal communication related to removal of the larynx
- Ineffective individual coping related to diagnosis, loss of voice after surgery, other factors (specify)
- Ineffective airway clearance due to inability to cough, raise secretions
- Social isolation related to change in body image, laryngectomy stoma, change in (laryngofissure) or loss of (laryngectomy) speech
- Potential for infection related to surgical procedure, poor physical condition
- Knowledge deficit of self-care of laryngectomy, nasogastric feedings, other treatment modalities

Planning and Implementation

The major goals of the patient include reduction of anxiety, reduction of pain, effective use of alternative methods of communication, acceptance of diagnosis and surgery, improved relationship with others, absence of infection, and understanding of laryngectomy care and other treatment modalities.

The major goals of nursing management include relief of pain and discomfort, maintenance of a patient airway, reduction in anxiety, absence of infection, and development and implementation of an effective teaching program.

Anxiety. It is not unusual to see anxiety and depression after surgery, when patients have had time to think about the changes in their bodies and their limited ability to communicate with others. Allowing these patients time to express (in writing) their concerns may help alleviate anxiety associated with communication difficulties.

Anxiety also may occur when suction is needed or when a dressing is changed by the surgeon. The nurse must assure the patient that the discomfort associated with suction is momentary.

Pain. Pain is relieved with analgesics; however, narcotic analgesics tend to depress respirations and the cough reflex. When needed, these drugs are usually given in low doses. Although all postsurgery patients experience varying degrees of pain, those with radical neck dissections usually have less pain because some sensory nerves are severed during surgery. These patients may respond to analgesics such as propoxyphene or pentazocine, especially after the first few postoperative days. Until the surgical dressings are removed, extreme movements of the head are avoided, and the patient's head is supported when moving or changing position. A small pillow or a folded towel placed under the patient's head and shoulders relieves tension of the suture line; full pillows are avoided.

Impaired Verbal Communication. After a total laryngectomy, patients are unable to speak. Once they appear interested in communicating, a pad and pen can be provided. Patients must be given time to convey their thoughts and questions. Pointing and nodding the head to yes or no questions are other ways to communicate. The nurse must ask questions that require as brief an answer as possible.

During the recovery period, a patient may be taught *esophageal speech,* a method of speaking by regurgitating swallowed air. A visit from a person who has had a laryngectomy and who has mastered esophageal speech often is the best way to convince a patient that such speech is possible. If a patient is unable to learn esophageal speech, an artificial (electronic) device may be used to produce speech. Several different portable models are available.

Ineffective Individual Coping. It can be difficult for the patient and family to accept the diagnosis and the type of surgery that must be performed. The nurse must allow them time to verbalize their feelings.

Instruction and emotional support help these patients learn to cope with the effects of surgery. Many cities have support groups of people who have had laryngectomies who help each other cope with the disability. Many group members visit others who are hospitalized for this surgery and distribute literature that offers practical help and encouragement. Patients can find out about the nearest group by contacting their local chapter of the American Cancer Society.

Respiratory Function. The laryngectomy tube opening is the way in which air passes into the lungs. On return from the operating room, patients are positioned as ordered by the physician until they are fully awake. Once awake, they are placed in a semi-

Fowler's or Fowler's position. A heavy pressure dressing may have been placed over the surgical area, although a minimal amount of dressing also may have been used. Drainage catheters may have been placed under the skin to remove excess fluid accumulation. These catheters are connected to a suction device as soon as the patient returns from surgery. The physician specifies the type and amount of suction to be used. A laryngectomy tube, which is similar to a tracheostomy tube but shorter and with a larger diameter, is in place. If a laryngofissure was performed, the patient usually has a tracheostomy tube.

During the immediate postoperative period, the patient must be assessed at frequent intervals for any signs of respiratory obstruction. The opening of the laryngectomy tube is checked for signs of crusting and the collection of thick, mucoid secretions. Auscultation of the chest usually detects the presence of excess secretions in the lower respiratory tract. Tracheal suctioning is performed every hour and as needed, and the area around the stoma is cleaned every 4 hours and as needed.

Suffocation is one of the biggest fears that patients have. The laryngectomy or tracheostomy tube must be kept patent and free of obstruction *at all times*. Tracheal suctioning is performed whenever mucus obstructs the tube. Suctioning must be attended to promptly lest the patient panic. All potential obstructions to the patient's air supply produce severe anxiety; therefore, the airway must be kept clear of crusts and mucus at all times. In time, these patients can be taught to suction with the aid of a mirror. To help thin secretions and reduce crust formation, the physician may order a mist collar to be placed over the stoma or a humidifier to be placed at the bedside. Once the surgical dressings have been removed, a dressing is placed under the laryngectomy tube to absorb secretions (Fig. 21-3). It is changed as often as necessary.

Usually, the patient is allowed to get up after the fourth or fifth postoperative day. At this time, teaching can begin. The patient is taught to administer nasogastric feedings (if a nasogastric tube is still used for nutritional intake), how to suction the laryngectomy (or tracheostomy) tube and oral cavity, how to change the gauze dressing used to catch secretions, and how to clean the inner cannula.

In 3 to 5 weeks, the edges of the stoma heal and the physician can remove the laryngectomy tube. Some conditions, however, require that the tube be kept in place permanently.

Social Isolation. Patients who have had laryngectomies may avoid social contact, especially with those outside of the immediate family. Once these patients learn that nursing personnel and the family accept this change in body image, they may begin to accept visitors. The process of acceptance by patients can be slow. Once rehabilitative speech therapy (esophageal speech, use of an electronic speech) begins, the patient often reestablishes social contact with close friends and relatives. It may take a long time before the patient feels comfortable during communication with strangers.

Potential for Infection. The surgical incision and edges of the stoma are potential areas of infection.

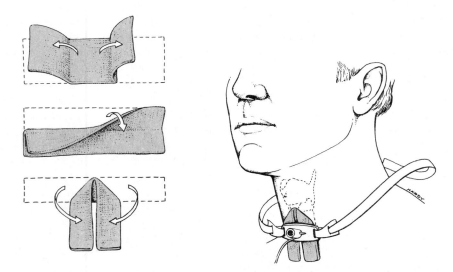

Figure 21-3. Gauze squares, slit halfway down, are placed around the tube to catch secretions. These dressings are changed by the nurse as often as necessary. Tapes hold the outer tube in place. They are tied in a knot at the back or the side of the patient's neck.

Pneumonia and inflammation and infection of the trachea and bronchi also may occur. Antibiotic therapy may be necessary. The patient is turned and encouraged to cough and deep breathe every 2 hours. The vital signs are monitored every 4 hours. Any rise in temperature or appearance of purulent drainage is reported promptly.

Knowledge Deficit. Patients and families often have many questions before and after surgery. The nurse must take the time to listen, answer questions, and, when necessary, refer questions to the appropriate professionals, such as the physician, social service worker, or dietitian.

An effective teaching program is one way to assure that patients will be able to care for their laryngectomy after discharge from the hospital. Teaching should begin as soon as patients appear able to take care of daily living activities. A structured program that teaches both patient and family in small steps and allows time for learning and adjustment to changes in lifestyle may improve the quality of home care. If any difficulty with home care arises, the nurse should evaluate the situation by asking questions and then determine which agencies may be needed for assistance with the problem.

The techniques to suction and clean the inner tracheostomy or laryngectomy tube are carefully taught to the patient and family. Patients should perform these tasks under the supervision of a nurse before discharge from the hospital. Additional treatment modalities, such as drug therapy and diet, are explained.

Patients may be informed of acceptable ways to camouflage the laryngectomy tube. A scarf or gauze dressing placed loosely over the tube helps to keep dust and dirt out of the trachea, as well as to make the opening less obvious. Fabrics or dressings that have fuzz must be avoided because small fibers can be drawn into the tube.

The patient with a laryngectomy tube must prevent water from entering the opening because it would flow down the trachea to the lungs. These patients can never go swimming and must be careful while taking a bath. Showers are usually avoided until the patient has experience with care of the stoma and can deflect water away from the stoma. Hand-held shower devices are less likely to cause a problem.

Nutrition. If the patient has been unable to eat a balanced diet and has lost weight, the physician may delay surgery for a short time in an effort to increase the nutritional intake. Nasogastric tube feedings or parenteral nutrition may be necessary during the preoperative period.

After surgery, the patient may be fed through a nasogastric tube. It remains in place until sufficient healing has occurred. When able to swallow, the patient usually is allowed sips of water. When able to swallow fluids without difficulty, the patient can have the nasogastric tube removed. The patient is permitted soft foods and fluids. Gradually, a regular diet is given if no difficulty with soft foods is found. Some surgeons do not use a nasogastric tube for feeding, and the patient is allowed to take oral fluids 1 or 2 days after surgery. Occasionally, a laryngectomy patient may require nasogastric feedings for a prolonged period of time. A patient fed this way can maintain good water and electrolyte balance and be well nourished. The amount and the type of tube feeding are ordered by the physician. Feedings may be ordered at 1-, 2-, or 4-hour intervals. Intake and output is measured to assure adequate fluid intake.

Caution must be used to avoid aspiration of food. Before feeding, the nasogastric tube is checked to make sure that the end is situated in the stomach (see Chapter 43).

Tube feedings are warmed to body temperature and allowed to flow by gravity. After the feeding is finished, it is followed by about 50 mL of clean water to rinse the tube and prevent food particles from lodging in the tube and turning sour. The patient is given mouth care and observed for irritation of the nostril through which the tube passes.

Oral medications may be given through the nasogastric tube. The liquid form, rather than a crushed tablet, is preferred. If a liquid form is not available, the tablet may be crushed thoroughly, mixed with water, and administered through the nasogastric tube. Water is always administered through the tube after the medication has been given, since small amounts of the medicine may cling to the sides of the tube.

Patients are taught to administer their own tube feedings as soon as they are able. They are instructed never to let the funnel become empty during the feeding (because this would allow air to enter the stomach) and to clamp the tube carefully after feeding. Many patients fold the tube over on itself and secure it with an elastic band. A heavy metal clamp is not desirable because its weight is uncomfortable and tends to pull the tube out.

Evaluation

- Anxiety is reduced
- Demonstrates ability to communicate needs to others
- Coping mechanisms are appropriate; patient and family demonstrate an attempt to cope with the diagnosis and results of surgery
- Nutritional needs are met
- Respiratory function is normal; airway is kept clear of

secretions; breathing pattern is normal; blood gas studies are normal
- Socializes with others in an appropriate manner
- No evidence of systemic or local infection
- Indicates a desire to enter a speech rehabilitation program
- The patient and family acquire adequate knowledge about care of the laryngectomy tube and stoma and are able to demonstrate the techniques of care

TREATMENT MODALITIES FOR AIRWAY OBSTRUCTION OR AIRWAY MAINTENANCE

Tracheostomy

A *tracheotomy* is the surgical procedure that makes an opening into the trachea. A *tracheostomy* is an opening into the trachea into which a tracheostomy or laryngectomy tube is inserted. A tracheostomy may be temporary or permanent. The physician may perform a tracheotomy for two reasons: to relieve upper airway obstruction and to create a permanent opening in the trachea. Upper airway obstruction may occur with the aspiration of food or a foreign object into the trachea, a severe allergic reaction, and infection or edema of the upper respiratory tract. A permanent opening in the trachea is required for certain disorders, such as cancer of the larynx that requires a laryngectomy (see earlier section). A tracheotomy for upper airway obstruction is best performed in the operating room but may be performed at the bedside, or even outside the hospital. In most instances, it is possible and preferable to prepare carefully for the procedure and perform it before respiratory distress becomes critical.

The long- and short-term complications of this procedure include infection, bleeding, airway obstruction due to hardened secretions, aspiration, damage to the recurrent laryngeal nerve, erosion of the trachea, fistula formation between the esophagus and trachea, and penetration of the posterior tracheal wall.

NURSING PROCESS —THE PATIENT UNDERGOING A TRACHEOSTOMY

Assessment

The patient's chart is reviewed for the medical, drug, and allergy history, laboratory or diagnostic tests, and the reason for the tracheostomy. Immediately after the procedure, the patient's vital signs are taken and the lungs auscultated for normal or abnormal breath sounds. A general assessment of the patient includes skin color, level of consciousness, and mental state.

Abnormal breath sounds may indicate conditions such as fluid collecting in the bronchi and lungs or pneumonia. The patient is also observed for signs of complications (see earlier discussion). Chart 21-1 summarizes the immediate postoperative nursing management of these patients.

Nursing Diagnosis

Depending on the presence of other diseases or disorders and whether the tracheostomy is temporary or permanent, one or more of the following diagnoses may apply to the patient with a tracheostomy:

- Ineffective airway clearance related to excessive tracheobronchial secretions
- Anxiety related to the change in breathing pattern, potential airway obstruction secondary to copious secretions, fear of abandonment, other factors (specify)
- Fear related to difficulty breathing, suctioning, abandonment, other factors (specify)
- Pain related to surgical procedure, tracheostomy tube
- Impaired verbal communication related to tracheostomy
- Potential for infection related to tracheostomy tube, presence of secretions
- Impaired swallowing related to presence of tracheostomy tube
- Altered nutrition: less than body requirements related to impaired swallowing
- Knowledge deficit related to suctioning and other procedures, care of (permanent) tracheostomy

Planning and Implementation

The major goals of the patient include an improvement in breathing, absence of infection, reduction of

---

Chart 21-1.   Immediate Postoperative Nursing Management of the Patient With a Tracheostomy

- ☐ Maintain patent airway.
- ☐ Suction as needed with a Y or vented catheter.
- ☐ Clear inner cannula as needed, usually every 2 to 4 hours.
- ☐ Administer heated mist to inspired air.
- ☐ Place bed in semi-Fowler's position.
- ☐ Clean skin around stoma every 4 hours and p.r.n. and replace dressing.
- ☐ Provide a means of communication: pen and pad, Magic Slate.
- ☐ Check vital signs every 4 hours or less, depending on the patient's condition.
- ☐ Measure intake and output.

fear and anxiety, a patent airway, and knowledge of care of the (permanent) tracheostomy.

The major goals of nursing management include maintenance of a patent airway, relief of pain and discomfort, prevention of infection, and effectively teaching the patient the techniques of (permanent) tracheostomy tube management.

Respiratory Function. The respiratory passages react to the creation of the new opening with inflammation and excessive secretion of mucus. Inspired air passes directly into the trachea, bronchi, and lungs without becoming warmed and moistened by passing through the nose. Copious respiratory secretions that occur immediately after the new opening has been made are life-threatening. The patient is frequently assessed for a patent airway, as secretions may rapidly clog the tracheostomy opening, an effect that can result in death by asphyxiation. To facilitate breathing during the immediate postoperative period, the patient is positioned as ordered by the physician until fully awake. When the patient has fully reacted and the blood pressure is stable, the head of the bed is elevated to about 45 degrees unless ordered otherwise. This position decreases edema and makes breathing easier. At first, patients are apprehensive and restless. The constant presence of the nurse, however, usually helps them feel more secure. Frequent suctioning of the tracheostomy and providing patients a means to communicate also are reassuring.

Patients should not be left unattended during the early postoperative period because they are unable to care for the tracheostomy. Leaving them alone may lead to panic, if not suffocation, and may frighten them so much that rehabilitation is difficult.

Humidification is necessary to prevent drying and incrustation of the mucous membrane in the trachea and the main bronchus. Crusts form easily as a result of drying of mucus secretions and can break off, obstruct the lower airway, and cause serious respiratory problems, such as atelectasis.

Tracheostomy tubes come in several sizes and differ from laryngectomy tubes in their length and diameter (Fig. 21-4). Before a tracheostomy tube is inserted into the tracheal opening, the obturator is placed in the tube and then removed as soon as the tube is in place. Most physicians prefer to use the cuffed tracheostomy tube, which has a cuff on the lower end that is inflated with air to provide a snug fit, thus preventing aspiration of liquids or the escape of air when a mechanical ventilator is used. The cuff is normally deflated *except* under the following circumstances:

- When mechanical ventilation is being used
- During and after eating

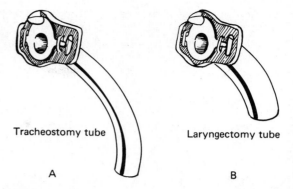

Tracheostomy tube   Laryngectomy tube

A   B

Figure 21–4. Both tracheostomy and laryngectomy tubes come in various sizes.

- When danger of aspiration is present
- During intermittent positive pressure breathing (IPPB) treatments
- During and for 1 hour after tube feeding
- When the patient is unable to swallow oral secretions

The physician specifies the amount of air to be injected into the cuff; the amount of air determines the seating of the cuff in the trachea. Many of the complications associated with a tracheostomy can be prevented when the cuff of the tube is kept at the proper inflation pressure. Normal pressure is 15 to 25 cm of water. If mechanical ventilation is used, the connection between the tracheostomy tube and the ventilator is checked at frequent intervals (Fig. 21-5).

An extra tracheostomy set always is kept at the patient's bedside because immediate change may be necessary if a patient's tube becomes blocked with mucus that cannot be removed. The correct size always must be at the bedside.

The outer tube is held snugly in place by tapes inserted in openings on either side of it and tied at the back or side of the patient's neck. These tapes always should be tied securely in a knot. A bow may be added if desired. If the knot is not tied securely, the patient can cough the tube out, a serious occurrence if the edges of the trachea have not been sutured to the skin, as may be the case in a temporary tracheostomy. If the outer tube accidentally comes out, the nurse immediately inserts a tracheal dilator to hold the edges of the opening apart until the physician arrives to insert another tube. A tracheal dilator is kept at the bedside at all times. The tube should never be forced back in. If force is used, the patient's trachea may be compressed (by pushing the tube alongside the trachea, thus compressing the trachea, rather than inserting the tube into the stoma). Such action could cause respiratory arrest. It is essential that the nurse remain calm if the patient's tube should come out and cannot be easily reinserted; the stoma must be held open with a tracheal dilator until the tube can be reinserted.

A gauze dressing is placed under the tube to absorb

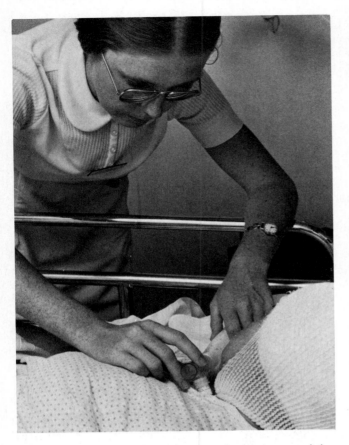

Figure 21–5. The connection between the respirator and the patient's tracheostomy is checked frequently for leaks or partial or total disconnection of the fitting. (Photograph by D. Atkinson)

secretions. Gauze squares usually are used for this purpose. A slit is cut halfway through the square so that the gauze can fit around the tube. This piece of gauze should be changed as often as necessary (see Fig. 21-3). If the material is kept damp, it helps to humidify the inspired air. The bib never should be made of the kind of gauze that has a layer of cotton inside, because bits of cotton are sucked into the tube easily. It is important not to let any material or clothing hide the opening of the tracheostomy tube, because a crusted tube that needs to be cleaned and changed may be overlooked. Many permanent tracheostomy patients who are able to care for their own tubes wear bibs of folded gauze or mesh placed loosely over the opening as a camouflage.

A suction machine is kept at the bedside at all times. Sterile equipment (eg, gloves, suction catheter, normal saline) is used for tracheal suctioning. Mucus is gently suctioned from the tracheostomy tube by a 10 to 14 F sterile disposable catheter, inserted gently into the lumen of the tube. Suction is *not* applied while the catheter is on the way down the trachea because it causes irritation to the lining of the trachea. Suction is commenced once the catheter has been passed. Suc-

tioning is continued while the catheter is withdrawn slowly. As the catheter is withdrawn, it is rotated so that the openings in the catheter can remove mucus more effectively. This procedure may be necessary at frequent intervals during the immediate postoperative period.

If the airway becomes completely obstructed, the patient becomes markedly cyanotic, restless, and frightened; he or she dies within a few minutes if the obstruction is not relieved. Relief of obstruction is of the greatest urgency, with the primary focus on establishing adequate ventilation by removal of the obstruction. The physician is notified immediately by one member of the nursing team while another remains with the patient and attempts to relieve the obstruction. The removal of the tracheostomy tube followed by suctioning may be lifesaving. The nurse should consult with the physician ahead of time about the emergency measures acceptable for each individual patient. The nurse then knows which patients may have their tubes removed as an emergency measure.

Normally, the tracheostomy tube is changed by the physician every 3 to 5 days. Once a firm stoma has developed, this responsibility may be the nurse's.

Anxiety and Fear. Constant assessment of the patient's respiratory status, especially during the immediate postoperative period, is necessary to keep the tube patent and reduce anxiety. Copious secretions are usually present and can quickly block the tracheostomy opening. The patient is usually aware of this possibility and often terrified of being left alone even for a moment. To reduce anxiety and fear of suffocation, the patient is assessed at frequent intervals. The suctioning procedure is explained, and the patient is assured before and during the procedure that insertion of the catheter takes only a few seconds.

Pain. The patient may experience discomfort or pain related to the surgical procedure or the tracheostomy tube. Pain or discomfort are minimized if care is exercised when working around and with the tracheostomy. If pain or discomfort occurs, the physician may order an analgesic. Narcotic analgesics are usually avoided because of the depressant effect on the respirations and cough reflex.

Impaired Verbal Communication. Patients who have had a tracheostomy without a laryngectomy can speak by taking a breath, briefly covering the tube with a finger, uttering a few words, and then removing the finger to resume breathing. The patient is taught this maneuver, beginning with one or two words and progressing to several words. In the immediate postoperative period, writing messages is the only means of communication available to the patient.

Potential for Infection.   The presence of a foreign body (the tracheostomy tube) in the trachea encourages the production of excess secretions as well as a localized inflammatory responses. Both situations, as well as other factors, can lead to infection. The secretions and the skin edges around the stoma are inspected for signs of infection, namely redness and thick, purulent drainage with or without an odor. The vital signs are monitored every 4 hours; any rise in temperature is reported to the physician.

Cleanliness of all equipment used in caring for the tracheostomy is essential. The hands are washed before suctioning the patient. Poor technique may lead to postoperative pneumonia by spread of infection to the lungs. If it is necessary to suction through the nose or the mouth, another catheter (not the one used for suctioning the tracheostomy) is used. Sterile disposable catheters are always used for suctioning to lessen the danger of introducing pathogenic microorganisms.

Impaired Swallowing and Altered Nutrition.   During the immediate posttracheotomy period, intravenous fluids are usually required. Once oral fluids are ordered, the patient is started on small, frequent amounts of clear liquids. If the patient appears able to swallow small amounts of liquids, the amount is slowly increased. Puréed and soft foods are then slowly added. If difficulty swallowing liquids or puréed foods is found, nasogastric tube feedings or total parenteral nutrition may be required to meet the patient's nutritional requirements.

Intake and output is measured, and the physician is notified if the urine output falls below 500 mL in 24 hours or the patient has difficulty taking oral fluids or food (when allowed).

Knowledge Deficit.   It is important to explain nursing tasks (eg, suctioning and the removal of the tracheostomy inner cannula for cleaning) to the patient and family. If the tracheostomy is permanent, the patient and family are taught to care for the tube and the suctioning techniques as soon as possible. Self-care is the patient's most effective defense against the fear of a blocked airway.

Evaluation

- Anxiety or fear is reduced or eliminated
- Comfort is attained and maintained
- Able to communicate needs to members of the health team
- Shows no evidence of local infection or other complications associated with a tracheostomy
- Food and fluid intake meet daily requirements
- Airway clear with no evidence of obstruction

Endotracheal Intubation

An endotracheal tube is inserted through the patient's mouth or nose and into the trachea. A laryngoscope is used to pass the tube. Endotracheal intubation is performed on those who cannot maintain an adequate airway on their own or who are having respiratory difficulty, such as patients who are comatose, who are under general anesthesia, who have extensive edema of upper airway passages, and who are awake but unable to breathe on their own.

An endotracheal tube can remain in place for up to 3 weeks. The cuff is inflated to provide a tight seal. An endotracheal tube can be attached to a respirator for controlled ventilation. Humidification is necessary because air going to the lungs through an endotracheal tube does not pass through the moist mucous membranes of the upper airway.

Accidental removal of an endotracheal tube must be prevented, because this can result in laryngeal edema or spasm (laryngospasm) and subsequent respiratory arrest. The endotracheal tube is secured by both its inflated cuff and the placement of tape around the tube and taping it to the patient's cheek. The proximal end of the tube is marked for determining if downward displacement has occurred.

The physician may order the tube removed when the patient's vital capacity, measured with an ventilometer, is adequate and the patient is able to breathe without assistance. Blood gas studies also are used as a guideline to removal. When the tube is to be removed, emergency equipment for respiratory support must be available. Depending on hospital policy, the removal of an endotracheal tube may, in certain instances, be done by the nurse. Before the cuff is deflated, the pharynx is aspirated so that secretions do not gravitate downward. The tube usually is removed with the patient in semi-Fowler's position. If laryngospasm occurs, air is given by positive pressure. Reinsertion of the endotracheal tube by the physician may be necessary if laryngospasm continues.

Complications that may be seen with the use of endotracheal intubation include ulceration and stricture of the trachea or larynx, atelectasis, and pneumonia.

NURSING PROCESS —THE PATIENT UNDERGOING ENDOTRACHEAL INTUBATION

Assessment
Vital signs are taken before insertion of the tube to provide baseline data and then at periodic intervals,

depending on the condition of the patient and the reason for endotracheal tube insertion. Blood gas studies are ordered periodically and changes reported to the physician. The lungs are auscultated every 30 to 60 minutes for normal and abnormal breath sounds.

Nursing Diagnosis

Additional nursing diagnosis may be appropriate for those with medical or surgical disorders that have resulted in respiratory insufficiency or failure.

- Anxiety related to inability to breathe, insertion of endotracheal tube, dependence on mechanical ventilation
- Fear related to dependence on mechanical support of respirations, being left unattended
- Impaired verbal communication related to endotracheal tube
- Ineffective airway clearance related to inability to cough, raise secretions
- Altered thought processes related to change in blood gas studies
- Altered oral mucous membrane integrity related to endotracheal tube, dry mouth

Planning and Implementation

The major goals of the patient are to improve respirations, maintain a patent airway, and communicate needs to others.

The main goal of nursing management is to provide respiratory support until such time as the patient is able to breathe effectively and respiratory activity and gas exchange are normal.

The patient is observed at frequent intervals for response to respiratory support and complications associated with endotracheal intubation. Vital signs are monitored at intervals based on the patient's condition.

Respiratory Function. Patients who are intubated endotracheally are unable to cough. Secretions are often thick and tenacious, and swallowing reflexes are depressed. The airway must be kept patent at all times. Suctioning technique is the same as for a tracheostomy (see earlier discussion). The frequency of suctioning depends on the patient and the amount of endotracheal secretions.

Auscultation of the lungs and observation of the symmetric rise and fall of the chest is observed every 30 to 60 minutes. If breath sounds are not detected bilaterally, the physician is notified immediately. Because inspired air must be kept moist, the T-piece is inspected for the presence of mist. The patient is hyperinflated (sighed) every hour; volume ventilators have built-in sigh mechanisms.

Altered Comfort and Anxiety. An endotracheal tube is uncomfortable. The patient may display anxiety or fear because of the tube, suctioning, and dependence on a machine for breathing. Each time suctioning is needed, the patient is reassured that the procedure takes only a short time. If the patient is fully or partially awake, attempts may be made to remove or pull on the tube; restraining measures may be necessary. If the patient is extremely restless, the physician is contacted.

Impaired Communication. Patients with endotracheal tubes are unable to talk and therefore are unable to communicate their needs. When they try to communicate, the nurse can ask questions requiring a yes or no answer, which the patient can give by a nod of the head.

Impaired Gas Exchange. An increase in P_{CO_2} caused by blockage of the endotracheal tube or malfunctioning of the ventilator may occur. The endotracheal tube may become blocked because of secretions or because the patient is biting on the tube. Suctioning is needed to clear the tube. If the patient is biting on the tube, a bite block or oral airway (inserted in the side of the mouth) may be inserted.

Altered Thought Processes. Some patients may appear confused as a result of abnormal blood gases or electrolyte imbalances. Restraints may be necessary if the patient attempts to pull at the tube or disturb nearby equipment. If the patient suddenly becomes restless and agitated, the endotracheal tube may be obstructed and immediate suctioning is required. Any change in the patient's mental status is carefully evaluated.

Oral Mucous Membranes. Oral care is given as needed to keep the mouth free of crusts and mucus. The oropharynx and mouth are suctioned as needed. The teeth may be cleaned with applicators. Any appearance of oral bleeding is noted and reported to the physician.

Postextubation Care. Once the endotracheal tube has been removed, the patient is placed in a high Fowler's or semi-Fowler's position to promote optimal chest and lung expansion. The posterior pharynx may be dry, and the voice may be hoarse. The patient is observed at frequent intervals for signs of laryngeal edema and increased respiratory distress.

Evaluation

- Comfort is maintained as much as possible
- Anxiety is reduced

■ Able to communicate needs with yes and no answers
■ Airway remains clear
■ Blood gas studies within normal range

■ Mentally clear; does not attempt to remove endotracheal tube
■ Oral mucous membranes intact with no evidence of bleeding, ulceration

General Nutritional Considerations

☐ Nasogastric tube feedings may be begun after a laryngectomy. These feedings are given slowly either at body or room temperature. The physician indicates the amount to be given in the first feeding and the temperature of the feeding. The amount given for each feeding is increased if the patient tolerates the amount given in the previous feeding. If the patient complains of gastric distress or has diarrhea, the physician is notified, because a change in formula may be necessary.

☐ Tube feedings may need additional supplements of certain vitamins and minerals. These may be added by the nurse at the time of the feeding or by the dietary department when the feeding is prepared.

☐ A diminished sense of taste and smell after a laryngectomy may result in a decreased desire to eat. When oral fluids and food are allowed, the patient is encouraged to eat and assured that some sense of taste and smell will return.

General Pharmacologic Considerations

☐ Antibiotics may be ordered for the patient with an upper airway infection; culture and sensitivity tests usually are done to identify the organisms causing the infection. Once the microorganisms are identified and the sensitivity to various antibiotics is determined, the antibiotic proved to be effective is prescribed.

☐ Antibiotics are of no value in treating the common cold but may be prescribed to prevent or treat secondary infections such as bronchitis or pneumonia.

☐ Preparations for treating the symptoms of a cold that contain multiple ingredients rarely are more effective than single-agent preparations.

☐ In some instances, one or more of the drugs contained in multiple-ingredient cold preparations may be contraindicated in certain disorders such as glaucoma, heart disease, hypertension, or prostatic enlargement. Patients with one or more known diseases and who are taking prescription drugs are encouraged to consult their physician before using nonprescription drugs for treatment of a cold.

☐ Indiscriminate use of nosedrops, which often contain an adrenergic agent that shrinks the nasal membranes, can lead to rebound congestion, which may be worse than the original problem.

☐ Aspirin is not given for the relief of pain or fever to children under age 12 because of the association of aspirin administration with Reye's syndrome.

☐ Profuse nasal bleeding may be controlled by the direct application of epinephrine, usually as a 1:1000 solution, to the nasal membranes.

General Gerontologic Considerations

☐ If an elderly patient requires a tracheostomy, the nurse must be alert to possible confusion after the procedure. If the patient is confused or does not understand the purpose of the procedure, attempts may be made to pull at the tube or to remove it. Restraining measures may be required.

☐ The common cold may be potentially serious for elderly patients, especially when they have other diseases such as a chronic respiratory disorder or heart disease. The elderly patient should be advised to see a physician if cold symptoms are severe or if breathing is difficult.

Suggested Readings

☐ Berkow R, Fletcher AJ, eds. Merck manual of diagnosis and therapy. 15th ed. Rahway, NJ: Merck & Co, 1987. *(In-depth coverage of subject matter)*

☐ Biggs C. The cancer that cost a patient his voice. RN April 1987;50:44. *(Additional coverage of subject matter)*

☐ Bowers AC, Thompson JM. Clinical manual of health assessment. 3rd ed. St Louis: CV Mosby, 1988. *(In-depth coverage of subject matter)*

☐ Carroll PF. Cyanosis: the sign you can't count on. Nursing '88 March 1988;18:50. *(Additional coverage of subject matter)*

☐ Clark WG, Brater DC, Johnson AR. Goth's medical pharmacology. 12th ed. St Louis: CV Mosby, 1988. *(In-depth and high-level coverage of subject matter)*

☐ Dennison RD. Managing the patient with upper airway obstruction. Nursing '87 October 1987;17:34. *(Additional and in-depth coverage of subject matter)*

☐ Dupuis VG. Ventilators: theory and clinical application. St Louis: CV Mosby, 1986. *(In-depth coverage of subject matter)*

☐ Feinstein D. What to teach the patient who has had a total laryngectomy. RN April 1987;50:53. *(In-depth coverage of subject matter)*

☐ Guzzetta CE, Bunton SD, Prinkey LA, Sherer AP, Siefert PC. Clinical assessment tools for use with nursing diagnosis. St Louis: CV Mosby, 1989. *(In-depth coverage of subject matter)*

☐ Handerhan B, Allegrezza N. Getting your patient off a ventilator. RN December 1989;52:60. *(Additional coverage of subject matter)*

☐ Kersten LD. Comprehensive respiratory nursing. Philadelphia: WB Saunders, 1989. *(In-depth, high-level coverage of subject matter)*

☐ Konz C. Action stat! Emergency intubation: how to reestablish a patent airway after a patient goes into respiratory arrest. Nursing '90 February 1990;20:33. *(Additional coverage of subject matter)*

☐ Lewis LW, Timby, BK. Fundamental skills and concepts in patient care. 4th ed. Philadelphia: JB Lippincott, 1988. *(Additional coverage of subject matter)*

☐ Luckmann J, Sorensen K. Medical–surgical nursing: a psychophysioloigic approach. 3rd ed. Philadelphia: WB Saunders, 1987. *(Additional and in-depth coverage of subject matter)*

☐ Mapp CS. Trach care: are you aware of all the dangers? Nursing '88 July 1988;18:34. *(Additional coverage and illustrations that reinforce subject matter)*

☐ Petty T. Drug strategies for airflow obstruction. Am J Nurs February 1987;87:180. *(Additional coverage of subject matter)*

☐ Wilkins RL, Sheldon RL, Krider SJ. Clinical assessment in respiratory care. 2nd ed. St Louis: CV Mosby, 1989. *(In-depth, high-level coverage of subject matter)*

Chapter 22

Disorders of the Lower Respiratory Airway

On completion of this chapter the reader will:

- List and discuss the symptoms, diagnoses, and treatment of infectious disorders of the lower respiratory airway

- Use the nursing process in the management of a patient with an infectious disorder of the lower respiratory airway

- List and discuss the symptoms, diagnoses, and treatment of disorders that result in decreased function of the lower respiratory airway

- Use the nursing process in the management of a patient with a disorder that results in decreased function of the lower respiratory airway

- Discuss the symptoms, diagnoses, and treatment of malignant disorders of the lower respiratory airway

- Use the nursing process in the management of a patient with a malignant disorder of the lower respiratory airway

- Discuss the symptoms, diagnosis, and treatment of thoracic trauma

- Use the nursing process in the management of a patient who incurs thoracic trauma

INFECTIOUS DISORDERS OF THE LOWER RESPIRATORY AIRWAY

Acute Bronchitis

Acute bronchitis is characterized by inflammation of the mucous membranes that line the major bronchi and their branches. Frequently, the inflammatory process also involves the trachea and is then referred to as *tracheobronchitis*. The most common cause of acute bronchitis is viral infection. Frequently starting as an upper respiratory infection, the inflammatory process extends into the tracheobronchial tree, with direct involvement of the mucous linings, the inflammation of which increases the amount of mucus produced by the secretory cells of the mucosa. Although acute bronchitis is most often related to an infectious process, chemical irritation due to noxious fumes (eg, sulfur dioxide, nitrogen dioxide, smoke, other air pollutants) also can cause acute bronchitis. The disease may be further complicated by the development of bronchial asthma.

Symptoms

Acute bronchitis is usually self-limiting, lasting several days. Symptoms initially include a dry, nonproductive cough that later becomes productive of a mucopurulent sputum, fever, and malaise. Acute bronchitis may be complicated by laryngitis with hoarseness and, occasionally, loss of voice and sinusitis. These secondary areas of infection usually subside as the bronchitis subsides.

Diagnosis

Diagnosis is made by a patient history and auscultation of the chest to rule out other respiratory pathology. A sputum sample for culture and sensitivity testing may be ordered to rule out bacterial infection. A chest radiograph also may be ordered.

Treatment

Acute bronchitis is treated with bed rest, salicylates, and a light, nourishing diet with plenty of liquids. Humidifiers are recommended because dry air aggravates the cough. Secondary bacterial invasion occasionally takes place, and the previously mild infection becomes a serious bacterial infection with the production of a thick, purulent sputum and a cough that may persist for several weeks. Although antibiotics are generally not ordered for the treatment of acute bronchitis of viral etiology, the physician usually interprets the establishment of a secondary invader in the tracheobronchial tree as an indication for culturing the sputum and starting antibiotic therapy. Obtaining results of a sputum culture report takes 2 or 3 days; the physician may order a broad-spectrum antibiotic immediately and may change the antibiotic medication later, depending on the results of the sputum culture.

Chronic Bronchitis

Chronic bronchitis is characterized by hypersecretion of mucus by the bronchial glands as well as a chronic or recurrent respiratory infection. A serious health problem, it has symptoms that develop gradually and often go untreated for many years until the disease is well established. A chronic cough, often attributed to smoking, may persist and gradually grow worse. The cough frequently is disregarded, and early treatment often delayed.

Multiple factors have been associated with the cause of chronic bronchitis. The development of the disease may be insidious or may follow a long history of bronchial asthma or an acute respiratory infection, such as influenza or pneumonia. Air pollution is a major cause, and the role of cigarette smoking cannot be overemphasized. Smoking characteristically causes hypertrophy of the mucous glands and hypersecretion. Many air pollutants, such as sulfur dioxide and smoke, have been shown to significantly alter the ability of the cilia lining the respiratory airway to propel secretions upward. Secretions are then retained in the lungs and form plugs within the smaller bronchi. These plugs become areas for bacterial growth and chronic infection, which results in greater increases in mucus secretion and, eventually, areas of focal necrosis and fibrosis. Although the disease may occur at any age, it is seen most frequently in middle age and is usually the result of many years of untreated, low-grade bronchitis.

Symptoms

The earliest symptom is a cough accompanied by the expectoration of thick, white mucus. The cough is ordinarily most marked on rising and before going to bed. Bronchospasm may occur during severe bouts of coughing. Acute respiratory infections are frequent during the winter months and may persist for several weeks or more. As the disease progresses, the sputum may become purulent and copious, and even may be streaked with blood after a severe paroxysm of coughing. Although a patient may have a sensation of heaviness in the chest, dyspnea usually is not a symptom of uncomplicated chronic bronchitis.

Diagnosis

The patient's history is important. The diagnosis usually is made by evaluating the duration of the patient's symptoms, the circumstances under which they started, the employment history, a history of previous respiratory diseases, and a smoking history. Physical examination, chest radiograph, and pulmonary function tests may be normal. Examination of the sputum, particularly the volume expectorated daily, may help to assess the severity of the disease. Sputum culture may be of value. All of these studies must be obtained to rule out bronchogenic carcinoma, bronchiectasis, tuberculosis, and other diseases in which cough is a predominant feature.

Treatment

In general, treatment is directed toward the prevention of recurrent irritation of the bronchial mucosa either by infection or chemical agents. Smoking should be discontinued immediately. Bronchodilators may be prescribed to dilate the bronchi and reduce airway obstruction and bronchospasm. Increased fluid intake and a well-balanced diet are recommended. Other treatment modalities include postural drainage to remove secretions from the bronchi and steroid therapy if other treatment measures prove ineffective. If a patient's work involves exposure to dust and chemical irritants, a change of occupation may be necessary. Air conditioning with filtration of incoming air may result in marked reduction of sputum production and cough. In the late stages of chronic bronchitis, the infection is usually persistent, and antibiotic therapy may become a lifelong therapeutic measure.

Bronchiectasis

Bronchiectasis is a chronic infectious disease in which structural changes in the walls of the bronchi and bronchioles result in saccular dilatations, which collect purulent material. The expulsive power of the affected areas is diminished, and the purulent material tends to remain in the dilated areas.

Bronchopneumonia and chronic sinusitis are possible precursors of bronchiectasis. Congenital weakness of the bronchi also may be a contributing factor. The disease often begins in early adulthood and progresses slowly.

Symptoms

Patients with bronchiectasis cough and expectorate copious amounts of purulent sputum. When left standing, the sputum settles into three layers. The top layer is frothy, the middle layer is clear, and the bottom layer appears purulent and contains clumps of particulate matter. This clumping is actually the thick sputum raised from alveolar sacs in the lungs. Coughing is most severe when a patient changes position, as on arising in the morning or lying down at night. The amount of sputum produced in one paroxysm varies with the stage of the disease and may be 200 mL or more. The expectoration of foul sputum leaves an unpleasant odor in the mouth and on the breath, making careful oral hygiene necessary. Fatigue, loss of weight, and anorexia are common. Hemoptysis may occur.

Diagnosis

The diagnosis is made by patient history and physical examination, bronchoscopy, chest radiograph, and a bronchogram.

Treatment

Treatment includes drainage of the purulent material from the bronchi. Antibiotics are used to control infection and may be prescribed for long periods. Humidification is often necessary to help raise thick, tenacious sputum.

Postural drainage is performed to remove secretions from the lungs. Postural drainage helps remove secretions by gravity (Fig. 22-1). The exact position of the patient during treatment depends on the location of the affected areas and is ordered by the physician. Treatment is usually 5 to 15 minutes three times a day in each prescribed position, while inhaling slowly and blowing the breath out through the mouth.

Patients are helped as necessary to assume each position and are encouraged to cough between position

changes. A sputum cup, tissues, and a call light are made available. Pulmonary physical therapy measures include gentle shaking or vibrating over the segment being drained and gentle but firm clapping or percussion with cupped hands on the chest wall over the segment while the patient exhales. These measures help loosen secretions that are then moved by gravity to the trachea where they can be coughed up or suctioned.

When bronchiectasis is confined to a relatively small portion of the lung, a cure may be achieved by the surgical removal of the diseased portion. Medical treatment includes administration of bronchodilators, antibiotics, mucolytics, and humidification of surrounding air or nebulizer therapy to thin secretions and help raise sputum.

Pneumonia

Pneumonia is an acute illness caused by inflammation or infection of the lungs and characterized by a productive cough, chest pain, and fever. When the inflammation is confined to one or more lobes of the lung, it is called *lobar pneumonia* (Fig. 22-2). Patchy and diffuse infection scattered throughout both lungs is called *bronchopneumonia*. Hypoventilation of lung tissue over a prolonged period—such as happens

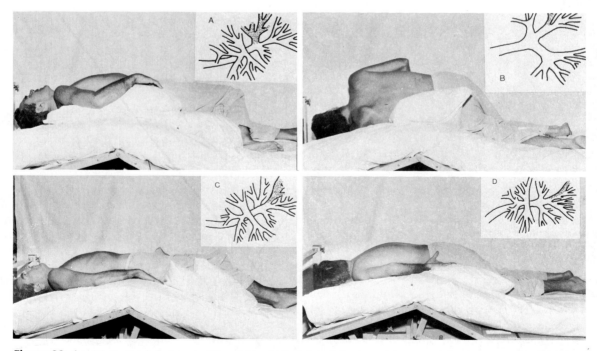

Figure 22–1. (*A*) Postural drainage of the right middle lobe of the lung. (*B*) Postural drainage of the lateral basal segment of the right lower lobe. The patient is placed on the unaffected side. (*C*) Postural drainage of the anterior basal segment of the right lung and the anterior and medial basal segments of the left lung. (*D*) Drainage of the posterior segments of the right or left lower lobe bronchi. (Ayers SM, Giannelli S. Care of the critically ill. New York: Appleton-Century-Crofts.)

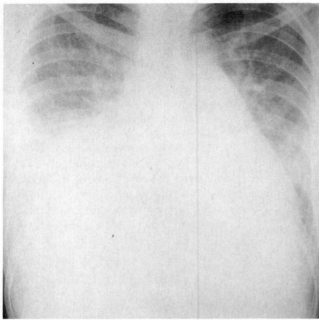

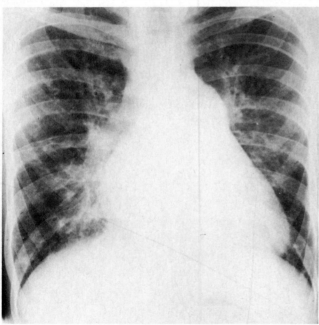

Figure 22-2. (*Top*) Right lobar pneumonia. Note the consolidation of the right lower lobe. The left lung field is essentially normal. (*Bottom*) Complete resolution of the pneumonia after 2 weeks of antibiotic therapy. (Department of Radiology, Methodist Hospital of Brooklyn)

when a patient lies quietly in bed, breathing with only a part of the lungs over a prolonged period—can result in the accumulation of bronchial secretions and cause *hypostatic pneumonia. Chemical pneumonia* may occur after inhalation of substances, such as volatile hydrocarbons (ie, kerosene, gasoline).

Pneumonia can be caused by many different types of microorganisms, such as viruses, rickettsiae, fungi, and bacteria. Pneumonia caused by the microorganism *Pneumocystis carinii* is often seen in people with acquired immunodeficiency syndrome. *Atypical pneumonia* describes pneumonia caused by mycoplasmas, viruses, psittacosis, and *Legionella pneumophila* (the causative agent of legionnaires' disease).

Symptoms

The onset of bacterial pneumonia is sudden. The patient experiences severe, sharp chest pain, rapid prostration, and often a shaking chill, which turns into a fever that may rise as high as 41.1°C (106°F). Irritation of the respiratory tract tissues produces a cough that is painful because it causes movement of the chest wall and, consequently, the rubbing together of the two pleural layers. The sputum often is rusty in color. Breathing causes pain, and the patient tries to breathe as shallowly as possible.

In bacterial pneumonia, the alveoli become filled with exudate. Bronchitis, tracheitis (inflammation of the trachea), and spots of necrosis (death of tissue) in the lung may follow. In pneumonia caused by mycoplasma, thickening of the alveolar septa and partial filling of the alveoli with exudate occur. As the inflammatory process continues, interference with the exchange of gases between the bloodstream and the lungs increases. With an increase in the carbon dioxide content of the blood, the respiratory center in the brain is stimulated, and breathing becomes more rapid and shallow. The patient is more comfortable and better able to breathe when sitting up.

If the disease process is not halted, the patient becomes increasingly ill. If the circulatory system is unable to maintain the burden of decreased gas exchange, the patient may die from heart failure or asphyxia.

The fever of mycoplasmal or viral pneumonia resolves by lysis; that is, it slowly returns to normal. Viral pneumonia also differs from bacterial pneumonia in that blood cultures are sterile, the sputum may be more copious, the chills are less frequent, and the pulse and respirations are characteristically slow.

The course of viral pneumonia usually is less severe than that of bacterial pneumonia, although the patient is far from comfortable. In viral pneumonia, the mortality is low but rises when bacterial pneumonia occurs as a secondary infection. A patient with viral pneumonia is often weak and ill for longer than the patient with successfully treated bacterial pneumonia.

Diagnosis

Diagnosis is made by patient history and physical examination, sputum culture and sensitivity studies, chest radiograph, and complete blood cell count. A blood culture also may be ordered.

Treatment

The antibiotics chosen for treatment depend on the sensitivity of the causative microorganism to their action. If the infecting microorganism has not been identified, broad-spectrum antibiotics may be ordered. Other treatment is mainly supportive, including bed rest and fluids in large quantities to replace those lost through increased respiration and perspiration. If a patient cannot tolerate oral fluids, intravenous fluids are given.

For cough and chest pain, codeine may be ordered. If the inflammatory process is far advanced, a patient may have considerable respiratory difficulty and may be cyanotic. Humidification of inspired air usually helps liquefy secretions and is best administered by a cool-mist vaporizer. A nasal catheter or cannula is usually ordered for supplementary oxygenation. In the presence of severe infection with thick, abundant secretions, the physician may perform endotracheal intubation or a tracheotomy.

Complications

The complications of pneumonia include congestive heart failure (which is more commonly seen in the elderly or in those with known heart disease), empyema (collection of pus in the pleural cavity), pleurisy, septicemia (infective microorganisms in the bloodstream), atelectasis, hypotension, and shock. Septicemia can lead to a secondary focus of infection and give rise to infectious disorders, such as endocarditis, pericarditis, and purulent arthritis. Recovery, especially from atypical pneumonia, also may be complicated by otitis media, bronchitis, or sinusitis that results from the spread of microorganisms to these organs or structures.

Pleurisy

Pleurisy is an inflammation of the visceral and parietal pleurae. Pleurisy is seen most commonly with pneumonia in which the inflammatory process spreads from the lung to the parietal pleura. Pleurisy also may develop with tuberculosis, lung cancer, cardiac and renal disease, systemic infections, and pulmonary embolism. The pleura becomes thick, swollen, and rigid. The visceral pleura has no pain fibers, but the parietal pleura does.

Symptoms

Sharp pain occurs when the two surfaces of the pleura rub together during respiration. As fluid is formed, pain gradually subsides, but the patient has a dry cough, fatigues easily, and may experience shortness of breath. Other symptoms include fever, malaise, dyspnea, and a friction rub heard when auscultating the chest.

Diagnosis

Diagnosis is made by a patient's symptoms, chest radiograph, microscopic sputum examination, and sputum culture. If the physician performs a thoracentesis, the specimen is usually sent to the laboratory for culture and sensitivity studies.

Treatment

If a great deal of fluid is found with respiratory difficulty, it can be removed by thoracentesis. Analgesic and antipyretic drugs are prescribed for pain and fever. More intense pain may require a narcotic analgesic, such as codeine, or an antiinflammatory drug, such as indomethacin. Severe cases may require an intercostal nerve block. In some cases, repeated thoracentesis may be necessary.

Pleural Effusion

In pleural effusion, large amounts of fluid are secreted and collect in the space between the pleural layers. The amount of fluid may be so great that the lung is partially collapsed on that side, and pressure on the heart and the other organs of the mediastinum occurs. Pleural effusion may be a complication of disorders such as pneumonia, lung cancer, tuberculosis, pulmonary embolism, and congestive heart failure.

Symptoms

Symptoms of pleural effusion include fever, pain, and dyspnea.

Diagnosis

Diagnosis is made by a history and physical examination, chest radiograph, computed tomographic (CT) scan, and removal of pleural fluid by thoracentesis for laboratory examination.

Treatment

The main goal of treatment is to eliminate the cause. Treatment includes administration of antibiotics, analgesics for pain, cardiotonic drugs to control congestive heart failure, removal of (excess) pleuritic fluid by thoracentesis, and surgery for the malignancy (lung, bronchiogenic cancers).

Lung Abscess

An *abscess,* a localized area of pus formation, may occur in the lung as a result of the aspiration of a foreign body, vomitus, or infectious material. A lung abscess also may follow pneumonia or a mechanical obstruction of the bronchi, such as that due to a tumor. Lung abscess can be prevented in the unconscious patient by avoiding aspiration of secretions, frequent changes of position, and by preventing or promptly treating obstructions and infections in the respiratory tract.

Symptoms and Diagnosis

Symptoms include chills, fever, weight loss, and a cough that produces purulent or bloody sputum. Clubbing of the fingers often occurs in chronic cases. Diagnosis is made by patient history, physical examination, chest radiograph, and other radiographic studies, such as a CT scan.

Treatment

Treatment of lung abscess involves drainage of the abscess, control of infection, and increasing the body's resistance. Postural drainage and antibiotics may prove sufficient; or, surgical drainage of the abscess may be necessary. The portion of the lung that contains the abscess may need to be surgically removed.

Empyema

Empyema is a general term used to denote pus in a body cavity. It refers most frequently, however, to pus within the thoracic cavity (thoracic empyema). Empyema results from infection, which causes the formation of pus. Infection may follow trauma or preexisting diseases, such as pneumonia, tuberculosis, or lung abscess.

Symptoms and Diagnosis

Symptoms include fever, pain in the chest, dyspnea, anorexia, and malaise. Diagnosis is made by chest radiograph and aspiration of purulent fluid by thoracentesis.

Treatment

Initial treatment often consists of antibiotics, given both parenterally and into the pleural space, and aspiration of pus by thoracentesis. Closed drainage of the empyema cavity is used occasionally. The drainage tubes are then connected to an underwater seal drainage bottle. Open drainage may be used when pus is thick and when the walls of the empyema cavity are strong enough to keep the lung from collapsing while the chest is opened. One or more tubes may be placed in the opening to promote drainage. The wound is then covered by a large absorbent dressing that is changed as necessary. The drainage of the pus results in a drop in temperature and general symptomatic improvement.

If empyema is inadequately treated, it may become chronic. A thick coating may form over the lung, preventing its expansion. Decortication (removal of the coating) allows the lung to reexpand.

Influenza

Influenza (flu) is an acute respiratory disease of relatively short duration caused by one of several related and yet distinct viruses. The three major strains of the influenza virus are A, B, and C. The virus is able to mutate and produce variants within a given strain. These variants are called subtypes. The viruses that cause influenza are transmitted through the respiratory tract.

Influenza occurs chiefly in epidemics, although sporadic cases appear between epidemics. Because the virus changes, antibodies produced by those who had influenza previously are no longer effective against a new subtype, and a different vaccine must be produced.

Symptoms

The incubation period is 2 or 3 days, and the onset is sudden, with considerable individual variation in symptoms. The patient looks ill and complains of chills, severe headache, muscular aching, and fever. Anorexia, weakness, and apathy, as well as respiratory symptoms, sneezing, sore throat, dry cough, nasal discharge, and herpetic lesions of the lips and mouth may be present. The gastrointestinal form usually begins with nausea, vomiting, and diarrhea, but symptoms may vary. For some, the symptoms are mild; for others severe. Fever of 37.8° to 39.5°C (100°–103°F) may persist for about 3 days, but other symptoms usually continue for 7 to 10 days. Cough may persist longer.

Diagnosis

Diagnosis is based on a patient's symptoms. Additional diagnostic studies, such as a chest radiograph or sputum culture and sensitivity tests, may be performed to rule out other diseases.

Treatment

Hospitalization is not necessary in uncomplicated cases. Vital signs are taken every 4 hours. Copious fluids, given frequently, include fruit juices and broths; a regular diet is begun as soon as the patient's appetite returns. Aspirin or acetaminophen may be given every 4 to 6 hours as circumstances require for fever, headache, and muscular aching. Steam or cool vapor inhalation eases a dry cough.

The patient is observed for signs of increasing fever, elevated pulse rate, difficulty breathing, change in the amount and the quality of the sputum (particularly, whether it is purulent or rusty), and for the sudden occurrence of chest pain.

Most patients recover. Fatalities are due usually to secondary bacterial complications, especially among pregnant women, the aged or debilitated, and those with chronic conditions, such as cardiac disease, and chronic pulmonary disorders, such as emphysema. During an epidemic, the death rate from pneumonia and cardiovascular disease rises.

Complications include tracheobronchitis caused by damage to the ciliated epithelium of the trachea and bronchi, bacterial pneumonia, and cardiovascular disease. Staphylococcal pneumonia is the most serious complication.

Pulmonary Tuberculosis

The presence of *Mycobacterium tuberculosis,* the tubercle bacillus, is necessary to cause pulmonary tuberculosis; it usually is not the only cause, however. In contrast to the number of people who have been infected with the tubercle bacillus, only a small proportion ever become ill from tuberculosis. Many factors predispose to the development of tuberculosis. When the body's resistance is lowered, through such factors as inadequate rest and poor nutrition, or when the organisms are sufficiently virulent and numerous, the clinical disease may develop. The highest incidence tends to occur in the most densely populated areas, as overcrowding and poor hygienic conditions make the spread of the disease more likely. The incidence of tuberculosis is especially high among alcoholics because of health and social problems associated with alcoholism (eg, malnutrition).

Tubercle bacilli are aerobic, gram-positive, and acid-fast. They are rod-shaped and can be identified by microscopic examination of sputum and other body substances. Although the bacilli can live in the dark for months in particles of dried sputum, exposure to direct sunlight kills them in a few hours. The organism is difficult to kill with ordinary disinfectants. Tubercle bacilli are killed by pasteurization (30 minutes at 62°C, 143.6°F), a process widely used in the prevention of the spread of tuberculosis by milk and milk products.

Tuberculosis infection is transmitted most commonly by direct contact with a person who has the active disease, through the inhalation of the droplets from coughing, sneezing, and spitting.

Symptoms

The onset of tuberculosis is insidious, and early symptoms vary from person to person. A patient may be asymptomatic for a long time; symptoms often do not appear until the disease is well advanced.

Early symptoms are often vague and may be readily dismissed. Fatigue, anorexia, weight loss, and a slight, nonproductive cough are all symptoms that can be attributed to overwork, excessive smoking, or poor eating habits; however, they are also early symptoms of tuberculosis. Temperature elevation, particularly in the late afternoon and evening, and night sweats are frequent as the disease progresses. The cough often becomes productive of mucopurulent and blood-streaked sputum. Marked weakness and wasting and hemoptysis are characteristics of later stages of the illness; dyspnea may be a late symptom. Chest pain may result from the spread of infection to the pleura.

Diagnosis

Diagnostic tests consist chiefly of tuberculin skin tests, chest radiographs, and examination of the sputum and other body fluids. A positive tuberculin skin test is evidence that a tuberculous infection has existed at some time, somewhere in the body. The chief value of these tests lies in case finding. The agent used for tuberculosis skin testing is tuberculin purified protein derivative. Intradermal (between the epidermis and the dermis) injection of this agent into the forearm is called a Mantoux test. Test results are read in 48 to 72 hours. The diameter of the indurated (raised) area is measured at its widest part. A measurement of 2 mm or more is significant and considered positive, and further diagnostic procedures may be performed.

Microscopic sputum examination may be ordered when tuberculosis is suspected, during and after a course of drug therapy, and after surgical removal of a diseased lobe of the lung. The patient is instructed to cough deeply so that the specimen does not consist mostly of saliva. Most patients find that it is easier to raise sputum when they first get up in the morning. Specimens obtained on several consecutive days may be necessary.

Gastric lavage or gastric aspiration may be used to determine the presence of organisms, particularly when a patient has had difficulty raising a sputum specimen for examination. Tubercle bacilli may reach the stomach from the lungs when sputum is raised and is not expectorated but swallowed.

When the tubercle bacillus is thought to have invaded other body areas, specimens may be obtained to confirm the diagnosis. If, for example, renal tuberculosis is suspected, 24-hour urine specimens may be ordered.

Treatment

Drugs have made recovery more rapid and have provided a chance for the arrest of the disease for those with advanced lesions, but they do not provide a guaranteed cure. Their usefulness lies in their ability to decrease the growth and multiplication of the tubercle bacillus, thus giving the patient's body a chance to overcome the disease. Two factors make drugs less than ideal: drug toxicity and the tendency of the tubercle bacillus to develop resistance to the drug. Combined therapy with two or more drugs decreases the problem of drug resistance, increases the tuberculostatic action of the drugs, and lessens toxic drug reactions.

Antituberculosis drugs are given for long periods and without interruption because healing is slow and resistance to drugs may be increased by interrupted treatment. Lapses in the administration of these drugs can be serious, and the patient must understand the importance of taking the drugs as prescribed by the physician. Resistance of the *Mycobacterium tuberculosis* to drugs is an important factor in lack of response to medical treatment.

Usually, drug therapy is carried out while the patient is at home. The patient must know that regular visits to the physician's office or clinic for follow-up care are necessary; this way the physician can assess the patient's progress. Culture and sensitivity tests may be performed, and the adverse effects of the drugs evaluated.

Surgical treatment may be used. When the disease is located primarily in one section of the lung, that portion may be removed by *segmental resection* (removal of a segment of a lobe) or by *wedge resection* (removal of a wedge of diseased tissue). If the diseased area is larger, a *lobectomy* (removal of a lobe) may be performed. In some cases, the entire lung is so diseased that a pneumonectomy is necessary.

NURSING PROCESS —THE PATIENT WHO HAS AN INFECTIOUS DISORDER OF THE LOWER RESPIRATORY AIRWAY

Assessment

A complete history of the symptoms is obtained, including when they first occurred, the severity, and what, if anything, made them better or worse. Vital signs are taken and the patient is weighed. The chest is auscultated for normal and abnormal breath sounds and for passage of air throughout the chest on inspiration and expiration. Laboratory and diagnostic test results are reviewed.

The following areas are also included in the assessment:

Cough—type (dry, productive of sputum, hacking, wheezing, severe)
Sputum production—amount, color, consistency (thick, thin)
Respirations—quality, rate, depth, wheezing or other respiratory noises or dyspnea (on rest or exertion)
Pain—location, pain present on inspiration or expiration, type of pain (dull, sharp, stabbing)

Skin—presence or absence of cyanosis, flushing, diaphoresis
Mental—confused, restless, alert

Nursing Diagnosis

The following nursing diagnoses may apply to a patient with an infectious disorder of the lower respiratory airway and depend on a patient's potential or actual diagnosis.

- Activity intolerance related to respiratory difficulty, malaise, fever, severity of illness
- Hyperthermia related to infectious process
- Pain related to pneumonia, pleurisy, pleural effusion, lung abscess, empyema (specify)
- Fluid volume deficit related to decreased oral intake and abnormal fluid loss secondary to profuse diaphoresis
- Potential for infection transmission related to coughing, contamination of environment, other factors (specify)
- Altered nutrition: less than body requirements related to anorexia, fever, mental confusion, severity of illness
- Ineffective airway clearance related to pain on coughing, thick secretions, inability to cough, abnormal respiratory rate, rhythm, and depth
- Ineffective breathing pattern related to infectious process, pain on inspiration and expiration
- Altered thought processes related to infection, fever
- Knowledge deficit of medical regimen, prevention, and prognosis

Planning and Implementation

The major goals of the patient include the relief of pain, maintaining an adequate oral food and fluid intake, maintaining a clear airway, attaining a normal breathing pattern, and acquiring an understanding of the treatment regimen and measures to prevent future infections.

The major goals of nursing management are to perform those tasks necessary to cure or control the infection, prevent transmission of the infection to others, meet the patient's fluid and nutritional requirements, and relieve pain and discomfort.

Activity Intolerance. Many patients with a respiratory disorder experience dyspnea (shortness of breath) on exertion. They tire easily and find that even small tasks require great effort. When possible, activities of daily living are planned and spaced so a patient has an opportunity to rest between each activity.

Hyperthermia. Vital signs are monitored every 4 hours. Fever is a symptom of many respiratory infections. An antipyretic agent, such as aspirin or acetaminophen, is usually ordered.

After administration of an antipyretic drug, a patient may have diaphoresis. The gown and bedding are changed as needed. The temperature is taken about 1 hour after the administration of an antipyretic to determine response to the medication. The physician is notified if a patient's temperature remains elevated.

Temperature changes to higher than 39.5°C (103°F) or lower than 37.0°C (98.6°F) should be reported to the physician immediately; these changes may be warnings of a drastic alteration in a patient's condition. A sharp increase or decrease in pulse rate warns of circulatory complications and is also reported to the physician.

Pain. Pain may be associated with lower respiratory infections, such as pleurisy and pneumonia. Coughing, as well as normal breathing, often intensifies the pain. Narcotics are usually avoided since they depress respirations, but small doses of codeine, which has less of a depressant effect on respirations, may be ordered.

The patient is assessed at frequent intervals for pain. Pain that suddenly intensifies is brought to the attention of the physician, as a more serious problem may exist.

When pain occurs as the patient coughs, the nurse may support the patient's chest with both hands and use firm pressure to splint the chest wall. This action decreases pain and make the patient more willing to cough. The infected sputum should not be swallowed. A sputum cup with a cover is provided if the sputum is to be saved for inspection or measurement. If not, disposable tissues and a paper bag may be used and kept within easy reach. The sputum cup or paper bag is changed at least twice a day, handled with great care, and sealed so that the infection is not spread.

Fluid Volume Deficit. Fever and profuse diaphoresis along with a decreased oral fluid intake can result in a fluid volume deficit. Mental confusion, malaise, pain, and the fact that the patient feels acutely ill can result in an insufficient fluid intake and failure to replace the amount of fluid lost. The patient must receive fluids in addition to those offered on the meal tray. Fluids are offered every 2 hours, and the patient is encouraged to take sips of water at frequent intervals. Intake and output are measured, and the physician is notified if the patient fails to take an adequate amount of fluid or if the urinary output falls below 500 mL/day. In some instances, intravenous fluids may be necessary.

Potential for Infection Transmission. Infectious disorders of the lower respiratory airway, such as influenza, a draining abscess of the lung, and pneumonia, may be transmitted to others. The physician may order those with certain types of a transmissible infection placed in isolation. Good hand washing technique is necessary to prevent the spread of the infection to self and other patients.

Antibiotics usually are ordered. These drugs must be given at the prescribed time intervals to maintain consistent blood levels.

Altered Nutrition. Patients may eat poorly because of anorexia, because they are too ill to eat, or because they are mentally confused. Meal trays are checked after each meal and the physician notified if the patient eats poorly. High protein and carbohydrate between-meal nourishments may be required. If the patient fails to maintain an adequate food intake, short-term intravenous fluids providing calories and electrolytes may be necessary.

Ineffective Airway Clearance. A patient with an infection of the lower airway is encouraged to cough and deep breathe every 2 hours while awake. Moderate to severe pain may keep a patient from effectively coughing and deep breathing, and thus the airway is not cleared of secretions. Infectious processes may begin in secretions that are thick, tenacious, and difficult to raise. Rapid, shallow respirations prohibit deep breaths and interfere with the ability to cough and raise secretions. Placing the patient in a semi-Fowler's position may help raise secretions and make breathing easier. Patients may require suctioning to remove secretions from the upper airway.

Postural drainage is ordered to clear the airway of secretions. Patients vary in their ability to tolerate this procedure. Special care and observation of elderly or weak patients are important during and after postural drainage. The patient should be observed frequently and assisted to resume a normal position when the treatment is over. The amount and type of sputum expectorated during and immediately after the treatment is recorded. Postural drainage should not be attempted after meals because nausea and vomiting may result.

Ineffective Breathing Pattern. Patients may have a tendency to splint or guard their respirations because of chest pain. Failure to take deep breaths or breathe normally may result in further complications, such as atelectasis. The patient is also observed for evidence of cyanosis, as oxygen administration may be necessary.

Altered Thought Processes.   A patient is observed closely for signs of restlessness or confusion that may occur in such instances as high fever, electrolyte imbalances, or a worsening of a patient's condition. The physician is informed if extreme restlessness or mental confusion should occur. A patient can be protected with padded side rails. If a patient is extremely confused and in danger of injury, the physician is notified. In some instances, restraints may be ordered.

Knowledge Deficit.   On discharge, a teaching plan includes a review for the patient and family of the prescribed medical regimen to be continued at home. The review may include areas such as drug therapy, diet, fluid intake, temperature monitoring, and postural drainage. If postural drainage has been recommended after discharge, the patient requires instruction or review on the method of performing this procedure.

Those who smoke and develop chronic bronchitis or other acute or chronic respiratory disorders must be told that smoking should be immediately discontinued; it is virtually impossible to prevent exacerbation and progression of the disease if a patient continues to smoke.

A patient with pulmonary tuberculosis must have the treatment program explained. Drugs for tuberculosis must be taken for a long period of time. Patients may fail to adhere to the prescribed drug regimen; the importance of continuous therapy is stressed, as lapses in taking the prescribed drugs can result in reactivation of the infection. The patient and family are also informed of the importance of routine follow-up care, periodic physical examinations and chest radiographs, and the importance of eating a well-balanced diet.

Evaluation

- Able to carry out activities of daily living with minimal assistance
- Attains normal body temperature
- Pain is eliminated or controlled
- Fluid volume deficit is corrected; maintains adequate fluid intake
- No evidence of spread of infection to others
- Attains and maintains adequate food intake
- Able to maintain a clear airway by effective coughing and deep breathing
- Breathing pattern is normal
- Remains oriented and mentally clear
- Understands treatment regimen, preventive measures or procedures to be carried out after discharge

Decreased Function of the Lower Respiratory Airway

Pulmonary Emphysema

Pulmonary emphysema is a chronic disorder of the lungs characterized by specific morphologic changes in lung tissue, namely, distention of the alveolar sacs, rupture of the alveolar walls, and destruction of the alveolar capillary bed. This process of lung destruction occurs over a long period.

In this disease, the alveoli of the lungs have lost elasticity, resulting in the trapping of air that normally should be expired. On microscopic examination, the walls of the alveoli have broken down, forming one large sac instead of multiple small air spaces. The capillary bed previously located within the alveolar walls is destroyed and much of the tissue replaced by fibrous scarring. This formation of fibrous tissue and the destruction of the alveoli prevent the proper exchange of oxygen and carbon dioxide during respiration. As the disease progresses, large air sacs (bullae, blebs) may be seen over the surface of the lung. These sacs can rupture, with the result that air enters the thorax, called *pneumothorax*, with each respiration. When this condition occurs, an emergency thoracentesis is performed to remove the air in the thoracic cavity. A chest tube may be inserted to keep further air from entering. Repeat episodes of pneumothorax may require thoracic surgery to correct the problem.

Symptoms

Shortness of breath occurring with minimal activity is called *exertional dyspnea.* It is often one of the first symptoms of pulmonary emphysema. As the disease progresses, the breathlessness may continue even at rest. A chronic cough is invariably present and is productive of mucopurulent sputum. Inspiration is difficult because of the rigid chest cage, and the patient must use the accessory muscles of respiration to maintain normal ventilation. Expiration is prolonged, difficult, and often accompanied by wheezing. In advanced emphysema, respiratory function is markedly impaired. The appearance of these patients is characteristic. They look drawn, anxious, and pale, and speak in short, jerky sentences. When sitting up, they often lean slightly forward and are markedly short of breath. Often the neck veins distend during expiration.

In advanced pulmonary emphysema, a patient may have loss of memory, drowsiness, confusion, and loss of judgment. These changes caused by the marked reduction in oxygen that reaches the brain and the increased amount of carbon dioxide in the blood. If untreated, the level of carbon dioxide in the blood may reach toxic levels, resulting in lethargy, stupor, and finally coma. This is called *carbon dioxide narcosis.*

Diagnosis

A thorough history usually reveals many of the symptoms of pulmonary emphysema, which can sometimes be diagnosed on the basis of the history alone. Physical examination may reveal classic signs that can be confirmed on radiographic films and by fluoroscopy. Tests of pulmonary function may indicate characteristic changes. Blood gas studies help assess the state of blood gas exchange across the lung.

Treatment

Symptomatic treatment is similar to that in chronic bronchitis. Efforts to increase pulmonary ventilation by reducing bronchospasm include the use of bronchodilators. Unfortunately, as patients reach advanced stages of the disease, they may respond poorly to bronchodilator therapy. The use of expectorants, humidity control, and postural drainage is necessary to remove excess respiratory secretions. The control of infection is important and may be achieved by increasing the patient's resistance, avoiding contact with people who have a respiratory infection, and using antibiotics. Oxygen may be necessary in severe obstructive disease if the arterial oxyhemoglobin saturation is significantly reduced. The use of oxygen in high concentrations, however, *can be dangerous* if the level of carbon dioxide in the patient's blood has increased.

The respiratory center of the brain usually is sensitive to the level of carbon dioxide in the blood; if the level increases slightly, the respiratory rate and depth increase to eliminate the excess carbon dioxide. If, however, the carbon dioxide level is chronically elevated, the respiratory center becomes insensitive to carbon dioxide changes. Under these circumstances, the level of oxygen in the blood becomes a regulatory factor—the hypoxic drive to respiration. As long as the level of oxygen saturation of the blood is low, a patient tends to breathe effectively to maintain oxygenation. Should a patient suddenly be given 100% (or any other high concentration) oxygen by mask or other means, the hypoxic drive to respiration is lost and the respiratory rate drops, leading to the further retention of carbon dioxide, apnea, and death.

If a patient with emphysema requires oxygen, the safest method of administration is by nasal catheter or cannula, with the oxygen flow rate set at no more than 2 or 3 L/min. If a patient's color improves but the level of consciousness decreases, oxygen administration should be discontinued and the physician notified; the patient may be approaching a state of respiratory arrest.

If a patient is not helped by the prescribed treatment regimen, progressive loss of sleep, appetite, weight, and physical strength may occur. A patient often has many complaints and may show signs of depression and anxiety based on fear of suffocation. As the disease progresses, these patients may need to curtail many of their activities.

Pneumoconiosis

Pneumoconiosis is an inclusive term that describes any disease of the lung caused by the inhalation of dust; however, it usually refers to diseases caused by the inhalation of silica (*silicosis*), coal dust, or asbestos (*asbestosis*). Exposure to asbestos particles has been implicated as a cause of lung cancer.

Pneumoconiosis is common among those who work in industries in which exposure to these substances is prolonged. Only the tiny particles of dust reach the lung; the larger ones are trapped in the respiratory passages. The tiny particles are the most hazardous, as they cause irritation and gradual fibrosis of lung tissue.

Symptoms

The lung tissue loses its elasticity, and its vital capacity is reduced. Dyspnea and cough are the most common symptoms.

Diagnosis

The diagnosis is based on the history of exposure, chest radiograph, and pulmonary function studies.

Treatment

Treatment is usually conservative because the disease is widespread rather than localized. Surgery is rarely of value. Infections, when they occur, are treated with antibiotics. Other treatment modalities include oxygen administration if severe dyspnea is present, improved nutrition, and adequate rest. Many people with an advanced form are permanently disabled.

The primary focus is on prevention, with frequent examination of those who work in areas where dust is present in high concentration. When possible, industry is encouraged to remove dust from the working area. Workers found to have early signs of the disease should change occupations.

Pulmonary Hypertension

Pulmonary hypertension exists when the pulmonary arterial pressure is greater than 30 mm Hg systolic and 10 mm Hg diastolic. Primary pulmonary hypertension is rare and has an unknown cause. Secondary pulmonary hypertension is usually related to heart or lung disease.

Symptoms

The most common symptom is dyspnea on exertion. Additional signs and symptoms are those of the underlying cardiac or pulmonary disease and include chest pain, fatigue, weakness, distended neck veins, and peripheral edema.

Diagnosis

Diagnosis is made by a patient's history and physical examination. Diagnostic studies include an electrocardiogram (ECG), cardiac catheterization, chest radiograph, and pulmonary angiography.

Treatment

Treatment of primary pulmonary hypertension includes administration of drugs such as nitroprusside (Nipride), hydralazine (Apresoline), and isoproterenol (Isuprel). The primary form of this disorder has a poor prognosis; thus certain patients may be considered as candidates for heart–lung transplantation. Treatment of secondary pulmonary hypertension includes management of the underlying cardiac or pulmonary disease. Oxygen administration is commonly used to increase pulmonary arterial oxygenation.

Pulmonary Embolism

An *embolus* is any foreign substance, such as a particle of fat or a clot, that travels in the bloodstream. A clot that has formed in a vein becomes dislodged and travels toward the heart and lungs. Often, the clot occludes one of the pulmonary vessels, causing infarction (necrosis or death), which is later replaced by scarring of the lung tissue. Most pulmonary emboli arise from venous clots in the lower extremities and pelvis. Emboli also may arise from the endocardium of the right ventricle when that side of the heart was the site of a myocardial infarction. Other conditions that cause pulmonary embolus include recent surgery, prolonged bed rest, fracture or trauma of the lower extremities, the postpartum state, and debilitating diseases.

Symptoms

When a smaller area of the lung is involved, symptoms are usually less severe and include pain, tachycardia, and dyspnea. Fever, cough, and blood-streaked sputum also may be seen. Larger infarcted areas produce more pronounced symptoms such as severe dyspnea, severe pain, cyanosis, tachycardia, and shock. Sudden death can also follow a massive pulmonary infarction.

Diagnosis

Pulmonary embolism almost always occurs suddenly. The most important nursing task is early recognition of this problem followed by an immediate report to the physician of the patient's symptoms and vital signs. Diagnostic studies, such as serum enzymes, chest radiographs, and ECGs, are ordered immediately. In addition, a lung scan, CT scan, or pulmonary angiogram also may be performed.

Treatment

An intravenous infusion is started as soon as possible to establish a patent vein before shock becomes profound. Hypotension requires administration of vasopressors such as metaraminol (Aramine) or levarterenol (Levophed). Oxygen is given for dyspnea and analgesics for pain and apprehension. Vital signs are monitored, and the patient is assessed at frequent intervals for changes. Continuous ECG monitoring is usually indicated, as right ventricular failure is a common problem. Intake and output are monitored, and frequent electrolyte and arterial blood gas studies are usually performed.

Treatment of a pulmonary embolus depends on the size of the area involved and a patient's symptoms. Intravenous heparin is usually ordered to prevent extension of the thrombus and the development of additional thrombi in veins from which the embolus arose. Other measures such as complete bed rest, oxygen, and analgesics also are used.

A pulmonary embolectomy, using cardiopulmonary bypass to support circulation while the embolus is removed, may be necessary if the embolus is lodged in a main pulmonary artery. Recurrent episodes of pulmonary embolism may be treated by insertion of an umbrella filter device in the vena cava. The umbrella filter is inserted by an applicator catheter inserted into the right internal jugular vein and threaded downward to an area below the renal arteries. Another surgical treatment is the insertion of Teflon clips on the inferior vena cava. These clips narrow the channel of the vena cava, allowing blood to pass through on its return to the right side of the heart but keeping back large blood clots.

Atelectasis

Atelectasis is the collapse of lung tissue. In some instances, the collapse may be limited to a small area of the lung. At other times, larger areas of the lung may be affected.

Atelectasis may be caused by aspiration of food or vomitus, a mucus plug, fluid or air in the thoracic cavity, or by compression on lung tissue by tumors, an enlarged heart, aneurysm, or enlarged lymph nodes in the thoracic or upper abdominal cavity. Common causes are the inability to breathe deeply and to cough and raise secretions plus prolonged bed rest.

Symptoms

A small area of atelectasis may cause few, if any, symptoms. When a larger area is affected, a patient experiences cyanosis, fever, dyspnea, increased pulse and respiratory rate, and increased pulmonary secretions. On auscultation, a crackling noise may be heard.

Diagnosis

Diagnosis is made by a patient's symptoms, chest radiograph, and auscultation of the lungs.

Treatment

Treatment includes improving ventilation and suctioning or instructing a patient to deep breathe and cough to raise secretions. Oxygen may be administered for dyspnea. When due to conditions such as tumors, infection, or fluid or air in the thoracic cavity, removal of the cause usually corrects the disorder.

The main focus should be on prevention of atelectasis, especially when due to failure to aerate the lungs properly. Deep breathing and coughing after any type of surgery can prevent atelectasis.

Bronchial Asthma

Bronchial asthma has been divided into two types. *Extrinsic asthma* occurs chiefly in response to allergens, such as pollen, dust, spores, or animal danders. *Intrinsic asthma* has been associated with upper respiratory infection or emotional upsets.

Asthma may occur at any period of life. A significant relationship has been noted between bronchiolitis (inflammation of the bronchioles) in the first year of life and the development of bronchial asthma in early childhood. Extrinsic asthma is the most common form noted in childhood and young adulthood. Intrinsic asthma, due to recurrent infection frequently related to chronic sinusitis or chronic bronchitis, is most often seen after age 40. Asthma may be limited to occasional attacks, and a patient is usually symptom-free between attacks.

The triad characteristic of the acute asthmatic state consists of spasm of the smooth muscle of the bronchi and the larger bronchioles, swelling of the mucosal lining, and thick bronchiole secretions. The degree of airflow obstruction is directly related to the severity of these mechanisms. Once the air has entered the alveoli, it is trapped because the bronchioles and bronchi are narrowed during the expiratory effort. The attempt to move air across a narrowed orifice results, and the wheezing typical of asthma is heard.

Symptoms

Bronchial asthma is typified by paroxysms of shortness of breath, wheezing, cough, and the production of thick, tenacious sputum. The onset and duration of the acute episode vary markedly among people. The duration may be brief, lasting less than a day, or extend into prolonged periods of several weeks.

The classic wheezing that is heard on auscultation of the chest also may be audible without the stethoscope. Patients are usually aware of the wheezing and report it as one of their symptoms. Every breath becomes an effort, and, during the acute episode, the work of breathing is greatly increased. A patient may suffer from a sensation of suffocation. Frequently, a classic sitting position is assumed with the body leaning slightly forward and the arms at shoulder height. This position facilitates expansion of the chest and more effective excursions of the diaphragm. Because life depends on the power to breathe, fear accompanies the symptoms. Unfortunately, fear and anxiety tend to intensify the symptoms.

The effort to move trapped air within the alveoli is accompanied by a marked prolongation of the expiratory phase of respiration. Coughing commences with the onset of the attack but is ineffective in the early stage. Only as the attack begins to subside is a patient able to expectorate large quantities of thick, stringy mucus. The skin is usually pale; if the attack is severe, however, cyanosis of the lips and nail beds may be noted. Perspiration is usually profuse during an acute attack. After spontaneous or drug-induced remission of the episode, examination of the lungs commonly reveals normal findings.

Occasionally, however, an acute attack can intensify and progress into *status asthmaticus* (persistent state of asthma).

Diagnosis

A complete patient history, including a detailed description of symptoms, may establish a diagnosis. Pulmonary function studies and chest radiograph may be performed to aid in the diagnosis. In some instances, it may be difficult for the physician to diagnose this disorder without observation during the acute attack.

Treatment

Symptomatic treatment is given at the time of the attack. Long-term care involves measures to treat as well prevent further attacks. Efforts must be made to determine the cause of the attacks. If a patient's history and diagnostic tests indicate that allergy is an important causative factor, treatment includes avoidance of the allergen, desensitization, or antihistamines.

Oxygen is usually not necessary during an acute attack because most patients with bronchial asthma are actively hyperventilating. Rarely, but particularly after a long bout of asthma, patients may develop cyanosis. Oxygen may be prescribed for a patient if cyanosis should occur. The physician specifies how the oxygen is to be administered (ie, by mask, nasal catheter, or other means) and the liter flow to be used.

A bronchodilator may be prescribed. Examples of bronchodilators include adrenergic drugs, such as epinephrine, isoproterenol, and terbutaline (Bricanyl), and the xanthine derivatives, such as aminophylline and theophylline. Adrenergic medications are most commonly used in the treatment of acute bronchial asthma. These agents tend to reduce bronchospasm by causing relaxation of the smooth muscle lining the bronchi and the larger bronchioles.

Adrenergic agents are extremely effective bronchodilators when given by nebulizer, which delivers the drug directly into the lung and has the advantage of providing maximal effect on the bronchial musculature. Although adverse drug effects do occur, they are limited compared to subcutaneous injection.

Aminophylline is effective in reducing bronchospasm. It is most useful when administered intravenously in a dose of 25 to 50 mg. The drug is injected slowly over a period of about 10 minutes to avoid a sudden drop in blood pressure, dizziness, faintness, palpitation, and headache. Aminophylline may be given over an 8-hour period in 500 to 1,000 mL of intravenous fluid. The use of aminophylline as a rectal suppository is valuable and effective. Most patients develop anorectal irritation, however, if the dose exceeds 0.5 g every 12 hours.

Corticosteroids are not generally used in the treatment of a patient with uncomplicated bronchial asthma. Should the disease progress, the physician may order these drugs by the oral route.

Humidification of the inspired air is valuable in the treatment of asthma. It has been shown that dehydration of the respiratory mucous membrane by itself may lead to attacks of bronchial asthma. The use of steam or cool vapor humidifiers has proved effective. Liquefaction of the secretions promotes more effective clearing of the airways and a rapid return to normal. Air conditioners may help eliminate offending allergens as well as control temperature and humidity.

Chronic Obstructive Pulmonary Disease

Chronic obstructive pulmonary disease (COPD) is a broad term used to describe a group of pulmonary disorders that affect the expiratory airflow. Asthma, chronic bronchitis, advanced bronchiectasis, and emphysema are disorders that ultimately can result in COPD.

The exact cause of COPD is unknown. The frequent association of chronic bronchitis with the development of severe COPD suggests more than a casual relationship. Causative factors cited in the section on chronic bronchitis are of obvious importance. These include smoking, respiratory infection, air pollution, and allergy. The constant irritation of the tracheobronchial tree and the suppression of normal cilia function in the respiratory airways predispose the respiratory tract to chronic infection. Repeated pulmonary infection can result in alteration of lung structure and destruction of pulmonary tissue. Pollutants, such as nitrogen dioxide and sulfur dioxide, can chronically irritate the tracheobronchial linings and cause permanent changes. Industrial exposure to coal dust, asbestos, cotton fibers, and molds and other fungi has resulted in COPD. Hereditary factors have also been incriminated. The disease is more prevalent and of greater morbidity and mortality in men than in women. Aging also may play a role in causing this disease. Normal manifestations of the aging process are overaeration of the lung and enlargement of the alveolar sacs. Destruction of alveolar walls and change in the pulmonary capillary bed have not been noted, however, as part of the aging process.

Symptoms

Symptoms include dyspnea (eg, on exertion, when at rest), increased pulse and respiratory rate, peripheral edema and distended neck veins (due to right-sided heart failure in the later stage of the disease), cyanosis, fatigue, anorexia, cough, and mental changes (due to a decreased supply of oxygen to the brain).

Diagnosis

Diagnosis is based on a patient's symptoms and medical history. A chest radiograph, sputum for microscopic examination, and pulmonary function studies may be used to establish a diagnosis.

Treatment

Treatment is aimed at relieving symptoms, improving respiratory function, and preventing further changes in lung tissue. Drug therapy may use one or several agents, including bronchodilators to improve breathing, diuretics to reduce peripheral edema, cardiotonic drugs to improve the strength of myocardial contraction, and oxygen therapy for severe dyspnea and cyanosis.

Preventive measures mainly focus on delaying further involvement of lung tissue by treating the original cause. For example, if a patient has chronic bronchitis due to smoking, stopping tobacco use would prevent recurrent irritation of the bronchi and, thus, progression of the disease.

RESPIRATORY FAILURE

Acute Respiratory Failure

Acute respiratory failure is a life-threatening condition in which alveolar ventilation cannot maintain the body's need for oxygen supply and carbon dioxide removal. This condition results in a fall in arterial oxygen (hypoxemia) and a rise in arterial carbon dioxide (hypercapnia). The many causes of acute respiratory failure include oversedation, anesthesia administration, head injury, chest trauma (including chest surgery), upper abdominal surgery, hemothorax, pneumothorax, and pneumonia. Neurologic diseases, such as myasthenia gravis, multiple sclerosis, and amyotrophic lateral sclerosis (AML), also may result in acute respiratory failure.

Symptoms

Apprehension, dyspnea, wheezing, and possibly cyanosis and use of the accessory muscles of respiration are usually seen in those with acute respiratory failure. If untreated or if treatment fails to relieve respiratory distress, cardiac dysrhythmias, hypotension, congestive heart failure, respiratory acidosis, and adult respiratory distress syndrome (see later discussion) can occur.

Diagnosis

Diagnosis of acute respiratory distress is based on symptoms and patient history (eg, surgery, a known neurologic disorder). Arterial blood gas studies also may be drawn.

Treatment

Treatment for acute respiratory failure is to establish a patent airway (if upper respiratory airway obstruction is present) by use of an oral airway, endotracheal intubation, or a tracheostomy. Additional treatments include administration of humidified oxygen by nasal cannula, Venturi mask, or a reservoir mask. Mechanical ventilation using intermittent positive pressure ventilation (IPPV) also may be used. When possible, the original cause of respiratory failure is treated.

Adult Respiratory Distress Syndrome

Patients that do not respond to treatment for acute respiratory failure may develop adult respiratory distress syndrome (ARDS). Other conditions that may result in ARDS include pneumonia, shock of any cause, drug overdose, pneumonitis that results from radiation therapy to the chest, drowning, uremia, pancreatitis, and smoke inhalation.

Symptoms

In a patient with ARDS, severe respiratory distress develops about 8 to 48 hours after the onset of illness or injury. The respiratory rate rises, breathing is shallow and labored, cyanosis occurs, and the intercostal muscles retract. The sternocleidomastoid muscles in the neck also may become prominent as the patient attempts to pull more air into the lungs. Distress is not relieved by oxygen administration, and the patient's condition becomes worse. The patient appears fearful and is extremely restless. Lack of oxygen to the brain (cerebral anoxia) ultimately develops and is followed by mental confusion, agitation, and finally drowsiness. Death may result if the condition is not recognized and treated.

Diagnosis

Diagnosis is based on a patient's symptoms, history, and arterial blood gas studies.

Treatment

The initial cause of ARDS must be identified and then treated. In addition, oxygen is administered along with humidification. A patent airway is established by means of tracheal intubation or a tracheostomy. Mechanical ventilation is often necessary. Positive end-expiratory pressure (PEEP), which means that the pressure in the respiratory airway is higher than atmospheric pressure, may be used if a patient is on mechanical ventilation. Normally, mechanical ventilators raise airway pressure during inspiration and let it fall to atmospheric (or zero) pressure during expiration (called IPPV). When a mechanical ventilator and PEEP are used, positive airway pressure exists on inspiration, expiration, and at the end of expiration. This process is also called continuous positive pressure ventilation. If a patient is able to breathe without mechanical assistance, PEEP also may be used; this process is called continuous positive airway pressure. A tight-fitting oxygen face mask is used, along with a PEEP device. Complications associated with the use of PEEP include pneumothorax and pneumomediastinum.

Although most patients benefit from the use of PEEP, some may succumb to complications associated with PEEP or the underlying cause of the disorder.

Chronic Respiratory Failure

Chronic respiratory failure is seen in those with chronic respiratory disorders, such as emphysema and chronic bronchitis. The difference between acute and chronic respiratory failure is that the lower respiratory airway is normal until the time acute failure occurs; whereas, in chronic failure, loss of lung function is progressive and, in most cases, irreversible.

Symptoms

Symptoms are those of the underlying cause (eg, symptoms of emphysema or chronic bronchitis).

Diagnosis

Diagnosis is based on a patient's symptoms, past history of a respiratory disorder, and arterial blood gas studies.

Treatment

Chronic respiratory failure requires long-term treatment of the underlying cause. In many cases, the disorder becomes progressive.

NURSING PROCESS —THE PATIENT WHO HAS DECREASED FUNCTION OF THE LOWER RESPIRATORY AIRWAY

Assessment

The patient with decreased function of the lower respiratory airway has varying degrees of respiratory distress. Initial assessment includes recognizing the degree of respiratory distress and evaluating the patient's status.

Unless a patient has severe respiratory distress, complete medical, drug, and allergy histories are obtained, vital signs are taken, and the patient is weighed.

Depending on the probable cause of decreased function and the condition of the patient, areas that may be involved in the initial assessment include the following:

Chest and Abdomen
- Respiratory rate, pattern, depth
- Evidence of trauma to the chest wall
- Abnormal shape of the chest (eg, barrel-chested)
- Auscultation of the lungs for normal and abnormal breath sounds

- Observation of chest movements during inspiration and expiration
- Evidence of abdominal distention
- Use of abdominal or intercostal muscles during respiration

Vital Signs
Skin and Accessory Structures (Lips, Nail Beds, Oral Mucosa)
- Color (eg, pale, cyanotic)
- General skin condition (eg, cool, warm, diaphoretic)

Head and Neck
- Use of neck muscles during inspiration
- Position of trachea (eg, midline, deviated)
- Distention of jugular veins
- Evidence of trauma to head, neck structures

Extremities
- Evidence of edema, clubbing of the fingers, toes

Mental Status
- Evidence of confusion, delirium, severe anxiety, restlessness, disorientation or other mental changes

General
- Physical appearance with respect to general body build and weight

The position that the patient assumes to facilitate breathing is noted. For example, a patient with emphysema often leans forward, placing the hands on the knees or arms of a chair in an effort to inspire and expire more air. The respirations are usually noisy, the cheeks may puff out, and the lips make a smacking noise as air is expired through the mouth.

Nursing Diagnosis

Depending on the severity and probable cause of decreased respiratory function, one or more of the following may be included in the nursing diagnoses. Causal relationships for each diagnosis may vary according to the patient's problem. Underlying medical conditions may require additional nursing diagnoses. If the patient requires a tracheostomy or endotracheal intubation, additional nursing diagnoses (see Nursing Process—Treatment Modalities of Airway Obstruction or Airway Maintenance) may be added.

- Anxiety related to inability to breathe, treatment modalities
- Fear related to inability to breathe
- Pain related to pulmonary embolus, pulmonary infection secondary to chronic respiratory disease
- Ineffective airway clearance related to thick secretions, inability to cough and raise secretions secondary to loss of lung elasticity
- Activity intolerance related to dyspnea, decreased respiratory function
- Feeding, bathing and hygiene, and dressing and grooming self-care deficits related to dyspnea, fatigue
- Potential for infection related to chronic respiratory disease

■ Fluid volume deficit related to decreased oral intake
■ Impaired skin integrity related to immobility
■ Altered oral mucous membrane related to mechanical ventilation, dry mucous membranes secondary to failure to take oral fluids, poor nutrition, other factors (specify)
■ Altered thought processes related to increased PCO_2, decreased PO_2, electrolyte imbalance
■ Knowledge deficit related to treatment modalities, prevention of infection, other (specify)

Planning and Implementation

The major goals of the patient include improvement of the breathing pattern, reduction of anxiety, prevention of infection, maintenance of an adequate fluid and food intake, and knowledge of ways to delay or halt progression of the disorder.

The major goal of nursing management is the improvement of pulmonary ventilation. Additional goals are based on patient assessment to determine individual needs.

Vital signs are monitored every 4 hours or at more frequent intervals if a patient is acutely ill. The respiratory rate, rhythm, and depth are closely monitored. Increased difficulty in breathing, cyanosis, and a change in pulse rate and rhythm are reported to the physician immediately.

If a patient suddenly appears acutely ill, has severe respiratory distress, is cyanotic, or has symptoms that indicate a possible pulmonary embolus or other severe lower respiratory problem, an intravenous line is established as an emergency measure (unless hospital policy dictates otherwise) and run to keep the vein open (*KVO*) until the physician sees the patient.

When drug therapy is prescribed for acute respiratory distress, it is important to note if symptoms are relieved. If symptoms are not relieved and the patient continues to have acute respiratory distress, the physician is notified.

Nursing Care Plan 22-1 is an example of nursing management of the patient with emphysema.

Anxiety and Fear. The inability to breathe or shortness of breath after mild activity may result in varying degrees of anxiety and fear. Patients can be easily discouraged for reasons such as poor response to therapy, poor prognosis, and the progression of their disease despite therapy. The nurse must first attempt to identify situations that cause anxiety and then try to modify those situations to improve the patient's emotional response.

A patient with acute respiratory distress or one on mechanical ventilation with a tracheostomy or endotracheal tube is often frightened. Either type of tube can quickly become obstructed with mucous. The patient is usually aware of this possibility and is often terrified of being left alone even for a moment.

To reduce anxiety and fear of suffocation, the patient is assessed at frequent intervals and tracheal suctioning is performed as needed.

When oxygen by mask or nasal cannula is administered to patients with a respiratory disorder, the nurse should explain the reason for the procedure. By providing an explanation, as well as by remaining with them until they are adjusted to the oxygen and equipment, the nurse helps to allay their anxiety and reduce the fear of suffocation.

Other methods of reducing anxiety include staying with patients (if possible) when severe respiratory distress occurs, listening to their concerns, and providing a way for them to signal for help.

Pain. When occurring suddenly, pain is brought to the attention of the physician; a change in the patient's status or a complication may have developed. Analgesics may be ordered for those with disorders such as pulmonary embolus or pneumonia associated with infection secondary to decreased function of the lower respiratory airway. The location, intensity, and type of pain is carefully evaluated, and the physician is informed if the pain is not relieved or becomes worse.

Respiratory Function. The airway of those with decreased lower respiratory function must be kept patent at all times. Depending on the patient's needs, the medical diagnosis, and the physician's orders, humidified oxygen, drug therapy, and suctioning may be used to keep the airway patent. The patient is observed at frequent intervals. Increased difficulty breathing, cyanosis, increased respiratory rate, or failure to cough and raise sputum effectively is reported to the physician.

Patients with decreased lower airway function may be candidates for impaired oxygen and carbon dioxide exchange in the lungs. Drugs, such as bronchodilators, increase the diameter of the bronchi and, therefore, increase the amount of inspired air as well as help the patient raise secretions. The administration of humidified oxygen also may be effective. Patients are also encouraged to take deep breaths at regular intervals. The physician may tell the patient to perform brief deep-breathing exercises as often as possible, such as every 15 to 30 minutes. The nurse must periodically remind the patient to do these exercises.

Breathing exercises may be prescribed for patients with emphysema. Therapeutic breathing exercises effectively use the diaphragm, thus relieving the compensatory burden on the muscles of the upper thorax. Patients are taught to let the abdomen rise as they take a deep breath and to contract the abdominal muscles as they exhale. They can feel the correct

Nursing Care Plan 22–1

Nursing Management of the Patient With Emphysema

Potential Problem and Potential Nursing Diagnosis	Nursing Intervention	Evaluation
Dyspnea *Altered respiratory function related to loss of lung elasticity*	Administer bronchodilating drugs, antibiotics, and other medications as ordered; instruct to avoid activities that result in severe dyspnea; encourage frequent rest periods; teach pursed-lip and diaphragmatic breathing; administer IPPB treatments as ordered	Respiratory rate reduced; patient feels in control of his breathing; activities spaced by patient to reduce exertional dyspnea
Difficulty in Raising Secretions *Altered respiratory function related to loss of lung elasticity*	Encourage an increased fluid intake (unless contraindicated) administer mucolytics as ordered; humidify surrounding air; teach and encourage use of postural drainage (if procedure can be tolerated)	Raises secretions with less difficulty
Fatigue *Altered respiratory function related to loss of lung elasticity*	Plan rest periods before and after activities (meals, morning care, ambulation, etc.); advise to rest during long activities; allow patient to perform activities at his own rate; work with physical or occupational therapist in planning and implementing an exercise program	Experiences less fatigue during activities
Anorexia; Poor Eating Habits; Weight Loss *Altered nutrition (less than body requirements) related to anorexia, dysphagia*	Offer interval feedings; have patient select foods that are liked; offer small, frequent meals instead of three large meals to increase dietary intake; alow rest period before meals; offer oral care before as well as after meals; weigh two or three times weekly; contact dietitian for discharge dietary planning of a well-balanced, nutritious diet	Maintains weight or gains weight; appetite improves
Infection *Potential for infection related to chronic respiratory disorder*	Instruct patient to avoid smoking, those with infections, temperature extremes, indiscriminate use of nonprescription drugs (especially those for respiratory disorders); personnel with infections are not given responsibility for patient care; family informed of importance of limiting patient contact if a member has an infection; advise of importance in contacting the physician if illness, infection, increased dyspnea, increased cough, sputum production or hemoptysis occur; advise patient of importance of a well-balanced, nutritious diet; monitor temperature one to four times per day; instruct patient in the signs and symptoms of an infection	Does not develop an infection during hospitalization; is able to list signs of infection
Progression of Disease *Altered health maintenance*	Instruct patient to avoid smoking, heavily polluted air, respiratory infections, environmental irritants; emphasize importance of adherence to the prescribed regimen and physician's recommendations; discuss signs and symptoms of an infection; include family in all teaching sessions	Able to list signs of infection, situations to be avoided

way to do this exercise by placing one hand on the chest and the other on the abdomen: during abdominal breathing, the patient's chest should remain quiet, and the abdomen should rise and fall with each breath. Other exercises include practice in blowing out candles at various distances and blowing a small object, such as a pencil or a piece of chalk, along a table top. Patients are encouraged to exhale more completely by taking a deep breath and then bending the body forward at the waist while they exhale as fully as possible. Pursed-lip breathing, that is, breathing with the lips pursed or puckered on expiration, helps patients control their respiratory rate and depth and slows expiration. Use of this maneuver helps control dyspnea and, in turn, reduces the anxiety that may be associated with breathing difficulties.

If a patient with emphysema requires oxygen, the safest method of administration is by nasal catheter or cannula, with the oxygen flow rate set at no more than 2 or 3 L/min. If the patient's color improves but somnolence increases, oxygen administration is discontinued and the physician notified; the patient may be approaching a state of respiratory arrest.

Activity Intolerance and Self-Care Deficits. Exertional dyspnea may make carrying out activities of daily living difficult. Management of patients with this condition can be planned so that these activities are spaced throughout the waking hours and the patient is given time to rest between each activity. Patients are encouraged to do as much for themselves as possible; however, they are assisted as needed. Allowing patients to perform easy tasks at their own pace offers encouragement and helps them feel that they are not totally dependent on others.

Potential for Infection. Patients with pulmonary disorders are subject to infections. Nurses or visitors with upper respiratory infections should avoid contact with the patient. The physician is notified if any symptoms of respiratory infection—fever, chills, chest pain, purulent sputum—are apparent.

The asthmatic patient's environment should be as free as possible of factors that contribute to respiratory infection. The patient should be protected from exposure to allergens that may have set off attacks or that may perpetuate them. Thorough cleanliness of all inhalation therapy equipment is essential.

Fluid Volume Deficit. An increased respiratory rate, frequent suctioning, or failure to take oral fluids can lead to a fluid volume deficit. Fluids are offered at frequent intervals, not only to prevent a fluid volume

deficit but also to loosen and thin respiratory secretions.

Intake and output are measured, and the physician is informed if the patient fails to take an adequate amount of oral fluids or the urinary output falls below 500 mL/day.

Impaired Skin Integrity and Altered Oral Mucous Membrane. A patient with acute respiratory distress or one on mechanical ventilation is relatively immobile and subject to skin breakdown and decubitus formation. To prevent skin breakdown, a patient's position is changed every 2 hours. If a patient cannot be turned, pressure points must be massaged and inspected for evidence of skin breakdown every 2 hours.

The oral mucous membranes also may be affected when mechanical ventilation is used or when a patient fails to drink sufficient fluids. Oral care for those with endotracheal intubation includes cleaning the mouth and teeth and lubricating the lips. Patients able to take oral fluids are encouraged to sip water frequently.

Altered Thought Processes. Patients may exhibit signs of mental changes due to hypoxemia or hypercapnia. They may become confused and disoriented and require supervision or frequent observation. If a patient suddenly becomes confused or confusion appears worse, the physician is notified.

Knowledge Deficit. Patients may be required to perform certain treatments at home. Education is an important part of therapy and is aimed at helping patients adjust to their present state of disability and adjust to the possibility of increased disability over time. The primary goal of patient and family education is to prevent (if possible) or delay progression of the disorder. Patients should be presented with individualized ways to slow disease progression and improve their present physical status. It is important to emphasize that successful results depend largely on cooperation and strict adherence to the treatment regimen prescribed by the physician. An approach that emphasizes day-to-day progress, however slight, often helps these patients adhere to the regimen. Highly motivated patients profit more from the treatment available and, despite their severely damaged lungs, make the best use of the remaining pulmonary function.

The importance of continued medical supervision is stressed. The patient is reminded to contact the physician if any of the following occur: adverse drug effects, failure of drugs to relieve symptoms, the appearance of new symptoms, increase in severity of symptoms.

When patients are prescribed nebulized bronchodilator therapy, specific instructions for use are given to them. The effectiveness depends on the dose and proper delivery of the drug into the lung. If the product encloses drawings and instructions, these are reviewed with the patient.

The tip of the nebulizer, whether a hand-bulb or pressurized aerosol, is placed in the open mouth. The lips are *not* closed around the nebulizer. While breathing in, the bulb of the nebulizer is squeezed or the lever is pressed on the aerosol. In this manner, the nebulized material is carried with the air stream into the trachea, bronchi, and bronchioles.

Depending on the diagnosis and prescribed treatment modality, a discharge teaching plan is developed. An example of a teaching plan is shown in Chart 22-1. Other lower airway disorders may require that additional information be added to the teaching plan.

Evaluation

- Anxiety and fear are reduced
- Maintains a clear airway by effective coughing, deep breathing
- Activity tolerance shows improvement
- Breathing pattern is normal
- Blood gas studies are normal
- No evidence of infection; temperature normal
- Remains mentally clear and oriented
- Able to perform some (or all) of the activities of daily living
- Maintains adequate fluid and diet intake

Chart 22–1. Education of the Patient Who Has Emphysema

Things to Avoid
- Respiratory irritants (fumes, smoking, air pollutants, smog)
- Contact with individuals with respiratory infections
- Extremely cold weather or sudden changes in temperature
- Dry, heated areas
- Hot or cold fluids
- Emotional stress, fatigue

Things to Do
- Take medications as ordered.
- Drink extra fluids
- Eat a well-balanced diet.
- Perform breathing exercises at intervals suggested by the physician.
- Try to cough and raise sputum after treatment or use of nebulizer.
- Report any sign of respiratory infection promptly.
- Take frequent rests during the day.

- Demonstrates ability to perform the prescribed treatments
- Discusses and shows understanding of the recommended ways to improve physical status and slow progression of disease

MALIGNANT DISORDERS OF THE LOWER RESPIRATORY AIRWAY
Cancer of the Lung and Bronchus

Cancers of the lung and bronchus have shown a marked increase in incidence. More accurate diagnosis may be partly responsible; the growing number of older persons in the population, cigarette smoking, and the increasing air pollution in industrial centers may be other factors that contribute to higher incidence. Exposure to asbestos and radioactive dust and gases has also been implicated as a cause. Cancer of these structures is more common in men than women; however, the rate in women is on the rise. Most patients are older than 40 when the disease is discovered.

The lung is a common site of metastasis of cancer that originates in another part of the body. When a tumor originates in the lung (or any other area), it is called a *primary tumor*; tumors due to metastasis are called *secondary* or *metastatic tumors.*

Symptoms

Bronchogenic carcinoma, a malignant tumor that arises from the bronchial epithelium, is the most common type of lung cancer. Bronchogenic tumors often produce no symptoms at first; however, as the tumor enlarges, the patient may experience a cough productive of mucopurulent or blood-streaked sputum. The cough may be slight at first and attributed to smoking or other causes. As the disease advances, the patient experiences fatigue, weight loss, and anorexia. Dyspnea and chest pain occur late in the disease. Hemoptysis is not uncommon.

Cancer of lung tissue also produces few symptoms. Early symptoms, which are vague and not indicative of lung cancer, include anorexia, weight loss, fatigue, and chronic cough. Pain may not be seen until late in the disease.

Diagnosis

Early diagnosis of cancer of the lung is difficult because symptoms often do not appear until the course is well established. Diagnostic tests that may be used to detect lung cancer include chest radiography, bronchoscopy with bronchial washings and tissue biopsy, lung and bone scans, CT scan, magnetic resonance imaging, sputum examination for malignant cells, lymph node biopsy, and mediastinoscopy.

Treatment

Treatment of lung cancer depends on several factors. One major consideration is the classification and staging of the tumor. Four major cell types of lung cancer exist: (1) the large cell or undifferentiated type, (2) the small cell or oat cell type, (3) the epidermoid type or squamous cell, and (4) adenocarcinoma. After classification of the tumor, the stage of the disease is determined. Staging basically refers to the extent of the tumor: its location and the absence or presence and extent of metastasis. Staging is determined by various methods, depending on the patient's symptoms and the physician's findings during a physical examination, as well as the results of the tests and procedures performed for diagnosis.

Other factors that determine the treatment of lung cancer are the age and physical condition of the person and the presence of other diseases or disorders, such as renal disease or congestive heart failure.

Surgical removal of the tumor offers the only type of cure and usually is successful only in the early stages of the disease. Depending on the size and location of the tumor, lobectomy or pneumonectomy may be performed. A lymph node dissection also may be performed at the time of surgery.

Radiation therapy may help slow the spread of the disease and provide symptomatic relief by reducing tumor size, thus easing the pressure exerted by the tumor on adjacent structures. In turn, pain, cough, dyspnea, and hemoptysis may be relieved. In a small percentage of cases, radiation may be curative, but, for most patients, it is a palliative measure. Use of radiation therapy is not without danger, and complications associated with radiation to the chest include esophagitis, fibrosis of lung tissue, and pneumonitis.

Chemotherapy may be used either alone or with radiation therapy and surgery. The principal effect of chemotherapy is to slow tumor growth, and, like radiation, reduce tumor size and the pressure exerted by the tumor on adjacent structures. Chemotherapy is also used to treat metastatic lesions of areas such as the bone and brain. Most chemotherapeutic regimens use a combination of drugs rather than a single agent and, while not curative, often make the patient more comfortable.

The prognosis is poor unless the tumor was discovered in its early stages and treatment begun immediately. Because cancer of the lung presents few early symptoms, mortality is high. Metastasis occurs to the mediastinal and cervical lymph nodes, liver, brain, spinal cord, bone, and opposite lung.

Mediastinal Tumors

Tumors of the mediastinum in adults are often malignant and metastatic. These tumors include tumors of the thymus, lymphomas, and neurogenic tumors.

Symptoms

Tumors of the mediastinum may be asymptomatic. If symptoms do occur, they include chest pain, difficulty in swallowing, dyspnea, and orthopnea. Symptoms are often related to pressure of the tumor on other structures of the chest.

Diagnosis

Diagnosis is made by physical examination, chest radiograph, CT scan, mediastinoscopy, and biopsy.

Treatment

Malignant tumors of the mediastinum are almost always inoperable but may respond to radiation and chemotherapy.

NURSING PROCESS —THE PATIENT WHO HAS A MALIGNANT DISORDER OF THE LOWER RESPIRATORY AIRWAY

Assessment

Assessment is based on a patient's general condition. The patient with advanced carcinoma of the lung with metastasis or a metastatic tumor of the mediastinum is usually seriously ill, but patients in the advanced stages may not appear to be acutely ill.

Assessment should contain a history, including all symptoms noted by the patient, vital signs, weight, and auscultation of the lungs for normal and abnormal breath sounds. The history should also include a smoking history or history of exposure to environmental or occupational hazards, such as radiation or asbestos. The patient is asked about appetite, recent weight gain or loss, and problems associated with breathing, such as wheezing, bouts of coughing, hemoptysis, dyspnea, or orthopnea. The patient's general physical condition is also noted.

Management of the patient with lung cancer or a tumor of the mediastinum is essentially the same as that for any patient with a malignant disease. See Chapter 19 for the nursing diagnosis, planning, implementation, and evaluation of the patient with cancer. If thoracic surgery is performed, see Chapter 23.

THORACIC TRAUMA

All chest injuries are serious or potentially serious. Any patient with a chest injury must be observed for dyspnea, cyanosis, chest pain, weak and rapid pulse, and hypotension—all signs of respiratory distress. The patient with a chest injury is examined by a physician as soon as possible after the injury.

Fractured Ribs

Fractured ribs are a common form of injury to the chest and may be caused by a hard fall or by a blow to the chest. Automobile accidents are a frequent cause. Although rib fractures are painful, they usually are not serious unless injury to other structures results; for example, the sharp end of the broken bone may tear the lung or blood vessels. If the injury involves fractured ribs without other complications, the patient often is permitted to return home after emergency treatment.

Symptoms
Symptoms consist primarily of severe pain on inspiration and expiration.

Diagnosis
Chest radiographs (usually from several angles) are necessary to confirm the diagnosis.

Treatment
Treatment includes supporting the chest with an elastic bandage or a rib belt. Because immobilization of the rib cage can lead to decreased lung expansion followed by pulmonary complications such as pneumonia or atelectasis, the use of these devices is usually limited to multiple rib fractures. Analgesics such as codeine or pentazocine may be prescribed for pain. A regional nerve block is sometimes necessary to relieve pain.

Blast Injuries

Injuries that result from compression of the chest by an explosion, for example, cause serious damage to the lungs by rupturing the alveoli. Death often results from hemorrhage and asphyxiation.

Symptoms
Severe respiratory distress with outward evidence of chest trauma.

Diagnosis
Diagnosis is made by physical examination and a patient's symptoms. Additional diagnostic tests, such as chest radiograph and lung scan, may be necessary.

Treatment
If the patient survives the trauma, treatment includes complete bed rest and the administration of oxygen. A thoracentesis to remove air or fluid may be necessary. Patients may require surgery and insertion of chest tubes if severe injury to lung tissue has occurred.

Penetrating Wounds

Penetrating wounds of the chest are serious since an opening into the thorax, which on inspiration is at negative pressure, creates continuous and direct communication with the outside, which is always at positive pressure.

Symptoms
An open wound permits air to enter the thoracic cavity, causing a pneumothorax. If the wound is large, a sucking noise may be heard as air enters and leaves the chest cavity. Depending on the size of the wound, it takes seconds to hours before the lung collapses as the pressure in the thorax reaches atmospheric pressure. Many chest injuries involve both pneumothorax and hemothorax (blood in the pleural space).

Diagnosis
Diagnosis is based on history of an injury and physical examination and auscultation of the lungs. Radiographs determine the degree of lung collapse or the amount of air or blood in the thoracic cavity.

Treatment
Emergency treatment of pneumothorax caused by a penetrating wound includes the application of a tight pressure dressing over the site of injury. Air and the blood are aspirated from the pleural space by thoracentesis. A chest tube may be inserted and attached to an underwater seal drainage system (see Chapter 23). Later, it may be necessary to perform a thoracotomy (surgical opening of the thorax) to repair the injury. Foreign bodies that have entered the chest are removed only by the physician. Their presence in the wound may prevent or slow the entrance of air. Removal before the patient is transported to the hospital may result in continuous sucking of air into the chest, collapse of the lung, compression of the heart and opposite lung, and death.

NURSING PROCESS —THE PATIENT WHO HAS THORACIC TRAUMA

Assessment

Because the patient has had a traumatic injury, assessment is focused on, first, the extent and type of injury and, second, additional injuries to other organs and structures of the body. The patient's respiratory status is first assessed by observing the skin color and respiratory rate and pattern. Auscultation of the lungs is performed to determine abnormal or absent breath sounds. The external chest wall is inspected for evidence of trauma, such as penetrating wounds (eg, gunshot, stabbing wounds, foreign objects such as glass or metal), deep cuts, or a crushing injury.

Nursing Diagnosis

Depending on the type, extent, and seriousness of the injury, one or more of the following nursing diagnoses may apply. Additional diagnoses may be added as emergency treatment is instituted.

■ Anxiety and fear related to injury, inability to breathe
■ Pain related to injury (internal, external)
■ Ineffective breathing pattern related to pain, pneumothorax, hemothorax
■ Knowledge deficit of home care of rib fracture

Planning and Implementation

A thoracic injury can be serious and even life-threatening. After a rapid assessment of the type and extent of injury, treatment modalities are instituted immediately.

The major goals of the patient are to improve breathing, restore normal breathing function, and reduce pain.

The major goal of nursing management is to assist in the emergency restoration of normal lung function and breathing pattern.

Anxiety and Fear. If conscious, a patient may appear anxious and frightened. Staying with the patient, assuming a calm attitude until respiratory distress is relieved, and explaining any necessary treatment may reduce emotional distress. If movement or transportation is necessary, move the patient slowly and provide support to the upper body.

Pain. The physician may order a narcotic analgesic for pain. Because many narcotics depress the respiratory rate to a significant extent, the respiratory rate is counted before the drug is administered and then rechecked in 30 to 45 minutes. The physician is informed if the analgesic does not provide relief.

Ineffective Breathing Pattern. Oxygen is administered as needed until a diagnosis has been established and treatment started. If blood or air has entered the chest, the physician may perform an emergency thoracentesis and insert chest drainage tubes. The patient must be closely observed for *any* changes in respiratory status until breathing is normal.

Knowledge Deficit. Patients with a rib fracture and no other pulmonary problem are normally treated on an outpatient basis. The following can be included in patient teaching:

1. During waking hours, take a few deep breaths every 30 to 60 minutes (it is natural to take shallow breathes in the presence of chest pain).
2. Take the analgesic as ordered to minimize pain, promote rest, and permit more normal breathing.
3. Breathing is more comfortable when sitting than when lying flat.
4. If sudden, sharp chest pain or difficulty in breathing should occur, call the physician at once.

Evaluation

■ Anxiety, fear are reduced or eliminated
■ Pain is reduced or eliminated
■ Breathing pattern is normal
■ Understands treatment regimen for home care

General Nutritional Considerations

☐ The patient with increased respiration is encouraged to drink extra fluids to replace those lost through increased respiration and perspiration.
☐ If the patient eats poorly, frequent feedings of juice, broth, and eggnog may supplement the patient's nutritional needs.
☐ Adequate fluid intake is of great importance in reducing tenacious secretions.
☐ Adequate nutrition is a key to maintaining good general health, which reduces the patient's susceptibility to recurrent infections.

General Pharmacologic Considerations

☐ Antibiotics may be ordered for the patient with a respiratory infection; a culture and sensitivity test usually are performed to identify the microorganisms that are causing the infection. Once the microorganisms are identified and the sensitivity to various antibiotics is determined, the antibiotic proved to be effective is prescribed.

☐ The indiscriminate use of nonprescription cough medicines may do more harm than good. Coughing is the way the body clears the respiratory passages of mucus; depressing the cough reflex may cause a pooling of secretions and lead to further problems.

☐ Nonprescription medications advertised for colds and allergies may benefit some but are not indicated for everyone, and in some instances may be harmful. These preparations may contain atropine or other cholinergic blocking agents that are contraindicated in those with glaucoma and prostatic hypertrophy. Patients are cautioned to avoid these drugs and consult their physicians if they require medication.

☐ Patients with respiratory disease are advised to check with their physician before using nonprescription antitussive preparations (drugs used to prevent coughing). These drugs suppress the cough reflex and are contraindicated in diseases such as bronchiectasis and emphysema.

☐ Bronchodilators, for example aminophylline, may be used in the treatment of bronchospasm associated with some lower airway disorders.

☐ Antibiotics may be necessary to control chronic infection in those with COPD.

☐ When a narcotic is administered, the respiratory rate is counted before and 20 to 30 minutes after the drug is given. If the respiratory rate falls below 10 at either time, the physician must be notified immediately.

☐ Antitubercular drugs are usually given over long periods of time. The importance of drug therapy, namely adhering to the dose schedule and not omitting the drug, must be emphasized during patient teaching. Drug therapy is of value *only* when medications are taken exactly as prescribed.

General Gerontologic Considerations

☐ The elderly are more prone to pneumonia than are healthy adults and may be more acutely ill with this infection because of concomitant health problems, such as heart disease and diabetes.

☐ Before the flu season, the physician may recommend that a vaccine be administered before the anticipated outbreak. Elderly and debilitated patients are more likely to contract the disease and develop complications.

☐ The elderly patient, who is often subject to falls, may fracture one or more ribs and may be more susceptible to pneumonia after a rib fracture.

☐ Advanced pulmonary emphysema may result in memory loss, drowsiness, confusion, and loss of judgment. Because these same symptoms also may be seen in elderly patients with cerebral arteriosclerosis, symptoms of advanced pulmonary emphysema with carbon dioxide narcosis may be difficult to identify unless blood gas studies are performed.

☐ Elderly patients may require detailed explanation and sufficient time to understand the instructions given for participation in the management of their disease.

Suggested Readings

☐ Berkow R, Fletcher AJ, eds. Merck manual of diagnosis and therapy. 15th ed. Rahway, NJ: Merck & Co, 1987. *(In-depth coverage of subject matter)*

☐ Burton GRW. Microbiology for the health sciences. 3rd ed. Philadelphia: JB Lippincott, 1988. *(Additional coverage of subject matter)*

☐ Caine RM, Buffalino PM, eds. Nursing care planning guides for adults. Baltimore: Williams & Wilkins, 1987. *(Additional coverage of subject matter)*

☐ Carroll P. ARDS pathophysiology and the resulting signs and symptoms. Nursing '88 October 1988;18:74. *(Additional coverage and illustrations that reinforce subject matter)*.

☐ Daeschner SA. Action stat! Pulmonary embolism. Nursing '88 September 1988;18:33. *(Additional coverage of subject matter)*

☐ Davis NB. Danger signs: pleural friction rub. Nursing '88 January 1988;18:70. *(Additional coverage of subject matter)*

☐ Dupuis VG. Ventilators: theory and clinical application. St Louis: CV Mosby, 1986. *(In-depth coverage of subject matter)*

☐ Eggland E. Teaching the ABCs of COPD. Nursing '87 January 1987;17:60. *(Additional coverage of subject matter)*

☐ Eubanks DH, Bone RC, House LR. Comprehensive respiratory care: a learning system. 2nd ed. St Louis: CV Mosby, 1989. *(In-depth, high-level coverage of subject matter)*

☐ Fuller J, Schaller-Ayers J. Health assessment: a nursing approach. Philadelphia: JB Lippincott, 1990. *(Additional coverage of subject matter)*

☐ Hahn K. Slow-teaching the COPD patient. Nursing '87 April 1987;17:60. *(Additional coverage of subject matter)*

☐ Karnes N. Don't let ARDS catch you off guard. Nursing '87 May 1987;17:34. *(Additional coverage of subject matter)*

☐ Kersten LD. Comprehensive respiratory nursing. Philadelphia: WB Saunders, 1989. *(In-depth, high-level coverage of subject matter)*

☐ Mayo J, Hammer J. A nurse's guide to mechanical ventilation. RN August 1987;50:18. *(Additional coverage of subject matter)*

☐ McFarland MB, Grant MM. Nursing implications of laboratory tests. 2nd ed. New York: John Wiley & Sons, 1988. *(Additional and in-depth coverage of subject matter)*

☐ Mims BC. The risks of oxygen therapy. RN July 1987;50:20. *(Additional coverage of subject matter)*

☐ Moorhouse MF. Critical care. In: Berkow R, Fletcher AJ, eds. Merck manual of diagnosis and therapy. 15th ed. Rahway, NJ: Merck & Co, 1987. *(In-depth coverage of subject matter)*

☐ Smith AJ, Johnson JY. Nurses' guide to clinical procedures. Philadelphia: JB Lippincott, 1989. *(Additional and in-depth coverage of subject matter)*

☐ Taylor MC, Lillis C, LeMone P. Fundamentals of nursing: the art and science of nursing care. Philadelphia: JB Lippincott, 1989. *(Additional coverage of subject matter)*

☐ Wilkins RL, Sheldon RL, Krider SJ. Clinical assessment in respiratory care. 2nd ed. St Louis: CV Mosby, 1989. *(In-depth, high-level coverage of subject matter)*

☐ Wilkins RL, Hodgkin JE, Lopez B. Lung sounds: a practical guide. St Louis: CV Mosby, 1988. *(Additional and in-depth coverage of subject matter)*

Chapter 23

The Patient Who Undergoes Thoracic Surgery

On completion of this chapter the reader will:

- Discuss the preoperative and postoperative management of a patient who undergoes thoracic surgery

- Use the nursing process in the preoperative and postoperative management of a patient who undergoes thoracic surgery

- Draw and label the three types of underwater-seal drainage bottles and describe the function of each bottle

Thoracic surgery may be performed for a variety of conditions. Surgery on structures of the chest such as the lungs and heart requires opening the thoracic cavity, thus exposing it to atmospheric pressure (see Chapter 20). After most thoracic surgeries, chest tubes and a closed drainage system are used to remove excess air and fluid (eg, blood, serous fluid) from the chest. The chest tubes usually remain in place for several days and are not removed until the lung has fully expanded and most fluid has been removed from the chest.

A thoracentesis may be performed as an emergency measure to remove blood, fluid, or air from the chest. In some instances, it is necessary to perform a thoracotomy with insertion of a tube or tubes (tube thoracotomy) to remove air or fluid from the chest. A patient with severe dyspnea due to fluid or air in the chest is in a state of emergency, and local anesthesia may be needed for the procedure. Other types of chest trauma also require measures such as the emergency thoracentesis or tube thoracotomy.

Before surgery, diagnostic tests, such as a chest radiograph, lung scan, and computed tomographic scan, are performed to determine the diagnosis and to evaluate the condition of the heart and lungs.

NURSING PROCESS —THE PATIENT UNDERGOING THORACIC SURGERY

Preoperative Period

Assessment

Assessment should include vital signs and auscultation of the chest for normal and abnormal breath sounds, as well as noting the presence or absence of breath sounds in any area of the chest. The history of the present disorder should include the symptoms, the length of time they have been present, and what (if anything) makes the symptoms worse or better. The patient history must also include the presence of other medical disorders, an allergy history, and a smoking history. The patient's general appearance, including the breathing pattern and the presence or absence of cyanosis, is noted. The extremities are examined for edema.

If surgery is an emergency, physical assessment may need to be limited to a general statement of the patient's condition, a list of emergency measures or treatment performed, and vital signs.

The preoperative preparation normal for a patient who undergoes surgery is also carried out (see Chapter 16).

Nursing Diagnosis

The nursing diagnoses are based on the data obtained during assessment and may vary, depending on the condition of the patient and the physician's diagnosis. The nursing diagnoses should state the exact cause of the problem (eg, ineffective breathing pattern related to hemothorax) and include the following:

- Anxiety related to diagnosis and surgery
- Ineffective airway clearance related to inability to cough and raise secretions secondary to lung disease, thoracic trauma, other factors (specify)
- Knowledge deficit of the surgical procedure, equipment present after surgery, other factors (specify)

Planning and Implementation

The major goals of the patient include a reduction in anxiety, an understanding of the preparations required for surgery, and an understanding and practice of the tasks required of the patient after surgery.

The major goal of nursing management is to prepare the patient physically and emotionally for surgery.

Anxiety. Preoperative anxiety is normal, but the patient with a respiratory disorder often has additional anxiety related to the actual or possible diagnosis, the anticipation of surgery, and the inability to breathe effectively. The nurse must take time to listen to these patients, answer their questions, and let them express their fears. These patients require assurance that they will be closely observed during the postoperative period.

Ineffective Airway Clearance. Patients with a chronic pulmonary disorder may have difficulty raising secretions and keeping the airway clear. To help these patients raise secretions during the preoperative period, the physician may order humidified oxygen administration and bronchodilating drugs.

Knowledge Deficit. The physician explains the surgery and what treatments or equipment, such as chest tubes and drainage bottles, will be present when the patient returns from the operating room. A patient, however, may need additional explanations from the nurse. Because of the specialized procedures in the postoperative period, and because patient participation is essential to the success of the postoperative regimen, careful instructions about what to expect are especially important. The array of special equipment required for postoperative care can be frightening if a patient does not understand its purpose. Patients must be aware that the use of

specialized equipment after chest surgery is normal and does not indicate a complication. The patient may be shown equipment (eg, an oxygen nasal cannula or mask or an incentive spirometer). The patient should be taught to use an incentive spirometer before surgery. The importance of coughing, deep breathing, and moving after surgery is emphasized. Coughing and deep breathing are practiced before surgery. The patient can also be taught to take a deep breath and then forcefully expel air through the open mouth. This maneuver helps to expand lung tissue and often causes less postoperative discomfort than coughing.

Evaluation

- Anxiety is reduced or eliminated
- Demonstrates an understanding of the surgical procedure
- Performs coughing, deep-breathing exercises
- Gas exchange improved
- Able to clear airway effectively

Postoperative Period

In addition to the general principles of postoperative care that apply to any patient who has had surgery, the opening of the thoracic cavity requires certain special postoperative nursing measures.

One particularly significant problem of chest surgery is its interference with normal pressure relationships within the thoracic cavity (see Chapter 20). When the chest is opened, air from the atmosphere rushes in because of the negative pressure that normally exists in the thoracic cavity. The entrance of air under atmospheric pressure collapses the lung. The anesthesiologist inserts an endotracheal tube after the patient is anesthetized and ventilates the patient with oxygen during surgery.

After chest surgery, it usually is necessary to drain secretions, air, and blood from the thoracic cavity. Accumulation of air, blood and other fluids within the chest prevents reexpansion of the lung. Drainage ordinarily must be carried out by the closed (underwater) method (Figs. 23-1 through 23-3). Closed drainage of the thoracic cavity is accomplished by means of a catheter placed in the pleural space. The catheter is securely connected to an underwater seal apparatus. More commonly used in thoracic surgery are the several types and variations of commercial underwater seal systems (Fig. 23-4); the type used is selected by the physician. The principles illustrated here are essentially the same even though different kinds of chest drainage apparatuses may be used.

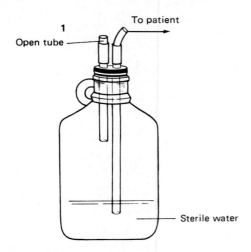

Figure 23–1. The one-bottle underwater seal drainage. The tube leading to the patient is always under water. As the patient inhales and exhales, the level of the water rises and falls in this tube.

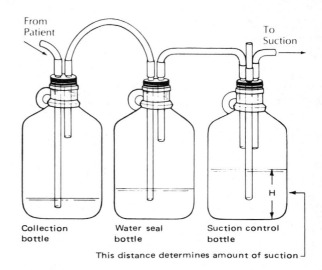

Figure 23–3. Three-bottle suction apparatus.

Chest fluid is allowed to drain underwater into a bottle or other device such as the Pleur-Evac system. When the one- or two-bottle system is used, the end of the drainage tube is kept underwater at all times to prevent air from being drawn up through the catheter into the pleural space. When the three-bottle system is used, the drainage tube in the collection bottle may or may not be placed underwater, depending on the surgeon's preference.

In the one-bottle system (see Fig. 23-1), fluid from the chest drains by gravity into a collection bottle. No suction is applied. In the two-bottle system (see Fig. 23-2), a sterile collection bottle, into which a measured amount of sterile water has been poured,

is used for collecting fluid from the chest. The collection bottle is connected by tubing to a trap bottle, which regulates the amount of suction being applied. The trap bottle is connected by tubing to a suction device. The physician regulates the amount of suction being applied by adjusting the position of a tube in the trap bottle—the length of tube that is submerged below the water level determines the amount of suction applied. The trap bottle lessens the degree of suction applied; therefore, it is used because the amount of suction applied by an ordinary suction device is too great to be applied to a chest catheter. The water in the trap bottle (in contrast to that in the chest drainage bottle) need not be sterile.

In the three-bottle system (see Fig. 23-3), the collection bottle is connected to a water seal bottle, which in turn is connected to a suction control bottle. The height of water in the suction control bottle regulates the amount of suction applied to the system.

Any break in the system, from either loose fittings or broken bottles, would possibly allow air to enter the tubing and be drawn up into the pleural space, collapsing the lung further. All connections of stoppers and tubing are taped carefully to minimize the possibility of a catheter end slipping off a connecting tip. Placing the drainage bottle in a holder is another precaution. The holder helps to protect the bottle from being knocked over and broken. More elaborate devices are also available to hold the bottles. Two or more large clamps must always be ready so that, if any break in the system occurs, the chest tube can be clamped immediately, as close to the chest wall as possible. The clamp is placed where it can be easily seen.

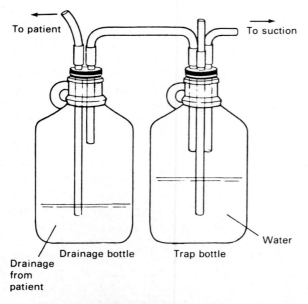

Figure 23–2. The two-bottle underwater seal.

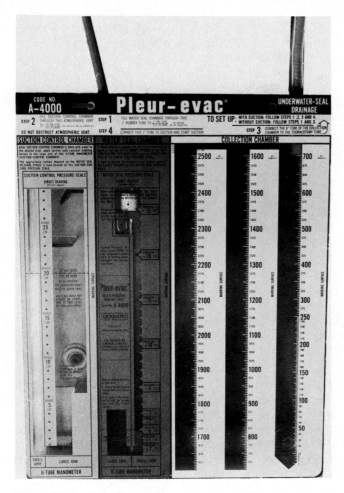

Figure 23–4. The Pleur-evac underwater-seal drainage system, in which the basic three-bottle setup is enclosed in one disposable unit. (Photograph by D. Atkinson)

Preventing fluids from flowing up through the catheter and entering the pleural space is also essential. While connected for drainage, the chest drainage bottle is *never* raised from floor level. Raising the bottle could result in a flow of fluid into the pleural space.

Often two chest catheters are used—one anteriorly and one posteriorly. In this instance, two bottles are used into which the chest drainage flows, and each is labeled "anterior" or "posterior." One clamp for each chest catheter is kept in readiness in case of a break in the drainage systems. The amount and character of the drainage in each bottle is noted and recorded separately.

The drainage tube must be patent to allow the escape of fluids from the pleural space. Clogging of the catheter, which may occur if a blood clot lodges in it or if it becomes kinked, causes drainage to stop. The lung does not expand, and the heart and great vessels may shift (mediastinal shift) to the opposite side. During the first hours immediately after surgery, the nurse must be constantly alert to the functioning of the drainage system so that if a malfunction occurs, it can be corrected immediately.

In the beginning, the fluid in the long glass tube in the drainage bottle of the one- and two-bottle system fluctuates with each respiration; bubbling occurs in the drainage bottle if the system is working properly. Failure of the fluid to fluctuate in the long glass tube may mean that the catheter is clogged or that the lung has completely reexpanded. During the early postoperative period, it is more likely that the catheter is clogged. In some hospitals, milking the drainage tube from the patient toward the drainage bottle to remove an obstruction is considered a nursing responsibility. If drainage is not reestablished by milking the tube, the physician should be notified at once. An radiographic film (taken by a portable machine) may be ordered to determine whether failure of the fluid to fluctuate is due to reexpansion of the lung.

It is important to check the color and amount of chest drainage frequently and note the condition of the dressings over the operative area. Although bloody drainage is expected through the catheter postoperatively, it should not be bright red or copious. In some hospitals, measuring and emptying the drainage bottles are nursing duties; in others, the physician assumes these responsibilities. To empty the drainage bottle, a clamp is placed on the chest catheter close to the patient's chest. The stopper is then removed from the bottle and the contents removed and measured. The amount of sterile water originally placed in the bottle must be subtracted from the total amount of drainage. Another sterile bottle with sterile solution is placed in position to cover the end of the drainage tube, the stopper is inserted and sealed tightly, and the clamp is removed from the chest catheter. Drainage must be reinstituted promptly so that the catheter does not become clogged and the necessary drainage is not delayed. The nurse should remain with the patient for a few minutes to make sure that the seal is effective and that no air is entering the chest. The patient should be checked at frequent intervals to ensure correct functioning of the underwater seal system.

On occasion, air escapes from the chest into the subcutaneous tissues, and an area of swelling may be noted above or below the dressing. This condition is called *subcutaneous emphysema*. On palpation, a crackling sensation (crepitation) is felt with the fingertips. Although a small amount of air in the subcutaneous tissues is not unusual, any increase should be reported to the physician. The area is marked with a pen for future comparisons.

Assessment

On arrival from surgery, vital signs are taken to establish baseline data. The underwater seal drainage system is checked, and observations are recorded. It is important to note the type and number of bottles or the type of commercial system used, the amount and color of drainage, and whether bubbling and fluctuation are present. The dressings are checked for drainage and firm adherence to the skin. The skin around the dressing is inspected for signs of subcutaneous emphysema. The patient's color, heart rate and rhythm, and the respiratory rate, depth, and rhythm are recorded. The chest is auscultated for normal and abnormal breath sounds.

Nursing Diagnosis

The number of nursing diagnoses depends on the condition of the patient, the type and extent of surgery, and additional medical problems (if any).

- Pain due to surgery, insertion of chest tubes
- Anxiety related to pain, respiratory difficulty, chest tubes
- Ineffective airway clearance related to anesthesia, pain, lung impairment
- Ineffective breathing pattern related to pain of surgery, chest tubes
- Potential fluid volume deficit related to surgery
- Impaired physical mobility (upper) related to surgery, pain, chest tubes
- Knowledge deficit related to prevention of further episodes of lung impairment, home care maintenance, postdischarge management, and rehabilitation

Planning and Implementation

The major goals of the patient include reduction of anxiety and pain, improvement in airway clearance, effective coughing and deep breathing, and acquisition of home care knowledge.

The major goals of nursing management are improvement of gas exchange and breathing pattern, reduction or elimination of pain and discomfort, effective airway clearance, and a return of normal lung expansion and function.

Pain. When the patient becomes fully awake after surgery, pain may be severe, especially with movement of the upper extremities and with deep breathing and coughing. Pain that is not controlled or lessened results in failure to perform coughing and deep-breathing exercises, a lack which can result in further complications, such as pneumonia. When a patient complains of pain or appears to have pain because of facial expression or movements, the severity, type, and location of the pain must be determined before an analgesic is administered.

Large doses of narcotics, and sometimes even normal doses, are avoided because respiratory depression can occur. The physician may prescribe smaller doses at frequent intervals. When an analgesic is administered, the respiratory rate is checked before and 20 to 30 minutes after the administration of the drug. As the patient's condition stabilizes and the lungs reinflate, a decision to remove one or more of the chest tubes is made by the physician.

Anxiety. Patients who have had chest surgery need nurses who are familiar with the equipment, who have operated it enough to be at ease with it, and who can center their attention on the patient. The nurse's confidence in performing necessary tasks can give the patient confidence and reduce anxiety.

Position changes depend on the type of surgery and the number of chest tubes. If only one lung is involved and one or two chest tubes are used, the position is changed every 2 hours, and the patient is encouraged to turn on the unoperated side (unless the physician orders a different position) as well as the back.

Airway Clearance. Deep breathing and coughing help ventilate and expand lung tissue and thus improve gas exchange and clear secretions from the tracheobronchial tree. The patient is encouraged to cough and deep breathe when the analgesic appears to have the greatest effect. Supporting the incision while deep breathing and coughing may relieve some discomfort, but the patient may still find these tasks painful.

Oxygen may be prescribed during the early postoperative period. The blood pressure, pulse, and respiratory rate and rhythm are monitored at frequent intervals, usually every 15 to 30 minutes during the immediate postoperative period and until vital signs are stable. After this time, vital signs are monitored as ordered or at least every 1 or 2 hours. The lungs are auscultated for normal and abnormal breath sounds every 1 or 2 hours. Incentive spirometry may be used to improve ventilation. A semi-Fowler's position is usually used to improve lung capacity and move air to the upper apex of the lung where it is removed by the anterior chest tube. Any sudden increase in the respiratory rate, evidence of respiratory distress, or cyanosis is reported to the physician immediately.

Excessive secretions often occur during the postoperative period. The patient may need to be suctioned until tracheobronchial secretions can be raised. The patient is encouraged to deep breathe at frequent intervals. If coughing is difficult (and it usually is) during the early postoperative period, the patient can take deep breaths and forcefully expel air through the mouth. When this and other breathing techniques are practiced before surgery, the patient is often more cooperative when doing these exercises during the postoperative period.

Patients may have a tendency to splint their respirations because of pain. Effective control of pain and discomfort with the administration of analgesics and supporting the incision when coughing and deep breathing may eliminate this problem.

Potential Fluid Volume Deficit. The intake and output are measured and recorded. Intravenous fluids are ordered until the patient is able to take a sufficient quantity of fluids by mouth. The infusion rate is monitored closely, as fluid overload places added stress on the heart and lungs. Once the patient is started on oral fluids, sips of water are given at frequent intervals.

Impaired Physical Mobility. The upper arm and shoulder on the operative side are usually held in a rigid position because movement causes pain. The patient is usually allowed out of bed the first or second postoperative day, and movement of the upper extremities is encouraged. Movement is begun slowly and increased as tolerated. After removal of the chest tubes, exercises are increased.

Knowledge Deficit. After discharge from the hospital, the patient may be instructed to continue upper extremity exercises to prevent stiffening and pain. The patient must fully understand how to perform these exercises and how often they are to be done.

Depending on the type of chest surgery, the patient may require information about, for example, the prevention of infection, avoidance of factors that may have caused the original problem, or prevention of further lung impairment. If drug therapy is prescribed, the dosage schedule and adverse effects are reviewed with the patient. The patient is encouraged to eat a well-balanced diet or follow the diet recommendations of the physician. Rest periods should be taken at periodic intervals throughout the day until fatigue is decreased.

Evaluation

- Pain is controlled or eliminated
- Anxiety is reduced
- Respiratory function is improved; coughs and deep breathing are performed; blood gas studies are normal
- Airway is cleared effectively
- Breathing pattern is normal
- Maintains adequate oral fluid intake
- Moves upper extremities; participates in upper extremity exercises
- Demonstrates upper extremity exercises; verbalizes importance of adhering to the physician's recommendations regarding preventive measures

General Nutritional Considerations

☐ Adequate fluid intake helps reduce tenacious tracheobronchial secretions.

☐ Those with a chronic lung disease or infection may have had decreased food intake before surgery and may require a diet high in calories and protein during the postoperative period.

General Pharmacologic Considerations

☐ When a narcotic is administered to patients who have had thoracic surgery, the respiratory rate is counted before and 20 to 30 minutes after the drug is given. If the respiratory rate falls below 10 at either time, the physician must be notified *immediately*.

☐ Analgesics are best given before pain reaches its maximum intensity. The patient is evaluated for drug effectiveness 30 to 45 minutes after administration. If an analgesic fails to provide pain relief, the physician is notified; a larger dose or a different drug may be needed or a complication of surgery may have occurred.

General Gerontologic Considerations

☐ During the postoperative period, the patient may be confused and may attempt to pull out the chest tubes. The physician is notified if the patient appears confused; an order for restraints may be needed.

☐ If confusion occurs, the patient requires more frequent observation and assessment of needs.

☐ The patient may require more detailed explanation of home care management. Adequate time and repeat demonstrations may be necessary.

☐ When possible, a family member should also be taught postsurgical exercises so that home care management is carried out.

Suggested Readings

☐ Berkow R, Fletcher AJ, eds. Merck manual of diagnosis and therapy. 15th ed. Rahway, NJ: Merck & Co, 1987. *(In-depth coverage of subject matter)*

☐ Brunner LS, Suddarth DS. The Lippincott manual of nursing practice. 4th ed. Philadelphia: JB Lippincott, 1986. *(Additional and in-depth coverage of subject matter)*

☐ Carroll P. Safe suctioning. Nursing '89 December 1989;19:48. *(Additional and in-depth coverage of subject matter)*

☐ Doenges ME, Moorhouse MF. Nurse's pocket guide: nursing diagnoses with interventions. 2nd ed. Philadelphia: FA Davis, 1988. *(Additional coverage of subject matter)*

☐ Dupuis VG. Ventilators: theory and clinical application. St Louis: CV Mosby, 1986. *(In-depth coverage of subject matter)*

☐ Erickson RS. Mastering the ins and outs of chest drainage: part 1. Nursing '89 May 1989;19:37. *(Additional coverage and illustrations that reinforce subject matter)*

☐ Erickson RS. Mastering the ins and outs of chest drainage: part 2. Nursing '89 June 1989;19:46. *(Additional coverage and illustrations that reinforce subject matter)*

☐ Gruendemann BJ, Meeker MH. Alexander's care of the patient in surgery. 8th ed. St Louis: CV Mosby, 1987. *(In-depth coverage of subject matter)*

☐ Hudak CM, Gallo BM, Benz JJ. Critical care nursing: a holistic approach. 5th ed. Philadelphia: JB Lippincott, 1990. *(In-depth coverage of subject matter)*

☐ Johanson BC, Wells, SJ, Hoffmeister D, Dungca CU. Standards for critical care. 3rd ed. St Louis: CV Mosby, 1988. *(In-depth coverage of subject matter)*

☐ Wilkins RL, Sheldon RL, Krider SJ. Clinical assessment in respiratory care. 2nd ed. St Louis: CV Mosby, 1989. *(In-depth, high-level coverage of subject matter)*

The Cardiovascular System

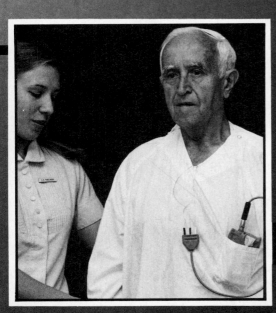

Unit 6

Chapter 24

Introduction to Cardiovascular Nursing

On completion of this chapter the reader will:

- Be familiar with the basic anatomy and physiology of the cardiovascular system

- List and discuss the areas covered during assessment of a cardiac patient

- Perform a physical assessment of a patient with a cardiovascular disorder

- List and discuss the tests performed for the detection of cardiac diseases and abnormalities

- Discuss patient preparation for diagnostic tests related to the cardiovascular system

- Use the nursing process in preparation of a patient for cardiovascular diagnostic studies

ANATOMY AND PHYSIOLOGY OF THE CARDIOVASCULAR SYSTEM

The heart is a four-chambered muscular pump about the size of a fist. Attached to this pump is a system of tubes for outflow and inflow: the aorta and pulmonary arteries, and the vena cava and pulmonary veins (Fig. 24-1).

The heart is anchored in the mediastinum, below and slightly to the left of the midline of the sternum. The heart's right ventricle is directly under the sternum, a location that is significant to the dynamics of external cardiac compression. The heart's lower border lies on the diaphragm and forms a blunt point extending to the left. This area is the *apex* of the heart.

Arteries and Veins

Arteries carry blood from the heart and *veins* carry blood back to the heart. The smallest arteries are called *arterioles* and the smallest veins, *venules*.

Arterioles branch into *capillaries*, which are microscopic branches that form a connecting network between venules and arterioles. They allow for the exchange of gasses (carbon dioxide, oxygen) and nutrients between the cells of the body and the blood and between the air in the lungs and the blood. Capillaries permeate the tissues of each organ and are in intimate contact with the cells of those tissues. Oxygen and metabolic substances are delivered to the cells through this complex circulatory network. The thin walls of the capillaries, their tremendous surface area, and their tiny size, all allow for rapid exchange of gases and metabolic substances between the blood and cells. After this exchange takes place, venous blood is transported back to the heart under low pressure by the veins.

Arterial walls are thicker than the walls of veins and consist of three layers. The outermost layer, the *tunica adventitia*, consists of connective tissue; the middle layer, the *tunica media*, is composed of smooth muscle; and the inner layer, the *tunica intima*, is composed of epithelial cells.

Veins that supply the extremities have valves that keep blood flowing in one direction only. Closure of successive sets of valves along the veins keeps the blood moving toward the heart.

Cardiac Muscle

Three distinct layers of tissue make up the heart wall. The bulk of the heart consists of specially constructed muscle tissue known as the *myocardium*. Covering the myocardium on the outside and adherent to it is the *pericardium*. The outermost layer is the *fibrous*

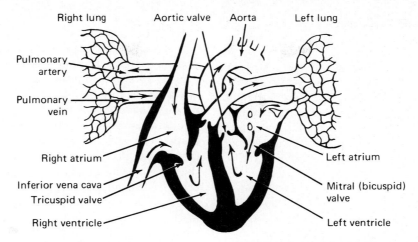

Figure 24-1. Diagram illustrating the flow of blood through the heart and lungs. The path can be observed by starting at the vena cava and following the arrows through the right atrium, right ventricle, pulmonary artery, lungs, pulmonary vein, left atrium, left ventricle, and into the aorta.

pericardium. The innermost layer, or that adhering to the myocardium, is the visceral layer, or *epicardium*. The pericardial space contains a small amount of pericardial fluid that lessens the friction between the myocardium and the pericardium. Because the pericardium does not stretch, overdilatation of the heart during diastole cannot take place.

Lining the inner wall of the heart and its valves is a delicate layer of endothelial tissue known as the *endocardium*. This layer of the heart is in direct contact with the blood passing through the heart.

Coronary Arteries

Blood is supplied to cardiac muscle by means of two main coronary arteries, namely the *left coronary artery* and the *right coronary artery*. The left coronary artery divides into the anterior descending coronary artery and the circumflex coronary artery. The right coronary artery supplies the right ventricle and, by its branches, the posterior wall of the heart (Fig. 24-2).

Chambers of the Heart

The heart has four chambers. The upper chambers are the left and right *atria* (singular, *atrium*). The lower chambers are the left and right ventricles.

Valves of the Heart

A series of thin but strong valves ensures that blood, in passing through the heart, does not seep back and reverse its direction of flow. A valve separates the atrium

from the ventricle on each side of the heart, preventing blood from passing back into the atrium each time the ventricle contracts. These valves are called *atrioventricular* valves. These two valves are cusped (leaflike) valves. The valve between the left atrium and left ventricle is the *bicuspid*—or two cusps—valve, also known as the *mitral* valve. The valve between the right atrium and right ventricle is the *tricuspid*—or three cusps—valve.

Two valves prevent blood that is pumped into the aorta and the pulmonary artery from flowing back toward the heart. The name of the artery is used to describe its valve; these valves are the *pulmonary* valve and the *aortic* valve.

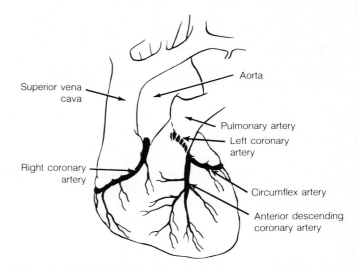

Figure 24-2. Anterior view of the heart, showing the right and left coronary arteries, which supply the myocardium with blood.

Chordae Tendineae and Papillary Muscles

Attached to the mitral and tricuspid valves are cordlike structures known as *chordae tendineae,* which in turn attach to two major muscular projections from the left ventricle known as *papillary muscles.* During contraction of the ventricles, these muscles also contract, providing tension on the atrioventricular valves that prevents prolapse or invagination of the valves into the atria.

Cardiac Cycle

The term *cardiac cycle* means a complete heartbeat, consisting of contraction (systole) and relaxation (diastole) of both atria and both ventricles. The two atria contract simultaneously; then, as they relax, the two ventricles contract and relax.

Though working toward different objectives and under different pressures, both sides of the heart work in unison. The left atrium receives newly oxygenated blood from the lungs by way of four pulmonary veins. Oxygenated blood flows during diastole into the left ventricle through the mitral valve; during atrial systole, a squeezing down of additional blood into the ventricle occurs before the valve closes.

During ventricular systole, blood is pumped through the aortic valve into the aorta, from which it then flows under pressure into many smaller arteries, and thence into the arterioles.

Veins from all organs of the body drain into the superior or inferior vena cava and, along with blood from the coronary veins, empty into the right atrium of the heart. Venous (unoxygenated) blood is then pumped into the right ventricle through the tricuspid valve. From this chamber, the blood is pumped through the pulmonary artery into the pulmonary circulation. The lungs are responsible for the exchange of oxygen and carbon dioxide. Blood leaves the right ventricle and flows through the pulmonary artery to the pulmonary capillaries. Here, carbon dioxide, which has built up in the venous blood from tissue release as a metabolic end product, is transferred from the blood into the alveoli and is exhaled. Venous blood takes on oxygen by coming in contact with inspired air. After this exchange of oxygen and carbon dioxide has taken place, oxygenated blood is transported through four pulmonary veins to the left side of the heart.

Conduction System of the Heart

In the posterior wall of the right atrium, a small area of specialized tissue, known as the *sinoatrial* (SA) node

(Fig. 24-3), has the ability to initiate an electrical impulse at the rate of about 72 times/min. In the following sequence of events, the cardiac impulse normally originates in the SA node and travels through the atria, causing them to contract. A few hundredths of a second after leaving the SA node, the impulse reaches the *atrioventricular* (AV) node, where it is delayed a few hundredths of a second while the ventricles fill with blood. The impulse then travels down the bundle of His, which divides into the right bundle branch and the anterior and posterior divisions of the left bundle branch. The left and right branches of the bundle of His further branch out and become Purkinje fibers. After the delay in the AV node, the cardiac impulse spreads rapidly down the bundle of His and into the Purkinje fibers, causing both ventricles to contract.

The SA node is called the *pacemaker* of the heart because it initiates the electrical impulse that causes the ventricles to contract. In certain types of heart disease, other areas of the heart may initiate an electrical impulse.

Cardiac muscle fibers are joined together in a kind of latticework formation. An electrical impulse that arises in any single fiber eventually spreads over the membranes of all of the fibers. The normal muscle cell has more negative than positive ions inside the cell membrane. The electrical cardiac impulse is caused by sudden transfer of ions through the membrane so that more positive than negative ions appear on the inside. This process is called *depolarization.* Once depolarization has occurred, another normal cardiac impulse cannot be carried out until the ions realign themselves to their original condition. This process is called *repolarization.* During this period, the cell is resistant to electrical stimulation and said to be *refractory.*

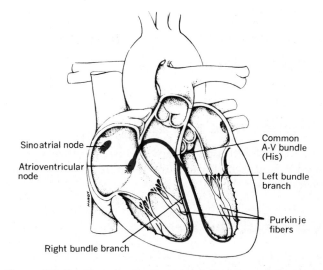

Figure 24-3.   The electrical conduction system of the heart. (Chaffee EE, Greisheimer EM: Basic physiology and anatomy. Philadelphia, JB Lippincott)

Depolarization and repolarization produce an electrical field. Because body tissues conduct current easily, this electrical potential can be detected by electrodes placed on the external surface of the body and recorded by a machine known as the *electrocardiograph* (ECG).

Normal heart rhythm can be disturbed in a variety of ways. Disturbances can be the result of disease or the harmless adaptations of normal functioning.

The heart adjusts its work to the changing needs of the body. It can increase the amount of blood that it pumps in two ways: by beating more rapidly and by increasing the volume of blood pumped with each beat. Sudden fright often causes the heart to beat faster and more forcefully, and we become aware of our heartbeat. These adjustments in heart action are beyond conscious control. The stimulation of the sympathetic nervous system quickens the heart; the stimulation of the parasympathetic nervous system slows it. Both systems constantly affect the heart. In fright, stimulation of the sympathetic nervous system causes a temporarily greater effect and, consequently, a faster heart rate.

Occasionally, in frightened or shocked people, however, vagal reflexes predominate and heart rate slows, cardiac output falls, and the person becomes weak or faint (vasovagal syncope). Such patients should be assisted to a supine position to encourage cerebral blood flow until equilibrium is restored.

Cardiac Output

In the normal person, cardiac output, or the amount of blood pumped by the ventricles, is about 5 L/min.

ASSESSMENT OF A PATIENT WHO HAS A CARDIOVASCULAR DISORDER
Patient History

The initial assessment must include the patient's (or family member's) description of all symptoms experienced before admission and during the admission assessment. An allergy history also is obtained, since diagnostic procedures may involve the administration of drugs or substances, such as radiopaque dyes, that may contain iodine. Any drug, food, or substance to which the patient is allergic is noted on the front of the patient's chart. An allergy to any type of seafood may mean an allergy to the iodine contained in the seafood.

General Appearance

An appraisal of the general appearance of the patient may identify problems, such as anxiety, depression, pain or discomfort, or an irregular breathing pattern, and help recognize areas that require further exploration.

Temperature

Fever is characteristic in some types of heart disease, particularly in acute myocardial infarction, rheumatic fever, and subacute bacterial endocarditis. Patients with these conditions should have their temperatures taken rectally because this method provides the most accurate reading. Oral temperatures might be ordered, however, to avoid vagal stimulation from the insertion of the rectal thermometer. Vagal stimulation can produce slowing of the heart (bradycardia) and other cardiac dysrhythmias, such as heart block, especially in the patient with acute myocardial infarction.

If rectal temperatures are necessary, care should be taken that the thermometer is well lubricated and inserted gently. Observing the ECG monitor or taking the patient's pulse reveals excess vagal stimulation. The physician is informed if this phenomenon occurs, and future temperatures taken orally unless directed otherwise.

Pulse

When taking the pulse, it is important to note not only its rate but also its rhythm and its quality.

A pulse deficit is taken during the initial assessment, and repeated as required. The numerical difference (if one exists) between the apical (heart) rate and the radial (pulse at the wrist) rate is known as the *pulse deficit*. It can be detected by taking an apical–radial pulse. One nurse counts the beats while listening over the apex of the patient's heart with a stethoscope. It is usually easiest to hear the heartbeat over the apex (the fifth intercostal space in the left midclavicular line). The stethoscope is placed near the left nipple or, in mature women, under the left breast. Simultaneously, another nurse counts the radial pulse. Both nurses count for at least 1 minute. Both figures are charted. If a pulse deficit exists, the number of beats at the radial artery is fewer than that at the apex. A pulse deficit can also be determined by one person. While listening to the apical rate with a stethoscope, the nurse places a finger on the radial artery. If no pulse deficit exists, a pulse is felt radially for every ventricular contraction heard. If ventricular contractions are heard but not palpated, a pulse deficit probably exists. Two nurses are then required to determine the exact difference between the apical and radial pulse.

The major arteries of the leg (Fig. 24-4) are palpated during the physical assessment. The radial pulse and

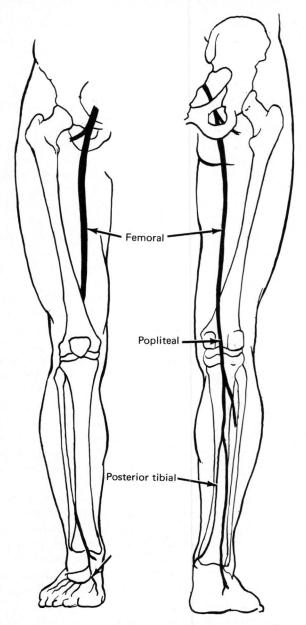

Figure 24–4. Major arteries of the leg that can be palpated for pulsation where they come close to the surface, such as in the popliteal area and immediately below the ankle.

the pulse in other areas, such as the carotid artery of the neck, also are palpated. The intensity and the presence or absence of a pulse are recorded.

The patient may be placed on continuous ECG monitoring. The monitor indicates the patient's heart rate and rhythm but not the quality of the beat; the quality can be ascertained by feeling the pulse. Correlating pulse quality is necessary, because the cardiac rhythm on the monitor may appear normal even when the pulse quality is abnormal.

Blood Pressure

These readings are important because diseases of the heart are often closely associated with changes in blood pressure. If the patient is not acutely ill, the blood pressure is taken with the patient in the standing, sitting, and lying positions. These three baseline determinations are necessary to monitor the effects of certain cardiac diseases and certain drugs that can alter the blood pressure during position changes.

The blood pressure is taken in both arms, on admission and once a day. A marked difference between the left and right arms is reported. In charting, it is necessary to identify the arm used to determine the blood pressure.

The patient should be questioned about dizziness or lightheadedness when changing positions, such as rising from a sitting or lying position. Occurrence of these symptoms may indicate postural (or orthostatic) hypotension, which may be seen in those with vasoconstrictor mechanisms. Drugs such as the antihypertensive agents also may cause postural hypotension.

Respirations

Careful observation of the rate and character of respiration is important. While counting the rate for a full minute, the quality and rhythm of the respirations are observed. It is important to note whether breathing is easy or labored (dyspneic), deep or shallow, wet or dry, wheezing or quiet. It should be noted if the neck or abdominal muscles are used during respiration.

Skin Color and Temperature

Many patients with cardiac disease show changes in skin color, namely, cyanosis and pallor. Cyanosis can be detected by carefully noting color changes in the mucous membranes of the mouth, as well as on the lips, ear lobes, skin, and nail beds. In white patients, extreme pallor is easy to detect, as the skin appears almost bloodless. In black patients, a grayish cast to the skin usually indicates the same effect as pallor. A good light is necessary to check skin color changes in all patients.

When assessing the skin, it is necessary to focus on the patient's initial problem. It is important to note whether the general skin area is warm to the touch, or whether it feels cold and clammy, and whether diaphoresis is present. If the patient has a problem related to peripheral vascular circulation, the skin over the area is inspected for color, differentiation of color and skin temperature between the affected area and other areas of the body, and the presence of varicosities (enlargement of veins).

Edema

Edema often accompanies congestive heart failure. In this disorder, blood is not pumped efficiently. Venous blood that returns to the heart by the large veins cannot be promptly received and pumped by the right side of the heart. As a result, the venous blood is returned to the heart pools in the veins, resulting in congestion in the veins and the collection of extra fluid in the tissues. Areas subject to edema are carefully examined, particularly in dependent parts of the body, such as the feet and ankles (Fig. 24-5). Other areas that are inspected for edema include the fingers, hands, and the area over the sacrum. If edema is noted in any area of the body, the examiner's fingers are gently pressed into the area and then quickly released. If the marks produced by the fingers remain, this effect is termed *pitting* edema.

Peripheral Pulses

The pulsations produced by each contraction of the ventricle can be detected in the arteries that lie close to the surface. A pulse rate is normally determined by the radial artery. In those with known or suspected cardiac disease, other peripheral pulses, namely, the dorsalis pedis (or pedal) pulse, the popliteal pulse, and the posterior tibial pulse (see Fig. 24-4), are palpated. The presence or absence of these pulses and their strength are noted.

Weight

Fluctuations in weight are important indications of edema. A gain in weight often means that edema is increasing. Loss in weight often reflects the desirable and needed loss of excess fluid that has collected in the tissues. If weight is recorded daily, the patient is weighed at the same time each day and with the same amount of clothing. The recording of weight should be as accurate as possible. One pound more or less may indicate that edema is increasing or decreasing.

Jugular Veins

Jugular vein distention seen with the patient in a supine position is usually considered normal. This distention should disappear when the patient is raised to a sitting position or a 45-degree angle. With the patient in a sitting position and the head turned to the left or right, the external jugular vein is inspected. Distention of this vein usually indicates increased filling and volume pressure of the right side of the heart.

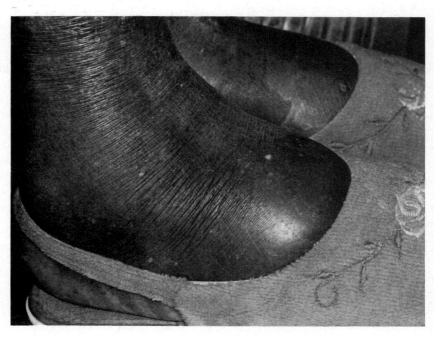

Figure 24-5. The patient with cardiac disease may have edema of the feet and ankles. (Photograph by D. Atkinson)

Sputum

Patients with cardiac disease may raise sputum in amounts that range from little to great. Others may cough yet raise no sputum. It is important to describe the amount as well as the appearance of any sputum that is raised by a patient. The type of cough and the frequency also are noted. The appearance of sputum may be important in diagnosing congestive heart failure or pulmonary embolus, a complication of prolonged bed rest.

Pain

When present, pain must be evaluated carefully. It is important to obtain as much information as possible about the pain experienced by a patient. This assessment includes the following points:

- Patient's description of the pain (eg, dull, sharp, squeezing, crushing)
- Exact location of the pain
- Duration of the pain; when did it start and end?
- Radiation of the pain to other areas (the pain may or may not radiate)
- Changes in the character of the pain (eg, increasing in severity, going from sharp to dull ache)
- Relationship of the occurrence of pain to any particular situation (eg, eating, exercise, emotions)

Mental Status

Although cardiac patients may be alert and oriented, they also may be confused and disoriented. When assessing the mental status of the patient, it is important to note the presence of anxiety, nervousness, depression, or fear. Any extremes of emotion are reported to the physician because they could interfere with diagnostic testing and the therapies prescribed for certain cardiac diseases. Any sudden occurrence of confusion or disorientation also must be reported; it could be caused by a decrease in the oxygen supply (cerebral anoxia) to the brain.

Heart and Lungs

Cardiac disease affects not only the heart but also the respiratory system. Auscultation of the heart requires practice as well as familiarization with normal and abnormal heart sounds. The first heart sound is the opening of the mitral and tricuspid valves and is referred to as S_1. The second heart sound is the closing of the aortic and pulmonic valves and is referred to as S_2. In addition to heart sounds, auscultation may reveal other abnormal sounds, such as murmurs and clicks, which are usually indicative of valvular disease. An-

other sound that may be heard is a friction rub, which is indicative of pericarditis (inflammation of the pericardium). This sound is similar to a heart murmur.

The lungs are auscultated for abnormal and normal breath sounds. Certain cardiac diseases, such as congestive heart failure, produce a crackling sound on auscultation. Other sounds that may be heard are wheezes and crackles. During auscultation of the chest, the respiratory rate, rhythm, and depth are noted.

DIAGNOSTIC TESTS
Laboratory Tests

Various general laboratory tests may be used in the diagnosis of heart disease and in monitoring the patient's progress during and after treatment. Laboratory tests may be performed daily or every few days. They may be used to monitor the results of therapy, for example, a daily prothrombin time for the patient who is receiving anticoagulant drugs.

Blood Chemistry

Laboratory tests that are not specific for heart disease are used to provide a general picture of a patient's physical status and the effect of the disease on other organs or structures of the body. Laboratory tests also may demonstrate abnormalities that are part of the overall condition of a specific cardiac disorder. Blood chemistries, such as fasting blood glucose, serum electrolytes, creatine, and serum cholesterol and triglyceride levels, may be used as part of the diagnostic analysis.

Serum Enzymes and Isoenzymes

Enzymes are complex proteins produced by living cells that function as catalysts. Catalysts are substances capable of producing changes in other substances without being changed themselves. An *isoenzyme* is one of several forms of an enzyme that may exist in cells and is capable of being separated from other isoenzymes by special laboratory techniques.

When tissues and cells break down, are damaged, or die, great quantities of certain enzymes are released into the blood stream and may be detected by laboratory methods. The enzymes of importance in cardiac disease are the following:

- Serum glutamic-oxaloacetic transaminase (SGOT)
- Aspartate aminotransferase (AST)
- Creatine phosphokinase (CPK) and its isoenzymes
- Creatine kinase (CK) and its isoenzymes
- Lactate dehydrogenase (LDH) and its isoenzymes

These enzymes also can be elevated in other diseases and disorders. The CK isoenzyme labeled CK-MB or CK₂ and the LDH isoenzymes LDH_1 and LDH_2 are more specific for cardiac muscle damage.

Radiographic and Radioisotope Studies

Chest radiographs and fluoroscopy may be used to determine the size and position of the heart as well as the changes in the lungs that may have occurred because of heart disease. These studies also may be used to determine the placement of catheters or wires, such as after the insertion of a cardiac pacemaker or central venous pressure line, or to guide catheters during cardiac catheterization and angiography. A computed tomographic scan and magnetic resonance imaging also may be used to detect heart size, lung involvement, and so on.

The radioisotope technetium 99m may be used to detect areas of myocardial damage. The radioisotope thallium-201 may be used to diagnose ischemic heart disease during a stress test.

Echocardiogram

Echocardiography uses ultrasound waves to detect the presence of cardiac disorders. The high-frequency sound waves, which cannot be heard by the human ear, pass through the chest wall and are recorded on an oscilloscope. Pictures are taken of the oscilloscope configurations for a permanent recording of the procedure. This procedure helps to determine the functioning of the left ventricle and to detect cardiac tumors, congenital heart disease, and pericardial effusion.

Phonocardiogram

A *phonocardiogram* is the graphic recording of heart sounds. This procedure is used in the diagnosis of heart valve and other cardiac disorders. Microphones are placed on the chest, and heart sounds are recorded graphically. The graphic recording enables the physician to differentiate between various heart sounds and murmurs.

Electrocardiogram

The *electrocardiogram* is a graphic record of the electrical currents generated by the heart muscle (Fig. 24-6). Connections are made between the machine and the patient by means of electrodes placed at various points on the patient's body. A special conducting jelly is placed on the electrodes, which are placed on the surface of the skin, usually on the wrists, ankles, and chest, in a number of combinations. The leads that go to the extremities are strapped in place. The chest lead is held in position by means of a suction cup. The ECG machines that are computerized immediately interpret the reading. The computerized interpretations

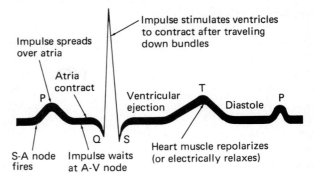

Figure 24–6. Electrical and mechanical events of basic ECG tracing. (Hewlett-Packard Co, Medical Electronic Division, Palo Alto, California)

serve as screening devices, and the ECG must be further interpreted by a physician.

The 12-lead ECG especially helps to determine the nature of myocardial damage and to interpret cardiac dysrhythmias. One lead of the ECG can be used to continuously monitor cardiac activity when changes in heart rate and rhythm or graphic changes in the ECG tracing need to be identified.

The ECG pattern consists of waves, intervals, segments, and complexes (Fig. 24-7). The *P wave* is produced at the time of depolarization of the atrial muscle. The *Q wave* is the first downward deflection of the P wave. The *QRS complex* is the time of depolarization of the ventricular muscle. The *ST segment* represents early repolarization of the ventricular muscle, and the *T wave* represents repolarization of the ventricular muscle. The *PR interval* is the measured distance between the P and the R waves and represents the time the electrical impulse travels across the atria to the conduction system and Purkinje fibers.

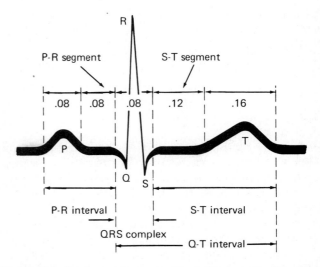

Figure 24–7. Basic electrocardiographic tracing. (Hewlett-Packard Co, Medical Electronic Division, Palo Alto, California)

Holter Recorder

One lead monitoring can also be used to record the patient's ECG on magnetic tape. The Holter recorder is a portable lightweight box that can be attached to a belt around the waist or carried over the shoulder by means of a strap. A single ECG lead is attached to the patient's chest and connected to the recorder. The patient keeps a log of activities throughout the day and makes an entry if any chest pain, palpitations, or other symptoms occur during activity or when at rest. The recorder is then returned to the hospital or physician, and a special scanning device is used to analyze the recording. The patient's log entries also are compared to the recording. The Holter recorder helps to detect dysrhythmias and myocardial ischemia during activity and rest. The advantage of the Holter recorder is that the patient need not be hospitalized. Cardiac activity can be monitored while the patient is carrying on normal daily activities.

Vectorcardiogram

Spatial vectorcardiography is a type of electrocardiography in which the heart's forces are represented by arrows and loops, rather than by the waves and complexes, as seen in a standard ECG. Heart damage can sometimes be inferred from the oscillographic loop when it is not readily apparent or questionable in the conventional electrocardiogram. The vectorcardiogram is obtained by a specially trained technician and interpreted by a cardiologist.

Stress Testing

The purpose of a stress test is to evaluate cardiac function, to determine patient response to drug therapy, and to identify cardiac dysrhythmias that occur during physical activity. This test enables the physician to evaluate the degree of cardiac ischemia and the amount of exercise required to produce angina.

To take this test, the patient walks on a treadmill, pedals a stationary bicycle, or climbs up and down a set of stairs. The physician determines the type of device to be used, since every patient cannot use them all.

Before the procedure, electrodes are attached to the patient's chest and then connected to an ECG monitor, and a baseline ECG is taken. During the test, the speed of the treadmill or the force required to pedal the bicycle is increased. Those climbing stairs are instructed to step up and down at an increasing pace. ECGs may be taken continuously or at periodic intervals during the test. Other tests monitor the blood pressure, pulse, and respiratory rate. The patient is closely observed and asked to report the first sign of chest pain or discomfort. Once the patient's predetermined maximum heart rate is reached, the test is discontinued and the results interpreted by the physician.

Cardiac Catheterization

Cardiac catheterization passes a long flexible catheter into the heart and great vessels. The most common use of cardiac catheterization is to determine the degree of blockage of the coronary arteries by performing an intravenous angiogram at the time the catheters are in place. Patients with coronary artery disease who are considered candidates for coronary bypass surgery almost always have a cardiac catheterization and intravenous angiogram before surgery.

Cardiac catheterization may be carried out on the left or right side of the heart (left or right cardiac catheterization). As the catheter enters the various chambers of the heart, the pressures are measured, and samples of the blood are obtained and analyzed for oxygen and carbon dioxide content. For example, the oxygen content of the blood in the right atrium is higher than normal when there is an atrial septal defect—a hole in the septum that separates the atria. The test is performed to aid in the diagnosis of congenital defects as well as other cardiac disorders.

The patient lies supine on a table in a special room equipped with radiography and fluoroscopy. The procedure usually takes one or more hours; the table is covered with a foam rubber pad, and the patient positioned as comfortably as possible.

Usually, the room is darkened at intervals during the test to facilitate the use of the fluoroscope. A device called a *fluoroscopic image amplifier,* or *image intensifier,* may make it possible to perform this test in a lighted room.

Ordinarily, the adult patient is not anesthetized (the walls of blood vessels have no fibers that transmit pain) but is given a sedative before the test. Breakfast is withheld on the morning of the test. The patient may have slight discomfort at first from the cutdown and the insertion of the catheter. As the catheter enters the chambers of the heart, irregularity of heart rhythm that resembles a feeling of fluttering may be experienced. If so, the patient is assured that the sensation will pass and that there is no cause for alarm. The patient may cough when the catheter is passed up the pulmonary artery. If so, the patient is told that the sensation will pass quickly. Despite sedation, the patient often is alert, apprehensive, and aware of the slightest sensation that is out of the ordinary. When the procedure is over, the catheter is withdrawn gently, and a small sterile dressing is placed over the site of the cutdown.

Introduction of catheters into the heart chambers can produce cardiac dysrhythmias, which may be fatal.

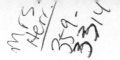

The patient is monitored by an ECG, and resuscitative equipment is on standby in case a serious dysrhythmia occurs. The patient's pulse is checked frequently after the procedure. A rapid or irregular pulse is immediately reported to the physician. The site of the cutdown is inspected for tenderness or inflammation. Pulmonary edema and air embolism are rare complications. The patient's temperature may be elevated for a few hours after the test. The patient usually is kept on bed rest for the rest of the day.

Angiography

An intravenous angiogram is a test in which a radiopaque dye is injected into a vein, and its course from the right heart to the lungs, back to the left heart and out the aorta is recorded by a rapid series of radiographic pictures. The pictures reveal not only the size and shape of these structures, but also the sequence and the time of their filling with blood. The angiogram is used particularly to diagnose certain congenital abnormalities of the heart and great vessels. This test usually is used when simpler diagnostic measures fail to provide the necessary information. Breakfast is omitted on the morning of the test, and sedative and antihistaminic drugs are usually administered before the patient is taken to the radiography department.

Arteriograms

Aortogram

Dye is injected into the aorta, and radiographic films are taken to outline the abdominal aorta and major arteries in the legs. Dye also may be injected into other vessels, such as the renal artery. An aortogram detects aortic abnormalities such as aneurysms (abnormal dilatation of a blood vessel wall) and blockage of an artery.

Peripheral Arteriogram

Dye is injected into an artery, and radiographic films are taken. This procedure may be used to diagnose occlusive arterial disease. After the procedure, a chance for bleeding is greater than after a venipuncture; therefore, a pressure dressing is applied and patient activity restricted for about 12 hours. The patient is observed for bleeding, cardiac dysrhythmias, and the adequacy of peripheral circulation by frequent checking of the peripheral pulses.

Hemodynamic Monitoring

Hemodynamic monitoring uses an invasive procedure to determine or evaluate factors such as cardiac function (especially the function of the left ventricle), the amount of oxygen used by the myocardium, cardiac output, and pulmonary vascular resistance. It also provides a survey of the patient's general physiologic status and can be used to evaluate responses to certain drugs.

Central Venous Pressure

Central venous pressure (CVP) is the measurement of the pressure of the blood in the right atrium. This measurement is used to detect early signs of congestive heart failure, to identify hypervolemia or hypovolemia (an increase or decrease in blood volume, respectively), and to determine the effectiveness of the heart's pumping action.

To monitor the CVP, a catheter is inserted into a large vein, usually the jugular vein (in the neck) or the antecubital vein of the arm. The catheter is connected to a three-way stopcock and a glass or plastic tube called a *manometer*. The stopcock is opened and the manometer filled with an intravenous solution. The stopcock is then rotated to the next position, and a reading is taken (Fig. 24-8). The height of the fluid in the manometer determines the CVP. Between readings, the three-way stopcock is turned so that intrave-

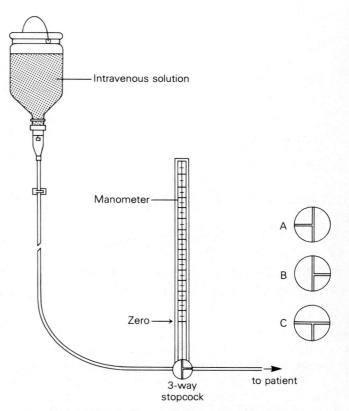

Figure 24–8. Central venous pressure measured by a water manometer. The arrow points to the zero mark, which must be at the level of the patient's right atrium. (A) Stopcock position for filling the manometer. (B) Position for measuring the central venous pressure. (C) Position for allowing intravenous solution to flow through the tubing to the patient, keeping the CVP line patent.

nous fluid runs through the catheter and into the patient. This process keeps the CVP line patent. Various types of CVP manometers exist, so the nurse must be familiar with the one being used.

The zero mark on the manometer *must* be at the level of the patient's right atrium; otherwise an incorrect reading is obtained. When a CVP measurement is taken, the patient is placed in a supine position. Between CVP measurements, the head of the bed can be raised or lowered. The physician orders the time intervals between CVP measurements.

Normal venous pressure is 4 to 10 cm of water. An increase in CVP usually indicates an impairment in cardiac contractions or an increase in blood volume (hypervolemia); a decrease indicates hypovolemia.

Systemic Intraarterial Monitoring

A catheter is inserted in an artery—usually the brachial, radial, or femoral artery—to draw arterial blood samples and obtain continuous blood pressure determinations. Intraarterial monitoring may be used intraoperatively and postoperatively on cardiac surgical patients as well as on those with severe and sustained hypertension or hypotension.

Pulmonary Artery Monitoring

The pressure in the left or right pulmonary artery may be measured by the insertion of catheters into the left or right atrium. A right pulmonary artery catheter is inserted in a large vein and threaded into the right atrium. To insert a left pulmonary artery, the chest must be surgically opened (thoracotomy).

The primary purpose of this type of hemodynamic monitoring is to determine left or right ventricular failure. The CVP can also be monitored when a right pulmonary artery catheter has been inserted.

NURSING PROCESS —THE PATIENT UNDERGOING DIAGNOSTIC TESTING FOR A CARDIOVASCULAR DISORDER

Assessment

A thorough initial assessment (see earlier discussion, Assessment of a Patient Who Has a Cardiovascular Disorder) is necessary to establish accurate baseline data for use before, during, and after a diagnostic procedure. Symptoms often change suddenly. Significant symptoms, such as changes in heart rate and rhythm, may occur only for brief intervals. *Any* change in the patient is reported immediately and recorded before the patient undergoes a diagnostic test.

Nursing Diagnosis

Depending on the condition of the patient and the potential or actual medical diagnosis, one or more of the following may apply to the patient scheduled for diagnostic tests. Additional nursing diagnoses may be appropriate, depending on the symptoms and needs identified during the initial assessment.

■ Anxiety related to diagnostic testing, results of tests, diagnosis
■ Pain related to coronary artery disease
■ Knowledge deficit related to purpose of test, how test will be performed, pain during or after the test, other areas (specify)

Planning and Implementation

The major goals of the patient include a reduction in anxiety, control of pain, and an understanding of the diagnostic procedure.

The major goals of nursing management are to reduce anxiety, assist in preparing the patient for a diagnostic procedure, and provide an basic explanation of the procedure.

Certain cardiac disorders, with or without pulmonary involvement, reduce a patient's tolerance to even slight activity. A patient may need help getting out of bed into a wheelchair or onto a gurney. A patient also may find it difficult to breathe while lying supine; pillows may be needed during transportation to other hospital areas. At all times, a patient is made as comfortable as possible before, during, and after the procedure.

Anxiety. Diagnostic tests may or may not be familiar to a patient. Many patients are concerned about the pain or discomfort that may be experienced during and after certain diagnostic procedures. Others may be afraid of death during the procedure. Anxiety may be reduced if the patient receives a full explanation of the procedure from the physician. The nurse may need to reinforce or reexplain what the physician has told the patient. Reassurance and understanding by medical personnel help reduce anxiety.

Pain. The acutely ill patient, such as one with a recent myocardial infarction, may have severe pain. The physician normally orders a narcotic analgesic for these patients, and the drug is given as needed. If pain is not controlled and the patient is scheduled for a diagnostic test, the physician is notified before the patient is transported to the testing area.

Other patients may have episodes of angina, which are brought on by activity or emotional stress. Anginal pain may occur in these patients before diagnostic testing. Usually, a medication to relieve anginal pain is ordered and is given whenever the patient experiences chest pain. If anginal pain occurs immediately before a scheduled diagnostic test or if the angina is not relieved by the prescribed medication, the physician is notified.

Knowledge Deficit. Patients and families often have many questions about a diagnostic procedure, such as what it will reveal, where it will be performed, and what may happen during and after the procedure. Although the physician explains the purpose and the procedure, a repeat explanation is often necessary: people with anxiety often fail to hear all of what has been told to them. The patient also is assured that he or she will be closely watched during the procedure. This assurance is especially important to those who need invasive tests, such as a cardiac catheterization.

Evaluation

■ Anxiety is reduced or eliminated
■ Pain is reduced or eliminated

■ Patient and family demonstrate understanding of the purpose of the procedure, how and where the procedure will be performed

Postprocedure Management and Observations

Invasive procedures, such as cardiac catheterization and hemodynamic procedures, require continued observation after the procedure. The blood pressure and pulse are monitored at frequent intervals, and the patient is observed for the development of cardiac dysrhythmias. Pain, changes in blood pressure, cyanosis, absence of a peripheral pulse, and other such symptoms are reported to the physician immediately. The dressing over the catheter insertion site is inspected for signs of bleeding, and the peripheral pulse of the artery used for insertion of dye or a catheter is checked at frequent intervals.

If a radiopaque dye that contains iodine was used during the procedure, the patient is closely observed for a delayed allergic reaction to iodine, which may be manifested by a drop in blood pressure, cold clammy skin, mental changes, difficulty breathing (due to edema of the larynx), fever, joint pain, and swelling of the lips and mouth.

General Pharmacologic Considerations

☐ A sedative may be given before invasive diagnostic procedures such as cardiac catheterizations. The sedative must be given at the time ordered to ensure adequate sedation during the procedure.

☐ Patients who have diagnostic studies that involve the use of contrast media are questioned about allergies, especially allergies to seafood (which contains iodine) and iodine. If the patient appears to have an iodine allergy, the physician must be notified *before* the test. An allergic reaction to iodine can be serious and occasionally fatal.

General Gerontologic Considerations

☐ The older patient may be confused and uncooperative during diagnostic tests, especially those involving an invasive procedure, such as insertion of a CVP line. Restraints may be necessary if the patient attempts to pull out catheters or intravenous lines or tries to remove ECG electrodes.

Suggested Readings

☐ Alfaro R. Applying nursing diagnosis and nursing process: a step-by-step guide. 2nd ed. Philadelphia: JB Lippincott, 1990. *(Additional coverage of subject matter)*
☐ Bates BA, Hoekelman RA. Guide to physical examination and history taking. 4th ed. Philadelphia: JB Lippincott, 1987. *(In-depth coverage of subject matter)*
☐ Becker KL, Stevens SA. Get in touch with cardiac assessment: part 1. Nursing '88 March 1988;18:51. *(Additional coverage of subject matter)*
☐ Durham CF. The no-fault way to assess carotid arteries. Nursing '88 November 1988;18:65. *(Additional coverage of subject matter)*

☐ Konick-McMahan J. Jugular vein distention: trouble in the heart's right side. Nursing '89 February 1989;19:100. *(Additional coverage of subject matter)*

☐ Memmler RL, Wood DL. Structure and function of the human body. 4th ed. Philadelphia: JB Lippincott, 1987. *(Additional coverage of subject matter)*

☐ Memmler RL, Wood DL. The human body in health and disease. 6th ed. Philadelphia: JB Lippincott, 1987. *(Additional coverage of subject matter)*

☐ Miracle VA. Get in touch with cardiac assessment: part 2. Nursing '88 April 1988;18:41. *(Additional coverage of subject matter)*

☐ Taylor DL. Assessing heart sounds. Nursing '85 January 1985;15:51. *(Additional coverage of subject matter)*

☐ Van Parys E. Assessing the failing state of the heart. Nursing '87 February 1987;17:42. *(Additional coverage of subject matter)*

☐ Yacone LA. Cardiac assessment: what to do, how to do it. RN May 1987;50:42. *(Additional coverage of subject matter)*

Chapter 25

Infectious and Inflammatory Disorders of the Heart and Blood Vessels

On completion of this chapter the reader will:

■ List and discuss the symptoms, diagnosis, and treatment of infective endocarditis, myocarditis, pericarditis, chronic constrictive pericarditis, rheumatic fever, and rheumatic heart disease

■ Use the nursing process in the management of the patient with an inflammatory or infectious disease of the heart and peripheral blood vessels

INFECTIOUS AND INFLAMMATORY DISORDERS OF THE HEART

Infective Endocarditis

Infective endocarditis (sometimes referred to as *bacterial* endocarditis) is an inflammatory condition of the endocardium caused by an invasion of microorganisms. Infective endocarditis may be classified as acute, subacute, or recurrent (chronic). The acute form has a more abrupt onset and more rapid course, whereas the subacute form has a gradual onset. In the subacute form, the infecting microorganisms tend to be less virulent.

The microorganisms that cause infective endocarditis include bacteria, fungi, and chlamydia. *Streptococcus viridans* and *Staphylococcus aureus* are two of the bacterial microorganisms frequently responsible for this disorder. Many patients who develop this disease have had rheumatic fever. This infection also may be seen with prolonged intravenous antibiotic therapy, insertion of cardiac pacemakers, cardiac catheterization, cardiac surgery, repeated genitourinary instrumentation, intravenous drug abuse, and in those with a surgically implanted prosthetic heart valve.

In infective endocarditis, vegetations form on the heart valves. These vegetations are friable (easily broken), and pieces are likely to break off and travel in the bloodstream. Called *emboli*, these pieces may damage other organs by occluding blood vessels, thus interfering with the organ's blood supply.

Symptoms

The disease often has an insidious onset, with slight fever, malaise, and fatigue. Patients may ignore early manifestations of the illness, attributing them to other causes. Early diagnosis and treatment are important. Patients—particularly those with rheumatic or congenital valvular defects—should see their physician if fever, malaise, or other symptoms of infection occur; they may have infective endocarditis or a recurrence of rheumatic fever.

As the condition advances, the patient often develops a muddy, sallow complexion, which has been described as the color of café au lait. Fever becomes marked and often is accompanied by chills and sweats. Pronounced weakness, anorexia, and weight loss are common. Petechiae, tiny reddish purple hemorrhagic spots on the skin and mucous membranes, are characteristic. Anemia and slight leukocytosis are common. Heart murmur is present in most patients. Embolism, which is the occlusion of a blood vessel by the emboli, may cause sudden disturbances in organs of the body, such as the brain, kidney, or lungs.

Clubbing of the fingers and toes may appear later in the course of the illness. The symptoms of congestive heart failure may appear, either during the active infection or afterward, as a result of damage to the valves of the heart.

Diagnosis

To establish a diagnosis, a patient's history is carefully taken, with particular attention to a history of rheumatic heart disease, congenital heart defects, or any recent surgery or illness. Blood cultures and sensitivity tests are ordered to identify the microorganism that is circulating in the blood. Several blood cultures may be required before the microorganism is found.

Treatment

Large doses of the antibiotic to which the microorganism is sensitive are given. Usually, the antibiotic is given by continuous or intermittent intravenous administration over a period of 2 to 6 weeks or longer. Bed rest is ordered. When the patient begins to improve, bathroom privileges may be allowed. As symptoms subside, the patient is allowed increased activity.

When antibiotic treatment is discontinued, the patient is observed for any recurrence of symptoms. Although the infection appears to be conquered, it may flare up again after drug therapy has been discontinued. In this case, treatment must be resumed and continued until the infection has been eradicated. If the heart valves have been severely damaged, surgical valve replacement may be necessary.

Patients with damaged heart valves, regardless of the cause, are given antibiotics just before and for a short time after any event that might cause bacteremia, such as an invasive diagnostic test or tooth extraction.

Complications

Congestive heart failure, development of emboli that may travel to vital organs such as the lungs or brain, and stenosis of the affected valves are complications of this disorder.

Myocarditis

Myocarditis is an inflammation of the myocardium (the muscle layer of the heart). This inflammatory disorder may be due to a viral, bacterial, fungal, or parasitic infection or may occur along with endocarditis or pericarditis.

Symptoms

Symptoms of myocarditis are often vague, but a patient may complain of general chest discomfort, dyspnea, fever, and anorexia.

Diagnosis

Diagnosis is made by a thorough patient history, chest radiograph, and throat and stool culture and sensitivity

tests. Myocardial biopsy and radioisotope studies also may be employed.

Treatment

Management is aimed at identification and treatment of the underlying cause. Bed rest, a sodium-restricted diet, and cardiotonic drugs (digitalis and related drugs) to prevent or treat heart failure are prescribed. Seriously ill patients with congestive heart failure or cardiac dysrhythmias may require continuous cardiac monitoring until their condition stabilizes.

Complications

Cardiomyopathy, a weakening and dilatation of the myocardium, is the most serious complication of myocarditis.

Pericarditis

Pericarditis, inflammation of the pericardium, can occur after an infection, chest trauma, or myocardial infarction. Other causes include malignant disorders, uremia, and connective tissue disorders, such as rheumatic fever. Blood, excess fluid, or pus can accumulate in the pericardial space and produce partial or complete cardiac tamponade (compression), resulting in a decrease in cardiac output and death.

Symptoms

A patient may feel sharp pain that is caused by the rubbing together of two inflamed surfaces (Fig. 25-1). Pain may be aggravated by moving and breathing, and dyspnea also may be present. A pericardial friction rub, which can usually be heard with a stethoscope, is

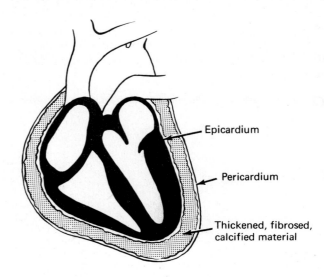

Epicardium

Pericardium

Thickened, fibrosed, calcified material

Figure 25–1. Pericarditis. Normally, the epicardium and the pericardium slide over each other easily. They are lubricated by a small amount of fluid, which is replaced in pericarditis by thicker material that can cause the surfaces to adhere to each other.

the most striking sign. The pain of acute pericarditis is similar to the pain of acute myocardial infarction— sudden, severe, beginning over the sternum, and radiating to the neck and left arm. The pain of the patient with pericarditis, however, is usually increased by rotating the chest or breathing deeply and relieved by sitting up and leaning forward. In contrast, the pain of acute myocardial infarction is not usually influenced by position, movement, or breathing. Chronic pericarditis may have few symptoms, but a friction rub can be heard during auscultation of the heart.

Diagnosis

Radiographs may show dilatation of the heart with pericardial effusion. A computed tomographic (CT) scan also may be performed. Serum enzyme changes are confusing because they are similar to those of acute myocardial infarction. If fluid in the pericardial space is sufficient to compress the heart, signs of congestive heart failure and a pulse that is weaker on deep inspiration (*paradoxical pulse*) may be found.

Treatment

Coronary precautions are usually taken until myocardial infarction is ruled out. Treatment depends on the underlying cause. Rest, analgesics, antipyretics, and other supportive treatments are usually prescribed. A pericardiocentesis, which removes fluid from the pericardium, may be performed. The fluid is sent to the laboratory for culture and sensitivity studies if the cause is suspected to be infection. A pericardiocentesis may be performed when fluid in the pericardial sac produces early symptoms of cardiac tamponade. Chronic accumulation of fluid may be treated by making a pericardial opening (window) that allows the fluid to drain into the pleural space. Constrictive pericarditis is treated surgically by removing the binding pericardium (pericardectomy or decortication) to allow more adequate filling and contraction of the heart chambers.

Complications

If untreated, pericarditis may progress to cardiac tamponade or severe congestive heart failure.

Cardiac Tamponade

Excess fluid in the pericardial sac has a constricting effect that does not allow full expansion of the chambers of the heart during diastole, resulting in reduced cardiac output. Ultimately, profound shock and death occur if the condition is not treated.

Symptoms

Symptoms include distant or muffled heart sounds, drop in blood pressure, dyspnea, and distended neck veins. The patient becomes confused and restless. Rapidly progressing cardiac tamponade must be recognized and treated as an emergency.

Diagnosis

Diagnosis is based on symptoms and auscultation of the chest. An emergency chest radiograph or CT scan may be performed to confirm the diagnosis.

Treatment

Treatment includes an emergency pericardiocentesis to remove the excess fluid. If trauma resulted in the collection of blood in the pericardial space, surgery is usually necessary to stop the bleeding.

Rheumatic Fever and Rheumatic Heart Disease

Rheumatic fever is most commonly found among children and young people between the ages of 5 and 15. It sometimes occurs in late adolescence or young adulthood, particularly in people with a history of the disease in childhood; it is rare after the age of 25 except when crowded living conditions favor streptococcal infections.

Rheumatic heart disease refers to the cardiac manifestations of rheumatic fever, either in the acute phase or the later stage of chronic damage.

The precise cause of rheumatic fever is unclear, but it is known to be related to an upper respiratory infection caused by the group A streptococci. A previous attack increases the risk of recurrent attacks after a streptococcal infection. It often follows such conditions as pharyngitis, tonsillitis, and scarlet fever.

Symptoms

Rheumatic fever often involves many body systems, such as the heart, joints, and nervous system. Carditis (inflammation of the layers of the heart), polyarthritis (inflammation of more than one joint), rash, subcutaneous nodules, and chorea (involuntary muscle twitching) are the classic symptoms. The occurrence of carditis may involve all three layers of the heart, the endocardium, myocardium, and pericardium, and lead to damage of the valves of the heart.

Symptoms of rheumatic heart disease depend on the type and extent of cardiac damage. If mitral stenosis is present, dyspnea is the most prominent symptom.

Diagnosis

Diagnosis of rheumatic fever is made by a history of recent infection, the presenting symptoms, and laboratory tests such as an ASO (antistreptolysin O) titer. No laboratory test is specific for diagnosis of rheumatic fever.

Rheumatic heart disease may be diagnosed by a patient history of rheumatic fever and other cardiac diagnostic tests, such as ECG and echocardiogram.

Treatment

Once rheumatic fever occurs, no treatment is specific. Penicillin is given to destroy any remaining group A streptococci. Aspirin and corticosteroids may be used to control other symptoms of the disorder.

Rheumatic fever can often be prevented if upper respiratory infections caused by the group A streptococci are promptly diagnosed and treated. Penicillin is the drug of choice; for people allergic to penicillin, another antibiotic may be prescribed. Long-term therapy with penicillin is indicated for patients with a history of rheumatic fever to prevent further streptococcal infections and, therefore, recurrences of rheumatic fever. Drug therapy is continued throughout childhood and may even continue throughout life if a high risk of exposure to streptococcal infections or evidence of rheumatic heart disease is present.

The treatment of rheumatic heart disease depends on the structure of the heart involved and the extent of damage to the structure. No treatment may be necessary or intensive treatment, such as surgery for mitral stenosis and drugs to treat heart failure, could be required.

Complications

Rheumatic fever often leads to permanent damage of the heart and valves with subsequent chronic valvular heart disease. About half of the patients with rheumatic heart disease have involvement of the mitral valve, called mitral stenosis.

NURSING PROCESS —THE PATIENT WHO HAS AN INFECTIOUS OR INFLAMMATORY DISORDER OF THE HEART

Assessment

In addition to the assessments performed on the cardiac patient (see Chapter 24), it is important to obtain a thorough history of the patient's symptoms as well as any past diseases or recent surgical procedures, including dental work. It also is important to determine what drugs the patient may have taken in the past 6 months. If the patient is unable to give an accurate history, a family member may be able to supply this information.

Nursing Diagnosis

Depending on the actual or potential medical diagnosis, the patient's presenting symptoms, and concurrent medical or surgical disorders, one or more of the following nursing diagnoses may apply:

- Activity intolerance related to symptoms of disease, seriousness of illness, decreased cardiac output
- Anxiety related to dyspnea, pain
- Hyperthermia related to infectious or inflammatory process
- Pain related to pericarditis
- Ineffective breathing pattern related to immobility
- Potential impaired skin integrity related to immobility
- Potential for infection at venipuncture site related to prolonged intravenous infusions
- Potential fluid volume deficit related to diaphoresis, inability to take oral fluids
- Altered nutrition: less than body requirements related to inactivity, anorexia, seriousness of condition
- Knowledge deficit of treatment regimen, home care

Planning and Implementation

The major goals of the patient include a reduction in anxiety, reduction of fever, relief from pain, improvement in respiratory function, prevention of skin breakdown, prevention of infection, attaining and maintaining adequate oral intake, improved nutrition, and acquiring knowledge of the treatment modalities and home care.

The major goals of nursing management are directed at elimination of the infectious or inflammatory process and recognition and prevention of complications related to prolonged inactivity.

Vital signs are taken every 4 hours. In the more acutely ill patient, the blood pressure, pulse, and respiratory rate may be taken more frequently. The patient is closely observed for signs of complications of the disorder or any change in status. In some instances, for example in a patient with pericarditis, constant awareness of the possibility of cardiac tamponade (see earlier discussion) must be kept in mind. Signs of complications are reported to the physician immediately because they can be life-threatening.

If antibiotics are administered, it is of critical importance that the drugs be given at the prescribed times. Omission of a drug dose or giving the drug late increases the chance that the infection will not remain under control. Adequate blood levels of these drugs must be maintained to destroy the infectious agent. The patient must also be observed for adverse drug reactions.

Activity Intolerance. Patients are often acutely ill. Complete bed rest may be mandatory if cardiac output is decreased and it is necessary to prevent added strain on the heart. Patients may require total assistance with most of their activities; or they may be allowed to participate in some activities but require assistance because of associated dyspnea, fatigue, and malaise.

Anxiety. Anxiety may occur for various reasons, such as pain, discomfort, concern over the prognosis, and difficulty breathing. If anxiety is apparent, the nurse makes an attempt to determine the cause. For example, if anxiety is due to pain or difficulty breathing, administration of the prescribed analgesic or oxygen may reduce anxiety as well as relieve the symptoms.

Hyperthermia. The temperature is monitored every 4 hours, and the prescribed antipyretic is given when the temperature is elevated. Prompt changes of perspiration-dampened bedding are required. If the antipyretic fails to lower the temperature, the physician is notified.

Pain. Pain can be severe and is usually controlled with the administration of an analgesic. Discomfort that suddenly progresses from mild to moderate or severe pain is reported to the physician immediately.

Respiratory Function. Shallow breathing can occur in relatively immobile patients. The patient is encouraged to take deep breaths every hour while awake to prevent respiratory complications, such as hypostatic pneumonia and atelectasis. The chest should be auscultated daily for normal and abnormal breath sounds. Difficulty breathing, rise in temperature, change in the rate or rhythm of respiration, sudden production of sputum, and pain in a different location or pain on inspiration are reported to the physician.

Potential Impaired Skin Integrity. Because patients on prolonged bed rest are prone to skin breakdown, good skin care is essential. The position is changed, and patients are encouraged to exercise and move their extremities every 2 hours. Early signs of skin breakdown (redness, soreness) are brought to the attention of the physician.

Potential for Infection. Prolonged administration of intravenous drugs can result in a localized or systemic infection. The intravenous line is changed according to hospital policy, and the insertion site is checked daily for redness (see also Chapter 13).

Potential Fluid Volume Deficit. The patient's intake and output are measured, and the physician is noti-

fied if the patient fails to take sufficient oral fluids or the output falls below 500 mL/day. Unless the physician orders fluid restrictions, the patient also is encouraged to drink fluids during waking hours.

Altered Nutrition. Prolonged inactivity may result in anorexia and weight loss. A special diet, such as one restricted in sodium, may be ordered if congestive heart failure is present. The tray should be checked after each meal, and the physician is notified if the patient fails to eat most of the food on the tray over a period of several days.

If the patient fails to eat because of a dislike of the prescribed diet, a dietary consultation may be necessary. The dietitian may be able to add certain foods or flavorings to make the diet more palatable.

Knowledge Deficit. The procedures required during therapy and the importance of each treatment modality must be explained to the patient and family, and they must be given time to ask questions.

Patients with endocarditis must be informed of the necessity of continued follow-up care after discharge from the hospital. Patients with damaged heart valves should be given antibiotics just before and for a short time after any event that might cause bacteremia, such as a tooth extraction or childbirth. Patients must understand that this precaution is necessary for as long as they live; they always will be vulnerable to episodes of endocarditis.

Those with other infectious or inflammatory disorders of the heart also may require continued drug therapy and follow-up care after discharge. The importance of continued treatment is stressed.

If a patient is discharged with a prescription, the importance of following the directions on the container regarding dosage and time intervals is stressed.

Evaluation

- The infection or inflammation is controlled
- Activity tolerance is increased
- Anxiety is reduced
- Body temperature is normal
- Pain is controlled
- Respiratory function is normal; breathing pattern is normal; takes deep breaths hourly while awake
- Skin remains intact with no signs of breakdown; changes position and moves extremities hourly while awake
- No evidence of localized infection at venipuncture site
- Fluid intake and urine output is normal
- Attains and maintains normal food intake
- Verbalizes an understanding of treatment modalities and importance of continued follow-up care

INFLAMMATORY DISORDERS OF PERIPHERAL BLOOD VESSELS
Thrombophlebitis *(+) Homan's sign*

Thrombophlebitis means inflammation of a vein accompanied by clot formation. Venous stasis predisposes to the development of thrombophlebitis. Factors that contribute to venous stasis are inactivity, heart failure, and pressure on the veins in the pelvis or legs. Elderly patients and those with heart disease, infections, or dehydration are susceptible to thrombophlebitis. Prolonged sitting has led to thrombophlebitis. The importance of changing position frequently and of exercising the legs at intervals cannot be overemphasized.

Symptoms

Symptoms include pain, heat, redness, and swelling in the affected region. The legs are usually involved. If interference with deep venous return is marked, the leg becomes swollen and may have a mottled, bluish color. A patient often has systemic symptoms of fever, malaise, fatigue, and anorexia.

Diagnosis

Diagnosis is based on the presenting symptoms and examination of the affected area. A positive Homans' sign (pain in the calf of the leg on dorsiflexion of the foot) may be elicited.

Treatment

Treatment usually includes complete rest of the leg and promotion of venous return by elevating the foot of the bed. The affected part *never* is rubbed; rubbing could dislodge a clot and result in an embolism to a vital organ.

Treatment for thrombophlebitis includes continuous warm, wet packs (or soaks) to ease pain and decrease inflammation. A thermostatically controlled device may be used to provide uninterrupted dry or moist heat. Anticoagulant therapy with heparin or oral anticoagulants also may be prescribed. People with repeated episodes of these disorders may be placed on long-term oral anticoagulant therapy.

On occasion, surgical intervention may be necessary when a large vein is occluded by a clot or danger of a pulmonary embolus arises. A thrombectomy, the surgical removal of a clot, may be performed if the clot interferes with a large area of venous drainage, such as in the femoral vein. With danger of pulmonary emboli, surgery on the vena cava may be necessary to reduce the possibility of a clot traveling from the lower extremity to the lungs. Several surgical procedures may be performed on the vena cava: ligation of the vena cava, insertion of an umbrellalike prosthesis in the vena cava, or a vena caval plication. A plication procedure changes the lumen of the vena cava from a single channel to several small channels through the use of suture or a Teflon clip.

When symptoms of thrombophlebitis have subsided, the patient gradually is permitted more activity. The leg is elevated for only part of the day, and the patient is allowed to walk. Usually, elastic bandages or elastic stockings are advised at first to give support and to promote venous return. The condition frequently subsides completely, and the patient may resume normal activities. The illness and convalescent period may last several weeks or even several months.

Prevention

Thrombophlebitis can be prevented. Unless leg exercises are contraindicated by a patient's condition, all patients who are unable to walk should perform leg exercises while in bed. Active exercises are preferable, such as bending the knee, rotating the foot at the ankle, and wiggling the toes. If a patient is unable to carry out active exercises, passive ones may be given. Pressure should not be applied to the legs, and pillows and blanket rolls should not be placed behind the knees for prolonged periods. Prolonged sitting is avoided because the chair may cause pressure behind the knees. Convalescent patients should alternate sitting with walking around the room or lying on the bed.

If a patient is on prolonged bed rest or is undergoing certain surgeries, elastic stockings may be applied to prevent thrombophlebitis. The stockings must be removed and reapplied at least twice daily. Elevating the foot of the bed also may be of value for these patients.

Anticoagulants may be given to patients who are especially susceptible to thrombophlebitis or who have had recurrent episodes of the disorder.

Thromboangiitis Obliterans (Buerger's Disease)

Thromboangiitis obliterans is an inflammation of blood vessels that is associated with formation of clots and fibrosis of the blood vessel wall. This condition leads to the obstruction of the blood vessels. This peripheral vascular disease affects primarily the arteries and the veins of the lower extremities. The upper extremities occasionally are involved. Thrombophlebitis also may be present.

The cause of thromboangiitis obliterans is not definitely established. It is far more common among men than women, and it usually has its onset during young adulthood.

Symptoms

The patient notes that one foot or both feet are always cold. Intermittent claudication (cramps in the legs after exercise) is a common symptom. Usually, the symptoms fluctuate in severity; attacks of acute distress are often followed by remissions during which few symptoms are present.

Cyanosis and redness of the feet and legs may be noted. Frequently, the color is a mottled purplish red. Ulcers that heal slowly or progress to the development of gangrene may occur, particularly at the toes and heels. Changes in the skin and nails are characteristic when circulation has been impaired for a considerable period. Phlebitis is common. Pain at rest occurs when circulation has been seriously impaired and particularly when ulcers have formed. Although the disease usually is most pronounced in one leg and foot, both legs usually are affected to some degree.

Diagnosis

Diagnosis is based on symptoms. Arteriograms of the affected extremity also may be used to identify the degree of occlusion of the involved arteries.

Treatment

Exercise helps stimulate circulation, provided it is not excessive and does not cause pain. Buerger-Allen exercises, walking, and active foot exercises may be prescribed by the physician. Analgesics may be required to ease pain. Because the disease is chronic, the physician attempts to control the pain without narcotics because of the danger of addiction.

The legs are kept horizontal or dependent, except during Buerger-Allen exercises or while the patient is on the oscillating bed, if these measures have been prescribed. Elevating the legs increases ischemia and therefore causes or increases pain.

A sympathectomy may be performed to relieve vasospasm. If ulcerations occur on the extremity and become infected, antibiotics are ordered to control the infection. If circulation becomes so impaired that gangrene results, amputation may be necessary.

NURSING PROCESS — THE PATIENT WHO HAS AN INFLAMMATORY DISORDER OF PERIPHERAL BLOOD VESSELS

Assessment

A thorough patient history is taken and includes the symptoms and the length of time the symptoms have been present. For those with thromboangiitis obliterans, a smoking history is especially important. If pain is present, a description of the type and degree of pain as well as factors that increase or decrease pain is recorded.

The affected areas are examined for redness, swelling, and other color changes, such as cyanosis or mottling. The nails and skin are inspected for changes, and the skin temperature above and below the affected area is noted.

Nursing Diagnosis

Depending on the type and severity of the disorder and the areas affected, one or more of the following may apply. Additional nursing diagnoses may be needed if the patient incurs other problems, such as loss of appetite or constipation due to inactivity.

- Activity intolerance related to inflammatory process
- Pain related to inflammatory process
- Impaired skin integrity related to inflammatory process, immobility
- Knowledge deficit related to treatment modalities, methods of prevention of repeat episodes (thrombophlebitis), importance of preventing infection and injury

Planning and Implementation

The major goals of the patient include an increase in activity tolerance, reduction or elimination of pain, prevention of trauma to the extremities, prevention of future episodes (thrombophlebitis), prevention of skin breakdown, and acquiring knowledge of home care.

The primary goals of nursing management are the prevention of complications and the relief of pain and other symptoms.

Activity Intolerance. Patients with thromboangiitis obliterans have difficulty walking. Buerger-Allen exercises may increase circulation to the extremities, thus increasing the amount of activity that can be performed without pain or discomfort. Patients are allowed to engage in activities as tolerated, and they should be assisted when pain is severe.

If Buerger-Allen exercises are prescribed, the patient requires a demonstration and explanation of the exercises followed by supervision until they are performed correctly. To perform these exercises, the patient first lies flat in bed with both legs elevated above the level of the heart for 2 or 3 minutes. Next, the patient sits on the edge of the bed with the legs dependent for about 3 minutes. At this time, the feet and toes are exercised by moving them up, down, inward, and outward. The last part of the exercise involves returning to the first position and holding it for about 5 minutes.

Pain. In patients with thromboangiitis obliterans, pain may be relieved by Buerger-Allen exercises. Elevation of the legs is avoided because it increases pain. Patients with thrombophlebitis experience no pain or varying degrees of pain, and a mild analgesic may be prescribed. If pain is experienced in an area other than the one affected by the thrombophlebitis, the physician is notified immediately; a part of the thrombus may have traveled to another area of the body.

Impaired Skin Integrity. Patients with thromboangiitis obliterans may develop gangrene of the extremity. The skin of the leg is protected from trauma and is inspected daily for any changes in color, breaks in the skin, or signs of infection.

Patients on prolonged bed rest must be encouraged to change their position at least every 2 hours. The skin over bony prominences is inspected for signs of skin breakdown.

Knowledge Deficit. In some cases, future episodes of thrombophlebitis can be prevented; thus, patient teaching assumes an important role in the prevention of this disorder. Thromboangiitis obliterans cannot be cured, but progression of the disorder can be delayed and symptoms relieved by patient adherence to the prescribed regimen.

THE PATIENT WITH THROMBOPHLEBITIS.   Patients with thrombophlebitis must be taught how to prevent future episodes. The measures that may be suggested include avoiding prolonged sitting, crossing the legs, tight garments that reduce venous return in the legs, and injury to the extremities, and weight reduction, exercise, and periodic elevation of the legs above the level of the heart. Patients who are prescribed long-term anticoagulant therapy are informed of the importance of taking the medication exactly as prescribed and of the importance of having the prescribed laboratory tests to determine the effectiveness of therapy.

THE PATIENT WITH THROMBOANGIITIS OBLITERANS.   Patients who are required to perform Buerger-Allen exercises at home must be thoroughly familiar with the sequence of the exercises. The exercises are performed under supervision until the patient has mastered them. The importance of doing these exercises as prescribed by the physician is stressed. Additional measures to teach include obtaining adequate rest, inspecting the skin and nails of the extremities daily, cleaning the extremities properly, avoiding trauma to and infection of the extremities, wearing proper fitting shoes and stockings (or socks), and avoiding prolonged exposure to the cold. When exposure to cold weather is necessary, warm socks and gloves are worn, and the feet are adequately protected from ice and snow.

The use of heating pads is avoided. The patient is instructed to avoid becoming chilled. Prolonged standing is avoided. The prevention of injury and infection of the extremities is important. Even mild injury or a slight infection can have serious consequences because of a decrease in circulation.

The use of tobacco in any form is contraindicated and should never be resumed, even if symptoms are relieved. It should be emphasized that smoking makes the disease worse.

Evaluation

- Able to perform activities of daily living within limits of tolerance or prescribed activity
- Pain is relieved or eliminated
- Demonstrates correct performance of Buerger-Allen exercises
- Verbalizes understanding of daily care of the affected extremities
- Verbalizes understanding of preventive measures
- Maintains skin integrity

General Pharmacologic Considerations

- ☐ Although patients with peripheral vascular disease usually have pain, narcotics are avoided. Nonnarcotic analgesics, such as salicylates, may be used.
- ☐ Heparin therapy may be instituted for a patient with thrombophlebitis. Heparin, an anticoagulant, prevents extension of the thrombus and the development of additional thrombi.
- ☐ Oral anticoagulants (eg, warfarin sodium) may be prescribed as part of the long-term management of venous thrombosis.
- ☐ Heparin is measured in units, and the dosage is regulated by venous clotting time determinations such as the Lee-White or the partial thromboplastin time. Optimum drug effect is reached when the Lee-White time is 2.5 to 3 times normal and the partial thromboplastin time is 1.5 to 2.5 times normal.
- ☐ Patients receiving any anticoagulant must be observed for signs of a tendency to bleed (eg, blood in the urine or stool, easy bruising, bleeding gums, excessive bleeding from minor cuts or scratches).

General Gerontologic Considerations

☐ When teaching the older patient how to increase the blood supply to an extremity and what situations to avoid, each point should be explained and then given in written form.

Suggested Readings

☐ Abrams AC. Clinical drug therapy: rationales for nursing practice. 2nd ed. Philadelphia: JB Lippincott, 1987. *(Additional and in-depth coverage of subject matter)*

☐ Andreoli KG, Zipes DP, Wallace AG, Kinney MR, Fowkes VK. Comprehensive cardiac care. 6th ed. St Louis: CV Mosby, 1987. *(Additional and in-depth coverage of subject matter)*

☐ Berkow R, Fletcher AJ, eds. Merck manual of diagnosis and therapy. 15th ed. Rahway, NJ: Merck & Co, 1987. *(In-depth coverage of subject matter)*

☐ Bowers AC, Thompson JM. Clinical manual of health assessment. 3rd ed. St Louis: CV Mosby, 1988. *(In-depth coverage of subject matter)*

☐ Burden LL, Rogers JC. Endocarditis: when bacteria invade the heart. RN December 1988;51:39. *(Additional coverage of subject matter)*

☐ Burton GRW. Microbiology for the health sciences. 3rd ed. Philadelphia: JB Lippincott, 1988. *(Additional coverage of subject matter)*

☐ Rodgers ML. Pericarditis: a different kind of heart disease. Nurs'90 February 1990;20:52. *(Additional coverage and illustrations that reinforce subject matter)*

☐ Solomon J. Introduction to cardiovascular nursing. Baltimore: Wilkins & Wilkins. 1988. *(Additional and in-depth coverage of subject matter)*

☐ Talkington S, Raterirk, eds. Every nurse's guide to cardiovascular care. New York: John Wiley & Sons, 1987. *(Additional coverage of subject matter)*

Chapter 26

Valvular Disorders of the Heart

On completion of this chapter the reader will:

- List the disorders of the aortic valve

- Discuss the symptoms, diagnosis, and treatment of aortic valve disorders

- List and discuss the disorders of the mitral valve

- Discuss the symptoms, diagnosis, and treatment of mitral valve disorders

- List and discuss the disorders of the tricuspid valve

- Discuss the symptoms, diagnosis, and treatment of tricuspid valve disorders

- Use the nursing process in the nursing management of a patient with a valvular disorder of the heart

DISORDERS OF THE AORTIC VALVE

The aortic valve has three crescent-shaped cusps and is situated between the aorta and the left ventricle. The two forms of valvular heart disease that affect the aortic valve are aortic stenosis and aortic insufficiency, or aortic regurgitation.

Aortic Stenosis

In aortic stenosis (a narrowing of the aortic valve), blood flow from the left ventricle is impaired owing to stiffened valve leaflets that fail to open properly. As a result, more force is needed to push blood through the narrowed opening. The work of the left ventricle is increased, causing the ventricular myocardium to thicken. The supply of blood passing through the narrowed valve may be insufficient to nourish the brain and the muscles of the heart.

The most common causes of this disorder are rheumatic fever and, in older patients, calcification of the aortic valve as a result of arteriosclerosis (Fig. 26-1).

Symptoms

A patient with aortic stenosis may experience dizziness, fainting, and anginal pain because of insufficient blood in the coronary arteries that arise from the aorta, immediately above the aortic valve. Dyspnea on exertion also may be noticed.

Diagnosis

Diagnosis is made by patient history and physical examination. Auscultation of the heart reveals a murmur during systole. An electrocardiogram (ECG) may reveal left ventricular hypertrophy. Left-sided cardiac catheterization may be used to determine the severity of the disorder.

Treatment

Medical management involves treating the symptoms of left ventricular failure. Digitalis, antiarrhythmic drugs, and diuretics may be prescribed. Antibiotics are prescribed before and after dental procedures and invasive procedures, such as urinary tract instrumentation, to prevent infective endocarditis.

Because medical management produces only temporary relief, valve replacement may be considered (see Chapter 31). Surgery, when possible, is performed before the patient reaches the late stages of the disease, when the left ventricle enlarges and heart failure occurs.

Aortic Insufficiency (Aortic Regurgitation)

In aortic insufficiency, the valve is incompetent and does not close tightly. Blood flowing through it during

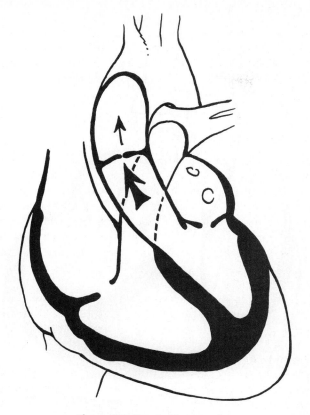

Figure 26–1. Aortic stenosis.

systole drops back into the left ventricle instead of moving forward through the aorta. This backflow decreases the amount of circulating blood, causes fluid overload in the ventricle, and may lead to left ventricular failure.

Valve damage usually is caused by rheumatic fever, endocarditis (especially when it is superimposed on a valve already damaged by rheumatic fever), and syphilis.

Symptoms
Pulse pressure usually is widened. The left ventricle ultimately hypertrophies and goes into failure. On palpation, the radial pulse is forceful, with quick, sharp beats followed by a sudden collapse of the force of the beat. This type of pulse is characteristic of aortic insufficiency and is called water-hammer (Corrigan's) pulse. The patient is aware of palpitation, a throbbing sensation in the head, and dyspnea related to left ventricular failure.

Diagnosis
Diagnosis is made by the patient history of symptoms and physical examination. Cardiac angiography also may be used.

Treatment
Treatment includes replacement of the aortic valve (see Chapter 31) as well as relief of symptoms asso-

ciated with left ventricular failure. Digitalis, antiarrhythmic drugs, and diuretics may be prescribed.

If the disorder is caused by endocarditis or rheumatic fever, prophylactic antibiotics are given before and after all dental procedures, instrumentation and surgery of the urinary tract, and any procedure that may cause bacteremia.

DISORDERS OF THE MITRAL VALVE

The mitral valve has two leaflets and is situated between the left atrium and the left ventricle. In healthy hearts, the leaflets open with each contraction of the atrium to allow blood to flow from the left atrium into the left ventricle. The mitral valve closes as the ventricle fills. The forms of valvular heart disease that affect that mitral valve are mitral stenosis, mitral insufficiency, and mitral prolapse.

Mitral Stenosis

The most common cause of mitral stenosis is inflammation and scarring of the leaflets as a result of rheumatic fever. The leaflets stick together and cannot open and close completely. They tend to become progressively thicker. The opening narrows, so that the left atrium cannot empty to receive a new full load of blood from the pulmonary artery and veins. To compensate, the left atrium contracts more forceably and enlarges. Pressure is then exerted backward through the blood vessels of the lungs and builds up in the pulmonary artery (pulmonary hypertension), which carries blood from the right ventricle to the lungs. Pressure also eventually increases in the right ventricle. Because it usually takes less force to pump blood through the lungs than through the rest of the body, the walls of the right ventricle are thinner than the walls of the left ventricle. In longstanding mitral stenosis, the walls of the right ventricle thicken. When the muscle walls can no longer meet the demands of the increased workload caused by the narrowed mitral valve, pressure is passed to the right atrium and to the entire venous system of the body. The liver and the lungs become congested; edema occurs in the legs. Because the ventricles are not receiving a normal amount of blood to pump through the body, the organs are not receiving sufficient oxygenated blood.

Symptoms
A patient with mitral stenosis tires easily, becomes short of breath even after slight exertion, has lowered systolic blood pressure, and may appear emaciated. Although weight may be gained because of edema, the

appetite is poor. As the disorder progresses, congestive heart failure (CHF) occurs.

Diagnosis

Diagnosis is made by the patient history and auscultation of the heart. Diagnostic tests may include ECG, phonocardiography, echocardiography, and cardiac catheterization.

Treatment

Relieving the symptoms of CHF often is an important part of the treatment of patients with mitral stenosis. Surgical treatment is possible; however, not all patients with mitral stenosis are suitable candidates for surgery. Usually excluded are those whose condition is so slight that it does not cause symptoms or so severe or of such long duration that profound changes in the heart and the lungs have occurred. The earlier in the disease process the surgery is performed, the greater the likelihood that the symptoms will be relieved. Surgical management of mitral stenosis includes commissurotomy, valvuloplasty, or valve replacement (see Chapter 31).

Mitral Insufficiency (Mitral Regurgitation)

In mitral insufficiency, the valve does not close completely. Consequently, blood from the left ventricle flows back (regurgitates) into the left atrium (Fig. 26-2). The left ventricle becomes overfilled with blood, and some blood is pushed back through the mitral valve into the left atrium. Because of overfilling, the ventricular walls become distended, and left ventricular failure occurs.

Insufficiency of the mitral valve may be caused by rheumatic fever or mitral valve prolapse (see later discussion).

Symptoms

Symptoms of mitral insufficiency include exertional dyspnea, palpitations, and cough caused by congestion in the lungs. Dysrhythmias, primarily atrial fibrillation, may occur. Atrial fibrillation may result in the formation of emboli.

Diagnosis

Diagnosis is made by a thorough patient history, auscultation of the heart, chest radiography, ECG, echocardiography, stress testing, and cardiac catheterization.

Treatment

Among the operations performed to correct mitral insufficiency are mitral commissurotomy and the im-

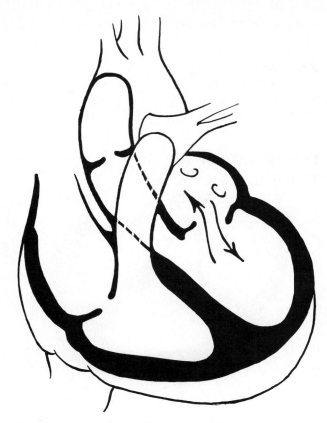

Figure 26–2. Mitral insufficiency. The inadequate valve allows blood to return to the left atrium.

plantation of a prosthetic valve to restore unidirectional blood flow (see Chapter 31). Medical treatment includes digitalis and anticoagulant therapy to correct dysrhythmias and prevent the formation of emboli.

Mitral Valve Prolapse

In mitral valve prolapse, the valve leaflets enlarge and bulge backward into the left atrium. Although the reason for this prolapse is not completely understood, it occasionally occurs in patients with some connective tissue diseases and in those with coronary artery disease. It is more common in young women and can be inherited.

Symptoms

Many patients with mitral valve prolapse are asymptomatic. When symptoms are present, they usually include chest pain, palpitations, and fatigue. Heart failure also may be present.

Diagnosis

Auscultation of the heart reveals a midsystolic click. Mitral insufficiency (see earlier discussion) also may be heard. Diagnostic studies include ECG, chest radiography, echocardiography, stress testing, and cardiac catheterization.

Treatment

Many patients require no treatment. Dysrhythmias may be controlled with antiarrhythmic drugs. If symptoms become severe, valve replacement may be considered.

DISORDERS OF THE TRICUSPID VALVE

The tricuspid valve has three leaflets and is located between the right atrium and the right ventricle. Two forms of valvular heart disease affect this valve: tricuspid stenosis and tricuspid insufficiency, or tricuspid regurgitation.

Tricuspid Stenosis

Stenosis (narrowing) of the tricuspid valve obstructs the blood flow from the right atrium to the right ventricle, causing the right atrium to dilate and hypertrophy.

The most common cause of this disorder is rheumatic fever.

Symptoms

Symptoms include a diastolic murmur and a noticeable pulse wave in the neck veins. Peripheral edema, ascites, and an enlarged liver may be seen. Mitral stenosis often is associated with tricuspid stenosis.

Diagnosis

Diagnosis is made by ECG and auscultation of the heart.

Treatment

When possible, surgical repair or replacement of the valve is attempted.

NURSING PROCESS —THE PATIENT WHO HAS A VALVULAR DISORDER

Assessment

In addition to the assessments performed on the patient with heart disease (see Chapter 24), it is important to obtain a thorough history of all past diseases and infectious disorders. Because rheumatic fever can affect one or more valves of the heart, a history of childhood diseases must be included. See Chapter 31 if the patient is scheduled for or has had valve replacement surgery.

Nursing Diagnosis

Depending on the severity of symptoms and the valve or number of valves affected, one or more of the following nursing diagnoses may apply:

- Activity intolerance related to dyspnea
- Fatigue related to dyspnea, CHF
- Anxiety related to dyspnea, scheduled diagnostic procedures, treatment, diagnosis
- Potential for infection related to past history of endocarditis or rheumatic fever, recent (invasive) diagnostic procedures
- Impaired home maintenance management related to inability to perform household duties
- Knowledge deficit of treatment modalities (home, hospital)

Planning and Implementation

The major goals of the patient include improvement in activity tolerance, reduction of anxiety, decrease in fatigue, absence of infection, and an understanding of postdischarge treatment.

The major goals of nursing management are to improve respiratory function, reduce anxiety, and recognize complications of the specific valve disorder (eg, CHF caused by failure of the left ventricle).

Vital signs should be monitored daily to every 4 hours, depending on the severity of the disorder. Any sudden change should be reported to the physician, as medical treatment (eg, drug therapy) may be necessary to stabilize the patient's condition.

Activity Intolerance.   Depending on their degree of exertional dyspnea, patients with valvular disease may require complete or partial assistance with activities of daily living. Patients should be allowed to participate in their activities of daily living according to the physician's orders as well as their degree of tolerance. Adequate time should be allowed for self-care, and activities should be spaced to reduce the workload of the heart.

Dyspnea may result in an impairment of oxygen–carbon dioxide exchange in the lungs. Oxygen therapy may be needed if dyspnea is severe. Mild exertional dyspnea may be controlled by promoting bed rest and spacing activities to reduce the workload of the heart.

Anxiety.   Anxiety may occur because of difficulty breathing, inability to care for self, or planned treatment (eg, surgery). Scheduling activities that are tolerated without inducing dyspnea may reduce anxiety. The nurse can reduce the patient's anxiety before an invasive diagnostic procedure by explaining the procedure and answering questions about it.

Because a valvular disorder can be serious, these patients often need time to talk about their disorder and the treatments proposed by the physician.

Potential for Infection. The patient's temperature should be monitored twice daily or as ordered. More frequent monitoring of the temperature may be necessary after an invasive diagnostic procedure such as angiography. A sudden rise in body temperature, chills, and inflammation of the area used for catheter insertion should be reported to the physician.

Impaired Home Maintenance Management. Some patients experience severe exertional dyspnea that interferes with their normal daily activities or ability to be employed. The extent of the problem should be identified and the appropriate agencies or individuals contacted in an effort to resolve the problem. For example, a mother who is having difficulty caring for her children and a household may be able to obtain help from other family members or from friends. If this is not possible, a community agency may be able to offer financial assistance as well as provide a home health care aide, which will partially or totally relieve the burden placed on her.

Knowledge Deficit. Before discharge from the hospital, the patient or a family member should receive a complete explanation of all treatment modalities prescribed by the physician. Treatment may include drug therapy, adequate rest, and a change in activities.

These patients should be advised to see their physicians before any dental or other invasive procedure is carried out, so that the appropriate prophylactic antibiotic therapy can be started.

Evaluation

- Activity tolerance is maintained or improved
- Anxiety is reduced
- No evidence of infection is present at site of invasive diagnostic procedure
- Patient's breathing pattern is improved; gas exchange is improved or remains stable
- Home maintenance problems are identified; appropriate agencies are notified and immediate needs are met
- Patient demonstrates understanding of treatment modalities
- Patient verbalizes understanding of importance of seeing the physician before dental or invasive procedures are performed

General Nutritional Considerations

☐ A low-sodium diet may be prescribed for patients with a valvular heart disorder to prevent edema or if the patient develops signs of CHF.

General Pharmacologic Considerations

☐ A cardiac glycoside such as digoxin may be prescribed for the patient with CHF resulting from valvular insufficiency.

☐ An anticoagulant may be prescribed to prevent the formation of emboli. Lifetime therapy with this type of drug may be necessary.

☐ Penicillin, as well as other antibiotics, may be prescribed to prevent (prophylaxis) a recurrent infection that could affect an already damaged heart valve.

☐ Dysrhythmias may require administration of an antiarrhythmic drug. Frequent monitoring of the effect of the drug may be necessary until heart rhythm returns to normal.

Suggested Readings

☐ Andreoli KG, Zipes DP, Wallace AG, Kinney MR, Fowkes VK. Comprehensive cardiac care. 6th ed. St Louis: CV Mosby, 1987. *(Additional and in-depth coverage of subject matter)*

☐ Baas L, Kretten C. Valvular heart disease: its causes, symptoms and consequences. RN November 1987;50:30. *(Additional coverage of subject matter)*

☐ Civetta JM, Taylor RW, Kirby RR. Introduction to critical care. Philadelphia: JB Lippincott, 1989. *(In-depth, high-level coverage of subject matter)*

☐ Cullen L, Laxson C. Ballooning open a stenotic valve. Am J Nurs July 1988;88:987. *(Additional coverage of subject matter)*

☐ Erickson B. Heart sounds and murmurs: a practical guide. St Louis: CV Mosby, 1988. *(In-depth, high-level coverage of subject matter)*

☐ Juleff GL. Cracking open a blocked heart valve. Nursing '89 July 1989;19:58. *(Additional coverage of subject matter)*

☐ Kretten C, Bass L. Valvular heart disease: surgery and postop care. RN December 1987;50:38. *(Additional coverage of subject matter)*

☐ Luckmann J, Sorensen K. Medical–surgical nursing: a psychophysiologic approach. 3rd ed. Philadelphia: WB Saunders, 1987. *(Additional and in-depth coverage of subject matter)*

☐ Mason CB, Davis JE. Cardiovascular critical care. New York: Van Nostrand Reinhold, 1987. *(In-depth, high-level coverage of subject matter)*

Chapter 27

Occlusive Disorders of Coronary and Peripheral Blood Vessels

On completion of this chapter the reader will:

- Distinguish between arteriosclerosis and atherosclerosis

- Discuss the major causes of coronary artery disease

- List and discuss the symptoms, diagnosis, and treatment of coronary artery disease

- List and discuss the symptoms, diagnosis, and treatment of angina pectoris

- List and discuss the symptoms, diagnosis, and treatment of myocardial infarction

- List the complications associated with myocardial infarction

- Use the nursing process in the management of a patient with an occlusive disorder of the coronary blood vessels

- List and discuss the symptoms, diagnosis, and treatment of Raynaud's disease

- List and discuss the symptoms, diagnosis, and treatment of thrombosis, phlebothrombosis, and embolism

- Use the nursing process in the management of the patient with an occlusive disorder of peripheral blood vessels

ARTERIOSCLEROSIS AND ATHEROSCLEROSIS

Arteriosclerosis and atherosclerosis commonly accompany the aging process. *Arteriosclerosis* refers to the hardening and loss of elasticity of the arteries. *Atherosclerosis*, the most common cause of arterial disease, refers to the accumulation of fatty deposits (chiefly composed of cholesterol) on the walls of the arteries. These deposits, called *plaques,* narrow the lumen of the artery, reducing the volume of blood flowing to areas served by the artery.

Arteriosclerosis and atherosclerosis affect many parts of the body (eg, the heart, brain, kidneys, and extremities) and cause a variety of disorders (eg, renal failure, myocardial infarction, and stroke).

The rate at which changes occur in various organs or structures varies. Patients with diabetes mellitus suffer these changes quite early in life. Other factors that may influence the age of onset and the severity of the condition are heredity and diet. Those with a family history of vascular disease may be prone to develop the condition.

OCCLUSIVE DISORDERS OF CORONARY BLOOD VESSELS

Coronary occlusion is the closing of an already narrowed coronary artery. It can reduce or totally interrupt blood supply to an area. The seriousness of the occlusion depends on the organ involved, the size of the blood vessel, and the degree of occlusion. Vital organs such as the heart, lungs, and brain often are affected by occlusive disorders.

Total or partial occlusion (obstruction) of a blood vessel can be caused by the following:

- Spasm of the blood vessel
- Narrowing of the lumen by atherosclerotic plaques
- Thrombus formation on the wall of the vessel
- Embolus consisting of fat, air, or blood that becomes lodged in the blood vessel lumen
- Tumor
- Scar tissue

Coronary Artery Disease

The myocardium has its own blood supply, which consists of a system of coronary arteries. Blood flows through these vessels and through branches over the outer surface of the heart, then into smaller capillaries in the cardiac muscle, and finally back to the systemic circulation through the coronary veins that empty into the coronary sinus in the right atrium.

The two main coronary arteries, the right and the left coronary arteries, originate from the aorta immediately above the aortic valve and receive the first supply of rich, oxygenated blood leaving the left ventricle. The myocardium is nourished with little overlap of vessels from one region to another. If a coronary artery is blocked, few other vessels can take over the blood supply to the area served by the blocked artery, and viability of myocardial tissue is threatened.

Like other arteries in the body, the coronary arteries may develop degenerative changes or disease. The pathologic change most responsible for coronary artery disease is atherosclerosis—the gradual deposition of substances such as lipids and calcium on the arterial walls, making them narrower.

Coronary artery disease is more common among people over age 50, but it may occur in younger people. A familial tendency toward early development of the condition has been noted. During early middle life, men are affected more frequently than women. The incidence of coronary artery disease rises in postmenopausal women and becomes similar to that in men.

During the course of slowly advancing atherosclerotic disease of the coronary arteries, or after an acute coronary occlusion, preexisting anastomotic (communicating) channels open up and grow into the involved area. This is called collateral circulation. In patients with coronary artery disease, the rate of development and the extent of new collateral circulation are of critical importance in the survival and viability of myocardial tissue.

A diminished oxygen supply to cells is one of the best stimulants to myocardial blood supply. A person with slowly progressive coronary atherosclerosis may have developed collateral circulation over the course of time that may be valuable if a major vessel suddenly becomes occluded. A young person who never had the need or opportunity to develop collateral circulation has a greater chance of dying instantly after coronary occlusion because of the effects of overwhelming oxygen deficiency in a critical portion of the myocardium.

At rest, normal myocardial blood flow may be maintained despite considerable coronary artery narrowing; the ability to increase this flow sufficiently during exercise to meet the increased metabolic needs of the heart may be markedly impaired, however. Beyond the narrowed segment, the vessels supplied by the artery dilate. Because of this vasodilation and the development of adequate collateral circulation, people with significant coronary artery atherosclerosis may be fairly asymptomatic, and the disease may go unrecognized, particularly if they have a sedentary lifestyle. During exercise or emotional stress, which increases cardiac workload, the coronary arterial vasodilation that usually allows myocardial blood flow to increase

proportionately can no longer occur because the local capillary bed is already in a maximally dilated state. Under these circumstances, the myocardial demand for oxygen and metabolic nutrients exceeds the ability of the coronary circulation to supply them, and clinical manifestations of coronary heart disease, such as chest pain of cardiac origin (angina pectoris), may then occur.

Epidemiology

Cardiovascular disease is the leading cause of death in the United States. Many deaths are premature, in the sense that the victims are young or middle-aged adults, in the prime productive years of life, with basically sound myocardiums. For each fatality, there are two nonfatal but disabling events.

Coronary artery disease is thought to be due to many factors, rather than a single cause. Risk factors include the following:

- Age
- Sex
- Family history of coronary disease
- Hypertension
- Rise in serum cholesterol and triglyceride levels
- Obesity
- Cigarette smoking
- Lack of physical activity
- Personality–behavior patterns
- Emotionally stressful situations
- Other diseases, such as gout and diabetes mellitus

Symptoms

Symptoms of coronary artery occlusion are caused by an insufficient supply of blood to the myocardium. Like other muscles, the myocardium requires more blood when it works hardest (ie, during physical exertion or emotional stress). Blood supply through narrowed arteries may be sufficient for a body that is at rest but inadequate for the more strenuous activities of daily living. If the normal vessels or collateral circulation cannot meet the needs of the heart during exertion, symptoms related to a lack of blood supply to the myocardium (myocardial ischemia) develop. The most prominent symptom is chest pain (angina) or discomfort; in some patients, however, coronary artery occlusion is asymptomatic (without symptoms).

Diagnosis

Diagnosis is made by patient history, resting electrocardiography (ECG), and exercise ECG, or stress testing. Coronary angiography may be used to identify the involved artery or arteries. Laboratory tests usually include the determination of serum cholesterol and triglyceride levels; elevation of these levels has been associated with the development and progression of coronary artery disease.

Treatment

Treatment of coronary artery disease includes relief of anginal pain with antianginal drugs and prevention of further arterial occlusion by lowering elevated cholesterol and triglyceride levels. Some physicians advise their patients to take one aspirin tablet daily to prevent thrombi from causing coronary occlusion. Surgical procedures used to relieve the obstruction include coronary bypass surgery and percutaneous transluminal coronary angioplasty (see Chapter 31).

Angina Pectoris

Angina pectoris (severe pain around the heart), a common symptom of coronary artery disease, is caused by a lack of adequate blood supply to the myocardium (*myocardial ischemia*).

Symptoms

Attacks of angina pectoris are characterized by sudden chest pain or pressure, which may be severest over the heart under the sternum (substernal). Pain may radiate to the shoulders and arms, especially on the left side, or to the jaw, neck, or teeth. Some patients deny that they have pain but describe other sensations, such as a burning, squeezing, or crushing tightness in the upper chest or throat and indigestion. Dyspnea, pallor, sweating, and faintness may be experienced. Although the intensity of pain and the apprehension that it arouses may make minutes seem like hours, the attack usually lasts for less than 5 minutes. The pain may cause some patients to stop whatever they are doing and wait, tense and motionless, for the pain to subside. Anginal pain often occurs during periods of physical or emotional stress. An attack may be brought on by a particular activity, or it may occur without any apparent relation to meals, activity, rest, excitement, or anything that is under the patient's control. Patients feel particularly helpless because there is little they can do to lessen the frequency of the attack. Because rest reduces oxygen requirements of the myocardium, the pain usually subsides as soon as the patient rests.

Recognition of the significance of chest pain may help to prevent serious illness or even sudden death. The possibility of sudden death in these patients is real. The underlying problems of atherosclerosis and diminished circulation make the heart especially vulnerable to dysrhythmias and myocardial infarction, both of which may cause sudden death.

Diagnosis

Diagnosis is made by a careful patient history of the symptoms. ECG and stress testing may help to identify coronary artery disease. Coronary angiography can reveal collateral circulation and the condition of the coronary arteries. Laboratory tests include determination of serum cholesterol and triglyceride levels.

Treatment

Antianginal agents, such as the nitrates (eg, nitroglycerin and isosorbide dinitrate), may be prescribed. Other drugs used for angina include calcium channel blocking agents, such as nifedipine (Procardia), diltiazem (Cardizem), and verapamil (Calan), and β-adrenergic blocking agents, such as nadolol (Corgard) and propranolol (Inderal). The physician selects the drug that produces the best results for the individual patient. Often selection is by trial and error, until the desired response is obtained.

When applicable, the physician advises the patient to stop smoking because of the association of smoking with the increased risk of coronary artery disease. Regular exercise, such as walking, often is beneficial in promoting collateral circulation, thus lessening the frequency and the severity of attacks. Overweight patients usually benefit from weight reduction.

For some patients, the symptoms remain the same for years, whereas for others the anginal attacks become more frequent and severe, despite treatment. The latter group of patients are so crippled by the severe interference with blood supply to the heart that everyday activities must be curtailed. A patient with angina must find his or her level of activity tolerance and then live within that level. Data obtained from the patient's performance on various tests in a cardiac work evaluation clinic are helpful to the physician.

The patient also has to learn to live with the ever-present possibility of an attack. For some patients the fear aroused by the attack is worse than the pain. Because the prognosis is so variable, a patient may live for years or die suddenly from an acute myocardial infarction.

Surgical attempts to correct the pathology caused by the diseases of the blood vessels that serve the muscle of the heart have been directed mainly toward improving vascularization. The techniques most commonly used are coronary artery bypass and percutaneous transluminal coronary angioplasty (see Chapter 31).

Myocardial Infarction

The reduction or occlusion of arterial blood flow to a portion of the myocardium often leads to necrosis (death) of that portion. The area of necrotic tissue is called a *myocardial infarction* (heart attack). The most common cause of myocardial infarction is atherosclerosis. *Coronary insufficiency* describes a clinical condition in which cardiac pain frequently is more severe than that of typical angina pectoris, but death of the heart muscle does not occur.

Myocardial infarction usually occurs in the left ventricle. The larger the affected area, the more serious the disorder, because a large infarcted area decreases the heart's pumping ability. The infarction may extend through the thickness of the myocardial wall to the subendocardium (transmural infarction), involve part of the myocardium, or just involve the subendocardial area. Different terms are used to describe the affected area. For example, in most people, the right coronary artery and its branches supply the posterior wall of the heart. Occlusion of this artery results in a *posterior myocardial infarction*. Heart block is more common with this type of infarction, since branches of the right coronary artery supply the sinoatrial and atrioventricular nodes. The left coronary artery and its branches supply most of the anterior and apical portions of the left ventricle. An infarction caused by occlusions of these branches is either an *anterior myocardial infarction* or an *anteroseptal myocardial infarction*, depending on the extent of involvement.

From the onset of the infarction until about the third day, there is acute tissue degeneration, and the infarct is soft, necrotic, and electrically inert. Dangerous dysrhythmias are most likely to develop during this time, since the affected areas and the areas surrounding them are electrically unstable. From the fourth to the seventh days, softening of the infarcted area is greatest, and there is danger of aneurysm formation on the ventricular wall. The weakened area in the ventricular wall may balloon out during systole. Rupture of the ventricle, which results in almost instant death, is likely to occur from the onset of the infarction to 2 weeks.

About the eighth to the 10th days, newly formed capillaries develop around the periphery of the infarct, but it takes 2 or 3 weeks before there is functionally significant collateral circulation. Collagen fibers begin to form around the 12th day. It is 3 or 4 weeks before the scar begins to grow firm, and 2 or 3 months before a scar of maximum strength is formed.

Symptoms

Symptoms vary but typically include sudden, severe pain in the chest. The pain usually is substernal and may or may not radiate to the shoulder, arm, teeth, jaw, or throat. The pain is more severe and of longer duration than anginal pain. Some patients describe it as squeezing or crushing pain. Unlike anginal pain, the pain of myocardial infarction is not relieved by rest or antianginal drugs. It may last for several hours or as long as 1 or 2 days. Finally, it becomes a soreness or an ache before it disappears entirely. Some patients experience little or no pain, and may never know that they

have had a myocardial infarction until it is detected weeks, months, or years later by ECG.

Additional symptoms may include pallor, sweating, faintness, a severe drop in blood pressure, nausea, and a rapid, weak pulse. Most patients are aware of the seriousness of chest pain, and are apprehensive. Symptoms of left-sided heart failure (ie, dyspnea, cyanosis, and cough) may appear if the pumping of the left ventricle is sufficiently impaired.

Diagnosis

Diagnosis is made by patient history, ECG, and elevated serum enzyme and isoenzyme levels. Changes in the ECG normally appear within 2 to 12 hours after the infarction but may take as long as 3 days to occur. The creatine phosphokinase (CPK) level begins to rise within 2 to 6 hours, and the isoenzyme CPK-MB is present in the blood (indicative of myocardial damage) about 2 hours after the infarction.

The patient usually is transferred as quickly as possible to a unit where specialized treatment protocols and medical management are available. A coronary care unit provides the necessary equipment and trained personnel (Fig. 27-1). Most deaths from acute myocardial infarction occur in the first hours after the onset of pain, so specialized care is essential. Sudden death usually is attributed to ventricular fibrillation, rupture of the ventricular wall, or irreversible cardiogenic shock.

Treatment

Treatment depends on such factors as the extent of the infarct, the degree of cardiogenic shock, the patient's age, and the coexistence of other medical diseases that may alter the form of treatment or the prognosis. Treatment is directed toward relieving pain, treating shock (if present), and recognizing and correcting dysrhythmias if they occur.

If the patient is seen within 6 hours of the onset of the infarction, treatment may include the administration of thrombolytic therapeutic agents. One such drug is recombinant alteplase (Activase), a tissue plasminogen activator, which is able to dissolve the thrombus occluding a coronary artery, thus restoring blood flow through the obstructed artery. Another drug that may be used is streptokinase, which produces essentially the same results. One risk factor in the administration of streptokinase is the occurrence of an allergic reaction, which may be fatal. More serious reactions appear to occur with the use of streptokinase than with the use of recombinant alteplase.

Drug therapy also may include analgesics for pain, tranquilizers to promote rest and reduce anxiety, anticoagulants to prevent additional thrombus formation, and antiarrhythmic drugs to treat dysrhythmias. Complete bed rest is initially prescribed; the amount of

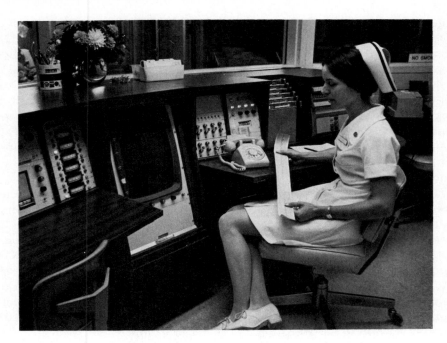

Figure 27–1.   The coronary care unit, phase I, at Sisters Hospital, Buffalo, New York. The console monitors the electrocardiogram of each patient in the unit. (Photograph by D. Atkinson)

activity allowed in the days after the onset of the infarction usually depends on the extent of the infarction, the occurrence of complications, and the patient's response to therapy.

Complications

A number of complications are associated with myocardial infarction.

DYSRHYTHMIAS.   A dysrhythmia may occur during the acute phase. More than half the deaths from myocardial infarction occur within 72 hours of admission to the hospital, many as a result of dysrhythmias (see Chapter 28). The abnormal rhythm typically occurs suddenly within the first 3 days after the infarction, and can be fatal within a few minutes. When dysrhythmias are detected as soon as they begin and are terminated as quickly as possible, the fatality rate associated with certain dysrhythmias decreases.

VENOUS THROMBOSIS.   Venous thrombosis arises mostly in the veins of the lower extremities and the pelvis. The use of antiembolism stockings, positioning pillows, and regularly scheduled foot and leg exercises helps to prevent thrombus formation. Anticoagulants also may be given.

PULMONARY EMBOLISM.   Most pulmonary emboli arise from venous thrombi in the lower extremities and the pelvis. They also may arise from the right ventricular endocardium when that side of the heart was the site of infarction. The onset of a pulmonary embolism usually is sudden, with chest pain, dyspnea, and cyanosis being the first symptoms. The sputum may be tinged

with blood. Treatment depends on the size of the infarcted pulmonary area, the age and condition of the patient, and the seriousness (or extent) of the myocardial infarction.

ARTERIAL EMBOLISM.   A clot can form in the left ventricular cavity overlying the infarcted area (mural thrombus). Part of it can break off, enter the systemic arterial circulation, and occlude the peripheral arteries, resulting in a mottled, cold, pulseless extremity. If the cerebral arteries become occluded, the result is a cerebrovascular accident, or stroke. Arteriotomy (opening of an artery) and embolectomy (removal of an embolus) may be necessary; a patient who has recently suffered myocardial infarction, however, is a surgical risk.

CONGESTIVE HEART FAILURE.   Onset of congestive heart failure may be sudden, or the condition may develop over a period of hours or days (see Chapter 30).

CARDIOGENIC SHOCK.   Cardiogenic shock has a high mortality. The earlier shock is detected and treatment instituted, the better the patient's chances of survival.

Because some experts believe that this mortality rate cannot be further reduced by conventional therapy, and because the size of the infarction is not always related to the extreme degree of shock, mechanical assistance devices such as the intraaortic balloon pump have been successfully used in some patients.

OTHER COMPLICATIONS.   Other complications include ventricular aneurysm, ventricular rupture, pericarditis, and pericardial effusion. A *ventricular aneurysm* decreases the pumping action of the heart. Some ventricular aneurysms can be surgically corrected. Those that cannot may rupture at any time. Rupture of the aneurysm is fatal.

Ventricular rupture occurs when a soft necrotic area gives way. Hemopericardium (blood in the pericardium), cardiac tamponade, and relatively sudden death ensue. There also can be rupture of the interventricular septum. Dyspnea, rapid right heart failure, and shock result; the prognosis is poor, although survival is possible.

Pericarditis may be mild or severe. The mild form may not require treatment. *Pericardial effusion*, a collection of fluid in the pericardial sac, may occur in a patient with pericarditis, congestive heart failure, or myocardial infarction. The patient should be closely observed for signs of cardiac tamponade and pericardiocentesis performed to remove excess fluid.

If invagination of the mitral valves occurs, as it sometimes does when the papillary muscles are involved in a myocardial infarction, blood would flow not only forward into the aorta, but also backward into the left atrium through an incompetent mitral valve (mitral insufficiency).

NURSING PROCESS —THE PATIENT WHO HAS AN OCCLUSIVE DISORDER OF THE CORONARY BLOOD VESSELS

Assessment

In addition to the assessments performed on the patient with cardiac disease (see Chapter 24), a thorough history from the patient or a family member is necessary to establish baseline data. The history should include a description of the pain, with regard to location, type, duration, and whether it radiates to other areas, such as down the arm or to the jaw. A medical history, including a drug history, also is important, because other disorders, such as diabetes mellitus and hypertension, may alter or require additional treatment modalities.

Vital signs should be taken, and if the patient appears acutely ill, a rapid assessment of the patient's status is necessary. The heart should be auscultated, and the cardiac rate and rhythm noted and recorded. Other symptoms, such as pallor, diaphoresis, cyanosis, and apprehension, are recorded. The lungs should be auscultated, with particular attention to normal and abnormal breath sounds. Crackling sounds at the base of the lungs may indicate congestive heart failure. The abdomen should be auscultated for bowel sounds.

The extremities should be examined for edema, which may be present if the patient has congestive heart failure. The extent and severity of edema are recorded. Peripheral pulses are assessed with particular attention to their amplitude, as weak peripheral pulses may indicate reduced cardiac output or the presence of a thrombus in the arteries of the lower abdomen or the legs.

It is important to determine whether the patient has been taking fluids, because a fluid volume deficit may be present. The recent voiding pattern with regard to color and amount also is important. Concentrated urine or a decrease in urine output may indicate a fluid volume deficit or a reduction in cardiac output, which reduces blood flow to the kidneys.

Nursing Diagnosis

Depending on the type of occlusion, the potential or actual medical diagnosis, and the condition of the patient, one or more of the following nursing diagnoses may apply. Additional nursing diagnoses may be added when specific patient needs are identified during assessment.

- Pain related to myocardial ischemia
- Anxiety related to pain, potential or actual diagnosis, fear of death
- Fear related to potential diagnosis and prognosis, current status, outcome of the illness, or death
- Activity intolerance related to impaired oxygen transport secondary to decreased cardiac output or anginal pain
- Impaired adjustment related to change in life-style (dietary changes, activity)
- Hypothermia related to cardiogenic shock
- Hyperthermia related to tissue necrosis (myocardial infarction)
- Colonic constipation related to bed rest, administration of narcotic analgesics
- Ineffective individual coping related to depression, diagnosis, uncertain future
- Altered family processes related to ill family member
- Fluid volume deficit related to decreased fluid intake, profuse diaphoresis
- Fluid volume excess secondary to decreased cardiac output, decreased renal perfusion, decreased urine output
- Impaired skin integrity related to immobility, edema
- Anticipatory grieving related to perceived losses (actual, potential) resulting from illness
- Impaired home maintenance management related to angina, inability to perform household tasks
- Ineffective breathing pattern related to congestive heart failure, fluid overload, pain, immobility
- Altered sexuality patterns related to coronary heart disease
- Sleep pattern disturbance related to cardiac monitoring, environment, treatments
- Knowledge deficit of prognosis, treatment modalities, postdischarge home care

Planning and Implementation

The major goals of the patient include relief of pain and anxiety; improvement in activity tolerance; absence of respiratory difficulties; attainment of normal temperature, bowel function, and fluid volume; knowledge and acceptance of the disorder; maintenance of skin integrity; and adherence to prescribed treatment modalities.

The main goals of nursing management are relieving pain, reducing anxiety, recognizing complications, and maintaining adequate tissue perfusion.

The physician may order cardiac monitoring for the patient. Vital signs should be measured and recorded at prescribed intervals, depending on the patient's condition.

EMERGENCY THROMBOLYTIC THERAPY. Thrombolytic therapy may be used as emergency treatment of a myocardial infarction. During and after administration of a thrombolytic drug, the patient should be closely observed for signs and symptoms of bleeding: blood in the urine or stool, bruising, epistaxis, abdominal pain (which may indicate intraabdominal bleeding), or change in the level of consciousness, mood, or behavior (which may indicate intracranial bleeding). The patient should be placed on a cardiac monitor and closely observed for development of a dysrhythmia. Intramuscular and intravenous injections and arterial punctures should be avoided during therapy and until such time as these procedures can be safely performed without excessive bleeding at the puncture sites.

COMPLICATIONS. Depending on hospital policy, evidence of shock or impending shock mandates the initiation of intravenous therapy to keep the vein open.

The presence of a thrombus or an embolus in a peripheral blood vessel is a complication of events such as myocardial infarction, or of prolonged bed rest. The nurse should listen carefully to the patient's complaint of pain in an extremity, and check for differences in temperature between the involved and surrounding areas. The patient also should be observed for severe pain in *any* part of the body, slurring of speech, change in level of consciousness, weakness, and paralysis, all of which may indicate the occlusion of a blood vessel in any part of the body.

If profound failure of the left ventricle occurs (eg, cardiogenic shock), an intraaortic balloon pump may be inserted into the left femoral artery and threaded up to the descending aortic arch. This device is connected to a mechanical system that is synchronized with the patient's heart rate. The balloon is inflated during diastole and deflated during systole. Inflation increases coronary artery and myocardium perfusion and decreases the workload of the left ventricle.

Pain. It is imperative to relieve pain, which is often severe, crushing, and the source of great fear. Dysrhythmias and shock can follow severe pain.

Patients with angina are closely watched for an increase in the type, duration, and intensity of pain as well as for evidence of the success or failure of antianginal drug therapy. Anginal pain is relieved by the administration of an antianginal drug such as nitroglycerin. The patient should be observed for the effectiveness of drug therapy; if the drug fails to relieve the pain, the physician should be notified immediately.

Often the pain of myocardial infarction is so severe that the analgesic does not completely relieve it, but makes it less intense and more bearable. An analgesic usually is given every 3 or 4 hours, as necessary, during the period when pain is severe. The blood pressure and pulse and respiratory rates are taken *before* a narcotic analgesic is given for pain. If the blood pressure is below 100 systolic or the respiratory rate is 10 or fewer breaths per minute, the drug is withheld and the physician immediately contacted, as an analgesic with less depressant effects may be required.

Dysrhythmias and hypotension can follow the administration of a analgesic. It is important to note any depression of respiration, nausea, dysrhythmias, and hypotension, particularly when morphine is given. Vital signs should be taken 30 to 45 minutes after the drug is given, and the patient closely observed. Any marked drop in the blood pressure or respiratory rate should be reported to the physician immediately, as a narcotic antagonist or other medical therapy may be necessary. The period during which narcotics are needed usually lasts about 1 or 2 days; during this period rest and the relief of apprehension are especially important.

Fear and Anxiety. The fear of death always present for the patient with angina or myocardial infarction. Exhibiting a calm and reassuring attitude and allowing time for the patient to express fears and concerns help to create a trusting relationship between the patient and members of the health care team.

Severe anxiety can place an added strain on the heart; therefore, it should be reported to the physician.

Ineffective Breathing Pattern. Bed rest reduces tissue demands for oxygen, and adequate oxygenation contributes to the relief of pain and the prevention of dysrhythmias. Patients who are dyspneic, tachycardic, or cyanotic are given oxygen as ordered. If the medical history indicates that the patient may have chronic obstructive pulmonary disease, oxygen given routinely at high concentration may result in respiratory arrest because the patient is deprived of the hypoxic stimulus to respiration. These patients may be prescribed oxygen at a lower than normal liter flow.

Congestive heart failure, pericardial effusion, unrelieved chest pain, and pulmonary embolism are examples of conditions that may alter the breathing pattern. The lungs should be auscultated at frequent intervals for normal and abnormal breath sounds. The patient should be encouraged and reminded to breathe deeply every 2 hours while awake. The peripheral pulses and the color and temperature of the skin of the extremities should be checked every 2 to 4 hours. Absence of peripheral pulses and cool cyanotic extremities may indicate lack of oxygen to these areas, and this should be immediately reported to the physician.

Activity Intolerance. Some patients require complete or partial assistance with their activities of daily living. Those with angina should be helped to understand what activities may or may not produce anginal attacks, so that they can pace their activities to reduce the incidence of anginal pain.

Objects should be placed within easy reach, so that the patient does not have to use effort to reach them. If the patient strenuously objects to certain activity restrictions, this problem should be discussed with the physician. Refusal to accept activity restrictions may be a manifestation of denial. Because this is an unconscious defense against anxiety, reasoning with the patient often does not help. Attempting to force restrictions can only increase the patient's anxiety and cardiac workload.

One of the hazards of bed rest is the Valsalva maneuver, which is performed when there is a forced expiration against a closed glottis. This can occur when straining to defecate or void, when lifting oneself up in bed, or during gagging, vomiting, or severe coughing. During the Valsalva maneuver, intrathoracic (within the thorax) pressure is increased and blood is trapped in the great veins, preventing blood from entering the chest and, ultimately, the right atrium. The heart becomes smaller in size, and, after an initial decrease in heart rate because of vagal stimulation, the heart rate increases. When the breath is released, blood gushes into the heart and rapidly distends it. This "overshoot" of blood results in increased blood pressure and tachycardia, which in turn stimulates pressure receptors in the carotid sinus and the aorta. Reflex bradycardia then ensues and can prove fatal. Patients should be instructed to avoid the Valsalva maneuver by exhaling, rather than holding the breath, when moving in bed.

Many physicians believe that the safest, quickest, and most effective way to help the patient resume activity is to observe the reaction to slightly increased amounts of activity and be guided accordingly in allowing increases in activity. The patient should be observed for dysrhythmias, chest pain, excessive fatigue, increased pulse and respiratory rates, and changes in blood pressure.

Impaired Adjustment. The patient with coronary artery disease may find that many changes are necessary. Weight reduction, maintenance of a diet low in saturated fats, cessation of smoking, and a change in occupation are some of the alterations in life-style that may be necessary. Some patients can accept these changes, others cannot. The patient should be helped to understand *why* these changes are necessary, what alternatives may be possible, and what may happen if these changes are not instituted.

Hypothermia, Hyperthermia. A decrease in body temperature may occur if the patient is in cardiogenic shock. Unless the patient complains of being cold, extra blankets are not necessary; this measure may dilate capillaries, resulting in a further decrease in blood pressure. Fever is common 1 or 2 days after myocardial infarction. It usually is low or moderate, and lasts for 4 or 5 days. Fever is one of the body's responses to necrosis of tissue. The physician should be informed of any temperature elevation.

Colonic Constipation. Constipation with consequent straining to have a bowel movement may occur when activity is limited. The physician may prescribe fecal softening agents to alleviate this problem. The use of a bedside commode often involves less energy expenditure than the use of a bedpan. Some physicians allow the patient with myocardial infarction to use a bedside commode several days after admission. The patient still requires assistance in cleaning the perineal area after defecation. To avoid straining and bladder distention, some physicians permit male patients to stand at the side of the bed to void if their condition has stabilized.

Fluid Volume Deficit or Excess. Profuse diaphoresis and lack of fluid intake may result in a fluid volume deficit. A decrease in cardiac output may occur in those patients with myocardial infarction. This in turn decreases renal blood flow and renal output, thus increasing the amount of fluid retained in body tissues. Edema may then occur.

Intake and output should be measured, and the physician notified if urine output falls below 500 mL in 24 hours. In critically ill patients, measurements may be required hourly. An intravenous volumetric controller normally is used to regulate the infusion of intravenous fluids.

If fluid volume excess occurs, signs of congestive heart failure and possibly pulmonary edema (see Chapter 30) may be noted.

Impaired Skin Integrity.   Patients who are on complete bed rest require a change in position every 2 hours. The bony prominences should be inspected for signs of skin breakdown. Various measures and supporting devices (eg, sheepskin padding, blanket rolls, a footboard, and an alternating pressure mattress) may need to be used if bed rest is prolonged.

Ineffective Individual Coping.   Patients with angina or myocardial infarction are beset by many fears. Fear of death and fear of living with impending death predominate. These patients must cope with these fears as well as with threats to their physical integrity, changes in body image and self-concept, loss of status at work, reduction of income or even loss of job, restriction of favorite activities, and permanent or temporary loss of the ability to care for their family.

Faced with many potential losses, these patients understandably experience a number of disturbing emotions—anxiety, anger, sorrow, depression, bitterness, and hopelessness. Helpful nursing action includes the capacity to confront the patient and family openly and humanly, to empathize with their situation, and to think and feel about it and not turn away or rush to intervene in this painful circumstance over which the nurse has little control. Supportive listening can assist these patients and their family members to acknowledge gradually the various problems that accompany coronary diseases.

Grieving.   Some patients believe that a normal life is no longer possible once advanced coronary artery disease has developed. They may think that the future is uncertain, that their condition is hopeless and nothing can be done. These patients should be allowed to discuss their fears regarding anticipated changes in lifestyle. Members of the health care team should correct misconceptions and help the patient to understand why some changes may be necessary.

Impaired Home Maintenance Management.   Some patients are unable to care for themselves and their home after discharge from the hospital. These concerns often are expressed after the acute stage of their illness has passed. The nurse should identify problem areas (eg, an inability to perform basic housework) and then seek appropriate consultation. The social service worker, along with the patient's family, may be able to resolve these problems. In addition,

cardiac rehabilitation programs can offer advice and assistance.

Altered Sexual Patterns.   Many patients have questions about resuming sexual activity. Some may be hesitant to ask questions on this subject. The nurse can detect clues that a patient may need help with this problem and can assist the patient and his or her sexual partner to formulate questions and seek the physician's advice. When the limitations are reviewed and understood, the couple are in a better position to make their own decisions. Depending on the degree of coronary artery obstruction and myocardial reserve, the physician may recommend no change in or a reduction of sexual activity. Some patients experience impotence because of fear and anxiety related to the strain of sexual activity on their hearts.

Sleep Pattern Disturbance.   The noise of the hospital and interruptions for diagnostic tests often interfere with the patient's ability to sleep. Lack of adequate sleep can result in mental changes, such as disorientation and confusion. When possible, lights should be dimmed during late evening and night hours, overhead lights turned off, the volume of sound on monitoring devices turned to low (providing the nursing staff is able to supervise these devices adequately), and talking kept to a minimum.

Knowledge Deficit.   Essential components in the management of coronary artery disease are relief of the symptoms and prevention of further development of the disorder. The patient with coronary artery disease needs to learn many things. The nurse should first establish what needs to be learned and then determine what the patient already knows.

Rehabilitation may be conducted in a cardiac rehabilitation program or carried out by the physician and other members of the health care team. Education about coronary artery disease is an effective way of promoting adherence to a rehabilitation program. Patients who understand their disorder and what can be done for them are more likely to adhere to a treatment regimen and the recommendations of the physician.

Depending on the physician's prescribed therapy, subjects that may be covered in a teaching program include the following:

- Medication regimen: importance of drug therapy, dose, time taken, adverse drug effects
- Type and amount of activity allowed; prescribed exercise program
- Rehabilitation programs: where located, types, cost
- Diet, how to read food labels, what food labels indicate

- How to monitor pulse rate and blood pressure
- Symptoms that should be reported to a physician as soon as possible
- How to avoid stressful situations
- Resumption of sexual activity
- Importance of continued medical supervision

Evaluation

- Patient tolerates increased activity as prescribed by the physician
- Patient demonstrates evidence of acceptance of changes required in life-style, activities, diet
- Fear and anxiety is reduced
- Body temperature is normal
- Defecation pattern is normal
- Pain is reduced or eliminated
- Family and patient demonstrate a positive attitude and ability to cope with the diagnosis
- Normal fluid balance is attained and maintained
- Home maintenance problems are identified and resolved
- Patient demonstrates a positive attitude and willingness to participate in a rehabilitation program
- Breathing pattern is normal; patient shows no signs of breathing difficulty
- Skin integrity is maintained
- Patient seeks physician's advice regarding sexual activity
- Normal sleeping pattern is attained
- Patient understands illness and preventive measures

OCCLUSIVE DISORDERS OF PERIPHERAL BLOOD VESSELS

Raynaud's Disease

Raynaud's disease is characterized by periodic constriction of the arteries that supply the extremities. The digital arteries of the hands and the feet usually are affected. The nose, ears, and chin are less commonly involved.

The underlying cause of Raynaud's disease is not entirely clear. The condition is much more common in young women than in men.

Symptoms

Attacks occur intermittently and with varying frequency but especially after exposure to cold. The hands become cold, blanched, and wet with perspiration. Numbness and tingling also may occur. Awkwardness and fumbling are noted, especially when fine movements are attempted. After the initial pallor, the hands, especially the fingers, become deeply cyanotic and begin to ache. The patient usually learns that the attack can be relieved by placing the hands in warm water or by going indoors, where it is warm. The warmth relieves the vasospasm, and blood rushes to

the part. The skin in the deprived areas becomes flushed and warm, and the patient has a sensation of throbbing.

In the early stages of the disease, the hands usually appear normal between attacks. The disease does not necessarily progress to cause severe disability. The symptoms often are mild and may even improve spontaneously. When the disease is severe and of long duration, cyanosis of the fingers may persist between the attacks and skin changes gradually may occur. Painful ulcers and superficial gangrene may appear at the fingertips. The fingers are especially vulnerable to infection. Healing of even minor lesions often is slow and uncertain.

Diagnosis

Diagnosis is made by a history of the symptoms and an examination of the involved extremities.

Treatment

Treatment involves avoiding factors that precipitate attacks. Smoking is contraindicated because it causes vasoconstriction. *avoid coldness!*

Drug therapy with peripheral vasodilators such as isoxsuprine (Vasodilan) may be tried, but results usually are disappointing. Other drugs, such as nifedipine (Procardia), are being used investigationally for this disorder.

Sympathectomy may be performed when the disease is severe and progressive, and when medical treatment fails to relieve the condition; long-term effects are disappointing. Gangrene may develop, requiring amputation of the affected areas.

Thrombosis, Phlebothrombosis, and Embolism

A *thrombus* is clot that obstructs the lumen of a blood vessel. *Thrombosis* is the formation of a clot within a blood vessel. Thrombi form relatively easily in arteries whose linings have become roughened and narrowed by atherosclerosis. An *embolus* is a mass (clot) of undissolved particles—either solid, liquid, or gas—that are present in blood vessels. *Phlebothrombosis* is the development of a clot within a vein without inflammation. Phlebothrombosis and thrombophlebitis have similar symptoms and treatment (see Chapter 25).

The basic difference between a thrombus and an embolus is the status of the clot. The term *thrombus* usually is used to identify the clot in its original place of formation, on the wall of an artery or a vein. A clot that is moving through blood vessels is termed an *embolus*. An embolus can become lodged in a smaller blood vessel and obstruct its lumen. When an embolus reaches a blood vessel that is too small to permit its passage, partial or total occlusion exists and blood is prevented from flowing through the vessel. The tissues that lie beyond the occlusion are deprived of their blood supply. *Deep vein thrombosis* is the presence of a thrombus in a deep vein rather than a superficial vein.

Thrombosis in the venous system most often occurs in the lower extremities and may be associated with disorders or circumstances such as prolonged bed rest, pregnancy, shock, lower-extremity paralysis, and trauma to the blood vessel wall. Arterial thrombosis may be caused by atherosclerosis, chronic congestive heart failure, and endocarditis. Arterial emboli may be caused by thrombi arising from one or more of the chambers of the heart. Emboli may arise from certain dysrhythmias, such as atrial fibrillation. They also may occur after myocardial infarction.

Symptoms

Symptoms of arterial thrombosis or embolism that affect the extremities arise from ischemia of the tissues that depend on the obstructed vessel for their blood supply. If *total* occlusion exists, the extremity suddenly becomes white, cold, and extremely painful. Normal arterial pulse is absent below the area of obstruction. Numbness, tingling, or cramping also may be present, and surrounding blood vessels go into spasm. These symptoms are followed by loss of sensation in the affected area and loss of the ability to move the part. Unless the obstruction is promptly relieved, tissue necrosis occurs and may necessitate amputation. Symptoms of shock frequently occur if a large vessel has been obstructed. When a small vessel is occluded, symptoms of ischemia, such as pallor and coldness, occur but are less severe.

Patients with *venous thrombosis* may be asymptomatic. When symptoms occur, they include edema and warmth and tenderness over the affected area (location of the clot). The leg suddenly may become swollen and cyanotic, calling attention to the condition. The patient may experience pain in the calf on dorsiflexion of the foot (positive Homans' sign). *Phlebothrombosis* may produce few, if any, symptoms because inflammation is slight or absent. The signs and symptoms of *deep vein thrombosis* usually include pain, swelling and tenderness of the affected extremity, and mild fever. A positive Homans' sign may be present.

Diagnosis

Diagnosis is made by examination of the affected extremity, palpation of peripheral pulses, and evaluation of the patient's symptoms. Phlebography may be performed to identify the point of obstruction. Doppler ultrasonography may be used to detect abnormalities in peripheral blood flow.

Treatment

Treatment depends on whether an artery or a vein is occluded and the degree of occlusion (partial, complete).

Arterial Occlusive Disease

If an artery is completely occluded, treatment must be *immediate.* To facilitate blood flow to the part, the extremity should be placed in a dependent position and kept at complete rest. The patient should be kept warm because chilling may lead to further vasospasm, which would decrease the blood supply to the extremity. The extremity may be wrapped to prevent radiation of heat. Direct heat should never be applied to ischemic tissues because it may burn the skin and accelerate the development of gangrene.

The physician may order an immediate intravenous injection of heparin to help prevent the development of further clots or the extension of those already present. An attempt may be made to improve circulation by administering vasodilative drugs. A sympathetic nerve block (injection of a local anesthetic into the sympathetic ganglia) may relieve vasospasm. Narcotic administration may relieve pain and ease the patient's apprehension.

If circulation to the extremity cannot be restored, a thrombectomy, embolectomy, endarterectomy (removal of the lining of an artery), or insertion of a bypass graft is necessary. The nursing management of thrombectomy, embolectomy, endarterectomy, and bypass grafting is discussed in Chapter 31.

Venous Occlusive Disease

Venous thrombosis is treated with bed rest, elevation of the extremity, analgesics for pain, and intermittent or continuous intravenous heparin (an anticoagulant) therapy. Laboratory monitoring for heparin therapy includes a partial thromboplastin time, prothrombin time, hemoglobin, and hematocrit. These tests initially may be performed every 6 to 24 hours, and the dose of heparin should be adjusted according to the results.

Continuous warm, moist heat may be applied to the affected extremity. Deep vein thrombosis may necessitate surgical removal of the clot (thrombectomy).

NURSING PROCESS —THE PATIENT WHO HAS AN OCCLUSIVE DISORDER OF PERIPHERAL BLOOD VESSELS

Assessment

A history of the symptoms should be obtained from the patient or family. The extremities should be examined for skin color and temperature and for abnormal changes. The peripheral pulses should be palpated and any absence or decrease in their intensity noted. The patient's activity tolerance should be assessed, and activities that produce pain or discomfort should be noted. Additional assessments may be required if the patient has a history of a cardiac disorder (see Chapter 24).

Nursing Diagnosis

One or more of the following nursing diagnoses may apply to the patient with an occlusive disorder of peripheral blood vessels. Additional nursing diagnoses may be necessary if the patient has concomitant cardiovascular disease.

- Activity intolerance related to pain, discomfort, exposure to cold
- Anxiety related to pain, discomfort, chronic status of disease, complications
- Pain related to occlusion or spasm of an artery or vein
- Impaired home maintenance management related to pain experienced with exposure to temperature extremes (Raynaud's disease), enforced rest of an extremity
- Impaired tissue integrity related to occlusive disorder of artery or vein and impaired oxygen transport to affected tissues
- Potential for infection of skin and underlying structures owing to impaired tissue integrity
- Altered tissue perfusion related to occlusive disorder
- Knowledge deficit of treatment modalities

Planning and Implementation

The major goals of the patient include increase in activity tolerance, reduction of pain or discomfort, reduction of anxiety, improved ability to manage the home environment, improved tissue perfusion, prevention of infection, and an understanding of the prescribed treatment modalities and prevention of complications.

The main goals of nursing management are directed toward establishing an increase in arterial or venous blood flow, relieving pain or discomfort, preventing complications, and providing effective and thorough patient teaching.

The patient with an acutely occluded blood vessel requires frequent assessments. Pain is severe, and the patient is apprehensive. The blood pressure should be monitored hourly or as ordered. The affected extremity should be inspected for changes in color and temperature, and the peripheral pulses should be checked every 30 minutes. The location of each peripheral pulse can be marked with a soft-tipped pen to facilitate measurement. Any change in the quality of a peripheral pulse or the sudden absence of a pulse should be reported immediately. In some instances of blood vessel occlusion, there is a decided color change (line of demarcation) above or

below the area of occlusion. This area can be outlined with a soft-tipped pen to establish a data base for future comparisons. Any increase in the area should be reported to the physician.

The nursing management for surgical procedures performed for occlusive disorders of peripheral blood vessels is covered in Chapter 31.

Activity Intolerance. The patient may require assistance to perform some or all routine activities of daily living. If exposure to cold results in pain, warm but loose-fitting socks can be worn by the patient when he or she is out of bed.

Anxiety. Anxiety may be caused by various factors, such as pain or discomfort, or the progressive disability that may accompany the disorder. Listening to the patient is one method of identifying a possible cause of anxiety. As problems are identified, one or more solutions can be proposed. Relieving pain, explaining the various tasks necessary to prevent complications or further episodes of pain, and answering questions may help the patient to understand the disorder and to comply with the physician's recommendations and prescribed treatments.

Pain. Narcotics usually are contraindicated if the patient has chronic pain. Preventive measures can be adopted to reduce the incidence of pain and discomfort (eg, the patient should wear warm socks and bedroom slippers while out of bed). Some of the discomforts associated with prolonged bed rest can be lessened if patients are encouraged to move their extremities and change position every hour while awake. Any sudden occurrence of severe pain in the affected area or other part of the body should be reported to the physician immediately.

Impaired Home Maintenance Management. Some patients find it difficult to carry out daily household activities because of pain or discomfort. Once the difficult activities are identified, the nurse may offer suggestions to help reduce the patient's discomfort while performing these tasks. Suggestions include wearing light cotton gloves at night if exposure to cold during sleeping hours causes pain, protecting hands from exposure to heat by wearing lined latex gloves while washing dishes, wearing warm socks when outdoors, and avoiding extremely cold temperature and wind as much as possible. Some patients may need to be referred to the social service worker for an evaluation of their circumstances possibly followed by referral to agencies that can provide housekeeping assistance.

Altered Tissue Perfusion; Impaired Tissue Integrity. While suitable management (eg, surgery and drug therapy) is directed toward improving blood flow to the affected extremities, the patient may increase tissue perfusion by exercising moderately, avoiding factors that cause pain, avoiding sitting for prolonged periods, and keeping the extremities warm.

Ischemia caused by occlusion of one or more peripheral blood vessels can result in tissue breakdown. The skin may become fragile and thin, and even the slightest injury may cause breaks in the skin that are slow to heal. Prolonged bed rest or periods of inactivity also can result in skin breakdown and decubitus formation.

The affected extremities should be inspected daily for signs of infection, any change in color, and signs of skin breakdown. The patient should be moved carefully, so that the skin of the affected extremities is not injured.

When a thrombus has totally or partially occluded a peripheral vessel, there remains the danger of the clot becoming detached and traveling to other areas, particularly the lungs. The patient should be observed for signs of pulmonary embolism, and the physician notified immediately if this complication occurs (see Chapter 22).

Potential for Infection. A break in the integrity of the skin may be followed by infection. Vital signs should be monitored every 4 hours or as ordered. Fever or the appearance of purulent drainage from open skin sites should be reported to the physician.

Knowledge Deficit. Patients with Raynaud's disease should be instructed to avoid becoming chilled and to dress warmly. The symptoms of Raynaud's disease may be controlled by avoiding events that precipitate arterial spasm. The patient may already realize what particular events increase pain but may still need advice regarding protection of the affected extremities. Injury to the affected extremities should be avoided, as such injuries heal slowly.

If a sympathectomy is performed, the areas from which sympathetic stimuli have been removed no longer perspire. The patient should be instructed to frequently apply cream to prevent excessive dryness of the skin.

Thrombosis, embolism, and phlebothrombosis often can be prevented, especially in those who are prone to develop these disorders, by avoiding prolonged periods of inactivity (especially sitting), elevating the legs during prolonged periods of sitting, breathing deeply every 1 or 2 hours, performing leg exercises when in bed, and, for the ambulatory patient, exercising moderately. If the patient is placed on almost complete bed rest when at home, the physician may prescribe antiembolism stockings for

the patient to wear while in bed. The patient should be instructed to remove and reapply the stockings twice a day or as recommended by the physician.

Evaluation

- Patient is able to tolerate minimal, some, or all activity without discomfort or pain
- Pain and discomfort are relieved or reduced
- Problems related to home maintenance management are resolved
- Oxygen transport to tissues is improved
- Skin of extremities remains intact
- Evidence of breakdown or infection in affected tissues is absent
- Patient demonstrates understanding of disease, preventive measures, and methods of reducing pain or discomfort

DISORDERS OF BLOOD VESSEL WALLS
Varicose Veins

Varicose veins are dilated, tortuous veins (varicosities). Blood collects in these veins and cannot be returned efficiently to the heart. The valves of the veins are incompetent, and close incompletely or not at all (Fig. 27-2). Rather than propelling it toward the heart, incompetent valves allow the blood to move back-

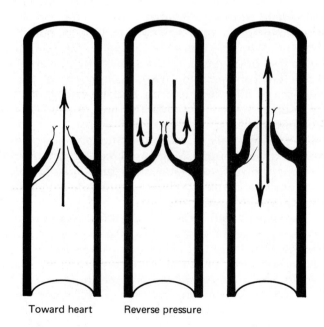

Toward heart   Reverse pressure

Competent valve   Incompetent valve

Figure 27-2. Competent valves in the veins permit the blood to flow toward the heart and prevent the flow of the blood in the opposite direction. Incompetent valves, by failing to close tightly, permit the blood to flow in both directions.

ward. This further congests the affected extremity with venous blood and further distends the veins. The saphenous veins of the legs commonly are affected. Varicose veins may occur in other parts of the body, such as the rectum (hemorrhoids) and the esophagus (esophageal varices).

Some people have a familial tendency toward varicose veins. The valves of the veins become incompetent early in life, resulting in the development of varicosities. Both sexes suffer from this disorder. Often the condition first manifests itself when other factors impair venous return. For example, pelvic tumors or pregnancy may exert pressure on the veins, causing interference with venous return. Prolonged standing aggravates the condition because venous return is further impaired by the force of gravity. The action of leg muscles during exercise, such as vigorous walking, aids venous return. Anything that constricts or puts pressure on the legs makes varicosities worse. Obesity contributes to inefficient venous return by placing excess weight on the legs. Thrombophlebitis sometimes leads to the development of varicose veins because the valves of the veins may be damaged during the inflammatory process. Several of these factors may combine to produce varicose veins.

Symptoms

When blood is not returned efficiently from the legs, it tends to collect in the saphenous veins. Because these veins are superficial and less well supported by surrounding tissues, they are prone to distention, whereas deeper veins of the legs are better supported by muscles. The veins become swollen and tortuous, and can be seen under the skin as dark blue or purple swellings. The legs feel heavy and tired and often become edematous, particularly after prolonged standing. There may be cramping pains. Inefficient venous return causes the tissues of the leg and foot to become congested. This congestion leads to diminished arterial blood supply and results in impaired nutrition of the tissues, with consequent reduction in their ability to resist infection and to allow wounds to heal. Minor injuries may readily readily infected and ulcerated. The healing of such lesions is slow and uncertain.

Diagnosis

Diagnosis is made by visual inspection of the extremity. The Brodie-Trendelenburg test also may be used for diagnosis. In this test, the patient lies flat and elevates the affected leg to empty the veins. A tourniquet is then applied to the upper thigh, and the patient is asked to stand. If blood flows from the upper part of the leg into the superficial veins when the tourniquet is released, the valves of the superficial veins are considered incompetent. Ultrasonography and phlebography also may be used in diagnosis.

Treatment

Surgical treatment for severe or multiple varicose veins consists of vein ligation and stripping. The affected veins are ligated, severed from their connections, and removed. The entire great saphenous vein, which extends from the groin to the ankle, may be removed. Treatment of mild varicose veins includes avoidance of prolonged periods of sitting, exercise (walking, swimming), weight loss (if needed), and the wearing of support stockings.

NURSING PROCESS —THE PATIENT UNDERGOING SURGERY FOR VARICOSE VEINS

Assessment

The legs should be inspected for evidence of superficial varicosities. Additional assessments may be required if there is a coexistent medical disorder.

Nursing Diagnosis

The following nursing diagnoses may apply during the preoperative and postoperative periods:

- Pain related to engorged varicosities, surgery
- Knowledge deficit of home care after surgery

Planning and Implementation

The major goals of the patient include relief of pain and an understanding of the care required after discharge from the hospital.

The major goals of nursing management include relieving pain and discomfort and providing instruction about care after discharge.

The patient returns from surgery with a compression stocking on the operative leg. The foot of the bed may be elevated in the immediate postoperative period to aid venous return.

Early ambulation is an important aspect of postoperative treatment because it stimulates circulation and helps to prevent venous thrombosis. Assistance is necessary the first few times, since the legs will feel clumsy and painful. This, plus the effect of preoperative medications and anesthesia, makes it especially important to protect the patient from falls. Antiembolism stockings should be removed and reapplied as ordered by the surgeon.

Pain. Preoperative pain is minimized by having the patient elevate the legs when sitting. Postoperative pain is controlled by analgesics prescribed by the physician.

Knowledge Deficit. Before discharge from the hospital, the patient may be instructed by the physician to continue wearing a compression stocking. The patient should be shown how to remove and reapply the stocking.

The postoperative period provides an excellent opportunity for the patient to learn how to minimize the possibility of the recurrence of varicosities or, if only one leg was affected, their development in the other leg. The importance of follow-up care at the physician's office or clinic should be emphasized, and the patient should be encouraged to follow the physician's directions concerning future care.

General instructions given by most physicians include elevating the legs while sitting, avoiding long periods of standing, and losing weight if the patient is obese.

Evaluation

■ Pain is controlled or minimized
■ Patient verbalizes importance of the physician's recommendations for preventing a recurrence of this disorder and the postoperative care required after discharge from the hospital

Aneurysms

The middle layer, or *media,* of the wall of an artery is elastic, allowing for pulsation with every heartbeat. When the elasticity is weakened by disease or trauma, an *aneurysm* (outpouching) of the wall is created (Fig. 27-3). Most aneurysms enlarge until they rupture. Other aneurysms lay down layer on layer of clots. Aneurysms of the aorta (aortic arch, thoracic, abdominal) are the most common, but aneurysms also can be found in other arteries, such as those of the leg.

On occasion the intima (inner layer of an artery) tears away from the media (middle layer of an artery). As a result, blood collects between the intima and the media (see Fig. 27-3), which further weakens the vessel wall. This type of aneurysm, called a *dissecting aneurysm,* can occur in the thoracic or abdominal aorta.

Dissection, or the tearing away of the intima, may result in the occlusion of one or more arteries that branch off the aorta. Blood flow through the involved artery or arteries then either decreases or stops. The aorta also can develop a tear, which causes a leakage of blood into the surrounding area, such as the thorax or abdomen.

Irrespective of whether a branching artery is occluded or a tear has occurred, the prognosis is grave. In some instances, a massive tear in the aorta causes death in a few minutes. Occlusion of an artery branching off the aorta has a widespread, profound effect on the organ or structure that depends on the blood flow provided by the occluded vessel.

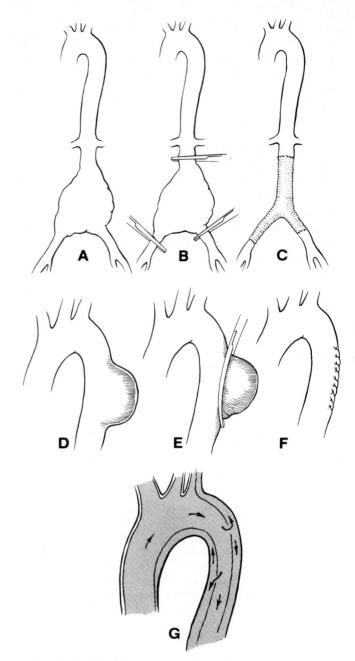

Figure 27–3.   Aneurysms. (*A*) Fusiform aneurysm of the abdominal aorta. (*B*) Aneurysm clamped off before removal. (*C*) Replacement with a graft. (*D*) Sacciform aneurysm; (*E*) Clamping before suturing. (*F*) Sutured vessel. (*G*) Dissecting aneurysm. In this instance, blood is seeping between the layers of the vessel wall through two holes.

Symptoms

Some aneurysms go undetected, producing no symptoms until they are found during a physical examination or the patient has a massive hemorrhage. Other aneurysms cause pain and discomfort and symptoms related to pressure on nearby structures. For example, a thoracic aortic aneurysm can cause bronchial obstruction, dysphagia, and dyspnea. An abdominal aortic aneurysm can produce nausea and vomiting from pressure exerted on the intestines, or it may cause back pain from pressure on the vertebrae or spinal nerves.

Symptoms of a dissecting aneurysm vary and depend on whether a branching artery has been occluded or a tear has occurred in the aortic wall. Many patients become suddenly and acutely ill. The blood pressure is taken in both arms and both legs. If the thoracic aorta is involved, there may be a marked difference in the blood pressures of the left and right arms. If the abdominal aorta is involved, there may be a marked difference in the blood pressures of the left and right legs. Severe pain and signs of shock usually are present, but symptoms can be less severe in some instances. Because symptoms vary, diagnosis may be difficult.

Diagnosis

When the walls of the aneurysm contain deposits of calcium, the exact location of the outpouching can be seen on radiographs. Aortography may be done to identify the size and exact location of the aneurysm. Some aneurysms of the abdominal aorta can be felt as pulsating masses.

Treatment

Aneurysms are treated surgically whenever possible; no other cure exists. They are repaired by bypass or replacement grafting. In some instances, removal of the aneurysm or repair of the weakened area is impossible. A dissecting aneurysm or rupture of an aneurysm is a surgical emergency. Medical treatment includes administering antihypertensive drugs to keep the blood pressure low until surgery can be performed.

See Chapter 31 for the management of a patient with an aneurysm.

General Nutritional Considerations

☐ A diet low in sodium, saturated fats, and cholesterol may be prescribed for patients with atherosclerosis.

☐ If the patient shows a dislike for the prescribed diet, a dietary consult is obtained, as other foods within the diet restriction may be suggested.

General Pharmacologic Considerations

☐ Aspirin, one tablet (0.33 g) daily, may be recommended by the physician for patients with coronary artery disease. It increases the prothrombin time and decreases the ability of the blood to clot, thereby reducing the possibility of thrombus formation in a coronary artery.

☐ When the patient with coronary artery disease requires rest and a reduction of anxiety, sedatives or tranquilizers may be prescribed. The physician should be notified if the patient becomes somnolent and no longer initiates deep breathing, leg exercises, or moving in bed.

☐ Nitroglycerin is available in several forms: as a sublingual tablet, sustained-release tablet or capsule, transdermal systems, and ointment that is applied to the skin.

☐ Sublingual nitroglycerin tablets are designed to dissolve quickly under the tongue, and are used at the first sign of an anginal attack. They usually relieve anginal pain in 2 or 3 minutes. The duration of effect is brief.

☐ The sustained-release form of nitroglycerin is used for prevention (prophylaxis) of anginal attacks, rather than for relief of the pain of an attack. This form is taken at 8- or 12-hour intervals. The transdermal systems are pads or disks that are applied to the skin. These systems slowly release nitroglycerin over a period of time (usually 24 hours), and are changed daily. With the topical ointment, a measured amount (in inches) is squeezed from a tube, applied in a uniform layer on the skin, and covered with a plastic wrap.

☐ Nitroglycerin can cause a throbbing headache, flushing, and nausea; usually these effects can be minimized by decreasing the dose. A patient who is not accustomed to taking nitroglycerin should remain seated for a few minutes after taking the medication because some people experience a feeling of faintness.

☐ Activase, a tissue plasminogen activator, may cause bleeding and dysrhythmias. The drug is administered intravenously over a period of several hours in divided doses.

General Gerontologic Considerations

☐ The incidence of arteriosclerosis and other vascular disorders rises with age.
☐ Older patients who take medication for angina should ask their pharmacists to dispense the drug in a container without a childproof cap. This type of cap usually is difficult to remove when the patient has arthritis, limited vision, or other disability.

Suggested Readings

☐ Adelman EM. When your patient's blood pressure falls . . . what does it mean? What should you do? Nursing '87 October 1987;17:66. *(Additional coverage of subject matter)*
☐ Boyd MD, Citro KM. Is your MI patient too scared to recover? RN May 1988;53:50. *(Additional coverage of subject matter)*
☐ Dudek SG. Nutrition handbook for nursing practice. Philadelphia: JB Lippincott, 1987. *(Additional coverage of subject matter)*
☐ Gerdes L. Recognizing the multisystemic effects of embolism. Nursing '87 December 1987;17:34. *(Additional coverage of subject matter)*
☐ Handerhan B. Action stat! Chest pain. Nursing '89 1989;19:33. *(Additional coverage of subject matter)*
☐ Klein DM. Angina: pathophysiology and the resulting signs and symptoms. Nursing '88 July 1988;18:44. *(Additional coverage and illustrations that reinforce subject matter)*
☐ McCann ME. Sexual healing after heart attack. Am J Nurs September 1989;89:1133. *(Additional coverage of subject matter)*
☐ Smith CE. Assessing chest pain quickly and accurately. Nursing '88 May 1988;18:52. *(Additional coverage of subject matter)*
☐ Solomon J. Introduction to cardiovascular nursing. Baltimore: Williams & Wilkins, 1988. *(Additional and in-depth coverage of subject matter)*
☐ Stoy DB. Controlling cholesterol with diet. Am J Nurs December 1989;89:1625. *(Additional coverage of subject matter)*
☐ Stoy DB. Controlling cholesterol with drugs. Am J Nurs December 1989;89:1628. *(Additional coverage of subject matter)*
☐ Swithers CM. Tools for teaching about anticoagulants. RN January 1987;50:57. *(Additional coverage of subject matter)*
☐ Thompson VL. Chest pain: your response to a classic warning. RN April 1989;52:32. *(Additional coverage and illustrations that reinforce subject matter)*
☐ Weinberg LA. Buying time with an intra-aortic balloon pump. Nursing '88 December 1988;18:44. *(Additional coverage and illustrations that reinforce subject matter)*
☐ Yacone LA. The nurse's guide to cardiovascular drugs. RN August 1988;51:36. *(Additional coverage of subject matter)*

Chapter 28

Cardiac Dysrhythmias

On completion of this chapter the reader will:

- Name and describe the major dysrhythmias

- Identify the basic parts of a normal electrocardiographic tracing

- Discuss the treatment of dysrhythmias with drug therapy

- Use the nursing process in the management of a patient receiving drug therapy for a dysrhythmia

- Discuss the treatment of dysrhythmias with elective cardioversion

- Use the nursing process in the management of the patient receiving elective cardioversion

- Discuss the treatment of dysrhythmias with defibrillation

- Use the nursing process in the management of the patient requiring defibrillation

- Discuss the treatment of dysrhythmias with a temporary or permanent pacemaker

- Discuss the types and uses of pacemakers

- Use the nursing process in the management of the patient with a temporary or permanent pacemaker

- Define cardiac arrest and describe the steps taken when it occurs

— what drugs are used
— don't need spec. details

To pump blood, the heart must alternately contract and relax, allowing blood to enter its chambers during the relaxation phase and forcing it out during the contraction phase. The alternate contraction and relaxation are provided by an inherent rhythmicity of cardiac muscle. In disease, the pacemaker of the heart can be too fast or too slow. The myocardial cells can become overexcitable or develop a shortened refractory period; the Purkinje system can be damaged, or blocks can develop in the conduction system.

A *cardiac dysrhythmia* is a disorder of the heartbeat that may include a change in the rate or rhythm, or both. Dysrhythmias (arrhythmias) can be life-threatening or relatively minor. Because of their irregularity, all dysrhythmias affect the rhythmic pumping action of the heart to some degree.

Many ambulatory patients receive treatment for dysrhythmias and live essentially normal lives. When their cardiac reserve becomes overtaxed by coexisting illness, they become subject to more dangerous dysrhythmias or more serious consequences of the underlying hemodynamic disturbances.

Sudden cardiac arrest is really not so sudden but often is heralded by less dangerous warning dysrhythmias. In a critically ill patient or a patient with heart disease, even minor changes in heart rhythm can compromise cardiac function by decreasing cardiac output, thereby reducing coronary artery blood flow. Dysrhythmias also increase myocardial oxygen need, lead to more dangerous complications, and make treatment of the patient's underlying disease more difficult and complex.

Many clinical states predispose to a dysrhythmia. Myocardial ischemia after infarction, disturbances in pH, inadequate ventilation, electrolyte imbalance, anxiety, and pain can disturb heart rate, rhythm, and conduction.

Although a dysrhythmia can be diagnosed from an electrocardiographic (ECG) rhythm strip, the effect of this phenomenon on cardiac output is the crucial factor. A person with a healthy heart who develops a sinus tachycardia (rate over 100 beats/min) after running up a flight of stairs is showing a normal physiologic response. A continued sinus tachycardia in a patient on bed rest can place an added work load on the heart already damaged by an acute myocardial infarction.

A cardiac monitor attached to a patient is useless unless accurate assessment and observations are made, interpreted correctly, and acted on appropriately.

Skill in dysrhythmia detection takes considerable study, supervised practice, and time to develop. Only one lead of the ECG usually is necessary to monitor and identify serious dysrhythmias. The cardiologist reviews the entire 12-lead ECG and, in addition to interpretation, makes other cardiac diagnoses, such as heart enlargement, electrolyte disturbance, ischemic tissue damage, necrosis, and intraventricular conduction delay.

323

TYPES

Figure 28-1 shows regular sinus rhythm. The sinoatrial (SA) node is the pacemaker, and impulses are conducted normally through the conduction system.

Examples of dysrhythmias are sinus bradycardia, sinus tachycardia, atrial fibrillation, complete heart block, and premature ventricular contractions.

Sinus Bradycardia

The pacemaker site in sinus bradycardia is the SA node, but the rate is below 60 beats/min (Fig. 28-2). The rhythm is regular. The heart can be slow in athletes and laborers, who have normally enlarged hearts from regular strenuous exercise and greater than normal stroke volume. Emotional states, such as fear or shock, can increase vagal tone and slow the heart, resulting in syncope. Bradycardia may occur in patients with increased intracranial pressure, hypothyroidism, or digitalis toxicity. Carotid sinus pressure, the Valsalva maneuver, and eyeball pressure result in vagal stimulation and slowing of the heart. Bradycardia can occur during anesthesia or after administration of certain drugs, such as narcotics.

In acute myocardial infarction, sinus bradycardia often is an ominous sign of reflex vagal mechanisms, and the slow rate may not be sufficient to maintain cardiac output. Escape ectopic beats or rhythms, such as idioventricular rhythm, may take over as the primary pacemaker if their inherent rate is faster. This can increase ventricular irritability, which is dangerous in myocardial infarction.

Sinus Tachycardia

In sinus tachycardia, impulses are initiated by the SA node, and the rate is regular but above 100 beats/min (Fig. 28-3). Sinus tachycardia occurs in patients with healthy hearts as a physiologic response to strenuous

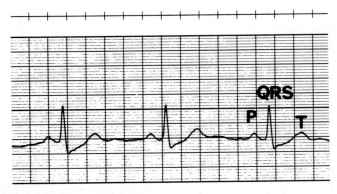

Figure 28-2. Sinus bradycardia.
Rate: Below 60; a relative bradycardia may exist at a faster rate if it is insufficient to maintain cardiac output.
Rhythm: Regular
P waves: Normal and precede each QRS complex
PR interval: Normal
QRS: Normal
Significance: Because cardiac output equals stroke volume times heart rate (CO = SV × HR), slow rate may not be sufficient for adequate cardiac output.
Treatment: Atropine sulfate IV may be ordered to override the vagal stimulus and increase sinus heart rate, thereby suppressing postbradycardia idioventricular beats. Isoproterenol (Isuprel) may be ordered to increase the heart rate by stimulation of the sinoatrial node.

exercise, strong emotion, pain, fever, hyperthyroidism, hemorrhage, shock, or anemia. The pulse rate can increase up to 150 beats/min; after that, cardiac decompensation can occur. A decrease in vagal tone or an increase in sympathetic tone, or both, can result in sinus tachycardia, which can be the initial evidence of heart failure.

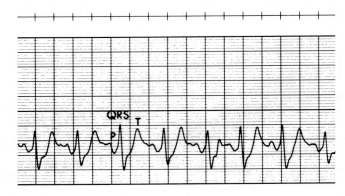

Figure 28-3. Sinus tachycardia.
Rate: 100 to 160
Rhythm: Regular
P waves: Normal, but may be obscured in T wave of previous cycle if rate is very fast.
PR interval: Normal
QRS: Normal
Significance: Can increase the work of the heart to the point of decompensation
Treatment: The underlying disease or the cause of the tachycardia must be treated. For example, anxiety is alleviated, fever is reduced, oxygen is given for hypoxia, or digitalis may be ordered for congestive heart failure. Keep the patient to minimum activity until rate decreases to compensated level.

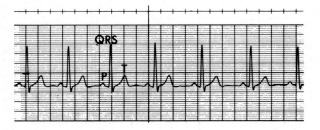

Figure 28-1. Normal sinus rhythm.
Rate: 60 to 100
P waves: Each has the same configuration and precedes the QRS complex
PR interval: 0.12 to 0.20 second
QRS: 0.07 to 0.10 second
Significance: Normal
Treatment: None

In patients with myocardial infarction or coronary artery disease, coronary insufficiency with chest pain can develop because coronary blood flow cannot keep up with the increased need of the myocardium imposed by the fast rate. With fast rates, diastole is shortened, and the heart does not have sufficient time to fill. Congestive heart failure, chest pain, or other symptoms of reduced cardiac output can occur.

Atrial Fibrillation

In atrial fibrillation, there is totally disorganized rapid atrial activity, and the atria quiver rather than contract normally (Fig. 28-4). The ventricles respond to the atrial stimulus in an irregular manner, depending on the sensitivity of the atrioventricular (AV) node and the conduction system. Some ventricular beats are so weak that they are ineffective in opening the aortic valve and propelling blood, and a pulse deficit exists. An apical–radial pulse should be taken.

Complete Heart Block

The atria and ventricles function without any relation to each other in complete heart block; therefore, P waves have no sequential relation to the QRS complex,

but the rhythm of each usually is regular (Fig. 28-5). The SA node functions normally; the main pacemaker in the heart is below the block in the AV node. What appears to be a PR interval changes with each complex; there really is no PR interval, however, because of the complete interruption in conduction from atria to ventricles.

Premature Ventricular Contractions

A premature ventricular contraction (PVC) is a ventricular ectopic beat that occurs before the ventricles have been depolarized by an atrial impulse (Fig. 28-6). Because it is not preceded by an atrial impulse and does not depend on an impulse from above, it also is called an *idioventricular beat.* A PVC usually is followed by a long *compensatory pause,* which occurs because the normally occurring atrial impulse finds the ventricle refractory because it has not recovered from depolarization by the PVC. The next normally occurring atrial impulse succeeds in depolarizing the ventricle. If the heart rate is very slow, the ventricles can repolarize after a PVC in sufficient time to receive the atrial stimulus precisely when it is due; there is an extra beat, but the basic rhythm is not interrupted. This is called an *interpolated* PVC.

Many people experience PVCs at one time or another. They often cause a flip-flop sensation in the

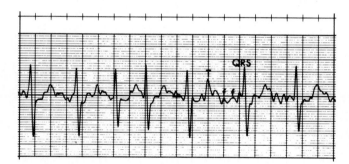

Figure 28–4. Atrial fibrillation.
Rate: 350 to 800 (atrial); ventricular rate varies but is irregular unless there also is a complete block at the atrioventricular node, in which case no atrial impulses are conducted and the lower pacemaker site produces a regular rhythm. In atrial fibrillation that is considered controlled either physiologically or by drugs, the ventricular rate is between 60 and 75/min. In uncontrolled atrial fibrillation, the ventricular rate is much faster.
Rhythm: Irregular
P waves: There are no P waves; there is an irregular rapid undulation of the baseline of the ECG; the atrial twitchings are called f waves.
PR interval: Because there are no P waves, the PR interval is not measurable.
QRS: Normal
Significance: Loss of atrial contraction diminishes cardiac output by about 15%. Irregular ventricular filling and rhythm diminish the pumping efficiency. Decrease in cardiac output can result in congestive heart failure.
Treatment: Digitalis may be given to slow the ventricular rate by its action on the atrioventricular node. If the patient's condition is potentially deteriorating, cardioversion is used.

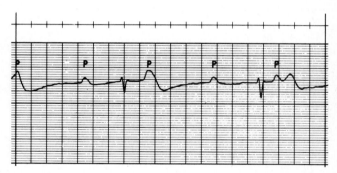

Figure 28–5. Third-degree atrioventricular block (complete heart block).
Rate: Atrial rate is normal; the ventricular rate is 20 to 40 beats/min.
Rhythm: Atrial and ventricular rhythms are regular.
P waves: Normal
QRS: Configuration is normal if pacemaker site is in atrioventricular node below block, but widened if pacemaker site is in ventricle.
Significance: The slow ventricular rate usually is ineffective in maintaining adequate cardiac output; angina, congestive failure, or Stokes-Adams syndrome from cerebral hypoxia can occur; ventricular standstill or ventricular fibrillation may ensue.
Treatment: Atropine or isoproterenol (Isuprel) may be ordered. Pacemaker is considered essential; adequate ventilation to correct hypoxia and treatment of other associated clinical conditions are necessary.

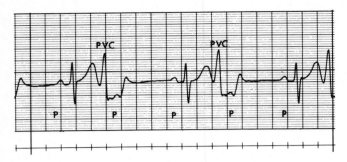

Figure 28–6. Premature ventricular contractions (PVCs).
Rate: Normal dominant rhythm
Rhythm: Irregular
P waves: Normal, but absent in idioventricular complexes
QRS: Bizarre in configuration; widened above 0.12 second in idioventricular complexes; T wave after PVC usually is opposite in direction to its QRS complex.
Treatment: Notify physician promptly. Digitalis may be withheld; myocardial depressant drug such as lidocaine is begun promptly if the patient has myocardial infarction, to prevent ventricular fibrillation.

chest. Some people describe it as a "fluttering" of the heart. The symptoms may be associated with pallor, nervousness, sweating, and faintness.

In healthy people, PVCs *usually* are harmless. They may be related to anxiety and stress, fatigue, or the excessive use of alcohol or tobacco. Although PVCs normally are not associated with organic heart disease, those who are frequently troubled by them should consult a physician. A thorough examination is important in making certain that no organic heart disease exists and in assuring these patients that their hearts are normal. Once these patients have received the physician's assurance that nothing is seriously wrong, they find it easier to ignore the symptoms. This in itself may cause the PVCs to occur less frequently and to disappear more quickly.

In the presence of acute heart injury, such as after surgery or in acute myocardial infarction, PVCs that occur in certain patterns are indicative of myocardial irritability, and are precursors of lethal dysrhythmias. These patterns or types are as follows:

■ More than six to eight unifocal PVCs per minute. A run of ventricular bigeminy (a normal beat followed by a PVC) also could meet this criterion.
■ Runs of PVCs, that is, two or more in a row
■ Multifocal PVCs, that is, from more than one location in the ventricle
■ A PVC whose R wave falls on the T wave of the preceding complex

TREATMENT

Treatment for cardiac dysrhythmias includes drug therapy and electrical modalities such as defibrilla-

tion, elective cardioversion, and a temporary or permanent pacemaker.

Drug Therapy

Drugs used in the treatment of dysrhythmias include the following:

■ Drugs that act primarily on tissues within the heart—myocardial depressants—such as lidocaine, procainamide, quinidine, propranolol, disopyramide, and bretylium tosylate
■ Drugs that increase cardiac rhythmicity (rhythmic activity) and contraction, such as isoproterenol
■ Drugs that depress conduction but increase contractile force, such as digitalis preparations
■ Drugs that act on the autonomic nervous system, such as atropine, which increases the heart rate

In some instances, the drug prescribed initially does not abolish the dysrhythmia or the patient experiences adverse reactions to the drug. In either case, another drug must be used. Other therapies, such as elective cardioversion, also may be necessary.

NURSING PROCESS —THE PATIENT UNDERGOING DRUG THERAPY FOR A CARDIAC DYSRHYTHMIA

Assessment
A systematic approach to dysrhythmia detection and treatment includes knowing certain norms, gathering data, comparing these data with a set of facts characteristic of certain dysrhythmias, and then gathering data about the clinical state of the patient. Additional assessments include those normally performed on the cardiac patient (see Chapter 24) as well as a complete medical history, including allergy and drug histories.

Nursing Diagnosis
The number and extent of the nursing diagnoses that apply depend on the seriousness of the dysrhythmia and the method of drug administration.

■ Potential activity intolerance related to the effects of the dysrhythmia on the cardiovascular and respiratory systems
■ Anxiety related to the symptoms of the dysrhythmia (eg, palpitations), treatment modalities, prognosis
■ Fear related to diagnosis, prognosis
■ Noncompliance to medical regimen related to anxiety, potential adverse reactions to treatment, knowledge deficit
■ Knowledge deficit of treatment regimen, adverse reactions

Planning and Implementation

The major goals of the patient include a reduction of fear and anxiety and an understanding of the treatment regimen.

The major goals of nursing management are restoring the heart to a normal sinus rhythm and decreasing the workload of the heart.

ORAL ADMINISTRATION. Before drug administration, the blood pressure and the pulse and respiratory rates are taken. Particularly important are the pulse rate and rhythm, and a comparison of these with previous findings. Also important is observing the patient for adverse drug reactions as well as response to therapy.

PARENTERAL ADMINISTRATION. Intravenous administration of antiarrhythmic drugs is used when an immediate effect is desired, when the patient is unable to take the drug orally, or when this is the only route of administration for a particular drug.

Intravenous administration usually necessitates placing the patient on a cardiac monitor. The dose of the drug may be repeated or adjusted according to patient response. The pulse rate and rhythm are checked both before and after administration. Appropriate references are checked before administration, as these drugs may be contraindicated in the presence of certain conditions such as shock, potassium imbalance, second- or third-degree AV block, and so forth.

Potential Activity Intolerance. The patient usually is placed on limited activities or complete bed rest until the dysrhythmia is abolished. When the patient is allowed to begin to resume ambulatory activities, he or she is carefully monitored for a return of the dysrhythmia. Dyspnea and fatigue may be signs of decreased cardiac output. Activities should be decreased, the pulse rate and rhythm monitored at frequent intervals, and the physician consulted.

Anxiety and Fear. Anxiety and fear may be caused by many internal and external factors, such as the symptoms of the dysrhythmia, the diagnosis and prognosis, and available treatment modalities. Anxiety may be reduced by allowing patients to verbalize their fears and emotions and by reassuring them that they are under constant supervision of the health care team.

Some patients find it difficult to cope with their diagnosis and possible lifetime treatment regimen. They may express concern or doubt, appear worried or depressed, or make statements that could indicate an inability to accept their treatment and diagnosis. For example, a patient may express concern over paying for the prescribed medication but not realize that certain resources would pay for some or all of the medication. The nurse should be willing to listen to these patients, help them work through their problems, and consult with the physician if the patient expresses concern over a certain problem.

Noncompliance, Knowledge Deficit. When drug therapy must be continued after discharge from the hospital, the patient should fully understand how and when to take the medication as well as the importance of the medication in controlling the dysrhythmia. Unless the patient fully understands the drug regimen, there is a potential for noncompliance and incorrect dosage. If the pulse rate is to be monitored before the medication is taken, the patient should be instructed in the correct method.

Also included in a patient-teaching plan are possible adverse reactions, the importance of continued medical follow-up, and what events necessitate the patient's contacting the physician before taking the next dose.

Evaluation

- Patient tolerates increased activity
- Anxiety and fear are reduced
- Patient demonstrates and verbalizes understanding of disorder, drug dosage regimen, adverse reactions, importance of follow-up care, and problems that necessitate contacting the physician

Elective Cardioversion

Elective cardioversion is a procedure performed by the physician to terminate rapid dysrhythmias such as atrial flutter, atrial fibrillation, and ventricular tachycardia, all of which decrease cardiac output to some degree. This procedure uses a defibrillator (or cardioverter), which consists of a monitor, a defibrillator unit (which is inside the defibrillator), and external electrodes (or paddles). The electrodes may be lubricated with a special jelly or with moist saline pads and applied to a specific area on the chest wall. By pressing the discharge button on the paddles, a specific amount of electric current is automatically delivered through the electrodes and passes through the heart. The defibrillator releases the electric current at a specific point in the QRS complex and at the point when the ventricles are depolarized. The delivery of an electric current completely depolarizes the entire myocardium at one time, so that the fastest normal pacemaker can regain control of the pacing function. Cardioversion avoids the time element and potential adverse effects encountered in the use of drug therapy.

The patient is anesthetized by intravenous administration of a tranquilizer (usually diazepam). Intubation usually is performed to control respirations and provide a patent airway. The desired response to elective cardioversion is a normal sinus rhythm, normal or adequate blood pressure, and strong peripheral pulses in all extremities.

NURSING PROCESS —THE PATIENT UNDERGOING ELECTIVE CARDIOVERSION

Assessment
Assessments include those normally performed on the cardiac patient (see Chapter 24) as well as a complete medical history, including allergy and drug histories.

Nursing Diagnosis
The following nursing diagnoses may be formulated before the procedure and amended or changed after the procedure:

- Activity intolerance related to dysrhythmia, decreased cardiac output (before and after the procedure)
- Anxiety related to cardioversion procedure, anesthesia, outcome of procedure
- Knowledge deficit of the procedure

Planning and Implementation
The major goals of the patient include the attainment of a normal sinus rhythm and the reduction of anxiety.

The major goal of nursing management is to prepare the patient physically and emotionally for elective cardioversion.

Digitalis and diuretics are withheld for 24 to 72 hours before cardioversion because it is believed that their presence in myocardial cells increases the chances of a fatal dysrhythmia's developing after cardioversion.

A 12-lead ECG usually is obtained immediately before the procedure. Preparations are the same as for any surgical procedure (ie, dentures are removed and the patient is asked to void). An intravenous line is inserted to administer the anesthesia and other drugs, as required.

Management after the procedure includes monitoring vital signs every 15 minutes for the first 1 or 2 hours and then as ordered. Continuous cardiac monitoring is used to evaluate heart rate and rhythm, and ECG changes are compared with those present before the procedure.

Activity Intolerance. Before the procedure, the patient's activities may be limited because of decreased cardiac output related to the dysrhythmia. After the procedure, the physician evaluates the patient's response to cardioversion and defines the amount of activity permitted. If dyspnea and fatigue occur during activity, the physician should be notified.

Anxiety, Knowledge Deficit. Most patients are apprehensive, even though the procedure has been explained by the physician. In elective cardioversion, there is time for the physician to explain the procedure. These patients usually are anxious as a result of the dysrhythmia and previous treatments for the disorder. The nurse may find it necessary to reinforce the physician's explanations as well as to reassure patients that the procedure is necessary and that they will be under constant surveillance immediately before, during, and after the procedure. The physician may order a sedative 30 to 60 minutes before the procedure.

Evaluation

- Normal sinus rhythm is attained and maintained
- Activity tolerance increases after termination of the dysrhythmia and increase in cardiac output
- Anxiety and fear are reduced
- Patient verbalizes understanding of the purpose and necessity of the procedure

Defibrillation

The only treatment for ventricular fibrillation is immediate *defibrillation*. Without it, the patient will die. This emergency procedure uses the defibrillator to completely depolarize the myocardium, which then allows the SA node to return to its role as the normal pacemaker.

Defibrillation must be instituted immediately after ventricular fibrillation has been detected. This procedure may be performed by a physician, or a nurse trained in the use of the defibrillator. After defibrillation, cardiopulmonary resuscitation is instituted if no pulse is present.

Even when cardiac activity is restored, the possibility remains that one or more organs have been affected, to a greater or lesser degree, because of being deprived of oxygen. Examples of problems include kidney failure and the effects of cerebral anoxia on certain areas of the brain (eg, paralysis, memory impairment, and comatose state).

The automatic implantable cardiac defibrillator is used on some patients with recurrent life-threatening dysrhythmias. This unit senses the heart rate (and thus the dysrhythmia) and then delivers an electrical impulse to correct the dysrhythmia.

NURSING PROCESS —THE PATIENT UNDERGOING DEFIBRILLATION

Assessment
Defibrillation is an emergency procedure, and therefore time for assessment is limited. Before institution of defibrillation, the nurse should quickly note the patient's level of consciousness, respiratory rate, and ECG pattern.

Nursing Diagnosis
Because defibrillation is an emergency procedure required to terminate a life-threatening dysrhythmia, there is no time to formulate nursing diagnoses. After the procedure, the nursing diagnoses depend largely on the patient's response to abolishment of the life-threatening dysrhythmia and any problems that arise from the procedure or from the effects of decreased to absent cardiac output.

Planning and Implementation
The major goal of the patient is the restoration of normal heart rate and cardiac output.

The major goal of nursing management is the restoration of cardiac activity and effective cardiac output.

After successful defibrillation, the patient's level of consciousness, ECG pattern, blood pressure, and pulse and respiratory rates are monitored at frequent intervals. Oxygen administration may be necessary to increase tissue perfusion. Laboratory tests such as arterial blood gas analysis and serum electrolytes may be ordered at prescribed intervals.

The paddle application sites are checked for redness and impaired skin integrity. The defibrillator usually is kept on standby, as repeat defibrillation may be necessary.

Evaluation

- Cardiac activity is restored
- ECG pattern is normal or near normal
- Prescribed postdefibrillation treatments are carried out
- Complications associated with cardiac arrest or ventricular fibrillation are absent

Pacemakers

A pacemaker (pulse generator) is a battery-operated electrical device that provides an electrical stimulus to the muscle of the heart. It is used to maintain the ventricular rate at a minimal level for effective cardiac output.

Types
There are two basic pacemaker designs: the temporary, or external, pacemaker and the permanent, or internal, pacemaker.

Temporary Pacemaker
The insertion of a temporary pacemaker may or may not involve an emergency situation, depending on the reason for insertion and the patient's physical condition. A temporary external pacemaker usually is inserted in the radiology department or a special room used for pacemaker insertion. Fluoroscopy and a cardiac monitor are used to determine the correct placement of the tip of the pacemaker lead. If the insertion is of an emergency nature, the procedure may be performed at the patient's bedside.

Continuous cardiac monitoring is necessary during and after the procedure. The pacemaker lead is inserted through a vein. The lead is threaded first into the right atrium and then into the right ventricle. The physician is able to determine the position of the lead by watching the cardiac monitor and the fluoroscope. Resuscitation equipment should be kept in the room, since ventricular fibrillation can be provoked mechanically by the tip of the pacemaker lead. Later, a radiograph or fluoroscopic examination of the chest may be ordered to determine exact placement of the pacemaker lead.

Permanent Internal Pacemaker
Insertion of a permanent pacemaker usually is performed under local anesthesia. The lead is inserted transvenously. After the pacing lead is properly seated in the right ventricle, the surgeon selects the correct pacing threshold and sets the voltage and rate. One type of pacemaker inserts leads into both the right atrium and the right ventricle.

The implantable pacemaker is then positioned under the skin (Fig. 28-7). The usual site of insertion is below the right clavicle, although the left side also can be used. The small incision is closed with suture.

Eventually the pacemaker lead becomes embedded in the right ventricular trabeculae (cords or bands attached to the inner walls of the ventricles that form a meshlike network). Immediately after insertion, the ECG display may show complexes with varying electrical potentials because the tip of the catheter may not touch the ventricular wall. PVCs are more frequent during the early postimplant period, and drug therapy may be ordered to suppress this dysrhythmia. The patient spends several days in a clinical unit in which a

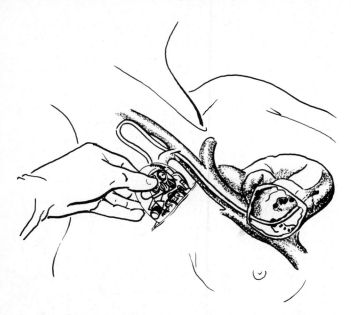

Figure 28–7. Implanted cardiac pacemaker. The battery and circuitry that make up the pulse generator are placed under the skin below the collarbone. Attached to the pulse generator is an electrode consisting of two encapsulated wires running through a vein to the right ventricle through which the electrical stimulus is carried to the heart.

defibrillator and other emergency equipment and drugs are available.

Some internal pacemakers are self-activating, and become operational when the patient's pulse falls below a preset level. These are called *demand* or *synchronous* pacemakers. Thus, if the physician sets this type of pacemaker at 72, the pacemaker unit is operational and produces an electrical stimulus only when the patient's pulse rate falls below 72. Battery life is prolonged with this type of pacemaker.

The *fixed rate* or *asynchronous* pacemaker is used less frequently than the demand or synchronous pacemaker. This type produces an electrical stimulus at a preset rate; its function is independent of the patient's cardiac rate. The battery life of this pacemaker is shorter.

Power for the pacemaker is provided by mercury–zinc, lithium, or nuclear-powered (plutonium) batteries. The mercury–zinc battery has the shortest life, and the nuclear-powered the longest. Externally charged batteries also are used.

Indications for Insertion

An external, temporary pacemaker may be indicated in patients with acute myocardial infarction complicated by heart block or other bradyrhythmias, in patients who have digitalis toxicity with heart block, and in patients with a slow heart rate and congestive failure who require treatment with digitalis. In some of these situations, the pacemaker is removed when normal sinus rhythm returns. This type of pacemaker is used as part of the emergency treatment of second- or third-degree heart block to correct the effects of this dysrhythmia until a permanent pacemaker can be inserted. Pacemakers also may be used to suppress rapid dysrhythmias, such as recurrent ventricular tachycardia, that do not respond to drugs or cardioversion.

The most frequent indication for insertion of a permanent pacemaker is to treat third-degree (complete) heart block associated with a variety of heart diseases, including coronary artery disease, rheumatic heart disease, and congenital malformations, or that occurs as a direct complication of cardiac surgery. A pacemaker also may be used to correct certain dysrhythmias that cause a marked decrease in cardiac output.

Complications

The most common complication of pacemaker insertion is improper functioning of the unit. Other complications include infection at the site of lead insertion (external pacemaker) or infection at the site of insertion of the internal pacemaker, perforation of the ventricular myocardium by the tip of the pacemaker lead, and development of dysrhythmias.

NURSING PROCESS —THE PATIENT WHO HAS A PACEMAKER

Assessment

In addition to a general assessment of the cardiovascular system (see Chapter 24), a medical history, including an allergy history, should be obtained from the patient or a family member. Any symptoms expressed by the patient, such as dizziness, faintness, or chest pain, also are recorded. The blood pressure and the pulse and respiratory rates are measured. If the patient is on a cardiac monitor, the dysrhythmia should be recorded to provide baseline data as well as documentation of its occurrence.

Nursing Diagnosis

One or more of the following nursing diagnoses may be stated for the patient with a pacemaker. These diagnoses usually are based on factors surrounding the dysrhythmia that were present before pacemaker insertion as well as factors associated with current or future treatment modalities.

- Anxiety related to symptoms of dysrhythmia, insertion of a pacemaker
- Activity intolerance related to symptoms, decreased cardiac output secondary to dysrhythmia
- Potential for infection related to internal or external pacemaker insertion
- Knowledge deficit of monitoring (permanent) pacemaker function, drug therapy, other factors (specify)

Planning and Implementation

The major goals of the patient include reduction of anxiety, improvement in activity tolerance, absence of infection, and an understanding of home care after pacemaker insertion.

The major goals of nursing management include identification of pacemaker malfunction, prevention of infection, and instruction of the patient in home care.

The pacemaker has its own characteristic tracing. The electrical artifact, or "blip," of the pacing stimulus should appear before the QRS complex of a ventricular pacer. It usually is identified as a thin, straight stroke. Absence of the artifact may mean faulty monitoring equipment or, more seriously, failure to pace because of malposition of the pacemaker lead, dislodgment of the pacemaker lead, pacemaker lead breakage, or rise of the pacing threshold due to tissue reaction to the pacemaker, or to infection. The location of the artifact is particularly important. If the paced rhythm competes with the patient's spontaneous rhythm, the artifact can fall in the vulnerable period of the cardiac cycle.

Cardiac monitoring usually is continued for several days. Vital signs are taken as ordered. Periodic ECG tracings may be ordered. These should be placed on the patient's chart along with the date and time of the recording.

TEMPORARY PACEMAKER INSERTION. Once the pacemaker lead is inserted, it is attached to the external pacemaker unit, which is firmly attached to the patient's forearm by means of tape or some other anchoring device. The unit is placed so that there is no tension on the pacemaker lead. Only grounded electrical equipment is used in the room. This means that all electrical plugs must have three prongs.

The pacemaker lead that was inserted into a vein is connected to terminals on the top of the external pacemaker. This connection should be checked several times each day because an improper connection or displacement of the wire from the terminal results in pacemaker malfunction. If the patient is on a cardiac monitor with an alarm system, the alarm sounds if the pacemaker malfunctions and the patient's pulse drops below the lowest level set on the alarm system.

Other causes of external pacemaker malfunction are battery failure, internal dislodgment of the pacemaker lead, and a break in the pacemaker lead. The battery of an external pacemaker is easily replaced, and one or more spare batteries should be readily available. Dislodgment of the pacemaker lead necessitates repositioning of the lead. This is performed by the physician. A break in the wire necessitates removal of the lead and insertion of a new one.

If the patient is confused or restless and movement disturbs the external pacemaker or its lead, the physician must be notified.

PERMANENT PACEMAKER INSERTION. Patients with implanted pacemakers also are placed on a cardiac monitor. Internal pacemaker malfunction has the same causes as external pacemaker malfunction; battery failure is not likely to occur on a new pacemaker unit, however. A pacemaker sometimes malfunctions shortly after insertion because of defective manufacture. Patients who have had an internal pacemaker inserted in the past may experience battery failure.

Anxiety. Anxiety may be related to the dysrhythmia or the necessity to insert an internal or external pacemaker. When the physician decides that a pacemaker is to be inserted, the reason for the procedure should be explained to the patient and family. A surgical consent is necessary. For most patients, the thought that their hearts require artificial electrical control produces anxiety. They need to talk about it and get used to the idea, but often there is little time for this. The nurse should listen to the physician's explanation to the patient and review, clarify, and correct any misinterpretations that the patient or family may have.

Activity Intolerance. After pacemaker insertion and correction of the dysrhythmia, the physician allows the patient to slowly resume normal activities. If fatigue or dyspnea occurs, the amount of activity should be decreased and then resumed at a slower pace. The physician should be kept informed of the patient's ability or inability to resume activity.

Potential for Infection. The venous insertion site of an external pacemaker should be inspected daily for signs of irritation, especially several days after insertion, because phlebitis or infection may occur. Any evidence of reddening near the site of insertion or along the pathway of the vein should be reported immediately. The dressing over the internal pacemaker insertion site should be changed daily and the incision inspected for signs of infection.

Knowledge Deficit. Education of the patient with a permanent internal pacemaker should include the following points:

1. Follow-up care is important. Clinic or physician's office appointments must be kept.
2. Check pulse rate daily or as ordered by the physician. Contact the physician *immediately* if the pulse rate is below or above the rate stated by the physician.
3. Take the prescribed drugs exactly as ordered.
4. Notify the physician if the suture line becomes inflamed or sore.

5. Avoid injury to the area where the pacemaker is inserted. Wear loose-fitting clothing over the area of pacemaker insertion.
6. Some pacemakers are sensitive to outside electrical interference, such as radiofrequency signals from diathermy machines and microwave ovens; proximity to these may interfere with the function of the pacemaker. Check with the physician regarding things to avoid.
7. Follow the physician's advice regarding activities such as lifting, sports, and exercise. Resume activities only at the pace recommended by the physician.
8. Carry an identification card, bracelet, or neck medallion indicating the presence of the pacemaker as well as the physician's name, type of pacemaker, and pacemaker settings (rate and electrical output). Medic Alert bracelets or medallions also carry this information plus a 24-hour toll-free answering service that will provide the physician's name, type of pacemaker, and other pertinent information. The pacemaker identification card provided by the manufacturer is to be carried on the person at all times.
9. Pacemakers can trigger alarm systems, such as those used in airports. Hand scanning should be requested and the pacemaker identification card shown to the inspectors.
10. A pacemaker change probably will be necessary in the future.

Evaluation

■ Anxiety is reduced
■ Patient tolerates increased activities after internal pacemaker insertion
■ Signs of localized infection are absent
■ Patient verbalizes understanding of home care program and self-evaluation of pacemaker function

Cardiac Arrest

Cardiac arrest is the sudden cessation of the heartbeat and effective cardiac output. The electrical mechanism of cardiac arrest can be ventricular asystole or ventricular fibrillation.

Care of the patient in cardiac arrest should encompass the following stages and maneuvers:

1. If the patient is on a cardiac monitor, respond to the monitor alarm and check ECG patterns.
2. Summon help.
3. If necessary and possible, the patient should be defibrillated immediately (if allowed by hospital policy).
4. Observe the ABC sequence of cardiopulmonary resuscitation: airway, breathing, circulation.

Airway. The first step is to create a patent airway by removing any material (eg, sputum or vomitus) from the mouth manually or by suction and then lifting the jaw forward. An oropharyngeal airway is then inserted. Only an experienced person should attempt endotracheal intubation. Establishment of an airway may be sufficient to permit spontaneous breathing.

Breathing. Mouth-to-mouth breathing done effectively delivers adequate oxygen to the patient. Because of the danger of transmission of infectious diseases, a bag-valve-mask device, such as the Ambu bag, is recommended.

Ten to 12 maximal insufflations should be given before chest compression is started, so that oxygenated blood will be circulated. With two rescuers, one inflation should be interposed after each five compressions without any halting of compression (1:5 ratio or 12 breaths/min). With one rescuer, two breaths are interposed after each 15 compressions. The breather should see the chest rise and fall, feel the resistance of the lungs as they expand, and hear the noise of air escaping during exhalation.

Artificial ventilation may cause distention of the stomach. This can lead to regurgitation, reduced lung volume, or the initiation of vagal reflexes. The physician may exert moderate pressure between the umbilicus and the rib cage to expel the air. The patient's head should be lowered and turned to one side to avoid aspiration of gastric contents.

Circulation: Cardiac Compression. Rhythmic pressure applied over the lower half of the sternum results in compression of the heart and pulsatile arterial circulation. A manual or automatic chest compressor may be used (if available) to perform external cardiac compression. External cardiac compression may be ineffective or contraindicated in such situations as crushing injuries of the chest and internal thoracic injuries, or in patients with advanced pulmonary emphysema with enlarged, fixed rib cages.

Closed cardiac massage is not without its dangers. Hands that are misplaced to one side may break ribs or rupture the liver or spleen.

Drug Therapy. During the resuscitation effort, various drugs are administered and may include one or more of the following:

Atropine—to correct vagus-induced bradycardia
Oxygen—to correct hypoxemia
Bretylium tosylate—to treat ventricular dysrhythmias
Calcium chloride—to strengthen cardiac contractions; to treat asystole
Dobutamine—to increase cardiac output
Sodium bicarbonate—to correct metabolic and respiratory acidosis

Vasopressors—to maintain adequate blood pressure

Epinephrine—to increase cardiac output; to treat ventricular asystole and fibrillation

Procainamide—to treat ventricular fibrillation

Lidocaine—to treat ventricular dysrhythmias

Other drugs also may be used, depending on the patient's medical history and response to resuscitative efforts.

The most important nursing responsibility is recognition of cardiac arrest. Once this has been identified, resuscitative efforts begin *immediately* and continue until the physician arrives. The nurse then assists in resuscitative measures and in the preparation and administration of drugs.

When resuscitative efforts are begun, the level of consciousness, skin color, breathing (if present) pattern, ECG pattern, and pupil size are noted. The patient's response should be evaluated during resuscitation by various members of the health care team. Because the pupils are the best index of brain oxygenation, pupillary response is evaluated at frequent intervals. Dilatation of the pupils begins 45 seconds after cardiac arrest and is complete in 1 or 2 minutes. Cerebral death begins in 30 to 90 seconds unless adequate cerebral oxygenation is restored. If the pupils begin to return to normal or near-normal size, efforts at cardiopulmonary resuscitation have been (currently) successful.

Peripheral pulses should be present during cardiac compression. Absence indicates ineffective compression. The patient's color also should improve.

After successful cardiac resuscitation, the patient should be closely observed. Vital signs should be taken frequently; the patient should be attached to a monitoring device.

Shock may have caused decreased renal perfusion with a reduction in urine output. In addition, fluids administered during resuscitation may not be excreted at a normal rate, resulting in a fluid volume excess. The output should be measured hourly and the physician notified if urine output remains low. Kidney dialysis or administration of an osmotic diuretic may be necessary.

A nasogastric tube may be passed to prevent gastric distention. Other complications for which the nurse should observe include pneumothorax, hematoma of the liver, brain damage, fractured ribs or sternum, and fat embolism.

Oxygen should be given to reduce the onset of dysrhythmias caused by hypoxemia. If resuscitative efforts are successful, the patient's color should improve and the breathing pattern return to normal.

General Pharmacologic Considerations

☐ Drug therapy for dysrhythmias includes myocardial depressants (antiarrhythmics), cardiotonics, adrenergic drugs, cholinergic blocking agents, and electrolytes.

☐ When drugs are used in the treatment of dysrhythmias, the patient's pulse rate and rhythm should be closely monitored. Patients who receive intravenous lidocaine, propranolol (Inderal), or bretylium tosylate (Bretylol) should be on a cardiac monitor during administration of the drug.

☐ Administration of lidocaine can result in serious adverse effects, including convulsions and cardiac arrest. An airway should be readily available. If hypotension or additional dysrhythmias occur during administration, the intravenous infusion should be adjusted to the slowest possible rate until the physician can examine the patient.

☐ The cardiotonics are digitalis and allied glycosides. The apical–radial rate should be taken before the drug is administered, especially during digitalization. Later, when the patient is fully digitalized, a radial rate may suffice.

☐ Drug toxicity can occur even when normal doses of digitalis and allied glycosides are administered. Signs of toxicity include anorexia, nausea, vomiting, halos around dark objects, diarrhea, abdominal discomfort, disturbance of green or yellow vision, and *dysrhythmias* such as bradycardia, tachycardia, and bigeminal pulse.

☐ The cholinergic blocking agent atropine may be used to treat the severe bradycardia of third-degree heart block or digitalis intoxication. An emergency dose of up to 1 mg may be given intravenously. Isoproterenol (Isuprel) also may be used to treat severe bradycardia. When either of these drugs is administered, the pulse rate should be closely monitored for drug response.

General Gerontologic Considerations

☐ In the elderly, stress, exercise, or illness may result in dysrhythmias as well as other cardiac disorders, such as congestive heart failure and myocardial ischemia.

☐ Sinus bradycardia and heart block are common dysrhythmias seen in elderly patients.

☐ To ensure patient compliance, the elderly patient should be given a thorough and detailed explanation regarding the drug regimen (eg, dose, time taken, and adverse effects).

Suggested Readings

☐ Blowers MG, Smith R. How to read an ECG. 4th ed. Oradell, NJ: Medical Economics, 1988. *(Additional and in-depth coverage of subject matter)*

☐ Burke LJ. Abnormal pulse rhythm: when is it cause for concern? Nursing '88 November 1988;18:117. *(Additional coverage of subject matter)*

☐ Burke LJ. Bradycardia: when is it life-threatening? Nursing '88 September 1988;18:102. *(Additional coverage of subject matter)*

☐ Caplan M, Ranieri C. What's his ECG telling you? A guide for nurses. RN February 1989;52:42. *(Additional coverage and illustrations that reinforce subject matter)*

☐ Conover MB. Understanding electrocardiography arrhythmias and the 12-lead ECG. 5th ed. St Louis: CV Mosby, 1988. *(Additional and in-depth coverage of subject matter)*

☐ Hahn K. About discharge medications. Nursing '88 November 1988;18:89. *(Additional coverage of subject matter)*

☐ Huang S, Kessler C, McCulloch C, Dasher L. Coronary care nursing. 2nd ed. Philadelphia: WB Saunders, 1989. *(In-depth coverage of subject matter)*

☐ Lubliner C. When to expect heart block. RN January 1990;53:28. *(Additional coverage and illustrations that reinforce subject matter)*

☐ Malseed R, Girton SE. Pharmacology: drug therapy and nursing considerations. 3rd ed. Philadelphia: JB Lippincott, 1990. *(Additional and in-depth coverage of subject matter)*

☐ Mason CB, Davis JE. Cardiovascular critical care. New York: Von Nostrand Reinhold, 1987. *(Additional and in-depth coverage of subject matter)*

☐ Molinari MA. Monitoring digoxin therapy in the elderly. RN November 1988;52:38. *(Additional coverage of subject matter)*

☐ Morton PG. About rate-responsive pacemakers. Nursing '88 May 1988;18:141. *(Additional coverage of subject matter)*

☐ Mutnick A, Fecitt S. Cardiac drugs: inotropic and chronotropic agents. Nursing '87 October 1987;17:58. *(In-depth coverage of subject matter)*

☐ Porterfield LM, Porterfield JG. How digoxin interacts with other drugs: a practical guide. Nursing '90 January 1990;20:50. *(Additional and in-depth coverage of subject matter)*

☐ Porterfield LM, Porterfield JG. What you need to know about today's pacemakers. RN March 1987;50:44. *(Additional coverage of subject matter)*

☐ Rhynsburger J. Action stat! third-degree heart block. Nursing '88 October 1988;18:33. *(Additional coverage of subject matter)*

☐ Schweisguth D. Setting up a cardiac monitor—without missing a beat. Nursing '88 November 1988;18:43. *(Additional coverage and illustrations that reinforce subject matter)*

☐ Sergeant LL. Tracking your patient's E.K.G. with a Holter monitor. Nursing '86 October 1986;16:47. *(Additional coverage of subject matter)*

☐ Teplitz L. Clinical close-up on lidocaine. Nursing '89 December 1989;19:44. *(Additional and in-depth coverage of subject matter)*

☐ Thaler MS. The only EKG book you'll ever need. Philadelphia: JB Lippincott, 1988. *(In-depth coverage of subject matter)*

☐ Yacone LA. The nurse's guide to cardiovascular drugs. RN September 1988;51:40. *(In-depth coverage of subject matter)*

Chapter 29

Hypertension

On completion of this chapter the reader will:

- Define hypertension
- Discuss the mechanisms responsible for systolic and diastolic blood pressure
- Discuss the physiologic control of systolic and diastolic blood pressure
- Name the two types of hypertension
- List some of the complications associated with hypertension
- Describe and discuss the symptoms, diagnosis, and treatment of essential hypertension
- Describe and discuss the symptoms, diagnosis, and treatment of secondary hypertension
- Describe and discuss the symptoms, diagnosis, and treatment of accelerated hypertension
- Describe and discuss the symptoms, diagnosis, and treatment of malignant hypertension
- Use the nursing process in the management of the patient with hypertension

The term *hypertension* refers to a disease entity characterized by sustained elevation of arterial pressure. In the elderly, slightly higher figures are used to determine hypertension.

ARTERIAL BLOOD PRESSURE
Systolic Blood Pressure

Systolic blood pressure is determined by the force and volume of blood ejected from the left ventricle, and the ability of the arterial system to distend at the time of ventricular contraction. The walls of the arteries normally are elastic, and yield to the force and volume of ventricular contraction. In the older person with a rigid, atherosclerotic aorta, systolic blood pressure may be quite elevated because of loss of elasticity. Systolic hypertension is a response to change in central hemodynamics.

Narrowing of the arterioles, either by arteriosclerosis or some other mechanism that causes vasoconstriction, increases peripheral resistance, which in turn increases systolic blood pressure. This resistance can be compared to the slight narrowing of a tube, such as a drinking straw or a garden hose. The narrower the lumen, the greater the pressure needed to push air or liquid through the hollow structure.

Diastolic Blood Pressure

Diastolic blood pressure is recorded during ventricular relaxation. It depends on peripheral resistance and the diastolic filling interval. If arterioles are constricted, blood pressure has to be increased to flow through the constricted area. On the other hand, if the arterioles are wide open, the blood flow is brisk, and diastolic pressure falls rapidly. Diastolic hypertension is a response to change in peripheral hemodynamics.

Pulse Pressure

The difference between the systolic and diastolic pressures is the pulse pressure. The magnitude of the pulse pressure largely determines the forcefulness and volume of the radial pulse felt at the wrist. Factors that increase the systolic pressure, such as a rigid, atherosclerotic aorta, or factors that decrease the diastolic pressure, such as a slow heart rate, increase (or widen) the pulse pressure. A strong, bounding pulse reflects a wide pulse pressure.

Factors that decrease the systolic pressure and increase the diastolic pressure decrease (or narrow) the pulse pressure. A rapid, weak, and thready pulse reflects a decreased or narrowed pulse pressure. This is the case in shock.

Physiologic Control of Arterial Pressure

Arterial pressure is regulated by the autonomic nervous system, the kidneys, and the endocrine glands. Normal blood pressure for adults ranges from about 100/60 to 140/90. The reasons for the changes in blood pressure in advancing age are not fully understood.

Blood pressure normally fluctuates with changes in posture, exercise, and emotion. It is lowest when a person is sleeping, slightly higher when awake but lying down, higher still when sitting up, and elevated even further when standing. These normal changes in blood pressure that occur with a change in position or consciousness are the reason the blood pressure of those with known or suspected cardiac disease is measured in the standing, sitting, and lying positions.

Exercise and emotional stress cause an elevation of blood pressure. These normal fluctuations show the importance of measuring blood pressure under similar conditions. For example, inaccurate results might be obtained if the blood pressure is taken one morning before the patient has been out of bed and again the next morning while the patient is sitting in a chair immediately after taking a shower. The nursing care plan should designate the circumstances for taking the patient's blood pressure so that conditions are most nearly duplicated.

Hypertensive Disease

Hypertension increases the workload of the heart and damages the arteries because of the increased resistance of the arterioles to the flow of blood. Congestive heart failure, myocardial infarction, cerebrovascular accident (stroke), and renal failure are serious complications associated with hypertension.

When a cardiac abnormality (demonstrated by electrocardiography [ECG] or radiographic evidence of enlargement of the left ventricle) is present with the elevated blood pressure, the term *hypertensive heart disease* is used. When extracardiac vascular damage is present without heart involvement, the term *hypertensive vascular disease* is used. When both heart and other pathology are present with hypertension, the appropriate term is *hypertensive cardiovascular disease.*

COMPLICATIONS

A increase in blood pressure that is sudden (over a few hours) or gradual (over days to months) and that re-

mains untreated can result in serious complications. Damage to many organs of the body, including the eyes, brain, heart, and kidneys, can occur. The heart may enlarge, and the patient may develop congestive heart failure. Many complications arise from hemorrhage or occlusion of blood vessels that supply important organs. The atherosclerotic process is exacerbated by hypertension. The hemorrhage of tiny arteries in the retina may cause marked visual disturbance or blindness. A cerebrovascular accident may result from hemorrhage or occlusion of a blood vessel in the brain. Myocardial infarction may result from occlusion of a branch of a coronary artery. Impaired circulation to the kidneys is believed to be related to the frequency of degenerative kidney disease among some hypertensive patients.

TYPES

Hypertension is divided into two main categories: essential (or primary) hypertension and secondary hypertension.

Secondary hypertension describes a variety of conditions in which elevation of blood pressure is secondary to some known cause. Pheochromocytoma (a tumor of the adrenal gland) is an example of a condition that causes secondary hypertension. Only 5% of people with hypertension are thought to have the secondary type.

Essential (Primary) Hypertension

Essential hypertension is characterized by sustained elevation of the diastolic pressure. A diastolic pressure of 90 mmHg or greater is usually accepted as a cutoff point for diagnosis.

The cause of essential hypertension is unknown. About 95% of hypertensive patients have this type of hypertension. Certain factors may play a role in the development of this disorder. Heredity, obesity, emotional stress, smoking, and increased serum cholesterol and sodium levels may be causative factors.

Measures to decrease the risk in susceptible populations may help to forestall the development of symptoms or curtail advancement of hypertension. People with a family history of hypertension or those who have transient elevations of blood pressure (considered to be indicative of a tendency to the disease) may be helped by the measures outlined in Chart 29-1.

Symptoms

The onset usually is gradual. Essential hypertension often is first discovered during a routine physical ex-

Chart 29-1. Measures to Reduce the Risk of Hypertension

□ Annual physical examination
□ Correction of obesity by eating a well-balanced and nutritious diet and engaging in a moderate program of physical exercise
□ Moderation of salt intake
□ Coping effectively with or avoiding problems or situations that produce stress whenever possible
□ Improvement of general health habits by obtaining adequate sleep and rest

amination. Because of its insidious onset, it is hard to say when the disease begins. People in their 30s and 40s may be discovered to have a sustained elevation in blood pressure without any symptoms. The condition may be present for 10 to 15 years before the patient experiences any discomfort or apparent complications.

One patient may experience no discomfort, whereas another with a similar blood pressure reading may complain of headache, dizziness, fatigue, insomnia, and nervousness. Headache is described as throbbing or pounding; nosebleeds and blurred vision also may be seen. Angina pain or shortness of breath may be the first clue to hypertensive heart disease. In some instances, hypertension may not be diagnosed until the patient becomes ill from its complications.

Diagnosis

Diagnosis is made by a thorough history and physical examination. Particularly important is a family history of hypertension or death caused by stroke or heart disease.

The blood pressure should be taken on both arms while the patient is standing, sitting, and lying down. Laboratory tests may be performed to detect damage to the kidneys and heart. An ECG may reveal abnormalities, such as enlargement of the left ventricle. Additional studies, such as chest radiography and excretory urography (intravenous pyelography), may be done to rule out damage to other organs or structures.

Treatment

The primary objective of medical care is sustained nutritional and pharmacologic management to prevent major complications. Initial management depends on the degree of pressure elevation and the individual patient. For mild elevations, weight reduction and decreased sodium intake may return the blood pressure to normal levels. If cholesterol and triglyceride levels

are increased, a diet low in saturated fats is recommended. Some physicians believe that certain patients fail to adhere to dietary restrictions after a time, and they prefer to initiate therapy with an antihypertensive drug as well as dietary measures and a weight reduction program.

Drugs do not counteract the cause of blood pressure elevation. Rather, they relax constricted arterioles so that the high arterial peripheral resistance is reduced. After careful evaluation of the patient, the physician prescribes a drug that will keep the pressure at a near-normal level. Depending on the degree of blood pressure elevation or patient response to the initial drug, a second antihypertensive agent may be added to the regimen. In some instances, poor response may necessitate discontinuing the original agent and trying one or two other antihypertensive drugs.

Secondary Hypertension

Secondary hypertension is due to a known cause, such as an adrenal tumor, renal artery stenosis, the use of oral contraceptives, and primary aldosteronism.

Symptoms

As with essential hypertension, the patient may be asymptomatic, and the elevated blood pressure discovered during a routine physical examination.

The physician, by means of a careful patient history and physical examination, should determine if the patient's elevated blood pressure is possibly due to a known cause. Diagnostic studies to determine the possible cause may include excretory urography, renal arteriography, determination of serum electrolyte levels, and funduscopic examination of the eye. The cardiovascular system should be evaluated for the presence of congestive heart failure and other cardiac abnormalities.

Treatment

When possible, secondary hypertension is treated by removing the cause. For example, if the cause is renal artery stenosis, a renal artery angioplasty has proved successful in some cases. When caused by the use of oral contraceptives, the patient is advised to discontinue the drug and use another form of contraception. A vasectomy for the man or tubal ligation for the woman may be recommended if other contraceptive measures fail and pregnancy is not desired. Surgery is advised for those with adrenal tumors.

The patient usually is prescribed an antihypertensive drug until the cause can be eliminated. The blood pressure is followed closely to ensure that it does not reach dangerously high levels.

Accelerated and Malignant Hypertension

Accelerated hypertension describes markedly elevated blood pressure accompanied by hemorrhages and exudates in the eye. If untreated, accelerated hypertension may progress to malignant hypertension. The term *malignant hypertension* describes markedly elevated blood pressure accompanied by papilledema (swelling of the optic nerve at its point of entrance into the eye).

Both types of hypertension usually have an abrupt onset and, if untreated, are rapidly followed by severe symptoms and complications. Malignant hypertension is fatal unless the blood pressure is quickly reduced. Even with intensive treatment, permanent damage may be done to the kidneys, brain, and heart.

Symptoms

A sudden, marked rise in blood pressure along with such symptoms as confusion, headache, visual disturbances, seizures, and, possibly, coma may be indicative of accelerated or malignant hypertension.

Diagnosis

Diagnosis is based on symptoms as well as the physical examination and patient history. Additional diagnostic studies may include chest radiography, computed tomographic scan, ECG, and kidney function studies.

Treatment

Rapid reduction of blood pressure is essential to prevent further organ damage. Depending on the patient's condition, an antihypertensive agent may be administered by the oral or parenteral route. Intravenous antihypertensive agents that may be used include nitroprusside sodium (Nipride) and labetalol (Normodyne). Oral agents include nifedipine (Procardia), verapamil (Isoptin), captopril (Capoten), and prazosin (Minipress).

NURSING PROCESS —THE PATIENT WHO HAS HYPERTENSION

Assessment

ESSENTIAL HYPERTENSION. Whether for routine screening, as part of the physical examination, or assessment of patients who suddenly develop a change in their condition, the blood pressure remains an important part of the assessment process. During an initial assessment of the patient newly diagnosed as having hypertension, the blood pressure should be taken in both arms with the patient in a standing, sitting, and then supine position. The pulse should be taken in both wrists. The apical pulse is taken with particular attention to the rate and rhythm as well as the presence of abnormal heart sounds. The lungs should be auscultated and abnormal breath sounds noted. The patient should be questioned regarding any symptoms that have occurred, and a complete medical and family history should be obtained.

The initial assessment of the hospitalized patient previously diagnosed and treated for hypertension should include questions about the treatment regimen prescribed by the physician. The patient should be asked to name the drug prescribed and to explain any restrictions or suggestions made by the physician about physical activity, diet, and weight management. Initial blood pressures should be taken on both arms, with the patient in the standing, sitting, and lying positions to establish a data base for future management.

Additional assessments may need to be performed on the cardiac patient (see Chapter 24), depending on the patient's medical history and current symptoms.

SECONDARY HYPERTENSION. Assessment of the patient with secondary hypertension is essentially the same as that for the patient with primary hypertension. Some of these patients are acutely ill, and therefore require more frequent appraisals of their physical status.

ACCELERATED AND MALIGNANT HYPERTENSION. Recognition of an abrupt onset of a markedly elevated blood pressure and the symptoms associated with its development is the most important part of assessment. The physician should be notified immediately and the patient closely monitored until treatment is instituted.

Nursing Diagnosis

Depending on the type and severity of hypertension, the age of the patient, and other factors, one or more of the following nursing diagnosis may apply:

- Activity intolerance related to symptoms, severity of hypertension, dyspnea secondary to cardiac involvement, other factors (specify)
- Anxiety related to symptoms, diagnosis
- Constipation related to adverse drug effects
- Diarrhea related to adverse drug effects
- Fluid volume deficit related to diuretic effect of drug
- Altered health maintenance related to lack of knowledge regarding health promotion, health maintenance, and treatment modalities
- Noncompliance related to lack of knowledge of prescribed treatment regimen, anxiety, negative side effects of treatment
- Altered sexuality patterns related to adverse drug effects
- Knowledge deficit of treatment regimen

Planning and Implementation

The major goals of the patient include maintenance of a normal blood pressure, reduction of anxiety, absence of adverse drug effects, and an understanding of and compliance with the prescribed treatment regimen.

The major goals of nursing management include a reduction of blood pressure, recognition of any sudden or marked increase in the blood pressure, and effective patient teaching.

Essential Hypertension. The results of drug therapy (ie, a decrease in blood pressure) as well as observation for the appearance of adverse drug effects are essential parts of the assessment process. When monitoring the patient's blood pressure, it is best to use the same arm and to place the patient in the same position each time a reading is taken.

Secondary Hypertension. The patient with secondary hypertension may receive an antihypertensive drug until the cause can be eliminated. If the patient is admitted to the hospital for treatment, the blood pressure and pulse rate should be monitored at frequent intervals. A sudden, marked increase or decrease in the blood pressure should be immediately reported to the physician.

Accelerated or Malignant Hypertension. The patient should be evaluated at frequent intervals before, during, and after the administration of an antihypertensive drug. The blood pressure and pulse rate should be monitored as ordered, and the physician informed if the blood pressure fails to respond to drug therapy. Intensive intravenous drug therapy may be necessary, and it is important to keep the intravenous line patent.

All patients with hypertension, regardless of the type, are observed for complications associated with this disorder. This is especially important if the blood pressure is or remains elevated despite medical therapy.

Activity Intolerance. Patients with longstanding, untreated hypertension may develop such complications as congestive heart failure. These patients may experience difficulty in performing routine daily activities and require assistance. They should be allowed to progress at their own pace and within the limits of their tolerance.

Because some antihypertensive drugs may cause postural hypotension, patients may feel weak, faint, or dizzy when they change position. To lessen discomfort, the patient should be instructed to rise from a sitting position slowly, and when getting out of bed to first sit on the edge of the bed for a few moments and then stand. Patients should be instructed to sit or, preferably, to lie down immediately if they feel faint. This helps the feeling to subside as well as to prevent injury from fainting and falling.

Anxiety. Newly diagnosed patients may show concern over their disorder and the treatment necessary to return the blood pressure to normal or near-normal levels, and awareness of complications associated with the disorder. Many patients seek repeated reassurance and explanation from the nurse. The nurse should allow these patients time to express their anxieties and fears, and offer reassurance. Presenting facts about the disorder and the effectiveness of medical treatment may help to dispel any doubts these patients may have and to create the positive attitude necessary for patient compliance.

Constipation or Diarrhea. Some oral antihypertensive drugs can cause constipation or diarrhea. The patient's bowel movements should be checked and recorded daily, and the physician notified if either problem should occur.

Fluid Volume Deficit. Administration of a diuretic for control of essential hypertension may result in excessive diuresis during initial therapy. The intake and output should be measured and the patient weighed daily. The skin and oral mucosa should be examined daily for changes associated with a fluid volume deficit (see Chapter 12). Complaints such as leg cramps and weakness may indicate an electrolyte imbalance caused by excessive fluid loss, and should be reported to the physician.

Altered Sexuality Patterns. Some antihypertensive drugs can cause sexual dysfunction; this usually is explained by the physician. If the patient verbalizes concerns over this matter, it should be brought to the attention of the physician.

Altered Health Maintenance, Noncompliance, Knowledge Deficit. Lack of knowledge about the disease and its treatment places the patient at risk for nonadherence to a treatment program. A thorough explanation of the prescribed treatment modalities (diet, exercise, medication, and weight reduction), why these must be followed, and what active role the patient must play in treatment may enhance patient compliance.

Working with hypertensive patients gives the nurse an opportunity to participate in long-term care that may help the patient to live longer and more comfortably. This care places a premium on the nurse's ability to teach, listen, and guide the patient in following a treatment program.

The importance of not omitting the prescribed medication as well as the necessity for lifetime medication should be emphasized. Many patients fail to adhere to their treatment program because they have few, if any, symptoms and feel well. The adverse effects of the prescribed medication should be explained as well as the importance of follow-up care. The patient also should know which adverse effects are serious and must be reported to the physician as soon as possible.

When diet restrictions are incorporated into the treatment program, a consultation with the dietitian may be necessary. The patient also is provided with a list of foods and food substances that are either excluded from the diet or taken in limited amount. The use of tobacco is discouraged, as nicotine use results in vasoconstriction and thus may increase the blood pressure.

If the patient expresses difficulty in adhering to a weight loss program, stopping smoking, or reducing stress, this should be reported to the physician. With physician approval, the nurse may recommend one or more of the various support programs available in the community for those who are having difficulty in these areas.

Self-monitoring of the blood pressure increases patient compliance. The patient or a family member should be taught how to monitor the blood pressure. Therapy can then be planned and adjusted according to multiple blood pressure recordings made in the patient's normal surroundings.

The following points may be included in a teaching program:

1. Reduce or increase physical exercise according to the physician's recommendations.
2. Take the prescribed medication exactly as ordered. Do not increase, decrease, or omit the dose unless directed to do so by the physician. Drug therapy normally is a lifetime necessity.
3. A lack of symptoms does not mean the problem is mild, does not require medical attention, or will not ultimately damage some body organs. Hypertension can be controlled by taking the prescribed medication.
4. The blood pressure and pulse rate are monitored (when recommended by the physician). The blood pressure is taken at the same time of the day. The same arm and body position (sitting, standing, or lying down) are used for each measurement. Keep a record of all blood pressure readings (date, time, arm used, body position, blood pressure reading), and give this record to the physician at the time of each office visit.
5. If salt or fat intake is to be reduced, read the labels of containers and packages carefully.
6. Alcohol may interact with some medications; therefore, alcohol should be avoided unless use has been approved by the physician.
7. If adverse drug effects should occur, these should be reported to the physician as soon as possible, preferably before the next dose is taken.
8. Do not use any nonprescription drug without first getting approval of the physician.
9. Always inform dentists and other physicians of the medication being taken.

Evaluation

- Patient is able to tolerate increased activity
- Anxiety is reduced
- Bowel elimination is normal
- Normal fluid balance is attained and maintained
- Patient verbalizes understanding of treatment modalities
- Patient verbalizes understanding of dietary restrictions
- Patient adheres to program of weight loss and dietary control of sodium and saturated fat intake
- Patient is able to explain drug regimen (dose, time)
- Patient demonstrates ability to monitor own blood pressure and pulse
- Patient demonstrates understanding of possible drug adverse effects and what to do if they occur
- Patient expresses interest in joining a support group to control weight and stop smoking
- Patient is willing to discuss concerns over a treatment regimen; asks questions regarding medical treatment

General Nutritional Considerations

☐ Patients with hypertension may be told to limit their sodium intake. This limitation may range from avoiding obviously salty foods and not using salt at the table to a sodium-restricted diet.

☐ The patient is shown how to check food labels for sodium that may be listed as "salt" or a form of "sodium" such as mono*sodium* glutamate.

☐ The amount of sodium allowed in a sodium-restricted diet may be stated as a 500-, 1,000-, or 2,000-mg sodium diet.

☐ The patient on a severe sodium-restricted diet should see a dietitian for an explanation of dietary allowances.

General Pharmacologic Considerations

☐ Patients who are receiving antihypertensive drugs for the first time should have the blood pressure taken every 1 to 4 hours, especially if hypertension is severe and a potent antihypertensive agent is administered. Those with mild to moderate hypertension may require blood pressure determinations only once or twice daily.

☐ Patients who are receiving antihypertensive drugs may experience postural hypotension early in therapy, and should be cautioned about this adverse effect. The patient can minimize symptoms of postural hypotension by rising slowly from a lying or sitting position.

☐ Drug therapy may include the use of a more potent antihypertensive agent, and the nurse should, therefore, acquire a thorough knowledge of possible adverse drug effects.

General Gerontologic Considerations

☐ Hypertension caused by arteriosclerosis or atherosclerosis, or a combination of both, is not uncommon in the elderly. This problem may go undiagnosed unless the patient sees a physician at regular intervals. Elderly people should be encouraged to have their blood pressure checked every 6 months.

☐ If the physician directs the patient to monitor his or her own blood pressure, a family member also should be taught how to take a blood pressure.

Suggested Readings

☐ Dudek SG. Nutrition handbook for nursing practice. Philadelphia: JB Lippincott, 1987. *(Additional coverage of subject matter)*

☐ Hill MN, Cunningham S. The last words for high BP. Am J Nurs April 1989;89:504. *(Additional coverage of subject matter)*

☐ Hill MN. Diuretics for mild hypertension: still the best choice? Nursing '87 September 1987;17:62. *(Additional coverage of subject matter)*

☐ Karch AN, Boyd EH. Handbook of drugs and the nursing process. Philadelphia: JB Lippincott, 1988. *(In-depth coverage of subject matter)*

☐ Malseed R, Girton SE. Pharmacology: drug therapy and nursing considerations. 3rd ed. Philadelphia: JB Lippincott, 1990. *(Additional and in-depth coverage of subject matter)*

Chapter 30

Failure of the Heart as an Efficient Pump

On completion of this chapter the reader will:

- Discuss the cause and pathophysiology of heart failure
- Distinguish between left- and right-sided heart failure
- List and discuss the symptoms, diagnosis, and treatment of left-sided heart failure
- List and discuss the symptoms, diagnosis, and treatment of right-sided heart failure
- Use the nursing process in the management of the patient with heart failure
- Discuss the cause and pathophysiology of pulmonary edema
- List and discuss the symptoms, diagnosis, and treatment of pulmonary edema
- Use the nursing process in the management of the patient with pulmonary edema
- Discuss the cause and pathophysiology of cor pulmonale
- List and discuss the symptoms, diagnosis, and treatment of cor pulmonale

Heart Failure

Heart failure develops when the heart is unable to meet the demands of body tissues for oxygen and nutrients. In effect, the heart becomes an inefficient pump. The term *congestive heart failure* (CHF) is used to describe this disorder because inefficient circulation leads to the congestion of many organs with blood and tissue fluid.

Heart failure can occur with varying degrees of severity. When symptoms are slight, the patient may be able to be up and about. In contrast, the patient in severe heart failure is critically ill. When patients show symptoms of heart failure, their condition is described as *decompensated*; that is, the heart is not able to compensate or make up for the demands placed on it. When treatment succeeds in enabling the heart to keep up with the circulatory load, the symptoms disappear, and the condition is described as *compensated*. The abnormality of the heart that led to heart failure often remains, however, and unless the patient has continued treatment, the symptoms of CHF may recur.

Etiology

Heart failure often develops gradually, as the result of strain placed on the heart by congenital defects, diseases of the heart and blood vessels, or other diseases that overburden the heart. Causes include rheumatic fever, hyperthyroidism, hypertension, and myocardial infarction.

In older age groups, heart failure frequently is brought about by a combination of factors. The blood vessels gradually may lose their elasticity (arteriosclerosis), and the lumen of the arteries may slowly grow smaller because of atherosclerosis. Elevation of the blood pressure is common among older people. These vascular changes can lead to heart failure by interfering with the blood supply to the heart muscle and by causing the heart to pump blood through vessels that have become narrowed and inelastic. The heart itself is not exempt from the process of aging. With advancing age, cardiac reserve is lessened, and the heart becomes less able to withstand the effects of injury or disease.

Pathophysiology

Disturbances of one part of the heart, if they are severe enough or last long enough, eventually affect the entire circulation. Using mitral stenosis as an example, the process of CHF is as follows:

1. Narrowing of the mitral valve impedes the flow of blood from the left atrium to the left ventricle.
2. Because it cannot empty completely, the left atrium enlarges, and the pressure within it increases.

3. Increased pressure in the distended left atrium, which has not emptied completely, creates a backward pressure in the pulmonary vascular bed. Because of increased pulmonary vascular bed pressure, fluid escapes from the capillaries surrounding the alveoli into the alveoli. The alveoli become filled with fluid and the lungs become congested.

4. Lung congestion results in inefficient oxygenation of the blood, since the fluid impairs gas exchange between the alveoli and the capillaries surrounding the alveoli. The patient develops dyspnea, cough, orthopnea, and, sometimes, hemoptysis. These are symptoms of left-sided, or left, heart failure.

5. Because of the congestion in the lungs and increased pressure in the pulmonary vascular bed, it becomes harder for the right ventricle to pump blood to the lungs. The right ventricle must pump more forcefully to overcome the resistance of the increased pulmonary vascular bed pressure.

6. The right ventricle eventually is unable to keep up with its work. As pressure increases in the right ventricle and incomplete emptying occurs, increased pressure in the right atrium now appears.

7. Venous blood returning to the right atrium by way of the superior and inferior vena cava cannot enter the right atrium in adequate amounts, and venous return is decreased. Congestion and increased pressure develop in the large veins leading to the vena cava and the heart, and eventually in other organs and tissues of the body, as the result of inefficient venous return.

8. Dependent edema, such as that of the feet and the ankles on standing, occurs. The abdomen may become distended with fluid (ascites). The liver may enlarge. Presacral edema may be present in the patient on bed rest. The neck veins become distended. These are symptoms of right-sided, or right, heart failure.

In each type of heart disease the process of CHF is somewhat different, depending on the location and severity of cardiac damage. One characteristic, however, is constant: Although one part of the heart and the circulation are primarily affected, the process, if it continues, eventually affects the entire circulation. The sequence in which symptoms appear reflects the sequence of physiologic disturbance. Symptoms of either right or left heart failure may appear first; eventually, symptoms of failure in both sides will be present.

LEFT- AND RIGHT-SIDED HEART FAILURE

Left-sided (left ventricular) heart failure and *right-sided (right ventricular) heart failure* describe the inability of the left or right ventricle to effectively meet the needs of body tissues. The left and right ventricles can fail separately, or they may both be in failure. Left ventricular failure often occurs first and then progresses to right ventricular failure. Left-sided heart failure produces respiratory effects, whereas right-sided heart failure causes systemic effects.

Left-Sided Heart Failure

When the left side of the heart is in failure, pulmonary symptoms occur and may progress to *pulmonary edema* (see section on pulmonary edema).

Symptoms

The symptoms of left-sided heart failure include cough, dyspnea, orthopnea, tachycardia, fatigue, and anxiety. Restlessness and confusion also may be seen. Moist crackles usually are heard on auscultation of the lungs.

Many patients notice unusual fatigue after activity that previously had not caused fatigue. Some find that dyspnea on exertion (exertional dyspnea) is their first symptom. Breathing difficulty while lying flat (orthopnea) also may be noted, and prompt the person to use two or even three pillows when in bed. Cough, occasionally productive of blood-streaked sputum, may occur.

Diagnosis

No one test is diagnostic for left-sided heart failure. Diagnosis is made by patient history and physical examination. Diagnostic tests include chest radiography, to detect cardiac enlargement and signs of fluid accumulation in the lungs, and electrocardiography (ECG). Laboratory tests include arterial blood gas analysis, complete blood count, and determination of serum electrolyte levels. If the patient is seriously ill, a pulmonary artery catheter may be inserted for hemodynamic monitoring.

Treatment

Medical management is directed toward reducing the work load of the heart and improving left ventricular output. The work load of the heart is reduced by bed rest. A low-sodium diet may be prescribed. Oxygen may be necessary to reduce dyspnea. In severe left ventricular failure, an intraaortic balloon pump may be inserted and used to maintain left ventricular function until the condition can be corrected.

Drug therapy aimed at improving cardiac output may include digitalis preparations, diuretics, and vasodilators. Each of these drugs has a specific action.

Digitalis Preparations (Cardiac Glycosides).

These drugs have inotropic action; that is, they increase the contractile force of the ventricles and slow the heart rate. When the contractile force of the ventricles is increased, cardiac output increases. Although these drugs do not have direct diuretic activity, diuresis occurs because of the increase in cardiac output and in renal perfusion.

Diuretics.   Diuretics increase renal excretion of water and sodium, thus reducing the fluid retention that may accompany heart failure.

Vasodilators.   Certain vasodilators have one or more of the following actions: (1) increase emptying of the left ventricle, (2) improve left ventricular output, (3) reduce peripheral vascular resistance, and (4) increase renal and cerebral blood flow. These activities enhance the effect of diuretics and digitalis preparations.

Right-Sided Heart Failure

When the right side of the heart is in failure, the end result is an accumulation of fluid (edema) in the extremities as well as in organs, such as the liver. Patients with this form of heart failure retain excessive amounts of sodium, which contributes to the edema by holding water in the tissues.

Symptoms

The patient may notice that the feet and ankles are swollen, particularly at the end of the day (Fig. 30-1). Swelling usually disappears during the night when the feet and legs are elevated, but the fluid can shift to the lungs or sacral region. Nocturia (excessive urination during the night) often is present.

The edema does not really disappear. It is just distributed differently because of the patient's posture and is, therefore, less noticeable. When the patient is standing or sitting, the ankles gradually swell again (dependent edema). By the time the edema becomes noticeable, the patient usually has retained 10 or more extra pounds of fluid in the tissues.

Edema of the feet and legs seldom causes pain, but it makes the legs feel heavy, clumsy, and tired. This usually is described as *pitting* edema because when pressure is exerted, the part that has been pressed becomes indented. The indentation gradually disappears after the pressure is released. Edema of other areas, although less visible, often causes symptoms of dysfunction of the involved organs. Distention of the liver and other abdominal viscera may cause flatulence, anorexia, and nausea. The collection of fluid within the lungs and the pleural space leads to dyspnea and possibly a persistent cough.

Diagnosis

Because right-sided heart failure can be caused by various diseases of the heart, any test or combination of tests used for cardiac patients may be ordered in an effort to discover the underlying cause. In addition to a history and physical examination, an ECG, chest radiograph, and various laboratory tests (eg, serum enzyme and electrolyte studies) may be ordered. The extremities should be examined for edema, and the liver palpated for enlargement (hepatomegaly). The neck veins often are distended when the patient is sitting or standing.

Treatment

Treatment involves following measures to help the heart function as effectively as possible and to relieve the symptoms produced by inefficient circulation:

1. The patient should be helped to rest. The heart may be able to meet the demands of the body at rest and yet be unable to cope with the demands placed on it by physical or emotional stress.

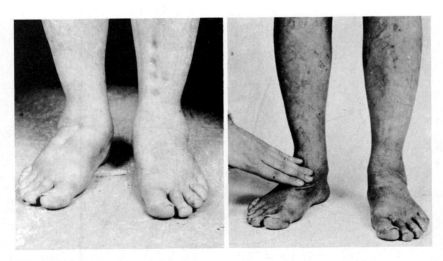

Figure 30–1.   (*Left*) Pitting edema of feet and lower legs. (*Right*) The same patient after treatment relieved the edema. (CIBA Pharmaceutical Company)

2. The abnormal retention of sodium should be treated by limiting the intake of sodium. Diuretics may be given to rid the body of the excess fluid and sodium that have been stored in the tissues. Sometimes paracentesis (removal of fluid from the abdominal cavity) is necessary to relieve ascites.

3. A digitalis preparation may be given to slow the heart rate and strengthen ventricular contraction. These two actions help the weakened, overburdened heart to pump blood more efficiently.

4. Oxygen may be ordered to improve ventilation when oxygenation is impaired by congestion and sluggish circulation through the lungs.

NURSING PROCESS —THE PATIENT WHO HAS HEART FAILURE

Assessment
Because one or both sides of the heart may be in failure, the initial assessment evaluates the patient's cardiac and respiratory status and includes a history of symptoms before admission. Incorporated in the cardiac and respiratory assessment are the vital signs, the type and appearance of the sputum raised (if any), the location and severity of edema (if present), skin color, and the patient's general physical appearance and mental status. Vital signs also include a thorough description of the cardiac and respiratory rates and rhythms. The lungs are auscultated for abnormal breath sounds. With the patient in a sitting position, the jugular veins are examined for distention. The mental state (alert, confused, or disoriented) is assessed. Additional assessments, based on the patient's medical history, may be necessary.

Nursing Diagnosis
Depending on the severity and type of heart failure (left- or right-sided or both), one or more of the following nursing diagnoses may apply:

- Anxiety related to dyspnea, diagnosis
- Activity intolerance related to dyspnea, fatigue secondary to decreased cardiac output
- Fluid volume excess related to decreased cardiac output, decreased renal perfusion, sodium retention
- Constipation related to immobility
- Potential impaired skin integrity related to immobility, decreased cardiac output, venous stasis
- Sleep pattern disturbance related to dyspnea, nocturia
- Noncompliance related to knowledge deficit, negative side effects of treatment, other factors (specify)
- Ineffective individual coping related to anxiety, inability to meet basic needs, changes in lifestyle, other factors (specify)

- Altered family processes related to an ill family member
- Knowledge deficit of disease process, treatment modalities

Planning and Implementation
The major goals of the patient include relief of anxiety, increase in activity tolerance, improved cardiac function, attainment of a normal sleep pattern, prevention of skin breakdown, and knowledge of and compliance with the treatment regimen.

The major goal of nursing management is a reduction in the work load of the heart followed by an increase in tissue perfusion and a decrease in respiratory difficulty.

Vital signs should be monitored at frequent intervals. The pulse rate should be checked before a digitalis preparation is administered. If signs of digitalis toxicity are present, such as an apical pulse below 60 or above 90 beats per minute, irregular rhythm, or premature ventricular contractions, the physician should be notified before the drug is given.

Ongoing assessments include the appraisal of the areas that were covered during the initial assessment. Patients admitted with mild CHF can become acutely ill in a short time, so the nurse must be alert to any increase in the severity of symptoms, such as increased dyspnea or a change in pulse rate or rhythm. A sample nursing care plan for the patient in CHF is shown in Nursing Care Plan 30-1.

Respiratory Function. To relieve respiratory distress and improve gas exchange, oxygen should be administered as ordered. The skin and nail beds should be inspected for evidence of cyanosis, and the respiratory rate checked at frequent intervals. The lungs should be auscultated for abnormal breath sounds, particularly moist crackles. Diuretic therapy and administration of drugs that increase the force of ventricular contractions may reduce pulmonary congestion.

Patients with right-sided heart failure may have hepatomegaly and ascites, resulting in discomfort and difficulty breathing when they assume certain positions in bed, especially a semi-Fowler's position. Several attempts may be necessary to find the most comfortable position that does not increase respiratory distress.

Anxiety. When a patient is admitted to the hospital in critical condition, the need for reassurance is especially great. Anxiety occurs because of difficulty breathing. In addition, reduced oxygenation of tissues, particularly cerebral tissues, results in restlessness and confusion. Correction of heart failure and

Nursing Care Plan 30-1
Management of the Patient Who Has Congestive Heart Failure

Potential Problem and Potential Nursing Diagnosis	Nursing Intervention	Outcome Criteria
Dyspnea	Elevate head of bed (do not raise knee gatch); administer oxygen if cyanosis present or respiratory rate increased markedly above data base; auscultate lungs q 1–4 hr (depending on severity of dyspnea); monitor BP, P, R q 2–4 hr, temperature daily to q 4 hr; allow patient to rest between allowed activities (eg, eating, grooming, ambulating); assist with those activities that result in dyspnea	Respiratory rate within normal range (12–18/min)
Edema	Administer diuretics and other cardiac drugs as ordered; measure intake and output; weigh daily; elevate feet/legs when out of bed in a chair; provide restricted sodium diet (if ordered); check areas of edema daily and compare with data base; give good skin care to edematous areas; observe for signs of hyponatremia or hypernatremia, hypokalemia, and dehydration (results of diuretic therapy)	Edema reduced or eliminated with patient attaining dry weight
Fatigue Activity intolerance related to congestive heart failure	Provide rest periods between activities; do not rush patient during morning care; begin ambulatory activities slowly and increase as tolerated; monitor pulse and respiratory rates before and after activity to determine tolerance; keep personal articles within easy reach; assist with getting in and out of bed, ambulation, as needed	Fatigue decreased; patient able to tolerate increased activity
Skin breakdown due to prolonged bed rest, inactivity Impaired skin integrity related to immobility	Change position q 2 hr; give good skin care to areas of edema and bony prominences; encourage well-balanced diet	Skin integrity maintained
Constipation Constipation related to immobility	Check for bowel movements daily; obtain order for a stool softener if patient has difficulty having a bowel movement; instruct patient to avoid straining at stool; encourage moderate fluid intake (unless physician orders otherwise); contact dietitian regarding use of brans, prune juice, etc. in the diet; encourage ambulation as tolerated	Constipation eliminated; bowel pattern normal

improvement in the respiratory status may reduce the anxiety associated with severe dyspnea.

Activity Intolerance. Physical and emotional rest reduce the work load of the heart and decrease the pulse rate and blood pressure. Severely ill patients should be placed on complete bed rest.

Activities are increased as the heart failure is corrected. At first, the patient requires assistance with activities of daily living. A call button should be kept within the patient's easy reach, and answered promptly. This reduces anxiety and reassures the patient that someone is always available. When the patient is allowed out of bed, assistance should be given until he or she can ambulate safely.

Fluid Volume Excess. Intake and output should be carefully recorded. If daily weight measurement is ordered, it should be performed at the same time every day (preferably before breakfast). Similar clothing should be worn by the patient each time the weight is measured.

Oliguria may be seen initially, but urine output should increase as a result of improved cardiac output and renal perfusion after therapy is started.

It is important to know the predicted time of effect of the diuretic given the patient. Diuretics administered intravenously may initiate diuresis in 5 to 10 minutes, with the peak volume in 30 to 60 minutes. Oral diuretics may produce a peak urinary volume in about 2 hours. Sudden diuresis can result in bedwetting or acute urine retention. The bedpan or urinal should be kept close by. If the patient is not voiding, or appears to be voiding in small amounts, the bladder is checked for distention, especially in those with known prostatic enlargement. Urinary frequency and urgency are tiring, especially on the first day of hospitalization. Women should be assisted in getting on and off the bedpan; men should be closely checked so that they have an empty urinal when they need it. Patients should be watched for signs of electrolyte depletion, especially potassium and sodium (see Chapter 12).

Constipation. Constipation may occur if prolonged bed rest is necessary. Straining to have a bowel movement should be avoided. A record of bowel movements should be kept, and the physician informed if constipation is apparent. A stool softener or laxative may be ordered.

Potential Impaired Skin Integrity. Patients with right-sided heart failure may have varying degrees of peripheral edema. When they are allowed out of bed, the feet should be elevated. The skin should be inspected daily for signs of tissue breakdown, as edematous tissues are especially prone to decubitus formation. Good skin care, along with a foam rubber pad, an alternating-pressure mattress, a flotation pad, or sheepskin, helps to prevent decubitus ulcers. These patients require a position change and encouragement to deep-breathe and perform leg exercises every 2 hours.

Because of the danger of thrombophlebitis in patients confined to bed, the knee gatch should not be raised. A footboard should be used to prevent footdrop and to keep the patient from sliding down in bed when the head of the bed is raised. Feet and legs should be maintained in good alignment. Elastic stockings may be prescribed to prevent thrombophlebitis.

Sleep Pattern Disturbance. Dyspnea, nocturia, anxiety, and general discomfort can interrupt the normal sleep pattern. If the patient wakens frequently during the night, the physician should be notified.

Ineffective Individual Coping. The nurse should be alert to signs that indicate that the patient is having difficulty coping with illness. The patient may appear anxious or depressed, and show concern over progress, potential changes in lifestyle, ability to return to work, or financial responsibilities. Problems such as these create stress, which in turn increases the work load of the heart.

The nurse should first identify areas of concern. An explanation of the measures necessary to prevent future episodes of heart failure may help some patients. work through and solve their problem. For others, referral to a member of the health care team (eg, the social worker or dietitian) may be necessary.

Altered Family Processes. Heart failure and the measures necessary to control symptoms as well as progression of the disorder may disrupt family routines, cause an additional financial burden, or create an alteration in family roles. The nurse should be alert to problems expressed by the patient or family and attempt to redirect thinking and possibly offer solutions.

Noncompliance, Knowledge Deficit. Some patients find it difficult to accept both an illness and the changes necessary to control the disorder. Others fail to adhere to a medical regimen and changes in lifestyle because of a lack of knowledge. Education plus active patient and family involvement in a program designed to control heart failure may encourage compliance.

Once heart failure is controlled and symptoms reduced or eliminated, the patient and family should be made aware of the treatment modalities necessary to prevent a recurrence of symptoms and progression of the disease. The following material, which can be modified to meet the patient's prescribed treatment or specific needs, may be included in a teaching plan:

1. Perform tasks with adequate rest periods to reduce or eliminate fatigue and dyspnea.
2. Learn to identify and then avoid occasions that produce stress.
3. Elevate the legs while sitting.
4. Follow the diet prescribed by the physician. Learn to read labels and identify products (foods, nonprescription drugs) that are high in sodium and saturated fats. Avoid using salt. When eating in a restaurant, select foods known to be low in sodium and saturated fats. Consult your diet plan when in doubt.
5. Increase activities gradually. If dyspnea should occur, cease the activity and rest.
6. Avoid extreme heat, cold, and humidity.
7. Take medications as prescribed and at the times per day as printed on the container label. Never omit a medication unless told to do so by the physician. Diuretics should be taken early in the day. The pulse rate should be monitored daily before taking a digitalis preparation. If the pulse rate is 60 or below, do not take the medication and contact the physician immediately.
8. Weigh yourself daily or as recommended by the physician. The weight should be measured at the same time each day while wearing about the same amount of clothing.
9. Contact the physician if symptoms return or there is a sudden increase in weight or swelling in the legs, ankles, or feet.
10. Continued follow-up care is an important aspect of treatment.

If the patient is taking a diuretic that is known to deplete potassium, the signs of hypokalemia should be explained. A list of foods high in potassium also can be provided. If a potassium supplement is ordered, the signs of hyperkalemia should be explained.

Evaluation

■ Anxiety is reduced
■ Patient increases daily activities without respiratory distress, fatigue, cough, or marked increase in pulse rate
■ Fluid volume excess is corrected
■ Skin color is normal; respiratory rate and rhythm are normal
■ Evidence of skin breakdown is absent
■ Peripheral edema is decreased
■ Bowel elimination is normal
■ Sleep pattern is normal
■ Patient verbalizes willingness to adhere to recommended treatment program
■ Patient shows signs of coping with disease and acceptance of treatment modalities

■ Family problems are identified and alternatives or solutions presented
■ Patient verbalizes understanding of medical and dietary regimens, adverse drug effects, importance of follow-up care, and self-participation in treatment

PULMONARY EDEMA

Pulmonary edema, which is an abnormal collection of fluid in the lungs, represents an acute emergency.

Etiology and Pathophysiology

Because the left ventricle may be weakened by such conditions as heart failure, acute myocardial infarction, arteriosclerotic heart disease, and cardiac dysrhythmias, the heart becomes incapable of maintaining sufficient output of blood with each contraction. The right ventricle, however, continues to pump blood toward the lungs. The pulmonary capillaries and the alveoli become engorged because blood is not adequately and promptly pumped into the systemic circulation by the left ventricle. Sometimes the lungs rapidly fill with fluid, and acute respiratory distress develops.

Acute pulmonary edema also can result from injury to the lung tissue, such as blast injuries that cause many small hemorrhages within the lung, and from conditions in which drainage of pulmonary secretions is impaired. For example, chronic pulmonary diseases such as emphysema may lead to obstruction of the respiratory passages when the patient is unable to cough up secretions. Pulmonary edema also may be caused by drug overdose or the inhalation of irritants such as ammonia.

Symptoms

Patients with acute pulmonary edema exhibit anxiety, restlessness, sudden dyspnea, wheezing, orthopnea, cough (often productive of pink, frothy sputum), cyanosis, bounding pulse, elevated blood pressure, and severe apprehension. Respirations sound moist or gurgling.

Diagnosis

Diagnosis usually is based on symptoms, but a chest radiograph, an arterial blood gas analysis, and an ECG may be ordered.

Complications

Cardiac dysrhythmias, heart failure, and cardiac and pulmonary arrest are complications of pulmonary edema.

Treatment

The relief of symptoms is urgent, as these patients literally can drown in their own secretions. Every effort should be made to relieve lung congestion as quickly as possible.

The physician's orders may include measures to provide physical and emotional relaxation, to relieve hypoxia, to retard venous return to the heart, and to improve cardiovascular function. An intravenous line should be established immediately (if one is not already in place) for administration of drugs.

PROVIDE PHYSICAL AND EMOTIONAL RELAXATION. Intravenous morphine or meperidine often is given to lessen apprehension. Morphine, in particular, seems to help relieve respiratory symptoms by depressing higher cerebral centers, thus relieving anxiety and slowing the respiratory rate. Morphine also promotes muscle relaxation to reduce the work of breathing. The patient should be permitted to stay in the position most comfortable for him, usually sitting up.

RELIEVE HYPOXIA AND IMPROVE VENTILATION. To raise the rate of oxygen diffusion across the edema fluid barrier in the alveoli, oxygen by intermittent or continuous positive pressure may be ordered. This helps to prevent further engorgement of the lungs with fluid. Later a nasal catheter or cannula may be substituted and oxygen given at a rate of 4 to 6 L/min. Oxygen should be humidified to prevent drying of secretions and further impairment of ventilation.

Intravenous aminophylline may be given to dilate the bronchi, improve breathing, and lessen pulmonary-capillary transudate.

RETARD VENOUS RETURN TO THE HEART. Measures to decrease the volume of circulating blood, which helps to relieve the congestion of blood and fluid in the lungs, include wet or dry phlebotomy (rotating tourniquets), the use of intermittent positive pressure or a mechanical ventilator with positive end-expiratory pressure (PEEP), and the administration of morphine. Wet phlebotomy (the removal of blood from a vein), with removal of about 500 mL of blood, or rotating tourniquets (dry phlebotomy) may be used to trap blood in the extremities, so that it is not returned to the already overburdened and congested heart and lungs.

OXYGENATION. Oxygen is given to relieve dyspnea, cyanosis, and hypoxia. Oxygen also may be given by intermittent positive-pressure breathing (IPPB). The physician determines flow rate, pressure, and inspiratory-expiratory ratio to arrive at an intrathoracic net positive pressure that will impede venous flow. If the patient is hypotensive, further reduction of venous return to the heart is contraindicated. IPPB has the additional benefit of assisting ventilation in all lung segments and is an effective means of administering oxygen.

If respiratory failure occurs despite treatment, a tracheostomy or endotracheal intubation along with mechanical ventilation may be necessary. The use of PEEP (see Chapter 22) with mechanical ventilation is effective in improving oxygenation.

IMPROVE CARDIOVASCULAR FUNCTION. When pulmonary edema is due to heart failure, other measures for treatment of this condition may be begun promptly, if the patient has not already been receiving them. For example, digitalization with a rapid-acting preparation and the injection of a rapid-acting, potent diuretic may be ordered.

Rotating tourniquets may be applied clockwise or counterclockwise, *provided they are always rotated in the same direction throughout the treatment.* A tourniquet is applied tightly enough to interfere with venous return but not so tightly as to cut off arterial circulation. If a rubber tourniquet is used, the pulse in the extremity should be checked after the tourniquet is applied. If the pulse has been obliterated, the tourniquet is too tight, and should be loosened. If blood pressure cuffs are used, each cuff should be inflated to a point between the patient's systolic and diastolic blood pressures.

The exact procedure to be used should be specified by the physician. Tourniquets may be rotated every 15 minutes, more frequent rotation is ordered in some instances. If 15-minute intervals are used, each extremity will have the tourniquet applied for 45 minutes and will be without a tourniquet for 15 minutes (Table 30-1 and Fig. 30-2).

The patient's extremities will become swollen, mottled, and uncomfortable because of engorgement with venous blood. The patient should be advised that the swelling will disappear when the tourniquets are removed. The pulse in the extremity should be frequently checked to ensure that the circulation to the part is adequate.

When the tourniquets are to be removed, the same rotation already established should be followed, and one tourniquet should be removed every 15 minutes, so that all tourniquets have been removed by the end of 45 minutes. *Tourniquets should never all be re-*

Table 30–1.   Plan for Rotating Tourniquets (Clockwise Rotation)

Time A.M.	Right Leg	Left Leg	Left Arm	Right Arm
9:00	Off	On	On	On
9:15	On	Off	On	On
9:30	On	On	Off	On
9:45	On	On	On	Off
10:00	Off	On	On	On

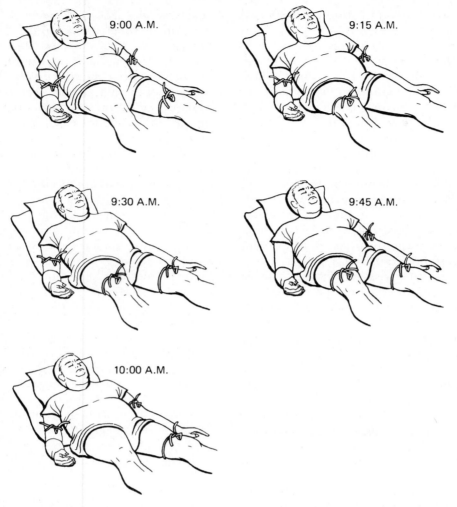

Figure 30–2. Rotation of tourniquets at 15-minute intervals in a clockwise rotation. (See Table 30–1.)

moved at the same time. This would cause a sudden increase in the amount of circulating blood, with a return of more blood to the heart and the lungs than they could handle, possibly causing another attack of pulmonary edema. If the extremities do not promptly regain their normal appearance after the tourniquets have been removed, the physician should be notified immediately.

NURSING PROCESS —THE PATIENT WHO HAS PULMONARY EDEMA

Assessment

Recognition of the early signs and symptoms of pulmonary edema is an important part of assessment. If pulmonary edema is suspected, the physician should be notified immediately so that treatment can be initiated before the acute form develops.

The blood pressure and pulse and respiratory rates are obtained to provide baseline data. Additional emergency assessments include skin color and temperature, auscultation of the lungs, determination of the level of consciousness and degree of apprehension, and the color and type of sputum raised.

Nursing Diagnosis

Depending on the degree and severity of pulmonary edema, one or more of the following nursing diagnoses may apply:

- Anxiety related to dyspnea
- Fear related to inability to breathe
- Pain related to dyspnea
- Ineffective airway clearance related to inability to remove airway secretions

- Fluid volume excess related to heart failure and low cardiac output, decreased renal perfusion, decreased blood pressure
- Impaired verbal communication related to severe dyspnea
- Self-care deficit: total, related to dyspnea, enforced (complete) rest
- Impaired home maintenance management related to disease process, degree of cardiac involvement
- Knowledge deficit of prevention of future episodes, treatment modalities, home management

Planning and Implementation

The major goals of the patient include improvement in respiratory function, reduction of anxiety and fear, relief of pain, effective airway clearance, reduction of fluid volume excess, improvement in communication, ability to manage the home, and knowledge of treatment modalities.

The main goals in the nursing management of pulmonary edema are to improve respiratory function, decrease the total circulating volume, and reduce the work load of the heart.

Respiratory Function. Treatment of pulmonary edema must be immediate. Once the condition is recognized, oxygen should be given and vital signs monitored at frequent intervals. After the patient has been seen by the physician, a determination is made regarding specific oxygen therapy (see section on treatment).

The head of the bed should be raised to an upright position and, when available, a footboard used to prevent the patient from sliding down in bed. If the patient is not critically ill, the legs can be dangled over the side of the bed to temporarily reduce venous return. The patient should be continually observed for improvement in color once treatment is instituted.

In acute pulmonary edema, respirations are labored and rapid. The patient frequently breathes through the mouth in an attempt to inspire more air. Frothy sputum, which cannot be effectively raised, is present in the alveoli and lower bronchi. Suctioning to clear the airway is of no value and only increases the patient's apprehension and fear. Once treatment measures become effective, the lungs are less congested and airway patency improves.

Anxiety and Fear. Fear and severe anxiety accompany acute respiratory distress. Morphine may reduce some anxiety, but the patient may still appear extremely apprehensive. Staying with the patient, briefly explaining procedures and treatments, and assuming a calm attitude are essential.

Pain. Patients with pulmonary edema are uncomfortable. They cannot breathe and may attempt to find a position that will improve breathing. They may thrash around in bed and pull at the covers or other nearby objects, which tends to make breathing more difficult. If rotating tourniquets are used, discomfort and anxiety are increased. Morphine may reduce anxiety and relieve some discomfort. The patient should be observed for relief of these problems after morphine administration.

Fluid Volume Excess. Fluid volume excess is treated with the administration of a diuretic, often by the intravenous route. If kidney function is normal, a large volume of urine may be produced shortly after administration of a diuretic. Intake and output are accurately recorded, and urine output is measured hourly. The physician may order an indwelling urethral catheter, because a large amount of urine may be produced after intravenous administration of a potent diuretic.

Unless ordered otherwise, intravenous solutions are run at a keep-vein-open (KVO) rate to prevent fluid overload. Intravenous control devices may be used to regulate the rate and amount of infusion.

Impaired Verbal Communication. During the acute stage of pulmonary edema, dyspnea, inability to clear the airway effectively, and the effects of hypoxemia on cerebral tissues reduce the patient's ability to communicate. The nurse should be alert to changes in expression and to hand and eye movements that the patient may use to communicate needs to others.

Self-Care Deficit. During the recovery stage, the physician may order limited patient activity, which is increased only as tolerated. The patient should be assessed daily to determine which tasks require assistance. If dyspnea occurs, the patient should be advised to rest before resuming an activity.

Impaired Home Maintenance Management. After correction of pulmonary edema and discharge from the hospital, the patient may still require certain activity restrictions, especially if the disorder was due to heart failure that cannot be completely corrected and controlled. The nurse should attempt to identify needs and concerns expressed by the patient or family and then provide information to help them comply with necessary changes in lifestyle.

Knowledge Deficit. Once symptoms of pulmonary edema are decreased or eliminated, the patient and the family should understand long-term management of the disorder. The following points may be included in a teaching plan:

1. Things to avoid include smoking, passive exposure to smoke, constipation, stress and emotional upsets, and contact with those with upper respiratory tract infections.
2. Long-term medical management and follow-up are necessary.
3. Take prescribed drugs exactly as ordered. Do not use nonprescription drugs without first consulting the physician.
4. Exercise as recommended by the physician. Avoid strenuous exercise.
5. Plan frequent rest periods throughout the day.
6. Be aware of symptoms that may require medical attention: dyspnea, sudden weight gain, swelling of the extremities, chest pain, decreased urine output, persistent cough, extreme fatigue. If these should occur, contact the physician.
7. Follow the diet prescribed by the physician. Read labels carefully, and avoid foods high in sodium.

The prescribed medication regimen should be reviewed with the patient, including the dose, the time of day taken, the purpose, and major adverse effects. A dietary consultation may be necessary to explain the foods to be avoided and how labels are read to determine if the food product can be included in the diet.

Evaluation

■ Airway is clear and pulmonary congestion reduced or eliminated
■ Breath sounds are normal; lung fields are clear; respiratory rate and rhythm are normal
■ Vital signs are stable
■ Anxiety and fear are reduced
■ Comfort is maintained as much as possible
■ Fluid volume excess is corrected; urine output is normal
■ Patient communicates effectively with medical team
■ Patient performs activities of daily living with minimal or no assistance
■ Patient verbalizes future problems with home maintenance management; situations are identified, and patient and family show interest in problem solving and seeking help from others
■ Patient verbalizes understanding of disease process, situations to avoid, drug therapy, diet restrictions, exercise tolerance, and necessity of long-term follow-up care

COR PULMONALE

Cor pulmonale is a disease of the heart (cor) and the lungs (pulmonale).

Etiology and Pathophysiology

In cor pulmonale, the right ventricle is enlarged because of a pulmonary disorder such as chronic obstructive lung disease. When a pulmonary disorder is present, certain physiologic events may occur. In the beginning, decreased oxygen–carbon dioxide exchange in the alveoli results in decreased arterial oxygen tension and increased carbon dioxide in the blood. By some unknown mechanism, pulmonary arterial vasoconstriction occurs, and the blood flow is redirected to pulmonary areas that are adequately ventilated (eg, have adequate oxygen–carbon dioxide exchange across the alveolar membrane). Prolonged pulmonary arterial vasoconstriction then results in pulmonary hypertension, with a mean pulmonary artery pressure above 25 mmHg. When pulmonary hypertension is present, right ventricular enlargement, and ultimately failure of the right ventricle, occurs.

Symptoms

Patients with cor pulmonale may be asymptomatic, and only experience symptoms of their chronic lung disorder. Symptoms of right-sided heart failure ultimately occur (eg, swelling of the feet and ankles, nocturia, weight gain, persistent cough, anorexia, nausea, and enlarged abdomen).

Diagnosis

Diagnosis is based symptoms of right-sided heart failure and known chronic pulmonary disease or other disease process known to result in cor pulmonale. A chest radiograph and ECG may reveal right ventricular enlargement. Additional tests may include a lung scan, pulmonary arteriography, and echocardiography.

Treatment

Management is aimed at treating the underlying cause of cor pulmonale. Drug therapy may include diuretics, bronchodilators, digitalis preparations, and oxygen administration when severe dyspnea is present.

The nursing management of the patient with cor pulmonale is essentially the same as for the patient with heart failure (see Nursing Process—The Patient Who Has Heart Failure) and obstructive pulmonary disease (see Chapter 22).

General Nutritional Considerations

☐ Patients with CHF usually are placed on sodium-restricted diets. The degree of restriction depends on the severity of the disease, the patient's response to other forms of therapy, and the presence of edema.

☐ Some patients may find a diet low in sodium unpalatable. Various books are available that contain information regarding seasoning of food with spices and herbs.

☐ Patients receiving diuretic therapy may be required to eat or drink food or fluids high in *potassium*. Examples of such foods are apricots, bananas, lima beans, liver, and celery. Orange juice also is high in potassium.

☐ Patients who must restrict the amount of sodium in their diets or who are on any other type of cardiac diet such as one that limits dietary intake of foods high in fat should meet with the dietitian before discharge from the hospital. They should receive a detailed explanation of (1) foods allowed, (2) foods to be avoided, (3) how to read food labels, (4) the various ways in which sodium and fats can be listed on a food label, and (5) seasonings that may be used in place of salt.

General Pharmacologic Considerations

☐ Digitalis preparations, which include digitalis, digoxin, and other related glycosides of digitalis, are indicated in the treatment of CHF. These drugs increase the force of contraction of cardiac muscle.

☐ Digitalis preparations are potent drugs that are capable of causing various toxic effects. The margin between a full therapeutic effect and drug toxicity is narrow. Thus, the patient should be observed for signs of digitalis toxicity, not only during the initial period of therapy, but also throughout the entire hospitalization.

☐ The signs of digitalis toxicity are anorexia, nausea, vomiting, epigastric discomfort, diarrhea, abdominal cramps, blurred vision, halos around dark objects, disturbance in green and yellow vision, headache, and change in pulse *rate* and *rhythm*. A patient with digitalis toxicity may have one or more of these signs.

☐ If signs of digitalis toxicity are noted, they should be reported at once and the drug withheld until the patient is seen by a physician.

☐ Patients receiving digitalis preparations should have an apical-radial pulse rate taken for 1 full minute before the drug is given. (If the patient is on a cardiac monitor, this is not necessary.) This method of determination is used during the first few days of therapy or until the patient is digitalized. Once the patient is on maintenance therapy, taking a radial pulse rate usually suffices. The drug should not be given if the pulse rate is below 60, unless the physician has indicated otherwise. The drug also is withheld if there is a change in cardiac rhythm or if there are signs of digitalis toxicity.

☐ Diuretic therapy often is necessary in patients with CHF. Patients receiving these drugs should be observed for signs of hyponatremia, hypokalemia, and dehydration.

☐ For patients taking diuretics, discharge instructions should include a discussion of the signs and symptoms of electrolyte and water loss and the importance of adhering to the medication schedule prescribed by the physician. The patient also may be instructed to eat foods high in potassium.

☐ Patients receiving emergency drug therapy for acute pulmonary edema should be observed for results of drug therapy and the adverse effects of the drugs administered. Many of the drugs given for this disorder are given by the intravenous route and occasionally in large doses, hence the importance of patient observation. Drugs that may be administered are morphine, amino-phylline, digoxin (or other digitalis preparations), and vasopressors for hypo-tension.

General Gerontologic Considerations

☐ Many elderly patients take digitalis preparations for cardiac disease. A thor-ough drug history from the patient or the family is essential.

☐ Patients who have been taking a digitalis preparation before admission usually receive a different dose than that ordered for the patient who has not pre-viously received one of these drugs. This is an important point to remember if the patient is admitted in acute CHF.

☐ If the elderly patient is prescribed a medication for cardiac disease for the first time, a detailed explanation of the drug regimen as well as a thorough expla-nation of its adverse and toxic effects are essential. For some patients this is best given in written as well as oral form.

☐ Some elderly patients have difficulty comprehending and following a diet restricted in sodium. Extra time may be necessary to explain the diet and the foods that are and are not allowed.

☐ If, for financial reasons, the patient is unable to adhere to the diet or to purchase needed medications, a social service worker or other community agent should be contacted for financial assistance.

Suggested Readings

☐ Loach J, Thonpson NB. Hemodynamic monitoring. Philadelphia: JB Lippincott, 1987. *(Additional and in-depth coverage of subject matter)*

☐ Mason CB, Davis JE. Cardiovascular critical care. New York: Von Nostrand Reinhold, 1987. *(Additional and in-depth coverage of subject matter)*

☐ Talkington S, Raterirk G. Every nurse's guide to cardiovascular care. New York: John Wiley & Sons, 1987. *(Additional and in-depth coverage of subject matter)*

☐ Thompson JM, McFarland GK, Hirsch JE, et al. Mosby's manual of clinical nursing. 2nd ed. St Louis: CV Mosby, 1989. *(Additional and in-depth coverage of subject matter)*

☐ Wilson DD. Acute pulmonary edema: how to respond to a crisis. Nursing '89 October 1989;19:34. *(Additional coverage and illustrations that reinforce subject matter)*

Chapter 31

Cardiovascular Surgery

On completion of this chapter the reader will:

- Describe the purpose of cardiopulmonary bypass

- List the complications associated with cardiopulmonary bypass

- Name some of the cardiac lesions that require surgical correction

- Describe the surgical correction used for disorders of the mitral valve

- Describe the surgical correction used for disorders of the aortic valve

- Describe the surgical correction used for disorders of the tricuspid valve

- Discuss the methods of restoring coronary artery blood flow

- Describe the surgical correction of a ventricular aneurysm

- Briefly discuss tumors of the heart

- Discuss the treatment of traumatic injury to the heart

- Discuss heart transplantation

- Use the nursing process in the management of the patient having cardiac surgery

- Use the nursing process in the management of the patient having central or peripheral blood vessel surgery

CARDIAC AND CORONARY BLOOD VESSEL SURGICAL PROCEDURES

Cardiopulmonary Bypass

A patient who requires surgery of the heart, heart valves, and thoracic aorta usually is placed on cardiopulmonary bypass (pump oxygenator). This procedure provides a mechanical method of circulating (cardio) and oxygenating (pulmonary) blood during surgery when the heart is stopped.

Once the chest is opened, cannulas are inserted in the aorta and vena cava. Blood flows from the vena cava to the pump, where it is oxygenated, and is then returned to the ascending aorta, immediately below the aortic arch. Blood may be returned to the femoral artery when surgery is performed on the aortic arch or thoracic aorta.

Intentional cardiac arrest provides direct visualization of cardiac structures and creates a bloodless field. Once surgery is completed, cardiac activity is restored and the cannulas are removed.

Complications

Use of cardiopulmonary bypass is not without complications and risk. Thrombus and embolus formation, fluid and electrolyte imbalances, tissue anoxia (including cerebral anoxia), and pulmonary complications may occur. If donated blood is used to prime the pump, there is a slight risk of transmitting infections such as hepatitis and acquired immunodeficiency syndrome, even though donated blood is tested for antibodies of these disorders.

Surgical Replacement or Repair of Heart Valves

Valves of the heart may become narrowed (stenosed) and necessitate surgical replacement or repair. Stenosis of a cardiac valve, such as the mitral valve, may reduce the valve lumen to pencil-point size (Fig. 31-1). The narrowed and scarred valve opens on cardiac contraction, but the reduced size of the lumen limits the amount of blood flowing through it.

As a result of the processes of scarring, fusion of the valve leaflets, and eventual calcification, the valves no longer close properly. Blood regurgitates backward through the incompetent (insufficient) valve. A damaged heart valve may be stenotic or incompetent, or both. Aortic insufficiency is the most serious of the valvular diseases.

Mitral Valve

There are several types of surgical approaches for mitral valve disease. One method of repair is mitral commissurotomy, which is done without direct visualiza-

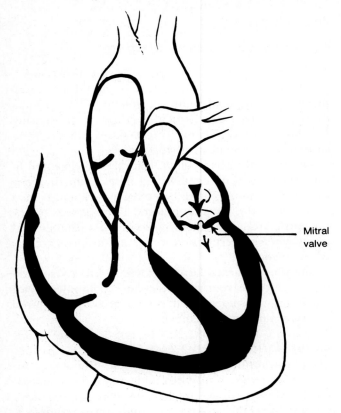

Figure 31–1. Mitral stenosis. The narrowed valve does not permit blood to flow freely from the left atrium to the left ventricle.

tion of the valve. This procedure is performed by means of a thoracotomy. A pursestring suture is placed in the wall of the atrium, an incision is made, and the surgeon's finger or a metal dilator is inserted through the incision. The pursestring suture is then pulled tight to prevent the escape of blood from the atrium. Dilatation of the valve is intended to release the scarred tissue that resulted in valvular stenosis. Cardiopulmonary bypass is not required for this surgery but usually is kept available for immediate use if complications occur or if direct visualization is required to repair the valve.

The mitral valve also may be replaced or repaired under direct vision by opening the heart and exposing the valve. A prosthetic valve, such as the Starr-Edwards valve, may be used for replacement. Repair of the valve may be accomplished by reconstruction of the valve leaflets and their attachment.

Aortic Valve

Aortic valve stenosis may be treated surgically by valve replacement. Prosthetic replacements include a porcine valve (an aortic valve from a pig), the Starr-Edwards valve, and the Bjork-Shiley valve. Cardiopulmonary bypass is required for aortic valve replacement.

Tricuspid Valve

Stenosis of the tricuspid valve, which lies between the right atrium and the right ventricle, may be surgically repaired by one of several procedures. Stenosis may be corrected by commissurotomy, and stenosis and valve insufficiency are corrected by means of reconstruction of the valve leaflets and their attachments. Cardiopulmonary bypass usually is required. Occasionally, the entire valve is replaced with a prosthetic device.

Coronary Artery Surgery

Atherosclerotic heart disease is the leading type of heart disease in the United States. Extensive surgical research techniques have been established in an effort to increase the amount of blood reaching the heart muscle and to redirect blood to the ischemic myocardium.

A widely used technique to increase the supply of blood to the myocardium is the saphenous vein revascularization procedure, also called a *coronary artery bypass* (Fig. 31-2). A section of saphenous vein is removed from the patient's leg and used to bypass the blocked or narrowed area of the coronary artery. One or more coronary arteries may require surgical repair.

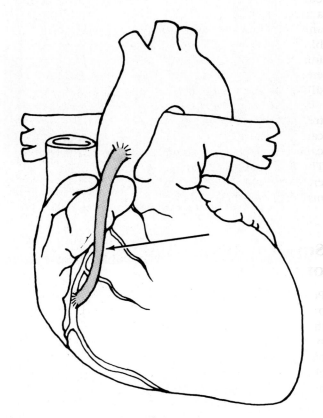

Figure 31–2. Section of saphenous vein is used to bypass a coronary artery.

An older method of coronary artery surgery is the Vineberg procedure, in which the branches of the internal mammary artery are implanted in the myocardium near the area of coronary artery stenosis.

An alternative method of treating coronary artery disease is *percutaneous transluminal coronary angioplasty*. In this procedure, a balloon-tipped catheter is inserted into a coronary artery under local anesthesia. Under fluoroscopy (cardiac cineangiography), the catheter is threaded to the area of stenosis and the balloon inflated with controlled pressure. Inflation of the balloon reduces the stenosis and increases blood flow through the narrowed portion of the artery. This procedure may be performed on selected patients with single, rather than multiple, coronary artery occlusion. Myocardial infarction and artery blowout (penetration of the arterial wall by the catheter tip) are complications of this procedure. Results have not been as good as with coronary bypass surgery, as it is often necessary to repeat the procedure after a period of time.

Repair of Ventricular Aneurysm

An aneurysm of the ventricular wall is the most lethal complication among those surviving the acute stage of a myocardial infarction. The frequency of ventricular aneurysms is increased with the presence of high blood pressure and overexertion after a myocardial infarction. The elasticity of the muscle wall is weakened, and an outpouching occurs. The diseased area dilates and produces a ballooning of the wall.

Suturing off the weakened area is an emergency treatment because the paradoxical motion of the myocardium may rupture the aneurysm. If possible, surgical correction is postponed until after the acute stage. The damaged tissue becomes necrotic and cannot tolerate surgical correction until scar tissue appears. This may take 4 to 8 weeks.

Surgical Removal of Tumors of the Heart

Primary tumors of the heart are rare and may be benign or malignant. The clinical course usually depends on the type of tumor and its location within the cardiac system (ie, whether it occupies space within the chambers of the heart or is contained within the muscle). Large tumors located on the left side of the heart may produce signs of mitral valve disease.

Surgery using cardiopulmonary bypass may be undertaken, because cardiac failure may occur and the potential of embolus formation often is present. Be-

nign tumors may stem from a base of a pedicle, and their removal usually is uncomplicated. Malignant tumors are more difficult to remove, and the prognosis extremely poor.

Surgical Treatment of Traumatic Heart Lesions

A nonpenetrating injury of the chest may include bruising of the heart. For example, a patient who has been crushed against the steering wheel of a car may have some bleeding of the muscle of the heart. Because the heart is enclosed by the pericardium, blood accumulates in the pericardial space, resulting in cardiac tamponade.

Most often the patient needs to have the fluid removed from the pericardial sac. The physician inserts a long needle into the pericardial sac (pericardiocentesis). During this procedure, the patient usually is placed at a 45-degree angle. One aspiration is sufficient in most patients, but if bleeding continues, an open thoracotomy may be indicated to control the bleeding site.

Direct trauma to the myocardium, such as a stab wound, also may cause leakage of blood into the pericardium; the tear in the pericardium often seals with a clot, whereas the tear in the myocardium continues to bleed. If the wound is large enough to cause immediate shock from hemorrhage, the prognosis is poor.

Sometimes traumatic cardiac tamponade is treated conservatively with bed rest and careful observation of the patient. The increased pericardial pressure may stop the leakage of blood and splint the wound. Larger tears require surgery.

Heart Transplantation

Heart transplantation is performed only when other medical and surgical treatment modalities fail or are inappropriate. The two major reasons for heart transplantation are cardiomyopathy (a severe weakness of cardiac muscle) and end-stage coronary artery disease.

Before a person can receive a donor heart, many factors must be considered. Included in these considerations are the general condition of the patient's other vital organs, the patient's age, the presence of other chronic diseases, the patient's emotional outlook, and the availability of support systems. Once a patient is considered a candidate for transplantation, his or her name and tissue type is placed on a computerized recipient list. Tissue typing is necessary to match the recipient with the donor.

Many problems are associated with heart transplantation, some of which are the availability of donors, rejection of the donor heart, postoperative infection, postoperative psychosis, and the cost of the procedure.

Transplantation recipients are given cyclosporine (Sandimmune) to prevent organ rejection in heart, kidney, and liver transplantation. This drug contributes to the increased rate in the success of transplantation procedures.

NURSING PROCESS —THE PATIENT UNDERGOING CARDIAC SURGERY

Preoperative Period

Assessment

When surgery is not an emergency, the patient who is to have heart surgery may be hospitalized 1 or more days before surgery, to undergo an extensive medical evaluation. A thorough review of all body systems and identification of the precise location of the lesion are necessary.

Cardiopulmonary evaluation may include chest radiography, electrocardiography (ECG), exercise ECG (stress test), pulmonary function studies, echocardiography, laboratory blood tests, and coronary angiography. Some or most of these studies may be performed on an outpatient basis.

If surgery is of an emergency nature, the required diagnostic tests are performed as rapidly as possible. A history should be obtained from the family if the patient is too ill to supply the necessary information.

On admission to the hospital, routine assessments such as height, weight, and vital signs should be obtained, followed by a thorough medical history. Unless the patient is acutely ill, a medical history should be obtained during the initial assessment and may include the following areas:

- A history of *all* past and current illnesses and the treatment prescribed for each
- A family history of illnesses and, when applicable, the cause of death (the current general health of all household members is included)
- Medications taken up to the time of admission, including *all* prescription and nonprescription drugs
- Tests performed before admission
- Allergy history
- Dietary history, including diet changes recommended by the physician (eg, low-sodium diet or diabetic diet)
- A history of use of tobacco, alcohol, or (illegal) drugs

The initial history is followed by a physical assessment as outlined in Chapter 24.

Nursing Diagnosis

The following nursing diagnoses may be used during the preoperative period. Additional diagnoses, such as fluid volume excess or impaired gas exchange, may be necessary if the patient is critically ill or has concurrent medical problems.

- Anxiety related to diagnostic tests, planned surgery
- Fear related to the surgical procedure, its outcome and future prognosis, threat to well-being, future health maintenance
- Knowledge deficit of diagnostic tests, preoperative preparations, postoperative period

Planning and Implementation

The major goals of the patient include a reduction of anxiety and fear and an understanding of preoperative tests and preparations.

The major goal of nursing management is to prepare the patient physically and emotionally for surgery.

The type of preoperative preparations vary, depending on such factors as the condition of the patient, hospital policy, reason for and type of surgery, and the operating surgeon's orders. Immediate preoperative preparations may include insertion of an indwelling catheter, a nasogastric tube, and an intravenous line.

Careful preparation of the skin over the operative site is important. Bacteria are found on all levels of the skin. An infection introduced while performing a thoracotomy could be serious, and can spread to the sternum and mediastinum and into the circulatory system. Usually a bacteriostatic soap scrub is ordered for 1 or 2 days before surgery. Patients who are able to shower without assistance may assume responsibility for the scrub. The nurse gives whatever assistance is required to those patients whose weakness prevents this activity. The operative area (chest) is shaved the evening before surgery. Medications usually are discontinued 1 or 2 days before surgery. To prevent postoperative infections, an antibiotic is ordered before surgery.

If the patient has suffered a traumatic injury to the heart, rapid preparation of the patient for surgery is necessary. During the short preoperative period, the patient is closely observed for signs and symptoms of increasing shock and cardiac compression, which include distention of superficial neck veins, cyanosis, dyspnea, hypotension, and changes in pulse rate and rhythm. The pulse should be taken frequently, as there may be inhibition of the vagus nerve, with a slowing pulse, and perhaps cardiac standstill. Cardiac and respiratory resuscitation equipment should be kept nearby, ready for instant use. The pain from a bruised heart may be masked by the pain from other chest injuries. Relaxation of the anal sphincter with fecal incontinence is a serious sign not found in other types of chest injury and should be reported to the physician immediately.

Fear and Anxiety. Although fear and anxiety may not be eliminated, the intensity of these emotions may be reduced. The patient and family should be allowed time to ask questions and verbalize their fears. During this time, the nurse can repeat or clarify information given by the physician.

Knowledge Deficit. Each diagnostic test should be explained to the patient, including the reason for the test, what will be done, and what is required of the patient before, during, and after the test. Every effort should be made to determine the patient's understanding of the test and answer questions raised by the patient or family.

The patient and family require explanations of other preparations for surgery, such as skin preparation and insertion of intravenous lines and an indwelling catheter.

The physician informs the patient what type of anesthesia will be used, but the nurse may need to repeat or clarify the physician's explanation. It should be remembered that the patient and family are under a great deal of stress at this time, and may not always understand what has been told to them by the physician.

If surgery requires cardiopulmonary bypass, anesthesia may begin the night before surgery with morphine or another narcotic added to a solution administered by slow intravenous drip. Anesthesia also may begin in the operating room with the patient sedated the night before surgery as well as the morning of surgery.

The physician also describes what will happen in the postoperative period, with explanations repeated by the nurse, when necessary. Included in this explanation is the need for endotracheal intubation and mechanical ventilation during the immediate postoperative period; the insertion of chest tubes during surgery, intravenous lines, and monitoring devices; the control of pain; and the postsurgical care unit. Deep-breathing and coughing techniques, leg exercises, and the use of the incentive spirometer are explained and demonstrated by the nurse. When possible, the patient should practice these techniques before surgery.

If surgery is an emergency, there may be little time for patient and family teaching. When possible, the nurse should spend some time with the family while surgery is being performed. At this time, some of the postoperative care can be explained.

Evaluation

- Fear and anxiety are reduced
- Patient and family verbalize fears and anxieties
- Patient and family demonstrate an understanding of the preoperative and postoperative period

Postoperative Period

Assessment
On return from surgery, the patient's chart is reviewed for the type of surgery performed and complications that may have occurred during surgery. The patient is thoroughly and systematically assessed to provide baseline data during the recovery period (Chart 31-1).

During the postoperative period, these assessments should be carried out at frequent intervals. The physician should be kept informed of all laboratory tests and any change in the patient's condition. The patient should be observed for complications such as shock, thrombus or embolus formation, cerebral anoxia, cardiac dysrhythmias, fluid overload, electrolyte imbalance, bleeding, respiratory failure, and cardiac tamponade.

Nursing Diagnosis
Depending on the type of and reason for surgery, prognosis, and complications encountered, the following nursing diagnoses may be stated. Additional diagnoses may be required, depending on the postoperative course.

- Anxiety related to pain, postoperative monitoring devices and technical equipment, other factors (specify)
- Pain related to the surgical procedure, invasive monitoring techniques, chest tubes
- Ineffective airway clearance related to chest pain because of surgery
- Fluid volume excess related to decreased cardiac output, decreased renal perfusion
- Potential fluid volume deficit related to blood loss during surgery
- Altered peripheral tissue perfusion related to presence of invasive lines, decreased venous return, anesthesia, immobilization, other factors (specify)
- Altered thought processes caused by complications of surgery (eg, cerebral embolus), surgical experience, intensive care unit
- Potential for infection related to surgical procedure
- Hyperthermia related to infection
- Altered family processes related to long rehabilitation program, prognosis
- Noncompliance to rehabilitation program related to anxiety, negative side effects of prescribed treatment, other factors (specify)
- Knowledge deficit of home care after discharge, rehabilitation program, postdischarge treatment modalities

Chart 31–1.   Assessment During the Recovery Period

Cardiac Status
☐ Blood pressure
☐ Pulse rate and rhythm
☐ Central venous pressure
☐ Arterial blood gas analysis results
☐ Pulmonary artery and pulmonary capillary wedge pressures

Respiratory Status
☐ Auscultation of the lungs for breath sounds (normal, abnormal)
☐ Inspection and location of chest tubes and drainage bottles
☐ Chest movement during inspiration and expiration
☐ Endotracheal tube patency
☐ Mechanical ventilator settings

Renal Function
☐ Urine output
☐ Urine color and specific gravity

Neurologic Status
☐ Level of consciousness
☐ Reaction to stimuli (light, sound, pain)
☐ Movement of extremities
☐ Pupil size, equality, and reaction to light

Peripheral Vascular Status
☐ Peripheral pulses
☐ Skin color and temperature

Fluid and Electrolyte Balance
☐ Fluid intake
☐ Output from all drainage tubes and indwelling catheter
☐ Observation for signs of electrolyte imbalance
☐ CVP measurement

Record Review
☐ Review of the surgical procedure
☐ Laboratory tests performed during or immediately after surgery
☐ Intraoperative administration of drugs such as heparin, analgesics, and antibiotics

Equipment
☐ Systematic inspection of all equipment and intravenous or intraarterial lines for function and placement

Planning and Implementation

The major goals of the patient include a reduction in anxiety, relief of pain, effective airway clearance, correction of fluid volume excess or deficit, improved cardiac output and tissue tissue perfusion, absence of complications, absence of infection, normal vital signs, and understanding of and compliance with postdischarge treatment modalities.

The major goals of nursing management include recognition of complications related to surgery, an increase in cardiac output, maintenance of adequate tissue and organ perfusion, maintenance of fluid and electrolyte balance, relief of pain, reduction of anxiety, maintenance of adequate gas exchange, effective airway clearance, and patient compliance to a rehabilitation program.

All parameters and mechanical devices should be closely monitored and assessments frequently performed during the immediate postoperative period. Examples of these tasks are vital signs and measurement of central venous pressure (CVP), urine output, and chest tube drainage.

Most patients require mechanical ventilation for 1 or 2 (or more) days after surgery. The patient's arterial blood pressure may be recorded directly and continuously. A small polyethylene catheter may have been left in place in the patient's femoral artery after the completion of cardiopulmonary bypass. The pressure in this artery is transmitted by way of the tip of the catheter through rigid plastic tubing to a pressure-sensitive device called a *transducer,* or *strain gauge.* The transducer converts the mechanical energy of pressure changes within the artery to electrical output. The output is calibrated and equated to equivalent changes in millimeters of mercury that can be displayed on an oscilloscope or recorder. Small fluctuations in arterial blood pressure can be recorded and are obtainable at times when cuff blood pressures cannot be obtained. The arterial line also serves as a direct means by which samples can be collected for blood gas analysis.

A Swan-Ganz catheter may be used to assess cardiac output by measuring pulmonary artery pressure. If this catheter is inserted, the CVP may be measured with this device. If a Swan-Ganz catheter is not used, a CVP line may be inserted.

Central venous pressure should be measured frequently. The CVP line also may be used to draw venous blood samples. The normal reading of the CVP in or near the right atrium is between 5 and 10 cm of water. The numeric value is not as important as the occurrence of a change (either increasing or decreasing). Because venous pressure is sensitive to increased pressure in the respiratory system, the patient should not be receiving mechanical ventilation at the time of the recording.

A nasogastric tube usually is inserted before surgery, and used to keep the stomach empty. Drainage from the nasogastric tube is recorded. Proper functioning of the tube is important because any abdominal distention may exert pressure on the diaphragm and move it upward, restricting respiratory movement.

The chest tubes should be frequently inspected, making sure that the tubes leading from the chest to the underwater-seal bottles are not compressed, that there is no leak, and that the drainage is flowing freely (see Chapter 23). Hourly observation of the amount of drainage is required. If it is copious, the amount should be recorded more frequently and the physician notified.

The patient is monitored by ECG for disturbances in heart rate and rhythm. The physician should be immediately notified of *any* change in the patient's condition or the development of complications, such as renal shutdown, shock, thrombus formation, cardiac dysrhythmias, and electrolyte imbalances.

Nursing management after heart transplantation is similar to that after open heart surgery. In addition, the patient should be closely observed for signs of organ rejection (eg, elevated white blood cell count, ECG changes, and fever). The patient should be placed in protective isolation to prevent infection, because even a mild infection can be life-threatening.

Anxiety. Anxiety caused by monitoring devices, noise, and technical equipment may be reduced by effective teaching during the preoperative period. During the postoperative period, the nurse should attempt to identify factors that cause anxiety. Explaining procedures and reassuring the patient, as well as controlling pain by administration of the prescribed analgesic, may help to reduce anxiety.

Patients with prosthetic valve replacements may hear or feel the prosthesis open and close. The sound or feeling may be disturbing at first and keep the patient awake. If extreme distress is noted, the physician should be informed.

Pain. Pain is controlled by administering analgesics as well as by instituting comfort measures such as proper positioning. Narcotic analgesics also have a sedative action, which in turn helps to reduce anxiety and promote sleep. The blood pressure and pulse and respiratory rates are monitored before and after the administration of a narcotic.

Ineffective Airway Clearance. While the patient is intubated, the endotracheal tube should be assessed for patency and suctioned as needed. The endotracheal tube should be properly secured, and tubing going from the endotracheal tube to the ventilator must be checked to be sure that it is tightly connected.

A respirometer may be used to evaluate the effectiveness of the breathing device and the patient's response. Blood gas analyses also are done. The color of the patient's nail beds and lips may be a clue to inadequate ventilation. Restlessness, flaring of the nostrils, and shallow respirations are causes for concern. The lungs should be auscultated hourly for normal, abnormal, or absence of breath sounds.

Once the patient is extubated, she or he should be encouraged to cough and deep-breathe every 1 or 2 hours, with support of the incision provided to decrease pain. The physician may order other methods of ventilating the lungs (eg, intermittent positive-pressure breathing, coughing and deep-breathing exercises, and the use of an incentive spirometer).

Fluid Volume Deficit or Excess. A fluid volume deficit resulting from blood and fluid loss during surgery may be present in the immediate postoperative period. A fluid volume excess may occur if cardiac output is decreased. To detect fluid volume changes, the CVP is closely monitored and accurate intake and output records kept. Drugs to increase the force of ventricular contraction, and thus increase cardiac output, also may be ordered.

The patient should be closely observed for signs of fluid and electrolyte imbalances (see Chapter 12), which should be promptly reported to the physician. Potassium imbalances are potentially dangerous, as they may precipitate cardiac dysrhythmias.

The type of intravenous solutions that are ordered depends on the patient's need for fluids and calories as well as laboratory determinations of serum electrolyte levels. An electronic infusion device should be used to regulate the infusion rate. The infusion rate may need to be adjusted because overloading the circulatory system would place an added strain on vital organs, especially the heart.

The major reason for the insertion of the indwelling catheter is to allow observation of kidney function, especially the early detection of renal shutdown—particularly if a problem with the kidneys is anticipated (eg, if there has been prolonged hypotension). An hourly output of 30 mL usually is adequate; output below this amount should be reported to the physician. Urine output on arrival in the intensive care unit often is increased if osmotic diuretics were used when the patient was on cardiopulmonary bypass. This situation corrects itself in a few hours. The patient also may have hemoglobinuria (hemoglobin in the urine) because lysis of blood cells can occur during prolonged cardiopulmonary bypass. Specific gravity should be measured to determine the patient's hydration and how well the kidneys are concentrating urine.

Altered Peripheral Tissue Perfusion. A decrease in tissue perfusion may occur if shock, venous stasis, or a decrease in cardiac output occurs. Vital signs should be monitored at frequent intervals and peripheral pulses palpated hourly. The color and temperature of the extremities also should be noted. When necessary, blood pressure may be maintained with the administration of vasopressors. Once the patient is awake and responding, venous return is enhanced by encouraging the performance of leg exercises every 2 hours. Antiembolism stockings also may be ordered. The patient should be assessed for signs of peripheral thrombus or embolus formation.

Altered Thought Processes.   Surgery and its complications, as well as environmental factors related to the intensive care unit, can result in confusion, restlessness, disorientation, and other behavioral changes. This condition is referred to as postcoronary surgery, or postcardiotomy, psychosis. Although the exact cause is not known, it is thought to be due to changes in the normal sleep pattern, sleep deprivation, and sensory experiences related to the noise of machines and other disturbances that occur in an intensive care unit. Any changes in behavior should be documented and the patient closely observed, because mental changes also can be a complication of surgery (eg, a cerebral embolus). Restraining measures may be necessary if the patient attempts to pull out tubes or catheters. Frequent personal contact, explanation of procedures, and conversation with the patient may reduce or eliminate this problem.

Potential for Infection, Hyperthermia.   The dressing over the incision as well as around chest tubes and other monitoring devices should be inspected for early signs of infection. The temperature should be monitored every 4 hours, and sudden elevation or the occurrence of chills should be immediately reported to the physician. Prophylactic antibiotic therapy should be given at the prescribed time intervals to attain and maintain adequate antibiotic blood levels.

Altered Family Processes.   A prolonged recovery and rehabilitation period may result in various types of difficulty for family members. Financial responsibilities and problems with home maintenance are two examples of problems that may be faced during recovery. The nurse should be alert to problems expressed by the patient or family and should identify current and future needs. Referral to various agencies or the social service worker may be necessary.

Noncompliance.   Some patients require a long rehabilitation program, changes in lifestyle, and possibly a change in employment. These alterations may be difficult without assistance and education. If the patient expresses concern over enrollment in a cardiac rehabilitation program or any changes in lifestyle, the nurse should identify areas of concern and help the patient work through the problem. The patient and family should be informed of their roles in the recovery process, and the importance of adherence to the physician's recommendations should be stressed.

Knowledge Deficit.   The patient may be discharged from the hospital 7 to 10 days after surgery. The patient and family may have many questions and concerns about the medical regimen required after discharge. An orderly teaching plan should be developed to establish a smooth transition from hospital to home. The following areas may be included in a teaching plan. Additional material may be added, depending on such factors as the type of surgery, the patient's degree of recovery, and the treatment regimen prescribed by the physician.

- Medication and dietary instructions
- Importance of follow-up care, periodic evaluation of progress, lifelong adherence to certain treatment regimens
- The purpose of a structured cardiac rehabilitation program (when prescribed and available)
- Monitoring of the pulse rate, blood pressure, weight
- Activity progression and exercise
- Weight control
- Stress reduction

Evaluation

- Anxiety is reduced
- Pain is controlled
- Respiratory function is normal; adequate gas exchange, normal breathing pattern, are patent airway maintained
- Fluid and electrolyte balance is normal
- Tissue perfusion is adequate
- Patient remains mentally clear and alert
- Infection is absent
- Body temperature is normal
- Family problems are identified; patient and family attempt to solve identified problems
- Patient verbalizes willingness to participate in the prescribed rehabilitation requirements
- Patient verbalizes understanding of treatment regimen after discharge from the hospital

SURGERY OF CENTRAL OR PERIPHERAL BLOOD VESSELS

Certain conditions such as aneurysm and thrombus formation found in blood vessels may necessitate surgery. Various surgical techniques may be used to correct the disorder.

Grafts

A graft may be used to *replace* or *bypass* a section of blood vessel. A replacement graft may consist of man-made material or be obtained from human donors (allografts).

When a graft is used to surgically replace a blood vessel, a clamp is placed above and below the affected area, and the diseased blood vessel is removed. The replacement graft is then sewn in place and the clamps removed. Depending on the area involved, cardiopulmonary bypass may be necessary.

Blood vessel grafts may be needed if the patient has an aneurysm or an obstructed blood vessel. Certain peripheral blood vessel disorders, such as Leriche's syndrome (arteriosclerotic disease of the lower aorta and iliac bifurcation), may necessitate blood vessel replacement. Figure 31-3 shows an aortoiliac replacement graft, which may be used to treat disorders of this area.

Embolectomy and Thrombectomy

When a major vessel has been occluded, embolectomy (surgical removal of an embolus) or thrombectomy (surgical removal of a thrombus) is indicated. When these procedures are performed, the vessel is opened above the clot, the clot is removed, and the vessel is sutured. This type of surgery may be an emergency, because complete occlusion results in loss of blood supply to an area.

Endarterectomy

Endarterectomy is the resection and removal of the lining of an artery. This surgery is commonly performed to remove obstructive atherosclerotic plaques from the carotid, femoral, or popliteal artery. A carotid endarterectomy is performed when cerebral circulation is impaired by atherosclerotic obstruction of the carotid artery. The femoral and popliteal arteries also may be affected by atherosclerotic plaques and require this type of surgery.

NURSING PROCESS —THE PATIENT UNDERGOING SURGERY ON A CENTRAL OR PERIPHERAL BLOOD VESSEL

Preoperative Period

Assessment

When surgery on a peripheral blood vessel is an emergency (eg, surgical repair of an aneurysm), assessment is brief and only vital baseline data are obtained. The patient's blood pressure, pulse and re-

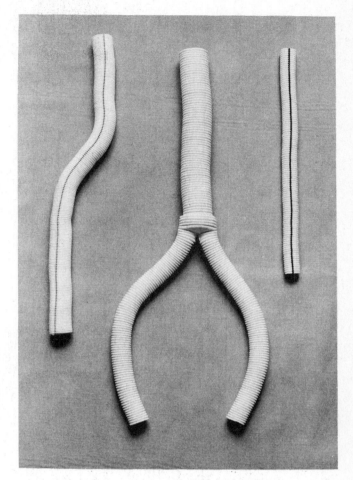

Figure 31–3. Teflon grafts. The lines on the left and right grafts are radiopaque and will show on radiographic examination. (Photograph by D. Atkinson)

spiratory rates, skin color, and general condition are quickly assessed while the patient is prepared for surgery.

When the situation is not an extreme emergency, a history of symptoms, past medical diseases, and allergies should be obtained from the patient or family. In addition to the assessments performed on the cardiac patient (see Chapter 24), the peripheral pulses should be identified, palpated, and marked with a skin pen. The presence or absence of a pulse as well as its intensity or weakness are noted. Additional assessments are based on initial findings, the patient's symptoms, and current medical disorders.

Nursing Diagnosis

One or more of the following nursing diagnoses may be used, depending on the gravity of the situation, the diagnosis, and the time interval between the medical diagnosis and the surgical procedure:

■ Anxiety related to pain, diagnosis, seriousness of the disorder, surgery

- Pain related to lack of blood supply to a part, pressure of the aneurysm on adjacent structures
- Knowledge deficit of surgery, preparations for surgery, postoperative exercises and activities

Planning and Implementation

The major goals of the patient include relief of pain and discomfort, reduction of anxiety, an understanding of the reason for surgery, and knowledge of postoperative exercises.

The major goal of nursing management is to prepare the patient physically and emotionally for surgery.

Profound shock during the preoperative period has a grave prognosis. Treatment modalities depend on decisions made by the physician regarding the advisability of the administration of drugs or intravenous fluids.

Anxiety, Pain. If the patient is conscious before surgical intervention, the seriousness of the situation is probably apparent because of the intense attitude displayed by members of the health care team. Although an emergency situation exists, the nurse may reduce fear and anxiety by reassuring the patient and staying at the bedside as much as possible.

The patient with severe pain is extremely apprehensive, and analgesics are administered as ordered. It is important to evaluate pain (location, type) before administration of an analgesic. The physician should be notified immediately if there is arm or leg pain or cramping that did not exist previously, a change in skin color or temperature of an arm or leg, or pain in a new area; these symptoms may indicate the occlusion of an artery or vein or other serious event.

In some instances, it is not possible or feasible to treat preoperative pain because an emergency situation exists or the blood pressure is rapidly falling.

When a peripheral blood vessel is obstructed, circulation must be restored as soon as possible. Rapid preparation for surgery, pain, and possible knowledge that an arm or leg may need to be amputated if circulation is not restored all create severe anxiety for the patient and family.

Knowledge Deficit. Before surgery, the physician will discuss with the patient or the family, or both, the reason for surgery, the type of surgery to be performed, the results expected, and the prognosis. If the patient or family does not appear to understand the situation, the physician should be contacted before the patient is prepared for surgery.

If there is time, the patient should be instructed in the techniques of coughing, deep-breathing, and leg exercises; however, these activities may be restricted after some surgical procedures.

Evaluation

- Pain is reduced or eliminated
- Anxiety is reduced
- Patient and family understand the reason for surgery, type of surgery, results expected, and the prognosis
- Patient demonstrates understanding of postoperative exercises

Postoperative Period

Assessment

On return from surgery, the patient's vital signs should be taken and the chart reviewed for the type and extent of surgery. Routine postoperative tasks should be performed (eg, checking tubes, catheters, drains, the surgical dressing, and intravenous lines). The general status of the patient should be evaluated.

Nursing Diagnosis

Depending on the location and type of surgery, the patient's condition, and problems encountered during surgery, one or more of the following nursing diagnoses may apply. If a thoracic incision was necessary to repair a thoracic aortic aneurysm, nursing diagnoses that apply to the patient having thoracic surgery (see Chapter 23) may be added.

- Pain related to surgery
- Hyperthermia related to surgery, infection
- Potential for infection related to surgery
- Fluid volume deficit related to abnormal fluid loss during surgery
- Ineffective airway clearance related to inability to cough, pain on coughing
- Bathing/hygiene and dressing/grooming self-care deficits related to surgery
- Potential impaired skin integrity related to immobility
- Knowledge deficit of postdischarge treatment modalities, home care

Planning and Implementation

The major goals of the patient include a reduction or absence of pain, absence of infection, normal respiratory function, effective coughing and deep-breathing exercises, correction of fluid imbalances, normal vital signs, ability to care for self, and knowledge of postdischarge treatment modalities.

The major goals of nursing management include a reduction of postoperative pain and discomfort, prevention of infection, restoration of a normal fluid volume, improved respiratory function, and instruction of the patient in the prescribed postdischarge treatment regimen.

If thoracic surgery was performed, the blood pressure and pulse rate should be measured in both arms. Although the blood pressure in the left arm usually is slightly higher than that in the right, any marked change should be reported to the physician immediately.

The abdomen should be inspected for signs of distention, and bowel sounds should be auscultated. Abdominal distention is an uncomfortable complication that may be caused by the handling of the intestines during surgery. A nasogastric tube may be passed (if one was not inserted before or during surgery) and attached to suction apparatus.

Depending on the type and location of surgery, the physician may order various positions, such as flat in bed, the head of the bed elevated, or the revascularized arm or leg positioned above the level of the heart, to improve venous and lymphatic drainage, reduce the formation of edema, and facilitate fresh arterial blood flow.

Postoperative exercise of the affected arm or leg should be not encouraged unless specified by the surgeon. Chilling of and pressure on the affected arm or leg should be avoided. The knees should not be elevated, and pillows should not be placed under the knees unless specifically ordered because pressure on the legs may impair circulation and lead to thrombosis.

The patient's position should be changed every 2 hours, and leg movement should be encouraged when leg exercises are ordered by the physician.

Shock that occurs during surgery is treated by administering whole blood and fluids. During the postoperative period, vital signs should be monitored at frequent intervals, intake and output measured hourly, and the patient observed for signs of electrolyte imbalance. A decrease in blood pressure, an increase in the intensity of abdominal or chest pain, narrowing of the pulse pressure, or a rise in the pulse rate may indicate internal hemorrhage at the graft site. A decrease in urine output may indicate occlusion of the renal artery. Changes should be reported to the physician immediately, as the patient may have to return to surgery for repair of a leak at the graft site.

The peripheral pulses (arms, legs) should be palpated every 15 to 30 minutes, or as ordered, during the first 24 to 48 hours and every 1 or 2 hours thereafter. The skin color and temperature of the arm or leg should be noted. The area where a peripheral pulse has been palpated should be marked with a skin pen. If a pulse cannot be detected or the arm or leg becomes cold, cyanotic, or mottled in color, the surgeon should be informed *immediately,* because a thrombus may be occluding the lumen of the graft. Heparin may be used during and after surgery to control thrombus formation, and the patient should be closely observed for bleeding episodes during the immediate postoperative period. When circulation

in the arm or leg has been reestablished, the part becomes warm, and color and sensation are normal.

A carotid endarterectomy necessitates a neurologic assessment (see Chapter 35) every 30 minutes, including evaluation of level of consciousness, movement in all four extremities, and thought processes.

Pain.   The correction of an aneurysm, or other reconstructive vascular procedures, frequently requires a long incision. The abdominal aorta is reached through a midline abdominal incision, and the intestines are retracted to one side. To reach the thoracic aorta, the chest cavity must be entered. The aneurysm may not be easily accessible, and the surgery may last for several hours. These patients have considerable incisional pain, which may interfere with their willingness to turn from side to side.

Before administration of a narcotic during the postoperative period, the location and type of pain should be carefully evaluated. Although pain after surgery is to be expected, sudden, intense pain that is greater than previous pain should be reported to the physician. Any pain or cramping in an arm or leg should be reported immediately because it may indicate occlusion of an artery or vein.

Back pain that occurs after the repair of an abdominal aortic aneurysm may indicate a hemorrhage or thrombosis at the graft site. Such pain should be reported immediately, because a return to surgery may be necessary.

Respiratory Function.   Unless ordered otherwise, the patient should be encouraged to cough and deep-breathe every 2 hours. The physician should be consulted about the advisability of incisional support with the hand or a pillow when the patient coughs. Pain may interfere with the patient's willingness to cough, deep-breathe, and turn from side to side; therefore, these tasks should be performed when the patient is experiencing the greatest effect of the analgesic.

When the surgery involves opening the thoracic cavity, postoperative assessment and management of the respiratory system are the same as for any patient who has had chest surgery (see Chapter 23).

Potential for Infection.   Prophylactic antibiotic therapy usually is ordered. The temperature should be monitored every 4 hours and the surgical wound inspected for evidence of infection. A marked rise in temperature or chills should be immediately reported to the physician.

Knowledge Deficit.   A teaching plan should be individualized to reflect the possible cause of the problem and what measures, if any, should be taken to prevent recurrence.

The patient and family require instruction in the medical treatment modalities necessary after discharge from the hospital. Some of the treatment modalities that may be prescribed or recommended include anticoagulant therapy, the wearing of support stockings, and dietary management to reduce elevated serum cholesterol and triglyceride levels. The importance of follow-up care and adherence to the medication schedule and treatment regimen prescribed by the physician is stressed. If the patient is placed on anticoagulant therapy to prevent future episodes of thrombus or embolus formation, instructions about the dosage regimen and the importance of immediately reporting any bleeding episodes to the physician should be emphasized.

In some instances—for example, when a graft is inserted in the lower abdominal aorta—the patient and family need to be informed of the measures to be taken to protect the legs from tissue damage (eg, avoiding injury and prolonged exposure to cold).

Evaluation

- Anxiety is reduced
- Pain is controlled or eliminated
- Localized or systemic infection is absent
- Skin color and temperature of extremities are normal
- Respiratory function is normal; lungs are clear to auscultation; patient coughs and deep-breathes effectively
- Urine output is normal
- Patient verbalizes understanding of the prescribed treatment modalities and the importance of avoiding injury to the extremities

General Nutritional Considerations

☐ Patients with atherosclerosis and elevated serum cholesterol and triglyceride levels should be placed on a low-cholesterol diet. Additional dietary recommendations, such as limiting sodium intake, depend on the type of disorder being treated.

General Pharmacologic Considerations

☐ Many types of drugs may be administered before and after cardiac or blood vessel surgery (eg, antibiotics, anticoagulants, vasopressors, diuretics, electrolytes, and cardiotonics). The nurse should be familiar with the dose, route of administration, and adverse effects of each drug given, as many of these drugs have narrow margins of safety.

General Gerontologic Considerations

☐ Many elderly patients are poor surgical risks, and have other concurrent medical problems, such as diabetes, heart failure, cardiac dysrhythmias, hypertension, and poor renal function. These problems require close observation during the postoperative period.

Suggested Readings

☐ Abels L. Critical care nursing: a physiologic approach. St Louis: CV Mosby, 1986. *(Additional and in-depth coverage of subject matter)*

☐ Dailey EK, Schroeder JS. Techniques in bedside hemodynamic monitoring. 3rd ed. St Louis: CV Mosby, 1984. *(Additional and in-depth coverage of subject matter)*

☐ Gruendemann BJ, Meeker MH. Alexander's care of the patient in surgery. 8th ed. St Louis: CV Mosby, 1987. *(In-depth coverage of subject matter)*

☐ Johanson BC, Wells SJ, Hoffmeister D, Dungca CU. Standards for critical care. St Louis: CV Mosby, 1988. *(In-depth coverage of subject matter)*

☐ Loach J, Thompson NB. Hemodynamic monitoring. Philadelphia: JB Lippincott, 1987. *(Additional and in-depth coverage of subject matter)*

☐ McConnell EA. Clinical considerations in perioperative nursing: preventive aspects of care. Philadelphia: JB Lippincott, 1987. *(Additional and in-depth coverage of subject matter)*

☐ Moorhouse MF. Critical care plans. Philadelphia: FA Davis, 1987.

The Hematopoietic and Lymphatic Systems

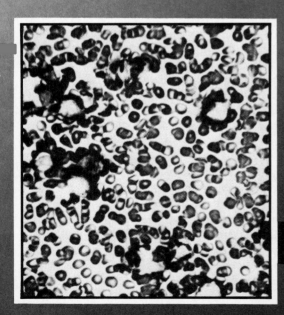

Unit 7

Chapter 32

Introduction to the Hematopoietic and Lymphatic Systems

On completion of this chapter the reader will:

- Be familiar with the basic anatomy and physiology of the hematopoietic and lymphatic systems

- Discuss the common tests used for diagnosing blood and lymphatic disorders

- Use the nursing process in the management of a patient having a diagnostic evaluation of the hematopoietic or lymphatic system

HEMATOPOIETIC SYSTEM
Anatomy and Physiology

Hematopoiesis is the manufacture and development of blood cells by the *hematopoietic system,* which consists of the bone marrow and lymph nodes.

Blood consists of cells that are suspended in a fluid called *plasma* (Fig. 32-1). There are different types of blood cells, each having specialized functions. They include *erythrocytes* (red blood cells), *leukocytes* (white blood cells), and *thrombocytes* (platelets).

Bone Marrow

Bone marrow is located in the interior of the long bones and spongy bones of the skeleton. There are two types of bone marrow: red marrow and yellow marrow. Red bone marrow is concerned with the manufacture of blood cells and hemoglobin. Yellow bone marrow, which consists primarily of fat cells and connective tissue, does not participate in the manufacture blood cells. Red bone marrow is primarily found in the ribs, sternum, and iliac crest.

Erythrocytes

Erythrocytes are flexible, anuclear (lack a nucleus), biconcave disks covered by a thin membrane that allows oxygen and carbon dioxide to freely pass through it. The flexibility of erythrocytes allows them to bend as they travel through capillaries. Their major function is to transport oxygen to the tissues and remove carbon dioxide from them.

Erythrocytes arise from *stem cells* in the red bone marrow, and go through several stages of maturation before they are released into the blood. In their early stage, they contain a nucleus and are called *erythroblasts*. As the cell matures, it loses its nucleus and then is released into the circulation. The normal number of erythrocytes is between 4.6 and 6.2 million/mm^3.

The red color of the blood is caused by *hemoglobin,* which is contained in the erythrocytes. The *heme* of the hemoglobin molecule consists of iron, which freely binds with oxygen. *Oxyhemoglobin* is the combination of oxygen and the heme of hemoglobin. Most of the iron in the body is contained in the erythrocytes. The normal amount of hemoglobin is 14 to 16 g/dL. As blood passes through the lungs, oxygen is taken up and carbon dioxide is released. Oxygenated blood is bright red, and is carried by arteries and capillaries to all tissues of the body. After oxygen has been released from the hemoglobin for use by the tissues, the hemoglobin is called *reduced hemoglobin*. The blood at this time is dark red, and is returned by the veins to the heart and the lungs, where the carbon dioxide is released and the blood reoxygenated.

Erythrocytes circulate in the blood for about 120 days. After this time, they are removed by the *reticuloendothelial system*, which are cells located throughout the body in such areas as the liver, spleen,

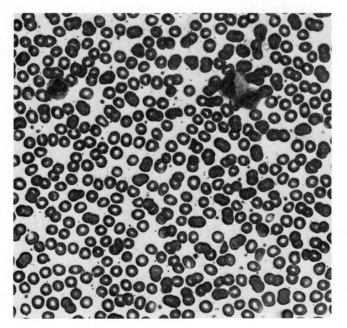

Figure 32–1. Normal blood cells (×450). (Photograph by D. Atkinson)

and lymph nodes (see Chapter 7). When erythrocytes are destroyed, the iron is used again.

Leukocytes

Leukocytes are divided into two general categories: granulocytes, which contain cytoplasmic granules, and agranulocytes, which do not contain cytoplasmic granules. The major functions of leukocytes are to protect the body from invading microorganisms and to manufacture antibodies.

Granulocytes. Granulocytes are divided into three subgroups: *eosinophils, basophils,* and *neutrophils.* Slightly immature neutrophils, called band cells, appear in peripheral blood. Granulocytes also are called polymorphonuclear leukocytes, because they contain multilobed nuclei.

Agranulocytes. Agranulocytes also are called mononuclear leukocytes, since they have nonlobular nuclei. They are divided into two groups: *lymphocytes* and *monocytes.* Lymphocytes are further divided into B lymphocytes (or B cells) and T lymphocytes (or T cells). The B lymphocytes produce antibodies against foreign antigens, and the T lymphocytes attack foreign cells or release a substance called lymphokine, which enhances the actions of phagocytic cells (see Chapter 7).

Platelets

Platelets are disklike, nonnucleated cells. They may be round, flat, or oval. Platelets are manufactured in the bone marrow and play a role in blood coagulation. When injury to a blood vessel occurs, platelets migrate to the injury site. A substance released from the platelet causes them to adhere and form a plug, or clot, that occludes the injured vessel. They have a short life span of about 7.5 days. The normal number of platelets is 150,000 to 350,000/μL.

Plasma

Plasma is the liquid form of blood without the suspended blood cells. Plasma contains proteins, as albumin and globulins, and other substances, such as prothrombin and pigments.

Albumin. Albumin is a protein that is formed in the liver. Because the albumin molecule cannot pass through a capillary wall, this protein aids in the maintenance of osmotic pressure that retains fluid in the vascular compartment.

Globulin. Globulins are divided into three groups: alpha, beta, and gamma. The gamma globulins also are called immunoglobulins. The major functions of globulins are as immunologic agents, but like albumin, they also help to maintain osmotic pressure in the vascular compartment.

Assessment

The cause of some hematologic disorders is unknown; causes of other hematologic disorders include exposure to chemicals, surgery, drugs, and a change in eating habits. At times, the cause of the disorder is evident, whereas at other times it is obscure.

A thorough patient history should include *all* symptoms noted by the patient, a thorough drug and dietary history (prescription and nonprescription), and an occupational history. In some instances, it is necessary to question the patient regarding when the symptoms first appeared and their severity and consistency. Recent events, such as exposure to or use of certain chemicals (including common household products), also should be covered in detail.

Physical examination includes inspection of the skin, with particular attention to skin color (normal, extreme redness, pallor) and the presence of ecchymosis or other skin lesions. A more detailed physical examination may be required if a certain hematologic disorder is suspected.

Laboratory Tests. A variety of laboratory tests are used in the diagnosis of hematopoietic disorders. Blood is obtained by venipuncture or finger puncture. The sample may be smeared on a glass slide and examined under the microscope or analyzed by various types of laboratory techniques. Examples of laboratory tests are a complete blood count, hemoglobin, prothrombin time, hematocrit, and white blood count and differential.

Diagnostic Tests.   Certain hematologic disorders, such as leukemia, may require an examination of the bone marrow for diagnosis. Under local anesthesia, a sample of bone marrow is aspirated from the sternum or iliac crest and examined under a microscope. If a bone marrow biopsy is performed, the iliac crest is used. The marrow is examined for the types and percentage of cells and their relative relation to those ready to be released into the circulation.

An example of a diagnostic test particular to a specific hematologic disease is the Schilling test. This test is used to diagnose pernicious anemia, macrocytic anemia, and malabsorption syndromes. Radioactive vitamin B_{12} is given orally, followed in 1 hour by an injection of nonradioactive B_{12}. All urine is collected for 24 to 48 hours after the patient receives the injected B_{12}. Low urine values indicate absence of the intrinsic factor, or defective malabsorption of vitamin B_{12} from the intestinal tract.

Other diagnostic tests include radiography, computed tomography, bone scan, and magnetic resonance imaging. These tests are not specific for hematologic disorders, but they may be used to rule out other disorders or note changes in organs or structures that may have a direct or indirect relation to the hematologic disorder.

LYMPHATIC SYSTEM
Anatomy and Physiology

Lymph is similar in composition to tissue fluid and plasma. A system of vessels called *lymphatics* (lymph nodes) carries tissue fluid from body tissues to the veins. Lymph nodes are located primarily in the axilla, groin, and neck, as well as along the large vessels of the thorax and abdomen. These nodes are connected by lymph ducts, through which lymph flows. Lymph enters the node by way of the afferent lymph duct, passes through the node, and leaves by the efferent lymph duct. The lymph node cortex is concerned with the production of B lymphocytes and antibody formation. The lymph node medulla contains T lymphocytes. As lymph passes through the node, macrophages, which are attached to a meshlike network, attack and engulf (phagocytose) antigens.

The primary functions of lymphatic tissue are to manufacture immune cells and remove foreign materials from the lymph.

Assessment

A thorough patient history should be taken, including all symptoms experienced and a past medical history. If an infectious process is evident, the patient should be asked when the infection was first noticed and the possible cause (eg, injury or untreated local infection). If there is painful or painless enlargement of the lymph nodes, the area of involvement is palpated and the size, location, and characteristics of each node are determined. The skin adjacent to the area is examined for redness, streaking, and swelling.

Laboratory Tests.   Depending on the disorder, various laboratory tests may be used. If an infectious process is suspected, a blood or lymph node culture may be performed. Nonspecific laboratory tests such as a complete blood count and white blood cell count and differential may be used for certain disorders to aid the physician in confirming a diagnosis.

Diagnostic Tests.   An examination of the lymphatic system may include lymphangiography. This procedure is performed to determine lymph node flow, and lymph node involvement in metastatic carcinoma, lymphomas, and infections. A radiopaque substance is injected into the lymphatics of the hands or feet. After injection of a contrast medium, radiographs are taken. Because lymph moves slowly through the lymphatic system, another radiograph is taken in 24 hours. Depending on the site of injection and the areas to be visualized, additional radiographs may be taken at 24-hour intervals.

A lymph node biopsy may be necessary, especially if a malignant process is suspected. Additional tests may include radiography, bone scan, computed tomography, and magnetic resonance imaging. These tests are not specific for lymphatic disorders, but may be used to rule out other disorders or note changes in organs or structures that may have a relation to the diagnosis.

NURSING PROCESS
—THE PATIENT UNDERGOING DIAGNOSTIC EVALUATIONS OF THE HEMATOPOIETIC OR LYMPHATIC SYSTEM

Assessment

If a diagnosis has not been established, the patient may be scheduled for a series of diagnostic and laboratory tests. A thorough patient history is important when the patient has a disorder of the hematopoietic or lymphatic systems. This is followed by a general physical appraisal and examination of specific areas, when indicated by the patient history. Vital signs and weight should be recorded.

Nursing Diagnosis

One or more of the following nursing diagnoses may apply to the patient with a disorder of the hematopoietic or lymphatic systems, depending on the patient's symptoms and possible diagnosis:

- Anxiety related to diagnostic tests, possible diagnosis
- Knowledge deficit of the tests to be performed, patient cooperation required during the test

Planning and Implementation

The major goals of the patient include a reduction of anxiety and an understanding of the cooperation required during specific tests.

The major goals of nursing management include a reduction of anxiety, correct preparation of the patient for scheduled tests, and adherence to hospital procedure in carrying out the test.

Care should be taken to use the correct container when a specimen of body fluid (blood, urine) is collected for laboratory examination. Certain tests require the addition of a preservative or other chemical to the collection bottle. If there is a question regarding the type of specimen container to be used, the laboratory should be consulted. Gloves should be worn when collecting body fluid specimens. After collection, the specimen should be checked to be sure it has been correctly labeled, and then it should be immediately taken to the laboratory.

After an invasive procedure such as a venipuncture or finger prick, the patient should be checked for signs of excessive bleeding, and pressure should be applied to the site as needed. Patients who are undergoing bone marrow aspiration require the application of pressure to the site for 2 or 3 minutes. If the iliac crest is used, a pressure dressing should be applied to the site. The patient should be observed every 30 minutes for several hours to be sure there is no further bleeding.

Anxiety. Many patients experience various emotional reactions before, during, and after a diagnostic procedure. The cause of the emotional response should be determined, and steps taken to relieve or eliminate anxiety and fear. Many times these emotional responses are due to a lack of knowledge, concern over the test results, and fear of pain or discomfort during and after the test.

If a bone marrow aspiration is performed, the patient requires emotional support during the procedure. Some discomfort may be experienced after the procedure, and a mild analgesic may be prescribed for discomfort.

Knowledge Deficit. To obtain optimal results from a diagnostic test, full patient cooperation is necessary. The nurse should determine what the patient already knows about the procedure. This should be followed by a basic explanation of the test, what tasks (if any) are necessary for participation in the test, and what discomforts (if any) may be experienced. The patient should be given time to ask questions.

Evaluation

- Anxiety and fear are reduced or eliminated
- Patient demonstrates understanding of procedure

Suggested Readings

☐ Alfaro R. Applying nursing diagnosis and nursing process: a step-by-step guide. 2nd ed. Philadelphia: JB Lippincott, 1990. *(Additional coverage of subject matter)*

☐ Fischbach FT. A manual of laboratory diagnostic tests. 3rd ed. Philadelphia: JB Lippincott, 1988. *(Additional coverage of subject matter)*

☐ Fuller J, Schaller-Ayers J. Health assessment: a nursing approach. Philadelphia: JB Lippincott, 1990. *(Additional coverage of subject matter)*

☐ Memmler RL, Wood DL. The human body in health and disease. 6th ed. Philadelphia: JB Lippincott, 1987. *(Additional coverage of subject matter)*

☐ Porth CM. Pathophysiology: concepts of altered health states. 3rd ed. Philadelphia: JB Lippincott, 1990. *(In-depth, high-level coverage of subject matter)*

☐ Tilkian SM, Conover MB, Tilkian AG. Clinical implications of laboratory tests. 4th ed. St Louis: CV Mosby, 1987. *(Additional coverage of subject matter)*

Chapter 33

Disorders of the Hematopoietic System

On completion of this chapter the reader will:

- Discuss the symptoms, diagnosis, and treatment of pernicious anemia, sickle cell anemia, acquired hemolytic anemia, and anemia caused by blood loss and iron deficiency

- Use the nursing process in the management of a patient with a decrease in erythrocytes and hemoglobin

- Discuss the symptoms, diagnosis, and treatment of polycythemia vera

- Use the nursing process in the management of a patient with an increase in erythrocytes and hemoglobin

- Discuss the symptoms, diagnosis, treatment, and prognosis of acute myelogenous leukemia, chronic myelogenous leukemia, acute lymphocytic leukemia, and chronic lymphocytic leukemia

- Use the nursing process in the management of the patient with leukemia

- Discuss the symptoms, diagnosis, treatment, and prognosis of agranulocytosis

- Use the nursing process in the management of the patient with agranulocytosis

- Discuss the symptoms, diagnosis, treatment, and prognosis of multiple myeloma

- Use the nursing process in the management of the patient with multiple myeloma

- Discuss the symptoms, diagnosis, and treatment of thrombocytopenia and hemophilia

- Use the nursing process in the management of the patient with a bleeding disorder

- Discuss cause, symptoms, diagnosis, treatment, and prognosis of bone marrow failure

- Use the nursing process in the management of the patient with bone marrow failure

The term *blood dyscrasias* (disease) describes a large group of disorders that affect the blood. Although blood dyscrasias affect the blood in some way, the disorders themselves are manifestations of many different pathologic processes. For instance, leukemia is believed to be caused by malignant changes, and anemia may be due to a variety of causes, such as blood loss, inadequate formation of red blood cells, or increased destruction of red blood cells. Regardless of the pathology, many disorders of the blood have similar symptoms and nursing problems, and require similar diagnostic tests.

DISORDERS ASSOCIATED WITH A DECREASE IN ERYTHROCYTES AND HEMOGLOBIN

The term *anemia* means that the patient has a decreased number of erythrocytes and a lower than normal hemoglobin level. The number of erythrocytes normally present varies with age, sex, and altitude. Infants have more erythrocytes per cubic millimeter than do adults. Women have fewer erythrocytes per cubic millimeter (about 4.5 million) than do men (about 5 million). This difference is most noticeable during the reproductive years. People who live at high altitudes have an increased number of erythrocytes.

Anemia can be caused by loss of blood and by destruction or faulty production of erythrocytes and hemoglobin. Blood loss can occur suddenly and copiously, as in severe hemorrhage from a severed artery, or it can occur slowly and persistently, as from bleeding hemorrhoids or a peptic ulcer. Bleeding also results in the loss of iron from the body because iron is contained in hemoglobin. By increasing its production of erythrocytes, the body can compensate for some degree of their loss or destruction; anemia becomes manifest only when the body is unable to sufficiently increase its production of erythrocytes to compensate for these losses.

Hemolysis (the destruction of erythrocytes) leads to a reduction in the number of erythrocytes. In hemolytic conditions, the erythrocytes do not survive as long as they normally do, and their increased destruction rate leads to anemia. Some of the causes of hemolysis are infection, transfusion of incompatible blood, and exposure to harmful chemicals.

Inadequate production of erythrocytes can result from an injury to the bone marrow (eg, by toxic effects of drugs) or the lack of necessary materials (eg, iron, folic acid, and vitamin B_{12}) for the formation of erythrocytes and hemoglobin. Anemia also may be caused by other diseases, such as cancer.

Irrespective of the cause, symptoms of anemia are similar, and are largely due to the inability of the blood to transport sufficient oxygen to the tissues. Fatigue, anorexia, faintness, and pallor are typical signs of anemia.

Anemia Caused by Blood Loss

The total blood volume is about one thirteenth of body weight. An adult who weighs 154 lb has about 6 qt of blood. The quantity of blood circulating in the body normally is kept relatively constant at all times.

Blood loss, either acute or chronic, causes anemia. Sudden severe bleeding leads to *hypovolemia* (diminished volume of circulating blood) and shock.

Symptoms

Acute and severe blood loss is evidenced by extreme pallor, tachycardia, hypotension, and other symptoms of hypovolemic shock (see Chapter 18). Chronic blood loss usually produces such symptoms as fatigue, anorexia, and pallor.

Diagnosis

Diagnosis of internal acute and severe blood loss is made by recognition of the symptoms of hypovolemic shock. Severe external blood loss is easily recognized. Laboratory confirmation of acute or chronic anemia is made by such tests as complete blood count, hemoglobin, and hematocrit. When blood loss is severe, a total blood volume determination may be performed to determine the amount of blood lost and then used as a guide for replacement therapy.

Treatment

Treatment of sudden severe bleeding involves the replacement of blood by transfusions. If blood loss is chronic, as may be the case in disorders such as uterine tumors or hemorrhoids, treatment is aimed at the underlying condition that is causing the bleeding. Depending on the amount of blood lost, treatment may include blood transfusion or administration of iron to help the body compensate for the blood loss and to correct iron deficiency anemia (see section on iron deficiency anemia). Continued care and observation are necessary for any patient who has experienced blood loss.

Iron Deficiency Anemia

Iron is necessary for the production of hemoglobin. Iron deficiency anemia occurs frequently among those whose need for iron is increased. Less than 10% of the iron obtained from food is absorbed. During periods of rapid growth, at the onset of the menses, and during pregnancy, the need for iron is increased; anemia often results unless additional iron is obtained. Sometimes it is difficult to provide for these increased needs by dietary measures alone, although correction of a faulty diet, if it exists, is an important aspect of treatment.

Iron deficiency anemia also occurs in conjunction with anemia caused by chronic blood loss (see section on anemia caused by blood loss).

Symptoms

Symptoms of iron deficiency anemia include fatigue, anorexia, and pallor. Severe forms of the disorder may produce tachycardia and exertional dyspnea.

Diagnosis

Diagnosis is made by laboratory tests such as complete blood count, hemoglobin, hematocrit, red cell indices, and serum iron level. A blood smear may be examined microscopically, since iron deficiency anemia is characterized by red blood cells that are microcytic (smaller than normal) and hypochromic (color lighter than normal).

To determine the cause of anemia, other laboratory and diagnostic tests (eg, stool samples for occult blood and barium enema) may be ordered.

Treatment

Treatment is first aimed at determining the cause of the anemia and, when possible, eliminating the cause. This type of anemia often is treated by administration of an oral iron preparation. Foods high in iron are added to the diet. The patient may have to make an effort to eat because anemia may cause anorexia.

DISORDERS ASSOCIATED WITH ERYTHROCYTE DESTRUCTION

A reduction in erythrocytes and hemoglobin may be caused by hemolysis, hence the term *hemolytic anemia*. The life span of the red blood cells is shortened.

Sickle Cell Anemia

Sickle cell anemia is caused by an abnormal form of hemoglobin (hemoglobin S). It is a hereditary disease found primarily in blacks, but it also may be seen in people from Mediterranean and Arab countries. Some of the red blood cells become deformed and sickle-shaped (Fig. 33-1). As a result of this deformity, these cells become lodged in small blood vessels, where they block the flow of blood. The reduction in blood flow caused by the blockage leads to ischemia or infarction of the area supplied by the blood vessel.

Symptoms

Patients with sickle cell anemia are anemic, and jaundice often is present. The bone marrow enlarges to compensate for the continuous need to produce more

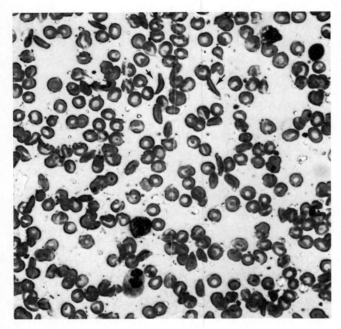

Figure 33–1. Blood cells found in sickle cell anemia (×450). (Photograph by D. Atkinson)

red blood cells, and the constant anemia causes tachycardia, dyspnea, enlargement of the heart (cardiomegaly), and cardiac dysrhythmias. Chronic leg ulcers may develop as a result of the blockage of the small blood vessels of the extremities.

Sickle cell crisis, a rapidly developing syndrome, results from the blockage of small blood vessels. These attacks occur suddenly and affect various areas of the body. Fever, pain, and swelling of one or more joints are common. Other symptoms also may occur, depending on the blood vessels involved. Sickle cell crisis may lead to such disorders as cerebrovascular accident, pulmonary infarction, shock, and renal failure.

Diagnosis

Diagnosis is made by a sickle cell screening test, which determines the presence of hemoglobin S. A positive result requires hemoglobin electrophoresis to determine whether the person has sickle cell disease or carries the sickle cell trait. Symptoms of the disease are not present in people who have the sickle cell trait, but some of their children may inherit the disease if the other parent has the same recessive gene pattern.

Treatment

There is no cure for sickle cell anemia, and treatment is only palliative. These patients are subject to infections that can be life-threatening; therefore, every infection, no matter now minor, should be treated promptly. If sickle cell crisis occurs, oxygen is given

for hypoxia, the patient is kept on complete bed rest, and blood transfusions are administered. Pain is controlled with analgesics, and fluid intake increased by the oral or intravenous route.

Acquired Hemolytic Anemia

A number of factors can cause acquired hemolytic anemia. The cause may be a physical factor that produces erythrocyte damage, for example the use of cardiopulmonary bypass during surgery. This type of anemia also may be caused by infectious agents or toxins. Poisoning by arsenic or lead, invasion of the erythrocytes by the malaria parasite, and the production of substances resulting in hemolysis, such as those generated by the bacterium *Clostridium perfringens,* are examples of causes of acquired hemolytic anemia. A third cause is the production of antibodies that destroy erythrocytes. Production of antibodies can be due to (1) the development of antibodies against antigens from another person, such as is seen in blood transfusion reactions, and (2) the development within the body of antibodies against its own erythrocytes. The latter form may develop from the use of drugs such as penicillin and phenylbutazone, as a consequence of diseases such as leukemia and lupus erythematosus, or for no known reason. When the reason for developing acquired hemolytic anemia is not known, the condition is called *idiopathic autoimmune hemolytic anemia.*

Symptoms

Symptoms may be so mild that they go unnoticed, or they may be severe and life-threatening. A positive Coombs test is seen, and in milder forms of the disorder, the patient may complain of symptoms usually associated with anemia. Patients with the severe form of the disorder may be jaundiced. Fatigue and dyspnea are severe, and a cardiac dysrhythmia may be present. The hemolysis may be so extensive that shock occurs.

Treatment

Treatment includes removing the cause (when possible) and administering corticosteroids. In some patients, the steroid dosage can be reduced and then discontinued after several weeks of therapy. Blood transfusions may be necessary. A splenectomy may be performed if the patient does not respond to treatment.

Thalassemia

One group of hereditary hemolytic anemias is referred to as *thalassemia.* The thalassemias are divided into two major groups: α-thalassemia and β-thalassemia.

The α-thalassemias are found in people from Southeast Asia and Africa, whereas the β-thalassemias are found in those from the Po valley in Italy and on islands in the Mediterranean.

Symptoms

Patients with α-thalassemia often are asymptomatic, as are those with minor forms of β-thalassemia. Those with Cooley's anemia, a severe form of β-thalassemia, exhibit symptoms of severe anemia and a bronzing of the skin due to hemolysis of red blood cells.

Diagnosis

Diagnosis is based on symptoms as well as hemoglobin electrophoresis.

Treatment

Treatment of the various forms of thalassemia is symptomatic. Frequent transfusions may be required.

ANEMIA CAUSED BY IMMATURE ERYTHROCYTE FORMATION
Pernicious Anemia

An intrinsic factor normally present in stomach secretions is necessary for the absorption of vitamin B_{12} found in food. Vitamin B_{12} is necessary for the normal maturation of red blood cells. Patients with pernicious anemia lack this intrinsic factor, and thus have many large, immature red blood cells.

The body requires such small amounts of vitamin B_{12} that most people have an adequate supply in their food. Those with pernicious anemia must have regular injections of vitamin B_{12} to control the disease because their lack of the intrinsic factor in gastric secretions prevents the adequate absorption of vitamin B_{12} from food.

Symptoms

In addition to the usual symptoms of anemia, patients with pernicious anemia occasionally develop a sore tongue and mouth, digestive disturbances, and diarrhea. The anemia may be so severe that the patient experiences dyspnea on the slightest exertion. Jaundice may occur. Personality changes are not unusual, especially when the disease is severe. Often the patient is irritable, confused, and depressed, but these changes usually disappear with treatment.

If the condition is not treated promptly, the patient develops degenerative changes in the nervous system. Numbness and tingling in the extremities and ataxia are common. Vibratory and position sense may be lost.

Symptoms of neurologic damage may improve somewhat, but sometimes permanent damage occurs before treatment is begun. The earlier the diagnosis and the more prompt the treatment, the greater the likelihood of escaping permanent neurologic damage.

Diagnosis

Diagnosis of pernicious anemia is established by the patient's history and symptoms and by studies of the blood and bone marrow. The Schilling test, which is specific for this disorder, may be used to confirm the diagnosis.

Treatment

Vitamin B_{12} is given intramuscularly in a dosage that is adequate to control the disease. Therapy must continue for life. No toxic effects have been noted from the use of vitamin B_{12}. Oral vitamin B_{12} is seldom effective, except for short intervals. Iron therapy is seldom needed, as once the condition is corrected, mature erythrocytes are manufactured and the hemoglobin is normal.

NURSING PROCESS —THE PATIENT WHO HAS A DECREASE IN ERYTHROCYTES AND HEMOGLOBIN

Assessment

The patient history should include a list of symptoms; a thorough dietary, medical, and allergy history; and a family history of any type of blood disorder. Because some anemias may be due to such causes as environmental factors, heredity, and drugs, a thorough history is especially important if the cause of the anemia has not been determined. It also is important to determine if the patient has noticed any change in the color of the stool or urine.

Physical examination includes examination of the skin and mucous membranes for pallor, dryness, and jaundice. A neurologic assessment (see Chapter 35) is important if pernicious anemia is suspected.

A cardiac assessment is performed (see Chapter 24), because severe anemia may result in cardiac dysrhythmias and congestive heart failure. Vital signs and weight should be taken, and the patient assessed for dyspnea on exertion or other signs of congestive heart failure.

Nursing Diagnosis

One or more of the following nursing diagnoses may apply to the patient with anemia, depending on the patient's age, length of time the disorder has been present, severity of the anemia, possible cause, and other factors. Additional nursing diagnoses may be added if the patient has another concurrent blood dyscrasia (eg, leukemia).

- Activity intolerance caused by decreased erythrocyte count, decreased hemoglobin
- Pain related to sickle cell crisis
- Altered nutrition: less than body requirements related to anorexia
- Potential for infection related to another concurrent blood dyscrasia, poor nutrition, other factors (specify)
- Knowledge deficit related to methods of prevention, signs and symptoms, treatment, complications, other (specify)

Planning and Implementation

The major goals of the patient include an increase in activity tolerance, a reduction of pain (sickle cell crisis), improved nutritional intake, prevention of infection, and an understanding of the disorder and its treatment methods.

The major goals of nursing management are to assist in attaining and maintaining a normal erythrocyte count, increase activity to a tolerable level, and relieve the symptoms associated with anemia.

Ongoing assessments evaluate the patient's response to treatment—an improvement in the patient's general condition and a decrease in the symptoms of the disorder. Vital signs should be taken every 4 hours or as ordered by the physician. Each stool passed should be examined for color; tarry or black stools should be saved until the physician is notified.

Patients with severe anemia should be protected from contact with those who have any type of infection.

Activity Intolerance.   Nursing management should be planned according to the ability of these patients to carry out their activities of daily living. Dypsnea and fatigue may decrease once the erythrocyte count approaches normal. Frequent rest periods and the spacing of activities may reduce dyspnea until the anemia is corrected.

A record should be kept of the activity level and goals established according to the patient's apparent ability to tolerate an activity. The prevention of falls is particularly important if the patient has neurologic symptoms associated with pernicious anemia or weakness caused by severe anemia. Patients with these symptoms should be assisted with activities such as getting out of bed, ambulating, and showering.

Patients with pernicious anemia and permanent neurologic deficits related to the disorder may benefit from physical therapy.

Pain.   The patient in sickle cell crisis often has severe pain in many areas. Proper positioning, assistance with activities, prevention of contractures, and the relief of pain by the administration of analgesics often are necessary. If pain is not relieved or suddenly becomes more intense, the physician should be notified. Whirlpool baths may be used to relieve pain. The patient should be closely observed for symptoms that may indicate the development of a serious complication, such as pulmonary infarction, cerebrovascular accident, and shock.

Altered Nutrition.   Despite anorexia, the patient should be encouraged to take easily digested, nutritious foods and fluids. Soft foods that are not highly seasoned are preferable, especially if the patient's mouth is sore.

Knowledge Deficit.   The short- and long-term treatment modalities necessary to correct the anemia should be explained to the patient and family. The importance of continued follow-up care and monitoring of the blood count should be stressed.

The addition of dietary iron and the use of iron supplements (when prescribed) should be explained in detail and a list of foods containing iron given. The patient should be informed that oral iron may color the stools black or dark green.

Patients with pernicious anemia are more likely to take the injections with the frequency recommended by the physician if a member of the family is taught to administer the medication. If such instruction cannot be arranged, the patient should return to the physician's office or clinic or have the injections given by a community health nurse.

Management of the patient with sickle cell anemia includes genetic counseling as well as testing for the sickle cell trait in family members. Management of the disease in its chronic form includes patient education regarding the avoidance of infections and the importance of seeking medical help when any illness or symptoms of a sickle cell crisis occur.

Evaluation

- Patient tolerates increased activities
- Pain of sickle cell crisis is reduced or eliminated
- Normal respiratory rate is attained and maintained
- Appetite improves; patient eats a well-balanced diet
- Patient demonstrates understanding of treatment modalities
- Evidence of infection is absent
- Patient verbalizes understanding of lifelong therapy for pernicious anemia
- Family members of patient with sickle cell anemia consent to genetic counseling and testing

DISORDERS ASSOCIATED WITH AN INCREASE IN ERYTHROCYTES AND HEMOGLOBIN

Polycythemia Vera

Polycythemia vera is characterized by excessive erythrocyte and hemoglobin production. The number of white blood cells also is increased.

There are three types of polycythemia: polycythemia vera (primary polycythemia), secondary polycythemia, and relative polycythemia. The cause of primary polycythemia is unknown. Secondary polycythemia is due to other causes that are thought to be such disorders as chronic obstructive pulmonary disease and some types of hemoglobin abnormalities. Relative polycythemia is seen in those living at high altitudes and usually requires no treatment.

Symptoms

The patient may have 10 million erythrocytes per cubic millimeter, rather than the normal 5 million. The increased number of cells in the blood makes it more viscous than normal, and leads to increased blood volume and a tendency to develop thrombi. Complications include gout, congestive heart failure, hypertension, peptic ulcer, and hemorrhage. When clots cut off the blood supply to the tissues, areas of infarction result. The thrombosis of cerebral vessels is common.

The face, especially the lips, is a reddish-purple. Fatigue, weakness, headache, exertional dyspnea, and dizziness are common. Pruritus may be seen. The patient may bleed excessively after minor injuries, perhaps because of the engorgement of the capillaries and veins. Constipation, anorexia, and epigastric distress also may be present. Splenomegaly commonly occurs. The condition usually has an insidious onset and a prolonged course.

Diagnosis

Diagnosis is based on symptoms as well as laboratory tests, which reveal a high erythrocyte count.

Treatment

Treatment of primary polycythemia involves measures to reduce the volume of circulating blood, lessen its viscosity, and curb the excessive production of erythrocytes. Frequent medical examinations are important to determine the course of the disease and the patient's response to therapy.

A phlebotomy may be performed at intervals. Usually 500 mL of blood is removed from the vein at a time.

Sometimes radiophosphorus and radiation therapy are used to decrease the production of blood cells in the bone marrow. Antineoplastic drugs (eg, mechlorethamine) may be administered to curb excessive bone marrow activity. The patient should be encouraged to continue activities as long as possible, and should be carefully observed for symptoms of thrombosis.

Secondary polycythemia may be relieved by eliminating the cause, if possible. If the erythrocyte count is excessively high, treatment is the same as for primary polycythemia. Relative polycythemia does not require treatment.

NURSING PROCESS —THE PATIENT WHO HAS AN INCREASE IN ERYTHROCYTES AND HEMOGLOBIN

Assessment

A patient history should be taken and all symptoms recorded. A general physical examination should include the appearance of the skin and an evaluation of the cardiovascular, gastrointestinal, respiratory, and central nervous systems, since any one or more of these systems may be affected by the disorder. Vital signs and weight should be taken.

Because thrombus formation may occur in any organ or structure or at any time, detailed assessments are necessary. Complaints or problems such as headache, chest pain, pain in the extremities, difficulty breathing, abdominal pain, and numbness, tingling, or paralysis in an extremity warrant further investigation and immediate notification of the physician.

Nursing Diagnosis

Depending on the type, severity, and presenting symptoms, one or more of the following nursing diagnoses may apply:

- Activity intolerance related to exertional dyspnea
- Impaired physical mobility related to gout, tissue hypoxia secondary to thrombus formation
- Constipation related to symptoms of disorder, impaired physical mobility
- Pain related to thrombus formation, gout, headache
- Altered nutrition: less than body requirements related to nausea, other gastrointestinal symptoms
- Potential for injury related to dizziness
- Knowledge deficit of treatment modalities, prevention of injury, signs of complications

Planning and Implementation

The major goals of the patient include an increase in activity tolerance, increase in physical mobility, normal bowel elimination, a reduction in pain or discomfort, improved nutrition, prevention of injury, and an understanding of treatment modalities.

The main goal of nursing management is to assist in relieving some, most, or all the symptoms related to polycythemia. Symptoms are evaluated and recorded at the time of initial assessment to provide a data base for future comparison. Vital signs should be monitored every 4 hours or as ordered. The patient should be observed for complications associated with primary polycythemia.

Activity Intolerance, Impaired Physical Mobility, Potential for Injury. These patients should be encouraged to participate in their activities of daily living only as tolerated. Frequent rest periods should be encouraged if dyspnea or other symptoms occur. If symptoms of gout occur, mobility may be impaired and assistance with ambulatory activities will be required. Ambulatory activities should be supervised if dizziness or other neurologic symptoms occur.

Constipation. Fluids and ambulation should be encouraged in an effort to eliminate constipation. A daily record of bowel movements should be kept and the physician informed if constipation is apparent, as a stool softener or other medication or treatment may be necessary.

Pain. The patient should be placed in positions of comfort, with proper support for the back and legs, and position changes made every 2 hours. Analgesics should be administered as ordered, and the physician notified if the analgesic or other comfort measures fail to relieve pain, if pain becomes severe, or if pain develops in a new area.

Altered Nutrition. Small, frequent feedings may be better tolerated than three large meals. Fluids between meals should be encouraged. A dietary consult may be necessary to provide foods that are better tolerated and liked.

Knowledge Deficit. The patient and family should be thoroughly familiar with the method and importance of treatments (eg, phlebotomy or the administration of radiophosphorus), as well as the importance of lifelong medical supervision.

The nurse should suggest ways to avoid trauma and bleeding tendencies caused by trauma, for example wearing properly fitted shoes, avoiding tight and restrictive clothing, avoiding clutter in areas of work or recreation, and avoiding those activities that may cause injury.

The patient should be reminded to plan frequent rest periods throughout the day and to avoid activities that are tiring. A dietary consult may be necessary if the physician has recommended a special diet. The patient should be reminded to avoid those foods that cause gastric distress and to drink extra fluids between meals.

If medication is prescribed, the patient and family should be informed of the type of medication, dose, time of administration, and adverse effects of the drug.

The signs and symptoms of complications and the importance of seeking immediate medical care if any new symptoms (regardless of how minor) arise should be emphasized.

Evaluation

- Activity tolerance increases; patient is able to assume responsibility for own care
- Pain and discomfort are relieved or eliminated
- Bowel elimination is normal
- Appetite improves; patient eats a well-balanced diet; fluid intake is increased
- Injury to self is not apparent
- Patient verbalizes understanding of the importance of treatment modalities, continued follow-up care, dietary restrictions, and the necessity of seeing the physician if symptoms of complications should occur

DISORDERS ASSOCIATED WITH AN INCREASE OR DECREASE IN LEUKOCYTES

There normally are between 5,000 and 7,000 leukocytes per cubic millimeter of blood. Fighting infection is one important function of the leukocytes, and they increase in number during most infections. This increase is called *leukocytosis.*

Leukemia is characterized by a rampant, unregulated proliferation of leukocytes (Fig. 33-2). This rampant increase is not useful to the body. The patient is less, rather than more, able to cope with infections. Although there are more leukocytes, many are immature, and therefore not effective in fighting infections. The rapid proliferation of leukocytes and of the tissues that produce them results in a decrease in the number of erythrocytes and platelets. The patient eventually suffers from severe anemia, and the reduction in platelets leads to bleeding. The cause of leukemia remains unknown, although certain factors, such as exposure to toxic chemicals and radiation, may result in leukemia.

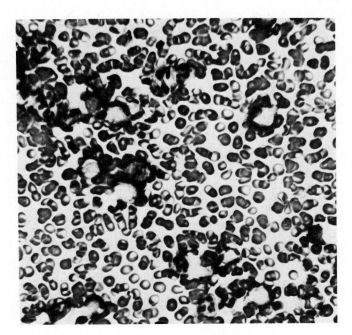

Figure 33–2. Blood cells found in chronic myelogenous leukemia (×450). (Photograph by D. Atkinson)

Chemotherapeutic agents used in the treatment of leukemia are highly toxic and can impair the formation of all blood cells. The patient's blood profile should be watched carefully while these drugs are being administered. Antibiotics should be given to treat the secondary infections that are the common complications of the illness. Although there is no cure, antineoplastic drugs that interfere with the multiplication of cells, particularly those undergoing rapid proliferation, may lessen clinical symptoms. This is called a remission.

The patient may develop a resistance to all forms of treatment, and become severely ill with weakness, fever, bleeding, and secondary infections such as pneumonia. Death may occur within a few weeks after the patient becomes resistant to drug therapy.

Bone marrow transplantation has been used to treat some patients with acute leukemia. Bone marrow for transplantation is obtained from a donor whose bone marrow closely matches the bone marrow of the recipient. Before transplantation is begun, the patient's body is irradiated to destroy the bone marrow (which is producing the abnormal leukemic cells). At this time, the patient is extremely vulnerable to infection and must be placed in a special isolation unit. After destruction of the leukemic bone marrow, the donor's bone marrow is injected into a peripheral blood vessel. The donated bone marrow finds its way to the patient's bone marrow by a process that is not completely understood. If transplantation is successful, the donated bone marrow takes over the production of

blood cells until the patient is able to produce normal bone marrow.

Another method is *autologous* bone marrow transplantation. The donor's own bone marrow is removed, the leukemic cells are destroyed, and the marrow is frozen with liquid nitrogen for later use. The patient is then prepared to receive his or her own treated bone marrow in the same manner as for those receiving bone marrow from another individual.

The leukemias are classified according to the white blood cells that are involved.

Acute Myelogenous Leukemia

Acute myelogenous leukemia (AML) affects the stem cells of the bone marrow. Stem cells are the original cells of the bone marrow that differentiate into (or become) monocytes, granulocytes, platelets, and erythrocytes.

Symptoms

Symptoms are caused by an insufficient production of normal blood cells. Anemia is seen because of an inadequate production of erythrocytes; infection may occur because of inadequate production of leukocytes; and bleeding tendencies develop because of inadequate production of platelets. The onset may be sudden, or it may occur over a period of several months. Peripheral blood smears show a decrease in erythrocytes and platelets. The white blood cell count may be low, normal, or high, but there is a decreased number of *normal* leukocytes.

Diagnosis

Diagnosis is made by examination of samples of peripheral blood and bone marrow.

Treatment

Drug therapy may include cyclophosphamide (Cytoxan), cytarabine (Cytosar-U), daunorubicin (Cerubidine), or mercaptopurine (Purinethol), either as single agents or in combination. Red cell and platelet transfusions may be used if anemia and thrombocytopenia occur.

Prognosis

The prognosis of AML is relatively poor, despite intensive therapy. Survival time averages about 1 year or less. Death usually results from an overwhelming infection that does not respond to antibiotic therapy.

Chronic Myelogenous Leukemia

Chronic myelogenous leukemia (CML) is milder than the acute form, and usually is seen in adults. There are fewer abnormal cells present in peripheral blood smears than are seen with the acute form. The onset is slow, and the patient may not experience symptoms for months to years.

Symptoms

The symptoms are basically the same as for acute myelogenous leukemia but are milder.

Diagnosis

Diagnosis is made by examination of samples of peripheral blood and bone marrow.

Treatment

Busulfan (Myleran) usually is the drug of choice, but other chemotherapeutic agents may include mechlorethamine (Mustargen), thioguanine, and uracil mustard.

Prognosis

The prognosis is fair, with some patients living 3 to 5 years. Bone marrow transplantation has increased survival time for some patients. Death usually results from hemorrhage, or an overwhelming infection that does not respond to antibiotic therapy.

Acute Lymphocytic Leukemia

Acute lymphocytic leukemia (ALL), which is more common in young children, is an increase in immature lymphocytes.

Symptoms

Symptoms include fever, bleeding tendencies, lymph node enlargement, fatigue, and weakness. Peripheral blood smears show a decrease in erythrocytes, leukocytes, and platelets. Anemia occurs and may be severe, causing pallor, weakness, and fatigue. Bleeding may be internal or external. Common sites from which bleeding occurs include the nose, mouth, and gastrointestinal tract. The tendency to bleed also may be reflected in the persistent oozing of blood after a minor injury such as a small cut or the administration of an intramuscular or subcutaneous injection. Fever often is present, especially as the disease advances. Infection is a cause for concern because it may not be controlled with antibiotic therapy, and can result in death.

Diagnosis

Diagnosis is made by examination of samples of peripheral blood and bone marrow.

Treatment

The patient may require repeated blood transfusions. Antineoplastic drugs—alone or in combination—are used to produce a state of remission. Some of the antineoplastic drugs that may be used are asparaginase (Elspar), daunorubicin (Cerubidine), methotrexate, mercaptopurine (Purinethol), prednisone, and vincristine (Oncovin).

Prognosis

The survival rate for ALL has improved. Many children survive 5 or more years, and some have had permanent remissions.

Chronic Lymphocytic Leukemia

Chronic lymphocytic leukemia (CLL) usually affects people who are age 40 or older. It is a milder form of acute lymphocytic leukemia.

Symptoms

The patient may be asymptomatic, or experience mild symptoms of anemia, weakness, and fatigue. There also may be lymph node enlargement. Many times symptoms go unnoticed, and the disorder is not discovered until the patient has a general physical examination and blood tests reveal lymphocytosis.

Diagnosis

Diagnosis is made by examination of samples of peripheral blood and bone marrow.

Treatment

Drugs used in treatment include chlorambucil (Leukeran), cyclophosphamide (Cytoxan), mechlorethamine (Mustargen), prednisone, and uracil mustard.

Prognosis

Survival time for CLL is about 7 or 8 years, although some patients live longer. On the other hand, an overwhelming infection that is unresponsive to antibiotic therapy may decrease survival time, especially if the patient has other medical problems.

NURSING PROCESS —THE PATIENT WHO HAS LEUKEMIA

Assessment

Initial assessment should include a list of symptoms experienced before as well as at the time of assessment. Physical appraisal should include noting the patient's general appearance, checking vital signs, and looking for any evidence of bleeding or excessive bruising. Additional assessments are based on the patient's symptoms. Patients who are acutely ill at the time of admission may be unable to describe their physical symptoms. If possible, the nurse should obtain the history from a family member.

Ongoing assessment depends on the symptoms manifested by the patient. Laboratory tests should be reviewed and the patient observed for any symptoms or changes that could be related to abnormal laboratory findings.

Nursing Diagnosis

Some patients with leukemia may be acutely ill, whereas others have few or no symptoms. One or more of the following nursing diagnoses may apply to the patient with leukemia:

- Activity intolerance related to anemia
- Self-care deficit (partial to complete) related to fatigue secondary to anemia
- Anxiety related to diagnosis, diagnostic tests, prognosis
- Fear related to diagnosis, prognosis, other factors (specify)
- Hyperthermia related to infectious process secondary to leukopenia, leukocytosis with many immature leukocytes
- Pain related to infiltration of leukocytes in systemic tissues
- Diarrhea related to toxic effects of antineoplastic drug therapy
- Ineffective individual coping related to the diagnosis, prognosis, inability to meet basic needs, other factors (specify)
- Potential for infection related to leukopenia, leukocytosis with many immature leukocytes
- Altered nutrition: less than body requirements related to anorexia, nausea and vomiting, secondary to administration of antineoplastic drugs
- Impaired swallowing related to altered oral mucous membrane and formation of ulcerations secondary to severe leukopenia
- Body image disturbance related to alopecia secondary to administration of antineoplastic drugs
- Knowledge deficit of treatment modalities, prognosis

Planning and Implementation

The major goals of the patient include reduction or elimination of anxiety and pain, improved activity tolerance, normal bowel elimination, absence of infection, improved coping ability, improved nutrition, elimination of stomatitis, improved self-concept, and understanding of treatment modalities.

The major goals of nursing management include helping the patient and family to cope with the diagnosis, treatment modalities, and prognosis, and reducing or eliminating the toxic effects associated with chemotherapy.

During and after treatment, nursing management should focus on the patient's needs, the drugs administered, the toxic effects that may or do appear during therapy, and response to treatment. For ex-

ample, patients with thrombocytopenia (below normal number of platelets) may experience episodes of bleeding that can be internal or external, or both. Whereas external bleeding can be evidenced by easy bruising or blood oozing from an area such as the nose or mouth, early signs of internal bleeding can be difficult to detect, as may be seen in the patient with hemorrhage into cerebral tissue, which may first be evidenced by restlessness. This may be followed by neurologic changes. Unless ongoing assessments are thorough and all complaints voiced by the patient carefully evaluated, early recognition of complications may go undetected.

Activity Intolerance, Self-Care Deficits. Many patients with leukemia experience extreme fatigue and require assistance with their activities of daily living. Time should be allowed for the patient to rest between activities.

Anxiety, Fear. The nurse should allow time for the patient and family to ask questions as well as discuss diagnostic and treatment modalities. Offering emotional support during procedures such as a bone marrow aspiration may help to reduce some of the anxiety associated with these procedures.

Although the physician explains the diagnosis and prognosis, the nurse should allow patients time to talk about their disorder and the effect it has had on them and their families. False hope should not be given, but encouraging and supporting the patient each day is part of nursing.

Hyperthermia. Patients with an increased leukocyte count usually have many immature white blood cells that are incapable of controlling infections. These patients are closely observed for early signs of decreased resistance to bacterial invasion. Vital signs are monitored every 4 hours or as ordered. Any rise in temperature should be reported to the physician. Acetaminophen to control fever may be ordered; aspirin should be avoided because of its affect on blood clotting mechanisms.

Pain. Joint pain and other symptoms associated with leukocyte infiltration of the central nervous system (eg, headache and confusion) can occur. Analgesics should be given as ordered. Pillows placed behind the back, knees, and other areas that require support may decrease discomfort.

Diarrhea, Impaired Swallowing, Altered Nutrition, Body Image Disturbance. Administration of antineoplastic agents may result in a variety of toxic effects, such as alopecia (loss of hair), nausea, vomiting, diarrhea, excessive bleeding, anorexia, stomatitis (inflammation of oral mucous membranes), and oral ulcerations. Some of these drug effects can be life-threatening, whereas others affect the patient's appearance. Life-threatening toxic drug effects, such as severe vomiting, diarrhea, and bleeding, should be reported to the physician immediately.

Anorexia may be severe. Ulcerations of the oral mucous membranes, nausea, vomiting, and diarrhea reduce the patient's ability to take, retain, and absorb food and fluids. Antiemetics usually are ordered to control nausea and vomiting. The oral mucous membranes should be inspected daily. Good oral care is essential to reduce oral discomfort. If severe, painful ulcerations appear, the physician may order an anesthetic gel that can be applied to or held in the mouth. Small, frequent feedings of bland food (which reduces oral irritation) and frequent sips of cool to cold water may help to maintain fluid and nutrition levels. If the patient is unable to meet and maintain normal food and fluid intake, intravenous fluids may need to be administered. Prolonged episodes of reduced food intake may require total parenteral nutrition (see Chapter 13). Intake and output should be measured, and the physician notified if the output falls below 500 mL/day. The patient should be weighed daily or as ordered, and significant weight loss brought to the attention of the physician.

If severe diarrhea occurs, the patient should be observed for signs of electrolyte imbalance (see Chapter 12). Treatment may be stopped until the mucous membrane of the bowel has had time to recover.

Changes in the hair, skin, and nails may occur during therapy. The most distressing change is alopecia, which may occur suddenly. The patient should be warned by the physician that this may occur. The nurse can advise the patient to consider wearing a cap, scarf, or wig until the hair grows back.

If the platelet count is low, easy bruising and excessive bleeding occur. When discontinuing intravenous therapy and after venipuncture and intramuscular and subcutaneous injections, prolonged pressure should be applied to the needle site. The skin should be inspected for signs of bruising and petechiae. Melena, hematuria, or nosebleeds should be immediately reported to the physician.

Uric acid levels may increase because of massive cell destruction during chemotherapy. The patient should be observed for signs of kidney, ureteral, or bladder stones (see Chapter 53). A high fluid intake should be encouraged to prevent crystallization of uric acid, which leads to stone formation.

Ineffective Individual Coping. The patient and family often experience great difficulty in coping with the diagnosis. The nurse should allow time for them to discuss their feelings, and offer emotional support and encouragement. Referrals to local support groups, the clergy, and various community and social service agencies may be necessary, as many patients and their families face emotional, financial, and spiritual crises during this time.

An atmosphere should be provided so family members can, if they wish, discuss some of their feelings and concerns with the patient, and also a place away from the bedside where the family can talk. At all times, the nurse should show concern and compassion as well as skillful care of the patient.

Potential for Infection. The newly diagnosed patient may have many immature leukocytes that are incapable of fighting infection. The white blood cell count also may drop to dangerously low levels during chemotherapy. The temperature should be monitored every 4 hours and the patient assessed for signs of infection, which may appear in any area or organ of the body. Some indications of an infection are fever, flushing, restlessness, headache, cough, pain in any area of the body, ulcerations in the oral cavity, cloudy urine, diarrhea, rash, increased respirations, and tachycardia.

Knowledge Deficit. The physician discusses with the patient and family the diagnosis, prognosis, and planned treatment modalities. Information regarding treatment should include the length of time treatment will take, results expected, alternatives if results are not as expected, and possible adverse drug reactions. Patients also should understand that every effort will be made to control symptoms associated with chemotherapy. The nurse may need to clarify some of the information given by the physician.

If medication is to be taken at home, the dosage schedule should be thoroughly explained, as patient compliance is essential when toxic drugs are prescribed.

The following information can be included in a patient teaching plan:

1. Frequent examinations of the blood and sometimes the bone marrow are necessary to monitor the results of therapy. (Emphasis should be placed on the importance of these examinations as an aid to staying well rather than on the possible complications from drug therapy.)
2. Precautions should be taken to avoid physical injury.
3. Avoid exposure to people who have an infection such as a head cold.
4. Seek medical care promptly if excessive bleeding or bruising or any symptoms of illness or infection occur.
5. Obtain sufficient rest and eat an adequate diet. These are important in preventing secondary infections.

6. When feeling well, continue usual activities unless the physician instructs otherwise.
7. If sores in the mouth occur, contact the physician as soon as possible. Do not self-treat this problem.
8. Contact the physician immediately if you experience any of the following: severe nausea with prolonged vomiting, severe diarrhea, fever, chills, excessive bleeding or bruising, cough, chest pain, cloudy urine, rash, blood in the stool or urine, severe headache, extreme fatigue, increased respirations or difficulty breathing, and rapid pulse.
9. Follow the recommendations of the physician, which may include tasks such as monitoring the temperature and weight.
10. Keep all clinic or office appointments.

Evaluation

■ Patient increases ability to carry out activities of daily living.
■ Anxiety is reduced
■ Temperature remains normal
■ Pain and discomfort are controlled; patient assumes positions that cause the least amount of discomfort; comfort measures are effective
■ Toxic drug effects are recognized and, when possible, controlled with the administration of prescribed drugs
■ Patient and family discuss their concerns and demonstrate an ability to try and cope with the diagnosis, treatment modalities, and prognosis
■ Patient maintains a positive self-image and verbalizes a desire to use methods to disguise alopecia or other skin changes
■ Patient is free of infection
■ Patient verbalizes understanding of treatment modalities and treatment regimen after discharge and is aware of the toxic reactions that may occur
■ Patient understands importance of continued follow-up care and monitoring of therapy
■ Patient discusses activities or situations to avoid during and after chemotherapy

Agranulocytosis

Agranulocytosis is characterized by decreased production of white blood cells. The most common cause is adverse drug effects. Drugs such as sulfonamides, chloramphenicol, and some tranquilizers have been implicated. Acute viral and bacterial infections also may cause agranulocytosis.

Symptoms

Symptoms include fatigue, fever, chills, headache, and the appearance of ulcers on the mucous membranes of the mouth, throat, nose, rectum, or vagina.

Diagnosis

Diagnosis is made by examination of blood smears to detect the abnormal decrease in agranulocytes. A careful patient history is necessary to determine the cause.

Treatment

Treatment includes removing the causative factor (eg, discontinuing the drug that is producing agranulocytosis). Severe infection usually occurs if the disorder is not detected and treated. Antibiotics are given to control infection. Careful medical aseptic technique is important in preventing the spread of pathogenic microorganisms to the patient, and reverse isolation techniques may be necessary. Ulcerations of body cavities, such as the mouth, rectum, and vagina, may or may not require specific treatment.

Prognosis

The prognosis is related to the cause and severity of the condition. When the cause can be determined and promptly removed, treatment can be started immediately and the patient usually recovers.

NURSING PROCESS —THE PATIENT WHO HAS AGRANULOCYTOSIS

Assessment

Assessment should include a thorough patient history of symptoms as well as the names of all drugs (prescription and nonprescription) used within the past 6 to 12 months. The patient should be made aware of the fact that an accurate drug history is vital in determining the cause of this serious problem. Physical assessment should include the taking of vital signs and an evaluation of the symptoms. For example, if the patient complains of mouth sores, the oral cavity should be examined thoroughly.

Nursing Diagnosis

Depending on the symptoms and the degree of agranulocytosis, one or more of the following nursing diagnoses may apply:

■ Hyperthermia related to infection secondary to agranulocytosis
■ Potential for infection related to agranulocytosis
■ Altered oral mucous membrane related to agranulocytosis
■ Fluid volume deficit related to inability to swallow secondary to ulcerations of the oral mucous membranes
■ Altered nutrition: less than body requirements related to inability to swallow
■ Knowledge deficit of the cause of the disorder and methods to prevent infection until the blood count is normal

Planning and Implementation

The major goals of the patient include an increase in the white blood cell count, normal body temperature, absence of infection, normal food and fluid intake, absence of ulcerations of the mucous membranes, and knowledge of the cause of the disorder and methods to prevent a future occurrence.

The major goals in nursing management are to reduce the symptoms associated with the disorder and prevent infection.

Vital signs should be monitored every 4 hours and the patient observed for early signs of infection.

Hyperthermia, Potential for Infection. Fever may be reduced by the administration of acetaminophen. Reverse isolation may be necessary if the white blood cell count is extremely low. Personnel with any type of infection (eg, bacterial or viral) should not be involved in close patient contact.

Altered Oral Mucous Membrane. The oral cavity should be inspected daily for signs of ulcerations. If ulcerations of the oral mucous membranes are noted, or if the patient complains of a sore mouth or throat, or pain or soreness in the nose, rectum, or vagina, the physician should be notified. Examination of the affected areas by a physician may be necessary.

Fluid Volume Deficit, Altered Nutrition. Fluids should be encouraged, and intake and output should be measured to be sure the patient is taking sufficient fluids. Ulcerations of the oral mucous membranes may be treated with topical anesthetics. Frequent oral hygiene and sips of ice water also may reduce oral discomfort. The diet should consist of soft, bland foods until the oral lesions have healed.

Knowledge Deficit. The patient should be made aware of the drug or other offending agent that has caused the agranulocytosis, and advised to inform all physicians and dentists who treat him or her of the effect the drug has on the white blood cell count so that the drug is not prescribed in the future.

Patients who are discharged before the white blood cell count is completely normal should be advised to avoid exposure to anyone with any type of infection until the blood count is normal. The importance of follow-up blood counts should be emphasized.

Evaluation

- Body temperature is normal
- No signs of infection are present
- Food and fluid intake are normal
- Mucous membranes are intact; soreness or ulcerations are absent
- Patient verbalizes understanding of the cause of the disorder, how a repeat episode is prevented, and the importance of follow-up examinations
- Patient verbalizes importance of avoiding exposure to infection until the blood count is normal

MULTIPLE MYELOMA

Plasma cells arise from B cells (B lymphocytes) and normally are not found in circulating blood. These cells are primarily concerned with antibody synthesis. Multiple myeloma is a malignant disease of plasma cells in which immature plasma cells proliferate in the bone marrow, forming single or multiple osteolytic (bone-destructive) tumors. Later, the neoplastic plasma cells infiltrate the liver, spleen, soft tissues, and kidneys.

Symptoms

The disease develops slowly. The first symptom usually is a vague pain in the pelvis, spine, or ribs. As the disease progresses, the pain may become more severe and localized. As bone marrow is replaced by tumors, pathologic fractures may occur. In addition, the patient may show a decreased resistance to infection and may have anemia caused by bone marrow destruction. Resistance to infection is decreased, probably because of a decrease in antibody formation. Renal calculi and renal failure may be seen.

Diagnosis

Diagnosis is made by skeletal radiographic studies that reveal punched-out bone lesions and bone marrow, and laboratory studies. Urine samples show the presence of M-type globulin (Bence Jones protein).

Treatment

Steroids, melphalan (Alkeran), and cyclophosphamide (Cytoxan) are used to decrease the tumor mass and lessen bone pain. Pain is controlled with analgesics, with the stronger analgesics reserved for the terminal stages of the disease. Radiation may be used to decrease the size of the lesions and relieve bone pain, and allopurinol (Zyloprim) prescribed to prevent uric acid crystallization and subsequent renal calculus formation.

Anemia is treated with blood transfusions, and infections managed with antibiotics. Back braces may be necessary when there is spinal involvement, and body casts (which usually are bivalved) are used when involvement is extensive and pathologic fractures are present.

Prognosis

The prognosis is poor, with an estimated survival of 1 to 3 years.

NURSING PROCESS —THE PATIENT WHO HAS MULTIPLE MYELOMA

Assessment

A history of the patient's symptoms should be obtained, and any areas that are tender or painful should be identified. Vital signs should be taken and the patient weighed. The apparent degree of illness should be evaluated to determine what assistance the patient needs with activities such as bathing, grooming, and ambulation.

Nursing Diagnosis

Depending on the stage (early, late, terminal) of the disorder, one or more of the following nursing diagnoses may apply:

- Pain related to osteolytic bone lesions, pathologic fractures
- Anxiety related to pain, diagnosis, prognosis
- Impaired physical mobility related to disease process
- Self-care deficits: partial (specify) to total related to pain, pathologic fractures, other factors (specify)
- Fluid volume excess related to renal failure, renal calculi
- Potential for infection related to decreased antibody formation
- Knowledge deficit of treatment modalities, home care after discharge

Planning and Implementation

The major goals of the patient include relief of pain, reduction of anxiety, improved physical mobility, improved ability to carry out activities of daily living, prevention of fluid volume excess, absence of infection, and knowledge of treatment modalities and home care.

The major goals of nursing management are to relieve pain and prevent the complications associated with the disorder.

Vital signs should be monitored every 4 hours, and the patient frequently assessed for signs of infection, excessive fatigue, or pain in a new area, all of which should be reported to the physician.

Pain. Pain is relieved with analgesics and by the patient's being able to maintain a position of comfort. Prescribed comfort measures include a back brace or bivalve cast.

The bivalve cast may be used in the terminal stages of the disease, when even the slightest injury can result in a pathologic fracture, which in turn increases pain. This type of cast is a full body cast that has been made and then cut along all the lateral aspects of the cast. Only one half of the cast—the part under the patient—is used at any one time. The patient should be turned every 2 hours, and the only possible body positions are supine and prone. When the patient is to be turned, one half of the cast is applied on top and fastened (with buckles or Velcro tape) to the bottom, and the patient turned to the next position. Then the top part of the cast is removed, and reapplied when it is time to turn the patient again. Two or more persons are needed to turn a patient in a bivalve cast.

In the terminal stage of the disease, the pain often is severe, and narcotic analgesics may be required at frequent intervals.

Anxiety. Although most of these patients are middle aged or older, they still have plans for the future, and may require time to express their doubts and concerns over their disease and its prognosis. The nurse should allow the patient time to verbalize anxieties and concerns. The nurse may discuss the patient's concerns with the physician, as a referral to an appropriate agency or group may be necessary.

Impaired Physical Mobility. The patient should be encouraged and assisted to ambulate because it is an important part of therapy. Immobilization can worsen osteoporosis (loss of calcium from the bone), which can lead to hypercalcemia and hypercalciuria (excess of calcium in the urine).

Any injury, no matter how slight, may result in a pathologic fracture. The patient should be instructed to take care when walking about and to obtain assistance as needed.

Self-Care Deficits. Depending on the degree and stage of illness, these patients may require some or complete assistance with their activities of daily living. Because some of these patients may experience a great deal of pain, any necessary activities should be carried out when an administered analgesic has reached its peak and the patient is experiencing the most relief from pain.

Fluid Volume Excess. An increase in fluid intake may prevent renal damage from hypercalcemia and the precipitation of protein in the renal tubules. *Ambulation and adequate hydration are important and should be stressed* during the hospital stay as well as when the patient is preparing for discharge.

Intake and output should be measured, and the physician informed if the output falls below 500 mL/day. The patient also is observed for signs of calculus formation in the kidney, ureters, or bladder (see Chapter 53) and weighed daily or as ordered. Any marked gain in weight should be reported to the physician.

Potential for Infection. The patient should be closely observed for early signs of infection, such as fever, chills, sore throat, and cough. The physician should be informed if early signs of infection occur, as immediate antibiotic therapy may be necessary.

Knowledge Deficit. Before discharge from the hospital, the patient should become thoroughly familiar with the treatment regimen. The drugs and their purpose, dose, adverse effects, and dosage schedule should be reviewed. It also is important to stress the need to avoid exposure to infections and injury. The importance of increasing fluid intake should be stressed. The patient should be instructed to contact the physician as soon as possible if chills, fever, increased pain, pain in a new area, decrease in urine output, concentrated urine, sore throat, cough, or adverse drug effects occur.

Evaluation

- Pain is relieved or eliminated
- Anxiety is reduced
- Patient increases ambulatory activities
- Patient is able to assume more self-care duties
- Normal fluid intake is attained and maintained
- Evidence of infection is absent
- Evidence of injury or fractures caused by injury are absent
- Patient verbalizes understanding of drug therapy regimen
- Patient understands importance of avoiding infections and injury

BLEEDING DISORDERS
Thrombocytopenia

Thrombocytopenia is characterized by a deficient number of platelets circulating in the blood. This phenomenon may occur when there is a decrease in platelet manufacture by the bone marrow, or when there is an increase in platelet destruction by the spleen. Some of the causes of thrombocytopenia are leukemia, severe infections, and certain drugs. *Idiopathic thrombocytopenia* is thrombocytopenia without a known cause.

Symptoms

Thrombocytopenia is evidenced externally by the appearance of purpura—small hemorrhages in the skin, mucous membranes, or subcutaneous tissues. Bleeding from other parts of the body, such as the nose, oral mucous membrane, and the gastrointestinal tract, also

may be seen. Thrombocytopenia may cause internal hemorrhage as well, which can be severe and even fatal.

Diagnosis

Diagnosis is based on symptoms, a platelet count, bleeding and clotting times, and a thorough patient history. In some instances, bone marrow aspiration is performed. If thrombocytopenia has been induced by drugs or other substances, a thorough patient history may reveal the cause.

Treatment

When possible, the cause of thrombocytopenia should be removed or treated. Corticosteroids may provide symptomatic relief until the platelet count is normal. Transfusion of platelets or whole blood may be necessary to supply additional platelets in a hemorrhagic emergency. If the patient does not recover spontaneously, splenectomy (removal of the spleen) may be performed. This operation is useful because the spleen (for reasons not fully understood) may be destroying too many platelets. The removal of the spleen often results in a rise in the platelet count and relief of symptoms.

Prognosis

Patients with idiopathic thrombocytopenia may recover spontaneously. Those in whom the cause of thrombocytopenia is known have a variable prognosis; if the cause can be removed or treated, prognosis usually is good. Those who have thrombocytopenia in conjunction with illnesses such as leukemia have a poor prognosis.

Hemophilia

Hemophilia is a hereditary clotting factor disorder characterized by a prolonged coagulation time, which results in persistent and sometimes severe bleeding. It occurs because of an absence of the antihemophilic factor normally present in blood plasma. The disorder is transmitted from mother to son as an X-linked recessive characteristic. Although women seldom develop the disease, they can inherit the trait, which, when passed on to a son, results in hemophilia.

Symptoms

Hemophilia occurs with varying degrees of severity. Mild forms may go unrecognized for years, until unusual bleeding is noted after an injury. Bleeding usually is noted in infancy and childhood. There is persistent oozing of blood after slight injuries, such as a pin prick or a tiny cut. Bleeding often occurs into joints, eventually damaging the joint and leading to deformity and limitation of motion. Relatively minor surgical procedures, such as tooth extraction, carry considerable risk and should be performed in a hospital.

Diagnosis

Diagnosis is based on the patient's history of symptoms, and laboratory tests such as a coagulant factor assay.

Treatment

Transfusions usually are necessary even when minor surgery is performed. Treatment also includes transfusions of fresh blood, frozen plasma, antihemophilic factor (for classic hemophilia A), antiinhibitor coagulant complex, factor IX complex, and the application of thrombin to the bleeding area. Other measures used to help control bleeding are direct pressure over the site of bleeding and the use of cold compresses or ice packs.

Prognosis

Life expectancy is considerably shortened by the disease; many patients do not reach adulthood. On the other hand, those with mild hemophilia may lead full and productive lives despite the illness.

NURSING PROCESS —THE PATIENT WHO HAS A BLEEDING DISORDER

Assessment

A thorough medical, drug, and allergy history is essential. Included in the history are any current symptoms and treatment for the bleeding disorder. The patient should be questioned regarding bleeding episodes (eg, when the last episode occurred, where it occurred [mouth, rectum, skin, and so forth], how long it lasted, and what treatments, if any, were necessary).

The skin should be inspected for purpura or hemorrhagic areas. Before the blood pressure is taken, the patient should be asked if the use of a blood pressure cuff ever produced bleeding under the skin or in the joints of the arm. The temperature should be taken orally, as insertion of a rectal thermometer may cause rectal bleeding.

Nursing Diagnosis

Depending on the type and severity of the bleeding disorder, one or more of the following nursing diagnoses may apply:

- Anxiety related to fear of uncontrolled hemorrhage
- Self-care deficits related to bleeding episodes

- Pain related to bleeding into joints and soft tissues
- Activity intolerance related to excessive bleeding, pain, discomfort
- Impaired tissue integrity related to bleeding episodes secondary to thrombocytopenia or lack of clotting factors
- Altered oral mucous membrane related to coarse foods, poor dental and improper oral hygiene
- Knowledge deficit of ways to prevent future bleeding episodes

Planning and Management

The major goals of the patient include control of bleeding episodes, reduction of anxiety, reduction of pain or discomfort, increased activity tolerance, prevention of injury to oral mucous membranes, prevention of tissue injury, and an understanding of ways to prevent further bleeding episodes.

The major goals of nursing management are to avoid tasks that may induce bleeding, reduce pain and discomfort associated with bleeding episodes, and help the patient evaluate daily tasks and ways of preventing future bleeding episodes.

Vital signs should be taken every 4 to 8 hours, and any change reported to the physician. Fever, increased pain in an area, rise in pulse rate, and decreased blood pressure may be early warning signs of internal bleeding. The urine and stools should be checked for overt signs of bleeding.

When transfusion of products such as whole blood, plasma, and antihemophilic factor are required for bleeding episodes, the patient should be closely observed for signs that bleeding has been controlled. The physician should be kept informed of the patient's progress, or lack of progress, as additional treatment modalities may be necessary.

If the patient with a bleeding disorder requires surgery or a dental procedure, close observation is required during and after the procedure. Those with hemophilia require special preparations for surgery or dental procedures, which are ordered by the physician and based on the patient's need for specific clotting factors.

Self-Care Deficit, Activity Intolerance. If bleeding episodes occur or anemia is present, patient assistance may be required for activities such as bathing, grooming, and ambulating. Tasks that may cause bleeding should be avoided whenever possible, and care should be taken to prevent excessive bleeding.

Impaired Tissue Integrity. The skin should be inspected daily or more often for the presence of new ecchymotic lesions. Old areas of ecchymosis should be checked for evidence of new or more extensive bleeding. Internal hemorrhage in the gastrointestinal tract may be evidenced by blood in the stool or vomitus that is bright red or has a coffee-ground appearance. Although epistaxis, vaginal bleeding, and bleeding from the mouth or gums are signs of external bleeding, there may be bleeding in other internal organs or structures that initially produces only vague symptoms.

The nurse should be alert to *any* complaint the patient may have (eg, abdominal discomfort or back pain) and report these findings to the physician promptly.

The patient should be be protected from even the slightest injury because extensive bleeding can occur with mild trauma. Intramuscular injections should be avoided whenever possible; however, if this route of administration is necessary, prolonged pressure should be exerted on the injection site. Venipuncture sites also require prolonged pressure on the vein after the needle is removed. Rectal temperatures and rectal drugs should be avoided because insertion can cause rectal bleeding.

Pain. Pain caused by bleeding into soft tissues and joints may be decreased by the use of pillows or other comfort measures. Analgesics, when ordered, should be administered as needed. The use of aspirin should be avoided, as this drug can increase bleeding tendencies. The nurse should carefully assess the patient's pain before administering an analgesic, as pain in a different area, such as the abdomen or chest, may indicate internal bleeding.

Altered Oral Mucous Membrane. The mucous membranes of the mouth may easily bleed. A soft diet may be necessary to decrease the chance of injury to the oral mucosa. Oral care with cotton swabs is necessary if use of a soft toothbrush causes bleeding. Oral rinses should be offered between and after meals.

Anxiety, Knowledge Deficit. Treatment modalities should be explained to the patient and family. In addition, anxiety may be reduced by a thorough explanation of how to prevent injury, which may result in bleeding episodes.

These patients should understand that they must anticipate each activity as one that may result in a bleeding episode and then plan to alter or avoid the activity. For example, shaving with a safety razor (which can produce minor skin cuts and abrasions) should be avoided; instead, an electric razor should be used. One method of helping these patients find ways to prevent injury is to have them list some of the activities that often are performed (eg, repairing the car, mowing the lawn, cutting up vegetables, and housework). Each activity should then be discussed

with regards to the need to perform the activity, if the activity can be done by someone else, and what steps may be taken to reduce or eliminate the possibility of injury.

Evaluation

- Anxiety is reduced
- Patient increases ability to perform own activities of daily living as bleeding episodes are controlled
- Bleeding episodes are controlled or eliminated
- Pain is reduced or eliminated
- Oral mucous membranes remain intact with no evidence of bleeding
- Patient demonstrates understanding of treatment modalities
- Patient is able to think through and plan activities that are less likely to result in injury and bleeding

BONE MARROW FAILURE

Aplastic anemia describes a condition in which bone marrow activity is depressed, and erythrocytes, leukocytes, and platelets are not produced in adequate numbers. It is a serious toxic manifestation of certain drugs, such as streptomycin, chloramphenicol (Chloromycetin), and mechlorethamine, as well as exposure to toxic chemicals and radiation. This condition also occurs without a known cause.

Aplastic anemia may be intentionally produced in patients with leukemia who are scheduled for bone marrow transplantation. Whole-body radiation is used to destroy malignant cells before bone marrow transplantation.

Symptoms

Major clinical signs of aplastic anemia are severe anemia, leukopenia, and thrombocytopenia. Symptoms include fatigue, weakness, exertional dyspnea, lowered resistance to infection, and a tendency toward bleeding.

Diagnosis

Diagnosis is made by a thorough patient history, general hematologic laboratory tests, and bone marrow biopsy.

Treatment

The objectives of treatment are to supply the elements missing in the blood and to prevent or treat infection or bleeding, in the hope that the patient will recover the ability to produce blood cells. The causative agent, if it is known, is removed.

Transfusions are given to supply erythrocytes, platelets, leukocytes, and hemoglobin. Antibiotics are administered to prevent or treat infection. High doses of corticosteroids also may be given. In some instances, withdrawal of the causative agent (when known) allows the bone marrow to regenerate and assume normal function. In patients with severe aplastic anemia, withdrawal of the causative agent may not produce results. In these cases, bone marrow transplantation is considered if a matching donor can be found.

Prognosis

Patients with aplastic anemia are very ill, and the death rate is high. If the bone marrow has been so damaged that recovery is impossible, death will result. Although false hope should not be given, the patient and family may be told by the physician that in some cases regeneration of the bone marrow is possible.

NURSING PROCESS —THE PATIENT WHO HAS BONE MARROW FAILURE

Assessment

Because bone marrow failure results in decreased production of all blood cells, the patient should be assessed for signs of severe anemia, infection, and bleeding tendencies. A general physical assessment should be performed to determine the overt effects of the disorder and the apparent severity of symptoms.

Nursing Diagnosis

Depending on the severity of aplastic anemia, one or more of the following nursing diagnoses may apply:

- Anxiety, fear related to severity of symptoms, treatment modalities, prognosis
- Activity intolerance related to severe anemia
- Ineffective individual coping related to the severity of symptoms, prognosis
- Hopelessness related to prognosis, failure of treatment
- Potential for infection related to leukopenia
- Altered oral mucous membrane related to tissue hypoxia secondary to anemia, thrombocytopenia, and leukopenia
- Altered nutrition: less than body requirements owing to fatigue, ulceration of oral mucous membranes
- Potential impaired skin integrity related to tissue hypoxia secondary to anemia, thrombocytopenia, leukopenia, and decreased activity intolerance
- Knowledge deficit of treatment modalities, home care

Planning and Implementation

The major goals of the patient include reduction of anxiety, increase in activity tolerance, effective coping mechanisms, absence of infection, improved nutrition, prevention of skin breakdown, and under-

standing of treatment modalities. If the patient is terminal and all medical efforts are failing, some of these goals may be unrealistic.

The main goals of nursing management are to prevent complications associated with aplastic anemia and help the patient and family cope with the seriousness of the disorder.

The patient with aplastic anemia usually is acutely ill. Once the diagnosis is established, treatment is planned. Because treatment also includes the prevention of severe hypoxia (owing to anemia), bleeding or hemorrhage (owing to thrombocytopenia), and infection (owing to leukopenia), preventive measures are begun immediately.

The skin, stools, urine, oral cavity, and intravenous line sites should be frequently assessed for evidence of bleeding and infection. Vital signs should be monitored every 4 hours. Rectal temperatures should be avoided, since bleeding may occur because of trauma to the rectal mucosa. Small-gauge needles should be used for injections, and pressure applied to the puncture site for 5 minutes. The patient's color and respiratory rate should be closely monitored. Oxygen administration may be necessary if cyanosis occurs or the respiratory rate rises.

Anxiety, Fear, Ineffective Individual Coping. The patient may know the seriousness of the disorder as well as the prognosis. The nurse may reduce anxiety by explaining the importance of treatment modalities (eg, reverse isolation) and offering emotional support to the patient and family. Allowing the patient time to express fears and concerns also may reduce anxiety and help the patient and family to cope with this disorder and its grave prognosis.

Activity Intolerance. Most of these patients are extremely weak because of severe anemia. Their needs should be identified and met. Total physical care or adequate rest periods between tasks often are necessary.

Hopelessness. Treatment may not be successful and bone marrow transplantation not possible because a donor match is not located or the patient is not a candidate for the procedure for any number of reasons. At times, all the nurse can do is listen and offer emotional support.

Potential for Infection. In treating the condition, every effort should be made to prevent infection. Reverse isolation may be ordered. If the white blood cell count falls extremely low, special isolation procedures, such as the use of a laminar airflow room, may be necessary.

The patient should be continually assessed for early symptoms of infection, such as chills, fever, sore throat, and cough. The presence of any of these should be reported to the physician immediately. Tasks that may cause injury to the skin, such as the removal of tape around an infusion site, should be avoided whenever possible, as these may become sites of infection. Good skin care is essential, as decubitus formation must be prevented.

Altered Oral Mucous Membrane.   Good (and gentle) oral care is essential to prevent oral lesions. The physician should be informed if severe stomatitis develops.

Altered Nutrition.   Food, between-meal supplements, and liquids should be offered throughout the waking hours. Liquids should be cool to room temperature, and hot, spicy, or coarse foods should be avoided. Small amounts of soft, bland foods offered at frequent intervals may be more easily taken. High-potency vitamin and protein supplements may be offered between meals. Intake and output should be measured, and an estimate of the amount of food eaten should be recorded.

Potential Impaired Skin Integrity.   Inactivity, general discomfort, fever, decreased protein intake, and other factors may lead to skin breakdown. The patient's position should be changed every 1 to 2 hours, and movement of the extremities encouraged. The skin over bony prominences should be inspected for early signs of decubitus formation as well as for abrasions and other breaks in the skin. Depending on the type of tissue injury, various nursing measures as well as application of prescribed ointments may be tried.

Knowledge Deficit.   The importance and method of treatment modalities should be fully explained to the patient. Some forms of isolation—for example a laminar air flow room—may be frightening; therefore, the area should be explained and described before the patient is placed in the special room.

Depending on the success of treatment, the patient and family should be informed of the prescribed home care and follow-up monitoring of the disorder. The nurse should obtain from the physician a list of prescribed medications as well as recommendations for home care. If the disorder was caused by a drug or a toxic chemical, the importance of avoiding these agents should be discussed with the patient and family.

Evaluation

- Anxiety is reduced
- Patient tolerates an increase in activities
- Patient and family discuss their fears and anxieties and possible fatal outcome of the disorder
- Infection is controlled; situations that may result in an infectious process are eliminated whenever possible
- Respiratory rate improves and approaches normal with no evidence of cyanosis
- Oral mucous membranes are intact with no evidence of bleeding or ulceration
- Normal food and fluid intake are attained and maintained
- Skin remains intact
- Patient verbalizes understanding of medication regimen and home care

General Nutritional Considerations

☐ Patients with iron deficiency anemia should be given a list of foods high in iron.

☐ Animal proteins, such as meat, milk, eggs, and cheese, contain vitamin B_{12}, and even a small daily intake of these foods ensures an adequate supply of this vitamin.

☐ Patients with a blood dyscrasia also may be anorexic. A list of the patient's food preferences should be given to the dietitian. If the patient still eats poorly, a dietary consult may be needed.

☐ A soft, bland diet is better tolerated by those with ulcerations of the oral mucous membranes.

☐ Patients who have nausea and vomiting should be offered clear liquids at frequent intervals. Once they are able to eat, a small amount of soft, bland food should be offered.

General Pharmacologic Considerations

☐ The importance of lifelong administration of vitamin B_{12} should be stressed to patients with pernicious anemia.

□ Oral iron preparations should be taken on an empty stomach. If gastric distress occurs, they can be taken with food or after meals.

□ Because some drugs (eg, antacids, tetracyclines, and vitamin C) interact with oral iron, the patient should consult the physician before taking other drugs.

□ The absorption of oral iron is decreased when the drug is taken with coffee, tea, eggs, or milk.

□ Antineoplastic agents have many serious adverse effects. The nurse should be thoroughly familiar with the dose, administration, and adverse effects to accurately administer these drugs and competently assess the patient for untoward reactions.

□ Patients who receive drugs that are capable of causing bone marrow depression should have their blood tested every 1 to 4 weeks.

General Gerontologic Considerations

□ Elderly patients who are receiving chemotherapy for leukemia should be given a detailed explanation of the drug regimen when an oral antineoplastic agent is prescribed on an outpatient basis. These patients may forget to take the medicine or take more than the prescribed amount. Instruction is important because most of the drugs used are extremely toxic, and adherence to the prescribed regimen is essential.

□ Anemia caused by a dietary iron deficiency may be seen in elderly patients. They may require a thorough evaluation of their dietary habits and education in the methods of treating iron deficiency anemia.

Suggested Readings

□ Berkow R, Fletcher AJ (eds). Merck manual of diagnosis and therapy. 15th ed. Rahway, NJ: Merck & Co, 1987. *(In-depth coverage of subject matter)*

□ Bowers AC, Thompson JM. Clinical manual of health assessment. 3rd ed. St Louis: CV Mosby, 1988. *(In-depth coverage of subject matter)*

□ Brown S. Behind the numbers on the CBC. RN February 1990;53:46. *(Additional coverage of subject matter)*

□ Brunner LS, Suddarth DS. Textbook of medical-surgical nursing. 6th ed. Philadelphia: JB Lippincott, 1988. *(Additional and in-depth coverage of subject matter)*

□ Caine RM, Buffalino PM (eds). Nursing care planning guides for adults. Baltimore: Williams & Wilkins, 1987. *(Additional coverage of subject matter)*

□ Farrant C. Multiple myeloma: controlling pain, prolonging survival. RN January 1987;50:38. *(Additional coverage of subject matter)*

□ Fischbach FT. A manual of laboratory diagnostic tests. 3rd ed. Philadelphia: JB Lippincott, 1988. *(Additional coverage of subject matter)*

□ Froberg JH. The anemias: causes and courses of action (Part I). RN January 1989;52:24. *(Additional coverage of subject matter)*

□ Froberg JH. The anemias: causes and courses of action (Part II). RN March 1989;52:52. *(Additional coverage of subject matter)*

□ Konradi D, Stockert P. A closeup look at leukemia. Nursing '89, June 1989;19:34. *(Additional coverage of subject matter)*

□ Moeller LL, Swartzendruber EJ. Suppressing the risks of bone marrow suppression. Nursing '87, March 1987;17:52. *(Additional coverage of subject matter)*

□ Simonson GM. Caring for patients with acute myelocytic leukemia. Am J Nurs March 1988; 88:304. *(Additional coverage of subject matter)*

□ Wallach JB. Interpretation of diagnostic tests: a handbook synopsis of laboratory medicine. Boston: Little, Brown & Co, 1986. *(In-depth, high-level coverage of subject matter)*

Chapter 34

Disorders of the Lymphatics

On completion of this chapter the reader will:

■ Discuss the symptoms, diagnosis, and treatment of lymphedema and elephantiasis

■ Discuss the symptoms, diagnosis, and treatment of lymphangitis and lymphadenitis

■ Discuss the symptoms, diagnosis, and treatment of infectious mononucleosis

■ Use the nursing process in the management of the patient with an occlusive, infectious, or inflammatory disorder of the lymphatics

■ Discuss the symptoms, diagnosis, and treatment of Hodgkin's and non-Hodgkin's lymphoma

■ Use the nursing process in the management of the patient with a malignant disorder of the lymphatics

OCCLUSIVE, INFLAMMATORY, AND INFECTIOUS DISORDERS
Lymphedema and Elephantiasis

Lymph is similar in composition to tissue fluid and plasma. A system of vessels called *lymphatics* carries tissue fluid from body tissues to the veins. An obstruction of lymph vessels causes accumulation of tissue fluid in the affected part. Edema (often massive) occurs, resulting in deformity and poor nutrition of tissues. This condition is called *lymphedema*. Lymphedema usually occurs in the legs but also may occur in other areas, such as the arms and genitalia. Lymphedema of the arm may be seen in patients who have had a radical mastectomy. Burns and excessive radiation may damage the lymphatics, which results in obstruction of lymph channels and, thus, lymphedema. Carcinoma often spreads by way of the lymph channels. The lymphatics often are damaged either by the cancer or by extensive surgery or radiation therapy.

Some children are born with inadequate lymph channels, although the edema may not manifest itself until puberty. Lymphedema also can follow repeated bouts of phlebitis and supervening streptococcal infection. With each attack, more permanent scar tissue accumulates, occlusion occurs, and fluid becomes trapped in small, "fibrous" lakes.

Elephantiasis is the invasion and obstruction of lymph channels by filarial worms, resulting in lymphedema. This disorder is seen primarily in the tropics.

Symptoms

Symptoms include enlargement owing to edema of the affected part, and tight, shiny skin. Sometimes the skin becomes thickened, rough, and discolored. Because tissue nutrition is impaired, ulcers and infection are common.

Diagnosis

Diagnosis is made by inspection of the involved area.

Treatment

Treatment consists in removing the cause, if possible. Rest, prevention of reinfection, and drug therapy (eg, diuretics) may be used. Sometimes the obstruction of lymphatics caused by such injuries as burns can be corrected by surgery.

Mild cases of lymphedema may respond to symptomatic treatment. The affected part is elevated at intervals to promote lymphatic drainage. An elastic stocking is worn when the part is dependent. Massage, starting at the toes or the fingers and moving toward the body, may be helpful. A mechanical pulsating air-pressure device can be applied to the extremity at prescribed intervals. The alternating filling and emptying "milk" the lymph upward. In some cases, treatment is ineffective and the lymphedema persists.

Lymphangitis and Lymphadenitis

Lymphangitis, or inflammation of lymph channels, may occur as a result of infection in an extremity by such microorganisms as the streptococci. When the lymph nodes near the lymph channels also are affected, this is called *lymphadenitis.*

Symptoms

Symptoms include red streaks that follow the course of the lymph channels and extend up the arm or leg. Fever also may be present. When lymphadenitis is present, the lymph nodes along the lymphatic channels are enlarged and tender on palpation.

Diagnosis

Diagnosis is made by visual inspection as well as palpation of lymph nodes in the affected area.

Treatment

Treatment consists of antibiotic therapy.

Infectious Mononucleosis

Infectious mononucleosis is caused by the Epstein-Barr virus. It affects lymphoid tissues as well as other organs, such as the spleen. This disorder most commonly affects young adults, especially those confined to close living quarters, such as in the armed services and college dormitories.

Symptoms

Fatigue, fever, sore throat, headache, muscle soreness, and cervical lymph node enlargement are common.

Diagnosis

Diagnosis is based on the patient's symptoms as well as laboratory studies such as white blood cell count and differential (which demonstrate many atypical lymphocytes), heterophil agglutination tests, slide agglutination test (Monospot test), and Epstein-Barr virus antibody test.

Treatment

The infection usually is self-limiting. Bed rest, analgesic and antipyretic agents, and extra fluids are recommended. A corticosteroid may be prescribed if complications, such as hepatic involvement or severe anemia, occur.

NURSING PROCESS —THE PATIENT WHO HAS AN OCCLUSIVE, INFLAMMATORY, OR INFECTIOUS DISORDER OF THE LYMPHATICS

Assessment

Vital signs should be taken if lymphangitis or lymphadenitis is present. The affected area should be examined for the extent of inflammation or edema and gently palpated for the presence of lymph nodes. If edema is present, the size of one or both of the affected extremities should be measured. If only one extremity is involved, the measurement is compared with that of the opposite extremity.

Nursing Diagnosis

The nursing diagnoses depend on the type, cause, and extent of the disorder, and one or more of following may apply:

- Anxiety caused by disfigurement (lymphedema of an extremity)
- Ineffective individual coping related to disfigurement
- Knowledge deficit of methods to reduce enlargement of the extremities (lymphedema), treatment modalities

Planning and Implementation

The major goals of the patient include reduction of anxiety, learning to cope with disfigurement (lymphedema), and an understanding of the prescribed treatment modalities.

The major goals of nursing management are to decrease discomfort, lessen anxiety, and reduce or eliminate symptoms associated with the disorder.

When the patient has lymphangitis or lymphadenitis, the area should be inspected two to three times per day and the response to antibiotic therapy noted. If the affected area appears to enlarge, additional lymph nodes become involved, or the temperature remains elevated, the physician should be notified. The patient should be encouraged to move and exercise the affected extremity to enhance the flow of lymph from the affected area.

Anxiety, Ineffective Individual Coping. When lymphedema responds poorly to therapy, the patient may have difficulty with social interactions. The nurse can help the patient find ways to disguise the abnormal enlargement of an extremity by suggesting the wearing of certain types of clothing. For women, long-sleeved dresses may hide lymphedema of the arms, and slacks may be worn to hide the legs. Men may need to avoid wearing shorts and short-sleeved shirts.

Knowledge Deficit. If treatment is to be carried out at home, the medication schedule or other treatments prescribed or recommended by the physician should be explained to the patient.

The patient with lymphedema may require instruction in the use of the mechanical, pulsating air-pressure device or the application of elastic stockings.

Evaluation

■ Anxiety is reduced
■ Patient demonstrates understanding of home care, use of devices to reduce lymphedema

MALIGNANT DISORDERS OF THE LYMPHATICS
Hodgkin's Disease

Hodgkin's disease is characterized by the painless enlargement of the lymph nodes. The cervical nodes usually are involved first; inguinal and axillary nodes may be affected later.

The cause of Hodgkin's disease is unknown. The disease is more common in men than in women, and most frequently occurs during young adulthood.

Symptoms

Early symptoms of Hodgkin's disease include the painless enlargement of one or several lymph nodes. As the nodes enlarge, they often press on adjacent structures, such as the esophagus or bronchi. Enlarged retroperitoneal nodes can cause a sense of fullness in the stomach and epigastric pain. Marked weight loss, anorexia, fatigue, and weakness occur. Chills and fever are common. Sometimes the patient develops marked anemia and thrombocytopenia, which results in a tendency to bleed. The resistance to infection is poor, and staphylococcal infections of the skin and respiratory tract infections often complicate the illness. Pruritus is a common symptom.

Diagnosis

The diagnosis is established by a biopsy of an affected lymph node. The pathologist notes the changes that are typical of Hodgkin's disease, including the presence of a particular type of abnormal cell (Reed-Sternberg cell). Additional diagnostic tests include chest radiography, bone scan, and lymphangiography. After diagnosis, the disease is staged, ranging from Stage I to Stage IV. Staging is based on the number of lymph nodes positive for Hodgkin's as well as involvement of

other organs and structures, such as bone marrow, lungs, and gastrointestinal system.

Treatment

Treatment includes radiation therapy, corticosteroids, and antineoplastic drugs. Antibiotics are given to fight secondary infections. Transfusions may be necessary to control anemia.

The involved lymph nodes may be subjected to intensive radiation therapy to reduce their size. Although irradiation of a node may be followed by remission, the disease may return and continue its progressive course.

Complications include a decreased resistance to infections, respiratory distress owing to enlargement of mediastinal lymph nodes and anemia, anorexia, gastrointestinal symptoms, and weight loss.

Prognosis

Some patients survive 10 or more years; others succumb in 4 or 5 years. Patients whose disease is localized to one section of the body may be cured with current treatment methods. Patients who receive treatment usually have remissions that last for months or even years. Symptoms may recur, however, and may cause death from respiratory obstruction, cachexia, or secondary infections.

Non-Hodgkin's Lymphomas

Non-Hodgkin's lymphomas are a group of malignant diseases that originate in lymph glands and other lymphoid tissue. Included in this group are lymphosarcoma, Burkitt's lymphoma, and reticulum cell sarcoma. These lymphomas are relatively rare in the United States.

Symptoms

Symptoms depend on the site of lymph node involvement. Lymph node enlargement, which usually is diffuse rather than localized, typically occurs in cervical, axillary, and inguinal regions.

Diagnosis

Diagnosis is made by lymph node biopsy.

Treatment

Treatment includes corticosteroids, radiation therapy, and chemotherapy with agents such as chlorambucil (Leukeran), vincristine (Oncovin), and doxorubicin (Adriamycin).

Prognosis

It is questionable whether patients are ever cured of Hodgkin's or non-Hodgkin's lymphomas. It is likely that even patients who experience long remissions eventually succumb to the disease.

NURSING PROCESS —THE PATIENT WHO HAS A MALIGNANT DISORDER OF THE LYMPHATICS

Assessment

A thorough patient history should be taken, including all symptoms and the length of time they have been present. Vital signs and weight also should be taken. A general physical appraisal and examination should be performed to detect any problems associated with the type of neoplastic disease, such as marked weight loss, bleeding tendencies, and skin infections.

Nursing Diagnosis

Some patients may be acutely ill or in a terminal stage of the disease, and require more intensive nursing management. Depending on the severity or stage of the disorder, one or more of the following nursing diagnoses may apply:

- Anxiety related to diagnosis, diagnostic tests, treatment modalities, prognosis
- Ineffective individual coping related to diagnosis, treatment modalities, prognosis
- Potential for infection related to decreased resistance to infection
- Altered nutrition: less than body requirements related to abdominal and gastrointestinal involvement and chemotherapy
- Impaired skin integrity related to pruritus, thrombocytopenia, radiation therapy
- Altered oral mucous membrane related to administration of antineoplastic drugs
- Ineffective airway clearance related to enlarged mediastinal node
- Self-care deficits related to anemia
- Knowledge deficit of treatment modalities, home care

Planning and Implementation

The major goals of the patient include reduction of anxiety, improved nutrition, absence of infection, improved coping mechanisms, absence of skin or oral mucous membrane lesions, effective airway clearance, increased ability to assume responsibility for activities of daily living, and an understanding of treatment modalities and home care.

The major goals of nursing management are to recognize and prevent or decrease complications associated with these disorders, and to help the patient and family cope with the seriousness of the diagnosis and necessary treatments.

Anxiety. The patient's level of anxiety should be assessed. When possible, the causes of anxiety should be identified and a plan developed to reduce or eliminate this emotional response. The patient should be allowed time to express concerns and ask questions. The nurse, by being a good listener, often can reduce the anxiety that occurs during the illness or prolonged schedule of antineoplastic treatments.

Ineffective Individual Coping. Because of many factors, the patient and family may find it difficult to cope with a malignant disorder. Families require time to deal with such a disorder, especially when it affects a young adult. The nurse should allow time for questions as well as attempt to determine existing problems. Once the problems are identified, possible solutions can be formulated.

Potential for Infection. Vital signs should be monitored every 4 hours, and the patient frequently assessed for early signs of infection, especially if leukopenia is present. Severe leukopenia may require reverse isolation procedures.

Altered Nutrition. Radiation therapy and chemotherapy may produce many distressing side effects, such as diarrhea, nausea, and vomiting. A soft, bland diet served in small portions four to six times per day is better tolerated than three large meals. The patient should be weighed daily. Severe vomiting and diarrhea and progressive weight loss should be brought to the attention of the physician.

The patient should be encouraged to eat as well as drink extra fluids. If the fluid intake appears low, intake and output should be measured. Failure to eat food or drink fluids should be brought to the physician's attention, as intravenous fluids or total parenteral nutrition may be necessary.

Impaired Skin Integrity. The condition of the skin should be assessed every 8 hours. If radiation therapy is being given, the irradiated area should be inspected for signs of redness or other skin changes. Good skin care is essential, especially if the patient is on bed rest. Itching (pruritus) may be relieved by cool sponge baths. When severe, the physician may order an oral or topical medication to relieve itching.

Altered Oral Mucous Membrane. Oral care should be given after each meal or interval feeding. The oral mucous membranes should be assessed during oral care. Painful ulcerations should be brought to the physician's attention, as a topical anesthetic may be necessary.

Ineffective Airway Clearance. When the mediastinal nodes are enlarged, the patient may have difficulty coughing and raising secretions. The respiratory rate should be assessed every 2 to 4 hours. The breathing pattern may be improved if the patient assumes a sitting position. Oxygen should be administered if respiratory distress or cyanosis is apparent.

Self-Care Deficits. Depending on the patient's condition, assistance may be needed with all or some self-care activities. Rest periods between activities may lessen fatigue.

Knowledge Deficit. All procedures and treatments should be explained, and the patient and family allowed time to ask questions. In preparation for discharge, continued treatment modalities are thoroughly explained and the patient is encouraged to resume normal activities as tolerated. The importance of avoiding exposure to infection, eating a well-balanced diet, and increasing fluid intake is emphasized. The patient should be informed that symptoms such as fever, cough, severe malaise, and the appearance of new enlarged lymph nodes require immediate medical attention.

Evaluation

- Anxiety is reduced
- Patient and family identify and attempt to solve problems related to diagnosis, treatment regimen, prognosis
- Signs of infection are absent; vital signs are normal
- Patient eats a balanced diet, maintains weight, and drinks extra fluids
- Skin remains intact with no evidence of bleeding, infection, or breakdown
- Oral mucous membranes are normal in appearance
- Breathing pattern is normal; patient coughs, deep-breathes at regular intervals
- Patient assumes role in or takes complete responsibility for own care; increases activities without excessive fatigue or dyspnea
- Patient verbalizes understanding of treatment modalities, home care, situations to avoid, and importance of continued follow-up care

General Nutritional Considerations

- A soft, bland diet may be better tolerated if the patient has ulcerations of the oral mucosa.
- Nausea and vomiting may accompany radiation therapy for a lymphoma. Food and fluid intake must be maintained. Small, interval feedings high in calories and protein should be offered. Clear liquids in the form of carbonated beverages, water, and flavored gelatin may be retained better than foods that are more difficult to digest.

General Pharmacologic Considerations

- A diuretic may be prescribed to reduce lymphedema. The patient should be informed of the signs and symptoms of electrolyte imbalance.
- Antineoplastic drug therapy for malignant disorders of the lymphatics may require a long period of therapy until remission occurs. Some combination drug regimens are given for about 6 months.

Suggested Readings

- Bates BA, Hoekelman RA. Guide to physical examination and history taking. 4th ed. Philadelphia: JB Lippincott, 1987. *(In-depth coverage of subject matter)*
- McConnell EA. Getting the feeling of lymph node assessment. Nursing '88, August 1988;18:55. *(Additional coverage and illustrations that reinforce subject matter)*

The Nervous System

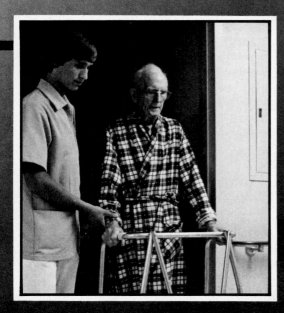

Unit 8

Chapter 35

Introduction to the Nervous System

On completion of this chapter the reader will:

- Be familiar with the basic anatomy and physiology of the nervous system

- Describe and perform a basic neurologic examination

- Discuss the common tests used in the diagnosis of disorders of the nervous system

- Use the nursing process in preparing a patient for diagnostic tests performed for neurologic disorders

ANATOMY AND PHYSIOLOGY

The nervous system consists of the brain, spinal cord, and peripheral nerves. It is responsible for coordinating many body functions and responding to changes in or stimuli from the internal and external environment.

The nervous system may be divided into two anatomic divisions: the *central nervous system* (CNS) and the *peripheral nervous system* (PNS). The basic structure of the nervous system is the nerve cell or *neuron* (Fig. 35-1). Neurons may be sensory or motor. Sensory neurons transmit impulses to the CNS, and motor neurons transmit impulses away from the CNS.

A neuron is composed of a cell body, a nucleus, and threadlike projections or fibers called dendrites. *Dendrites* conduct impulses to the cell body, and are called afferent (to or toward) nerve fibers. A nerve fiber that projects from the cell body, which usually is (but not always) larger than the dendrites, is called an *axon*. The axon conducts impulses away from the neuron, and therefore is called an efferent (away from) nerve fiber.

Some axons in the CNS and PNS are covered with a fatty substance called *myelin*, and are called myelinated, or white, nerve fibers. The myelin is covered by a sheath called the *neurilemma*. Myelin serves as an insulating substance for the axon. Axons without myelin are called unmyelinated, or gray, nerve fibers.

Central Nervous System

The CNS consists of the brain and spinal cord. The major structures of the brain are shown in Figure 35-2 and those of the spinal cord are shown in Figure 35-3.

Brain

The brain is divided into three parts: the cerebrum, cerebellum, and brain stem. The brain is protected by the rigid bones of the skull, and covered by three membranes or *meninges*: (1) the *dura mater*, the tough, outermost covering; (2) the *arachnoid*, or middle membrane lying directly below the dura; and (3) the *pia mater*, a delicate layer that adheres to the brain and spinal cord. The *subarachnoid space* is between the pia mater and the arachnoid membrane.

Within the brain are four hollow structures called *ventricles* (Fig. 35-2). The ventricles manufacture and absorb the cerebrospinal fluid (CSF) circulating in the subarachnoid space. CSF produced in the ventricles passes down into the spinal subarachnoid space, up through the basilar cisterns, and over the cerebral hemispheres to the region of the dural venous sinuses, where most of the absorption takes place. By acting as a cushion, it protects these structures and helps to maintain relatively constant intracranial pressure.

The *cerebrum* consists of two hemispheres that are connected by the *corpus callosum*, a band of white fibers that acts as a connecting bridge for transmitting

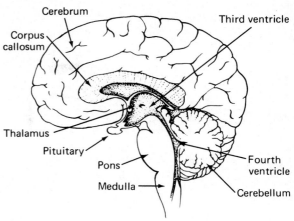

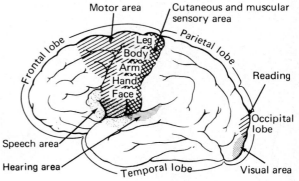

Figure 35-2. (*Top*) Major structures of the brain. (*Bottom*) Diagrammatic representation of approximate areas of the brain that control various functions.

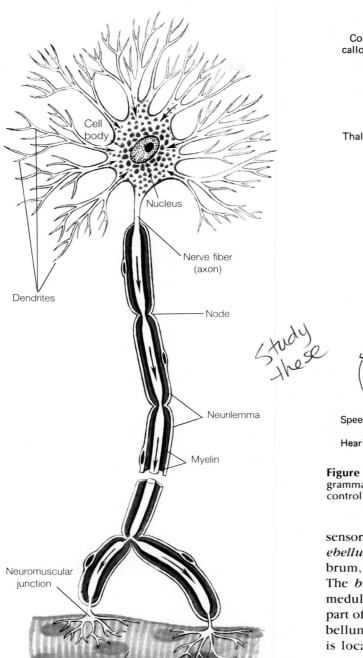

Figure 35-1. Diagram of a motor neuron. The break in axon denotes length. The arrows show the direction of the nerve impulse.

impulses between the left and the right hemispheres. Each hemisphere has four lobes: frontal, parietal, temporal, and occipital. The location and primary functions of each lobe are shown in Figure 35-2. The cerebral cortex is the surface of the cerebrum, and contains motor neurons that are responsible for movement and sensory neurons that receive impulses from peripheral

sensory neurons located throughout the body. The *cerebellum*, which is located behind and below the cerebrum, controls and coordinates muscle movement. The *brain stem* consists of the midbrain, pons, and medulla oblongata. The *midbrain* forms the forward part of the brain stem and connects the pons and cerebellum with the two cerebral hemispheres. The *pons* is located between the midbrain and medulla, and connects the two hemispheres of the cerebellum with the brain stem, spinal cord, and cerebrum. The *medulla oblongata* lies below the pons, and transmits motor impulses from the brain to the spinal cord and sensory impulses from peripheral sensory neurons to the brain. The medulla contains vital centers concerned with respiration, heartbeat, and vasomotor activity controlling smooth-muscle activity in blood vessel walls.

Spinal Cord

The spinal cord is a direct continuation of the medulla, and is surrounded and protected by the vertebrae (or vertebral column). The spinal cord ends between the

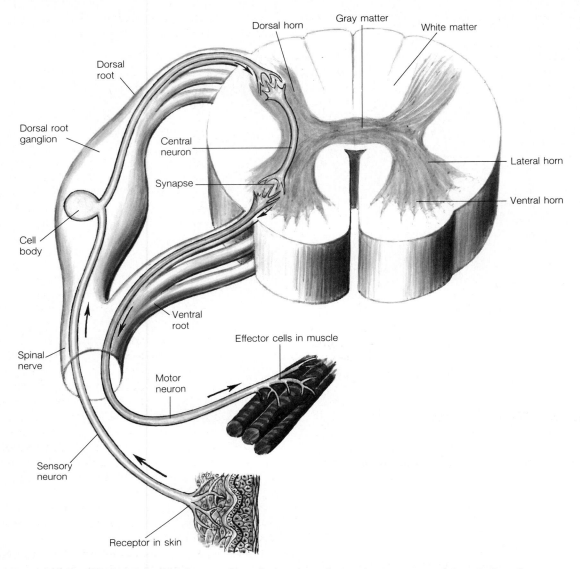

Figure 35–3. Reflex arc showing the pathway of impulses and cross section of the spinal cord.

first and second lumbar vertebrae, where it divides into smaller sections called the *cauda equina*.

The spinal cord functions as a passageway for ascending sensory and descending motor neurons. It also acts as a center of reflex action, for example the knee jerk reflex. Reflex action involves sensory input and motor output without the impulse traveling to the brain.

The two main functions of the spinal cord are (1) to provide centers for reflex action and (2) to provide a pathway for impulses to and from the brain. The *sensory fibers* enter the *posterior* portion of the cord (called the *posterior horn*); the nerve fibers that transmit *motor* impulses run outward to the peripheral nerves from the *anterior* portion of the cord (called the *anterior horn*).

Peripheral Nervous System

The PNS consists of all nerves outside the CNS.

Cranial Nerves

The 12 pairs of cranial nerves, which are identified according to Roman numerals, are as follows:

I—Olfactory nerve: sense of smell
II—Optic nerve: sight
III—Oculomotor nerve: contraction of eye muscles
IV—Trochlear nerve: eye movement
V—Trigeminal nerve: sensory nerve to face, chewing
VI—Abducens nerve: eye movement
VII—Facial nerve: facial expression, taste, secretions of salivary and lacrimal glands

VIII—Vestibulocochlear (or auditory) nerve: hearing, balance

IX—Glossopharyngeal nerve: taste, sensory fibers of pharynx and tongue, swallowing, secretions of parotid gland

X—Vagus nerve: motor fibers to glands producing digestive juices, heart rate, muscles of speech, gastrointestinal motility, respiration, swallowing, coughing, vomiting reflex

XI—Accessory (or spinal accessory) nerve: head and shoulder movement

XII—Hypoglossal nerve: movement of the tongue

Spinal Nerves

There are 31 pairs of spinal nerves: 8 cervical, 12 thoracic, 5 lumbar, 5 sacral, and 1 coccygeal. Spinal nerves have two roots, the dorsal (anterior) root and the ventral (posterior) root. Dorsal nerve fibers are sensory, and ventral nerve fibers are motor. Peripheral sensory nerve fibers in various areas of the body transmit impulses to the spinal nerves, which in turn transmit impulses up the spinal cord to the brain. Motor impulses traveling from the brain and down the spinal cord leave by the ventral root and travel to areas of the body.

Autonomic Nervous System

The autonomic nervous system consists of the *sympathetic nervous system* and the *parasympathetic nervous system*. This part of the PNS is concerned with those functions essential to the survival of the organism.

Sympathetic Nervous System

This division of the autonomic nervous system regulates the expenditure of energy, and is operative when the organism is confronted with stressful situations, such as danger, intense emotion, and severe illness. The two neurohormones (or neurotransmitters) of this system are epinephrine and norepinephrine.

Parasympathetic Nervous System

This division of the autonomic nervous system works to conserve body energy, and is partly responsible for such activities as slowing the heart rate, digesting food, and eliminating body wastes.

ASSESSMENT OF A PATIENT WHO HAS A NERVOUS SYSTEM DISORDER *Read*

A neurologic examination is performed to identify and, in some instances, locate disorders of the nervous system. The scope and extent of the neurologic examination often depend on the patient's symptoms and the probable or actual diagnosis.

Patient History

A thorough history of all symptoms is essential. Also included in the patient history is a record of trauma (no matter how slight) to the head or body within the past 6 to 12 months, a drug history, an allergy history, and a family medical history. If the history is obtained from the patient, the nurse should observe the patient's speech pattern, mental status, intellectual functioning, reasoning ability, and movement or lack of movement.

Physical Examination *Read*

The physical examination consists of assessment of the cerebral, motor, and sensory areas. Intellectual function and the speech pattern may be initially assessed during the patient history by noting the way the patient responds to questions. Additional testing of intellectual function may include asking a variety of questions such as those concerned with current events. The patient also may be asked to perform mental tasks, such as simple arithmetic or counting backward. People who have certain disorders of the nervous system may have difficulty with the easiest tasks, be unable to answer simple questions, or have an abnormal speech pattern.

The body posture should be evaluated, and any abnormal position of the head, neck, trunk, or extremities noted.

If head trauma has occurred, the ears and nose should be examined for evidence of bleeding or other type of drainage. The head should be carefully examined for bleeding, swelling, or wounds. The head should not be moved during this part of the assessment.

Cranial Nerves. Evaluation of the 12 cranial nerves may be performed by the experienced examiner. All or some of the following tests may be done. The appropriate cranial nerves are in parentheses.

- Asking the patient to identify specific odors (I) *olfactory*
- Examining visual acuity (II) *optic*
- Testing eye movements (III, IV, VI)
- Eliciting sensations of pressure, light touch, warmth, cold to the forehead, cheek, jaw; testing ability to chew (V)
- Checking for equal movements of facial muscles as the patient frowns, smiles, closes eyes, purses lips; ability to identify substances such as salt and sugar placed on the anterior two thirds of the tongue (VII)

- Checking hearing and equilibrium or balance (VIII)
- Testing ability to identify substances placed on posterior third of tongue (IX)
- Eliciting the gag reflex, evaluating vocal ability and symmetrical movement of the soft palate (X)
- Assessing strength and movement of head and shoulder muscles (XI)
- Evaluating movement of tongue (XII)

Motor Function. Assessment of motor function includes tests for muscle movement, size, tone, strength, and coordination. Large muscle areas are examined for evidence of atrophy, and opposing muscles examined for equality of size and strength. The patient is asked to perform tasks such as pushing the palm or sole against the examiner's palm. Picking up small and large objects, grasping the objects firmly, and resisting removal from the fist or fingers are ways of evaluating muscles of the shoulder, arm, and hand.

The patient can be asked to walk away from the examiner, turn, and walk back while gait, movement, and balance are noted. Other tests include climbing a small set of stairs, walking and then turning abruptly, and walking heel to toe. In the Romberg test, the patient stands with feet close together and eyes closed. If swaying is noted and there is a tendency to fall, this is considered a positive Romberg, indicating a problem with equilibrium. When this test is performed, the nurse should stand fairly close to the patient, in case loss of balance occurs.

Tests to evaluate motor and cerebral function include the finger-to-nose test with the eyes closed, writing words, and identifying common objects. The choice of tests depends on the original complaints and, possibly, the findings of diagnostic tests.

The sudden occurrence of sensory or motor changes is an important neurologic finding, and should be brought to the physician's attention at once. Lack of movement (paralysis), muscle rigidity, muscle weakness, tremors, and patient complaints of sensory changes such as numbness and tingling are examples of significant findings. Additional observations include changes (from the normal) in body position or posture, and extreme restlessness.

Sensory Function. Tests of the extremities evaluate sensitivity to heat, cold, touch, and pain. Various objects, such as cotton balls, tubes filled with hot or cold water, and sterile pins, may be used to check sensation in the extremities.

Level of Consciousness. Depending on the patient's symptoms, it may be necessary to assess level of consciousness. The following classification of levels of consciousness applies to altered consciousness from any cause. Sometimes it is difficult to differentiate between each of the levels; some patients may show characteristics of two or more levels.

CONSCIOUSNESS. The patient responds immediately, fully, and appropriately to visual, auditory, and other stimulation.

SOMNOLENCE OR LETHARGY. The patient is drowsy or sleepy at inappropriate times but can be aroused only to shortly fall asleep. Questions may be answered, but the response may be delayed or inappropriate. The speech may be incoherent. The patient may respond to verbal commands, but the response is slow. There usually is a response to painful stimuli.

STUPOR. The patient can be aroused only by vigorous and continuous stimulation, usually by manipulation or perhaps by strong auditory or visual stimuli. Such stimulation may result in answers to simple questions with one or two words, or the response may be only restless motor activity or purposeful behavior directed toward avoiding further stimulation.

SEMICOMA. The patient is unresponsive except to superficial, relatively mild painful stimuli, to which some purposeful motor response is made to evade stimulation. Spontaneous motion is uncommon, but the patient may groan or mutter.

COMA. The patient is unresponsive to all but very painful stimuli, to which a response is made by fragmentary, delayed reflex withdrawal; in deeper stages, all responsiveness usually is lost. There is no spontaneous movement, and the respiratory rate may be irregular.

The patient's level of consciousness often is determined after injury to the head or neck, cranial surgery, a cerebrovascular accident (acute phase), a ruptured cerebral aneurysm, and other neurologic disorders. This assessment is made hourly unless the physician orders otherwise or a change in the patient's condition has been noted.

Eyes. The size and equality of the pupils and their reaction to light are an assessment of the third cranial (oculomotor) nerve. Pupil size (normal, pinpoint, dilated), equality (equal, unequal in size), and reaction to a bright light (normal, sluggish, no reaction, fixed) are noted. When the pupils are examined, any abnormal movement or position of one or both eyes is noted.

Assessment of the pupils is carried out in dim light. The pupils are first checked for size and equality and then observed for reaction to light by the use of a bright flashlight. Unequal pupils (one pupil larger than the other), dilated or pinpoint pupils, and failure of the pupils to respond quickly to light are, in most instances, abnormal findings. *Any sudden change in pupil size, equality, or reaction to light is an important neurologic finding and should be reported to the physician at once.*

Neck. The neck is examined for stiffness or abnormal position. The presence of rigidity is checked by moving the head and chin toward the chest. This maneuver should *not* be performed if a head or neck injury is suspected or known.

Vital Signs. The blood pressure, pulse and respiratory rates, and temperature are closely monitored on all patients with a potential or actual neurologic disorder. The frequency of these determinations may be ordered by the physician or may depend on the nurse's assessment of the patient's condition. The temperature may have to be monitored every hour because CNS disorders can affect the temperature-regulating ability of the hypothalamus. A sudden increase or decrease in any of the vital signs may indicate a change in the patient's neurologic status, and the physician should be notified immediately.

DIAGNOSTIC TESTS
Imaging Procedures

Imaging procedures have largely replaced invasive procedures such as ventriculography and pneumoencephalography. Computed tomography (CT), magnetic resonance imaging (MRI), and positron emission tomography (PET) may be used in the diagnosis of disorders of the nervous system.

The advantage of imaging procedures is threefold: (1) there is neither discomfort (other than having to lie on a table or having the head immobilized) nor pain during the procedure; (2) the procedure is safe; and (3) it is a highly effective method of detecting lesions and abnormalities. Imaging procedures are particularly useful in the diagnosis of neurologic disorders such as brain tumors, Alzheimer's disease, intracranial bleeding or hemorrhage, and cerebral infections.

A radiopaque dye may be used during a CT scan to emphasize or highlight a certain area. Use of a radiopaque dye entails a risk, and therefore decreases the safety of the procedure.

Lumbar Puncture

A lumbar puncture (spinal tap) is performed to obtain samples of CSF from the subarachnoid space for laboratory examination and to measure spinal fluid pressure. A lumbar puncture also may be performed to inject a drug into the subarachnoid space (intrathecal injection), to administer a spinal anesthetic, to withdraw spinal fluid for the relief of intracranial pressure, or to inject air, gas, or dye for a neurologic diagnostic procedure. In health, the CSF is clear and colorless,

with a pressure of 80 to 180 mm of water; a pressure over 200 mm of water is considered abnormal.

Changes in the CSF occur in many neurologic disorders. Bacteriologic tests on specimens of CSF may reveal the presence of pathogenic organisms. Strict aseptic technique is required during the procedure.

Sometimes a *cisternal puncture* is performed to remove CSF. The back of the neck is shaved, the skin washed with an antiseptic, and a needle inserted just below the occipital bone of the skull. The patient lies on the side, with a small firm pillow or sandbag placed under the side of the head and the head flexed forward. This procedure is more commonly performed on children. Headache appears to occur less frequently with cisternal puncture than with lumbar puncture.

Contrast Studies

Cerebral angiography, *ventriculography*, *pneumoencephalography*, and *myelography* (Fig. 35-4)

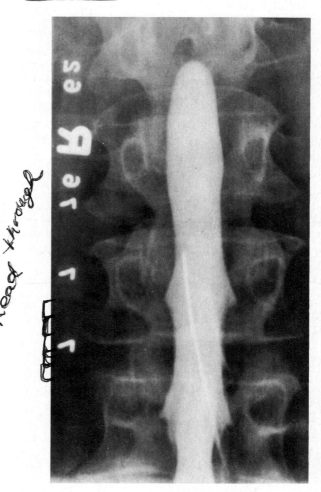

Figure 35–4. A normal myelogram. (Courtesy of H. Revollo, MD. Photograph by D. Atkinson)

are contrast studies; that is, radiopaque dye or air is injected for radiographic visualization of cerebral or spinal structures. Cerebral angiography, ventriculography, and pneumoencephalography have been largely replaced by CT scans, PET, and MRI.

Cerebral angiography detects distortion of cerebral arteries and veins, indicating an aneurysm, a tumor, or other vascular abnormality. A radiopaque dye is injected into the right or left carotid artery, the brachial artery, or the femoral artery. A rapid sequence of radiographs is taken as the dye circulates through the cerebral arteries and veins.

A pneumoencephalography is an air contrast study performed when there is a suspected abnormality such as a brain tumor. The patient may be given a local or general anesthetic. CSF is removed by means of a lumbar puncture, followed by injection of air or gas. A series of radiographs is taken. The procedure for ventriculography is similar to that for pneumoencephalography, except that the air is injected into the ventricles of the brain through burr holes made in the skull. Ventriculography is used when pneumoencephalography is not possible. —sickness afterward

A lumbar puncture is required to perform myelography. A radiopaque substance is injected through the spinal needle into the spinal canal. Radiographs are taken to demonstrate abnormalities of the spinal canal, such as tumors or a ruptured intervertebral disk. After the radiographs have been taken, the dye is removed through the spinal needle to prevent irritation of the meninges. Movement of the spinal needle is necessary to remove the dye.

Electroencephalography ✓

Electroencephalography records the electrical impulses generated by the brain. Electrodes are placed on the patient's scalp, and the graph is recorded by a machine. The procedure is not painful.

Brain Scan ✓

A brain scan may be ordered if an abnormality of the brain is suspected. The brain scan may identify such disorders as a brain tumor, hematomas in or around the brain, cerebral abscess, cerebral infarction, and displacement of the ventricles. A radioactive material is injected before the procedure. This procedure can take as long as 1 hour or as little as a few minutes. It may be necessary for some patients to return for follow-up scans at 24-, 48-, or 72-hour intervals. The procedure is not painful.

Electromyography ✓

Electromyography studies the changes in the electrical potential of muscles and the nerves supplying the muscles. Needle electrodes are placed into one or more skeletal muscles, and the results recorded on an oscilloscope. This test is useful in determining the presence of muscle disorders.

NURSING PROCESS —THE PATIENT UNDERGOING DIAGNOSTIC TESTING FOR A NEUROLOGIC DISORDER

Assessment
A patient history should be obtained and may direct the examiner to the area or areas that require more detailed investigation and examination. Some radiopaque contrast media contains iodine. If the allergy history reveals a possible or known history of iodine allergy, the physician should be informed and the cover of the patient's chart labeled.

A neurologic examination should be performed. During the patient history and examination, the patient should be closely observed for any mental or physical deviations from the normal. Vital signs should be taken and the patient weighed.

Nursing Diagnosis
Depending on the presenting symptoms, the condition of the patient, and other factors, nursing diagnoses in addition to those that follow may be necessary:

- Anxiety related to possible diagnosis, diagnostic tests
- Pain after a diagnostic procedure
- Knowledge deficit of the diagnostic procedure

Planning and Implementation
The major goals of the patient include reduction of anxiety, relief of pain or discomfort, and an understanding of the scheduled diagnostic procedure.

The major goals of nursing management include proper preparation of the patient for the diagnostic procedure and relief of anxiety and pain. Nursing management depends on the signs and symptoms noted during the initial assessment as well as the diagnostic tests performed.

Some procedures require a fasting state, or a sedative may be ordered before the procedure. If a lumbar puncture is performed, samples of CSF usually are sent to the laboratory. It is essential that the tubes containing the specimens be properly labeled and that request slips clearly identify the patient and the tests desired. Loss or breakage might necessitate repeating an uncomfortable procedure. A firm container for holding CSF samples should be provided as a precaution.

When a diagnostic procedure is completed, the physician may order specific observations or tasks such as vital signs or keeping the patient flat in bed for 6 to 8 hours. The patient's neurologic status should be evaluated and the results recorded.

After myelography, the patient should rest flat in bed for a few hours or as ordered by the physician. The patient should be observed for signs of meningeal irritation (eg, stiffness of the neck and pain when an attempt is made to bend the head forward).

If a radiopaque dye containing iodine was used for a contrast study, the patient should be observed for signs of a severe iodine allergy (severe hypotension, tachycardia, profuse diaphoresis, and a sudden change in the level of consciousness).

Anxiety. Most patients experience anxiety when a diagnostic test involves the brain or spinal cord. When assisting the physician with a diagnostic test, the necessary equipment should be brought to the patient's room immediately before the procedure. Leaving the equipment in the room, even for a short time, can create unnecessary anxiety. If severe anxiety is noted, the physician should be informed of the problem before the procedure.

Pain. After a lumbar puncture, some patients experience a "spinal" headache that is thought to be due to the removal of CSF. Keeping the room dark and quiet and administering analgesics usually relieve discomfort. If no pillow is allowed, a small towel covered with a pillowcase will provide some support for the head and take the strain off the neck muscles.

Knowledge Deficit. Some patients experience apprehension simply because they have been misinformed about the procedure. Before a diagnostic test, the purpose of the procedure and how the procedure will be performed should be explained by the physician. Although invasive procedures are first explained by the physician, the nurse may explain noninvasive procedures (eg, the participation of the patient during a CT scan, which would include information such as the importance of holding still and not talking during the test).

Evaluation

■ Anxiety is reduced
■ Pain and discomfort are reduced or eliminated
■ Patient demonstrates understanding of the procedure or diagnostic test

General Pharmacologic Considerations

☐ Patients who are allergic to iodine cannot receive radiopaque dyes that contain this substance. A thorough allergy history is an essential part of the neurologic examination. Seafood allergies may indicate an allergy to iodine.
☐ Some narcotic analgesics, particularly morphine, can affect the size of the pupils and their reaction to light.
☐ Drug abusers may have taken morphine, heroin, or other narcotic or CNS depressant shortly before a neurologic examination. The effects of these drugs should be kept in mind when the patient undergoing a neurologic examination is suspected of using illegal drugs.

General Gerontologic Considerations

☐ Elderly patients may have difficulty following directions during a neurologic examination or diagnostic procedure. Instructions should be brief and repeated as needed. They may best follow directions if the directions are given one at a time during each step of the examination or diagnostic procedure.
☐ Elderly patients may have difficulty remembering recent or past events, symptoms, drug and medical history, and other facts necessary for a patient history. If this is apparent, information should be obtained from a family member or friend.

☐ Elderly patients may respond poorly to questions because of a failure to understand what physical or verbal response is desired. Their poor response may be due to a hearing or sight disability, rather than a neurologic problem.

Suggested Readings

☐ Bates BA, Hoekelman RA. Guide to physical examination and history taking. 4th ed. Philadelphia: JB Lippincott, 1987. *(In-depth coverage of subject matter)*

☐ Coburn KL. High-tech maps of the brain. Am J Nurs November 1988;88:1500. *(Closely related to subject matter)*

☐ Fisher J. What you need to know about neurologic testing. RN January 1987;50:47. *(Additional coverage of subject matter)*

☐ Memmler RL, Wood DL. Structure and function of the human body. 4th ed. Philadelphia: JB Lippincott, 1987. *(Additional coverage of subject matter)*

☐ Memmler RL, Wood DL. The human body in health and disease. 6th ed. Philadelphia: JB Lippincott, 1987. *(Additional coverage of subject matter)*

☐ Mitchell M. Neuroscience nursing: a nursing diagnosis approach. Baltimore: Williams & Wilkins, 1989. *(In-depth coverage of subject matter)*

☐ Plankey ED, Knauf J. What patients need to know about magnetic resonance imaging. Am J Nurs January 1990;90:27. *(In-depth coverage of subject matter)*

☐ Porth CM. Pathophysiology: concepts of altered health states. 3rd ed. Philadelphia: JB Lippincott, 1990. *(In-depth, high-level coverage of subject matter)*

☐ Stevens SA, Becker KL. A simple, step-by-step approach to neurologic assessment, (Part I). Nursing '88, September 1988;18:53. *(Additional coverage and photos that reinforce subject matter)*

☐ Stevens SA, Becker KL. A simple, step-by-step approach to neurologic assessment, (Part II). Nursing '88, October 1988;18:51. *(Additional coverage and photos that reinforce subject matter)*

Chapter 36

Central and Peripheral Nervous System Disorders

On completion of this chapter the reader will:

- List the symptoms, diagnosis, treatment, and complications of increased intracranial pressure

- Use the nursing process in the management of a patient with increased intracranial pressure

- Discuss the etiology, symptoms, and treatment of meningitis, encephalitis, Guillain-Barré syndrome, and brain abscess

- Use the nursing process in the management of a patient with an infectious or inflammatory disorder of the nervous system

- List the symptoms, diagnosis, treatment, and complications of multiple sclerosis, myasthenia gravis, muscular dystrophy, and amyotrophic lateral sclerosis

- List the symptoms, diagnosis, and treatment of trigeminal neuralgia, Bell's palsy, and temporomandibular joint syndrome

- Use the nursing process in the management of a patient with a cranial nerve disorder

- List the symptoms, diagnosis, treatment, and complications associated with Parkinson's disease and Huntington's disease

- Use the nursing process in the management of a patient with an extrapyramidal disorder

- List the various types of convulsive disorders and their symptoms, diagnoses, and treatments

- Use the nursing process in the management of a patient with a convulsive disorder

- List the symptoms, diagnosis, treatment, and complications of brain tumors

- Use the nursing process in the management of a patient with a brain tumor

INCREASED INTRACRANIAL PRESSURE

Tumors, cerebral edema, brain abscess, or severe head injury with bleeding within the cranial vault may result in a rise in intracranial pressure (ICP). This disorder is extremely serious and can result in death.

Symptoms

The signs and symptoms of increased ICP are prominent.

Changes in the Level of Consciousness. A change in the level of consciousness (LOC) is often one of the earliest signs of increased ICP. The change may occur within a period of a few minutes or over many hours or days. A decrease in the LOC means that a person's wide range of responses to stimuli from the environment is diminished. The terms used to describe a decrease in responsiveness include *lethargic, semicomatose*, and *comatose*.

Confusion, restlessness, periodic disorientation, and drowsiness may or may not be signs of an impending change in the LOC. Because alterations may be difficult to determine, any sudden change in a patient's mental status is reported immediately to the physician.

The Glasgow Coma Scale (Table 36-1) is a measure of the LOC. It consists of three parts: eye opening response, best verbal response, and best motor response. To evaluate responses correctly, several verbal and motor responses are noted, and the best response is recorded.

The eye opening response is determined by talking to the patient and calling his or her name. If no response is noted, a painful stimulus is introduced and the response noted. The best verbal response is an evaluation of the patient's verbal reply to questions. The motor response is the ability of the patient to follow commands, such as "wiggle your toes" or "move your left hand." If the patient does not respond, a painful stimulus is introduced and the response noted. The responses are assigned numbers, and the numbers are totaled. A normal response is 14. A score of 7 or less is usually considered coma. The evaluations can be recorded on a graphic sheet. Connecting lines show an increase or decrease in the LOC (Fig. 36-1).

Headache. Pain is usually intermittent. Constant headache usually indicates that the patient's prognosis is grave. Actions that increase ICP, such as coughing, sneezing, or straining at stool, increase the headache. Lying quietly in bed—especially if the head of the bed is elevated—tends to reduce ICP and thus helps relieve the headache.

Vomiting. Vomiting usually occurs without the forewarning of nausea and without any relation to eating. It may be projectile.

Table 36–1. Glasgow Coma Scale	
Eyes Open	
Spontaneously	4
To speech	3
To pain	2
Do not open	1
Best Verbal Response	
Oriented	5
Confused	4
Inappropriate words	3
Incomprehensible sounds	2
None	1
Best Motor Response	
Obeys commands	5
Localizes pain (tries to remove painful stimulus)	4
Flexion to pain (moves arm or leg in response to pain)	3
Extension to pain (elbow or knee extends and may rotate internally)	2
None	1

Papilledema.   Edema of the optic nerve (papilledema) at the point at which it enters the posterior eye is caused by obstruction of venous drainage from the eyeball as a result of increased ICP. This condition can only be noted with an ophthalmoscope.

Vital Signs.   When ICP increases, the vital signs respond. The body temperature rises, the blood pressure rises, and the pulse pressure widens. The pulse rate may be increased initially but later usually becomes slow (40 to 60/min), full, and bounding. The respiratory rate may be irregular or Cheyne-Stokes respirations (shallow, rapid breathing building in intensity and depth, then decreasing, followed by a period of apnea) may be seen. Often, changes in vital signs occur after an alteration in the LOC has occurred.

Pupils.   Pressure on the oculomotor nerve usually occurs with increased ICP. The size of the pupils (in dim light) and the reaction of the pupils to strong light is evaluated. Normally, pupil response to strong light is rapid. In patients with rising ICP, the response may be sluggish or nonexistent (fixed pupils). The nurse should note whether pupil sizes are equal and, if not, which pupil is larger (or smaller).

Diagnosis

Diagnosis may be based on the presenting symptoms and a patient history. Diagnostic tests include a skull radiograph, computed tomographic (CT) scan, lumbar puncture, and cerebral angiography.

Treatment

Treatment, which must begin immediately, varies according to the probable or known cause of the disorder. Treatment is aimed primarily at removing the cause, when possible. Osmotic diuretics (mannitol, glycerol) and corticosteroids may be given to reduce cerebral edema. Emergency surgery may be performed if increased ICP is due to a head injury. Depending on the cause, other treatments include the restriction of fluids (oral, intravenous), repeated lumbar punctures to remove small amounts of cerebrospinal fluid, and hyperventilation therapy by means of mechanical ventilation. This latter maneuver causes respiratory alkalosis, which produces vasoconstriction of the cerebral arteries followed by a decrease in cerebral blood volume and a reduction in ICP.

A hollow screw or bolt inserted into the subarachnoid space or a catheter inserted into one of the lateral ventricles may be used to monitor ICP. These devices are connected to an oscilloscope to record changes in ICP.

Complications

Impaired respiratory function and cerebral damage that results in neurologic deficits, such as permanent paralysis and mental changes, may occur. Death may occur when herniation of the brain through the foramen magnum (Fig. 36-2) results in pressure on the brain stem and suppression of vital functions.

NURSING PROCESS —THE PATIENT WHO HAS INCREASED INTRACRANIAL PRESSURE

Assessment

A complete patient history is obtained and includes all symptoms as well as a medical, drug, and allergy history. A complete neurologic examination is performed, including assessment of the LOC (see Chapter 35) and signs of increased ICP. A neurologic flow sheet and the Glasgow Coma Scale may be used for a data base and ongoing assessments.

Nursing Diagnosis

Depending on the cause and degree of increased ICP, one or more of the following may apply:

- Self-care deficit: total (if partial, specify) related to decreased LOC, other neurologic involvement
- Ineffective airway clearance related to pressure on the brain stem secondary to increased ICP

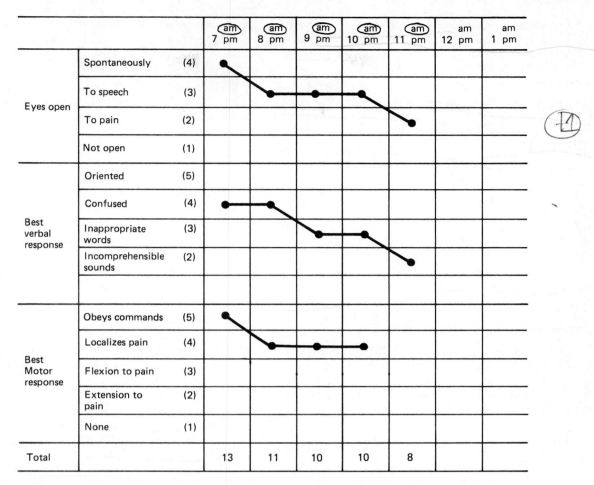

			am/7 pm	am/8 pm	am/9 pm	am/10 pm	am/11 pm	am/12 pm	am/1 pm
Eyes open	Spontaneously	(4)	●						
	To speech	(3)		●	●	●			
	To pain	(2)					●		
	Not open	(1)							
Best verbal response	Oriented	(5)							
	Confused	(4)	●	●					
	Inappropriate words	(3)			●	●			
	Incomprehensible sounds	(2)					●		
Best Motor response	Obeys commands	(5)	●						
	Localizes pain	(4)		●	●	●			
	Flexion to pain	(3)							
	Extension to pain	(2)							
	None	(1)							
Total			13	11	10	10	8		

Figure 36–1. Example of a graphic record of hourly evaluations using the Glasgow Coma Scale.

- Fluid volume deficit (intentional) related to fluid restriction, vomiting, administration of osmotic diuretic
- Bowel incontinence related to decreased LOC, neurologic effects of increased ICP
- Potential for infection related to surgery, invasive diagnostic or monitoring procedures, original head injury
- Impaired verbal communication related to decreased LOC
- Altered nutrition: less than body requirements related

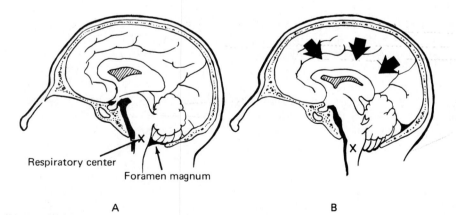

Respiratory center   Foramen magnum

A   B

Figure 36–2. (A) The normal brain. (B) Herniation of the lower portion of the brain stem (medulla) through the foramen magnum, caused by increased intracranial pressure. Note the position of the respiratory center.

to vomiting, inability to take oral food secondary to decrease in LOC
■ Impaired skin integrity related to immobility secondary to decreased LOC

Planning and Implementation

The major goals of the patient include a patent airway, improvement in ability to take care of self, correction of a fluid volume deficit, normal bowel function, absence of infection, improved ability to communicate with others, and improved nutrition.

The major goal of nursing management is to administer the prescribed drugs and therapies that are intended to reduce ICP, prevent infection, improve nutrition, prevent skin breakdown, prevent constipation, maintain a patent airway, and meet the patient's physical needs.

Neurologic assessments are performed and recorded on a flow sheet every 30 minutes or as ordered. *The physician must be notified immediately should any change occur.* Vital signs are monitored at the prescribed intervals. An increase in ICP can affect the temperature-regulating mechanism of the brain; hyperthermia may be seen. Any change in vital signs is immediately reported to the physician. A persistent, high fever may require the use of hypothermia measures, such as a cooling blanket, if the temperature does not respond to antipyretic drugs.

Depending on the degree and cause of increased ICP, the physician may order insertion of an indwelling catheter, a stool softener to prevent straining at stool, mechanical ventilation to produce respiratory alkalosis, and intravenous fluid and calorie supplementation. The patient's head is kept in a midline (straight) position, and the head of the bed is slightly elevated as ordered by the physician. Patients with basal skull fractures may be kept flat. In no instance should the patient's head be allowed to rest below the level of the body.

Elevating the head of the bed (if ordered), limiting patient movements, spacing tasks, such as oral care, and reducing or eliminating environmental stressors, such as loud noises and bright lights, help reduce ICP.

Self-Care Deficit. All self-care needs of the patient must be met; complete bed rest and limitation of movement are necessary to prevent an increase in ICP.

Ineffective Airway Clearance. The lungs are auscultated for normal and abnormal breath sounds. Turning the patient on the side (if allowed) may help maintain a patent airway. An oral airway may be inserted if the patient is comatose and the tongue obstructs the oropharynx. Suctioning should only be

performed when absolutely necessary; this maneuver usually results in coughing, which momentarily raises ICP. Oral secretions can be gently removed with the fingers wrapped in a plain compress (ie, one without a cotton layer). Mild respiratory difficulty may require administration of oxygen; severe respiratory depression requires contacting the physician immediately, as mechanical ventilation may be necessary.

Fluid Volume Deficit and Altered Nutrition. In those with increased ICP, a fluid volume deficit may be part of treatment. Unless a written order states otherwise, patients with increased ICP are not given oral fluids for two reasons: restricted fluid intake helps to decrease cerebral edema; and oral fluids may be aspirated or cause vomiting with danger of aspiration. Vomiting and coughing usually increase ICP.

Fluids may be given intravenously. With a marked increase in ICP, the physician may order a fixed amount of intravenous fluid to be administered over a specific period of time. The rate of infusion is calculated so that the total amount of fluid is administered at an even rate over a 24-hour period.

Special attention is given to the skin turgor and the oral mucous membranes for evidence of a fluid volume deficit and to the patient for signs of electrolyte imbalances (see Chapter 12).

Bowel and Bladder Elimination. Intake and output are measured. Because fluid intake may be restricted, hourly measurements of fluid intake, urine output, and urine specific gravity determinations may be necessary. If corticosteroids are ordered, the urine is tested for glucose and the stool is tested for blood.

A stool softener may be ordered to prevent straining at stool. The abdomen is checked for distention and auscultated for normal, abnormal, or absent bowel sounds.

Potential for Infection. Infection related to invasive monitoring procedures or depressed skull fracture also may cause a rise in temperature. The temperature is monitored every 4 hours or more frequently if markedly elevated.

Aseptic technique is used to handle any part of the intracranial monitoring devices or to change dressings that cover the intraventricular catheter or subarachnoid screw.

Impaired Verbal Communication. If the LOC is decreased, patients are unable to communicate their needs. The nurse must look for signs, for example a facial grimace or moan, that indicate discomfort, pain, or another problem, such as bladder distention or abdominal discomfort. An attempt must be made to determine what the patient is trying to convey, and then, when possible, the problem is corrected.

Impaired Skin Integrity. From the beginning of treatment, skin care is essential because a patient may remain immobile for a long time. If the physician allows the patient to be turned on the side, position changes are made every 2 hours. If the physician orders the patient to remain in a supine position, an alternating pressure mattress, flotation pad, or other device is necessary. The skin is inspected daily for signs of skin breakdown.

Evaluation

- Intracranial pressure returns to normal or near normal levels
- Self-care needs are met
- Breathing pattern is normal; airway clear; lungs clear to auscultation
- Fluid volume deficit maintained as ordered
- Intravenous fluids administered at the (hourly, daily) rate ordered by the physician
- Nutritional needs are met
- Takes oral fluids once conscious and able to swallow
- Bowel and urine elimination are normal
- Temperature is normal; no evidence of infection
- Skin remains intact; no evidence of skin breakdown
- Able to communicate needs to others when consciousness returns

INFECTIOUS AND INFLAMMATORY DISORDERS OF THE NERVOUS SYSTEM
Meningitis

Meningitis is an inflammation of the meninges. The meningococcus, streptococcus, staphylococcus, and pneumococcus are the most common causative microorganisms of meningitis. They reach the meninges by way of the bloodstream or by direct extension from infected areas, such as the middle ear or the paranasal sinuses.

Symptoms

Symptoms, which may develop at a slow or rapid rate, include fever, pain and stiffness of the neck (nuchal rigidity), nausea, vomiting, aversion to light (photophobia), headache, restlessness, irritability, and, in some instances, convulsions. Severe irritation of the meninges may cause opisthotonus—an extreme hyperextension of the head and arching of the back. The patient with meningococcal meningitis may have multiple petechiae on the body.

Diagnosis

Diagnosis is based on the patient's history and physical examination. A lumbar puncture may be performed and samples of cerebrospinal fluid (CSF) obtained for glucose, cell count, and culture and sensitivity studies. The physician may request a CT scan, blood culture, complete blood cell count, and other laboratory tests to rule out other possible disorders.

Treatment

Intravenous fluids and antimicrobial therapy are started immediately. The antibiotic may be changed, if necessary, once the causative microorganism is identified and the results of sensitivity tests obtained. Drug therapy may be continued after the acute phase of the illness to prevent the recurrence of infection. Anticonvulsants may be necessary if convulsive seizures occur.

Those having recent contact with a patient with meningococcal meningitis are placed on prophylactic sulfonamide therapy. Medical personnel caring for a patient also may be prescribed a sulfonamide.

Complications

Most adults with bacterial meningitis recover without permanent neurologic damage or dysfunction, owing to the use of antibiotics. When complications occur, however, they are usually serious. The infection may be overwhelming, and the patient may not survive. Neurologic complications, such as damage to cranial nerves and, especially, visual and auditory deterioration, may take place. Cerebral edema, irreversible coma, seizure disorders, brain abscess, and neurologic changes also may occur.

Encephalitis

Encephalitis is an infectious disease of the central nervous system characterized by pathologic changes in both the white matter and gray matter of the spinal cord and brain. Severe, diffuse inflammation of the brain with intense lymphocytic infiltration, especially around the blood vessels of the brain, is found. In some patients, extensive nerve cell destruction occurs.

Encephalitis can be caused by bacteria, fungi, or viruses. Poisoning by drugs and chemicals, such as lead, arsenic, or carbon monoxide, may closely resemble encephalitis clinically.

The disease can occur after any viral infection elsewhere in the body, such as measles, or after vaccination. The viruses that cause encephalitis that have been identified include the St. Louis virus, the Western equine virus, and the Eastern equine virus. Some viruses are transmitted by ticks, others by mosquitoes.

Symptoms

The onset of viral encephalitis is often sudden with symptoms such as fever, severe headache, stiff neck, vomiting, and drowsiness. Lethargy is a prominent symptom, and coma or delirium may be present. Other symptoms include tremors, convulsions, spastic or flaccid paralysis, irritability, incoordination, and muscular weakness. Incontinence and eye symptoms, such as photophobia, involuntary eye movements, double vision, or blurred vision, also may be seen.

Diagnosis

Diagnosis is made by the patient history and physical examination. Because the patient is most always acutely ill, the history is obtained from a family member. A lumbar puncture, blood cultures, CT scan, brain scan, and electroencephalogram (EEG) may be performed.

Treatment

Because no specific antiviral measure has yet been developed, treatment for encephalitis is mainly supportive.

Complications

Cerebral edema, neurologic deficits, such as paralysis and speech changes, increased ICP, respiratory failure, seizure disorders, and shock, may occur in those with encephalitis.

Guillain-Barré Syndrome

Guillain-Barré syndrome (acute postinfectious polyneuropathy) is a disorder that affects the peripheral nerves and spinal nerve roots. Though the exact cause of the disorder is unknown, many patients give a history of a recent infection, particularly of the respiratory tract.

Symptoms

Although symptoms may vary, motor weakness, usually in the extremities, is often the first symptom. The weakness may be progressive and may move to upper areas of the body, where the muscles of respiration may be affected. Sensory disturbances, such as numbness and tingling, also may be present. Cranial nerve involvement makes chewing, talking, and swallowing difficult.

Diagnosis

Diagnosis may be difficult but may be made by patient history and physical examination as well as by ruling out other possible central nervous system disorders. A lumbar puncture may be performed, as CSF protein is usually elevated in this disorder.

Treatment

Treatment is primarily supportive and depends on symptoms. If the muscles of respiration are involved, a tracheostomy and mechanical ventilation may be necessary. Difficulty with chewing and swallowing requires intravenous fluids, and, if the condition persists, total parenteral nutrition or nasogastric tube feedings may be needed. Plasmapheresis, which has shown to shorten the course of the disease, may be used within the first 2 weeks.

Most patients begin to show signs of recovery about a month after the progression of symptoms ceases. Recovery may be slow and take 1 or more years.

Complications

Paralysis or mild to severe muscle weakness may be permanent. Death occurs in about 5% of the cases.

Brain Abscess

A brain abscess is a collection of purulent material within the brain. It may occur as an extension of an infection in nearby structures, such as the middle ear, sinuses, or teeth, or it may result from an infection in other organs or structures, such as the lungs. Brain abscess also may occur after intracranial surgery or trauma to the head.

Symptoms

Signs of increased ICP (caused by cerebral edema), fever, headache, and neurologic changes, such as paralysis, seizures, muscle weakness, and lethargy, may be seen.

Diagnosis

Diagnosis is made by patient history and physical examination, CT scan, and brain scan. Laboratory tests may show an elevated white blood cell count.

Treatment

Antimicrobial therapy is started once the diagnosis is confirmed. Surgery is often indicated to drain the abscess. Cerebral edema may be treated with corticosteroids and seizures treated with anticonvulsant therapy. Additional treatment, such as the control of fever, may require additional therapy.

Complications

Complications include paralysis, mental deterioration, seizure disorders, and visual disturbances. Complications depend on the site of the brain abscess.

NURSING PROCESS —THE PATIENT WHO HAS AN INFECTIOUS OR INFLAMMATORY DISORDER OF THE NERVOUS SYSTEM

Assessment

A complete history is obtained, including all symptoms and a medical, drug, and allergy history. Because the patient may be acutely ill, most of the history may be obtained from the family.

A complete neurologic examination is performed, including assessment of the LOC (see Chapter 35). Vital signs are taken, and the patient is assessed for signs of increased ICP. A neurologic flow sheet may be used for a data base and comparison with ongoing assessments.

Nursing Diagnosis

Depending on the severity of symptoms, one or more of the following may apply:

- Ineffective airway clearance related to inability to raise secretions secondary to decreased LOC, motor weakness
- Potential for aspiration related to decreased LOC, motor weakness (cranial nerves)
- Potential altered body temperature: hyperthermia related to infectious process, damage to temperature regulating mechanism of brain
- Fluid volume deficit related to decreased oral intake, vomiting, other factors (specify)
- Altered nutrition: less than body requirements related to inability to chew, motor weakness, decreased LOC
- Potential impaired skin integrity related to petechiae (meningitis), immobility
- Constipation related to immobility, diet, other factors (specify)
- Pain (headache) related to cerebral edema, irritation of the meninges
- Self-care deficit: total related to decreased LOC, enforced bed rest
- Knowledge deficit of home care

Planning and Implementation

The major goals of the patient include maintaining a patent airway, attaining normal body temperature, achieving normal bowel elimination, attaining and maintaining an adequate food and fluid intake, relief of discomfort, maintaining skin integrity, and acquiring knowledge of self care after discharge.

The major goals of nursing management include identifying complications associated with the disorder, maintaining a patent airway, relief of pain or discomfort, maintaining skin integrity, attaining and maintaining an adequate food and fluid intake, and providing knowledge of care after discharge.

Vital signs are monitored every 4 hours. If a change in any one or more of the vital signs occurs, the physician is notified and the patient monitored at more frequent intervals. The physician may order an antipyretic for an elevated temperature. If the temperature fails to respond to the drug, the physician is notified because other measures (eg, a cooling blanket) may be necessary.

A neurologic assessment is performed as ordered. The Glasgow Coma Scale may be used to evaluate the LOC. All neurologic assessments are recorded on a flow sheet, and the physician informed is if changes occur.

Because convulsive seizures are a possibility, the room is kept dimly lit and activities and noise kept to a minimum. An oral airway is kept at the patient's bedside. In some instances, the physician may order an anticonvulsant to prevent seizures. These drugs must be given at the times ordered; an adequate blood level of the drug must be maintained to be effective.

For a discussion of the procedure to care for a patient who develops a neurologic deficit, see Chapter 39. Nursing management of the patient after surgery for a brain abscess is the same as for a patient with a craniotomy (see Chapter 38).

Respiratory Function. The lungs are auscultated every 4 to 8 hours, and the patient is suctioned as needed. If the ICP is increased, the patient should not be suctioned unless there is a specific order to do so. The physician may order the head of the bed raised to increase the depth of respirations.

Any change in the respiratory status or the development of cyanosis is immediately reported to the physician. Respiratory difficulty due to involvement of the muscles of respiration may require an emergency tracheostomy or endotracheal intubation as well as mechanical ventilation.

Fluid Volume Deficit and Altered Nutrition. Intake and output are measured. If increased ICP occurs, fluid intake may be limited in an attempt to control cerebral edema.

Oral fluids are given with caution to a semiconscious patient or a patient with cranial nerve involvement because aspiration may occur. Unconscious patients require intravenous fluids until they are reasonably alert and able to swallow without difficulty. Prolonged inability to take oral fluids or food may require total parenteral nutrition.

Potential Impaired Skin Integrity. The patient is turned every 2 hours and bony prominences inspected for signs of skin breakdown. Various nursing measures (eg, a foot board or sheepskin pads) may be used to preserve skin integrity and loss of muscle tone. If prolonged immobility occurs or the skin shows signs of redness, the use of a flotation mattress or other device is discussed with the physician. Passive exercises may be instituted if approved by the physician.

Constipation.   A record of bowel movements is kept. Straining at stool is avoided because this increases ICP. The physician may order a stool softener (if the patient is able to swallow) or a suppository to encourage a bowel movement.

Pain.   Cerebral edema or meningeal irritation may result in headache. Depending on the diagnosis and other factors, the physician may order an analgesic. If given orally, the patient is closely observed for the ability to swallow the drug. Any sudden occurrence of a headache or an increase in the severity of the headache is reported to the physician immediately; either may be a sign of a complication of the disorder.

Self-Care Deficit.   Most patients require complete care during the acute stage of the illness. If there is a danger of seizure, the patient is disturbed as little as possible and only when necessary. When bathing a patient, the nurse must be gentle to reduce the possibility of a seizure. As patients recover, they may be able to perform some bathing and grooming tasks.

Knowledge Deficit.   Before a patient is discharged from the hospital, the nurse discusses with the physician the anticipated postdischarge treatment modalities and then develops a teaching plan.

The home care regimen may include instructions for physical exercise, visits to a physical therapist, drugs (eg, prophylactic antibiotic, anticonvulsant) respiratory therapy, and special diet.

Evaluation

- Airway is patent; able to raise secretions; lungs clear to auscultation
- No evidence of aspiration; able to swallow fluids and food
- Temperature remains normal; vital signs are stable
- Fluid volume deficit corrected
- Nutrition is adequate
- Skin remains intact; no evidence of breakdown
- Bowel elimination is normal
- Pain (headache) and discomfort reduced or eliminated
- Able to participate in own activities of daily living; assumes more responsibility for own care
- Demonstrates understanding of the prescribed home care regimen

Poliomyelitis

Poliomyelitis (polio) is an acute infectious disorder caused by three different viral strains, namely, poliovirus I, II, and III. If the virus reaches the central nervous system, the anterior (motor) horn of the spinal cord or the brain stem (including the cranial nerves) is affected and paralysis occurs. This condition is known as *paralytic poliomyelitis* or *bulbar (brain stem) poliomyelitis*. A nonparalytic form of poliomyelitis also may be seen in which paralysis does not occur, even though the virus reaches the central nervous system. This infectious disorder is rare today because of widespread immunization of children.

Prevention and Treatment

Immunization against poliomyelitis is achieved with the Sabin (live attenuated virus) or Salk (killed virus) vaccine. Unless all children are adequately immunized, this infectious disorder cannot be totally eliminated. If poliomyelitis should occur, treatment is supportive.

Herpes Zoster

Herpes zoster (shingles) is an acute viral infection caused by reactivation of the varicella-zoster virus, which lies dormant in sensory ganglia after a previous infection of chickenpox (varicella). Those who have never had chickenpox and are in contact with someone who has herpes zoster appear to be susceptible, as are those who have lost their naturally acquired immunity to chickenpox. Immunocompromised people, for example those with leukemia or those who are undergoing chemotherapy for a malignancy, also are susceptible.

could die from it

Symptoms

Initial symptoms include a blotchy appearance of the affected area, itching, numbness, or pain. In about 24 to 48 hours, vesicles appear and follow the path of sensory nerves of the head, neck, or trunk. Usually the eruptions are unilateral (on one side). At this time, the person experiences severe pain along the affected nerve pathways. The vesicles rupture in a few days and crusts form. Intense pain and itching may persist for several weeks to months. Scarring or permanent skin discoloration can occur. The infection is contagious until the crusts have dried and fallen off the skin.

Diagnosis

Diagnosis is made by examination of the lesions and symptoms.

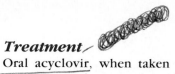

Treatment

Oral acyclovir, when taken within 48 hours of the appearance of symptoms, may reduce the severity of symptoms and prevent the development of additional lesions. Topical acyclovir also may be applied to the lesions. A brief course of corticosteroid therapy may reduce pain. Lesions of the ophthalmic division of the trigeminal nerve require immediate examination and treatment by an ophthalmologist. Additional treatment is symptomatic. Analgesics and liquid preparations that have a drying or antipruritic effect may be applied to the affected area once the crusts have fallen off.

Complications

Pain (postherpetic neuralgia) and itching may persist for months or as long as 2 or more years. Secondary skin infections may occur from scratching the area.

If the ophthalmic branch of the trigeminal nerve is affected, acute eye involvement may occur. Cerebral vasculitis (inflammation of cerebral vessels) is the most serious complication since involvement of the internal carotid arteries may result in hemiplegic strokes. Rarely, the virus spreads to the brain, resulting in encephalitis.

NURSING PROCESS —THE PATIENT WHO HAS HERPES ZOSTER

Assessment

A patient history of symptoms is obtained and the lesions examined. Nursing personnel who have not had chickenpox should not be assigned to examine or care for a patient with herpes zoster.

Nursing Diagnosis

Depending on the location and number of lesions, one or more of the following may apply:

- Pain related to involvement of sensory nerve pathways
- Potential for infection transmission
- Knowledge deficit of medication schedule, methods of relieving pain and itching

Planning and Implementation

The major goal of the patient is to relieve pain and itching.

The major goal of nursing management is to keep the patient as comfortable as possible.

Pain, Intense Itching. A narcotic analgesic such as codeine sulfate is often necessary during the first few days to weeks. The skin may be so sensitive that any clothing or application of topical drugs may intensify pain or itching. Application of cool or warm com-presses or warm showers may relieve these symptoms. It may be necessary to experiment with both to determine which best relieves the discomfort.

Potential for Infection Transmission. The patient is instructed to avoid contact with immunocompromised people and people who have not have chickenpox until the crusts fall off.

Knowledge Deficit. The patient is instructed to wear loose clothing and to avoid scratching the area. If oral acyclovir is prescribed, the dose regimen, as printed on the prescription label, is reviewed with the patient. Methods to relieve pain and itching are offered.

Evaluation

- Pain, itching is reduced or relieved
- Demonstrates understanding of importance to avoid contact with immunocompromised people and those who have not had chickenpox
- Demonstrates understanding of drug therapy regimen, importance of not scratching the affected area, and other methods that may be used to relieve discomfort.

NEUROMUSCULAR DISORDERS

A neuromuscular disorder is one that involves the nervous system and indirectly affects the muscles. Patients with these disorders have a neurologic deficit that causes the nervous system—for any number of reasons—to fail to operate in a normal manner. The nursing process for a patient with a neurologic deficit is covered in Chapter 39.

Multiple Sclerosis

Multiple sclerosis (MS) is a chronic, progressive disease of the nervous system. It also is called a *demyelinating* disease because it causes a permanent degeneration and destruction of myelin. Myelin is thought to act as an insulator, enabling nerve impulses to pass along a nerve fiber. Loss of myelin and subsequent degeneration and atrophy of nerve axons interrupt transmission of impulses along these fibers.

Multiple sclerosis is a disease of youth and early middle life. The highest incidence occurs between the ages of 20 and 40, with about equal incidence in men and women. The disease is more common in northern temperate zones than it is in warm climates. The cause of multiple sclerosis is unknown.

Symptoms

Usually, symptoms appear gradually, and early symptoms vary greatly from patient to patient. Often the seemingly minor symptoms are dismissed as a result of fatigue or strain. Just as the symptoms themselves vary, their intensity and duration differ. Some patients have severe, long-lasting symptoms early in the course of the disease; others may experience only occasional and mild symptoms for several years after onset.

Common symptoms of multiple sclerosis include blurred vision, diplopia (double vision), nystagmus (involuntary movement of the eyeball), weakness, clumsiness, numbness and tingling of an arm or leg, ataxia (motor incoordination), paralysis (usually of lower extremities), disturbance of bowel and bladder function, intention tremor, mood swings (emotional lability), and slurred, hesitant speech. The patient may feel ecstatic one minute, and soon afterward appear depressed. Usually, the patient gradually develops more severe symptoms and shorter remissions. Weakness of a limb may progress gradually to paraplegia. Bowel and bladder incontinence may ultimately develop, and slight visual disturbances may progress to total blindness.

Symptoms often subside during early phases of the illness, and the patient may seem to be perfectly healthy for several months or even years. With each reappearance, however, the symptoms tend to be more severe and last longer. These periods of getting better and then worse again are called *remissions* (getting better) and *exacerbations* (getting worse). They may form a characteristic pattern. Although many patients experience gradual worsening of their symptoms, not all do. A few patients have the disease in a mild form and do not experience an increase in severity of symptoms.

Diagnosis

Early diagnosis may be difficult since symptoms can be vague and temporary. Patient history, CT scan, magnetic resonance imaging (MRI), myelography, and lumbar puncture and examination of the CSF for increased white blood cell count and γ-globulin level may be used to confirm the diagnosis.

Treatment

There is no cure for multiple sclerosis nor any single treatment that relieves symptoms. Symptomatic treatment may be complicated by the uneven and unpredictable course of the disorder. Infections and emotional upsets may precipitate exacerbations.

People can live a long time with multiple sclerosis. Living for 20 years after the diagnosis has been established is not unusual.

Complications

Patients may show symptoms of impaired intellectual functioning late in the course of the illness. Loss of memory, difficulty in concentrating, and impaired judgment may occur. As the disease progresses, the patient is subject to many complications. It is not unusual for pneumonia to be the immediate cause of death. The patient is susceptible to infection because of limited activity, shallow breathing, and general debility. Additional complications include decubitus ulcers, cachexia, deformities, and contractures.

Myasthenia Gravis

Myasthenia gravis is a neuromuscular disorder characterized by severe fatigue of one or more groups of skeletal muscles. Although the exact cause of the disease is unknown, skeletal muscle fatigue is due to a defect in the transmission of nerve impulses from nerve endings to muscles. This transmission defect is apparently due to a decrease in the production of acetylcholine (ACh) at the neuromuscular junction.

Symptoms

Symptoms are caused by muscle weakness and may vary, depending on muscles affected. The most common symptoms include ptosis of the eyelids, difficulty with chewing and swallowing, double vision, voice weakness, a masklike facial expression, and weakness of the extremities.

Diagnosis

Diagnosis is made by patient history and physical examination. Confirmation of the diagnosis may be made by intravenous administration of an anticholinesterase drug, such as edrophonium (Tensilon), which produces relief of symptoms in a few seconds. An electromyogram also may be performed.

Treatment

Treatment includes the administration of an indirect-acting cholinergic (or anticholinesterase) drug, such as pyridostigmine bromide (Mestinon) or ambenonium chloride (Mytelase). The dose of the drug must be adjusted upward or downward according to patient response. Patients who receive drug therapy are observed for signs of drug overdose, such as abdominal cramps, clenched jaws, and muscle rigidity. These signs indicate that the dose is too high for this particular patient at this particular time. Atropine, a cholinergic blocking agent, may be given if overdose symptoms are severe. Other treatments include surgical removal of the thymus gland, prednisone, and plasmapheresis for those not responding to other methods of therapy.

Complications

Poor response to treatment can result in respiratory distress, pneumonia, poor nutrition because of inability to chew and swallow, and aspiration of food or liquids.

Muscular Dystrophy

Muscular dystrophy (or dystrophies) is a group of neuromuscular disorders that are hereditary, chronic in nature, and characterized by progressive skeletal muscle weakening and wasting.

Symptoms

Varying degrees of muscle weakness and wasting are characteristic of the disorder.

Diagnosis

Diagnosis is made by patient history, physical examination, electromyograph studies, and muscle biopsy. Laboratory tests include a serum creatine phosphokinase, which is usually elevated.

Treatment

There is no treatment for this disorder except for the management of complications that arise from the disease process, such as pneumonia, contractures, decubitus formation, deformities, and fractures.

Amyotrophic Lateral Sclerosis

Amyotrophic lateral sclerosis (ALS; Lou Gehrig's disease) is a progressive, fatal neurologic disorder of unknown cause that is characterized by degeneration of the motor neurons of the spinal cord and brain stem.

Symptoms

Symptoms include progressive muscle weakness and wasting of the arms, legs, and trunk. Episodes of muscle fasciculations (twitching) may be experienced, and, if the brain stem is affected, the patient may experience difficulty when speaking and swallowing. Periods of inappropriate laughter and crying also may occur.

Diagnosis

Diagnosis is made by patient history and physical examination. The disorder may be difficult to diagnose in the early stages.

Treatment

There is no specific treatment, and in many cases death occurs several years after diagnosis. The patient is encouraged to remain active as long as possible. Death usually occurs from respiratory arrest or overwhelming respiratory infection.

CRANIAL NERVE DISORDERS
Trigeminal Neuralgia (Tic Douloureux)

The fifth (trigeminal) cranial nerve has three major branches: mandibular, maxillary, and ophthalmic (Fig. 36-3). It is a sensory and motor nerve important to mastication, facial movement, and sensation. For reasons not fully understood, it occasionally becomes painful, hence the term *neuralgia* (nerve pain).

Symptoms

The pain comes in paroxysms, each lasting about 2 to 15 seconds. During a spasm, the face may twitch and tears may come to the eyes. Certain trigger spots (or areas that provoke the pain) may cause an attack when they receive the slightest stimulus (eg, the vibration of music, a passing breeze, or a change of temperature). Patients are understandably reluctant to wash that side of the face, and men may remain unshaven. The forehead over the eyebrow is a common trigger spot when the ophthalmic branch of the nerve is affected.

Diagnosis

Diagnosis is made by patient history.

Treatment

Mild analgesics rarely relieve pain. Narcotic analgesics may be necessary, although continued use can result in addiction. Phenytoin (Dilantin) and carbamazepine (Tegretol) have proved of value for the relief of symptoms for some patients.

After diagnosis, the physician may recommend that the patient consult a dentist for examination of the teeth, since some cases of trigeminal neuralgia have been relieved by correction of dental deformities.

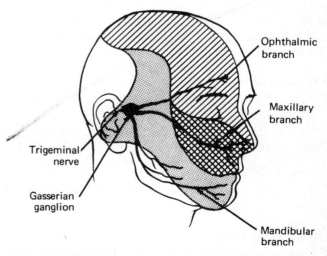

Figure 36–3. Areas innervated by the three branches of the trigeminal nerve. These are the areas that become painful in tic douloureux.

If medical management is unsatisfactory, surgical intervention may be necessary. Surgical division of the sensory root of the trigeminal nerve provides permanent relief. Other surgical procedures include: (1) a percutaneous radio-frequency rhizotomy, which uses heat to destroy the nerve; (2) an intracranial approach for decompression of the trigeminal nerve, which involves the insertion of a small prosthetic device between the nerve and the artery pressing on the trigeminal nerve root; (3) alcohol or phenol injection into one or more branches of the trigeminal nerve root; and (4) a temporal or suboccipital craniotomy for sectioning of the trigeminal nerve root. Additional treatment is supportive.

Bell's Palsy

Bell's palsy is due to involvement of the seventh cranial nerve. The etiology is unknown.

Symptoms

Bell's palsy usually occurs on one side of the face, resulting in weakness and paralysis of facial muscles, often including the muscles of the eyelid. Symptoms develop in a few hours or during a period of 1 or 2 days. Facial pain, pain behind the ear, numbness, diminished blink reflex, ptosis of the eyelid, and tearing of the affected side may occur. Speech difficulty also may occur.

Those who recover usually begin to show improvement in a few weeks. Those whose paralysis is permanent fail to show improvement after 3 or more months.

Diagnosis

Diagnosis is based on the patient's symptoms and physical examination. In some instances, it may be necessary to rule out other neurologic problems, such as brain tumor or stroke, that may have comparable symptoms.

Treatment

Short-term prednisone therapy may be prescribed. Other treatment is supportive.

Temporomandibular Joint Syndrome

Temporomandibular joint (TMJ) syndrome results when the meniscus between the condyle of the mandible and the temporal bone becomes displaced, causing muscle spasm and compression of nerves and arteries in the area.

Some of the causes of TMJ include degenerative arthritis of the mandibular joint, malocclusion of the teeth, and excessive movement of the jaw at the time of endotracheal intubation for general anesthesia.

Symptoms

Symptoms include jaw pain, headache, tinnitus, ear pain, clenching of the jaw, inability to open the mouth, pronounced spasm, and tenderness of the masseter and temporalis muscles. At times, these symptoms may be confused with disorders such as trigeminal neuralgia, migraine, and other neurologic disorders.

Diagnosis

Diagnosis is based on the patient's symptoms. Special dental radiographs often reveal displacement of the meniscus.

Treatment

Treatment may be conducted by a dentist who has experience with the disorder. Analgesics may be prescribed, and a custom-fitted mouth guard may be worn during sleep. Transcutaneous electrical nerve stimulation (TENS), injection of a local anesthetic to relieve muscle spasm, and ice water oral irrigations may be used. Analgesics may be prescribed or recommended for pain. Reconstructive surgery of the mandibular joint may be necessary if conservative treatment is ineffective.

NURSING PROCESS —THE PATIENT WHO HAS A CRANIAL NERVE DISORDER

Assessment

A complete patient history is taken; it may be necessary to rule out other neurologic disorders. A general medical and allergy history also is obtained. Examination of the cranial nerves (see Chapter 35) also may be carried out by the experienced examiner.

Nursing Diagnosis

Depending on symptoms, one or more of the following may apply:

- Anxiety related to symptoms
- Altered nutrition: less than body requirements related to pain, inability to chew
- Pain related to cranial nerve involvement
- Impaired verbal communication related to facial paralysis, pain
- Altered oral mucous membrane related to loss of sensation in the mouth, paralysis of chewing muscles, or pain
- Knowledge deficit of home care, treatment regimen

Planning and Implementation

The major goals of the patient include relief of pain, improved ability to chew and swallow, protection of oral mucous membranes, and an understanding of the treatment regimen.

The major goals of nursing management include relief of pain, improved nutrition, prevention of injury to oral mucous membranes, and developing an effective patient teaching plan.

BELL'S PALSY. If ptosis of the eyelid and a diminished blink reflex occurs, the eye must be protected; corneal ulceration and infection may develop. The physician may order application of an eye patch to keep the eyelid closed and a protective eye shield to be applied at night. An antibiotic ophthalmic ointment may be prescribed. The affected eye is inspected daily for signs of inflammation or purulent drainage.

TRIGEMINAL NEURALGIA. Surgery may be necessary to relieve pain. If the ophthalmic branch was severed, the eye on the operative side is bandaged for 1 or 2 days. When the dressing is removed, eye irrigations with sterile saline may be ordered.

If the mandibular branch was severed, eating becomes a problem. The tongue may be bitten without realizing it, food gets caught in the mouth, and the jaw deviates toward the operative side. Until the patient becomes used to the altered sensation, swallowing also may be difficult. Especially if the patient is elderly and aspiration of fluid or food may lead to a fatal pneumonia, supervision after the operation is necessary when the patient first begins to swallow. The patient is encouraged to take small sips and to concentrate on chewing, eating, and swallowing.

Anxiety. Once a diagnosis of Bell's palsy is confirmed, the patient is assured that a more serious problem (eg, stroke, tumor) has not occurred. The patient with trigeminal neuralgia is assured that every effort will be made to reduce or eliminate those factors that result in attacks of pain.

Altered Nutrition. The patient is instructed to chew on the unaffected side. A soft diet is often tolerated better than a regular diet. Temperature extremes may precipitate an attack of pain when the patient has trigeminal neuralgia. Food and fluids are served at room temperature, and the patient is given food that is easy to chew and swallow. The older patient should be reminded to drink fluids at frequent intervals.

Pain. Mild analgesics may be prescribed if a patient with Bell's palsy has pain. In those with trigeminal neuralgia, every effort is made to reduce the possibility of causing an attack of pain. When drugs such as phenytoin or carbamazepine are used to relieve pain, the patient is observed for the effectiveness of therapy and for adverse drug effects. Because pain relief is neither sudden nor dramatic, it becomes necessary to ask the patient to describe the pain currently experienced and compare the intensity of the present pain with the pain experienced in the past.

Mouth rinses or cleaning the mouth with cotton tipped applicators is attempted if the patient can tolerate these measures. The patient should talk as little as possible because facial movement can precipitate an attack of pain. Ventilation of the room is important: breezes and drafts must be avoided. A sign should be placed on the patient's bed that it is not to be jarred. The face should not be touched in any way.

Altered Oral Mucous Membrane. After the patient has eaten, the inside of the mouth is checked for particles of food that may remain and lead to infection. The oral cavity is gently inspected daily for signs of bleeding, soreness, infection, or breaks in the mucous membrane.

Impaired Verbal Communication. The patient is instructed to speak slowly and in short sentences. If severe pain persists, the patient may need to write questions rather than attempt to speak.

Knowledge Deficit. A teaching plan is developed according to the diagnosis and instructions of the physician or dentist.

BELL'S PALSY. The patient with Bell's palsy may require instruction and demonstration in the application of an eye patch, eye shield, and ophthalmic ointment. Placing the finger on the paralyzed lid and drawing it gently downward before the patch is applied usually keeps the eye closed. Excessive tearing requires frequent changes of the eye patch.

TRIGEMINAL NEURALGIA. During drug therapy, the patient is instructed to keep a record of attacks so the physician may have a guideline for dosage adjustment. Before surgery for this disorder, the physician explains that some loss of sensation may occur and the loss can be permanent. If surgery was performed, the patient is instructed to inspect the mouth daily for signs of breaks in the oral mucous membrane, to chew on the opposite side, to avoid eating hot foods, and to use mouth rinses after eating. The importance of regular dentist visits is stressed because the warning pain of a cavity, abscess, or other dental problem may not be felt.

TEMPEROMANDIBULAR JOINT SYNDROME. The patient is instructed to follow the treatment modalities recommended by the physician or dentist. If a TENS unit is used, the patient is instructed in its use by the physician or dentist. The patient may require a review of what has been explained or shown. If muscle spasm and clamping of the jaw are severe, the patient is encouraged to drink nourishing liquids until able to chew solid food.

Evaluation

- Anxiety is reduced
- Attains and maintains a normal food and fluid intake
- Pain or discomfort is controlled or eliminated
- No evidence of bleeding, infection, or injury to the oral mucous membrane
- Communicates effectively with others
- Demonstrates understanding of home care, treatment modalities

EXTRAPYRAMIDAL DISORDERS
Parkinson's Disease

Parkinsonism (Parkinson's disease, paralysis agitans) was first described by Dr. James Parkinson in 1817. The term *parkinsonism* is used more often because it encompasses the various causes of the disorder, including drugs, head injuries, encephalitis, and so on.

Parkinson's disease affects primarily the basal ganglia and their connections. The main pathway of the basal ganglia is the extrapyramidal tract, which is composed of the system of motor nerves responsible for automatic movements like blinking, walking, eating, posture, muscle tone, and the movements of facial expression. Idiopathic parkinsonism is thought to be due to a deficiency of dopamine, a neurohormone, in the basal ganglia of the brain.

Symptoms

Parkinson's disease usually begins after age 50. Early signs include stiffness, tremors of the hands that are described as "pill-rolling" (a rhythmic motion of the thumb against the fingers), and difficulty performing movements. Usually tremors decrease when movement is voluntary, for example, when picking up an object. Patients may experience the reverse effect, however, when tremors increase during voluntary movements. This type is called an *intention tremor.*

As the disease progresses, tremors of the head, masklike expressions, stooped posture, monotonous speech, shuffling gait, and weight loss are seen. The shuffling gait, with difficulty turning or redirecting forward motion, is a typical manifestation of the disease. Arms rarely swing while walking. Parkinsonism caused by certain drugs is characterized by symptoms similar to those of Parkinson's disease. Rhythmic and involuntary movements of the tongue, the jaw, the neck, and the extremities, along with facial grimaces may be seen.

Symptoms of the disorder progress so slowly that years may lapse between the time of the patient's first symptom and the time of diagnosis. The symptoms may start on only one side of the body and later become bilateral. The spread to the other side may occur quickly or it may be delayed for as long as 15 years.

Rigidity is more widespread through the muscles of the body than is tremor. There is a slight but continuous flexion of all limbs. Reflexes and the power of contraction are not affected but speed of movement is.

In late stages of the disease, when jaw, tongue, and larynx are affected, the speech becomes slurred, and food is chewed inadequately and swallowed with difficulty. Rigidity that is not controlled by drug therapy, physical therapy, or surgery, can lead to contractures. Increased salivation occurs and may be accompanied by drooling. In a small percentage of patients, the eyes roll upward or downward and stay there against the patient's will (oculogyric crises), perhaps for several hours or even a few days.

Diagnosis

Diagnosis is based on symptoms, patient history, and neurologic examination.

Treatment

Treatment is aimed at prolonging independence and preventing dependence. Drugs such as levodopa (Larodopa) and anticholinergiclike agents such as benztropine (Cogentin) and procyclidine (Kemadrin) often reduce the intensity of symptoms. Rehabilitation measures, such as physical therapy, occupational therapy, patient and family education, and counseling, are employed concurrently with drug therapy. Surgery (stereotaxic thalamotomy) has been performed in selected cases; it destroys part of the thalamus so that excessive muscle contraction is decreased.

Complications

Because of their disability, patients are susceptible to respiratory disease. Additional complications are related to problems of immobility and other symptoms of the disorder, including contractures, decubitus, and decreased nutritional intake.

Huntington's Disease

Huntington's disease is a hereditary disorder of the central nervous system, namely, the basal ganglia and portions of the cerebral cortex.

Symptoms

Symptoms occur slowly and include mental apathy and emotional disturbances, choreiform movements (uncontrollable writhing and twisting of the body), facial grimaces, difficulty with chewing and swallowing, speech difficulty, intellectual decline, and loss of bowel and bladder control. Severe depression is not uncommon and may lead to suicide.

Diagnosis

Diagnosis is based on symptoms as well as a family history of the disorder. In some instances, diagnosis is difficult until the symptoms become prominent.

Treatment

No specific treatment exists for this disorder. Tranquilizers and antiparkinsonism drugs have relieved the choreiform movements in some patients. Other treatment modalities are aimed at meeting patient and family needs, such as assistance with home care, rehabilitation, physical therapy, and counseling. Because this disorder is inherited, genetic counseling is advised.

Complications

Pneumonia, contractures, aspiration of food or fluids, falls, and decubitus formation are some of the complications of the disorder.

NURSING PROCESS —THE PATIENT WHO HAS AN EXTRAPYRAMIDAL DISORDER

Assessment

A complete neurologic examination (see Chapter 35) is performed to determine the effects of the disorder on the patient's ability to function. Activities, such as walking, eating, talking, and picking up objects, are evaluated and listed according to whether the patient is able to perform them without help.

Nursing Diagnosis

Depending on the stage of the disease, one or more of the following may apply. As neurologic deficits occur, additional diagnoses may be added when certain needs and problems are identified (see also Chapter 39).

- Activity intolerance related to fatigue
- Impaired physical mobility related to muscle rigidity or abnormal involuntary movements
- Anxiety related to inability to care for self, tremors
- Constipation related to immobility, failure to drink fluids, diet
- Impaired verbal communication related to inability to articulate words secondary to involvement of speech muscles
- Ineffective individual coping related to diagnosis, symptoms, progression of disease

- Altered family processes related to illness of family member, progression of disease, prognosis, uncertain future, dependence of patient on others
- Impaired swallowing related to impairment of cranial nerves that control swallowing
- Potential fluid volume deficit related to difficulty with swallowing, inability to take fluids without help
- Altered nutrition: less than body requirements related to difficulty with chewing, swallowing, inability to handle utensils
- Potential for injury related to muscle rigidity, tremors, unsteady gait, involuntary movements
- Self-care deficit: total or partial (if partial, specify areas) related to muscle rigidity, tremor, abnormal muscle movements
- Impaired skin integrity related to immobility
- Impaired home maintenance management related to inability to care for self, home, and others
- Social isolation related to immobility, difficulty communicating with others
- Knowledge deficit of medication regimen, other treatment modalities

Planning and Implementation

The major goals of the patient include increased activity tolerance, improved physical mobility, reduced anxiety, improved communication skills, improved nutrition and fluid intake, prevention of injury, improved ability to care for self, prevention of skin breakdown, improved social interactions, learning to cope with the illness, and understanding the treatment regimen.

The major goal of nursing management is to encourage independence and prolong dependence.

Many people with extrapyramidal disorders are admitted to the hospital for other problems or because of the debilitating effects of the disease, such as severe contractures, fractures from falling, pneumonia, or extensive decubitus ulcers. Rehabilitation in the advanced stages of the disease is difficult, and usually only minor progress is achieved. Decreased debilitation and prevention of secondary problems, such as pneumonia and decubitus ulcers, are often the main goals of treatment in advanced cases. Patients in less advanced stages of the disease are usually more amenable to rehabilitation. A sample nursing care plan is shown in Nursing Care Plan 36-1.

Drugs administered for parkinsonism are capable of causing a wide variety of adverse side effects that require careful observation of the patient, especially when therapy is first instituted.

Activity Intolerance, Self-Care Deficit, Impaired Physical Mobility. Although it cannot halt progression of the disease, physical therapy can help the patient maintain self-care activities. Physical therapy is not indicated for tremor but is of value in the rigidity of

Nursing Care Plan 36–1
Nursing Management of the Patient Who Has Parkinsonism

Potential Problem and Potential Nursing Diagnosis	Nursing Intervention	Outcome Criteria
Muscular Rigidity (Bradykinesia) *Impaired physical mobility related to muscle rigidity*	Administer antiparkinsonism agents as ordered; work with physical and occupational therapist to plan for active and passive exercises, followed by supervision of active exercises; perform passive exercises of extremities; offer encouragement when patient able to perform exercises	Experiences some decrease in muscle rigidity; demonstrates increased ability to carry out ADL
Tremors *Impaired physical mobility related to muscle rigidity, abnormal involuntary movements*	Administer antiparkinsonism agents as ordered; teach patient how to perform ADL with minimal interference from tremors (holding glass with both hands, wearing slip-on shoes instead of those with laces, using straws to drink, etc.)	Experiences decrease in interference with ADL
Dependence on Others for Care and ADL *Self-care deficit related to muscle rigidity, tremors*	Encourage patient to do as much for himself as possible; allow ample time to perform ADL; adapt clothing, eating, and grooming utensils for ease of use; set realistic goals and encourage and praise patient for each goal attained	Demonstrates decreased dependence on others
Contractures; Muscle Atrophy; Deformities	Encourage ambulation; provide cane, walker for ambulation as needed; encourage active ROM exercises while in bed; change position when in bed q 2 hr	Has no contractures, muscle atrophy or deformities
Anorexia; Weight Loss	Offer small frequent high-caloric, high-protein feedings; allow patient to select foods that are preferred (unless prohibited by special dietary orders); provide food that is easy to chew, follow each meal with good oral care	Maintains weight; appetite improves
Constipation *Altered bowel elimination; constipation related to immobility*	Check daily for bowel movement; note consistency of stool; encourage fluids hourly; obtain order for stool softener; obtain order for laxative or enema if needed; contact dietitian for dietary consult and possible inclusion of foods that prevent constipation in daily menu	Reports constipation prevented or relieved
Difficulty in Communication With Others *Impaired verbal communication related to inability to articulate words*	Advise patient to speak slowly; avoid impatience when patient unable to communicate; provide pad and pen or pencil for patient to communicate needs (some patients are unable to write because of tremors); anticipate patient's needs; decrease occurrences of frustration by working with patient in communicating with others	Demonstrates improvement in communication
Depression, Withdrawal	Encourage interaction with others; promote independence by having patient participate in ADL; encourage active participation and interest in a hobby or other forms of entertainment; discuss current events or subjects of interest with patient	Attempts to communicate with others; is interested in self and others; shows desire to make decisions

ADL, activities of daily living; ROM, range-of-motion.

parkinsonism and may be of limited value for those with Huntington's disease. Early and consistent treatment is most beneficial. Chart 36-1 describes the rehabilitation of a patient with parkinsonism.

Physical activity and ambulation are encouraged. As activity is increased, the ability to tolerate activity also may increase. Depending on the stage of the disease, partial or total assistance may be necessary when the patient is ambulating, bathing, or eating, but self-care activities should be encouraged and sufficient time allowed to perform them.

Active or passive range-of-motion (ROM) exercises help prevent muscle contractures. The nurse must work with the physical and occupational therapist to plan additional active and passive exercises.

The patient should be helped by family, friends, or the professional staff only when unable to perform a movement. It is important that stress, anxiety, and fatigue, all of which make the symptoms worse, be kept to a minimum.

Anxiety, Ineffective Individual Coping. The patient may experience anxiety and frustration when unable to perform routine tasks. Ample time must be allowed for these patients to participate in their own care. These patients move slowly or find it difficult to move and perform routine tasks and cannot be hurried. To do so only increases stress.

Drooling, which often occurs in the later stage of parkinsonism, disgusts the patient, the blank face and the slowed movements make social interaction difficult, and muscle rigidity is anxiety-provoking and frustrating. Every effort must be made to keep the patient clean and well groomed. Tissues are kept available so the patient can remove saliva from the face.

Patients with a neuromuscular disorder may realize what is wrong with their body but be unable to cope with the symptoms. Emotional outbursts may occur as the patient tries to fight the changes occurring in the body. The nurse must offer emotional support, encouragement, and understanding, which in turn may help the patient cope with the disability.

Constipation. If constipation is a problem, stool softeners may be necessary. A record of bowel movements is kept, and the physician is informed if constipation occurs.

Impaired Verbal Communication. The patient is encouraged to speak slowly to improve communication with others. Patients who have great difficulty communicating their needs may use gestures such as pointing or nodding the head to answer questions. Patience is always necessary when communicating with patients who have speech problems. A speech therapist may be able to help the patient improve the quality of speech and communication.

Altered Family Processes, Impaired Home Maintenance Management. Extrapyramidal disorders are discouraging for patients and their families. The affliction is long-term, without remission of symptoms. If a patient is responsible for the financial or physical support of others, the family must be encouraged to work together to solve immediate and long-range problems.

The nurse must evaluate a patient's ability to care for self and home. A patient who lives alone particularly may experience many difficulties with managing a household and may require assistance from relatives, friends, or a social agency. If a patient does not ask for assistance but evaluation reveals that help would most likely be needed, further investigation is necessary. A referral may be made to a social service worker or the problem discussed with the family.

In time, the patient's physical care may become difficult to carry out at home, and admission to a hospital, nursing home, or skilled nursing facility may be necessary. The family must be given emotional

---

Chart 36–1. Rehabilitation of the Patient Who Has Parkinsonism

Minimal Physical Disability
- Physical activity and ambulation is encouraged.
- Exercise of the extremities is important. The type of exercise may be suggested by the physical therapist and must be demonstrated to the patient.
- Self-care activities are encouraged but must be done gradually. The patient should sit for activities such as shaving, grooming, bathing, and so on.

Moderate Physical Disability
- The patient is assisted with ambulation several times a day.
- Exercises of the extremities is necessary; passive exercises should be done if the patient is unable to move or exercise his legs.
- Participation in daily self-care is encouraged, with assistance when needed.

Advanced Disability
- The patient is allowed to do as much as possible even though participation in any activity is minimal.
- Total dependence is avoided as long as possible.
- If eating is difficult, a soft diet and ample time to eat will be necessary.
- If feeding becomes necessary, the patient is fed slowly.
- A suction machine is placed in the room because difficulty in chewing and swallowing poses the threat of aspiration.

support when a decision is being made about admission to a health care facility.

Impaired Swallowing, Potential Fluid Volume Deficit, Altered Nutrition. Patients may have poor appetites, but a well-balanced diet is necessary to maintain nutrition. Adequate fluid intake is important, especially for those in advanced stages of the disease who may neglect to take fluids because tremors make it difficult to hold a glass. Fluids are offered hourly, and a record of intake and output is kept. If tremors are severe, the drinking glass must be held for the patient.

If chewing and swallowing is difficult, a soft diet and ample time to eat is necessary. Food containers are opened and, when necessary, food cut into small pieces. Fluids are offered with meals. A suction machine is kept in the room because of the threat of aspiration. In the advanced stages of these disorders, a patient may need to be fed.

Potential for Injury. When necessary, assistance is given when the patient is allowed to ambulate. Patients with a tendency to have ambulatory difficulties are instructed to ask for help before attempting to get out of bed or to walk.

Impaired Skin Integrity. Patients largely confined to bed require a position change every 2 hours. Pressure points are examined for signs of skin breakdown.

Social Isolation. When possible, the patient is encouraged to participate in events that provide recreation, diversion, and interaction with others. Planned periods of activities help the patient become involved in meaningful endeavors, reduce depression and boredom, and increase awareness of the environment.

Knowledge Deficit. Many patients are diagnosed and started on medical management in a physician's office or clinic. The initiation of rehabilitation and patient and family education rests with the physician, who may delegate some teaching responsibility to other professional staff members in these facilities.

The patient is encouraged to lead as normal a life as possible, with emphasis on the importance of exercise and self-care. The medical regimen is explained to the patient and family.

The patient can be taught to perform some tasks with minimal difficulty, such as using both hands to hold a drinking glass, using a straw to drink, and wearing slip-on shoes instead of those with laces.

Evaluation

- Demonstrates less anxiety when performing motor tasks
- Tolerates increased activity
- Self-care needs are met
- Makes effort to increase mobility
- Shows evidence of being able to cope with the effects of the disorder
- Attains normal bowel elimination pattern
- Demonstrates improvement in speech
- Family demonstrates willingness to cope with the symptoms of the disorder
- Family participates in plans for home care
- Takes fluids at regular intervals
- Attains and maintains an adequate food intake
- No evidence of injury
- Socializes with others
- Patient and family demonstrate understanding of treatment modalities

CONVULSIVE DISORDERS

Convulsive disorders (or seizures) involve abnormal motor, sensory, or psychic activity. These abnormalities may occur alone or in combination. A seizure is an abnormal electrical disturbance in one or more specific areas of the brain. If the electrical disturbance involves the entire brain, a generalized seizure occurs.

Convulsive disorders are generally classified as idiopathic or acquired. Idiopathic seizures have no known cause. The causes of acquired seizures include high fever, electrolyte imbalances, uremia, hypoglycemia, hypoxia, brain tumors, and some drug withdrawal reactions. Once the cause is removed (if it can be removed), the seizures theoretically cease.

Epilepsy is a permanent, recurrent convulsive disorder. The known causes of epilepsy include brain injury at birth, head injuries, and inborn errors of metabolism. In some patients, the cause of epilepsy is never determined.

Each different type of convulsive disorder is characterized by a specific pattern of events. Table 36-2 lists the international classification of epileptic seizures.

Partial Seizures

Partial or focal seizures begin in a specific area of the cerebral cortex. In some instances, a partial seizure may progress to a generalized seizure. The two general types of partial seizures are those with elementary (or simple) symptoms and those with complex symptoms. A patient who has a partial seizure with elementary symptoms generally does not lose consciousness, and the seizure rarely lasts longer than 1 minute. A patient who has a partial seizure with complex symptoms may have a variety of sensory or motor manifestations.

Table 36–2. International Classification of Epileptic Seizures

I. Partial Seizures (seizures beginning locally)
   A. Partial seizures with elementary symptomatology (generally without impairment of consciousness)
     1. With motor symptoms (include jacksonian seizures)
     2. With special sensory or somatosensory symptoms
     3. With autonomic symptoms
     4. Compound forms
   B. Partial Seizures With Complex Symptomatology (generally with impairment of consciousness; temporal lobe or psychomotor seizures)
     1. With impairment of consciousness only
     2. With cognitive symptomatology
     3. With affective symptomatology
     4. With psychosensory symptomatology
     5. With psychomotor symptomatology (automatisms)
     6. Compound forms
   C. Partial seizures secondarily generalized
II. Generalized Seizures (bilaterally symmetrical and without local onset)
     1. Absences (petit mal)
     2. Bilateral massive epileptic myoclonus
     3. Infantile spasms
     4. Clonic seizures
     5. Tonic seizures
     6. Tonic–clonic seizures
     7. Atonic seizures
     8. Akinetic seizures
III. Unilateral Seizures (or predominately unilateral)
IV. Unclassified Epileptic Seizures (incomplete data)

(Modified from Gastaut H. Clinical and electroencephalographical classification of epileptic seizures. Epilepsia 1970;11:102.)

These also rarely last longer than 1 minute, but some alteration of consciousness usually occurs. After the seizure, the patient may experience a period of confusion.

The terms *Jacksonian, focal motor,* and *focal sensory* have been used to describe partial elementary seizures. The terms *psychomotor* and *psychosensory* have been used to describe partial complex seizures. On occasion, these terms are still used.

Partial elementary seizures with motor symptoms include uncontrolled jerking movements of a body part, such as a finger, mouth, hand, or foot. Partial elementary seizures with sensory symptoms include hallucinatory sights, sounds, and odors (which are often unpleasant), mumbling, and the use of nonsense words. Partial complex seizures often include automatic repetitive movements (automatisms) that usually are not appropriate to the immediate situation,

such as lip smacking or picking at clothing or objects (real or imaginary). Other manifestations of this type of seizure include emotional reactions, such as fear or anger, distorted visual or auditory sensations, and memory impairment.

Generalized Seizures

Generalized seizures involve the entire brain. Consciousness is lost, and the seizure may last from several seconds to several minutes. The various types of generalized seizures are discussed below.

Absence Seizures. Absence seizures, also referred to as *petit mal* seizures, are more common in children. They are characterized by a brief loss of consciousness during which physical activity ceases. The person stares blankly, the eyelids may flutter, the lips may move, and slight movement of the head and extremities may occur. These seizures usually last for a few seconds, and the person rarely falls to the ground. Because of their brief duration and relative lack of prominent movements, these seizures often go unnoticed. Patients with absence seizures may have them many times a day.

Myoclonic Seizures. These seizures are characterized by sudden excessive jerking of the extremities or the body. In some instances, the muscle activity may be so severe that the patient falls to the ground. These seizures are usually brief.

Tonic-Clonic Seizures. These seizures, also referred to as *grand mal* seizures, are characterized by a sequence of events that begins, in some patients, with a prodromal (or preictal) phase. The prodromal phase consists of vague emotional changes, such as depression, anxiety, or nervousness. This phase may last for minutes or hours and then may be followed by an aura, which usually precedes the seizure by a few seconds. The aura may be sensory, that is a hallucinatory odor or sound, or it may be a sensation, such as weakness or numbness. In those who experience an aura, the aura is almost always the same. The aura is related to the anatomic origin of the seizure.

The aura is followed by the so-called epileptic cry, which is caused by spasm of the respiratory muscles and muscles of the throat and glottis. This cry immediately precedes the loss of consciousness and the ensuing tonic and clonic phases of the convulsion. In the tonic phase, the muscles contract rigidly; in the clonic phase, the muscles alternate between contraction and relaxation, resulting in jerking movements and thrashing of the arms and legs. The skin becomes cyanotic, and breathing is spasmodic. Saliva mixes with air, resulting in "frothing" at the mouth. The jaws are tightly clenched, and the tongue and inner cheek may be bitten. Urinary or fecal incontinence usually occurs. The clonic phase may last up to a minute or more; it then gradually subsides and is followed by the postictal state. This phase of the seizure may vary; headache, fatigue, deep sleep, confusion, nausea, and muscle soreness may be experienced. Many fall into a deep sleep for several hours.

Other Types of Seizures. Atonic (loss of muscle tone) seizures are those that affect the muscles. In this type of seizure, a brief loss of consciousness causes the patient suddenly to fall to the ground; however, the patient then rises and resumes normal activity. An akinetic (loss of movement) seizure is similar because muscle tone is briefly lost and the muscles completely collapse. The patient may or may not fall to the ground, and recovery from the seizure is rapid. Clonic seizures are spasms of the muscles, and tonic seizures are characterized by muscle rigidity. Infantile spasms affect only infants.

Status Epilepticus. Status epilepticus refers to a series of tonic-clonic seizures that a patient experiences without regaining consciousness between them. This is an extremely dangerous condition that can lead to a patient's death unless it is terminated. Status epilepticus may occur spontaneously and for no known reason but also may occur if anticonvulsant medications are suddenly stopped. Intravenous barbiturates or diazepam (Valium) may be administered to terminate the attack.

Diagnosis

A convulsive disorder may be the easiest or most difficult to diagnose, depending on the symptoms, the patient history, and the results of diagnostic tests. The most accurate diagnosis is made when the seizure is observed by medical personnel or when an accurate description of the seizure is given by a family member. Along with observation, a thorough medical history (including a history of all previous illnesses and injuries), a history of the onset of the seizures and the seizure pattern, and a family history are important. A neurologic examination and an EEG may be performed, and other laboratory or diagnostic studies, such as a CT scan, serology, and serum electrolytes, may be used to confirm the diagnosis and, in some instances, to determine the cause of the convulsive disorder. Although the EEG is a useful diagnostic tool, it may not be abnormal in the epileptic patient, especially the first time the EEG is performed. Abnormal EEGs also may be seen in those who do not have epilepsy. When epilepsy is suspected, a series of EEGs may be necessary if the first one is normal.

Treatment

Once a diagnosis of a convulsive disorder is confirmed, the physician selects one or more anticonvulsant agents to control the seizures (eg, phenytoin [Dilantin], phenobarbital, carbamazepine [Tegretol], ethosuximide [Zarontin], and valproic acid [Depakene]). Drug therapy may control the seizures or reduce their frequency or severity. A small number of patients do not respond to any type of drug therapy. In addition, patients may experience adverse drug effects (some of which can be serious) and may require another agent, which could be less effective.

When drug therapy is instituted, the dosage often has to be adjusted over a period of several weeks. The drug may need to be changed or another drug added to the regimen to obtain optimum control. Serum levels of some anticonvulsant drugs may be ordered to allow for more accurate adjustment of dosage and the prevention of toxicity. Serum levels also identify patients who are not taking the drug as ordered.

Convulsive disorders due to brain tumor, brain abscess, or other cerebral disorder may require surgical intervention. Surgery for epilepsy is usually not considered unless the patient does not respond to drug therapy and seizures are frequent and serious in nature. Even then, surgery may not be possible, since the area of the brain that is the focus of the seizure must be first identified and then amendable to surgical removal.

NURSING PROCESS —THE PATIENT WHO HAS A CONVULSIVE DISORDER

Assessment

A complete patient and family history, including a drug and allergy history, is obtained. The patient is questioned regarding events or symptoms that occurred before and after the seizure. A description of the seizure is obtained from an observer. Additional information should include a family history of seizures and any injury that may have occurred in the past (from birth to the present). If the patient has been treated for a seizure disorder in the past, it is important to determine if the medication has been taken as prescribed. A neurologic examination (see Chapter 35) also is performed.

Nursing Diagnosis

Depending on the type of convulsive disorder, one or more of the following may apply:

■ Anxiety related to diagnosis, occurrence of more seizures, social stigma

- Potential for injury related to uncontrolled movements during seizure
- Social isolation related to stigma attached to epilepsy
- Altered oral mucous membrane related to drug therapy, injury during seizure
- Knowledge deficit of treatment regimen, community agencies that offer assistance

Planning and Implementation

The major goals of the patient include reduced anxiety, improved social interactions, and knowledge of treatment regimen and adverse drug effects. Goals of the newly diagnosed epileptic may be to learn more about the disorder and to obtain information about community agencies that offer information and assistance to those with epilepsy.

The major goals of nursing management are to work with the medical team to control the seizures and to help the patient understand and adjust to the disorder.

The patient with a convulsive disorder is closely and frequently observed, especially when the patient has frequent seizures, when the seizures are severe in nature, and when the diagnosis of a convulsive disorder is uncertain. It also is important that the prescribed medication not be omitted because status epilepticus could occur.

Observations of a patient's seizure include the length of the seizure, the patient's behavior immediately before and after the seizure, the type of body movements (if any), whether consciousness was lost, whether the patient was incontinent, and whether any apparent injury has occurred. It is most important that the observations be as complete as possible and that every detail of patient behavior is recorded. The patient's condition after the seizure (eg, sleepiness or confusion) also is recorded.

Care of the patient during and after a tonic-clonic seizure is given in Chart 36-2. The patient who has a petit mal seizure usually requires no special care during or after the seizure.

Anxiety. The patient is assured that drug therapy most likely will reduce the number of seizures. A diagnosis of a seizure disorder often produces feelings of helplessness, anxiety, fear, and depression. The patient is concerned about the effects the diagnosis will have on others and is faced with the worry that another seizure may occur at any time. Depending on state and insurance laws, a person with a seizure disorder may not be able to drive or work in certain industries. With this diagnosis, the patient and family are often faced with many problems.

The patient and family must be given time to talk about the disorder and the effects it has on themselves and others. Many patients and families require

---

Chart 36–2. Management of a Patient During and After a Tonic–Clonic (Grand Mal) Seizure

During the Seizure

- The patient should be turned on the side to keep the airway patent and to prevent aspiration of saliva and vomitus. Remove oral secretions by suctioning, if possible.
- Any objects that may obstruct breathing must be removed: pillows, bedding, clothing.
- Restrictive clothing should be loosened, if possible.
- It is necessary to protect the patient from injury, but *it is dangerous to restrain the extremities or the head forcibly.*
- The nurse must *stay with the patient.*

After the Seizure

- The bed is kept flat and the patient turned on the side until awakening. The room should be dim and noise kept to a minimum.
- Restrictive clothing should be loosened if this could not be done during the attack.
- Vital signs must be taken immediately and every 30 min until the patient is awake.
- The lips, the tongue, and the inside of the mouth should be checked for injury.
- If the patient is incontinent, the bedding should be changed with as little disturbance as possible.

---

counseling to cope with the obstacles associated with the disorder. In some instances, the family becomes overprotective.

After a seizure, the patient may need reassurance. Even though unaware that a seizure has occurred, patients may be aware of the extra attention they received during or after a seizure.

Potential for Injury. The patient must not be forcibly restrained during a generalized seizure because fractures of the arms, legs, or shoulders may result. If a nurse is present *before* the tonic phase (the rigid or stiffening part of the seizure), an oral airway can be inserted. Keeping these patients on their side prevents the tongue from obstructing the pharynx.

The side rails can be padded and raised while the patient is on bed rest. Those who have atonic or akinetic seizures should be checked for injury if falling has occurred. These patients may benefit by wearing a rigid helmet or another type of padded head gear when seizures are frequent.

If confusion occurs after a seizure, the patient should remain in bed with the side rails raised. After a tonic-clonic seizure, the patient may sleep for several hours.

Social Isolation. Many epileptics suffer more acutely from the stigma attached to epilepsy than from the symptoms. Every life situation is tinged with the dread of an attack and the fear of what others will think. The family often is ashamed that the patient has epilepsy. Because some types of epilepsy have a familial predisposition, family members often feel that a relative's disorder is a reflection on their health, and they may make every effort to conceal it. The patient and family may require counseling, which can help them understand the disorder and the potential limitations imposed by it and can help them cope with problems as they arise.

Altered Oral Mucous Membrane. After a generalized seizure, the oral cavity and teeth are checked for signs of injury. The physician is notified if profuse bleeding, cuts on the surface of the tongue, or loose or broken teeth are present. If the teeth are injured, an examination and treatment by a dentist may be necessary.

Gingival hyperplasia (overgrowth of gum tissue) can occur with the prolonged administration of the hydantoins (phenytoin, ethotoin, mephenytoin). Good oral hygiene and dental checkups every 3 to 6 months may control advanced gum disease in these patients.

Knowledge Deficit. Discharge teaching and public education are two important nursing responsibilities. The newly diagnosed epileptic needs a thorough explanation of the disorder. The physician initially instructs them about the type of epilepsy they have, the medications necessary, and the precautions, if any, to be taken. In some patients, seizures may be precipitated by strong stimuli, such as flashing or blinking lights, or by other factors, including stress or lack of sleep.

The teaching plan can include the following points:

- Medication regimen and the importance of medication, which in most instances must be taken daily throughout one's life
- The dangers associated with omitting or stopping the medication unless told to do so by the physician
- Adverse effects of the medication, which should be reviewed after the physician's original explanation
- Necessity of routine visits to the physician's office or clinic
- Hazards of operating a motor vehicle or performing potentially dangerous tasks until seizures are under control with medication
- Importance of wearing Medic-Alert tags or other medical identification
- Importance of avoiding situations known to produce a seizure

Questions of marriage and children may arise. The patient may be helped by personal and genetic counseling.

Finding and keeping a job may be difficult for a person with epilepsy. There is a false impression that epileptics are of subnormal intelligence. Although some epileptics experience alteration in their mental functioning, many nevertheless cope satisfactorily with work, home, and community responsibilities. The number of epileptics who have severe impairment of intellectual functioning, due to brain damage, and who, therefore, are unable to function adequately in work and other community situations is small. Persons with epilepsy who have frequent, severe seizures can be employed only in controlled situations, such as sheltered workshops.

The Epilepsy Foundation of America, which has chapters in many large cities, provides services to epileptics and their families, including counseling, low-cost prescription services, and referral to agencies that are geared toward vocational rehabilitation, job opportunities, and sheltered workshops.

Evaluation

- Seizures are controlled
- Anxiety is reduced
- No evidence of injury noted
- Socializes with others; states desire to return to routine daily activities
- Demonstrates understanding of disorder and treatment modalities
- Makes appointment for counseling
- Talks openly about epilepsy and asks questions

BRAIN TUMORS   *causes ↑ICP (×1)*

A brain tumor, whether malignant or benign, can result in death because, as it expands within the narrow confines of the skull, it encroaches on brain tissue that is vital for life. Tumors may be extracerebral, that is, they are situated outside the brain but within the cranium. These tumors, such as meningiomas (tumors of the meninges), press on the brain tissue from without. Tumors may arise from cerebral tissue, such as gliomas and glioblastomas, which are malignant neoplasms; or they may arise from blood vessels, such as angiomas, which are benign. The brain also is the site of metastatic lesions from primary tumors, especially tumors of the lungs and breast.

Brain tumors are seen in all age groups. Some types are more common in people younger than 20 years of age, whereas others more frequently strike older people. About half of all brain tumors are gliomas. *astrocytoma*

Symptoms

Because tumors take up space and because they may block the flow and, thus, the absorption of CSF, symptoms of increased ICP occur. The classic triad of headache, vomiting, and papilledema is common. Headache is most common early in the morning, when the patient gets out of bed. Headache becomes increasingly severe and frequent as the tumor grows. Vomiting occurs without nausea or warning. Convulsions also may occur. In addition to symptoms of generalized cerebral irritation and increased ICP, other symptoms of disturbed neurologic function may be observed, depending on the location of the tumor. Thus, symptoms such as speech difficulty, paralysis, and double vision may be seen.

The progression of symptoms is characteristic of brain tumors. As the tumor grows and exerts increasing pressure, symptoms intensify. When the ICP is greatly increased, the brain stem is forced through the foramen magnum (see Fig. 36-2) and the patient is in grave danger; the vital centers that control respiration and heart rate are compressed. Respirations become deeper, labored, and noisy, and then slow and only periodic. Unless the condition is relieved, the patient dies of respiratory failure. In the early stages, bradycardia appears; tachycardia appears near the end. Blood pressure may remain relatively stable, but hyperthermia may occur as the temperature-regulating center in the brain is affected. Coma becomes progressively deepened.

Diagnosis

Diagnosis is made by a history of the patient's symptoms, a neurologic examination, CT scan, MRI brain scan, and cerebral angiography.

Treatment

The treatment of a brain tumor depends on several factors, including the location of the tumor, the age of the patient, the type of tumor (primary or metastatic), and the physical condition of the patient. Brain tumors may be treated by surgery, radiation, or chemotherapy. In some instances, a combination of two or all three of these treatment methods may be used. A newer method of removing brain tumors involves the use of a laser beam directed at the tumor site. This surgical technique has enabled the physician to reach tumors that were previously considered inoperable because of their location.

Brain tumors are sometimes still inoperable, and radiation or chemotherapy is the remaining treatment of choice. Patients may be unable to withstand treatment with surgery, chemotherapy, or radiation and thus are kept as comfortable and pain-free as possible.

Some brain tumors can be removed without damage to nearby brain tissue; others cannot be removed without causing permanent brain damage. If healthy brain tissue has to be traumatized or removed to reach the tumor, some of the patient's postoperative symptoms are determined by the location and function of the damaged or removed tissue. Brain tissue does not regenerate.

Surgery for operable brain tumors is performed by means of a craniotomy (incision through the skull) or craniectomy (excision of part of the skull). A bone flap may be made by sawing the skull to reach the brain. After the tumor is removed, the dura is reapproximated (the cut edges are lined up and sewn together), the bone flap is replaced, and the skin sutured. On occasion, the bone fragment is not reinserted, but the space is left free so that the brain has room to expand. This procedure may be followed when increasing ICP or tumor growth is expected, as in cases in which not all the tumor can be removed.

Complications

Increased ICP, paralysis, mental changes, infection, and problems associated with prolonged immobility are some of the complications of brain tumors.

NURSING PROCESS —THE PATIENT WHO HAS A BRAIN TUMOR

Assessment

A patient history is taken, and a neurologic examination (see Chapter 35) is performed. Additional assessments depend on the patient's symptoms and general condition. For example, the patient with no motor or sensory involvement requires different additional assessments than the debilitated patient with inoperable lung cancer and cerebral metastasis.

Nursing Diagnosis

Depending on the type and location of the tumor, treatment modalities, and other factors, one or more of the following may apply. At various stages of the disorder or after surgery (see Chapter 38), additional nursing diagnoses may be added as needed. If temporary or permanent neurologic deficits occur as the result of surgery or tumor growth, additional nursing diagnoses, as outlined in Chapter 39, may be added.

- Anxiety related to diagnosis, surgery and its complications, prognosis
- Ineffective individual coping related to diagnosis, treatment modalities, prognosis
- Altered family processes related to nature of disorder, prognosis, change in family roles
- Self-care deficit: total or partial (if partial specify deficit) related to effect of tumor on motor or sensory areas of the brain

- Pain related to pressure of tumor on brain tissue
- Altered nutrition: less than body requirements related to decreased LOC, pain, nausea and vomiting associated with chemotherapy or radiation therapy, vomiting associated with increased ICP
- Potential fluid volume deficit related to vomiting secondary to increased ICP, decreased LOC
- Impaired physical mobility related to effect of tumor on motor areas of the brain
- Anticipatory grieving related to uncertain future, actual or perceived loss of function, prognosis
- Impaired tissue integrity related to immobility
- Altered oral mucous membrane related to chemotherapy, radiation therapy
- Knowledge deficit of treatment modalities, home care

Planning and Implementation

The major goals of the patient include relief of pain, reduction of anxiety, improved nutrition and fluid intake, improved physical mobility, ability to care for self, prevention of oral mucous membrane and skin breakdown, learning to cope with the disorder, and an understanding of treatment modalities and home care.

The major goals of nursing management are to meet the patient's basic needs, relieve discomfort and pain, recognize symptoms of increased ICP and other complications associated with the disorder, and help the patient and family cope with the disorder.

If the patient has a craniotomy, see Chapter 38.

Anxiety, Ineffective Individual Coping, Grieving. The impact of the diagnosis and proposed treatment modalities result in pronounced emotional responses in the patient and family. The nurse must allow them time to verbalize their concerns, talk about the situation, and ask questions. Questions that cannot (or should not) be answered by a nurse are referred to the physician.

The patient and family most likely will have difficulty coping with the situation. The patient with cerebral metastases may incur psychological changes, such as depression, euphoria, and anxiety. These changes often deeply affect family members, making it more difficult for them to cope with the fact that the cancer has spread to the brain.

The patient and family may experience grief over the diagnosis, uncertain future, and possibly death. The family must be assured that their loved one is receiving the best possible care, the most modern methods of treatment, and, when needed, help and advice from appropriate personnel. Clergy, family, friends, and other professionals and support groups that deal with terminal malignant disorders or motor disabilities can be of benefit to the patient and family. Knowing that other people and agencies can offer emotional and perhaps financial support can help patients and families deal with present and future problems.

Altered Family Processes. Surgery, radiation therapy, and chemotherapy may result in profound and, in some cases, permanent physical and mental changes. These changes may affect the patient's ability to totally or partially assume physical, financial, and emotional responsibility in the family structure. The burden of these responsibilities may shift to others who may or may not be able to assume them adequately. In addition, the patient may become totally dependent on the family for physical care—another role they may not be able to assume.

The nurse must be alert to problems articulated by the patient and family. Once a problem is identified, plans of action can be proposed to the family.

Self-Care Deficit. Assessment reveals what a patient can and cannot do. At all times, patients are encouraged to participate in personal care as much as possible, giving a feeling of independence and control over their lives.

Immediately before discharge from the hospital, the ability of the patient or members of the family to carry on activities of daily living is evaluated. It may be necessary for the family to obtain assistance with home care.

Pain. The patient with an inoperable brain tumor is kept as pain-free as possible. Pain often increases as the tumor expands. Intravenous morphine has relieved intractable pain in these patients.

Altered Nutrition and Potential Fluid Volume Deficit. While some patients may be able to tolerate a regular diet, others find it difficult to maintain an adequate food and fluid intake. Food should be offered at a time when the patient is rested and relatively free from pain. Accurate intake and output records are kept and meal trays checked. The physician is informed if the patient fails to eat or take fluids; intravenous fluids or total parenteral nutrition may be necessary.

Impaired Physical Mobility. Even when the prognosis is grave, it is important to encourage mobility for as long as possible. Whenever the patient is unable to safely ambulate, assistance is always given.

Respiratory Function. Patients may experience increased ICP that results in an alteration in their respiratory rate, rhythm, and depth. The patient is closely observed for respiratory changes, and the physician is notified if they occur. Respiratory support, such as oxygen administration or mechanical ventilation, may be necessary.

Impaired Tissue Integrity. Patients confined mostly to bed must have their position changed every 2 hours, and their skin must be inspected for early signs of breakdown and decubitus formation. Contractures are prevented by proper positioning and, when ordered, active or passive ROM exercises.

Altered Oral Mucous Membrane. Patients who receive radiation or chemotherapy may develop oral lesions. These lesions may develop because of xerostomia (dry mouth), the effects of radiation on the parotid glands, or as a direct result of chemotherapy. Treatments to relieve discomfort include topical anesthetics, meticulous oral care, and frequent sips of water and mouth rinses. If the patient is able, a visit to the dentist for evaluation and treatment may be of value.

Knowledge Deficit. All treatment modalities are explained to the patient and family by one or more members of the medical team. Faced with many decisions, the patient and family may find it difficult to decide which treatment would have the best results. The nurse must allow them time to ask questions and make decisions and must direct them to appropriate professionals to discuss possible alternatives; some treatment modalities carry potential risks and leave permanent physical changes.

The patient and family require an individualized teaching plan that is developed and instituted before discharge from the hospital. Before developing a plan, the patient and family or support group must be evaluated to identify immediate and potential long-term needs. Once these needs are identified, a plan of action can be developed and proposed to the family. Areas included in a teaching plan are the medication regimen, appointments for chemotherapy or radiation treatments, the adverse effects of these treatments, and financial assistance. The nurse must not be afraid to ask questions and explore situations or possible problems that arise during conversations with the patient or family.

Evaluation

- Anxiety is reduced
- The patient and family demonstrate an attempt to cope with the illness
- The patient and family show evidence of moving through the grieving process with effective coping measures
- The family attempts to make plans for the patient's return home and make decisions regarding changes necessary for home care
- Patient demonstrates willingness to participate in some or all personal care
- Self-care needs are met
- Pain is controlled
- Attains and maintains a normal food and fluid intake
- Attempts to ambulate and perform other motor activities
- Respiratory rate, rhythm, and depth is normal
- Oral mucous membranes intact
- Family and patient ask questions relevant to future care

General Nutritional Considerations

☐ A low protein diet appears to enhance the effect of L-dopa and carbidopa in patients who respond poorly and have daily fluctuations in response to these antiparkinsonism medications.

☐ If the patient eats poorly, meals should be served in small, attractive portions. Between meal supplements of easily digested food or fluids may improve nutrition and correct fluid deficits.

☐ The patient with a neuromuscular disorder may have difficulty chewing and swallowing. A soft diet, with food cut into small portions, may improve the ability to chew and swallow food.

☐ The patient who must be fed or who has difficulty eating is given ample time to eat. Rushing the patient only creates frustration and possibly a refusal to eat.

General Pharmacologic Considerations

Read

☐ A stool softener, such as docusate calcium (Surfak), may be ordered to prevent constipation and straining at stool.

☐ Aspirin and acetaminophen are antipyretics that may be used to treat hyperthermia. If bleeding from any cause is suspected or known, acetaminophen is preferred because aspirin can affect the clotting mechanism.

- ☐ Sulfadiazine, sulfisoxazole, or sulfamethoxazole are sulfonamide preparations recommended for treatment or prophylaxis of meningococcal meningitis.
- ☐ Carbamazepine (Tegretol), a drug used in treatment of trigeminal neuralgia, is taken with meals. The dose is gradually increased until relief is obtained. Phenytoin (Dilantin), also used in the treatment of trigeminal neuralgia, requires periodic laboratory evaluation for signs of bone marrow depression. This drug also has been implicated in birth defects and, therefore, should not be taken by pregnant women or those planning a pregnancy.
- ☐ Drugs capable of causing parkinsonism include the phenothiazine derivatives, such as chlorpromazine (Thorazine) and thioridazine (Mellaril), reserpine, and haloperidol (Haldol).
- ☐ Acyclovir (Zovirax) prescribed for herpes zoster requires 50 doses taken as one capsule every 4 hours while awake for a total of 5 doses per day for 10 days.
- ☐ Topical anesthetics such as lidocaine (L-Caine Viscous) may be held in the mouth to relieve the pain and discomfort associated with oral lesions.
- ☐ The hydantoins include phenytoin (Dilantin), mephenytoin (Mesantoin), and ethotoin (Peganone). These drugs may cause hyperplasia of gum tissue.
- ☐ Mannitol and glycerol are osmotic diuretics that may be used to treat cerebral edema and lower ICP.
- ☐ Corticosteroid administration may produce hyperglycemia and gastrointestinal bleeding, both complications of therapy with this group of drugs.
- ☐ Narcotic analgesics depress the respiratory center and raise CSF pressure. Their use is contraindicated in those with a head injury or increased ICP, unless administration is absolutely necessary.

General Gerontologic Considerations

- ☐ The elderly patient has a tendency to drink less water and, therefore, may incur a chronic fluid volume deficit.
- ☐ The elderly patient is more susceptible to the complications of prolonged bed rest and inactivity. These patients are watched closely for problems such as hypostatic pneumonia, decubitus, contractures, and deformities.
- ☐ Because Parkinson's disease is seen more frequently in the older age groups, the nurse must work closely with the relatives when planning for the patient's discharge to the home environment.

Suggested Readings

- ☐ Berkow R, Fletcher AJ (eds). Merck manual of diagnosis and therapy. 15th ed. Rahway, NJ: Merck & Co, 1987. *(In-depth coverage of subject matter)*
- ☐ Brunner LS, Suddarth DS. Textbook of medical–surgical nursing. 6th ed. Philadelphia: JB Lippincott, 1988. *(Additional and in-depth coverage of subject matter)*
- ☐ Callanan M. Epilepsy: putting the patient back in control. RN 1988;51:48. *(Additional coverage of subject matter)*
- ☐ Clark WG, Brater DC, Johnson AR. Goth's medical pharmacology. 12th ed. St Louis: CV Mosby, 1988. *(In-depth and high level coverage of subject matter)*
- ☐ Coderre CB. Meningitis: dangers when the Dx is viral. RN 1989;52:50. *(Additional coverage of subject matter)*
- ☐ Doenges ME, Moorhouse MF. Nurse's pocket guide: nursing diagnoses with interventions. 2nd ed. Philadelphia: FA Davis, 1988. *(Additional coverage of subject matter)*
- ☐ Friedman D. Taking the scare out of caring for seizure patients. Nursing '88 1988;18:52. *(Additional coverage of subject matter)*
- ☐ Johnson GE, Hannah KJ. Pharmacology and the nursing process. Philadelphia: WB Saunders, 1987. *(Additional coverage of subject matter)*
- ☐ Lewis S, Collier I. Medical–surgical nursing: assessment and management of clinical

problems. 2nd ed. New York: McGraw-Hill, 1987. *(Additional and in-depth coverage of subject matter)*

☐ McBride EV, Distefano K. Explaining diagnostic tests for MS. Nursing '88 1988;18:68. *(Additional coverage of subject matter)*

☐ Rhynsburger J. How to fight myasthenia's fatigue. Am J Nurs 1989;89:337. *(Additional coverage of subject matter)*

☐ Swearingen PL (ed). Manual of nursing therapeutics: applying nursing diagnosis to medical disorders. 2nd ed. St Louis: CV Mosby, 1990. *(Additional and in-depth coverage of subject matter)*

☐ Talotta D, Lisanti P. Countering Parkinson's assault on your patient's will. RN 1989;52:34. *(Additional coverage of subject matter)*

☐ Vallerand AH, Russin MM. Taking the bite out of TMJ syndrome. Am J Nurs 1989;89:688. *(Additional coverage of subject matter)*

Chapter 37

Cerebrovascular Disorders

On completion of this chapter the reader will:

- Discuss the symptoms, diagnosis, and treatment of headache disorders, transient ischemic attacks, stroke, cerebral aneurysm, and Alzheimer's disease

- Use the nursing process in the management of a patient with transient ischemic attacks, stroke, cerebral aneurysm, and Alzheimer's disease

HEADACHE

Headache (cephalgia) is a common ailment of humankind. It is a symptom and not a disease in itself. It may be due to emotional tension, allergies, temporomandibular joint (TMJ) syndrome, sinusitis, or brain tumor—to name only a few possible causes.

Tension Headache

Tension headache is the most common type of headache and is due to tension or emotional or physical stress.

Symptoms

Symptoms may vary from a mild ache to severe disabling pain.

Diagnosis

Persistent headache may require tests such as computed tomographic (CT) scan, brain scan, angiography, and laboratory and diagnostic tests to rule out a possible medical disorder, such as a brain tumor, TMJ syndrome, and infected sinuses.

Treatment

Treatment for severe, recurrent headache starts with determining the cause and, when possible, removing or correcting those factors or situations that result in headache. Therapy may involve prescription of glasses, drainage of an infected sinus, or psychotherapy. Occasional headaches that result from fatigue or emotional stress are usually relieved by rest and a mild analgesic such as aspirin.

Migraine

Migraine is a particular type of headache believed to be due to initial constriction and subsequent dilation of cerebral arteries. The underlying cause of the condition is not fully understood, but it has been noted that emotional stress may play a part in precipitating attacks. Certain foods, chemical additives, and fatigue also may precipitate attacks. A marked familial tendency toward the disorder has been found.

Symptoms

The attack may begin with feelings of malaise, irritability, and fatigue. Pallor and puffiness of the face may occur. Just before the headache begins, some patients experience visual disturbances such as an irregular pattern (scintillating scotomata) before their eyes. The headache usually starts on one side, but it may involve the entire head before the attack is over. Patients describe the pain as "throbbing" or "bursting." The headache is severe and often accompanied by nausea and vomiting. A patient may be incapacitated for a day or more. Often light increases the pain, and many find that lying in bed in a darkened room relieves the symptoms.

Diagnosis

Diagnosis is based on the patient's description of symptoms.

Treatment

Treatment should include a thorough medical and neurologic examination, as well as investigation of the patient's social and personal background. After evaluation, the physician may prescribe drugs such as ergotamine and caffeine (Cafergot), methysergide (Sansert), or propranolol (Inderal). Antiemetics may be necessary if nausea and vomiting become acute during an attack. Ergotamine derivatives (ergotamine tartrate, dihydroergotamine mesylate) may be prescribed to abort an attack but must be taken as soon as symptoms begin.

→ dilates the blood vessels

Cluster Headache

The term *cluster* is used to describe a certain type of headache in which the attacks seem to occur in clusters or groups and last for several days or weeks then disappear. The headaches may not recur for months or years. Though the cause of cluster headaches is unknown, some believe them to be related to migraines.

Symptoms

The headache is usually on one side of the head and may be accompanied by tearing of the eye on the affected side, nasal congestion, and pain behind the eye.

Diagnosis

Diagnosis is based on the patient's description of symptoms and the pattern of headache occurrence.

Treatment

Symptoms may be controlled with administration of an ergotamine derivative or methysergide.

NURSING PROCESS —THE PATIENT WHO HAS A HEADACHE

Assessment

Those with chronic headaches or headaches that result in a variety of symptoms require a complete medical and allergy history as well a record of frequency and description of the pain experienced during an attack. Descriptions should include the location of the pain, whether it is in one area or over the entire head; factors that appear to bring on, make worse, or relieve the headache; how long the pain lasts; and symptoms such as tearing, nausea, or vomiting.

Vital signs are taken. A neurologic examination may be performed if the cause of the headache is unknown.

Nursing Diagnosis

Depending on the severity of the headache and symptoms associated with the attack, one or more of the following may apply. Additional diagnoses, for example fluid volume deficit because of prolonged vomiting, may be necessary under certain circumstances.

- Pain related to constriction and dilatation of cerebral arteries
- Knowledge deficit of treatment modalities

Planning and Implementation

The major goals of the patient include relief of pain and understanding the treatment modalities and methods to minimize pain.

The major goal of nursing intervention is to relieve pain and discomfort. Depending on the possible cause of the headache, nursing management also is geared toward helping the patient possibly eliminate those factors that may cause headache.

Pain. Pain may be relieved by administration of a mild analgesic. Patients with a serious medical disorder, such as a brain tumor, may require a narcotic analgesic. Environmental factors that appear to intensify pain, such as bright light or noise, are eliminated as much as possible.

Knowledge Deficit. Possible adverse drug effects and the dosage regimen are explained to the patient who receives methysergide or an ergotamine derivative.

Patients with migraine and cluster headaches are instructed to keep a record of their attacks, their activities before the attack began, and any environmental or emotional circumstances that appear to bring on the attack or increase or decrease pain during the attack. With this information, the factors that cause or intensify an attack may be identified and possibly modified or eliminated.

The patient is taught how to modify headache pain when an attack occurs. Suggestions include lying down in a darkened room and avoiding noise and movement.

Evaluation

- Pain is relieved or eliminated
- Demonstrates understanding of drug dosage regimen and possible adverse drug effects

CEREBROVASCULAR DISORDERS

Cerebrovascular disorders are one of the major medical problems that affect adults, and their frequency increases with age.

Cerebral nerve cells are extremely sensitive to a lack of oxygen; in about 3 to 7 minutes complete ischemia leads to the destruction of cells that have been deprived of oxygen. These changes are irreversible because cerebral nerve cells do not regenerate. Thus, any disorder that decreases the supply of oxygenated blood to the brain can have serious consequences.

Transient Ischemic Attacks

Transient ischemic attacks (TIAs) are brief, fleeting attacks of neurologic impairment that result from disease (usually atherosclerosis) of cerebral blood vessels or the carotid arteries. Impaired circulation momentarily deprives part of the brain of an adequate supply of oxygen. A TIA may be a warning that a stroke could occur in the future.

warning of stroke

Symptoms

Symptoms vary but include lightheadedness, speech disturbances, visual loss in one eye, diplopia, variable changes in consciousness, and numbness, weakness, or paralysis on one side. Symptoms may last for a few moments to as long as a day, followed by complete recovery from the symptoms.

Diagnosis

Diagnosis is based on the patient history and neurologic examination. Additional tests include a CT scan, magnetic resonance imaging (MRI), and carotid arteriogram.

Treatment

Anticoagulant therapy may be prescribed. If narrowing of the carotid artery by atherosclerotic plaques is the cause, a carotid endarterectomy may be considered. A balloon angioplasty, a procedure similar to a percutaneous transluminal coronary angioplasty (see Chapter 31), also may be performed.

NURSING PROCESS —THE PATIENT WHO HAS TRANSIENT ISCHEMIC ATTACKS

Assessment

A complete history of symptoms, and a medical, drug, and allergy history are obtained. A neurologic examination (see Chapter 35) is performed.

Nursing Diagnosis

Depending on the cause and subsequent treatment, one or more of the following may apply

- Anxiety related to TIA episode
- Potential for injury related to transient motor changes
- Knowledge deficit of treatment modalities

Planning and Implementation

The major goals of the patient include a reduction in anxiety, prevention of injury, and an understanding of the prescribed treatment.

The major goals of nursing management are to reduce anxiety, prevent injury, and immediately detect neurologic changes should they occur.

SURGERY.   If carotid artery surgery is performed, the patient is closely observed after surgery for signs of neurologic impairment. A flow sheet may be used for recording assessments. Any change in the patient's neurologic status, such as paralysis, increased confusion, facial asymmetry, or aphasia, is reported to the surgeon immediately; a thrombus or other problem may be decreasing the blood supply to the brain. The patient also is observed for the development of a cardiac dysrhythmia.

Because surgery is performed on structures of the neck, swelling may occur. The patient is observed closely for difficulty breathing, difficulty swallowing, or hoarseness. A tracheostomy set is kept at the bedside should airway obstruction occur.

Anxiety.   Anxiety may occur because TIAs are frightening and develop without warning. The patient is assured that treatment may prevent or decrease the number of future attacks.

Potential for Injury.   Many of these patients are in the older age group. The family should be warned that falls and other injuries may occur at the time of a TIA.

Knowledge Deficit.   The medical regimen is explained to the patient or family. If frequent and repeated attacks occur, the family is advised to observe the patient closely, attempt to prevent falls or other injuries, and contact the physician regarding any change in the patient's condition.

Evaluation

- Anxiety is reduced
- Patient shows no sign of injury
- Patient and family understand medical regimen
- Family members discuss importance of preventing injury, observing the patient, and continued medical follow-up

Stroke (Cerebrovascular Accident)

The most common cerebrovascular disease is a cerebrovascular accident (CVA) or *stroke*. The most common causes of a stroke are cerebral embolus and cerebral thrombus (Fig. 37-1). Atrial fibrillation accompanied by embolus formation is a common cause of stroke in the elderly. Embolus formation also may be seen after insertion of a heart valve prosthesis. Atherosclerosis and arteriosclerosis may contribute to the formation of a cerebral thrombus. Cerebral hemorrhage is another cause of stroke (Fig. 37-2). Common causes of cerebral hemorrhage (also called *intracranial hemorrhage*) are rupture of cerebral aneurysms, usually in circle of Willis, rupture of a cerebral vessel, hemorrhagic disorders such as leukemia, aplastic anemia, and tumors of the brain. The role of hypertension in stroke is not entirely clear, but it is thought to involve the narrowing of cerebral vessels, which reduces the amount of blood traveling through them and which, ultimately, may result in cerebral ischemia and infarction.

Symptoms

Symptoms of stroke are highly variable and depend on the area affected: numbness, tingling, weakness, paralysis, speech difficulty, or blurred vision may be seen. Patients may have no warning and the symptoms occur suddenly, or they may experience transient ischemic attacks (see above) for days, weeks, or years before a stroke occurs.

In most instances, the onset of a stroke is sudden; the level of consciousness may range from lethargy and mental confusion to deep coma; the blood pressure may be severely elevated, but symptoms of shock may be present in some instances. A patient also may experience a severe headache along with nausea and vomiting. Breathing may be difficult, and paralysis, speech disturbance, and memory impairment may be experienced. Occasionally, symptoms may be milder: headache, fatigue, dizzy spells, weakness, numbness and tingling of an extremity, speech or visual disturbances, and mental confusion may be present. Symptoms may occur days, weeks, months, or just immediately before the stroke.

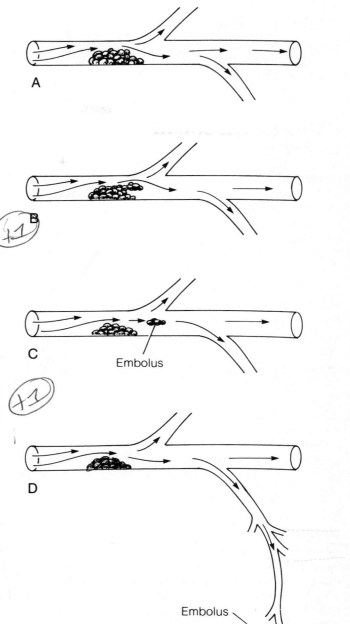

Figure 37–1. (*A*) A thrombus forms in a vessel. (*B*) The force of the flowing blood over the clot helps to break off a piece from it. (*C*) The embolus is loose in the bloodstream and can travel to any tissue fed by connecting blood vessels. (*D*) The embolus is pushed into a small terminal vessel, completely occluding it and causing anoxia of the tissue served by the occluded vessel.

Immediately after a severe cerebral hemorrhage, the patient is unconscious, the face is often brick red, and breathing is noisy and sometimes labored. On the paralyzed side, the cheek blows out with each respiration.

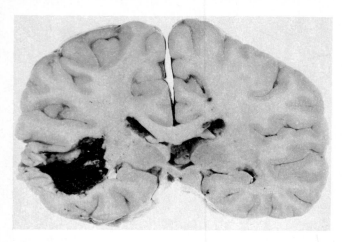

Figure 37–2. Postmortem specimen of a cerebral hemorrhage of the right temporal lobe. (Courtesy of P. S. Milley, MD. Photograph by D. Atkinson)

The pulse usually is slow but full and bounding. Initially, blood pressure is likely to be elevated. The patient may proceed into deeper and deeper coma until death occurs. Coma may persist for days or even weeks, and then consciousness may begin to return. The longer the coma, however, the poorer the prognosis and the less likely it is that consciousness will return. Pneumonia is the most common cause of death during prolonged coma.

When the stroke is due to a cerebral embolism, neurologic symptoms are seen usually without loss of consciousness, although the state of consciousness may be altered.

If the patient survives a major stroke, the neurologic deficit that remains (if any) depends on the extent and the severity, as well as the location, of the resulting brain damage. Areas of the brain may have suffered from hypoxia and may then recover as the supply of oxygen and other essential elements carried by the blood improves; other areas may have died from anoxia. During the early stage, it is often not possible to tell whether the symptoms will be permanent or temporary. Improvement in neurologic symptoms can occur for at least 6 months after the accident; this fact should both encourage the patient and motivate the nurse to do everything possible to prevent deformities and to help the patient maintain and improve contact with others and orientation to the surroundings.

The most common neurologic sequela of a stroke is hemiplegia. A hemorrhage or clot in the right side of the brain causes the patient to have a left hemiplegia because nerves in the pyramidal tract crossover as they lead from the brain down the spinal cord. A right-handed person usually is left-brain dominant, and a left-handed person usually is right-brain dominant. Aphasia, the inability to use or understand spoken and written language, and hemianopia are neurologic

symptoms associated with stroke. Hemianopia is a condition in which the patient can see only half of the normal visual field. When looking straight ahead, the patient cannot see with either eye anything to the right or left. This condition is caused by damage to the visual area of the cerebral cortex or its connections to the brain stem (optic radiations). This symptom, like other symptoms that result from stroke, may subside completely, partially, or not at all. Confusion and emotional lability also are characteristic symptoms.

Diagnosis

Diagnosis of a stroke is often made after a neurologic examination of the patient, a review of past illnesses, such as hypertension, diabetes, and so on, and a history of events before the illness. Additional diagnostic studies include CT scan, MRI, brain scan, cerebral angiography, transcranial Doppler ultrasonography (to diagnose a stroke due to emboli and thrombi), and lumbar puncture.

Treatment

Treatment varies and is directed toward the cause, if known. If atherosclerosis of the carotid artery is the cause, the plaque may be removed (carotid endarterectomy).

For cerebral thrombosis and emboli, anticoagulant therapy may be used in selected patients, with the hope that the drug will discourage further formation of thrombi. An osmotic diuretic may be administered during the first few days of the acute phase to treat cerebral edema. The thrombolytic enzymes urokinase and recombinant alteplase (tissue plasminogen activator [TPA]) are being used experimentally in the treatment of stroke due to a thrombus or embolus. Anticoagulants are always contraindicated in cerebral hemorrhage. Some forms of intracranial hemorrhage, such as ruptured cerebral aneurysm, can be treated surgically.

In many cases, treatment is supportive because, once brain tissue dies, no medical or surgical intervention can repair the damage. The best treatment available involves an intensive medical program aimed primarily at rehabilitation and, when possible, the prevention of future strokes. The emphasis on rehabilitation after a stroke has made it possible for patients to live fuller lives than they had previously.

Prevention

Strokes may be prevented by reducing certain risk factors. The control of hypertension, weight reduction, treatment of cardiac dysrhythmia (especially atrial fibrillation in the elderly), the lowering of blood cholesterol levels, prophylactic anticoagulant therapy (including daily aspirin) in selected people, and proper treatment of medical disorders, such as diabetes mellitus and cardiovascular disease, may prevent a stroke.

NURSING PROCESS —THE PATIENT WHO HAS A STROKE Read!

Assessment

A history of symptoms and a complete medical, drug, and allergy history are obtained from the family. If able to communicate and not acutely ill, the patient may provide some or all of the medical history. Vital signs are taken, and a complete neurologic assessment (see Chapter 35) is performed. A neurologic flow sheet is used to record the findings.

Nursing Diagnosis

The symptoms depend on the areas of the brain that have been deprived of oxygen. One or more of the following may apply. Additional diagnoses may be added or deleted as the patient progresses from the acute to rehabilitative stages of the disorder. If the patient incurs a permanent neurologic deficit, see Chapter 39 for additional nursing diagnoses.

- Ineffective airway clearance related to decreased level of consciousness
- Hyperthermia related to effect of stroke on temperature-regulating center
- Impaired physical mobility related to paralysis, muscle spasticity, loss of balance
- Impaired skin integrity related to immobility
- Colonic constipation related to immobility
- Total incontinence related to brain damage, flaccid bladder
- Impaired verbal communication related to aphasia
- Self-care deficit: total or partial (specify areas) related to brain damage secondary to stroke
- Potential for disuse syndrome related to damage to motor areas of the brain
- Altered thought processes related to brain damage secondary to stroke
- Ineffective individual coping related to permanent neurologic deficit (eg, aphasia, paralysis)
- Potential fluid volume deficit related to inability to take oral fluids, impaired swallowing
- Altered nutrition: less than body requirements related to inability to chew and swallow food
- Altered family processes related to patient's neurologic deficit, burden of care, financial losses, other factors (specify)

Planning and Implementation

The major goals of the patient include improving mobility, attaining normal bowel and bladder elimination, establishing and improving communication, improving thought processes, improving ability to carry out activities of daily living, maintaining an adequate nutrition and fluid intake, maintaining a patent airway, preventing skin breakdown, and striving to cope with disability.

The major goals of nursing management include maintaining a patent airway, recognizing and preventing complications, helping the patient regain optimum neurologic function, and helping the family restore normal family processes.

Because the number and severity of symptoms vary with each patient, nursing management is based on the needs identified during the initial and ongoing assessments. Additional material that concerns the management of a patient with a neurologic deficit is discussed in Chapter 39.

Ineffective Airway Clearance. Patients may be comatose or semicomatose after a stroke. The airway must be kept patent at all times. Suctioning may be necessary to maintain a patent airway until the patient is more alert and able to cough, deep breathe, and swallow. Once able to perform these tasks, the patient is encouraged to take deep breaths hourly.

The lungs are auscultated daily. A rise in temperature, abnormal lungs sounds, difficulty breathing, and noisy respirations are examples of problems that must be reported to the physician.

Hyperthermia. Vital signs are monitored every 4 hours. More frequent determinations may be necessary if there is an increase or decrease in any one or more of the measurements.

Fever may be reduced by administration of the prescribed antipyretic drug, which may be given by suppository if the patient is unable to swallow. The temperature is monitored hourly after administration of an antipyretic. Failure to respond to antipyretic administration is reported to the physician; other measures, such as a cooling blanket, may be necessary.

Impaired Physical Mobility, Impaired Skin Integrity. During the acute phase, one of the major goals of management is the prevention of contractures and joint deformities. The patient's position is changed every 2 hours, and the prone position is used, if tolerated by the patient, several times a day. Care is given each time the patient is turned. Devices such as foot boards, trochanter rolls, pillows, and wrist splints may be used to maintain body alignment. The physical therapist also may recommend specific devices tailored to the patient's needs.

Range-of-motion exercises are performed as soon as prescribed and are performed on both the affected (paralyzed) and unaffected sides. Physical therapy may be ordered as soon as the acute phase has passed. The nurse works with the physical therapist by continuing exercises between physical therapy treatments. The patient is encouraged to use and exercise the unaffected side. Once alert and able, the patient is shown how to perform passive exercises to the affected upper extremities.

The skin is inspected, and special attention is paid to the bony prominences. Early signs of skin breakdown require special care to the area. The physician is consulted because devices such as sheepskin padding or a flotation mattress may be necessary.

Colonic Constipation, Total Incontinence. Intake and output are measured. An indwelling urethral catheter may be ordered at the time of admission and may be removed once the acute phase has passed. After removal of the catheter, the bedpan or urinal is offered at regular intervals, usually every 1 or 2 hours, and the patient is encouraged to void. Each voiding is measured. Voiding in small amounts, dribbling, and complaints of suprapubic pain or discomfort may indicate urinary retention. The physician is notified; it may be necessary to reinsert an indwelling catheter.

If the patient is incontinent of feces, the perineal area must be thoroughly cleansed after each bowel movement. A record of bowel movements is kept. If constipation occurs, the physician may order a daily suppository to encourage a regular pattern of bowel elimination.

Potential Fluid Volume Deficit, Altered Nutrition. Initially, a patient may require intravenous fluids. Once able to swallow, a liquid to soft diet is ordered. When first taking oral fluids, the patient is closely observed for difficulty swallowing because aspiration may occur. A suction machine is kept at the bedside until the patient is able to take fluids and food without difficulty. Prolonged inability to take oral fluids or food may require total parenteral nutrition.

Impaired Verbal Communication. A variety of speech defects may occur and may range from slightly slurred speech to total loss of speech. When a deficit occurs, the nurse must attempt to find the best method of communication. Total loss of speech may require that the patient be asked yes or no questions, with the patient responding by nodding the head. If speech is present but difficult to understand, the patient is asked to speak more slowly. Other methods include pointing or writing (if the dominant side is not paralyzed).

As soon as the acute phase has passed, speech therapy may be prescribed. The nurse works with the speech therapist by using words or phrases that are practiced during therapy sessions.

Self-Care Deficit. The patient's ability to participate in care is evaluated at regular intervals. As soon as the patient appears able to perform some tasks, encouragement is given to participate in activities such as bathing and grooming. The physical or occupational therapist also may involve grooming and bathing activities as part of therapy. In some instances, devices can be purchased or made to facilitate active participation in self-care activities. A homemade device, such as a toothbrush inserted and cemented into a foam rubber ball, can be useful.

Altered Thought Processes. Confusion, emotional outbursts, and disorientation are examples of mental changes that may occur in patients. Depending on severity, the physician may order a psychologic evaluation followed by institution of a training program that includes areas such as reality orientation and cognitive retraining by appropriate specialists. Once the patient's problems have been identified and a treatment regimen instituted, the nurse may reinforce certain parts of therapy such as reality orientation by repeating the day of the week, month, and year during each patient contact.

Ineffective Individual Coping. Once these patients are aware of the deficits that have occurred, they often have difficulty coping with the changes to their bodies. Depression and withdrawal may be seen. Emotional support and encouragement from medical personnel as well as the family are necessary. Each time the patient has shown even the slightest improvement, encouragement is given. This encouragement, in turn, may motivate patients to continue to compensate for and accept their loss as well as to strive for any new improvement.

Altered Family Processes. The family is confronted with many short- and long-term problems when a member has had a stroke. In some instances, the patient achieves full or almost full recovery and is able to resume an active and normal role as a member of the family. Other times, a permanent neurologic deficit creates many burdens, requiring a variety of decisions.

The family is encouraged to openly discuss the problems created by a member's illness. Once a problem is identified, the nurse may be able to help the family work toward a solution. Examples of family problems include home care, decisions about placement in a nursing home or skilled nursing facility, and financial burdens imposed by the illness. If approved by the physician, referrals to appropriate agencies and social service workers can be made.

Evaluation

- Airway remains patent; lungs are clear to auscultation
- Takes deep breaths hourly
- Temperature is normal
- Improved mobility is achieved
- Skin remains intact; no evidence of skin breakdown
- Achieves a normal bowel elimination pattern
- Attains normal bladder elimination; voids at regular intervals
- Drinks an adequate amount of liquids
- Eats an adequate amount of solid foods
- Improves ability to communicate with others
- Achieves self-care alone or with assistance
- Appears oriented to date, time, and place
- Shows cognitive improvement
- Demonstrates an ability to cope with illness, neurologic deficits
- Family openly discusses problems associated with postdischarge management

Cerebral Aneurysms

Aneurysms are formed by the ballooning of blood vessel walls, which may occur in cranial vessels. Most cerebral aneurysms occur in circle of Willis (Figs. 37-3 and 37-4) and are called *berry aneurysms.* These are thought to be congenital and may rupture at any time, often without warning.

Symptoms

Symptoms include severe headache, dizziness, nausea, and vomiting, which may be followed by loss of consciousness. Bleeding from a berry aneurysm results in blood in the subarachnoid space with grossly bloody cerebrospinal fluid.

Diagnosis

Diagnosis is based on the symptoms and a neurologic examination. Diagnostic tests include a CT scan, MRI, lumbar puncture, and cerebral angiography.

Treatment

As the danger of further hemorrhage from the weakened sac is great, particularly in the first weeks after the initial hemorrhage, surgical repair may be attempted. The operation is not without hazard; manipulation of the small cerebral vessels may result in increased vasospasm or thrombosis and cerebral infarction. Usually, the risks of surgery are less serious than the dangers of recurrent hemorrhage.

Surgery involves a wrapping or clipping of the aneurysm in an attempt to control further episodes of bleeding. Aneurysms that are inoperable because of their anatomical location must be treated medically. Medical treatment, which includes a reduction in blood pressure and complete bed rest, is usually employed until the bleeding has stopped.

An alternative to direct repair of the aneurysm when collateral circulation is believed to be adequate is li-

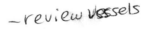

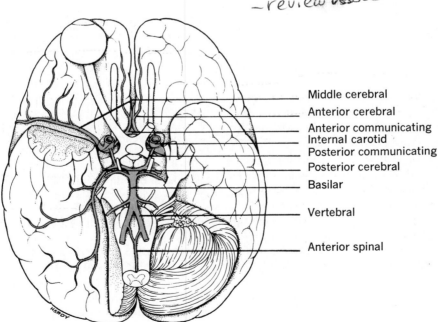

Figure 37–3. Cerebral arteries that form the circle of Willis. (Chaffee EE, Lytle IM. Basic physiology and anatomy. 4th ed. Philadelphia: JB Lippincott)

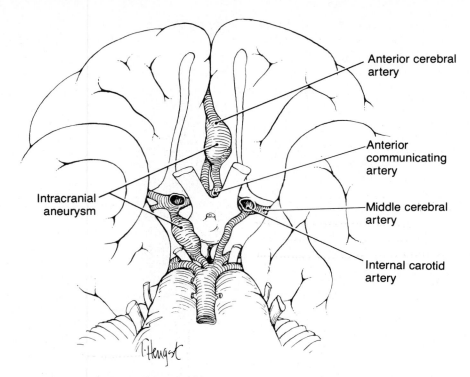

Figure 37–4. Intracranial aneurysm in the circle of Willis. (Brunner LS, Suddarth DS. Textbook of medical-surgical nursing. 5th ed, Philadelphia: JB Lippincott, 1982:1340)

gation of one of the carotid arteries. The purpose is to obstruct the blood flow to the vessel that has an aneurysm and thus reduce the pressure in the aneurysm and prevent rupture.

An alternative to carotid artery ligation is the application of a clamp to the carotid artery. The purpose of this surgical procedure is basically the same as a ligation of the carotid artery. Usually, the clamp is tightened gradually over a period of several days in the hope that collateral circulation will have a chance to develop. Medical treatment includes absolute bed rest in a quiet area, preferably a private room. Visitors are restricted, except for family members. The head of the bed is elevated to reduce intracranial pressure and cerebral edema. If the patient is hypertensive, antihypertensive agents are used to reduce the blood pressure. Because convulsive seizures may occur, prophylactic anticonvulsant therapy may be instituted. Tranquilizers also may be prescribed to keep the patient relaxed. Increased intracranial pressure may be managed with osmotic diuretics and corticosteroids.

NURSING PROCESS —THE PATIENT WHO HAS A CEREBRAL ANEURYSM

Assessment
Most cerebral aneurysms are not detected until they have begun to bleed. At this time, neurologic symp-

toms are present. A complete neurologic examination (see Chapter 35) is performed. A history must often be obtained from a family member or friend because the patient may be comatose or semicomatose.

Nursing Diagnosis
Depending on the type and severity of symptoms and the treatment employed, one or more of the following may apply. If temporary or permanent neurologic deficits occur, additional nursing diagnoses, as outlined in Chapter 39, may be added.

- Anxiety related to diagnosis, symptoms, enforced bed rest, impending surgery
- Constipation related to immobility
- Pain related to meningeal irritation secondary to intracranial bleeding
- Self-care deficit: total, related to imposed limitation on physical activity
- Impaired tissue integrity related to enforced immobility
- Knowledge deficit of diagnostic tests, treatment modalities, home care

Planning and Implementation
The major goals of the patient include a reduction of anxiety, relief of pain (headache), normal bowel elimination, improved nutrition, improved airway clearance, and knowledge of the proposed diagnostic tests, treatment, and home care.

The major goals of nursing management are to aid in the prevention of further bleeding and other complications related to immobility and to detect neurologic changes, should they occur.

A neurologic flow sheet may be used to record the results of the neurologic assessments. The patient is closely observed for signs of increased intracranial pressure. Should *any* neurologic change occur, the physician is notified immediately.

If clamping of the carotid artery has been performed, the patient is observed frequently for neurologic changes. Should *any* neurologic change occur, the physician must be notified immediately; changes may indicate inadequate circulation to the brain and usually require loosening of the carotid clamp. The patient is not out of danger until after the clamp has been tightened for 48 or more hours. Patients with a carotid artery ligation require the same assessments. Should a neurologic deficit occur, the physician is notified immediately.

Surgical repair of the aneurysm requires a craniotomy. See Chapter 38 for the postoperative management of a patient with a craniotomy. The patient is observed for signs of increased intracranial pressure, which may mean intracerebral hemorrhage or cerebral edema, and for neurologic symptoms on the side of the body opposite the site of the surgery. The neurosurgeon usually writes specific postoperative orders about the administration of intravenous fluids, the position of the patient in bed, whether turning is allowed, and so on. Although deep breathing exercises may be performed, coughing, which increases intracranial pressure, is not encouraged.

Anxiety. Anxiety raises the blood pressure, which in turn may cause further leakage of blood from the aneurysm. Keeping the room dimly lit, limiting the number of visitors, explaining the purpose of treatments, and administering a tranquilizer may relieve anxiety and encourage complete rest.

Constipation. The patient is instructed not to strain to have a bowel movement because straining increases intracranial pressure. The physician may order a stool softener to prevent constipation.

Pain. The conscious patient may experience a severe headache because of increased intracranial pressure or meningeal irritation due to blood in the subarachnoid space. Narcotics are avoided whenever possible; they affect the level of consciousness and, in some cases, the pupil size, making accurate neurologic assessments difficult. If nonnarcotic analgesics fail to control pain, the physician may order codeine, which has little or no effect on pupil size

but may cause drowsiness and make evaluation of the level of consciousness somewhat difficult.

Self-Care Deficit. Unless ordered otherwise, absolute bed rest is maintained. All physical care must be performed by nursing personnel. Sudden jarring and excessive movement are avoided. The physician may order limited bathing and grooming activities for the first several days.

Impaired Tissue Integrity. The physician is consulted about turning a patient. If a patient is not to be turned, a flotation mattress may be used to prevent pressure on bony prominences. The skin is inspected daily for signs of breakdown. Passive exercises and back rubs are not given unless specifically ordered by the physician.

Elastic stockings may be used to prevent thrombophlebitis, a complication of prolonged bed rest.

Respiratory Function. If conscious, the patient is reminded to (slowly) take deep breaths hourly. The lungs are auscultated for normal and abnormal breath sounds. Coughing is not encouraged and suctioning is not performed unless specifically ordered by the physician. These maneuvers may increase intracranial pressure and possibly may cause further bleeding from the aneurysm.

Knowledge Deficit. Diagnostic tests and treatment modalities are explained to the family as well as to the alert patient. The physician must also inform the family of the possible results of surgery, that some permanent neurologic deficits may occur.

If conscious, the patient is instructed to remain quiet and not to attempt to change position in bed. The purpose of complete bed rest and what it entails is explained to the patient. The rationale for visitor limitations is explained to the patient and family. The family is reminded to disturb the patient as little as possible.

Discharge teaching depends on the treatment used, the results of treatment, and the recommendations of the physician. Usually, these patients are instructed to avoid heavy lifting, straining at stool, extreme emotional conditions, and other circumstances that may raise the blood pressure or increase intracranial pressure. Depending on the results of treatment, the patient may find it necessary to limit many activities. In some instances, a major and permanent neurologic deficit may require severe limitation of all activities, including employment. When these restrictions occur, the nurse must be aware that the changes may affect the financial, physical, and social obligations of the patient and family. Appropriate referrals to a social service worker, counselor, or social service agency may be necessary.

Evaluation

- Anxiety is reduced
- Bowel elimination is normal
- Pain is controlled or eliminated
- Self-care needs are met
- Skin remains intact; no evidence of skin breakdown or decubitus formation
- Lungs are clear to auscultation
- Patient and family demonstrate an understanding of treatment modalities and home care

ALZHEIMER'S DISEASE

Alzheimer's disease is a progressive, deteriorating brain disorder that has profound effects on the patient and family. The cause of this disorder is unknown, but some evidence for a genetic relation has been found.

The disease is marked by a decrease in the size of the cerebral cortex along with degeneration of nerve cells primarily in association and memory areas.

Symptoms

"tangled" nerve cells in post-mortem examination

The onset is usually insidious. Early symptoms often include memory loss, particularly of recent events and names, and disturbances in behavior. As the disease advances, memory, cognition, awareness, and self-care ability begin to show marked deterioration. Other symptoms include a problem with language and learning skills, personality changes, and difficulty in making judgments or solving problems.

Diagnosis

Diagnosis is based on symptoms and physical examination. Positron emission tomography (PET) may be used to detect a decrease in cerebral perfusion. A CT scan may show a marked shrinking of the cerebral cortex.

Treatment

Treatment is mainly supportive. Antidepressants or tranquilizers may be prescribed to make the agitated or depressed patient more manageable. If a patient is in the advanced stage of the disease, a nursing home or skilled nursing facility may provide the best care.

NURSING PROCESS —THE PATIENT WHO HAS ALZHEIMER'S DISEASE

Assessment

A patient history is obtained. Because the patient may not be able to give a reliable history, the family needs to supply most of the necessary information. Assessment should include evaluation of the patient's behavior and emotional status, their cognitive and motor skills, their ability to carry out activities of daily living and to socialize, and their orientation. A neurologic examination (see Chapter 35) also is performed.

Nursing Diagnosis

Depending on the stage of the disorder and the degree of mental impairment, one or more of the following may apply. Unless otherwise stated, the diagnoses are related to decreased mental functioning and associated symptoms secondary to degenerative changes of the cerebral cortex. Additional diagnoses may be necessary if the patient is in the advanced stage of the disease and is totally dependent on others for care.

- Anxiety
- Impaired adjustment
- Altered thought processes
- Impaired physical mobility related to ataxia
- Potential for injury
- Self-care deficit: total or partial (specify)
- Potential fluid volume deficit related to inability to obtain fluids by self
- Altered nutrition: less than body requirements related to inability to obtain food by self
- Impaired verbal communication
- Impaired social interaction
- Sleep pattern disturbance
- Altered family processes related to responsibilities necessary for care of patient
- Knowledge deficit (family) of treatment modalities, prevention of problems (eg, injury, wandering)

Planning and Implementation

The major goals of the patient, which may not be realistic for all patients, include a reduction of anxiety, prevention of injury, improved ability to carry on activities of daily living, improved nutrition and fluid intake, improved verbal communication and social interactions, and a normal sleep pattern.

The major goals of nursing management are to improve the patient's quality of life, maintain optimal mental functioning and physical safety, and assist the family in making decisions about the care of the affected person. Nursing management of these patients is primarily supportive.

Anxiety. The nurse may be able to reduce anxiety in patients by maintaining a structured daily routine and removing or changing situations or people that upset the patient. It is not always possible to determine what, if anything, is causing anxiety because anxiety could be due to mental changes rather than environmental situations.

Impaired Adjustment. Depending on the patient and the degree of mental deterioration, the nurse may find it necessary to guide the patient in making decisions about daily activities. Patients who are completely unable to make decisions need to have them made for them. At times, patients cooperate; at other times they do not. Each situation must be handled differently and depends on the patient's response. Forcing patients to comply may only make them more angry, hostile, and uncooperative. It may be necessary to delay or change a situation until the patient becomes more willing to accept it.

Altered Thought Processes. The patient's behavior must be accepted because the progress of the disease cannot be halted. Certain measures may be taken, however, to improve or modify behavior. Reducing confusing stimuli, following structured routines, checking reality orientation, giving gentle reminders to perform tasks such as drinking fluids, and providing a quiet and pleasant environment may help the patient maintain contact with reality.

Impaired Physical Mobility, Potential for Injury. Assistance must be given if the patient appears to have difficulty walking or the gait is unsteady. Hazards, such as footstools and small tables, are removed from the ambulatory area. Side rails are raised when the patient is in bed, and calls for assistance are answered as soon as possible. The bed should be kept in a low position except when administering nursing care.

Because it is against fire safety laws to lock exit doors, frequent observation is necessary when the patient is confused and has a tendency to wander. Physical restraints are avoided as much as possible. The patient who lives at home may need constant attendance to prevent injury. Patients who smoke should not be allowed to keep matches on their person or smoke unless someone is present in the same room.

Self-Care Deficit. When able to do so, the patient is encouraged to participate as much as possible in personal care, such as bathing, grooming, and toileting. Patients who are unable or unwilling to participate must have their needs met by nursing personnel.

Patients able to participate must be given time to do so. Explanations or directions are kept short and simple, and the patient is supervised as needed.

Potential Fluid Volume Deficit, Altered Nutrition. Depending on the degree of cerebral impairment, the patient may need help eating and drinking. Patients who are unable to take control of their nu-tritional and fluid needs must be fed and offered fluids at regular intervals throughout the day. If a patient appears able to eat without assistance, the food may need to be prepared. Meat is cut, containers are opened and the contents poured out, and eating utensils are placed where the patient can see them.

If a patient eats or drinks poorly, intake and output are measured. The patient should also be weighed weekly; weight loss is reported to the physician.

Impaired Verbal Communication and Social Interactions. Some patients fail to communicate; others communicate poorly and have difficulty making their needs known. Time must be taken to understand what the patient is trying to say. Questions are abbreviated and, when necessary, should require simple answers. The patient is given time to answer. Directions should be short and easy to understand. Patients are encouraged to be with others and join social activities even if they appear to have no interest in those around them.

Sleep Pattern Disturbance. When physical activity is limited and the patient responds poorly to stimulation in the environment, there is a tendency to sleep during the day and remain awake at night. Keeping the patient active (when possible) during daytime hours may promote longer periods of sleep during the night. Although extreme fatigue due to uninterrupted activity is avoided, short naps instead of long periods of daytime sleep reduce fatigue and also may induce sleep at night. When the patient is ready for bed, noise and lights must be reduced to a minimum. Limiting fluids during the later evening hours may reduce the need to waken and void at night.

Altered Family Processes. If the patient is to return home, many changes are usually necessary. Because the patient should not be left alone or unsupervised, a family member must be present at all times. The family may find it necessary to modify the home environment so that injuries and falls are prevented. Although each home is different, the family is alerted to situations that could cause injury or falls, such as loose throw rugs, furniture (eg, footstools, floor lamps) in or near walking areas, and open cupboard doors.

A patient should not be allowed to leave home alone because confusion often results in getting lost. Doors may need to be kept locked in addition to constant family supervision.

Knowledge Deficit. Once a diagnosis has been established, most families have many questions and require much explanation about the disease process and how they should handle problems as they arise. It is most important that gentleness, patience, and understanding be conveyed when talking with family members.

When approaching the family, it is necessary to evaluate what the patient can and cannot do, what problems may be anticipated, and what home modifications may be necessary.

The family is encouraged to contact community agencies for assistance in home management, financial support, and nursing care. Many communities have Alzheimer's disease support groups that share common problems and supply information and suggestions for solving problems. Group sharing often helps the family work through their frustrations, anger, and feelings of helplessness.

Evaluation

- Anxiety appears reduced
- Shows improvement in decision making
- Behavior and cooperation improve
- Performs simple tasks when asked
- Ambulatory activities improve; makes an effort to walk and engage in purposeful motor activities
- No apparent injury occurs
- Increases participation in self-care activities
- Attains and maintains an adequate food and fluid intake; weight remains stable
- Participates in social activities; interacts and communicates with family, friends, nursing personnel
- Sleeps through all or most of the night and remains awake during most of the day
- Family seeks advice and actively participates in home care plans

General Nutritional Considerations

- ☐ The patient with a cerebrovascular disorder may eat poorly. The meal tray should be checked after each meal. If an appreciable amount of food is left, the nurse must try to find out why the patient is not eating.
- ☐ Some causes of poor eating in the elderly include lack of dentures, poor repair of teeth, and foods that are hard to chew.
- ☐ Patients unable to take oral food may require nasogastric tube feeding or total parenteral nutrition.

General Pharmacologic Considerations

- ☐ Anticoagulant therapy with heparin, which is given parenterally or with an oral anticoagulant, may be indicated for some patients who have had a stroke.
- ☐ If the patient is receiving heparin, the dose may be ordered after each clotting time determination (Lee-White, partial thromboplastin time).
- ☐ If heparin is administered by the subcutaneous route, the site of injection *should not be massaged before or after* the drug is given.
- ☐ The most notable adverse effect of heparin is hemorrhage. Protamine sulfate should be available in case it becomes necessary to counteract the effects of heparin.
- ☐ If the patient is receiving oral anticoagulants, the dose is adjusted according to the prothrombin time determination. Optimum therapeutic results are obtained when prothrombin levels are one and a half to three times the normal control value.
- ☐ Bleeding can occur at any time, even when the prothrombin level appears to be within safe limits. The patient is observed for evidence of bleeding, such as easy bruising, nosebleeds, excessive bleeding from small cuts, and blood in the urine or stool. The antidote for oral anticoagulants is vitamin K, which should be available in parenteral form.
- ☐ Stool softeners may be ordered to prevent constipation and straining. Straining increases intracranial pressure, which must be avoided in some neurologic disorders.

General Gerontologic Considerations

- ☐ The elderly patient is more susceptible to the complications of prolonged bed rest and inactivity. Because the rehabilitation period after a stroke may be prolonged, patients are watched closely for problems such as hypostatic pneumonia, decubitus, contractures, and deformities.

☐ After discharge from a hospital, older patients with cerebrovascular disease may be unable to care for themselves. The spouse also may be unable to assume responsibility for home care. Referral to a home care agency may be necessary.

☐ Older patients with strokes that have resulted in moderate to severe incapacitation may place a financial and physical burden on their spouse or children. The nurse must work closely with the family and social service agencies to ease the burden of their responsibilities and help the family assume, to the extent of their ability, the care of the patient.

☐ After a stroke, depression (which is not uncommon in any patient with a chronic disability or illness) may occur. Depression and other mental changes may influence the patient's participation in a rehabilitation program.

Suggested Readings

☐ Fode NC. Subarachnoid hemorrhage from ruptured intracranial aneurysm. Am J Nurs 1988;88:673. *(Additional coverage and drawings that reinforce subject matter)*

☐ Gray-Vickey P. Evaluating Alzheimer's patients. Nursing '88 1988;18:34. *(Additional and in-depth coverage of subject matter)*

☐ Hahn K. Left vs right: what a difference the side makes in stroke. Nursing '87 1987;17:44. *(Additional coverage of subject matter)*

☐ Hickey J. The clinical practice of neurological and neurosurgical nursing. 2nd ed. Philadelphia: JB Lippincott, 1986. *(In-depth coverage of subject matter)*

☐ Hufler D. Helping your dysphagic patient eat. RN 1987;50:36. *(Additional coverage of subject matter)*

☐ Lewis S, Collier I. Medical–surgical nursing: assessment and management of clinical problems. 2nd ed. New York: McGraw-Hill, 1987. *(Additional and in-depth coverage of subject matter)*

☐ Thompson JM, McFarland GK, Hirsch JE, Tucker SM, Bowers AC. Mosby's manual of clinical nursing. 2nd ed. St Louis: CV Mosby, 1989. *(Additional and in-depth coverage of subject matter)*

☐ Zastocki DK, Rovinski CA. Home care: patient and family instructions. Philadelphia: WB Saunders, 1989. *(Additional coverage of subject matter)*

Chapter 38

Head and Spinal Cord Trauma

On completion of this chapter the reader will:

- List the types of head injuries

- Discuss the symptoms, diagnosis, and treatment of head injuries

- Differentiate between an epidural and subdural hematoma

- Use the nursing process in the management of a patient with a head injury

- Discuss the types of intracranial surgeries

- Use the nursing process in the management of a patient undergoing intracranial surgery

- Discuss the types of spinal cord trauma

- Discuss the symptoms, diagnosis, treatment, and complications of spinal cord trauma

- Use the nursing process in the management of a patient with a spinal cord injury

- Discuss the symptoms, diagnosis, and treatment of spinal nerve root compression

- Use the nursing process in the management of a patient with spinal nerve root compression

HEAD INJURIES

The bony casing of the skull protects the brain. Because of this protection, slight injuries do not affect the brain. A severe blow to the head, however, can cause lacerations, bruises, hemorrhage, and edema of the brain and the tissues that surround the brain.

Concussion

A concussion results from violent jarring of the brain and may be seen after a blow to the head.

Symptoms

Concussion may result in a loss of consciousness, which may be followed by headache, irritability, dizzy spells, confusion, and an unsteady gait.

Diagnosis

Diagnosis is made by history of a head injury followed by the occurrence of symptoms. A radiograph of the skull may be taken to rule out a more serious head injury.

Treatment

Treatment involves observation of the patient for several days and a mild analgesic (usually acetaminophen) for headache. If the patient is discharged from the hospital, a family member is instructed to closely observe the patient for changes in behavior, speech, gait, or other abnormalities and return the patient to the physician or emergency department should any change occur.

Complete recovery is usual; however, recovery may take months, particularly in older people.

Contusion

A contusion is more severe than a concussion. In this type of injury, bruising and possible hemorrhage of superficial cerebral tissue are found.

Symptoms

Symptoms may resemble those of a concussion. An examination may reveal one or more neurologic changes. The blood pressure may be low, the pulse rapid and weak, and the skin pale and cool to the touch. The patient may be unconscious but may respond to strong stimuli.

Diagnosis

Diagnosis is based on a patient's symptoms as well as a history of a head injury. A radiograph of the skull, computed tomographic (CT) scan, or magnetic resonance imaging (MRI) may be performed to rule out more serious injury, such as epidural or subdural bleeding.

Treatment

Treatment includes close observation of the patient and bed rest until symptoms diminish. On rare occasions, permanent damage may result, causing impaired intellect, speech difficulties, epilepsy, paralysis, impaired gait, and continuing stupor.

Epidural Hematoma

An epidural (extradural) hematoma usually is caused by arterial bleeding and occurs on top of the dura (*epi* means above; Fig. 38-1). Bleeding occurs rapidly, separating the dura from the cranium.

Symptoms

Characteristically, the patient has a momentary lapse of consciousness and then may appear perfectly alert and clear after the injury. Within a period of time, which varies from a few minutes to several hours, drowsiness may be seen. This is one of the first signs of increasing intracranial pressure (ICP) due to arterial bleeding. Later, the patient becomes comatose. Death may occur if the symptoms are not recognized and the bleeding is not stopped.

Diagnosis

This condition is a true surgical emergency. Unless the increased ICP is relieved immediately, destruction of brain tissue takes place. A radiograph of the skull and emergency CT scan may be used for diagnosis. In most cases, a history of a head injury and rapid change in neurologic symptoms—namely, signs of increased ICP—usually prompt emergency surgical intervention.

Treatment

Treatment consists of drilling holes (burr holes) in the skull to relieve pressure, remove the clot, and stop the

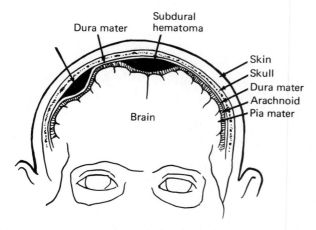

Figure 38–1. Anatomic sites of epidural and subdural hematomas.

bleeding. If the source of bleeding cannot be located by means of burr holes, a craniotomy is performed immediately.

Subdural Hematoma

This condition occurs as a result of venous bleeding in the space below the dura (see Fig. 38-1). Bleeding is usually slower than it is with an epidural hematoma. Subdural bleeding may occur as a result of a head injury, but it also may be seen after rupture of a cerebral aneurysm (see Chapter 37) and with various bleeding disorders, such as those associated with leukemia or aplastic anemia. Subdural bleeding may be acute, subacute, or chronic.

Symptoms

Symptoms may occur immediately or may not be present for as long as several months. In the chronic form, the clot that gradually develops is walled off. Often the clot is absorbed by the body, and no treatment is necessary. When absorption fails to occur, the patient experiences symptoms of compression of the brain, including periodic episodes of memory lapse, confusion, drowsiness, or personality change.

The acute and subacute forms have more pronounced symptoms that occur more rapidly. The patient may be comatose or semicomatose, and neurologic symptoms are more pronounced.

Diagnosis

Diagnosis is based on patient history, neurologic examination, radiograph of the skull, and CT scan.

Treatment

Burr holes are made into the cranium, and the hematoma is aspirated. Like an epidural hematoma, the acute and subacute forms are surgical emergencies. Despite rapid surgical intervention, mild to severe brain damage may follow a subdural hematoma.

Skull Fractures

A skull fracture occurs because of a blow to the head. Most simple skull fractures are not serious, but fractures at the base of the skull and injuries to the skull that cause bone fragments to penetrate the contents of the skull (depressed skull fractures) are serious and may be life-threatening.

Symptoms

Simple skull fractures cause few if any symptoms and tend to heal without trouble. In a depressed skull fracture, however, the broken bone is pushed inward, injuring underlying cerebral tissue. Symptoms depend on what area of the brain has been injured; for example, a bone fragment that is pressing on the motor area may cause hemiplegia. Characteristically, symptoms are not progressive but tend to remain static until the bone is elevated and the pressure is relieved. Epilepsy is a common late complication.

Trauma to the base of the skull may cause edema of the brain near the origin of the spinal cord (foramen magnum) and may interfere with the circulation of cerebrospinal fluid; it may injure the nerves that pass into the spinal cord; or it may create a pathway between the brain and the middle ear that can result in meningitis.

Diagnosis

Diagnosis is based on patient history and neurologic examination as well as a radiograph of the skull. A CT scan also may be performed.

Treatment

Simple skull fractures require no treatment other than bed rest and close observation of the patient for signs of increased ICP. Depressed skull fractures require surgical intervention that consists of a craniotomy to remove bone fragments and control bleeding, elevation of the depressed fracture, and repair of damaged tissues.

NURSING PROCESS —THE PATIENT WHO HAS A HEAD INJURY

Assessment

A head injury, no matter how mild it may appear, is treated as an emergency. A history of the injury is obtained and should include information about the time of the injury and the cause. A summary of the patient's condition from the time of the injury to the present is essential and should include information about the level of consciousness (LOC), vital signs (if taken), and any indications of paralysis in one or more extremity.

A neurologic examination (see Chapter 35) is performed with particular attention to vital signs, the LOC, the presence or absence of movement, pupil size, equality, reaction to light, and signs of increased ICP. The external surfaces of the head are examined for bleeding, cuts, abrasions, or other forms of injury.

Nursing Diagnosis

Depending on the type and degree of injury, one or more of the following may apply. Additional nursing diagnoses based on the patient's LOC, seriousness

and length of injury, and the presence of rising ICP (see Chapter 36) may be added as needed. If temporary or permanent neurologic deficits occur as a result of the injury, additional nursing diagnoses, as outlined in Chapter 39, may be added.

- Altered nutrition: less than body requirements related to decreased LOC
- Fluid volume deficit related to decreased oral intake secondary to decreased LOC
- Potential for infection related to depressed skull fracture
- Ineffective airway clearance related to decreased LOC
- Self-care deficit: total related to decreased LOC
- Altered thought processes related to head injury, increased ICP
- Potential for injury related to disorientation, confusion
- Knowledge deficit (family) of home care management

Planning and Implementation

The major goals of the patient include maintaining a patent airway, maintaining adequate food and fluid intake, and preventing further injury.

The main goals of nursing management are to prevent infection, maintain a patent airway, institute nursing measures to reduce or prevent a rise in ICP, and recognize changes in the patient's condition.

Patients are usually detained in the hospital for 24 hours or more after a significant head injury. The patient is closely monitored for signs of increased ICP (see Chapter 36). A neurologic flow sheet may be used to record the results of each neurologic assessment. Vital signs may be taken as often as every 15 minutes. The patient is closely observed for changes in the LOC, dilatation or unequal size of the pupils, convulsions, and muscle paralysis or weakness. The patient also must be closely monitored for seizures, since they may occur.

Since patients may have increased ICP due to intracranial bleeding, the nursing management also includes those tasks applicable to this disorder (see Chapter 36).

Altered Nutrition, Fluid Volume Deficit. If ICP increases, fluids may be restricted. Intravenous fluids are usually given since oral fluids pose a danger of aspiration, especially if a patient is confused or has a change in the LOC. Intake and output are measured, and the patient is closely observed for electrolyte imbalances (see Chapter 12). If recovery is prolonged, tube feedings may be ordered to provide nutrition.

Potential for Infection. The temperature is monitored every 4 hours, and the physician is notified of any increase. Antipyretics and cooling measures may be necessary.

Ineffective Airway Clearance. A patent airway is essential. The head of the bed is elevated to about 30 degrees or as ordered to decrease ICP. The physician is consulted about other positions for the patient; certain types of head injuries require that the patient not rest on the injured side. If responding, the patient is instructed to deep breathe every hour; coughing, however, is avoided. Suctioning is not performed if the patient has increased ICP due to intracranial bleeding. Mechanical ventilation may be necessary if respirations are shallow and irregular.

Self-Care Deficit. Complete bed rest and strict limitation of activities are usually ordered. All care, including bathing and oral care, must be done for the patient. The patient is disturbed as little as possible, and tasks are spaced to provide optimum rest.

Altered Thought Processes, Potential for Injury. The patient may be confused and disoriented. The confused patient who attempts to get out of bed may fall or incur other injuries. Although restraints should be avoided whenever possible because they add to disorientation and confusion, they may be necessary for some patients.

Mental changes may reflect a worsening of the patient's condition, but they also may be indicative of other problems, such as nausea, a full bladder, or pain—problems that the patient is unable to communicate to others. The nurse must attempt to determine whether the cause of mental change is related to the patient's neurologic condition.

Knowledge Deficit. A patient with a concussion may be sent home, and the family is instructed to closely observe the patient for 2 or 3 days. The physician may recommend that the patient's LOC and ability to move and talk be assessed every hour while awake and every 2 hours while asleep. During the night, the patient must be aroused to determine the LOC and response to questions. Many hospitals issue an instruction sheet for these observations. The nurse must review this material with the family to make sure they understand the instructions.

If surgery or invasive monitoring of ICP is necessary, these procedures are explained to the family.

Evaluation

■ Demonstrates evidence of improvement
■ Vital signs remain within normal range
■ Fluid volume deficit corrected or deficit maintained according to physician's order
■ Nutritional needs are met
■ No evidence of electrolyte imbalance
■ No evidence of infection
■ Respiratory rate, rhythm, and depth is normal

■ Attains and maintains effective airway clearance
■ Personal care needs are met
■ Is oriented to time and place; shows evidence of improving thought processes
■ No evidence of injury
■ Family demonstrates understanding of treatment modalities

INTRACRANIAL SURGERY

A *craniotomy* is a surgical opening of the skull to access the structures below the cranial bones. A craniotomy may be performed, for example, to remove a tumor, stop intracranial bleeding, repair damage to tissues beneath the skull, repair a cerebral artery aneurysm, and remove a blood clot. A *craniectomy* is the removal of a portion of the skull, and a *cranioplasty* is the repair of a defect in the skull. In the latter procedure, a metal or plastic plate is used to replace the removed bone.

Two approaches may be used for a craniotomy. The supratentorial (above the tentorium) approach and the infratentorial (below the tentorium) approach. The tentorium consists of the section of the dura mater that separates the cerebrum and the cerebellum.

In cranial surgery, burr holes are made in the skull, and a section of bone is cut. The bone flap is removed and then usually replaced after surgery is completed. In some instances, such as an inoperable tumor, the bone flap is not replaced, allowing the tumor to expand and, thus, preventing increased ICP. Two examples of cranial incisions are shown in Figure 38-2.

Complications

Complications associated with intracranial surgery include cerebral edema, infection, shock, fluid and electrolyte imbalances, venous thrombosis (especially in the extremities), increased ICP, convulsive disorders, leakage of cerebrospinal fluid, and gastrointestinal ulceration (stress ulcers) and hemorrhage.

NURSING PROCESS —THE PATIENT UNDERGOING INTRACRANIAL SURGERY

Preoperative Period

Assessment

A neurologic examination (see Chapter 35) is performed to provide a preoperative and postoperative data base. The results of diagnostic tests are reviewed.

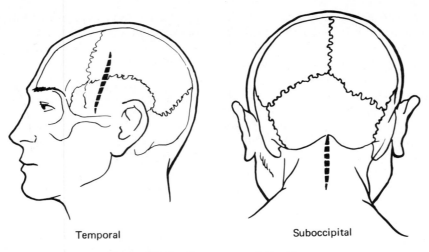

Temporal   Suboccipital

Figure 38–2.   Common cranial incisions.

Nursing Diagnosis

Depending on the condition of the patient, the diagnosis, and the reason for surgery, one or more of the following may apply:

- Anxiety related to diagnosis, impending surgery
- Ineffective individual coping related to diagnosis, impending surgery
- Knowledge deficit of preoperative preparations, the surgical procedure

Planning and Implementation

The major goals of the patient include a reduction in anxiety, an ability to (begin to) cope with the diagnosis and impending surgery, and an understanding of preoperative preparations.

The main goal of nursing management is to physically and emotionally prepare the patient and family for surgery.

The following preoperative preparations may be ordered: an anticonvulsant such as phenytoin (Dilantin) to reduce the risk of convulsive seizures before and after surgery; restricted fluids, an osmotic diuretic, and a corticosteroid to reduce cerebral edema and ICP; the insertion of an indwelling urethral catheter and intravenous line; and the shaving of the scalp.

Anxiety.   Depending on the diagnosis, general condition, and LOC, a patient may exhibit emotional reactions to the impending surgery as well as the preoperative preparations, such as shaving of the head. Time must be allowed for the patient and family to ask questions and talk about the surgery and preparations.

Ineffective Individual Coping.   The patient and family may have difficulty coping with the diagnosis and

the possibility of neurologic deficits after surgery. Listening to the patient and family may help the medical personnel identify problems and develop plans for immediate and long-term rehabilitation and care.

Knowledge Deficit.   The surgical procedure and preoperative preparations are explained to the patient (when possible) and family. Many times questions and concerns arise after the surgeon has talked to the family. Unless an emergency situation exists, the family must be given time to ask questions about the impending surgery and the preparations required before surgery.

Evaluation

- Anxiety is reduced
- The patient and family begin to show an ability to cope with the potential or actual diagnosis and impending surgery
- The patient and family demonstrate an understanding of the surgical procedure and preoperative preparations

Postoperative Period

Assessment

Immediately after surgery, a complete neurologic examination is performed to provide a data base (see Chapter 35). The patient's surgical records are reviewed. The patient's room should be equipped with a suction machine, oral airways, sterile dressings, emergency tracheostomy tray, a ventricular puncture tray, and materials with which to perform neurologic assessments. Other equipment or materials may be ordered by the neurosurgeon.

Postoperative assessments are performed at frequent intervals and include all areas of neurologic function: vital signs, LOC, motor and sensory responses, pupils, speech, body posture, and reflexes. These assessments are usually made every 15 to 30 minutes during the immediate postoperative period and then extended to hourly intervals. A neurologic flow sheet may be used to record data obtained during assessments. Cranial surgery may cause cerebral edema or intracranial bleeding; the patient is observed closely for any possible complications.

Nursing Diagnosis

Depending on the postoperative diagnosis, the type and extent of surgery performed, and the condition of the patient, one or more of the following may apply. The nursing diagnoses for disorders such as cerebral edema and brain tumor also may be added. If temporary or permanent neurologic deficits occur as the result of surgery, additional nursing diagnoses, as outlined in Chapter 39, may be added.

- Pain related to surgery
- Impaired verbal communication related to decreased LOC, cerebral damage
- Impaired physical mobility related to surgery, brain tissue trauma
- Potential for infection related to surgery
- Ineffective individual coping related to postsurgical diagnosis, neurologic deficits after surgery
- Hyperthermia related to infection, cerebral edema, damage to temperature-regulating mechanisms of brain
- Ineffective airway clearance related to decreased LOC
- Sensory and perceptual alterations (specify type) related to cerebral edema, results of surgery
- Self-care deficit: partial to total related to surgery, LOC
- Impaired skin integrity related to prolonged immobility
- Knowledge deficit of postdischarge treatment regimen, prognosis, other factors (specify)

Planning and Implementation

The major goals of the patient include relief of pain, effective communication with others, improved physical mobility, absence of infection, improved coping mechanisms, maintenance of a patent airway, maintenance of skin integrity, deceased sensory and perceptual alterations, improved ability for self-care, and an understanding of home care.

The major goals of nursing management are to achieve neurologic equilibrium, improve cerebral tissue perfusion, and recognize overt and covert changes in the patient's condition. Neurologic assessments are performed at regular intervals. Edema around the eyes (periorbital edema) may make examination of the pupils difficult. Ecchymosis also may

be present. The Glasgow Coma Scale (see Chapter 36) may be used to determine the LOC. Anticonvulsant drugs may be administered prophylactically to prevent convulsive seizures.

The main goals in the rehabilitation of a patient with a poor prognosis (eg, someone with an inoperable brain tumor) are to keep the patient as comfortable as possible and to prevent complications of prolonged inactivity, such as decubitus, contractures, and pneumonia.

Surgery on the central nervous system may result in a temporary or permanent neurologic deficit, that is, the loss of one or more functions of this system, such as aphasia or paralysis of an extremity. Long-term rehabilitation goals are formulated and based on (1) what neurologic deficit (if any) has occurred, (2) whether the loss is believed to be temporary or permanent, and (3) the patient's prognosis. Patients who are not expected to return to full activity are given every chance and encouragement for the return of as much function as possible. As soon as a patient returns from surgery, rehabilitation begins. At this time, it is geared toward the prevention of complications, such as decubitus or contractures, that would alter the course of recovery. Physical and occupational therapies are planned and coordinated so that the patient can work toward realistic and attainable recovery goals.

After surgery and a return to the hospital room, the patient is positioned either in a supine position or turned on the unoperative side. A small pillow is placed under the head, and the head of the bed is elevated. The surgeon specifies the degree of elevation and the positions allowed. Corticosteroids and limitation of fluids may be used to control cerebral edema and, thus, increase cerebral perfusion.

To prevent thrombophlebitis and deep vein thrombosis, which may develop because of prolonged immobility during neurosurgery, antiembolitic stockings are usually applied before surgery. These stockings may be left in place for several days after surgery or as long as the patient is immobile. The stockings are removed and reapplied as ordered.

Pain. Pain, which can be minimal, is controlled by the use of analgesics such as codeine or pentazocine (Talwin). Opiates, such as morphine, are usually not ordered because these drugs depress respirations, affect pupil size, and mask signs of increased ICP. Aspirin or drugs that contain aspirin are avoided because they can increase bleeding tendencies.

Hyperthermia. The temperature is monitored every 2 to 4 hours. More frequent monitoring may be necessary if the temperature rises and antipyretic measures are used. If the temperature does not respond to antipyretic drugs, a cooling blanket may be ordered.

Impaired Verbal Communication.   Unconscious patients are totally dependent on others for their needs as well as for anticipation or recognition of problems that may occur. During assessment, the patient is closely observed for signs (eg, facial grimacing, pulling at a catheter, moaning) that may indicate a problem.

If aphasia occurs after surgery, the conscious patient has difficulty conveying needs to others. If the patient tries to communicate but is unable to, the nurse can ask a series of yes or no questions to establish communication with the patient.

Potential for Infection.   The surgical dressing is reinforced as necessary. Sterile dressings and aseptic technique are used for dressing reinforcement because the moist area can introduce microorganisms into the meninges. The appearance of bleeding or straw-colored fluid on the dressing is reported immediately. Aseptic technique is used when monitoring ICP by means of a ventricular catheter or other device.

Ineffective Individual Coping.   Intracranial surgery may result in temporary or permanent neurologic changes. Once patients are awake and aware of the surroundings, they also may be aware of any body changes (neurologic deficits). Depression and withdrawal may be seen. Although each patient's problem may require a different approach, the nurse must be aware of similar ineffective coping mechanisms. Encouragement and praise when a task is accomplished, for example, may help a patient begin to cope with the disability and develop self-confidence, especially during active rehabilitation.

Fluid Volume Deficit.   Oral fluids are withheld until the patient is fully conscious and swallowing and gag reflexes return. The physician may order an intentional fluid volume deficit. Oral and intravenous fluids are given in specified limited amounts to control cerebral edema. Depending on the patient's postoperative course, fluid restrictions may be necessary for 3 to 5 days or more after surgery. The patient also is observed for signs of electrolyte imbalances (see Chapter 12).

An indwelling catheter may be inserted before surgery. The urinary output is measured every 8 hours. If an osmotic diuretic is given for treatment of cerebral edema, the urinary output is measured at more frequent intervals.

The syndrome of inappropriate secretion of antidiuretic hormone (SIADH), which is a secretion of excess antidiuretic hormone (ADH) by the pituitary gland, may occur after surgery and result in water retention, hyponatremia, and serum hypoosmolarity. Symptoms of this syndrome include water retention, low urinary output despite adequate intake, and symptoms of hyponatremia. Frequent and accurate intake and output measurements and monitoring of the urine specific gravity are necessary to recognize this syndrome in its early stages. It is treated by limiting the fluid intake and, possibly, administering diuretics.

Ineffective Airway Clearance.   An ineffective breathing pattern or depressed respirations may require the use of mechanical ventilation. When the conscious patient is able to breathe without mechanical assistance, deep breaths are encouraged every hour. Elevation of the head of the bed also increases the depth of respiration. Suctioning is used with caution because this procedure increases ICP.

Sensory and Perceptual Alterations.   Visual, auditory, and speech changes may occur after surgery. Edema around the eyes may interfere with the patient's sight, resulting in confusion and sensory deprivation. Talking to the patient when entering the room and touching the patient's arm or hand while talking may reduce confusion. Depending on the surgical site and extent of surgery, hearing and speech difficulties also may occur and produce confusion and disorientation. An increase in stimuli (eg, voices of medical personnel, leaving a radio on at low volume) often helps patients maintain contact with reality and reduces disorientation and confusion.

Self-Care Deficit.   All personal care is performed for the patient until active rehabilitation begins. Once disabilities (if any) are determined, plans are made to help the patient assume responsibility for personal care. Occupational and physical therapists can develop special devices that help disabled patients attain self-reliance and the ability to carry out some or most of their activities of daily living.

Impaired Physical Mobility, Impaired Skin Integrity.   The patient's position is changed every 2 hours. The physician may prohibit turning the patient on the operative side, for example, if a large tumor has been removed. Special attention is given to areas subjected to pressure, such as the bony prominences.

If limited movement or paralysis of one or more extremities is noted, the extremity is positioned to prevent contractures and joint deformities. Passive exercises are not instituted until ordered by the physician. The physician may order physical therapy once the patient's condition has stabilized.

Knowledge Deficit. The family should be informed of the swelling and discoloration around the eyes, the head dressing, and the presence of monitoring devices before they see the patient for the first time after surgery. The family also is encouraged to ask questions of the physician when they have any concern about the surgery, the results of surgery, and the patient's future condition and prognosis.

Once an active rehabilitation program is instituted, discharge teaching is planned. Depending on the eventual condition of the patient as well as other factors, the teaching program includes the medication regimen, techniques of home care management, importance of physical and occupational therapies, and agency referrals, for example, for financial problems, home nursing care, and transportation.

Evaluation

- Achieves neurologic stability; begins to move extremities, responds verbally and physically to commands, answers questions
- Pain is controlled or eliminated
- Demonstrates improved ability to verbally communicate with others
- No evidence of infection at surgical site, lungs, or other organs or structures
- Attains and maintains normal vital signs
- Patient and family begin to cope with disabilities related to surgery or diagnosis
- Fluid volume deficit maintained (to correct or prevent cerebral edema) or corrected
- No evidence of electrolyte imbalance
- Cerebral edema prevented or corrected
- No evidence of thrombosis, thrombophlebitis
- Becomes oriented to time and place
- Self-care needs are met
- Skin remains intact; no evidence of skin breakdown
- Family demonstrates understanding of postdischarge care

SPINAL CORD INJURIES AND DISORDERS
Trauma

Spinal cord trauma is serious and sometimes fatal. Causes of spinal cord injuries include automobile accidents, falls, and gunshot wounds. The cervical and lumbar spines are the most common sites of injury.

Violence to the back may fracture or collapse one or more vertebrae. A bone fragment pressing into the cord can interfere with the transmission of nerve impulses. Even if no fracture has occurred, momentary compression of the cord can lead to edema, which further compresses the cord. In this instance, symptoms may disappear gradually as edema subsides.

Trauma may lead to bleeding within the cord; because the blood has no place to drain, it forms a hematoma that occupies space and compresses the nerve roots. An injury to the cord also may sever spinal cord nerve fibers. When this kind of injury occurs and complete severance of the cord results, the patient is permanently paralyzed and loses sensation below the site of the injury to the cord. Because the tracts of the nerves are cut, no effective nerve regeneration occurs. The term *paraplegia* refers to paralysis of both lower extremities and *quadriplegia* to paralysis of all four extremities (Fig. 38-3).

A variety of diseases, such as multiple sclerosis, metastatic lesions of the spine, and poliomyelitis, may result in a degree of paraplegia or quadriplegia. When the injury comes from disease, the paralysis is likely to develop gradually. The paralysis caused by fracture or dislocation of vertebrae due to an injury most often occurs suddenly.

Symptoms

The degree and location of the injury determine the symptoms that occur immediately after a spinal cord injury. The patient may complain of symptoms such as pain in the affected area, difficulty breathing, numbness, or inability to move. If the injury is high in the cervical region, respiratory failure and death follow paralysis of the diaphragm. Midcervical injuries result in paralysis of the muscles of the upper thorax; hence, breathing can be accomplished only by diaphragmatic movement. The fifth and sixth cervical vertebrae and the first and fifth lumbar vertebrae are especially vulnerable to injury; injury at these levels is more frequent than injury to other levels of the spinal cord.

The degree and location of the injury also determine the extent of the disability and the loss of function (Table 38-1). When the cord is completely severed, function is lost permanently below the level of the injury. If the damage to the cord is partial, function may be maintained or, possibly, regained.

Diagnosis

Diagnosis is made by history of the trauma and neurologic examination. Radiographs, myelography, MRI, and CT scan may be used to identify the location and extent of injury.

Treatment

Emergency management at the scene of injury is crucial because improper removal from the accident

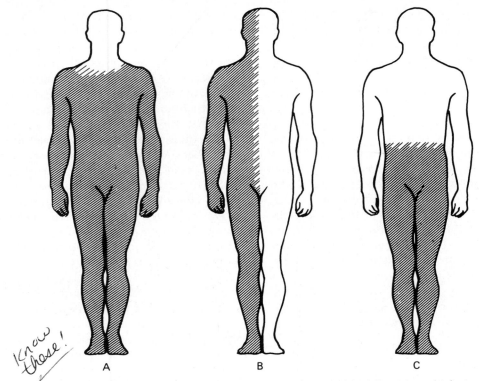

know those!

Figure 38–3. Body areas affected in three common types of disability: (*A*) quadriplegia, (*B*) hemiplegia, and (*C*) paraplegia. The location and extent of the paralysis depend on the location and the severity of the injury. The diagrams are oversimplified. A patient may have some remaining function in an affected part.

scene and transportation to the hospital may cause further damage to the spinal cord. *The head and back must be immobilized* by means of neck support (cervical collar) and transfer board (a rigid stretcher) at the scene of the accident. An intravenous line is inserted to provide access to a vein should shock occur. During diagnostic evaluation in the hospital, these immobilization devices are left in place until their removal is ordered by the physician.

Vital signs are stabilized. Corticosteroids may be given to reduce spinal cord edema. When the patient has a known or suspected spinal cord injury, proper alignment of the spine must be maintained at all times to prevent further injury to the spinal cord.

Cervical Spine Injuries. After diagnostic evaluation, those with cervical spine injuries may be moved to a regular hospital bed or Stryker frame. The head is immobilized with a cervical collar or cervical traction, such as Crutchfield, Vinke, or Gardner-Wells traction tongs or a halo vest traction. Burr holes must be made to insert the pointed end of the Crutchfield or Vinke traction tongs or the halo traction apparatus. The Gardner-Wells traction does not require burr holes. Traction by means of weights and pulleys is applied to the tongs to provide correct cervical vertebrae alignment and increase the space between the vertebrae.

Additional weight may be added over a few days to increase the space between the vertebrae.

Depending on the extent of cervical injury, it may be necessary to surgically remove bone fragments or to stabilize the cervical spine.

Lumbar Spine Injuries. After diagnostic evaluation, patients with injuries to the lumbar spine may be transferred to a special bed, such as a Stryker frame. Surgery may be performed immediately if diagnostic studies show compression of the spinal cord. If spinal instability remains a problem after several weeks of immobilization, surgery may be performed to stabilize the injured area. The vertebrae may be fused with bone obtained from the iliac crest, and the spine may be stabilized with a steel rod.

Thoracolumbar Injuries. Patients with these injuries also are transferred to a special bed such as a Stryker frame. Surgery may be necessary to stabilize the spine. Various types of rods or other special devices such as Weiss springs may be used. The patient also may require external immobilization with devices such as a Jewett brace or plastic molded shell.

Spinal Shock. This phenomenon involves a sudden depression of reflex activity below the level of injury.

Table 38–1.   Level of Injury to Spinal Cord and Neurologic Findings*

Injury to	*Findings*
Cervical Spine	
C1, C2, C3	Usually fatal
C4	Quadriplegia, respiratory difficulty
C5 to C8	Variable function of neck, shoulder, and arm muscles; no function in lower extremities
Thoracic Spine	
T1 to T11	Paraplegia—leg braces occasionally can be used when injury is to lower thoracic spine
Thoracic–Lumbar Spine	
T12 to L3	Paraplegic; wheelchair with leg braces

* Complete transection of the cord results in symptoms additional to those of partial transection, which may produce only sensory or motor loss or hemiplegia.

Pronounced hypotension, bradycardia, decreased respiratory rate, decreased temperature, flaccid paralysis, and warm, dry skin are seen. If the level of injury is in the cervical or upper thoracic region, respiratory failure may occur. Bowel and bladder distention may be seen. The patient does not perspire below the level of injury; therefore, hyperthermia may occur. Depending on the level of injury, treatment includes support of respiratory and cardiac activities, gastrointestinal decompression to relieve bowel distention, an indwelling urethral catheter to keep the bladder empty, suctioning, and mechanical ventilation. Spinal shock may persist for up to 6 weeks or until the body readjusts to the damage imposed by injury.

Autonomic Dysreflexia (AD).   This acute emergency may be seen in those with a cervical or high thoracic spinal cord injury, usually after spinal shock subsides. The cause of AD is an exaggerated response to sympathetic stimuli, such as a full bladder or impacted fecal mass. The primary symptoms are severe hypertension, bradycardia, pallor, blurred vision, and nausea. Convulsive seizures and death may occur.

Treatment includes the removal of the sympathetic stimuli that may have caused the condition.

Complications

Spinal shock, permanent paralysis below the level of injury, AD (cervical to mid-thoracic area), and respira-

tory arrest may occur. Long-term complications are those associated with prolonged immobility and include decubitus formation, contractures, respiratory infections, loss of calcium from the bones, urinary tract calculi, and decreased cardiac output.

Prognosis

The level of the cord injury, the occurrence of complications, the patient's motivation and perseverance, and the quality of care received by the patient are important influences on prognosis. Many paraplegic patients are able to go home to care for themselves and, in some instances, to resume work. The quadriplegic patient also may return home but requires extensive physical care.

NURSING PROCESS —THE PATIENT WHO HAS A SPINAL CORD INJURY

Assessment

On arrival, the type of injury incurred is obtained from the family or witnesses. The physician may perform an immediate neurologic assessment to prioritize diagnostic and treatment modalities. The nurse reviews the physician's assessments and record of neurologic deficits.

Vital signs are taken, and the patient's breathing pattern is evaluated. A neurologic flow sheet is used to record initial and subsequent findings.

Nursing Diagnosis

Depending on the type and location of injury, one or more of the following may apply. Additional nursing diagnoses that pertain to permanent neurologic deficits are discussed in Chapter 39 and may be added as needed.

- Impaired physical mobility related to spinal cord injury (state level of injury if known)
- Pain related to spinal cord trauma, other injuries
- Impaired skin integrity related to immobility
- Colonic constipation related to bowel atony secondary to spinal cord injury
- Ineffective airway clearance related to spinal cord injury
- Dysreflexia related to spinal cord injury (at T7 or above)
- Total incontinence related to spinal cord injury
- Ineffective individual coping related to neurologic deficits after spinal cord injury
- Knowledge deficit of short- and long-term treatment modalities

Planning and Implementation

The major goals of the patient include improvement of mobility, relief of pain, maintenance of skin integrity, attainment of normal bowel and bladder elimination, maintenance of a patent airway, improved coping mechanisms, and an understanding of short- and long-term treatment modalities.

The major goals of nursing management include the prevention of further injury to the spinal cord, prevention of contractures and joint deformities, and recognition and prevention of complications.

The patient may be placed in traction. When traction is applied, the weights must hang free and are *never* lifted, removed, increased, or decreased except by order of the physician.

The nursing process for the patient with a neurologic deficit is discussed in Chapter 39.

Ineffective Airway Clearance.   A patent airway must be maintained at all times, especially if the injury is high in the spinal cord. Suctioning may be necessary. If respiratory distress occurs, the physician is notified immediately; a tracheostomy with or without mechanical ventilation may be required.

Impaired Physical Mobility.   Proper body alignment must be maintained at all times with devices such as footboards, trochanter rolls, and pillows. Whenever these devices are used, it is important that their application follow the principles of body alignment and that their use be approved by the physician.

When the acute phase had ended, the physician may prescribe physical therapy. Areas above and below the level of injury receive therapy. In time, patients who have use of their upper extremities are taught to use overhead bars or a trapeze to increase the physical strength and movement of the upper extremities.

Pain.   Analgesics may be ordered for pain. When administered by the intramuscular or subcutaneous routes, the injection is given above the level of paralysis because areas below this level absorb drugs poorly.

Impaired Skin Integrity.   Decubitus formation is often a problem, mainly because patients in certain types of traction cannot be turned on their sides. Frames, such as the Foster or Stryker frame, may be used to turn the patient from supine to prone and back every 2 hours. Once the patient is turned and the top part of the frame removed, special skin care can be given.

The skin is kept well lubricated. Powders are avoided because caking may occur. Pressure points can be gently massaged, unless the physician orders otherwise.

Colonic Constipation.   A paralytic ileus (cessation of peristalsis of the bowel) may be seen shortly after injury. The physician may order insertion of a nasogastric tube to empty the contents of the stomach and relieve gastric distention. The abdomen is auscultated daily for bowel sounds. Once peristalsis returns, the physician may order removal of the nasogastric tube. A stool softener or rectal suppository may then be ordered to encourage daily bowel elimination.

Dysreflexia.   If this problem occurs, the physician is notified immediately. An antihypertensive drug may be ordered and administered intravenously to immediately bring down the blood pressure. Placing the patient in a sitting position also may help reduce the blood pressure. Autonomic dysreflexia may occur at intervals over a period of many years after spinal cord injury.

Total Incontinence.   An indwelling urethral catheter usually is inserted shortly after admission. Depending on the level of injury, the patient may permanently require a catheter or use intermittent catheterization to empty the bladder.

Intake and output are measured, and the physician is informed if the urinary output falls below 500 ml per day. The catheter is changed as ordered by the physician or according to hospital policy. Periodic urinalysis usually is ordered to detect bladder infections.

Ineffective Individual Coping.   One of the most difficult problems the nurse must deal with is the effect of the injury on the patient. When the injury results in a permanent neurologic deficit, medical science can do nothing to return the patient to normal neurologic function. Patients are well aware of this fact and usually have difficulty coping with the disability that has changed their lives.

Because each patient responds differently, each approach the nurse takes must be different. The nurse must be willing to listen and offer encouragement as the patient progresses through rehabilitation.

Knowledge Deficit.   As soon as the acute phase has ended, patients often have many questions about their conditions, future treatments, and prognoses. While these questions are answered by the physician, the nurse is responsible for explaining treatments such as insertion of a suppository, use of a trochanter roll, or special skin care.

Once active rehabilitation is prescribed, the therapists explain the purpose of the program and the patient's participation. These explanations may be reinforced by the nurse.

A teaching plan for patients who do not incur permanent disability is developed according to the postdischarge regimen prescribed by the physician. The nurse reviews these recommendations or treatment modalities with the patient and family.

A more extensive discussion of patient and family teaching for people with neurologic deficits is covered in Chapter 39.

Evaluation

- Demonstrates improved physical mobility or demonstrates improved strength and mobility of the upper extremities
- Pain is relieved or eliminated
- Shows no signs of skin breakdown
- Attains a normal bowel elimination pattern
- Maintains a patent airway; is able to cough and raise secretions
- Dysreflexia identified and treated according to physician's orders
- Attains normal urinary elimination
- Demonstrates beginning of ability to cope with the effects of the injury

- Demonstrates understanding of treatment modalities, rehabilitation, postdischarge home care

Spinal Nerve Root Compression

Lesions of the spinal cord are of two basic types: those that involve the spinal cord, or *intramedullary* lesions, and those of the tissues that surround the spinal cord, or *extramedullary* lesions.

Pressure on spinal nerve roots may be caused by trauma, herniated intervertebral discs, and tumors of the spinal cord and surrounding structures (Fig. 38-4).

Discs are composed of cartilage that act as cushions between the vertebrae. Their spongy center (nucleus pulposus) is encased in a fibrous coat. When stress, age, or disease weakens an area in the coat or in a ligament attachment to the vertebra, and the nucleus pulposus becomes thickened and hardened, the disc may herniate (protrude), causing pressure on the nerves. The most common site of the protrusion is one of the three lower lumbar discs. Because the spinal cord ends at the level of the first or the second lumbar vertebra, herniated lumbar discs compress spinal nerve roots rather than the cord itself. Pain along the distribution of the sciatic nerve is a common symptom.

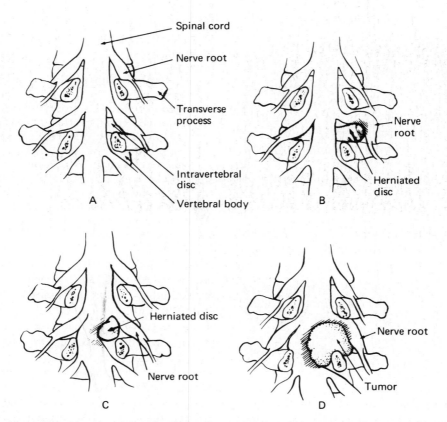

Figure 38–4. (*A*) Diagram of the normal spinal column. (*B*) Herniated disc pressing on a spinal nerve root. (*C*) Herniated disc pressing on the spinal cord. (*D*) Tumor compressing both the spinal cord and a spinal nerve.

Whatever causes increased pressure within the spinal cord (eg, straining, coughing, lifting a heavy object) intensifies pain. Pain is more severe when the nerves are stretched, such as when the patient, while lying supine, tries to lift a leg up without bending the knee. Also, weakness and changes in sensation may be seen. In the beginning, symptoms tend to be recurrent rather than steady. Herniated intervertebral discs also may be seen in the cervical spine.

Tumors of the spinal cord and surrounding areas may be malignant or benign. Malignant tumors may be primary or metastatic.

Symptoms
Whatever the type of lesion, it is the pressure on the cord that causes the symptoms. Symptoms vary depending on the cause of the compression and the level involved and include one or more of the following: numbness, tingling, weakness, paralysis, pain, and paresthesia, all of which appear below the level of the lesion.

Diagnosis
Diagnosis is based on the patient's symptoms and one or more diagnostic test. The tests performed depend on the probable diagnosis and include radiograph, CT scan, MRI, myelogram, and electromyogram.

Treatment
When a patient has a herniated intervertebral disc, conservative therapy may be tried first. Metastatic spinal cord tumors also are treated conservatively, as removal is not feasible. Surgery is the treatment of choice for benign and primary malignant spinal cord tumors. Surgery for a primary malignant tumor is usually followed by radiation therapy.

Conservative therapy includes one or more of the following:

Bed Rest. Bed rest with a firm mattress and bed board may be used for those with a lumbar herniated disc.

Immobilization. The patient with a herniated cervical disc may be treated by means of immobilization of the cervical spine with a cervical collar or brace. Later, as inflammation subsides, the collar or brace may be worn intermittently, such as when the patient is walking or sitting in a chair.

Traction. Buck's extension or pelvic traction for a lumbar herniated disc, or a cervical halter or tongs implanted in the skull for a cervical herniated disc, may be used to decrease severe muscle spasm. Trac-

tion also increases the distance between adjacent vertebrae and may be continuous or intermittent. Five to 30 pounds of weight may be applied. Traction keeps the patient in bed with good alignment, and some patients find that it relieves pain. Treatment may be so effective that the patient remains symptom free for a long time. Pelvic traction or a cervical halter may be used at home, provided the patient has been thoroughly instructed in its set-up and use.

Drug Therapy. Skeletal muscle relaxants may be prescribed for those with an intervertebral disc. Diazepam (Valium), a tranquilizer with skeletal muscle relaxing ability, may be used for its twofold effect—the reduction of anxiety associated with the pain and discomfort of a herniated disc and the relaxation of skeletal muscle. Drugs such as aspirin, phenylbutazone (Butazolidin), and corticosteroids may be used to treat inflammation. Reducing inflammation and muscle spasm reduces pain, but additional analgesics also may be required.

Patients with an inoperable spinal cord tumor are given analgesics to control pain.

If conservative therapy fails to relieve the symptoms of a herniated disc, surgery usually is considered. The operative procedure for removal of a spinal cord tumor is a laminectomy, which may or may not be followed by a spinal fusion (see below). Surgical procedures for a ruptured intervertebral disc include the following:

1. *Discectomy.* This procedure involves removal of the ruptured disc.
2. *Laminectomy.* This procedure involves removal of the posterior arch of a vertebra to expose the spinal cord. The surgeon can remove whatever lesion is causing compression: a herniated disc, tumor, or clot, bone spur, or broken bone fragment.
3. *Discectomy with spinal fusion.* After removal of the ruptured disc, a piece of bone is taken from another area, such as the iliac crest, and grafted onto the vertebrae to fuse the vertebral spinous process. Bone also may be obtained from a bone bank.

Fusion stabilizes the spine weakened by degenerative joint changes, such as osteoarthritis, and further weakened by the laminectomy. Fusion results in a firm union; mobility is lost, and the patient must become accustomed to a permanent area of stiffness. When a portion of the lumbar spine is fused, the patient usually doesn't feel the stiffness after a short time because motion increases in the joints above the fusion. When the area of fusion is in the cervical spine, motion usually is more limited. Spinal fusion also may be performed for spinal cord tumors, fractures and dislocations of the spine, and Pott's disease (tuberculosis of the spine).

NURSING PROCESS —THE PATIENT WHO HAS SPINAL NERVE ROOT COMPRESSION

Assessment

A history of symptoms and a complete medical and allergy history are obtained. If the disorder occurred as a result of an accident, a complete history of the trauma is recorded.

A neurologic examination is performed (see Chapter 35), and any limitation of motion and the type of movement that causes pain are noted. When the patient has spinal compression, whatever the cause, specific observations of function and sensation are made.

Nursing Diagnosis

Depending on the type of disorder, treatment modalities, and other factors, one or more of the following may apply. Additional nursing diagnoses related to conservative treatment modalities (eg, immobilization or drug therapy) may be necessary.

- Pain (acute or chronic) related to compression of sensory nerve roots, surgery
- Impaired physical mobility related to pain, surgery, conservative treatment (immobilization)
- Anxiety related to pain, diagnosis, impending treatment (surgery, conservative), other (specify)
- Impaired skin integrity related to immobilization
- Knowledge deficit of drug therapy, treatment at home (eg, application of traction, cervical collar)

Planning and Implementation

The major goals of the patient include a relief of pain or discomfort, improved physical mobility, a reduction of anxiety, prevention of skin breakdown, and an understanding of postdischarge treatment modalities.

The major goals of nursing management are to relieve pain and improve function in the affected areas.

CONSERVATIVE THERAPY.   Once treatment is started, the patient's response to therapy is periodically evaluated. It is important to note the activities and positions that increase pain and the gain or loss in motion or sensation since the last observation. Comparison of present symptoms with those first experienced provides an evaluation of response to therapy. It also is important to note any change in symptoms if the patient is allowed out of traction.

Traction may be continuous or intermittent. The physician prescribes the time intervals in which the patient on intermittent traction is allowed out of traction. The physician may allow bathroom privileges, but the patient is assisted when getting out of

bed. When reapplying traction, the weights should be supported and lowered gently so that the patient does not experience a sudden and strong pull by the traction apparatus. A pillow may be placed under the legs to prevent the heels from rubbing on the sheets.

When out of traction and able to move in bed, the patient is reminded to roll from side to side without twisting the spine; sudden movement that strains or twists the spine is avoided. When first getting out of bed, the patient is instructed to stand straight, walk slowly, and avoid bending forward. Help putting on slippers and bathrobe as well as with getting in and out of a chair is given.

The traction apparatus must be checked several times a day for the proper application and use.

1. The belt (pelvic traction), cervical collar or brace, cervical traction with use of a sling or halter, or Buck's extension must be applied properly.
2. Traction weights must hang free.
3. Ropes must be seated in pulley grooves.
4. The position of the patient must allow correct pull of the traction apparatus.
5. Padding, when needed, must be correctly applied around the cervical collar, brace, sling, or halter.
6. The cervical tongs must be in correct position and the tips firmly inserted in the skull.

A cervical collar or brace must not be removed unless ordered by the physician. When the collar or brace is removed for short periods, for example, to check the skin, instruct the patient to keep the head relatively still and in the same alignment as when the cervical collar or brace was in place. When the collar or brace is removed for longer periods, the patient is advised to avoid extreme hyperextension of the neck or side-to-side rotation of the head.

SURGERY.   Before surgery, the care of the patient is similar to that of conservative treatment. Preoperative instructions include deep breathing exercises and the technique of log-rolling, which will be used to change position from side to side after surgery.

Postoperatively, vital signs are monitored until stable and the temperature is monitored every 4 hours. Deep-breathing exercises are performed hourly while awake. Although breathing exercises are an important part of care, the patient should cough only when necessary; coughing increases pressure within the spinal canal.

The dressing is examined for leakage of spinal fluid and bleeding. The patient is observed for signs of compression due to edema or hemorrhage at the operative site. Compression of the cord causes changes of motility or sensation from that point downward.

Voiding may be a problem after surgery. For this and other reasons, many surgeons order the patient out of bed the evening of the day of surgery. Intake and output records are kept, and the physician is notified if the patient cannot void.

If the patient is kept in bed after surgery, it is necessary to use a fracture bedpan with a bowel movement. If a regular bedpan is used, the patient should roll onto the bedpan with the back supported with pillows.

One of the most important principles of care after a lumbar laminectomy is for the patient to rest the back as much as possible. Twisting, turning, and jerking the back are not conducive to healing. The bed is kept flat until ordered otherwise. Postoperative orders vary. Some patients are kept flat the first postoperative day, and pillows are used to support the back when turned. When in bed, the patient is instructed or helped to turn using the log-roll method.

After a cervical discectomy, a cervical collar is put in place before the patient leaves surgery. The patient is instructed to turn the body when moving, as the neck must be kept in a straight (midline) position until healing takes place. When allowed out of bed, the head, neck, and upper shoulders are supported as the patient moves from a lying to a sitting then standing position. Support also is provided when the patient gets into or out of a chair.

Pain. Pain experienced preoperatively or during conservative therapy may be treated with analgesics, tranquilizers, or muscle relaxants. If pain is not relieved, the physician is notified.

Incision pain is managed with narcotics for the first few days after surgery. Surgery for a herniated disc abolishes the pain that was due to compression of the nerve root, but a few patients continue to have backache, especially after standing for long periods. When the nerve has been irritated by pressure exerted by the herniated disc or by surgery, the pain may last for some time after surgery.

Impaired Physical Mobility. Evaluation of impairment in physical mobility in the extremities reveals what tasks may need to be performed for the patient. The patient may require assistance with personal care, eating, and walking, for example.

Anxiety. Anxiety may be experienced during the period of conservative treatment or before and after surgery and may be due to concern over the effectiveness of treatment or the postoperative diagnosis. The nurse must allow time for the patient to discuss any concerns and, when necessary, must refer questions about treatment to the physician.

Impaired Skin Integrity. In Buck's extension traction, special attention is paid to the skin on the legs; in pelvic traction, however, attention is given to the skin beneath the harness around the waist and hips. Patients who wear a cervical collar or brace or who are in cervical traction require attention to the skin under each apparatus as well as the areas where pressure is placed on the skin by these devices.

Because the patient may spend a great deal of time in a supine position, special attention is given to the heels, elbows, sacral area, and other bony prominences. Good skin care is essential. Sheep-skin padding may be needed to protect areas subject to skin breakdown. These areas should be checked daily for signs of redness or superficial abrasions.

Knowledge Deficit. Many patients who have surgery for a cervical or lumbar disc are discharged in 2 to 3 days. A discharge teaching plan includes information about care at home, medication (if prescribed), and proper back or head alignment until healing has taken place. The patient with a lumbar laminectomy is told to wear proper fitting shoes (rather than slippers) and to avoid uneven surfaces until healing has taken place. The importance of performing the exercises recommended by the physician is emphasized.

The patient with a cervical laminectomy is told to follow the physician's recommendations about wearing the cervical collar and to avoid turning, flexing, or extending the neck. Usually these measures are necessary for 6 or more weeks after surgery.

If conservative treatment has been employed and is to be continued at home, the patient requires instructions about the set-up and use of the prescribed type of traction.

Patients scheduled for radiation therapy require instructions about the time of the first treatment. The importance of following the radiologists suggestions after the first and subsequent treatments is emphasized.

Evaluation

- Pain is reduced or eliminated
- Mobility is improved
- Skin remains intact with no evidence of breakdown, decubitus formation
- Anxiety is reduced or eliminated
- Verbalizes understanding of instructions and recommendations to be followed after discharge from the hospital

General Nutritional Considerations

☐ High fluid intake is necessary for the immobilized patient with a spinal cord injury.

☐ To increase the fluid intake, liquids other than water may be offered. If the diet has not been restricted, the patient also may have carbonated beverages, ice cream, broths, and flavored gelatin.

General Pharmacologic Considerations

☐ Skeletal muscle relaxants, such as carisoprodol (Soma) or the tranquilizer diazepam (Valium), may be prescribed for the patient with a herniated intervertebral disc, back strain, and spasms of the muscles of the back.

☐ Phenytoin (Dilantin) is commonly used before and after cranial surgery to prevent seizures. Other drugs with anticonvulsant activity also may be ordered.

☐ Codeine, in low doses, has a minimal effect on the respiratory center and pupil size even though it is an opiate.

Suggested Readings

☐ Berkow R, Fletcher AJ (eds). Merck manual of diagnosis and therapy. 15th ed. Rahway, NJ: Merck & Co, 1987. *(In-depth coverage of subject matter)*

☐ Chadwick AT, Oesting HH. Caring for patients with spinal cord injuries. RN 1989;52:52. *(Additional coverage of subject matter)*

☐ Hickey J. The clinical practice of neurological and neurosurgical nursing. 2nd ed. Philadelphia: JB Lippincott, 1986. *(In-depth coverage of subject matter)*

☐ Reimer M. Head-injured patient: how to detect early signs of trouble. Nursing '88 1988;18:34. *(Additional coverage of subject matter)*

☐ Romeo JH. Spinal cord injury: nursing the patient toward a new life. RN 1988;51:31. *(Additional coverage of subject matter)*

☐ Romeo JH. The critical minutes after spinal cord injury. RN 1988;51:61. *(Additional coverage of subject matter)*

☐ Wells T, Sunderlin D. Action stat! Closed head injury. Nursing '88 1988;18:33. *(Additional coverage of subject matter)*

Chapter 39

The Patient Who Has a Neurologic Deficit

On completion of this chapter the reader will:

■ List the physical problems associated with a neurologic deficit

■ Discuss the emotional problems associated with a neurologic deficit

■ Discuss the role of the medical team and family in the rehabilitation of a patient with a neurologic deficit

■ Use the nursing process in the management of a patient with a neurologic deficit

The patient with a neurologic deficit is faced with many problems. While the cause of the deficit may vary, the results are essentially the same: the patient is unable to perform tasks in the same manner as before the deficit occurred.

When a neurologic deficit occurs, one or more body systems are affected. The patient may be unable to walk, talk, or perform simple tasks like feeding and bathing. A temporary deficit is difficult; when the changes are brief, however, the patient often is able to accept the disability, knowing that soon it will disappear. On the other hand, a permanent disability creates many emotional, financial, and physical problems. Some patients, ultimately, can accept the changes in their body, while others cannot.

Neurologic deficits may occur immediately, for example, when a patient has a spinal cord injury or stroke, or they may be progressive, as seen in multiple sclerosis.

NURSING PROCESS —THE PATIENT WHO HAS A NEUROLOGIC DEFICIT

Assessment
To establish baseline data, a thorough patient history, including all symptoms and a medical and allergy history, is obtained from the patient or a family member. A general neurologic assessment (see Chapter 35) is performed, and the extent of neurologic involvement and the physical capabilities and limitations are carefully noted. The initial assessment includes an evaluation of the airway, breathing, circulation, and level of consciousness. Vital signs are taken. The alert patient may be able to answer questions about the symptoms and medical history. Because neuromuscular and central nervous system disorders and spinal cord injury can affect bowel and bladder tone, the abdomen is auscultated for bowel sounds, the bladder area is palpated for distention, and evidence of bowel and bladder incontinence is noted.

Nursing Diagnosis
Depending on the type and severity of symptoms, one or more of the following may apply. The nursing diagnoses may require change, modification, additions, and deletions. The relation between the nursing diagnoses and the known or potential cause of the problem also may change during various stages of the illness.

■ Anxiety related to diagnosis, symptoms, present and future problems associated with the neurologic deficit
■ Fear related to loss of body function
■ Pain related to injury, overuse of opposite extremity, other factors (specify)

- Potential fluid volume deficit related to hyperthermia, inability to take oral fluids, difficulty swallowing, inability to obtain fluids by self
- Impaired swallowing related to lethargy, effects of disease process on the central nervous system
- Altered nutrition: less than body requirements related to decreased level of consciousness, inability to swallow, anorexia, inability to chew, swallow, or feed self
- Altered nutrition: potential for more than body requirements related to lack of expenditure of physical energy
- Ineffective airway clearance related to effects of disease on the central and peripheral nervous system, prolonged immobility, decreased level of consciousness
- Hyperthermia due to infection (specify site), effect of disorder on temperature-regulating mechanism of the brain
- Potential for infection related to ineffective airway clearance, invasive procedures, decreased resistance to infection, other (specify)
- Impaired skin integrity related to immobility, incontinence, other factors (specify)
- Constipation or diarrhea (specify) related to prolonged immobility, tube feedings, decreased fluid intake, effect of the disease or injury on the spinal cord nerves
- Urinary incontinence or retention (specify), related to effects of disease or injury on the nervous system or spinal cord nerves, loss of bladder tone
- Impaired verbal communication related to decreased level of consciousness, involvement of muscles of speech or respiration, damage to speech area of brain
- Sensory and perceptual alterations related to increased or decreased sensitivity to external stimuli
- Altered thought processes related to brain damage
- Potential for injury related to muscle weakness, unilateral paralysis, seizure disorder, loss of calcium from the bone, other (specify)
- Impaired physical mobility related to muscle weakness, paralysis
- Activity intolerance related to muscle weakness, fatigue, paralysis
- Self-care deficit: partial to total (specify areas) related to weakness, paralysis, immobility, decreased level of consciousness
- Powerlessness related to inability to control situation, complete dependence on others for care
- Hopelessness related to prognosis
- Dysfunctional grieving due to loss of body function, inability to function at an adequate level, inability to assume family responsibilities, dependence on others, other factors (specify)
- Impaired adjustment related to inability to accept the physical changes associated with the disorder
- Ineffective individual coping related to diagnosis, symptoms
- Impaired home maintenance management related to symptoms of the disorder, inability to care for self, inadequacies such as housing, care, financial resources (specify)

- Altered family processes related to changes in health status, disability of family member
- Diversional activity deficit related to immobility, depression and withdrawal, inability to participate in social activities, monotonous environment
- Impaired social interaction related to aphasia, immobility
- Social isolation related to immobility, lack of transportation, other (specify)
- Altered sexuality patterns related to effect of disease on sexual activity, disturbance of nerve supply to the genitalia
- Sexual dysfunction related to disturbance of nerve supply to the genitalia
- Knowledge deficit of tests, treatments, home care, other (specify)

Planning and Implementation

The major goals of the patient include the following:

- A reduction of anxiety and fear
- A relief of pain and discomfort
- Adequate fluid and nutrition intake
- Maintenance of a patent airway
- Normal body temperature
- Absence of infection
- Prevention of skin breakdown
- Normal bowel and bladder elimination
- Improved verbal communication
- Absence of injury
- Improved physical mobility and activity tolerance
- Improved thought processes
- Improved ability to assume care for self
- Effective coping mechanisms and adjustment to illness
- Improved social interactions
- Engagement in diversional activities
- Sharing of concerns over sexuality
- Understanding of tests, treatments, home care

The major goals of nursing management include the following:

- Recognition of serious or life-threatening problems associated with a neurologic deficit
- Identification and meeting of the patient's needs
- Preventing complications
- Helping the patient compensate for the neurologic deficit
- Improving quality of life as much as possible
- Maintaining and prolonging independence and delay dependence
- Helping the patient and family cope with the disorder
- Engaging in a cooperative effort with all members of the medical team to rehabilitate the patient to the fullest potential

Disorders that cause a neurologic deficit may begin slowly, have few or vague symptoms, and progress through stages of remission and exacerbation. The disorder may begin with a chronic phase, but then periodic episodes of an acute phase may be seen. Other neurologic disorders begin with an injury or a patient appearing acutely ill and then may progress from an acute phase to a recovery phase to a chronic phase.

Acute Phase

During the acute phase, a patient is often critically ill. Neurologic assessments may be recorded on a flow sheet. The extent and frequency of the neurologic assessments depend on the cause of the disorder and the original symptoms.

Neurologic changes may indicate a need for immediate medical or surgical intervention to prevent further neurologic damage; therefore, *any* change in a patient's condition is reported immediately to the physician. Continued neurologic assessments by all members of the medical team are necessary to evaluate a patient's status and response to treatment.

VITAL SIGNS. Blood pressure; pulse rate, quality, and rhythm; respiratory rate, depth, and rhythm; and temperature are taken every 4 hours. More frequent assessment may be necessary. If a cervical injury has occurred, the respiratory rate is carefully assessed at frequent intervals.

The blood pressure must be maintained to ensure adequate cerebral oxygenation. Any marked rise or drop in blood pressure or change in the respiratory rate, rhythm, or depth is reported to the physician immediately.

ASSESSMENT OF THE LEVEL OF CONSCIOUSNESS. The Glasgow Coma Scale (see Chapter 35) or other form may be used to record the level of consciousness. This assessment is important when a cerebral injury, such as in head trauma and stroke, has occurred.

MOTOR AND SENSORY ASSESSMENT. The presence or absence of voluntary movement, speech, response to pain or discomfort, pupil size, equality, and reaction to light are determined and recorded.

FLUID AND ELECTROLYTE BALANCE. Intake and output are measured, and the patient is observed for signs of electrolyte imbalances.

ABNORMAL NEUROLOGIC SIGNS. The patient is assessed for development of nuchal rigidity, tremors, convulsive seizures, and changes in posture.

Recovery Phase

After the acute phase, the physician usually performs a neurologic examination to determine what deficits are present, the degree of each deficit, and an opinion as to whether the deficits are most likely permanent or temporary. Even though deficits may be temporary, a prolonged period of time and enrollment in a rehabilitation program may be necessary before a patient regains full use of the affected area.

When a neurologic deficit is identified, a rehabilitation program is planned and instituted. Although rehabilitation usually begins as soon as the patient is admitted to the hospital, a more formalized and intense program usually begins after the acute phase has passed. Psychological counseling also may begin during the recovery phase and extend into the rehabilitation and chronic phase.

Rehabilitation

Rehabilitation is designed to meet the patient's immediate and long-term needs and to create environmental changes that help the patient adapt to the disability and fully use any remaining abilities. An important part of the nurse's role in rehabilitation is to help these patients avoid complications so that they can profit from a rehabilitation program.

A successful rehabilitation program includes many members of the medical team, such as physicians, nurses, speech and occupational therapists, the prosthetist, and the social worker. When all members work as a unit, sharing information and following through on each member's suggestions and rehabilitation tasks, the patient receives optimum benefit from the program.

Members of the rehabilitation team may recommend devices or procedures to prevent complications as well as enhance the patient's remaining abilities. Devices that help a patient walk, eat, groom, and perform other motor skills may be recommended or devised to suit a patient's particular needs. Flotation pads for wheelchairs, walkers, sheepskin boots, and range-of-motion (ROM) exercises are examples of the many appliances and procedures employed in rehabilitation. Once the patient is ready for discharge, the patient and family members may require training in the use of devices or the performance of procedures. When the patient leaves the hospital, continued evaluation and training may be carried out by home health care personnel.

The prosthetist may fit patients who have a lower extremity weakness or paralysis with braces that ultimately enable them to walk. The patient or a family member can learn to put on the braces. Because of the tremendous effort required to walk (the patient must raise the entire weight of the body, plus the weight of the braces, with the arms), most paraplegic patients use the wheelchair most of the time and walk only short distances. A trapeze over the bed enables the paraplegic or the patient with unilateral paralysis to move in bed.

It is important for paraplegic patients to assume an upright posture at intervals during the day, whether or not they are able to walk. Quadriplegic patients who cannot stand or walk may be placed in an upright position with the aid of a tilt table or a Circ-Olectric bed. The upright position helps the patient breathe deeply and relieves pressure on the sacral region. The patient often feels dizzy and faint the first few times an upright position is assumed. The pooling of blood in the abdominal area is one cause of these symptoms, and the patient is watched carefully and protected so that a fall or other injury does not occur. The application of an abdominal binder and elastic stockings before the patient gets up may prevent dizziness and faintness. When a tilt table is used, the patient is strapped to it, and it is tilted gradually to an erect position.

Parallel bars help support the patient whose upper extremities are unaffected. Body weight can be supported by grasping the bars. With the help of parallel bars, patients can learn to balance themselves and to practice skills that are useful in walking with crutches.

Many jobs do not require full use of all four extremities; therefore, patients may benefit from vocational rehabilitation. The occupational therapist, social worker, vocational guidance counselor, and others may work with the patient to determine areas of interest and available opportunities for training and education.

Chronic Phase

Patients with a neurologic deficit may enter the chronic phase. In this part of the disorder, the patient shows little or no further evidence of improvement, and the neurologic deficit remains stationary or may become progressively worse. Physical and psychological rehabilitation is continued in the chronic phase, primarily to prevent complications such as decubitus and muscle contractures.

Patients in the chronic phase may be admitted to a hospital for treatment of complications associated with the deficit (eg, decubitus formation, pneumonia, kidney stones). Patients also may be admitted to a skilled nursing facility or hospital when family members can no longer manage their care, or when the disease has become progressively worse so that hospitalization is mandatory.

Anxiety, Fear.

The symptoms associated with a neurologic deficit, during any phase of the disorder, often produce varying degrees of fear and anxiety. These patients recognize their partial or complete dependence on others and are fearful because they can no longer help themselves. If the patient is a quadriplegic, helplessness is extreme. The mind is active, even if the body is not.

Frequent patient contact and reassurance may reduce these emotional responses. The nurse may be able to help by being a good listener. When these patients are ready to talk about how angry or discouraged they are, they need someone to listen and accept their feelings.

Anxiety and fear also may occur when certain treatments are performed (eg, suctioning). Gentleness when giving care, an explanation of the procedure or treatment, and skilled performance of a procedure may help reduce anxiety.

Pain.

After a spinal cord injury, the patient may have pain in the affected area, even though sensation in the usual sense has been lost. The pain is associated with scar formation or irritation around a nerve root. In most patients, the pain decreases gradually with recovery from the initial injury. Analgesics may be ordered for pain. Narcotic analgesics are avoided during the acute phase, as they may interfere with such neurologic assessments as the level of consciousness or the pupil size. Their use also is avoided during the recovery and rehabilitation periods because prolonged use can cause addiction.

When possible, intramuscular injections for pain or other treatments are given above the level of the paralysis. Because capillary circulation is sluggish below the injury, the medicine is absorbed poorly, and injury to the tissues from the injection is more likely to occur.

Pain or discomfort also may be experienced in the unaffected extremities when these are used to compensate for or assist the affected areas. For example, patients with left-sided paralysis after a stroke may experience muscle soreness as they attempt to overuse their right side. These discomforts may require rehabilitation training to help the patient compensate for the deficit without incurring discomfort.

Potential Fluid Volume Deficit, Impaired Swallowing.

In the acutely ill patient, an intravenous line is established for the administration of drugs as well as for fluids and calories. After recovery from the acute phase, inability to take oral food and fluids may require total parenteral nutrition or nasogastric tube feedings.

When the patient has difficulty swallowing or the danger of aspiration exists, a suction machine is kept at the bedside. Oral fluids are given with extreme care. Once the patient appears able to take oral fluids, the physician may order clear liquids given in small amounts.

Patients who are unable to reach for or hold drinking containers must be offered fluids at periodic intervals throughout the day. Fluids are best taken when offered in small amounts every hour. Patients who can take fluids on their own must be encouraged to drink and must have an adequate supply of a variety of fluids at the bedside.

Intake and output are measured, and the patient is weighed weekly. The physician is informed if a patient fails to take a sufficient amount of fluids or if the urinary output falls below 500 mL/day.

Altered Nutrition.   Adequate nutrition must be maintained. High-protein foods are important for the control of decubitus ulcers because they help to keep tissues healthy and increase the ability of tissues to heal.

Patients who are unable to chew or swallow require parenteral nutrition until oral food and fluids can be given safely. When patients can take oral food, they must be fed slowly. A suction machine is kept at the bedside until the patient can eat safely without danger of aspiration. If they can feed themselves, patients must be allowed ample time to finish the meal. A soft diet, food cut into small portions, and foods that the patient likes and tolerates may improve nutrition. Since patients are physically inactive, a better food intake can be maintained by small meals served at frequent intervals rather than large meals served three times a day.

During rehabilitation, as well as during the chronic phase, patients may eat foods that are extremely high in calories but low in nutritional value that have been brought by visitors. Because physical activity is limited, so are the daily caloric requirements. Excessive weight gain can interfere with a patient's ability to move from a wheelchair to bed or chair or to walk with a walker or cane. In addition, obesity places an added strain on the heart and may cause hypertension.

If a patient shows an appreciable weight gain or loss, it is necessary to investigate the cause. A special diet or a dietary consultation may be necessary.

Ineffective Airway Clearance.   Symptoms, such as difficulty breathing and swallowing, can create intense fear. The patient is reassured that someone is nearby and that attention is paid to any problem that develops.

Respiratory distress or arrest may occur in patients with a neurologic disorder. It may occur suddenly and without warning. When a patient is unable to move and breathing is shallow, respiratory secretions are not coughed up and a predisposition to respiratory complications, such as pneumonia, exists. The respiratory rate and rhythm are monitored frequently if the patient is acutely ill or shows early signs of respiratory distress. The temperature is monitored every 4 hours, and any elevation is reported to the physician.

A patent airway is maintained by keeping the patient on the side (unless the physician orders otherwise or the patient has a head or neck injury) and slightly elevating the head of the bed. The patient is turned every 2 hours, and the airway is suctioned as needed. The lungs are auscultated for abnormal and normal breath sounds several times per day (see Chapters 20 and 22). Extreme respiratory difficulty may require endotracheal intubation or a tracheostomy and mechanical ventilation.

Patients who are alert and cooperative are encouraged to cough and deep breathe hourly. Coughing may be contraindicated, however, in patients with increased intracranial pressure. Changing a patient's position frequently and encouraging deep breathing and coughing are important for the prevention of respiratory complications. Suctioning may still be necessary if a patient is unable to raise secretions. IPPB treatments may be indicated for some patients. Oxygen by mask or nasal catheter also may be ordered.

Potential for Infection, Hyperthermia.   Strict aseptic technique is used when performing invasive procedures, such as catheterization, insertion of intravenous lines, and suctioning.

The temperature is monitored every 4 hours during the acute phase and usually once or twice per day during the recovery or chronic phase of the disorder. The patient is assessed for signs of infection that may arise from such areas as an indwelling catheter, decubitus, and the lungs (pneumonia). Antibiotic therapy may be necessary if an infection should occur.

Antipyretic drugs and a cooling blanket may be necessary to reduce an elevated body temperature. The temperature is monitored more frequently if the response to cooling measures or antipyretic therapy is poor.

Impaired Skin Integrity.   When nerve impulses to the skin are interrupted, the skin's normal response to injury is diminished. In the normal person, constant movement during waking and even sleeping hours protects the skin from pressure sores. People with limited movement or paralysis cannot engage in movement and, therefore, are subject to skin breakdown.

Skilled nursing management is essential if rehabilitation is to be uncomplicated by decubitus formation, contractures, and other problems related to prolonged immobility. Decubitus ulcers may become infected easily and heal slowly (Fig. 39-1); contractures, which develop unless preventive measures are taken, may result in permanent deformity (Fig. 39-2). Footdrop, a frequent complication, requires use of a footboard from the beginning for its prevention. Elastic stockings may be ordered to improve circulation and enhance venous blood return to the major veins. The stockings are removed and reapplied at least twice a day.

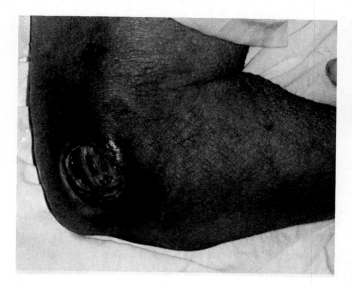

Figure 39-1. Decubitus ulcer of the elbow in a patient with a cerebrovascular accident cared for at home. This patient was admitted to the hospital for treatment of multiple decubitus ulcers. (Photograph by D. Atkinson)

The patient's position is changed every 2 hours, and pressure areas are inspected for signs of skin breakdown. A flotation mattress or pad may be used to prevent undue pressure on bony prominences. The paraplegic, quadriplegic, or patient with a head injury may be placed on a Stryker frame or other device to be turned from a prone to supine position and back every 2 hours. When patients with head or neck injuries are placed in a regular bed and turning is allowed, they must be log-rolled. (The hands are placed on the chest, a pillow is positioned between the legs, the head and neck are supported, the head pillow is removed, and the patient is turned.) The areas affected by paralysis are checked for beginning signs of pressure sores whenever the patient is turned. The bottom sheet must always be free of wrinkles. Patients who are allowed out of bed part of the day still need frequent position changes when in bed.

Patients who spend part of their day in a wheelchair or regular chair may need flotation or sheepskin pads or other devices to prevent skin breakdown.

Constipation, Diarrhea, Altered Patterns of Urinary Elimination.   Bowel and bladder incontinence pose physical and social problems. Early in life, we are taught to maintain high standards of personal cleanliness and the control of excretory functions. Adults who become unable to control these functions often feels shamed and disgraced, even though intellectually they may understand the reason for the lack of control.

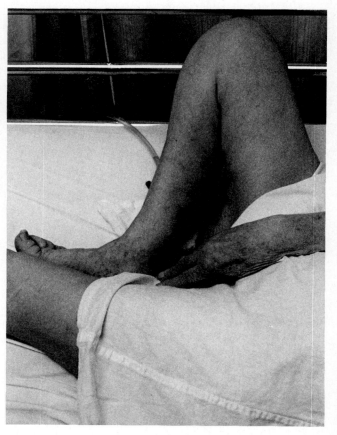

Figure 39-2. Contracture of the right leg in a patient cared for at home after a cerebrovascular accident. The patient was brought to the hospital after development of extensive decubitus ulcers. (Photograph by D. Atkinson)

Bowel and bladder rehabilitation are crucially important to help patients move toward independence. Some patients can achieve self-controlled emptying of the bowel and bladder, provided that they and those who care for them exert the persistent effort required to achieve this goal. Bowel control usually is easier to achieve than control of the bladder.

A bowel and bladder training program is often instituted as soon as the acute phase of the disorder has passed. Rehabilitation is important not only for physical reasons, such as preventing decubitus ulcers, but also for reasons of morale.

BOWEL.   A record of bowel movements is kept. Each stool is inspected for evidence of bleeding; severe, prolonged illness can result in the development of stress ulcers and upper gastrointestinal (GI) bleeding. The physician is informed if diarrhea, constipation, or tarry stools occur. Constipation may be treated with administration of a stool softener, increase in fluid intake, insertion of a suppository that promotes evacuation, addition of fiber to the diet, or establishing a regular evacuation pattern. Diarrhea may be caused by factors such as diet, nasogastric feeding formulas, medications, or fecal impaction. Adding dietary fiber or eliminating foods or drugs that may cause diarrhea also can be attempted. Often, a trial and error method is used to find the best solution. When GI bleeding is evident, frequent complete blood cell counts and hemoglobin determinations may be ordered. In some cases, blood transfusion or ulcer therapy may be necessary.

The following steps may be used in bowel rehabilitation:

1. Encourage liquids throughout the day. Foods that produce bulk, such as fresh fruits and vegetables, should be included in the diet. Foods that cause loose stools are avoided.
2. Help the patient go to the bathroom at a certain time each day. Select a time that will later fit into a personal schedule for self-care after discharge from the hospital. Allow the patient privacy and sufficient time to have a bowel movement.
3. When and if able, encourage the patient to go to the bathroom rather than use the bedpan. The physical activity involved in getting out of bed often helps the patient to have a bowel movement. Using the bathroom has psychological value, too, because it suggests self-help rather than helplessness.
4. Enemas and suppositories may be needed at first. The physician may order a suppository inserted or a small enema given each day at the same time. Later, bowel function may become regulated so that the patient can have a bowel movement without these aids. Giving an enema to a paraplegic or quadriplegic patient requires skill. The temperature of the solution must be checked because a patient cannot feel if the solution is too warm. Gentleness is required when inserting the rectal tube. Only small amounts of liquid are allowed to flow because the patient is unable to consciously retain fluid in the lower colon. The fact that these patients cannot feel means that they are more, not less, vulnerable to trauma. Leakage of the solution may occur during the enema; therefore, pads are placed under the buttocks to absorb the fluid that is not retained.

URINE. Control of the bladder is more difficult to establish, but some patients can achieve it. Many patients with a neurologic deficit that affects their control of voiding constantly are fearful that an embarrassing accident will occur while they are with others, or that others will detect odors from catheters and urinals.

Intermittent catheterization may be employed for urinary retention and incontinence. This procedure, which in some instances is preferable to the use of an indwelling urethral catheter, is usually performed about every 4 hours throughout waking hours, before going to sleep, and on waking in the morning. It may be used until the patient begins to sense the urge to void. When and if able to void, the patient is usually catheterized for residual urine immediately after each voiding. A residual urine of more than 200 mL requires recatheterization every 8 hours, regardless of how often the patient voids. A residual urine of 150 mL or less usually indicates that bladder-emptying control is being regained. One or 2 days are allowed to lapse before again checking residual urine. For some patients, intermittent catheterization may be carried on at home, providing a family member or nurse is available to perform the procedure.

Urinary retention also may be managed by creating a voiding schedule. The patient is encouraged to void every 30 minutes to 2 hours while awake. If the patient is able to use the bedpan or urinal, these are kept readily available, and the patient's call light is answered when assistance is required.

The unconscious patient, the patient with a spinal cord or head injury who must remain immobile until healing has taken place, or patients who are not responding to other methods may require insertion of a urethral catheter. If bladder training is unsuccessful and incontinence remains a problem, or the use of an indwelling catheter results in a severe, chronic urinary tract infection, other methods may be tried. Male patients may wear a condom sheath appliance for urine collection. Urinary diversion surgery, such as a permanent cystotomy for male or female patients, may be also considered.

Urinary tract irritation and infection may occur with an indwelling catheter, permanent cystotomy, and intermittent catheterization. Irritation of the penis may be seen with the condom sheath.

Patients are encouraged to drink extra fluids; people who remain relatively immobile for the rest of their lives are subject to bladder infections and calculus (stone) formation in the urinary tract.

Impaired Verbal Communication. The loss of the usual ability to use or to understand spoken and written language is called *aphasia*. Types of aphasia include the following:

Receptive
■ Auditory aphasia (difficulty in understanding the spoken word)
■ Alexia (difficulty in reading)
Expressive
■ Motor (difficulty in speaking)
■ Agraphia (difficulty in writing)

Aphasia may exist with or without intellectual impairment. In one type of aphasia, a patient may know what a pencil is, if shown one. If placed in the hand, the patient writes with it but cannot think of the word *pencil*. The patient may use another word, which may be clearly pronounced, but which has an entirely different meaning. The patient may be able to conceive the symbol but cannot express the word *pencil*. This type of aphasia is expressive aphasia.

It is not uncommon for the hemorrhage or clot responsible for the stroke patient's hemiplegia to cause aphasia by cutting off the blood supply to the speech center. Any type of vascular disorder, brain tumor, and some types of neuromuscular disorders can cause aphasia if the speech center in the brain is involved. (The speech center of a right-handed person is located in the left side of the brain, and the speech center of a left-handed person is in the right side of the brain.) The patient may find that, along with loss of the power of speech, *auditory aphasia* occurs; words spoken by people with normal speech cannot be understood and are as garbled as an unfamiliar language.

Lethargy or an effect of the neurologic disorder on the respiratory or speech muscles can result in speech problems, such as slurred speech. Although the speech center remains intact, the patient's speech is difficult to understand.

Communication problems create feelings of anxiety, anger, frustration, and hopelessness. Communication can be improved by encouraging patients to speak slowly and in short sentences or by instructing them to take several breaths between every couple of words. Questions that only require yes or no answers also may be asked.

Patients may be able to write questions or answers. Hand muscle weakness or other neurologic deficits, however, may make writing impossible. Computer programs and devices are available for people with limited ability to speak or write. With a computer speech synthesizer program, people who can use their hands type material that is then "vocalized" by the computer. Other computers synthesize speech by reading pointers that are held between the teeth and used with a special chart to identify pictures or words. Although somewhat expensive, funds for purchase may be available to certain people.

When aphasia has occurred, the speech therapist may help the patient regain some or almost all original speech. The nurse must work with the patient and therapist so that speech rehabilitation is a continuous process, rather than limited only to the time spent with the therapist.

Sensory and Perceptual Alteration, Altered Thought Processes. Patients may require a quiet environment and a slightly darkened room to reduce stimuli that may precipitate convulsive seizures or cause mental confusion. For these patients, sudden, forceful movements are avoided whenever possible, and gentleness is used when moving the patient. Dis-

comfort associated with photophobia is reduced or eliminated by closing curtains or blinds on sunny days, keeping the room dimly lit, and avoiding the use of overhead lights.

Patients may become confused, disoriented, or experience mental impairment such as memory loss, emotional lability, or blunted affect. These changes may be temporary or permanent. After assessment and evaluation of the changes in thought processes, the medical team develops a plan of action. The confused patient may require frequent observation and, in some instances, the application of restraints to prevent injury. Additional therapies include socialization with others, recreational therapy, and the use of reality orientation (see Chapter 3).

The role of the nurse is supportive. Patience and understanding are an important part of nursing management.

Potential for Injury. During rehabilitation, a patient may require assistance with walking or may be trained by the physical therapist to use a walker or cane. Assistance is given when a patient is allowed to ambulate either alone or with a device such as a walker. The patient is encouraged to stay out of bed as much as possible; walking helps strengthen unaffected muscles and prevents contractures in weakened muscles.

Prolonged immobility, as seen in patients with paraplegia, quadriplegia, or a debilitating neuromuscular disorder, may result in a loss of calcium from the bone. These patients are subject to fractures. Care is taken when moving and lifting the patient who has been immobile for a long period of time.

Disorders of the central nervous system, such as head injuries or brain tumors, can cause a temporary or permanent seizure disorder. Side rails are raised at all times, and the patient is observed at frequent intervals for seizures. Padding of the side rails may be necessary, and an oral airway and suction machine are kept at the bedside. The patient's room should be dimly lit, quiet, and free from excitement because seizures can be caused by strong stimuli.

Impaired Physical Mobility. One goal in the management of patients with a neurologic deficit is to prevent *further* disability, which can occur when the patient is immobile. The development of contractures and muscle atrophy in the affected and unaffected extremities may prevent optimal response to a rehabilitation program. To prevent contractures and muscle atrophy, active or passive ROM exercises (Figs. 39-3 and 39-4) are performed on the affected and unaffected extremities as soon as possible. A physician's order is obtained, however, before any exercises are instituted because active intracranial

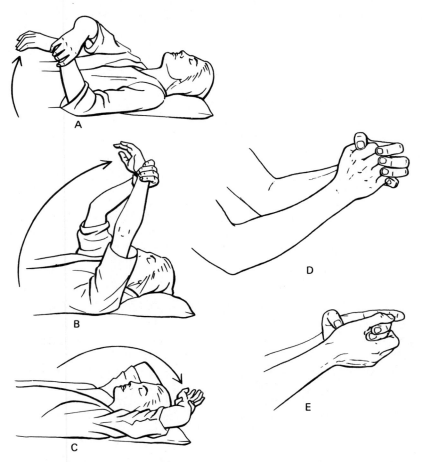

Figure 39–3.   Exercises of the affected hand and arm that hemiplegic patients should learn to do themselves. (*A–C*) The affected arm is grasped at the wrist by the unaffected hand and is raised over the head. (*D* and *E*) The unaffected hand is slipped into the spastic hand, and each finger is extended slowly in turn.

bleeding or other neurologic disorders may be a contraindication for ROM exercises. If these patients are able, they are encouraged to perform ROM exercises on their own.

The patient's position is changed every 2 hours, and the principles of good body alignment are used to promote comfort as well as prevent contractures and skin breakdown. Pillows, pads, trochanter rolls, splints, and other devices may be necessary to maintain proper body alignment.

In the patient with a spinal cord injury, flaccid paralysis is usually seen at first, and later it becomes spastic. Severe uncontrollable reflex spasms of the muscles are frequent; the muscle movement is spasm and not the return of voluntary function. Physical activity may help decrease spasm. Passive exercises and changes of position, when they are used regularly, also reduce spasms.

Before rehabilitation begins, the patient is evaluated for the type and extent of neurologic deficit. In those potentially capable of regaining some mobility in the lower extremities, ambulatory training in the physical therapy department is started as soon as the patient is able to stand with assistance. Patients with only upper extremity mobility and permanent lower extremity paralysis receive training to strengthen the muscles of the upper extremities, which ultimately help them move from bed to chair or wheelchair.

Once a rehabilitation program is begun, various types of devices may be constructed or purchased to improve physical mobility when performing tasks such as eating, brushing the teeth, or retrieving objects. A fork with an added curved handle that can be placed over the hand below the knuckles is an example of a device that has been developed for people with limited use of their hands.

A trapeze over the bed can be used to help movement for people with good upper extremity mobility. Small battery-operated carts and motorized wheelchairs can be used to enable the patient to move about in the environment. The latter can be adapted with special controls for people with limited or no

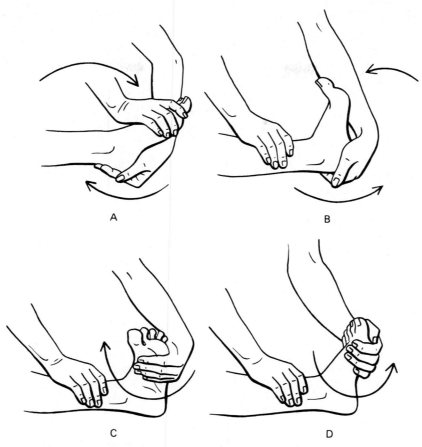

Figure 39–4. Range-of-motion exercises for the affected foot in hemiplegia. The motions should be conducted slowly and smoothly, with a momentary pause when spasticity causes resistance. As soon as the patient has movement, these exercises should be done actively rather than passively. In the beginning of the regaining of function, the patient may start the exercises, with the nurse completing the movements. As the patient gains strength, he or she should do them without assistance.

use of the upper extremities. Financial assistance may be available for the purchase of the more expensive devices.

Activity Intolerance. The patient's activity tolerance must be assessed frequently; activity must be limited to avoid extreme fatigue. When patients have gained some mobility, they are advised to rest between activities and not continue tasks to the point of fatigue. Activities are planned so that patients can have periods of rest. They are encouraged to continue activities that are enjoyable but to find ways to make them less strenuous.

Patients who are immobile also require consideration. Daily activities, such as bathing and oral care, must be spaced with rest between each one. Even though tasks are being performed for them, patients still can become tired when all daily activities are grouped together.

Self-Care Deficit. Depending on a patient's condition, partial or total assistance with activities of daily living is necessary. The skin must be kept clean and dry. Mouth care is given as needed, and the oral cavity is inspected for dryness, injury, or infection.

After the acute phase, an evaluation of abilities determines what tasks can be performed. Patients are allowed to do as much as they can, and they are given help with those tasks they find difficult. The immediate environment is arranged so that self-care is encouraged (eg, with feeding devices, by keeping personal grooming devices handy). Self-care skills are extremely important for when the patient returns home. Learning them well may mean the difference between needing someone present at all times and being able to be left alone.

Quadriplegics may have limited use of one or both of their upper extremities. Various tools, such as pointers and spoons, may be custom-fitted to the patient's needs. Specially developed computerized and robotic equipment enables patients to use a special telephone, drink fluids, eat, and execute other tasks. This equipment is expensive, however, and limited in availability. Research is in progress to help paraplegic and quadriplegic patients become more self-sufficient and less dependent on others.

Powerlessness. Patients who are dependent on others for care often feel a loss of control. Patients can be helped to regain control over their environment by allowing them, when possible, to participate in decision-making. For example, a patient could select a daily menu or decide when to be out of bed or have a bath. Although the nurse or caregiver may need to guide patients toward the best decisions or establish guidelines, providing an opportunity for active participation gives them a sense of control over their environments.

Dysfunctional Grieving and Hopelessness. The psychological trauma is intense as patients begin to recover and gradually or suddenly become aware of the physical changes that have happened, that they are no longer whole, healthy people. At first, the alert patient may react with depression and withdrawal, starring into space and showing no interest in people and events around him. During this period, the nurse should emphasize quiet presence, empathy, and attention to physical needs. Recovery from the psychological as well as the physical hurt associated with the changes to the body takes time.

Patients who often cannot talk to their family because of the emotional response to their illness may find it easier to talk to a nurse. Although grieving and feelings of hopelessness are normal, patients may be helped by understanding, by allowing them to voice their concerns, and by being aware of and accepting their feelings, emotions, and behavior. The nurse must offer emotional support, take time to listen, and encourage them each step of the way through rehabilitation.

Patients with a neurologic deficit may feel that their situation is hopeless, the future uncertain, and problems insurmountable. These feelings may diminish as patients progress through a rehabilitation program; however, they may persist and remain permanent. A patient's response to the deficit might be determined by the emotional stability and general outlook on life before the neurologic deficit occurred.

Ineffective Individual Coping, Impaired Adjustment. During the acute phase, the family needs frequent assurance that optimal care is being given and that the patient is being monitored frequently.

Once the diagnosis and prognosis have been understood by patients, many express varied reactions to their present and future. They may find it difficult to accept the temporary or permanent changes in their bodies. No easy solution to this problem is available. Some patients eventually accept their disability; others do not. The nurse must constantly encourage and praise each patient during rehabilitation. Showing personal interest and pleasure in each accomplishment, no matter how small, may help patients accept what they cannot or never will be able to do.

Patients must be given time to talk about their problems, fears, and concerns. Once needs are identified, the nurse can encourage the patient to set goals, which may help maintain independence as long as possible. The nurse should then work with the patient and family to develop solutions and possible alternatives. Developing possible solutions establishes a bond between the patient, the family, and the medical team. It helps the family meet each problem as it arises, understand the limitations, establish goals, and work toward a solution. Referral to a social service worker or a publicly funded agency may be necessary. Patients often face a multitude of problems that involve, for example, financial and family support, purchase of equipment, such as wheelchairs, and home nursing care.

With rehabilitation comes the patient's awareness of progress or lack of progress. At times, improvement is slow and barely noticeable. A patient may have difficulty coping: discouragement, depression, withdrawal, and anger are not unusual. The patient is encouraged to persevere and is helped to cope when progress can no longer be made. Various support groups are often available for those with neurologic deficits. A visit from a member of one of these organizations may offer encouragement and support and help the patient cope with the disability. After discharge from the hospital, contact with a support group can be maintained for emotional, physical, and social support.

Impaired Home Maintenance Management. Patients who are responsible for the physical or financial support of a household and its members may encounter many problems. These problems need to be recognized, however, before solutions can be found. The nurse must listen and be alert to subtle hints given by the patient or family. Questions, always posed with tact, may be asked to identify problems and needs. Once identified, appropriate steps can be taken to help the patient attain and maintain a near-normal home life. Certain associations, such as the Muscular Dystrophy Association, may be able to offer suggestions or assistance. Family members or hospital personnel may contact these organizations for patient services, clinical care, and financial assistance in the purchase of supplies, such as braces, wheelchairs, and ramps.

Before discharge, the nurse or social worker must evaluate the patient's ability to administer self-care, assume the role of a member of the family, and, when needed, have an available support system. While some patients recover sufficiently to assume responsibility for their own care, at least partly, others do not. An older patient may have a spouse who is unable to administer the necessary home care; the burden of care, then, falls on the children, who may or may not be available or willing to share this responsibility.

An assessment of the available facilities, the family support system, physical aids required (eg, a wheelchair or walker), and the amount of assistance required with activities of daily living help plan for the changes or modifications necessary to care for the patient at home. The family is encouraged to help plan for the patient's return home, ask questions about care, and seek assistance from those agencies that can provide emotional, physical, and financial support.

Patients with spinal cord injury face many problems once they are eligible for discharge to their home. The physical environment may require changes to accommodate a wheelchair or special bed. Wide doorways, ramps instead of stairs, special fixtures in the bathroom for bathing and bowel and bladder elimination are examples of changes that are usually necessary.

In addition to physical and emotional needs, the injured patient also may have been the sole, or at least the major, wage earner. Financial resources may have been strained during hospitalization and may continue to be so after discharge. Patients may be able to enter a training program that allows them to find employment. Others learn a skill that enables them to be employed at home. Some patients, however, because of age or extreme physical disability, may never be able to earn money.

Home care, in whole or in part, may need to be administered by nursing personnel. Public and private agencies can provide the personnel, but the family may be unable to pay for the service. Once discharge is planned, the nurse and social worker must discuss these problems with the family and offer possible solutions. Families may find it necessary to seek public assistance to meet their financial obligations.

Altered Family Processes.   The family faces many disruptions because of the permanent disability of a family member. Lifestyles are altered, financial re-

sources are strained, conflicts arise, and people must accept new responsibilities. The family requires time and guidance to deal with and accept these changes. They need a chance to talk and openly express their anger, fears, guilt, and helplessness.

Although no single perfect solution to any problem exists, the following may help the family adjust to present and future changes:

- Explain the nature of the dysfunction
- Include the family in the patient's rehabilitation
- Give encouragement and praise when a family member is able to help with a part of home care or shows interest in becoming involved in the patient's care
- Explain the purpose of each segment of rehabilitation (eg, ROM exercises, positioning)
- Teach each procedure or task slowly, giving the family time to practice under supervision
- Prepare a list of public or private agencies that may assist with home care, transportation, financial support, and so on

Diversional Activity Deficit.   These patients may exist in a monotonous environment. The nurse must make every attempt to alter the pattern of daily activities and provide physical and mental stimulation. Television, radio, interaction with other patients, and encouraging family members to visit as much as possible may help relieve boredom. Patients who are physically unable to participate in diversional activities may be helped by volunteers who can read or talk to them. For patients with few visitors, volunteers perform an invaluable service, and they should be used as much as possible.

Impaired Social Interaction, Social Isolation.   As soon as patients are able to respond to those around them, they are encouraged to socialize. At first, socialization may be limited to medical personnel and family. The family is encouraged to talk to the patient, discuss current events, and motivate the patient to respond to questions. The support given by family and friends is most important.

Patients who are allowed out of bed in a wheelchair are encouraged to be up and about, get dressed, and become more mobile. These activities are fatiguing, especially at first, and patients must have planned rest periods along with periods of activity.

Patients with speech difficulties often have trouble socializing with others and tend to become withdrawn and depressed. Visitors are instructed to talk to the patient and ask questions that require a yes or no response. The patient may be able to write questions or information for the family. Family members are encouraged to use patience when trying to understand the patient.

Occupational therapy and diversional and recreational activities are part of the rehabilitation program and require a team effort. In the beginning, occupational therapy may be designed to help strengthen muscles that are under voluntary control. Later, certain tasks may be learned or relearned to help the patient interact with others. Participation in these therapies increases socialization time and helps the patient interact with others.

Altered Sexuality Patterns, Sexual Dysfunction. Patients experience varying degrees of difficulty with sexual identity and ability to function as a sexual partner. Whereas some patients openly discuss and ask questions about their problems, others do not. The nurse must be alert to subtle references to a sexual dysfunction or problem and discuss the problem with the physician.

Paraplegic men may be impotent. Women may be able to have children. Questions about sexual function must be answered individually by each patient's physician; the degree of return to normal sexual function is determined by the particular nature and extent of the neurologic deficit. Both patients and their sexual partners should have an opportunity to discuss this subject with the physician. A sexual therapist may be used to help the patient and partner adjust to changes in their sexual life. Penile implants may be inserted to provide the male with an erection during sexual activities.

Knowledge Deficit. Home is the normal environment—and usually the best one—provided that these patients have a home and a family who wants them. Going home is a major step in rehabilitation. It presents the challenge of helping the disabled patient adjust to the home and community.

The patient and family must be allowed time to ask questions about tests, treatments, prognosis, complications, and home care. Many times, these questions must be referred to the physician. During hospitalization, treatment modalities and the expected results are explained to the patient and family.

Home care management requires a teaching plan that depends on the therapies prescribed by the physician as well as the extent of the neurologic deficit. The patient and family usually have many questions during the acute as well as the recovery phase. The type of questions asked may reveal what information and instructions must be given before discharge from the hospital. Teaching must begin long before discharge so that the patient and family have sufficient time to learn and understand home care management.

The home situation may need evaluation. The physical environment (eg, the stairs, the bathroom) as well as the attitude of the family toward the return of the patient are part of a home evaluation.

Often, the family may not have considered certain factors, and the nurse must initiate discussion of the problem. For example, the residence of a patient who uses a wheelchair must be able to accommodate this device, and special fixtures may be required in the bathroom for showering and use of the toilet. The patient with a spinal cord injury or the patient with advanced neuromuscular disease with maximum disability requires extensive home care management, such as special beds, mechanical ventilation, a suction machine, tube feedings, and home nursing care.

The teaching plan must be individualized and depends on the amount and extent of care necessary. The following areas may be included in a teaching plan.

SKIN CARE.   Because the patient cannot feel the discomfort caused by a beginning decubitus ulcer, daily inspection of the skin of paralyzed areas is essential. The patient and family are taught skin care and how and when to change positions so that pressure on bony prominences is relieved at periodic intervals. Patients may be able to manage part of their skin care and may only require that certain areas such as the sacrum and buttocks be cared for by others. Other patients require complete skin care by a family member or care giver.

MAINTAINING BODY ALIGNMENT.   Good body alignment is essential. The joints are put through a full range of motion: flexion, extension, abduction, adduction, internal rotation, external rotation, pronation, and supination. Range-of-motion exercises must be performed several times per day or as ordered by the physician or physical therapist. Various devices, such as rolled blankets or pillows, can be used to support or align areas of the body, such as the back, hips, and legs. A footboard or other type of device is used to prevent footdrop when the patient is in bed. When in a chair, the feet must be kept at right angles to the legs.

NUTRITION AND FLUIDS.   Meal planning is an important aspect of home care. A high fluid intake is essential to prevent urinary tract complications. A well-balanced diet is essential. The diet must also be planned so that the patient does not gain or lose a great deal of weight. Small meals and interval feedings may be easier than three large meals.

The patient who must be fed needs time to chew the food and take fluids. Patients sometimes feel that they are taking time away from the family when they need to be fed, so they begin to eat and drink less. If this occurs, the patient must be encouraged to take fluids and nourishment at frequent intervals.

BOWEL AND BLADDER. Careful aseptic technique is used when irrigating, changing, or inserting catheters. If an external sheath is worn by the male patient, the penis is cleansed daily to remove urine and dried secretions. The urine is inspected for cloudiness (which may or may not indicate a urinary tract infection), blood, and offensive odor. Chills and fever also may indicate a urinary tract infection and must be brought to the attention of the physician.

Skin care of the genitalia and around the perineal area is important. Special care must be given to the anal area after defecation. The genitalia are washed thoroughly and dried.

ACTIVITY. The physician determines the type, amount, and limitations of activity that are allowed. Social contacts, hobbies, and changes in the daily routine are encouraged because they relieve boredom. The importance of avoiding fatigue and exposure to infection is emphasized.

Patients whose activities are limited are advised to take deep breaths every 1 or 2 hours while awake and to cough to raise secretions.

GENERAL MANAGEMENT TECHNIQUES. The family may need to be taught such tasks as monitoring vital signs, catheterization and catheter irrigation, moving and lifting, and suctioning, when they assume responsibility for the patient.

THERAPIES. Therapy such as physical and speech therapy may be carried on at home or on an out-patient basis. The family is instructed to work with the therapists and to follow their advice about performance or practice of the therapies.

COMMUNITY SERVICES. The patient and family are made aware of services available for home care, such as provision of financial assistance, home nursing care, and transportation services.

EQUIPMENT. The equipment necessary for care may be purchased, rented, or borrowed. Financial assistance may be required and obtained from a public or private agency or organization. Some community organizations have loan closets that allow people who need certain types of equipment to borrow these materials. Modified cars or vans that enable paraplegics to drive are available.

Evaluation

The evaluations vary, depending on the original goals and nursing diagnoses. All of the following may not apply to each patient.

- Anxiety and fear are reduced
- Pain or discomfort is controlled or eliminated
- Attains and maintains a normal fluid and food intake; body weight stable; fluid and nutritional needs are met
- Swallows without difficulty; no evidence of aspiration of food or fluid
- Respiratory rate, rhythm, depth is normal; no evidence

of cyanosis, respiratory distress, pulmonary congestion or infection
- Vital signs within normal range
- Coughs and deep breathes at regular intervals; maintains clear airway
- Attains and maintains a normal body temperature
- No evidence of infection
- Skin and mucous membranes remain intact with no evidence of breakdown, decubitus formation, contractures
- Achieves bladder and bowel control
- Attains and maintains a normal defecation pattern
- Attains a normal urinary elimination pattern
- Able to communicate effectively and makes needs known to others
- Appears oriented to time and place; carries on a meaningful conversation
- No apparent injury to self
- Able to tolerate increased physical activity
- Shows improvement in physical mobility; maintains maximum physical mobility within limitations of disease process
- Begins to use trapeze, wheelchair, and other methods of increasing mobility
- Able to stand and walk with assistance
- Shows increased sensory and motor improvement in the affected side
- Self-care needs are met; participates in some (or all) self-care activities
- Participates in decision-making
- Patient and family begin to show acceptance of disability
- Patient and family members demonstrate a more positive attitude and ability to cope with the diagnosis, treatment modalities, prognosis, complications of disorder
- Demonstrates adjustment to disease, limitations, and prognosis
- Demonstrates effective coping mechanisms
- Demonstrates ability to accept illness, prognosis, physical limitations
- Takes part in and expresses a desire for diversional activities
- Interacts socially with others
- Begins to talk about sexual activity, role with sexual partner
- Discusses problems related to sexuality
- Patient and family demonstrate understanding of information presented during teaching sessions
- Patient and family demonstrate understanding of diagnostic tests, treatment modalities, disease process, limitations, home care management, postdischarge treatment modalities
- Patient and family actively participate in planning for home maintenance management and the shifting of certain responsibilities to others
- Patient and family make an attempt to assist in decisions about home maintenance
- Discusses potential problems that may arise at home
- Financial, social, emotional, home management problems identified and discussed

General Nutritional Considerations

☐ When encouraging an adequate fluid intake, water as well as other fluids are offered. These include carbonated beverages, ice cream, flavored gelatin, fruit juices, punch, and milk shakes.

☐ Foods that provide bulk, including fruits, vegetables, bran, and other cereals, are usually included in the diet of the patient on a bowel rehabilitation program.

☐ If the patient appears to have a problem with excessive gas when drinking carbonated beverages, the beverage can be allowed to stand open for several hours and then served cold. This process eliminates some of the carbonation.

☐ A high-protein diet is essential to the prevention of skin breakdown.

☐ The hospital dietitian may be needed to help the patient select foods high in protein. The dietitian can also plan meals that are appetizing and include the patient's own food preferences.

General Pharmacologic Considerations

☐ Bowel rehabilitation of the paraplegic or quadriplegic patient may include the use of suppositories or enemas. Examples of suppositories are glycerin suppositories, which soften the stool in the lower rectum, and bisacodyl (Dulcolax), which stimulates peristalsis in the terminal section of the large colon. Enemas may be plain water, glycerin, and Fleet Brand enema.

☐ Patients are placed on their sides, and a suppository is gently inserted past the rectal sphincter. If the patient expels the suppository soon after insertion, it may be necessary to tape the patient's buttocks together to keep the suppository in place. The tape is then removed at the time the suppository is expected to work.

☐ Enemas are given slowly because paraplegic and quadriplegic patients are unable to *voluntarily* retain the enema solution. If a small amount (about 1 to 2 oz) of the fluid is given, followed by a waiting period (which varies from patient to patient), the patient may be able to retain a sufficient amount of the enema solution.

☐ Patients with impaired swallowing may have difficulty taking pills or capsules. Whenever possible, medications are given in liquid form.

☐ If a patient must take solid medications at home, the family is advised to check with their physician or pharmacist before crushing or breaking tablets or opening capsules; some medications must not be crushed or opened.

General Gerontologic Considerations

☐ The elderly patient has a tendency to drink less water and, therefore, may incur a chronic fluid volume deficit.

☐ Financial circumstances or the availability of someone to prepare nutritious meals may influence the nutritional status.

☐ The elderly patient with a neurologic deficit may lack an adequate support system once they are discharged from the hospital.

Suggested Readings

☐ Brannon M. A hands-on rehab technique that really works. RN 1989;52:65. *(Additional coverage of subject matter)*

☐ Buchanan LE, Nawoczenski D. Spinal cord injury: concepts and management approaches. Baltimore: Williams & Wilkins, 1987. *(In-depth coverage of subject matter)*

☐ Ferguson JM. Helping the MS patient live a better life. RN 1987;50:22. *(Additional coverage of subject matter)*

☐ Hickey J. The clinical practice of neurological and neurosurgical nursing. 2nd ed. Philadelphia: JB Lippincott, 1986. *(In-depth coverage of subject matter)*

☐ Matthews P, Carlson C. Spinal cord injury: a guide to rehabilitation nursing. Rockville, MD: Aspen Publishers, 1987. *(Additional and in-depth coverage of subject matter)*

☐ Moorhouse MF. Critical care plans. Philadelphia: FA Davis, 1987. *(Additional and in-depth coverage of subject matter)*

☐ Passarella P, Gee Z. Starting right after stroke. Am J Nurs 1987;87:802. *(Additional coverage of subject matter)*

■ Introduction to the Special Senses
■ Disorders of the Eye and Ear

The Special Senses

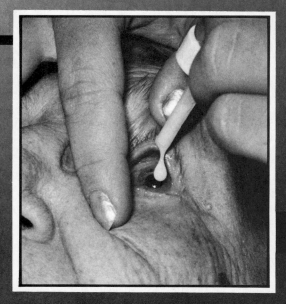

Unit 9

Chapter 40

Introduction to the Special Senses

On completion of this chapter the reader will:

- Be familiar with the basic anatomy and physiology of the eye and ear

- Discuss the common tests used for diagnosing eye and ear disorders

- Use the nursing process to prepare a patient for diagnostic studies related to the eye and ear

THE EYE
Anatomy and Physiology

The eye is the sense organ for sight. The eyeball is located in a protective bony cavity of the skull. Fat and muscle protect the posterior, superior, inferior, and lateral parts of the eyeball. The eyelid and tears protect the anterior surface of the eye. The basic structures of the eye are shown in Figure 40-1.

The Retina, Choroid, and Sclera.   The three layers of the eye are the retina or innermost layer, the choroid or middle layer, and the sclera or outer layer. The *sclera*, the white part of the eye, is composed of connective tissue. The *choroid* contains blood vessels, connective tissue, and a dark pigment which prevents light from scattering off the inner layer of the eye. The *retina,* the innermost layer of the eye, lies inside the choroid. The retina is composed of a pigmented outer layer and an inner sensory layer. The two layers are held closely together. The sensory layer of the retina receives visual stimuli that are then transmitted to the brain by the optic nerve. The pigmented layer is in close contact with the choroid, through which both layers of the retina receive their blood supply.

The retina contains nerve cells called rods and cones. The rods function in dim light. The cones function in bright light and are sensitive to color. Three types of cones largely respond to either red, blue, or green. When an image is perceived, the color depends on which cone or combination of cones is stimulated. People who lack cones are color-blind.

Optic Nerve.   The optic nerve receives and transmits images to the occipital lobe of the brain.

Cornea.   The cornea is a continuation of the sclera. Since it is transparent, light passes through the cornea to the retina.

Lens.   The lens, which is located in the anterior chamber of the eye, is a small transparent structure that lies behind the iris and is enclosed in an elastic membrane called the *capsule.* The lens is one of the refractive media through which light passes. Normally, the lens is not visible; we see only the dark spot that is the opening (pupil) through which light passes. To allow the eye to focus on near and far objects (accommodation), the shape of the lens is changed by the ciliary muscles.

Iris and Pupil.   The iris is the colored part of the eye, and the pupil is the central opening in the iris. The circular and radial muscles control the size of the pupil, which changes according to the amount of light that enters the eye. Drugs may also affect the size of the pupil.

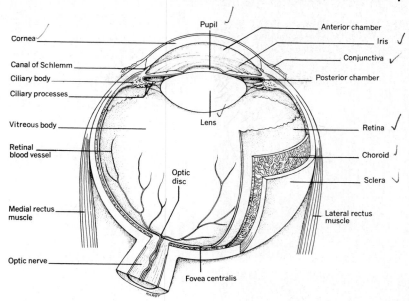

Figure 40–1. Transverse section of the eyeball. The cornea, aqueous humor, lens, and vitreous body are the refractive media.

Aqueous and Vitreous Humor. The aqueous humor, which is a watery substance, fills the anterior chamber of the eye. The vitreous humor, which is more firm and gelatinous, fills the posterior chamber of the eye. Aqueous humor maintains ocular pressure. Vitreous humor maintains shape to the eye. Both substances are transparent, thus allowing light to pass through the eye to the retina.

Canals of Schlemm. These small canals allow for the movement of aqueous humor to the anterior ciliary veins. Closure of these canals results in increased intraocular pressure (pressure within the eye).

Eyelids. The eyelids are lined with a sensitive mucous membrane called the *conjunctiva*. The inner and outer canthus are the corners or edges of the eyelids.

Tears. Tears, which keep the conjunctiva moist, are produced by lacrimal (tear) glands located beneath the bony orbital ridge. Tears flow across the eye and drain into the nasolacrimal duct, a tiny opening in the inner canthus of the lid margin, and into the nose.

Diagnostic Tests

Tonometry. A tonometer is used to test pressure within the eyeball. Increased intraocular pressure is a sign of glaucoma. Two methods of tonometry are available (Fig. 40-2), but applanation tonometry is the most commonly used because of its greater accuracy and ease of use. Before use of either apparatus, a local anesthetic ophthalmic solution, such as tetracaine or benoxinate with fluorescein (Fluress), is instilled in the eye. Anesthesia begins almost immediately and lasts a few minutes. The patient does not feel the application of the tonometer while the eye is anesthetized.

Although not as accurate, a machine that blows a puff of air against the cornea can also measure intraocular pressure. No local anesthetic is required.

Slit Lamp Examination. The applanation tonometer is also equipped for slit lamp examination. A narrow beam of light is directed on the cornea, allowing examination of the anterior segments of the eye. This examination may identify disorders such as corneal abrasions, iritis, conjunctivitis, and lens opacities (cataracts).

Visual Fields. This examination is performed by the ophthalmologist to determine peripheral vision or detect blind spots. Certain disorders, such as a stroke or retinal detachment, may produce changes in the visual field.

Vision Testing. A Snellen eye chart may be used as a screening test to determine visual acuity. Visual acuity may also be determined with a computerized refractor that records the strength and type of lens necessary to correct the refraction error. The printed readout is used by the examiner to prescribe corrective lenses.

Visual acuity is expressed as a fraction and is based on a standard of normal vision. For example, to the person with 20/200 vision, letters readable to the

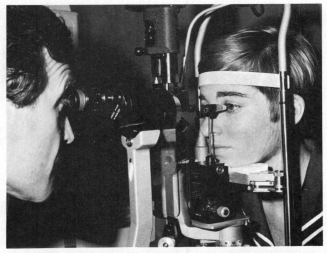

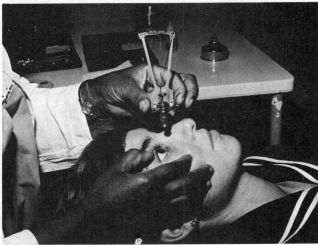

Figure 40–2. (*Top*) Intraocular pressure measured with the Goldmann applanation tonometer. (*Bottom*) Intraocular pressure measured with the Schiotz tonometer. (Courtesy of Raymond Harrison, MD)

normally sighted at 200 feet are readable at distances no greater than 20 feet. If you have 20/70 vision, to read the letters you must be within 20 feet of letters large enough for one with normal vision (20/20) to read at 70 feet. The Snellen test for visual acuity is based on these values.

Echography. Two types of echography are used: the A-scan and the B-scan. The A-scan is one dimensional and the B-scan is two dimensional. After instillation of anesthetic ophthalmic drops, an ultrasound probe is placed on the cornea and a recording is made on an oscilloscope. Echography is used to detect eye lesions (both the A- and B-scan) as well as to measure for an intraocular lens implant (A-scan).

Fluorescein Angiography. This test is used to determine retinal circulation and to detect disorders such as diabetic retinopathy and eye tumors. Sodium fluorescein is injected into a peripheral vein, and a special camera photographs the appearance of the dye in the retinal arteries, capillaries, and veins.

Fluorescein Eye Drops. Fluorescein is a dye that may be instilled in the eye to detect foreign bodies and corneal abrasions.

THE EAR

Anatomy and Physiology

The ear is the sense organ for hearing and equilibrium. The ear is divided into three areas: the outer, middle, and inner ear. The structures of the ear are shown in Fig. 40-3.

Outer Ear. The outer (or external) ear consists of the pinna (outer projection of the ear, ear lobe) and the external acoustic meatus (or canal). The tympanic membrane (eardrum) is at the end of the external acoustic canal and forms the boundary between the outer and middle ear. The external acoustic meatus extends from its own orifice to the tympanic membrane, is about an inch long, and contains the ceruminous (wax) glands.

Middle Ear. The middle ear is a small, air-filled cavity in the temporal bone. Stretched across the middle ear cavity from the tympanic membrane to the oval window lies a chain of small bones called *ossicles*—the *malleus*, the *incus*, and the *stapes*—joined together by small ligaments and attached to the tympanic membrane by the handle of the malleus. The footplate of the stapes fits into the oval window, held in position by a ligament that allows free motion for the transmission of sound. The medial wall of the middle ear has two openings that communicate with the inner ear, the oval window (fenestra ovalis) and the round window (fenestra rotunda). Sound waves pass into the external ear and its canal and strike the tympanic membrane, causing it to vibrate. The vibrations are transmitted by way of the mechanical linkage of malleus, incus, and stapes to the oval window. The motion of the footplate of the stapes in the oval window agitates the perilymph and endolymph, thus stimulating the sensitive sound receptors of the organ of Corti, in the inner ear.

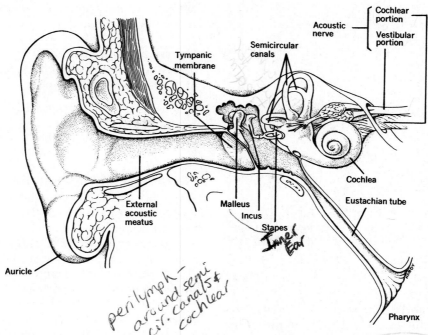

Figure 40–3.   Diagram of the ear, showing the external, middle, and internal subdivisions.

The eustachian tube extends from the floor of the middle ear to the pharynx and is lined with mucous membrane.

Inner Ear. The inner ear, or labyrinth, is a complicated structure that lies deep in the temporal bone. It consists of a series of cavities and canals. The bony canals and spaces constitute the bony labyrinth. These canals and spaces are lined with periosteum and enclose the much smaller membranous labyrinth. The space between the two is filled with perilymph. The membranous labyrinth is filled with endolymph. The movement of this fluid stimulates the nerve endings of both branches (vestibular and cochlear) of the vestibulocochlear (eighth cranial, auditory) nerve. The inner ear has two sections: an anterior portion, the cochlea; and a posterior portion, the semicircular canals. Nerve fibers of the vestibular portion of the vestibulocochlear nerve are located at the base of the semicircular canals and transmit information about the position of the head. The function of the semicircular canals is to maintain equilibrium or balance.

The perception of sound results in a flow of vibrations that start with a movement of the tympanic membrane. This is followed by the vibration of the three bones of the middle ear. The foot of the stapes, which rests on a window in the cochlea, transmits the vibration to the fluid contained in the cochlea. Receptors connected to fibers of the cochlear portion of the vestibulocochlear nerve then transmit the impulses to the brain.

Diagnostic Tests

Audiogram. An audiogram detects the degree and type of hearing loss and is usually performed by an audiologist.

Tuning Fork Tests. A tuning fork test is a screening test to detect hearing loss (Fig. 40-4).

Tympanometry. This test evaluates the functioning of the tympanic membrane and the middle ear.

NURSING PROCESS —THE PATIENT UNDERGOING TESTS FOR AN EYE OR EAR DISORDER

Assessment
The type and scope of assessment performed on a patient with an eye or ear disorder depends on the symptoms.

Patient History
A list of symptoms, the length of time they have been present, and a complete medical, drug, and allergy history are obtained from the patient or a family member. It is also important to determine if the patient has used any nonprescription eye or ear drops. Medical disorders may affect the eye or ear; there-

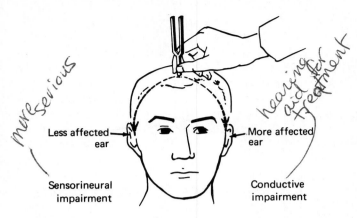

nurse serious

hearing aid for treatment

Less affected ear

More affected ear

Sensorineural impairment

Conductive impairment

Figure 40–4. When a vibrating tuning fork is placed against the forehead of a patient with conductive hearing loss, the tone sounds louder in the more affected ear; to the patient with sensorineural hearing loss, the tone sounds louder in the less affected ear.

fore, a thorough medical history is essential. Traumatic injuries to the eye are often painful, and a patient may be unable to give a detailed history.

Physical Examination

Physical examination of the eye includes inspection of the sclera, iris, pupil, eyelids, and skin around the eye. Any evidence of infection, trauma, drainage, swelling, or discoloration is noted. The experienced examiner may use an ophthalmoscope to examine the interior of the eye.

Eye muscle movement is checked by having the patient look up, down, left, and right, without moving the head. The pupils are checked for size, equality, and reaction to light. The patient is asked if contact lenses are being worn or have been worn in the past. A routine visual acuity screening test may be performed.

Physical examination of the ear includes examination of the external ear for signs of infection, swelling, redness, drainage, and evidence of trauma. Excessive ear wax (cerumen), foreign bodies, and the appearance of the tympanic membrane can be visualized with an otoscope. The areas in front of and behind the ear lobe are palpated for tenderness and

swelling. When applicable, a basic hearing test may also be performed.

Nursing Diagnosis

Depending on the patient's symptoms, one or more of the following may apply:

- Anxiety related to symptoms, diagnostic tests, possible diagnosis
- Pain related to injury, infection
- Knowledge deficit of tests to be performed

Planning and Implementation

The major goals of the patient include a relief of pain, a reduction of anxiety, and an understanding of the tests to be performed.

The major goals of nursing management are to relieve pain or discomfort and to explain the type of test being performed and what procedure will be followed before and during the test.

Anxiety, Knowledge Deficit. The test to be performed is thoroughly explained to the patient; most of these tests require full patient cooperation.

Patients are assured that the anesthetic drops instilled in the eyes are effective and that little or no discomfort will be felt. They are told to follow the directions of the physician when the eyes are being examined. Most tests for ear pathology are not painful, but some may result in momentary dizziness or mild discomfort. If a patient has a hearing loss, the instructions are given slowly, and the patient is asked to repeat what has been said. If patients understand the procedure, anxiety usually decreases.

Pain. Certain ear disorders, such as infection and trauma, produce mild to severe pain. If trauma to the eye or ear has occurred, the patient usually has severe pain. The physician is contacted immediately.

Evaluation

- Anxiety is reduced
- Pain is reduced or eliminated
- Demonstrates understanding of the testing procedure and cooperation required during the procedure

Suggested Readings

☐ Memmler RL, Wood DL. Structure and function of the human body. 4th ed. Philadelphia: JB Lippincott, 1987. *(Additional coverage of subject matter)*

☐ Memmler RL, Wood DL. The human body in health and disease. 6th ed. Philadelphia: JB Lippincott, 1987. *(Additional coverage of subject matter)*

☐ Porth, CM. Pathophysiology: concepts of altered health states. 3rd ed. Philadelphia: JB Lippincott, 1990. *(In-depth, high-level coverage of subject matter)*

Chapter 41

Disorders of the Eye and Ear

On completion of this chapter the reader will:

- Use the nursing process in the management of the visually impaired patient

- List the types of trauma to the eye

- Use the nursing process in the management of the patient with an eye injury

- Discuss the symptoms, diagnosis, and treatment of infectious and inflammatory disorders of the eye

- Use the nursing process in the management of the patient with an infectious or inflammatory disorder of the eye

- Discuss the symptoms, diagnosis and treatment of macular degeneration and glaucoma

- Use the nursing process in the management of the patient with glaucoma

- Discuss the symptoms, diagnosis, and treatment of cataracts

- Use the nursing process in the management of the patient with a cataract

- Discuss the problems associated with hearing impairment and methods of helping the hearing impaired

- Use the nursing process in the management of the patient with a hearing impairment

- List common disorders of the external, middle, and inner ear and describe the symptoms, diagnosis, and treatment of each

- Use the nursing process in the management of the patient with a disorder of the external ear

- Use the nursing process in the management of the patient with a disorder of the middle or inner ear

- Use the nursing process in the management of the patient who is having ear surgery

The following terms are used to describe the professions associated with eye care.

An *optician,* like a pharmacist, fills prescriptions written by an optometrist or ophthalmologist. In this instance, the prescription is for glasses. The optician has the prescribed lenses made and sees that the glasses are properly fitted.

An *optometrist* has special training in testing vision for refractive errors and in prescribing and fitting glasses to correct such errors. Because optometrists are not physicians, they are not permitted to prescribe medications for the eye or to diagnose or treat eye diseases.

An *ophthalmologist* is a physician who has had special training in the diagnosis and treatment of eye diseases, including refraction and the prescription of glasses.

REFRACTIVE ERRORS

The cornea, the aqueous humor, the lens, and the vitreous body constitute the *refractive media* of the eye. Ocular refraction is the bending of light rays so that they focus on the retina. Normally, all of the refractive media are transparent.

Refractive errors are the most common type of eye disorder that results when the refractive media do not focus light rays on the retina (Fig. 41-1). Refractive errors may be inherited.

Myopia (nearsightedness) usually results from elongation of the eyeball. Because of the excessive length of the eyeball, light rays focus at a point in the vitreous humor before they reach the retina.

Hyperopia (farsightedness) results when the eyeball is shorter than normal, causing the light rays to focus at a theoretical point behind the retina.

Astigmatism results from unequal curvatures in the shape of the cornea or, sometimes, of the lens. Vision is distorted. For example, a straight object may appear to be slanted. Often a person has both astigmatism and myopia or hyperopia. Astigmatism is corrected by cylindrical lenses.

Presbyopia is caused by the gradual loss of the elasticity of the lens, which leads to decreased ability to accommodate to near vision. The shape of the lens of the eye is changed by the action of the ciliary muscle, thus providing the eye with a focusing mechanism. This process is known as *accommodation*. The lens is elastic and pliable in youth and early adult life. In middle life and old age, it becomes more rigid. The loss of accommodation begins in youth and progresses gradually. By age 40 to 50, the loss is sufficiently marked and may interfere with reading and other close work.

Myopia, hyperopia, and astigmatism can cause diminished and blurred vision. People with myopia must bring things close to their eyes to see them,

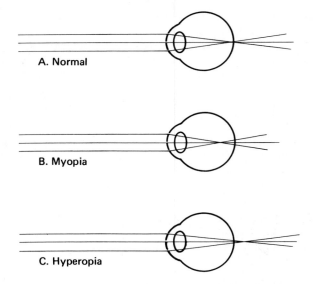

Figure 41–1. Ocular focusing of parallel light rays.

whereas people with hyperopia usually can see objects better at a distance.

Corrective Lenses

The above conditions may be corrected by the prescription of glasses that contain corrective lenses that bend light rays to compensate for a patient's refractive error.

Bifocals are prescribed for presbyopia. The lower part of the glass is for near vision, the upper part for distance vision. These glasses permit the wearer to see both near and distant objects clearly. A further refinement uses trifocals (three kinds of lens in one glass), which some patients find even more effective for viewing objects at various distances. Other people who have never needed glasses previously use reading glasses that enable them to see close objects. Bifocals with a plain upper portion are sometimes used by people who do not require distance correction, so that glasses do not have to be removed and replaced constantly. Others prefer full reading glasses, especially people who work on a computer or who do extensive reading that requires movement of the eyes up and down the page.

Contact Lenses

Contact lenses are tiny, almost invisible plastic lenses that fit directly on the cornea and are separated only by the tear film from the eye itself. They are worn by people who object to the appearance of conventional glasses in frames and by those with special needs that are better met by contact lenses.

Several different types of contact lenses are available. The hard contact lens is made of rigid plastic (polymethyl methacrylate, or PMMA). The wearing time must be increased gradually, to allow the wearer to become accustomed to the lens. The hard contact lens corrects astigmatism and is easy to care for but may be somewhat less comfortable than the soft contact lens. The soft contact lens is made of a hydrophilic plastic, which is more flexible. This type of lens usually requires a shorter adjustment period. Soft contact lenses are more difficult to care for and have a shorter life than the hard contact lens. Gas-permeable (extended wear) lenses, made of a variety of materials that allow oxygen and carbon dioxide to pass freely through the lens, may be worn for up to 2 weeks before removal. They are more fragile than the other lenses. One advantage of these lenses is that they can be used by elderly people after cataract removal. Another type of contact lens is disposable. At the end of the wearing period, the lens is discarded and a new set of lenses is inserted. Contact lenses also are available in different colors. The wearer can change eye color by inserting these tinted lenses.

Contact lenses require an adjustment period. They usually feel uncomfortable in the beginning, and the patient may experience tearing, eye irritation, and increased blinking. Occasionally, visual blurring may occur. Not everyone can wear contact lenses; people with a history of repeated eye infections, low tear production, or severe allergic reactions especially have trouble with them.

The greatest danger with the use of any type of contact lens is the possibility of injury to or infection of the cornea, both of which can permanently affect the vision.

Radial Keratotomy

This surgical procedure, which is usually done on an outpatient basis, is used to correct myopia and astigmatism. Under local anesthesia, incisions that resemble the spokes of a wheel are made in the cornea. These incisions start near the center of the cornea (the clear zone) and extend outward to the edge. The incisions are made by a special knife that can be calibrated to cut at a predetermined depth. After the cuts are made, pressure in the anterior chamber of the eye reshapes the cornea to a normal or near-normal curvature.

This surgery is not without hazards. Infection and failure to produce anticipated results may be seen. Some patients report a worsening of their vision after the surgery, whereas others achieve complete success.

THE VISUALLY IMPAIRED

Poor vision affects a person's emotional, social, and vocational life. Visual disorders are extremely common, and the incidence of visual impairment rises markedly with increasing age.

Enough people wear corrective glasses that the need for them is not usually considered a disability. Some people's vision, however, cannot be improved by glasses or by any other type of treatment. Their defective vision may have been caused by injury or disease. For some, impaired vision is only temporary, as in the case of a patient with cataracts who is awaiting surgery. Others have a permanent visual impairment that cannot be corrected.

The term *blindness* is used for many legal purposes when central visual acuity is 20/200 or less in the better eye, even when corrective glasses are worn. People who have visual acuity between 20/70 and 20/200 in the better eye, with the use of glasses, are often referred to as partially sighted. People with severe restrictions in the field of vision (or visual fields) also are referred to as blind.

The only thing that visually impaired people have in common is the inability to see. They differ from one another in other ways, just as sighted people do. These patients must be helped to maintain their individuality and must not be expected to conform to a nebulous personality considered appropriate for the blind. Blind people rely on us, not for pity, but for help to resume independent lives despite the impairment.

NURSING PROCESS —THE VISUALLY IMPAIRED PATIENT

Assessment

The visually impaired person may be partially sighted or blind. The amount of vision a patient has is evaluated either by questioning the patient or by performing a basic visual evaluation.

If partially sighted, a patient's visual acuity and the types of aids that may improve vision or the ability to function are evaluated. If a patient is blind or nearly blind, it is important to determine the level of independence and whether the patient has participated in a rehabilitation or training program.

Nursing Diagnosis

The nursing diagnosis depends on the degree of vision loss, the length of time vision loss has been present, the possibility of treatments that either restore or improve vision, and other factors. Restatement of the relationship of the nursing diagnosis to causative factors may be necessary because each patient encounters different problems with visual impairment or blindness.

- Self-care deficit (specify areas) related to impaired vision or vision loss

- Potential for injury related to impaired vision or vision loss, unfamiliar surroundings
- Dysfunctional grieving related to recent vision loss
- Self-esteem disturbance related to vision loss, inability to adapt to vision loss
- Impaired adjustment related to change in vision
- Altered family processes related to recent or sudden loss of vision of family member
- Impaired home maintenance management related to indifference, lack of rehabilitation, other factors (specify)
- Diversional activity deficit related to vision loss
- Knowledge deficit of assistance agencies

Planning and Implementation

The major goals of the patient include prevention of injury, acceptance and adjustment to vision loss, improvement in ability to care for self and home, participation in recreational activities, improvement in self-esteem, and knowledge of agencies that offer assistance to the partially sighted and blind.

The major goals of nursing management of partially sighted people whose vision cannot be improved are preserving the remaining sight, when possible, and making the fullest possible use of remaining vision. The major goals of nursing management of the blind patient are directed toward helping the patient adjust to hospitalization, assisting the patient as needed, and making the fullest possible use of the remaining senses.

Nursing management largely depends on many factors, such as the degree of vision loss, the functioning level of the person, the length of time partial or total vision loss has been present, and whether vision possibly can be restored.

Courtesies that are helpful to patients who are blind or have extremely poor vision include the following:

- Introducing yourself each time you enter their room because many voices sound similar
- Orienting them to the location of the water pitcher and glass, grooming articles, urinal, and so forth on admission to the hospital and keeping these objects in about the same place at all times
- Calling these patients by name when others are present and the conversation is directed toward them; they cannot see the speaker look in their direction when conversation is directed to them
- Speaking to them before touching them so they realize you are present
- Telling them that you are leaving the room so that they are not embarrassed by carrying on a conversation with someone who is no longer present
- Guiding them around the room or adjacent areas by allowing them to place their arm in yours; holding them firmly when ambulating is usually unnecessary unless they have other physical problems
- Walking slowly when guiding them; if they have used a

cane for guidance in the past, allow them to continue to do so if possible

The nurse can assist or begin rehabilitation for patients who have recently lost most or all of their vision and have not attained an adequate level of functioning in their activities of daily living. The following can be part of a basic rehabilitation program in the hospital setting:

1. After evaluation of the visual loss and level of function, the required amount of supervision and assistance can be determined. Patients are taught at the same time they are being helped. It is important to remember to keep all articles the patient needs (eg, bed pan, urinal, towel, face cloth, toothbrush) in the same place each day.
2. At mealtime the patient is told where the food is on the plate. The number positions on the face of a clock may be used to describe the location; for example, the meat is at 9 o'clock and the baked potato at 3 o'clock. Eating utensils, napkins, cups, and salt and pepper shakers are shown by guiding the patient's hand to their locations. Removing dishes and eating utensils from the tray and placing them on a larger surface area gives the patient more room to use the hands to locate everything. At first, help may be needed in buttering bread, cutting meat, and pouring beverages, but, at the same time, the patient is taught to accomplish these tasks without assistance.
3. Patients are encouraged to gradually assume responsibility for their own care. As each task is mastered, another is introduced.
4. Patients may be willing and able to try to master several tasks simultaneously, or they may only attempt to learn one task at a time. It is important to avoid creating frustration and repeated failure. Giving the patient time to accomplish a task as well as encouragement and support throughout this period creates a positive atmosphere that is conducive to learning.

Self-Care Deficit, Potential for Injury. The visually impaired person must be oriented to the room and helped to form a mental image of the surroundings. Knowing where objects are helps them move about the room with minimal assistance.

To prevent injuries, objects in the room are always kept in the same place. The patient is told when something has been moved or is different from usual. Doors should be left wide open or completely closed because the patient is more likely to bump into a partly closed door.

Dysfunctional Grieving. Newly blind people or people who have suddenly lost much of their vision typically experience grief. With assistance and support, they may gradually move through the stages of grief to the point where they are ready to learn to become as independent as possible.

Self-Esteem Disturbance, Impaired Adjustment. Visually handicapped patients may have difficulty adjusting to a loss of vision and may experience negative feelings about the disability. They may express feelings of doubt about their ability to assume an active role in society, be independent, support themselves and their family, and manage their affairs. While some patients adjust well to a loss of vision, other do not.

The nurse must listen to the patient and identify areas of concern. Helping the patient adjust to a vision loss includes understanding the feelings and emotional reactions as well as formulating and instituting a plan of rehabilitation. In addition, early recognition of potential problems may allow for the development of plans of action that, along with the help of others, nurture self-confidence and independence in the patient.

The hospitalized patient who has been blind for a period of time and who has a seeing-eye (or guide) dog may find the separation distressing because of the dependence on the dog for guidance and companionship.

Altered Family Processes. The visually impaired patient may have been the sole financial support of the family. Role reversals may be necessary as one or more family members find it necessary to assume this role.

Vocational preparation or rehabilitation for the person who must be self-supporting or contribute to the support of a family is undertaken after evaluation of the patient. If financial obligations cannot be met through employment, financial assistance from government or social service agencies may be necessary.

Impaired Home Maintenance Management. Patients who have recently lost their sight or who have poor vision may require training to learn to manage the home environment. Every effort is made to encourage independence. A home visit by a public health nurse may be necessary to ensure that all hazards that could result in falls or other injuries are removed from the environment and that the activities of daily living can be performed with minimum difficulty. When the patient lives alone, it may be necessary to ensure that a support system, composed of family members, relatives, or friends, is available for activities such as shopping, banking, and visits to the physician's office.

Diversional Activity Deficit. For the partially sighted, books and magazines are available in large print editions, and special magnifying lenses may be used to read labels, telephone books, and other printed matter that is in small type. The blind can read print set in Braille, a system of raised dots that the patient feels with the fingertips. The dots are arranged in specific patterns that signify the alphabet and punctuation marks. Learning Braille requires time and patience. Special typewriters that type Braille make it possible for blind people to write to one another.

Radio, records, and tapes also provide enjoyment for many who are visually impaired. Talking books (records, cassettes) are available for loan from many public libraries. For people who wish to purchase talking books, many classic and contemporary books are available on cassette tape at reasonable cost. Many bookstores and general merchandise stores carry these cassettes.

A reading aid, which is available in limited areas, uses optical scanning and a synthesized voice process to "read" printed material to the listener. This device is especially valuable for students, for example, who wish to read texts and other books normally not available as talking books.

In some areas, community activities for the visually impaired are organized. Transportation, when needed, can often be provided.

Knowledge Deficit. Families and the patients who have recently lost their sight or who have become visually impaired require information about available services and agencies.

Agencies such as the local chapter of the American Foundation for the Blind are invaluable resources that can provide information about special schools, teachers of Braille, the purchase of special equipment and apparel (eg, Braille watches), seeing-eye dogs, activities, transportation, sources of aids (eg, talking books), and assistance with personal and financial matters.

Evaluation

Evaluation not only depends on the effectiveness of nursing management but also on the degree of vision loss, the length of time visual impairment has been present, the level of functioning, and the amount of rehabilitation. Not all of the following may apply to each patient, and some may require reformulation.

- Begins to perform self-care activities, improves ability to perform self-care activities, or performs self-care activities with minimal assistance
- No evidence of injury
- Demonstrates evidence of acceptance of visual disability
- Appears self-confident when performing activities
- Develops positive feelings about visual loss and a desire to compensate for the loss in other ways
- Expresses a desire to engage in vocational rehabilitation

- Moves from dependence to independence
- Expresses a desire to assume responsibility for home management
- Engages in meaningful activities; expresses a desire to use aids that provide recreation
- Patient and family express interest in obtaining information about public and private agencies that supply assistance to the visually handicapped

TRAUMA TO THE EYE

Injury to the eye and surrounding structures can result in a decrease in or total loss of vision. Children and adults are subject to eye injuries, such as those resulting from chemical sprays, direct blows to the eye, and flying objects, such as bits of metal or wood.

The importance of protecting the eyes by wearing glasses with shatter-resistant lenses or safety goggles while working or handling substances that could cause eye injury cannot be overemphasized.

NURSING PROCESS —THE PATIENT WHO HAS AN EYE INJURY

Assessment

An immediate history of the type or cause of injury is obtained from the patient or family member. If a chemical has been splashed or sprayed into the eyes, it is important to know the name or type of substance and if any treatment, such as washing out the eye, was given.

The eye and surrounding structures are immediately examined for evidence of bleeding, swelling, and cuts. Because severe pain may be present and the patient unable or unwilling to open the eye, the initial examination may need to be performed by a physician.

Great care must be taken in wiping away blood or debris or everting the eyelids. When a foreign body is present, any pressure on the eye may push the object into the tissues of the eyeball. Because eye injuries may require immediate treatment, examination of the eye may be carried out as treatment is begun.

Nursing Diagnosis

Depending on the type of injury, one or more of the following may apply:

- Anxiety related to pain, possible loss of vision, procedures necessary to treat the injury
- Pain related to injury of the eye or surrounding structures
- Potential for infection related to injury

- Impaired tissue integrity related to injury
- Knowledge deficit of care of the eye after treatment

Planning and Implementation

The major objectives of the patient include a relief of pain or discomfort, a reduction of anxiety, absence of infection, and an understanding of home care after treatment of the injury.

The major objectives of nursing management are to institute emergency treatment (when applicable), relieve pain or discomfort, and reduce anxiety.

The physician is contacted immediately if the eye has been seriously injured. An eye tray that contains materials such as topical anesthetics, antibiotic ointments, irrigating solutions, and fluorescein strips and drops is immediately placed at the patient's side. All labels are checked before use to be sure they read "ophthalmic." A light with a magnifying lens is brought to the patient's side.

Emergency treatment, when applicable, is begun immediately.

Foreign Bodies

Foreign bodies are best removed by a physician. An attempt to remove a foreign body may be performed by a nurse if it is not on the cornea, it has not penetrated the tissues of the eye, and it has only been present for a short time.

In a darkened room, the patient is asked to close the eyes and a flashlight is directed at the eye. If a foreign body is present, the patient may see a black spot. The lower lid is everted, and the patient is instructed to look up. The inferior conjunctival sac is inspected using direct vision or a magnifying lamp. If nothing is seen, the upper lid is everted and the patient directed to look down.

When the foreign body is located, it is touched gently with a sterile swab moistened in sterile saline. After the particle has been removed, the patient usually continues to feel irritation. If the particle is not removed, the patient must be treated by a physician who may place fluorescein drops or strips in the eye to locate the foreign body.

Chemicals

An irritating chemical splashed into the eye is an emergency that requires immediate treatment. If the accident occurs in the home or work, the person is taken to the nearest sink or water fountain and instructed to hold the eyes open while running water cleanses them. The person is taken immediately to an ophthalmologist or to a hospital emergency department for further treatment.

When brought to the emergency department, the patient's eye is immediately flushed copiously with sterile saline or water to remove the chemical as promptly as possible. The importance of speed cannot be overemphasized; the longer the chemical is in contact with the eye, the more damage can occur.

The flow of solution is directed from the inner canthus to the outer canthus, so that it does not flow into the other eye. If both eyes must be irrigated, it is preferable to have two people work simultaneously. If two people are not available, the irrigation flow is switched from one eye to the other, so that both eyes are flushed as quickly and thoroughly as possible. Eye irrigation is carried out for 10 to 15 minutes. A physician must examine the patient as soon as possible. After the eye has been irrigated, the physician may order an application of an ophthalmic ointment and eye pad. The patient is instructed to close the eye, and an eye pad is applied over the lid and held in place with tape.

Contusions and Hematoma

A blow to or near the eye can result in swelling and bleeding into soft tissues with ultimate discoloration (black eye) of the area. To reduce swelling, ice or a cold pack is gently applied to the injured area until the patient is examined by a physician.

Abrasions and Lacerations

Cuts that involve the eyelid are serious and require treatment by an ophthalmologist; an untreated cut can produce scarring and misalignment of the lid margins. To repair a laceration of the eyelid, the physician injects a local anesthetic and the lid margins are approximated with sutures. A cut on the eyeball, especially the cornea, is serious and requires immediate treatment by an ophthalmologist.

The patient is instructed to keep the hands away from the eyes until examined by a physician. If bleeding from a laceration of the eyelid occurs, the blood can be wiped from around the eye, but pressure is not exerted on the bleeding lid margins since a foreign body also may be present.

Anxiety.   Assure the patient that everything possible is being done to relieve pain and treat the injury. Because pain may be severe, the patient may have difficulty cooperating with treatment.

Pain.   Pain is most severe when the eyeball has been injured. The physician usually instills anesthetic drops to relieve pain or discomfort.

Potential for Infection.   When possible, sterile solutions are used to irrigate the eye. An antibiotic ointment may be prescribed to prevent infection. After treatment, an eye dressing with or without a protective shield may be ordered.

Impaired Tissue Integrity. Whenever an injured eye is examined by the nurse, it must be remembered that a foreign body also may be present even though a liquid or spray has been splashed into the eye. Great care is always used when examining the eye.

The physician may prescribe ointments or drops to be used until healing has occurred. Corticosteroid ointments may be instilled to reduce inflammation.

Knowledge Deficit. If an ophthalmic drug has been prescribed, the patient or a family member requires instruction in its use. If a dressing is put on the eye and is to be changed by the patient, instruction about its application is needed.

If a foreign body was removed, the patient is instructed not to rub the eye and, if it is not completely comfortable within a short time, to visit an ophthalmologist or return to the emergency department.

The importance of follow-up visits to check the condition of the eye or surrounding structures is emphasized.

Evaluation

■ Anxiety is reduced
■ Pain is reduced or eliminated
■ No evidence of infection on return visits
■ Verbalizes understanding of the application of an eye dressing, medication schedule, and technique of instilling eye drops or applying eye ointment
■ Verbalizes understanding of the importance of not rubbing the eyes and importance of follow-up care

INFECTIOUS AND INFLAMMATORY DISORDERS
Conjunctivitis

Conjunctivitis is an inflammation of the conjunctiva that results from a bacterial, viral, or rickettsial infection. Conjunctivitis also may be due to allergy or trauma caused by chemicals or foreign bodies in the eye.

Symptoms
Symptoms include redness, excessive tearing, swelling, pain, and possibly purulent drainage and itching.

Diagnosis
Diagnosis is made by visual inspection of the conjunctiva. Cultures may be taken to identify the causative microorganism.

Treatment
Treatment includes antibiotic ointments or drops. Warm soaks or sterile saline irrigations may be used to remove purulent drainage, reduce swelling, and relieve pain or itching.

Uveitis

This disorder is an inflammation of the uveal tract, which consists of the iris, ciliary body, and choroid. Uveitis may be seen with diseases or infections such as juvenile rheumatoid arthritis, ankylosing spondylitis, tuberculosis, and herpes zoster. The cause also may be unknown.

Symptoms
Symptoms include eye congestion, pain, reduced vision, and a small pupil that reacts poorly to light.

Diagnosis
Diagnosis is made by slit lamp examination.

Treatment
Treatment includes oral or topical corticosteroids, mydriatic eye drops such as atropine, or antibiotic eye drops.

Keratitis and Corneal Ulcer

Keratitis is an inflammation of the cornea. Trauma to the cornea and bacteria, fungus, or viral infections are causes of keratitis.

Symptoms
Symptoms of keratitis include pain, photophobia, blurred vision, tearing, possibly a purulent discharge, and redness of the sclera. Keratitis may result in a corneal ulcer. Symptoms of a corneal ulcer depend on the stage of the disorder. Early symptoms include blurred vision, pain, tearing, possibly a purulent discharge, and redness of the sclera, all of which are similar to the symptoms of keratitis. Later, when the ulcer heals and scar tissue forms, visual changes are noted. The degree of visual change depends on the size of the corneal scar tissue.

Diagnosis
Diagnosis of keratitis is made by examination and patient history. Diagnosis of a corneal ulcer is made by examination, patient history, and the use of fluorescein drops or strips to identify the ulcer or scar tissue.

Treatment
Treatment of keratitis includes topical anesthetics, mydriatics, and antibiotics. Systemic antibiotics also may be used. Dark glasses can be worn to relieve photophobia. Treatment in the early stages of a corneal ulcer is the same as for keratitis. Once corneal scar

tissue has formed, the only treatment is corneal transplantation (keratoplasty).

Blepharitis ✓

This disorder is an inflammation of the eyelids. Causes include excessive dryness of the eyes and infection of the lid margins.

Symptoms

The lid margins appear inflamed and purulent drainage may be present. This disorder may coexist with conjunctivitis.

Diagnosis

Diagnosis is made by visual examination of the eyes.

Treatment

Treatment includes careful cleansing of the eyelids once or twice per day. Because seborrhea (excessive oiliness of the skin) of the face and scalp also may result in blepharitis, daily cleansing of the skin and frequent washing of the hair may be recommended. A topical antibiotic ointment applied to the lid margins also may be prescribed.

Hordeolum (Sty) and Chalazion ✓

A sty is an inflammation and infection of an oil gland of the eyelid. A chalazion is a cyst of one or more meibomian glands, which are sebaceous glands located at the junction of the conjunctiva and inner eyelid margins.

Symptoms

Symptoms of a sty include an area of the eyelid that has become tender, red, and swollen. A chalazion cyst is usually painless and results from an infection of the gland.

Diagnosis

Diagnosis of both conditions is made by visual inspection of the area.

Treatment

Treatment of a sty includes warm soaks of the area and a topical antibiotic. Severe cases may require incision and drainage.

Treatment of a chalazion is not necessary if the cyst is small and causes no interference with vision. An incision and drainage may be necessary if the cyst is large, becomes infected, or interferes with vision or closure of the eyelids.

NURSING PROCESS —THE PATIENT WHO HAS AN INFECTIOUS OR INFLAMMATORY DISORDER OF THE EYE

Read through!

Assessment

The eye and surrounding structures are examined for signs of inflammation and infection. A history of symptoms and a general medical and allergy history are obtained. It is important to note if the patient has worn or is wearing contact lenses, has suffered recent trauma to the eye, or has a history of repeated eye infections.

Nursing Diagnosis

Depending on the symptoms and type of infection or inflammation, one or more of the following may apply:

- Pain related to inflammation, infection, swelling
- Anxiety related to discomfort, pain
- Potential for infection transmitted to other eye related to rubbing the eyes
- Knowledge deficit of treatment regimen

Planning and Implementation

The major goals of the patient include a relief of pain, reduction of anxiety, prevention of transmission of infection to other eye, and an understanding of the treatment regimen.

The major goals of nursing management include the relief of pain, reduction of anxiety, and effective teaching of the patient about home care and follow-up treatment.

The materials necessary for examination and treatment by a physician are prepared and placed next to the patient. A lighted magnifying lens also is made available.

See the later discussion under Nursing Process— The Patient Undergoing Eye Surgery for management of the patient who is undergoing corneal transplantation.

Pain, Anxiety.   The examination and treatment procedures are explained to the patient. The patient is assured that treatment usually produces relief from pain and discomfort. These explanations also usually help to relieve anxiety. If severe pain is present, the physician may order anesthetic eye drops. Warm soaks or eye irrigations also may be ordered to relieve discomfort or pain.

The technique of eye drop instillation (Fig. 41-2), the application of the prescribed drug or other treatment modalities (eg, soaks, cleansing of the

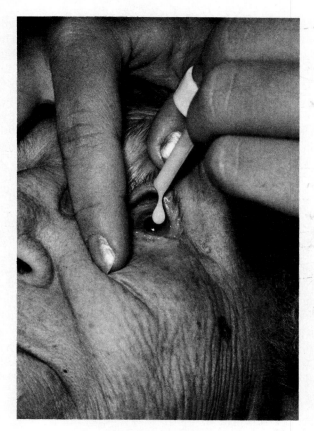

Figure 41–2. When eyedrops are instilled, the patient looks up. The lower lid is gently everted as the drop is placed just inside of it. (Photograph by D. Atkinson)

eyelids), and the dosage regimen are explained and demonstrated.

Potential for Infection, Knowledge Deficit. Because it is important to prevent the spread of infection (when applicable) to the other eye, the following teaching points are emphasized: *Know these:*

1. A full course of treatment with the prescribed drug must be completed to achieve satisfactory results.
2. The hands must be washed thoroughly before cleansing the eyelids, instilling eye drops, or applying an eye ointment.
3. The eyes must not be rubbed, and hands must be kept away from the eyes.
4. Nonprescription eye products must not be used during or after treatment unless use has been approved by the physician.
5. The physician's recommendations regarding follow-up visits, how to avoid future infections, and so on must be followed.

Evaluation

- Pain or discomfort is reduced or eliminated
- Anxiety is reduced

- Inflammation and infection are reduced or eliminated
- No evidence of spread of infection to other eye
- Demonstrates understanding of prescribed dosage regimen, treatments, methods of avoiding future infections

MACULAR DEGENERATION

Macular degeneration is breakdown or damage to the macula, which is the point of the retina where light rays meet as they are focused on the cornea and lens of the eye. The patient loses vision in the center of an image but is still able to see to the side. Macular degeneration does not affect peripheral vision.

The most common form of macular degeneration, accounting for about 70% of the cases, is involutional macular degeneration, which is associated with the aging process. Other forms of this disorder include exudative macular degeneration and injury, infection, or inflammation that damages the macula.

straight lines tend to jump around

Symptoms

Blurred vision may be the first symptom of macular degeneration. Other symptoms include disturbance in color vision (colors become dim), difficulty in reading and doing close work, distortion of objects (especially those with lines), and an empty area in the field of vision.

Diagnosis

The ophthalmologist can detect early macular degeneration by means of an ophthalmoscope. A fluorescein angiogram, which is an injection of fluorescein dye into the patient's arm followed by photographs of the retina and macula, may be used to confirm the diagnosis.

Treatment

The laser may be used to seal off leaking membranes and destroy new blood vessels in exudative macular degeneration. The patient with involutional macular degeneration does not respond to laser therapy. Optical aids, such as magnifying glasses, may be of value, and high-intensity reading lamps have helped people. The ophthalmologist may refer patients to a low-vision center for evaluation and selection of devices that will be the most useful to them.

For management of the patient with macular degeneration, see the earlier discussion under Nursing Process—The Visually Impaired Patient.

GLAUCOMA *very imp!*

The anterior chamber of the eye lies between the cornea anteriorly and the iris posteriorly. The anterior chamber is filled with aqueous humor, a transparent fluid that nourishes the lens and the cornea. At the outer margin of the anterior chamber, between the iris and the cornea, lies the angle of the anterior chamber. It is at this angle that the aqueous humor drains through sievelike structures into Schlemm's canal and from there into the general circulation. A balance is achieved between the amount of aqueous humor formed by the ciliary body and the amount drained out of the eye. This balance helps to maintain normal intraocular pressure.

Glaucoma is a condition that results from increased intraocular pressure (IOP) due to a disturbance of the normal balance between the production and the drainage of the aqueous humor that fills the anterior chamber. Although glaucoma can occur at any age, it is most common after age 40. Anatomic abnormalities and degenerative changes partially cause glaucoma. Glaucoma is more common among people who have a family history of the disorder. Glaucoma is the second most common cause of blindness in the United States.

Although glaucoma has no cure, it can be controlled, and blindness can be prevented. Early diagnosis and treatment are of the utmost importance to prevent loss of vision. Everyone should be examined regularly for early indications of glaucoma. Persons older than 40 years of age should have annual eye examinations.

In general, glaucoma is classified as angle-closure, open-angle, congenital, and secondary.

Angle-Closure (Acute) Glaucoma

This form of glaucoma occurs less often than open-angle glaucoma and requires immediate recognition and treatment. A delay in treatment may result in partial or total loss of vision in the affected eye.

Symptoms

The symptoms of this form of glaucoma are easier to recognize because they are dramatic and appear suddenly. Symptoms include severe pain in and around the eyes, blurred vision, and the appearance of halos (rainbow-colored rings), particularly around lights. Nausea and vomiting also may occur.

Diagnosis

Diagnosis is based on symptoms and a marked increase in IOP.

Treatment

Unless the condition is relieved promptly, blindness may occur in 1 or 2 days. Miotics (drugs that constrict the pupil) are given at once to pull the iris away from the drainage channels (Schlemm's canal) so that drainage of aqueous humor can resume, thus reducing the IOP and relieving the symptoms. Acetazolamide (Diamox), a carbonic anhydrase inhibitor, may be given to slow the production of aqueous fluid, thus helping to decrease the IOP. Drugs are likely to be used just before and during surgery to lessen IOP and make the operation safe. Analgesics are given to relieve pain, and the patient is kept at complete rest.

Early surgical intervention usually is indicated to relieve acute glaucoma and to prevent further attacks. An iridectomy is performed to relieve the symptoms. A section of iris is removed, thus preventing it from bulging forward, crowding the chamber angle, and obstructing the drainage of aqueous fluid. This way, a permanent entrance to the drainage canal is achieved. Two types of iridectomy are performed: the peripheral, in which a small section of iris is removed at the periphery, and the sector or keyhole, in which a larger segment of iris is removed (Fig. 41-3).

The laser also may be used to burn holes in the iris (nonsurgical iridectomy). This treatment is performed under topical anesthesia on an outpatient basis.

Open-Angle Glaucoma

Open-angle glaucoma, also called chronic glaucoma, occurs more frequently than acute glaucoma. The onset of this form of glaucoma is slow, and it may be several years before the patient begins to experience any noticeable symptoms.

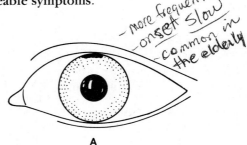

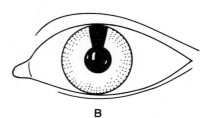

Figure 41–3. (A) Appearance of the eye after peripheral iridectomy. (B) After keyhole (sector) iridectomy.

Timoptic
Diamox
Glaucoma (oral & systemic)

Symptoms

Often, symptoms are absent, mild, or intermittent. Because they are not so dramatic, they are more readily ignored. When symptoms do occur, they include discomfort and aching of the eyes, occasional temporary blurring of vision and the appearance of halos around lights, reduced peripheral vision, and a frequent need to change eyeglasses.

Many patients experience no symptoms of chronic glaucoma, and the condition is not discovered until the patient has a routine ophthalmologic examination.

Diagnosis

Diagnosis is made by measurement of the IOP.

Treatment

Patients with this form of glaucoma also require prompt medical treatment. As in acute glaucoma, miotics, such as carbachol or pilocarpine, may be prescribed. The disadvantage of these agents is that they need to be instilled 2 to 4 times or more per day. Pilocarpine, however, is available as an ocular therapeutic system inserted by the patient and replaced every 7 days.

Other drugs that may be used for lowering the IOP include echothiophate iodide (Phospholine), epinephrine, dipivefrin (Propine), and timolol maleate (Timoptic). All of these agents are instilled in the eye. A systemic drug that also may be used to lower the IOP is acetazolamide (Diamox).

When patient compliance is poor (eg, failure to instill the eye drops as directed), when drug therapy is no longer effective, or when a patient develops severe adverse reactions to the drug, an iridectomy may be considered. The laser also may be used. In this procedure, the laser beam is directed at the trabecular network, which lies near Schlemm's canal, thus facilitating the drainage of aqueous humor. Another surgical procedure makes a small hole at the junction of the cornea and sclera (corneal trephine) to encourage drainage of aqueous humor. The opening is then covered by a flap of the conjunctiva.

mydriatics = dilate the pupil

Other Types of Glaucoma

Congenital glaucoma is present at birth. Treatment depends on the amount of damage to the vision. Many people with this type of glaucoma are born blind, and no treatment can restore vision.

Secondary glaucoma occurs as a result of such conditions as trauma, infection, cataract surgery, and swelling of the lens of the eye. The treatment of secondary glaucoma is managed in the same manner as open-angle glaucoma. Swelling of the lens may require surgical removal.

NURSING PROCESS —THE PATIENT WHO HAS GLAUCOMA

Assessment

A history of symptoms and a general medical and allergy history are obtained. If the patient has symptoms that may indicate acute glaucoma, the physician examines the patient and determines the IOP.

If the patient has a history of glaucoma, it is important to determine when the condition was diagnosed, the medications that have been prescribed, and if the patient has been adhering to the prescribed medication schedule.

If a vision loss has occurred, it is important to determine about how much vision remains.

Nursing Diagnosis

Depending on the type of glaucoma, one or more of the following may apply. If vision loss has occurred, additional nursing diagnoses may be needed (see earlier discussion, Nursing Process—The Visually Impaired Patient).

- Pain related to increased IOP
- Anxiety related to symptoms, diagnosis, proposed treatment, possible loss of vision
- Self-care deficit (specify type) related to loss of vision
- Noncompliance to medical treatment modality related to anxiety, indifference, knowledge deficit, other factors (specify)
- Knowledge deficit of treatment modality

Planning and Implementation

The major goals of the patient include a relief of pain, reduction of anxiety, improvement in ability to care for self, compliance with treatment modalities, and an understanding of treatment prescribed by the physician.

The major goals of nursing management are to relieve pain and discomfort by instituting prescribed therapies, to inform the patient of the importance of the prescribed treatment regimen, and to reduce anxiety.

Acute closed-angle glaucoma is an emergency; treatment is instituted *immediately*, as vision loss may occur in 1 or 2 days. If the patient has chronic open-angle glaucoma, one or more drugs are prescribed to lower the IOP.

When the patient with glaucoma is hospitalized, it is absolutely essential that the prescribed drugs be administered, regardless of what other disease or illness is being treated.

Extreme care must be taken when administering eye drops to any patient but, especially, to patients with glaucoma. Usually, a miotic is ordered to constrict the pupil. If a mydriatic such as atropine is given in error, the resulting dilation of the pupil can further obstruct drainage of aqueous humor, precipitating an acute attack that could result in permanent blindness. *No amount of caution is too great to prevent such a tragedy.* The physician's order is read carefully as to which eye is to receive the medication. The physician's order and the label on the bottle are checked carefully, and the patient is identified before instilling the medication into the eye.

If surgery is performed, see the later discussion under Nursing Process—The Patient Undergoing Eye Surgery.

Pain. An analgesic may be prescribed for the patient with acute closed-angle glaucoma. The patient is reminded frequently that once treatment begins to take effect, pain begins to diminish. The patient is evaluated at frequent intervals for relief of pain and other symptoms of the disorder, and the physician is informed immediately if the patient states that the pain has worsened, despite current treatment.

Anxiety. The methods of treatment are carefully explained to the patient. The physician also discusses with the patient and family the expected outcome of treatment.

The nurse must allow time for the patient or the family to ask questions about the prescribed treatment regimen.

Self-Care Deficit. On occasion, a patient did not seek immediate treatment for acute closed-angle glaucoma, and blindness or a marked visual impairment occurred. Also, people with undetected chronic open-angle glaucoma may not have had an eye examination until some vision loss occurred. Patients with decreased visual acuity may need partial assistance with their activities of daily living.

Noncompliance. The nurse must stress that adherence to the treatment regimen of prescribed eye drops and oral medication (if applicable) is *absolutely essential* if vision loss or blindness is to be prevented. Blindness due to glaucoma is in most instances preventable, but *only* when the patient complies with the prescribed regimen.

Knowledge Deficit. All patients with glaucoma (even those who have had surgery) require continued care and examinations as recommended by the ophthalmologist. Because these patients are instilling eye drops or inserting ocular therapeutic systems, the technique of each is explained and demonstrated.

Certain general measures also can help to control the condition. The patient is instructed to do the following:

1. Obtain assistance from a family member, relative, or friend if instilling eye drops is difficult.
2. Avoid *all* drugs that contain atropine, including prescription as well as nonprescription drugs. Preparations advertised as beneficial for symptoms of a cold or an allergy may contain atropine. It is best to check with a physician or pharmacist before using any nonprescription drug.
3. Maintain regular bowel habits; straining at stool can raise the IOP.
4. Avoid heavy lifting and emotional upsets (especially crying) because these increase the IOP.
5. Limit activities that make the eyes feel strained or fatigued.
6. Keep an extra supply of prescribed drugs on hand for vacations, over holidays, or in case some is lost or spilled.
7. Seek medical attention *immediately* if pain or any type of visual disturbance occurs.
8. Always inform all physicians of this disorder and the treatment prescribed by the ophthalmologist. A card or Medic-Alert bracelet that states that the person has glaucoma informs medical personnel of the problem in the event of illness or injury.

Evaluation

- Pain is reduced or eliminated
- Anxiety is reduced
- Self-care needs are met
- Demonstrates understanding of medical regimen, situations to avoid, and symptoms that require immediate notification of the physician
- Verbalizes understanding of importance of drug therapy to control IOP and prevent visual loss or blindness
- Demonstrates the correct technique of eye drop instillation

CATARACTS

A cataract is a condition in which the lens of the eye becomes opaque, thus reducing the amount of light that reaches the retina. When the lens becomes opaque, a white or a gray spot is visible behind the pupil. Vision diminishes as the lens becomes more opaque. The process usually advances slowly and, eventually, may lead to loss of sight unless surgery is performed. If both eyes are severely affected, the patient becomes blind.

Cataracts may be congenital, caused by injury to the lens, secondary to other diseases of the eye, or be a part of the aging process. When cataracts occur in response to injury, they usually develop quickly. Most cataracts, however, are caused by degenerative changes associated with the aging process and tend to

Halo = glaucoma
or cataracts

glaucoma = pain
cataracts = no pain

Chapter 41 — Disorders of the Eye and Ear 499

-hard for
the elderly

develop slowly. Although people do develop cataracts in earlier life, the incidence rises steadily with age. Cataracts are especially common among people in the seventh, eighth, and ninth decades of life. A high incidence of cataracts occurs among patients with certain disorders, such as diabetes. A family history of cataracts often exists. Prolonged exposure to ultraviolet rays (eg, sunlight, tanning lamps) and radiation, as well as to certain drugs (eg, the corticosteroids), has been associated with cataract formation.

Symptoms

One of the earliest symptoms a patient may notice is a halo around lights. Bright lights that shine directly into the eye may cause a halo with spokes or rays. Additional symptoms include difficulty reading, a change in visual acuity, changes in color vision, a glaring of objects in bright light, and distortion of objects. As the lens becomes more opaque, visual acuity markedly decreases.

Diagnosis

Diagnosis is made by ophthalmoscopic and slit lamp examination and tests for visual acuity.

Treatment

The treatment of a cataract involves surgical removal of the lens when vision is sufficiently impaired. Removal of the lens is necessary because its opacity prevents light rays from reaching the retina. The lens may be removed by the intracapsular method (removal of the lens within its capsule) or by the extracapsular method (removal of the lens, leaving the posterior portion of its capsule in position). Phacoemulsification, which uses ultrasound to break the lens into minute particles that are then removed by aspiration, may be employed with the extracapsular method. The method of removal is chosen by the surgeon after considering the patient's age, the degree of opacity of the cataract, and other factors.

Vision may be restored after surgery by three methods. The first and oldest is the prescription of cataract glasses. The correcting lens for the aphakic (without a lens) eye causes the patient to see objects about one third larger than a normal eye sees them. These lenses distort peripheral vision, and the patient must learn to turn the head to the side to see objects that are not in the center of vision. If the lens has been removed from both eyes, the patient can continue to use both eyes simultaneously. If the lens has been removed in only one eye, however, the patient must use only one eye at a time. Usually a coating is applied to the eyeglasses so that only the aphakic eye with a corrective lens is used for seeing.

The second method is the wearing of a contact lens. An advantage of the contact lens is that peripheral vision is not lost and objects are relatively the same size. The disadvantage is the need to remove, clean, and reinsert the lens, which may be difficult for the elderly patient who possesses poor manual dexterity or who has a cataract in both eyes.

A third method is the insertion of an intraocular lens (IOL) at the time of cataract surgery (Fig.41-4). The lens may be inserted in front of or behind the iris. Several different types of lenses are made, and the type is chosen by the ophthalmologist. An A-scan is performed before surgery to determine the size and prescription of the lens implant.

Intraocular lens implants are usually recommended for people 60 years old or older or for those who would experience difficulty with a contact lens or cataract glasses. Not everyone is a candidate for an IOL implant, and the choice to use this type of vision correction after cataract surgery is made by the ophthalmologist. One of the newer types of lens implants is a foldable, soft IOL. When phacoemulsification is used to remove the cataract and a foldable lens inserted, a smaller incision is required, and the patient usually returns to full activity in a shorter time than with the other methods.

Surgery is often performed under local anesthesia. A tranquilizer also is given before and during surgery to relax the patient. General anesthesia is sometimes used and has certain advantages, especially with an overly apprehensive patient.

Before surgery, the physician discusses with the patient the advantages and disadvantages of the procedure and the method (cataract glasses, contact lens, lens implant) used to restore vision.

Complications after cataract surgery include eye infection, loss of vitreous humor, intraocular hemorrhage, retinal detachment, and, when applicable, slipping of the lens implant. Loss of vitreous humor can occur during or after surgery and is serious because vitreous humor does not regenerate. Its loss may cause serious damage to the eye. Hemorrhage can injure the delicate structures of the eye.

If surgery is performed, see the later discussion under Nursing Process—The Patient Undergoing Eye Surgery.

hemorrhage cause ↑IOP and/or blindness

DETACHED RETINA

In a detached retina, the sensory layer becomes separated from the pigmented layer of the retina. The separation of the two layers of the retina deprives the sensory layer of its blood supply. Vision is lost in the affected area because the sensory layer can no longer receive visual stimuli. Fluid (vitreous humor) flows between the separated layers of the retina, holding the layers apart and causing further separation.

Types of Implants

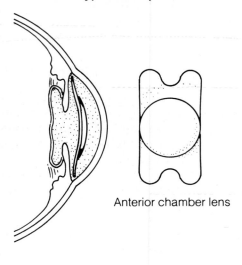

Anterior chamber lens

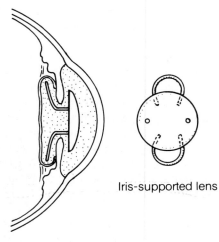

Iris-supported lens

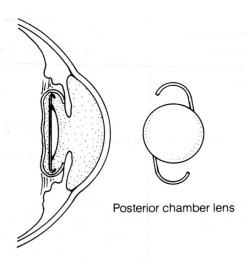

Posterior chamber lens

Retinal separation usually is associated with a hole or a tear in the retina that results from stretching or from degenerative changes in the retina. Retinal detachment may follow a sudden blow, a penetrating injury, or surgery on the eye. Tumors, hemorrhage in front of or behind the retina, and loss of vitreous fluid are particularly liable to lead to retinal detachment. It also may be a complication of other disorders, such as advanced diabetic changes in the retina. In many instances, the cause of retinal detachment is unknown. Retinal separation occurs more commonly among people older than 40 years.

Symptoms

Patients often notice definite gaps in their vision, or areas that they cannot see. They may have the feeling that a curtain is being drawn over their field of vision, and they often see flashes of light. The sensation of spots or moving particles before the eyes is common. Complete loss of vision may occur in the affected eye. There is no pain, but the patient usually is extremely apprehensive.

Diagnosis

Diagnosis is made by symptoms and ophthalmoscopic examination of the eye.

Treatment

Prompt diagnosis and treatment are essential. After examining the patient's retina with the ophthalmoscope and establishing the diagnosis, the physician usually recommends prompt admission to the hospital. The physician's orders on admission usually include bed rest, application of an eye patch (with or without an eye shield), and the use of mydriatics to dilate the pupil and facilitate further examination of the retina.

The patient is kept on complete bed rest until surgery is performed. Depending on the location of the detachment, the surgeon determines if the patient can or cannot lie on either side or on the back to encourage reattachment of the retina to the choroid. Sedation also may be ordered.

The following methods of surgical intervention are used to reattach the separated retina:

CRYOSURGERY.   This method uses a supercooled probe, which is applied to the sclera. The sclera, choroid, and retina then adhere to one another as a result of scar tissue formation. (pulls 3 parts of eye together)

ELECTRODIATHERMY.   An electrode needle is inserted into the sclera so that the fluid that has collected underneath the retina escapes. The retina ultimately adheres to the choroid. This method is rarely used.

LASER.   A laser beam is focused on the damaged area of the retina, causing a small burn. The exudate that forms between the retina and choroid results in adhesion of the retina to the choroid. Laser therapy can only be used when the retinal separation involves a small area.

SCLERAL BUCKLING. This procedure shortens the sclera, thus allowing contact between the choroid and retina. A section of the sclera is exposed, opened, and retracted from the choroid. A laser beam or cryosurgery probe is then used to produce adhesion of the retina and choroid. A small silicon patch is placed between the sclera and choroid, and the sclera is pulled over the patch and sutured. The inward displacement of the choroid allows for reattachment of the retina to the choroid.

The amount of sight regained depends on the extent of the detachment and the success of the surgery.

See the later discussion under Nursing Process— The Patient Undergoing Eye Surgery for the management of a patient with a detached retina.

ENUCLEATION

Removal of the eye may be necessary when the eye has been destroyed by injury or disease or if a malignant tumor develops. Fortunately, malignant tumors of the eye are not common. Removal of the eye is necessary, however, when a tumor, such as a retinoblastoma, is discovered. The eye also may be removed to relieve pain when it has been severely damaged by injury or disease, or if it is sightless.

The following terms are used in association with eye surgery. *Enucleation* means removal of the entire eyeball. *Evisceration* means removal of the contents of the eyeball, leaving the sclera in place. *Exenteration* is the removal of the entire eyeball as well as tissues in the bony orbit.

When enucleation is performed, a ball made of metal or plastic usually is buried in the capsule of connective tissue from which the eyeball has been removed. After the tissues have healed, a glass or plastic prosthesis, shaped like a shell, is placed over the buried ball. The shell is painted to match the patient's remaining eye, and it is the part that is sometimes referred to as a glass eye.

NURSING PROCESS —THE PATIENT UNDERGOING EYE SURGERY

Cataract surgery is often performed on an outpatient basis, using local anesthesia and intravenous sedation. Other eye surgeries, such as enucleation and detached retina, require hospitalization and general anesthesia. Cataract surgery may be performed under general anesthesia, especially if the patient has severe anxiety over the impending surgery.

Preoperative Period

Assessment
A complete medical, allergy, and drug history is taken. It is particularly important to know the name and dose of any prescription eye drops used before admission. When applicable, the patient's visual acuity is determined.

Nursing Diagnosis
Depending on the type of surgery, the diagnosis, and preoperative symptoms one or more of the following may apply:

- Anxiety related to vision loss, impending surgery, results of surgery, discomfort or pain (if present)
- Pain related to increased IOP
- Potential for injury related to decreased visual acuity
- Knowledge deficit of preoperative preparations

Planning and Implementation
The major goals of the patient include a reduction in anxiety, decrease of pain, absence of injury, and an understanding of the preparations for surgery.

The major goals of preoperative nursing management are to prepare the patient for surgery, reduce anxiety, and reduce pain or discomfort (when applicable).

Depending on the type of surgery, eye drops may be instilled at regular intervals the evening before and the morning of surgery. Other special orders may include an enema or laxative, a soap scrub around the eyes, hair shampoo, and a shower. If surgery is performed on an outpatient basis, preoperative preparations are done by the patient before coming to the hospital. The nurse must review the prescribed tasks with the patient or a family member to be sure they have been completed.

A tranquilizer or antiemetic may be administered 30 to 45 minutes before surgery. Patients with a detached retina received minimal physical preoperative preparations.

Anxiety. Any eye disease, injury, or operation can be upsetting and even frightening because of its possible effect on vision. Preoperative anxiety may be reduced by careful explanation of the preparations for surgery. If a patient appears extremely apprehensive, the physician is contacted.

flat on back (maybe c̄ a pillow)

Pain.   An analgesic or tranquilizer may be ordered for a patient with increased IOP.

Potential for Injury.   If a patient has decreased visual acuity and is allowed out of bed before surgery, assistance may be required with ambulatory activities as well as with preoperative preparations, such as showering and shampooing.

Knowledge Deficit.   If a preoperative instruction sheet is given to a patient in the physician's office, time is allowed for the patient or family member to read the material and ask questions. The importance of taking nothing by mouth after the time stated on the instruction sheet is stressed. If a patient is hospitalized, preoperative preparations are explained.

Evaluation

- Anxiety is reduced
- Pain or discomfort is relieved
- Shows no evidence of injury
- Verbalizes understanding of preoperative preparations

Postoperative Period

Assessment
On return from surgery, the patient's chart is reviewed for specific postoperative orders. Vital signs are taken. The eye dressing may be covered by a plastic or metal shield. The tape of the dressing is checked to make sure the dressing and shield are held in place.

Nursing Diagnosis
The number and extent of the following nursing diagnoses depend on the type of surgery performed:

- Anxiety related to anticipated results of surgery
- Pain related to surgery
- Potential for injury related to decreased visual acuity secondary to eye dressing, decreased vision in unoperated eye
- Noncompliance related to postoperative treatment modalities, physical restrictions (specify)
- Potential for infection related to surgery, contamination of eye (by patient)
- Impaired home maintenance management related to impaired ability to perform activities of daily living
- Dressing and grooming and bathing and hygiene self-care deficits related to impaired vision, restriction of physical activities
- Knowledge deficit of postdischarge treatment regimen

Planning and Implementation
The major goals of the patient include a reduction of anxiety and pain, absence of injury, compliance with

the prescribed treatment regimen, absence of infection, and an understanding of the postdischarge treatment regimen.

The major goals of nursing management include a reduction of anxiety, relief of discomfort or pain (when applicable), and a review of the physician's postoperative instructions.

Vital signs are monitored every 15 minutes until the patient is awake and responding. When awake, the patient is reminded not to touch the eye dressing. Depending on the type of surgery, the patient may not be allowed to lie on the operative side.

Mental confusion may occur during the postoperative period if the patient is elderly. Side rails are raised at all times, and the patient's mental status is assessed frequently. If a patient appears confused, is extremely restless, or attempts to remove the eye dressing, the surgeon is contacted immediately. Restraints may be necessary, but they also can increase confusion. Restlessness in an overly confused patient may indicate pain or pressure in the eye, a sign of possible hemorrhage or other complication. The nurse can help identify the problem by giving an accurate description of the pattern of the patient's movements (eg, trying to reach the eye or forehead) to the physician.

Postoperative orders for patients who have had surgery for a detached retina vary. After surgery, the patient is usually kept on complete bed rest for several days. The physician may order sandbags placed on both sides of the head for immobilization. The patient should not be turned or moved without orders. If both eyes are covered, the patient should always have a call light within reach.

After enucleation, a pressure dressing is applied to control hemorrhage, a complication of enucleation. The patient is observed carefully for any symptoms of bleeding or infection. The dressing is changed by the surgeon. Usually, the patient is allowed out of bed the day after the operation.

When healing is complete (about 2 to 4 weeks), the patient is fitted with the shell and must be taught how to insert and remove the prosthesis. Usually, the prosthesis is removed before going to bed at night and inserted the next morning. The patient is instructed to hold the head over a soft surface, such as a bed or a well-padded table, when removing or inserting the prosthesis so that the shell does not break if it is dropped. The shell is cleansed gently after removal and is kept in a safe place where it will not be scratched or broken.

Anxiety.   The patient may exhibit anxiety over the possible results of surgery. The cataract patient may be concerned with the restoration of vision and the patient with glaucoma concerned with the effectiveness of the surgery to lower IOP and reduce pain. The patient is encouraged to discuss any concerns or questions with the physician.

Depression is common after surgery for removal of an eye. No amount of explanation or reassurance erases the fact that the patient has lost an eye and that the loss is irretrievable. Most patients are gradually able to accept the result of enucleation, and they become interested in acquiring a prosthesis.

Pain.   Pain may occur after surgery for a detached retina and enucleation. Analgesics are usually ordered. Cataract surgery or surgery for glaucoma (iridectomy) is not painful, but discomfort due to the eye sutures may be experienced. If the patient had surgery for cataracts or glaucoma and experiences pain, the physician is notified immediately; pain may indicate intraocular hemorrhage or rising IOP, both of which are serious problems that require immediate medical intervention.

Potential for Injury.   Once the patient is allowed out of bed, assistance with walking may be needed, especially if the unoperated eye has decreased visual acuity.

People who have outpatient surgery are reminded to exercise care when walking, especially the first few days after surgery. People with decreased visual acuity in the unoperated eye should receive assistance from a family member until vision in the operated eye is restored.

Potential for Infection.   Pain and fever may indicate an infection. Patients discharged the day of surgery are instructed to keep the hands away from their eye and to wash the hands thoroughly before changing the eye dressing or instilling eye drops. Another source of infection may come from contamination of the eye drops when the patient is home.

Self-care Deficits, Impaired Home Maintenance Management.   Physical restrictions imposed on a patient may make it difficult to carry out normal daily activities, such as meal preparation, laundry, and shopping. People who live alone or in a household where others are unable to perform these functions require a support system to assist them. The nurse must ask if assistance is available. If help is not available, it should be discussed with the physician, and a social worker should be contacted for assistance and advice. It may be necessary for the nurse to contact friends or relatives to provide help. Services such as a home health aide or a social service agency also may be suggested.

When one eye is removed, covered with a dressing, or has limited visual acuity, the binocular vision and, therefore, depth perception are lost. The patient needs to learn to adjust to this loss of depth perception when carrying out activities of daily living. Driving an automobile, for example, requires practice and getting used to the lack of depth perception.

Knowledge Deficit, Noncompliance.   The importance of adhering to the physician's postoperative instructions is emphasized. Patients who have eye surgery are usually restricted in such activities as bending over, lifting, and driving a car. The length of time that the restrictions are imposed varies with the physician and the type of surgery.

If a patient expresses concern over the restrictions or makes statements that indicate that the recommendations would be difficult or impossible to follow, this information is reported to the physician. The patient should be told that irreparable eye damage can occur if the physician's recommendations are not followed.

Patients with detached retinas remain hospitalized and on complete bed rest for several days. Usually, they are advised to wear dark glasses for several weeks, thereby preventing the discomfort from bright light that occurs after treatment with mydriatics.

Depending on the type of surgery, one or more of the following may be included in a teaching plan. The nurse should review these instructions with the patient or family member.

1.   Avoid straining, such as straining at stool, and sudden movement or jarring of the head, which might lead to hemorrhage in the eye or opening of the incision. For patients with a repaired retinal detachment, a reoccurrence of the detachment is possible.
2.   Do not bend over or lift heavy objects (usually those over 5 pounds) until permitted to do so.
3.   Leave a night light on in the bedroom and bathroom to prevent falls and other injuries during nighttime hours.
4.   Replace the cap of the eye medication immediately after instilling the eye drops.   *photophobia*
5.   If strong light causes discomfort, wear dark glasses. (Note: On the first postoperative visit, the eye surgeon may provide the patient with dark glasses that may be comfortably worn over an eye shield or eyeglasses).
6.   Contact the physician immediately if sudden pain or a drastic change in or loss of vision should occur.
7.   Follow the physician's instructions about instilling eye drops, applying the eye shield (which may be worn all the time or only at night), not bending or lifting, and so on. If questions about any of the instructions arise, always ask the physician for clarification.

8. Patients who have had cataract surgery and a lens implant have blurred vision for a week or more, usually until corrective lenses (if needed) are prescribed. If near perfect vision is achieved with an implant, reading glasses are usually necessary. Patients who need cataract glasses or a contact lens can only see light and shadow until the contact lens or special eyeglasses are prescribed.

9. Continued follow-up by the physician is necessary. In some cases, the patient must be seen periodically for 2 or more years after surgery.

Evaluation

- Anxiety is reduced
- Pain or discomfort is relieved
- Shows no appearance of injury; asks for assistance with activities
- Shows no appearance of infection; temperature is normal
- Assistance given with activities of daily living as needed
- Verbalizes understanding of postoperative orders, physical restrictions, medication schedule, technique of eye drop instillation, importance of follow-up care
- Family or friends state willingness to assist patient at home

HEARING IMPAIRMENT

Hearing loss may be divided into two types: conductive and sensorineural (see Chapter 40, Fig. 40-4). Conductive hearing loss or conduction deafness is caused by any disease or injury that interferes with the conduction of sound waves to the inner ear. For example, an accumulation of cerumen in the external acoustic meatus or the failure of the ossicles to vibrate may cause conductive hearing loss. Sensorineural hearing loss or sensorineural deafness (sometimes called nerve deafness) results from a malfunction of the inner ear, the vestibulocochlear nerve, or the auditory center in the brain. The prognosis is better in conductive hearing loss because often its cause can be treated, for example, by removing excess cerumen from the external acoustic meatus or by performing surgery to restore the ability of the ossicles to vibrate. People with conductive deafness benefit more from the use of hearing aids because the organs that perceive sound, such as the vestibulocochlear nerve and the brain, are able to function.

Causes of sensorineural deafness include arteriosclerosis, a tumor of the eighth cranial (vestibulocochlear) nerve, infections, and drugs that are toxic to the cochlea, eighth cranial nerve, or vestibule of the ear. Examples of drugs that are ototoxic are neomycin, kanamycin (Kantrex), and gentamicin (Garamycin). Another recently identified cause of sensorineural deafness is prolonged exposure to loud music. This type of deafness is seen in musicians as well as those who listen to loud music.

Sensorineural deafness is usually irreversible and, thus far, is beyond surgical correction. Unfortunately, these patients frequently have difficulty understanding speech and, therefore, are helped to a limited degree by hearing aids. Some patients have mixed hearing loss, a combination of conductive and sensorineural elements.

Problems Associated With Hearing Impairment *Read*

Hearing loss can seriously impair people's ability to protect themselves and to communicate with others. A sound can be a warning of danger as with, for example, a smoke detector alarm or the sound of an approaching car. Listening to what others say is a vital element in all human relationships. Everyday life is accompanied by background sounds that we hear without being aware of them. Besides keeping us in tune with the world, auditory background noises serve as cues to changes that are occurring in the environment.

People with hearing impairments are sensitive to the attitudes of others. Some refuse to admit that they have the disability and, in so doing, deprive themselves of the help that they require.

The age at which hearing loss occurs, as well as the severity of the impairment, affects rehabilitation. If a person has been born deaf, education and opportunities for marriage, friendship, and career may be jeopardized unless the person is helped to learn to compensate for the impairment. Even with special training, people born deaf may have difficulty communicating with hearing people for several reasons. Most hearing people do not understand sign language, and the speech of people born deaf is often difficult to understand because they have never heard the spoken word.

People who become deaf later in life have several advantages; they have learned to speak normally, acquired an education, and may have started a home and found a job before the onset of deafness. Older people may find it difficult to adjust to loss of hearing, especially if it occurs quite suddenly. People who develop hearing impairment early in life usually become accustomed to the use of a hearing aid or acquire skill in speech reading or signing. Developing these capabilities entails considerable new learning and adaptation for older people.

Help for the Hearing Impaired *Read*

People with hearing impairments can get help in many ways. The type of help depends largely on the degree of hearing loss and the age of the person.

The seriously impaired person can learn speech reading (also known as lip reading). The term *speech reading* is preferred by many to *lip reading* because the skill encompasses not only reading lips but also noting facial expressions and gestures. People who speech read require others to face them when they speak, so that they can see the lip movements and facial expressions. Often they do not catch every word, but they understand enough to be able to follow the conversation.

For people with little or no hearing even with the use of a hearing aid, signing may be used. Signing (or sign language) is a method of spelling words as well as portraying words or ideas. Signing uses the fingers to spell out the letters of the alphabet. Signing also includes the use of standardized gestures or movements of the hands, arms, or body to indicate words such as *mother* or *I*. The person who uses signing can only communicate with those who are able to understand these finger movements or gestures. Many people use signing and speech reading simultaneously to convey their thoughts.

A newer surgical procedure called a cochlear implant has helped some people who are deaf or profoundly deaf and cannot benefit from a hearing aid. This system consists of a microphone to collect sound, a processor which amplifies and filters sound, a transmitter, and a receiver. The microphone and processor are worn externally, usually attached to the clothing. The transmitter is magnetically attached to the receiver, which has been surgically implanted in the mastoid bone. The receiver has two wires, one of which was surgically inserted into the cochlea and the other attached to nearby muscle. Although the person does not hear sounds in the same manner as a hearing person, they are able to distinguish various types of sounds and understand the speech of others. Time is required to become accustomed to the device as well as to learn to distinguish sounds.

Advancing technology has helped the deaf and hard of hearing communicate with others and understand what is being communicated. Many television programs have closed caption inserts. By means of a special converter, the conversation is printed on the bottom of the screen. Another method that allows the deaf or hard of hearing to understand the spoken word on television uses an insert in the corner of the screen where a hearing person conveys the conversation in sign language. This method usually is used for special events such as speeches, news announcements, or religious programs. These inserts do not require a special converter for the television set.

Another device for people with severe hearing impairments is a telecommunication device for the deaf (TDD). This device is a combination special typewriter and telephone. After dialing a number, the sender types a message. The receiver, who must also have this machine, is able to read the printed message on a small screen. With a TDD, two people can communicate by telephone. Businesses that have a TDD give deaf people the opportunity to place orders for merchandise by telephone. Computers also allow the deaf to communicate with one another. Both must have a compatible computer, telephone, and modem to transmit and receive messages.

Many other products allow the hearing impaired to perceive (rather than hear) sound. For example, light-activated alarms (eg, smoke detectors, alarm clocks), doorbells, and telephones flash a light when sound is produced. Hearing dogs, like seeing-eye dogs for the blind, are specially trained to warn their masters when certain sounds occur, such as doorbells, telephones, or smoke alarms.

Modern hearing aids are battery-operated sound amplifiers with a transistor circuit. Adjustable volume and tone controls are provided so that the wearer can adapt the aid to changing conditions. Some of these devices fit into the ear and are practically invisible.

Although hearing aids have helped many people, they do not restore normal hearing. In addition, time and effort are required to learn to use the hearing aid. The failure to understand these facts has led many people to become discouraged and abandon the use of the aid.

Because sound is considerably modified as it passes through the aid, it approximates—but does not duplicate—the sound that the patient remembers hearing before the hearing loss occurred. The range of tone is greatly reduced. The sounds are sufficiently similar, however, to be interpreted correctly by most patients. The aid has the disadvantage of amplifying background noise as well as the sounds the patient wants to hear. Amplified background noises are distracting, particularly to patients who have not become accustomed to the aid.

Despite these disadvantages, the modern hearing aid provides new opportunities for many people with hearing losses. Constant improvements are being made in these devices, so that they are not only less conspicuous but more efficient. Their efficiency even poses a problem in adjustment. Patients sometimes find that the sudden increase in their ability to hear is quite startling. They must become accustomed to the sounds of everyday experiences all over again.

NURSING PROCESS —THE PATIENT WHO HAS A HEARING IMPAIRMENT

Assessment
Information about the degree of hearing impairment and the methods used to understand the speech of

others is obtained from the patient or family member. The clarity and sound level of the patient's speech also are determined.

Nursing Diagnosis

Depending on the degree of hearing impairment, the length of time the impairment has been present, the age of the patient, and the methods used for communication with hearing people, one or more of the following may apply:

- Anxiety related to potential difficulty in communication with hearing people
- Impaired verbal communication related to hearing impairment, deafness since birth
- Impaired adjustment related to hearing impairment
- Social isolation related to hearing impairment
- Knowledge deficit of methods of improving hearing (hearing impaired people), instructions given by medical personnel

Planning and Implementation

The major goals of the patient include a reduction of anxiety, improved communication with others, adjustment to a hearing impairment, improved social interactions, and an understanding of the methods to improve hearing and the instructions given by medical personnel.

The major goals of nursing management are to reduce anxiety, improve communication between the patient and the medical team, and help the patient explore new avenues of communication.

The degree of hearing impairment and the methods used to communicate with hearing people are noted in the Kardex and on the front of the patient's chart. All members of the health team must be aware of the patient's hearing impairment.

Anxiety. Anxiety may result when the hearing impaired patient experiences difficulty communicating with hearing people. The best way to communicate with the hearing impaired patient is determined at the time of assessment. Shouting is seldom a help; often it confuses and embarrasses the patient.

Impaired Verbal Communication. If speech reading is used, it must be remembered that some words are more difficult to read than others. Changing the wording may help the speech reader understand what is being said. Another way to help those who use speech reading is to mention briefly and tactfully the topic of the conversation. If the patient does not understand, the thought can be restated in different words. New or unfamiliar words are pronounced with special care or written down. It must be remembered that the person speaking must always face the person who is speech reading.

Although almost all patients who sign also are able to speech read, a few patients, because of lack of training or a visual disorder, are unable to speech read. In this case, the patient is given paper and a pen or pencil. The medical team also needs to write (in large letters if the patient's vision is impaired) to communicate with the patient. If the patient is unable to write, effort is made to locate a person who understands sign language.

If the patient uses a hearing aid, the family is asked to bring it to the hospital, along with an extra set of batteries. In the stress of illness, the aid may be forgotten, and its absence can make the adjustment to the hospital all the more difficult.

To prolong battery life, many people turn off the hearing aid when they are not engaged in conversation or listening to the radio or television. Patients must be given time to adjust the device, if necessary, before speaking to them. When the patient is not wearing the hearing aid, it must be protected from loss or injury. The acutely ill patient or those scheduled for surgery should have the hearing aid given to the family until the aid can be used again.

Impaired Adjustment, Social Isolation. When unable to communicate effectively with others, for any reason, patients may have difficulty adjusting to hospitalization. When effective lines of communication are established, patients are better prepared to adjust to the changes in their environment.

The patient who has recently or gradually lost the ability to hear and who has not sought medical advice may experience difficulty adjusting to this disorder. Depression, withdrawal, and a refusal to socialize with others may be seen. The patient must be encouraged to have the hearing problem professionally evaluated and then to follow the recommendations of the physician to obtain the type of device that may improve hearing.

Knowledge Deficit. People who have recently developed a hearing impairment are encouraged to see a physician for an evaluation. The best possible results are obtained when hearing is evaluated by an audiologist or otologic clinic. It can then be determined if an aid is likely to be of benefit and what type of aid would be most useful. Mail order hearing aids or those sold by salesmen that come to the home are to be avoided.

A knowledge deficit also may occur when the hearing impaired patient does not understand the instructions of the physician or nurse. If it appears that the teaching plan may not be fully understood, a family member is included in the discharge teaching program or the material is given in writing.

Evaluation

- Anxiety is reduced
- Effective lines of communication are established between all members of the medical team and the patient
- Socializes with others
- Shows evidence of adjusting to hospitalization, recent hearing loss
- Understands instructions, points included in a teaching plan
- Patient with a recent hearing loss verbalizes need to seek medical advice

DISORDERS OF THE EXTERNAL EAR

The external acoustic meatus is subject to a variety of disorders. Usually, these are discomforts rather than threats to life or hearing. If they are not carefully and adequately treated, however, they may involve the middle ear and become serious problems.

Impacted Cerumen (Ear Wax) ✓

Some people produce an excessive amount of ear wax that eventually may partially or completely occlude the external acoustic meatus. Unskilled attempts at removing cerumen or foreign bodies may perforate the eardrum and push the material into the middle ear.

Symptoms

Symptoms include a mild to moderate hearing loss and ear pain.

Diagnosis

Diagnosis is made by inspection of the external acoustic meatus with an otoscope.

Treatment

Cerumen may be softened by instilling 1 or 2 drops of hydrogen peroxide, warm glycerin, or mineral oil. Several products on the market use a combination of agents, such as carbamide peroxide, glycerin, and triethanolamine. If these agents are ineffective, the physician may remove the wax with a cerumen spoon. Irrigation of the external canal also may be attempted, but this procedure can cause dizziness (especially if the solution is too hot or too cold) and discomfort. In addition, contamination of the middle ear is possible if the patient also has a perforated ear drum, which may not be detected if the cerumen blocks a direct view of the ear drum.

Foreign Bodies ✓

Insects occasionally enter the external ear. Although they usually fly out, they do not always.

Symptoms

Symptoms include a buzzing sound in the ear (if the insect is still alive) and a feeling of movement in the ear canal.

Diagnosis

Diagnosis is made by inspecting the ear with an otoscope.

Treatment

Holding a flashlight to the ear may draw a live insect out by attracting it to the light. A few drops of mineral oil may be effective in killing the insect; turning the head to the side may help the dead insect float out of the ear canal. If these measures are not successful, the physician needs to remove the insect with a small forceps.

Although children are usually the ones to insert foreign bodies in their ears, adults also use a variety of objects, such as toothpicks or hairpins, to remove ear wax. These objects must be removed by the physician.

Furuncle ✓

A furuncle or boil is an infection of the skin and underlying subcutaneous tissue.

Symptoms

When found in the external acoustic meatus, the symptoms include ear pain, headache, enlargement of local lymph nodes, and fever.

Diagnosis

Diagnosis is made by inspection with an otoscope.

Treatment

Treatment includes warm soaks to the side of the head and antibiotic ear drops.

External Otitis ✓ ** made go along c̄ a middle ear infection develops from the mid-ear infec.*

Infections of the external ear and adjacent skin may be caused by fungi or bacteria. The most common cause is contact with contaminated water (swimmer's ear).

Symptoms

Symptoms include pain, redness, and swelling of the affected area.

Diagnosis

Diagnosis is made by examination of the external ear structures and by otoscopic inspection of the external acoustic meatus. Culture and sensitivity studies may be performed.

Treatment

Treatment includes warm soaks, analgesics, and antibiotic ear drops (when the external canal is affected). If the pinna is involved, soaks with Burow's solution may be prescribed.

NURSING PROCESS —THE PATIENT WHO HAS A DISORDER OF THE EXTERNAL EAR

Assessment

A history of the disorder is taken. If an infectious or inflammatory disorder is present, a medical history should be obtained; some medical disorders, for example diabetes mellitus or disorders that require drugs that depress the immune system, may affect the healing process or the patient's own natural ability to fight an infection.

The external structures of the ear are inspected for signs of redness, swelling, or injury. The experienced examiner may use an otoscope to examine the external acoustic meatus for signs of infection, cerumen, or the presence of a foreign body. The temperature is taken if an infectious process is suspected.

Nursing Diagnosis

Depending on the disorder, one or more of the following may apply:

- Anxiety related to symptoms, examination, treatment
- Pain related to infection, inflammation, foreign body in the ear canal
- Hyperthermia related to infectious process
- Knowledge deficit of treatment regimen, prevention of recurrence

Planning and Implementation

The major goals of the patient include a reduction of anxiety, elimination of pain or discomfort, maintenance of normal body temperature, and an understanding of the prescribed treatment regimen and preventive measures.

The major goal of nursing management is to relieve symptoms associated with the disorder.

If irrigation or instillation of liquids is ordered, the liquid must be warm (body temperature). Cold and hot liquids can cause dizziness, and injury may occur if the liquid is hot. Ear drops may be warmed by holding the container in the hand for a few moments or by placing it in warm water. An antipyretic is usually recommended to reduce fever and discomfort.

Anxiety, Pain. Examination and treatment procedures are explained to the patient. The patient is assured that treatment relieves some or all of the symptoms.

Knowledge Deficit. If ear drops or warm soaks are prescribed, the patient is taught the procedure.

Measures to prevent recurrence may need to be explained and include one or more of the following:

1. Complete the prescribed course of treatment. Do not stop taking or using the medication even though symptoms are relieved.
2. Avoid swimming in contaminated water. Always wear soft plastic ear plugs when swimming if they have been recommended by the physician.
3. Do not insert anything into the ear canal, including cotton plugs, unless recommended by the physician as part of treatment.
4. If excessive ear wax is a continuous problem, the ears should be checked by a physician on a periodic basis.
5. Avoid the use of nonprescription remedies unless they have been approved by the physician.
6. Contact the physician if symptoms are not relieved in a few days.

Evaluation

- Anxiety is reduced
- Pain is reduced or eliminated
- Body temperature is normal; no evidence of infection
- Verbalizes understanding of treatment modalities, preventive measures

DISORDERS OF THE MIDDLE AND INNER EAR

A disorder of the middle ear may be serious because it can result in a partial or total loss of hearing. Inner ear disorders also can result in a loss of hearing. Inner ear disorders also may be distressing and, in some instances, may result in a temporary or permanent disability.

Otitis Media

Otitis media is an infection in the middle ear. The middle ear connects with the nasopharynx by way of the eustachian tube, which serves to equalize the air pressure on either side of the tympanic membrane. Upper respiratory infections spread readily from the nose and throat to the ear through the eustachian tube. Children are especially vulnerable because of the more nearly horizontal position of the eustachian tube during childhood. Adults can and do develop ear infections, however, and suffer from the same consequences of ear infections as do children. Before the development of antibiotics, ear infections often caused considerable damage to the ear. Use of antibiotics has created another problem: microorganisms are becoming resistant to them, and, for some infections, the available antibiotics are of limited benefit.

There are three types of otitis media: serous otitis media, acute otitis media, and chronic otitis media.

Serous Otitis Media   *fluid behind eardrum*

The secretory form of serous otitis media is found primarily in children. Aerotitis media, which occurs as a result of a sudden change in barometric pressure, occurs during rapid descent in an airplane or high elevator. Measures that help prevent aerotitis media include avoiding flying while suffering from a head cold and chewing gum, yawning, or repeated swallowing during descent, which open the eustachian tubes. Valsalva's maneuver, which is done by pinching the nostrils while simultaneously trying to blow air through the nose, is usually successful in equalizing the pressure on both sides of the eardrum. *popo ears*

Acute Purulent Otitis Media

This acute infection of the middle ear usually results from the spread of microorganisms to the middle ear through the eustachian tube during upper respiratory infections. Pus collects in the middle ear, causing increased pressure, which, in turn, causes bulging of the eardrum.

Symptoms ✓

Symptoms, which vary according to the severity of the infection, include fever, ear noises, malaise, severe earache, and diminished hearing. *fluid behind eardrum*

Diagnosis

Diagnosis is made by patient symptoms and otoscopic examination of the eardrum, which appears red and bulging. Sometimes it has perforated, and pus is present in the external acoustic meatus.

Treatment

Prompt treatment usually can avoid rupture of the eardrum. Rupture often causes a jagged tear that heals slowly, sometimes incompletely, and with considerable scarring. Such scarring can interfere with the vibration of the drum, causing diminished hearing. To prevent spontaneous rupture, the physician may perform a myringotomy, which is an incision into the ear drum, to allow the purulent material to drain. This eases the pressure and relieves the throbbing pain. The incision heals readily with little scarring. At first, the

discharge from the ear is bloody, and then it becomes purulent. Culture and sensitivity studies are usually obtained. A loose cotton plug may be inserted into the end of the external ear canal to collect drainage; it is changed when it is moist or as directed by the physician. The external ear must be cleaned frequently. Antibiotics are given to control the infection. Fluids are encouraged.

Complications

Complications include mastoiditis (the middle ear connects with the mastoid process by complex passages through which infection can travel), scarring or permanent perforation of the eardrum, and hearing loss. The infection also may spread to the meninges, causing meningitis, or it may become chronic (see later discussion). Other complications include labyrinthitis (inflammation of the labyrinth of the inner ear), indicated by nystagmus, vertigo, nausea, and vomiting, and lateral sinus thrombosis (spread of the infection to the large veins at the base of the brain), causing clot formation and septicemia. Infection may injure the facial nerve and cause facial paralysis. Brain abscess may result from the extension of the infection to the brain. These complications almost always occur when otitis media goes untreated. With prompt and correct treatment, complications are rare.

Patients with perforated eardrums are prone to repeated infections throughout life. Often a chronic infection develops that is difficult to cure and that spreads throughout the ear and the mastoid process.

Plastic surgery (myringoplasty) is usually successful in repairing the perforated drum. In one technique, the edges of the perforation are cauterized, and a patch of bloodsoaked Gelfoam is used as a scaffolding over which new tissues grow until they have completely filled in the defect. Repeated chronic infections, which can spread to involve the brain and can lead to loss of hearing, may be prevented if the drum can be repaired.

Chronic Otitis Media   *— where infection never really clears up!*

This preventable condition usually results from neglect, incomplete treatment of acute otitis media, or repeated attacks of acute otitis media with microorganisms that are resistant to antibiotic therapy.

Symptoms

The patient usually has a chronic discharge from the ear, a reduction of hearing, and sometimes a slight fever.

Diagnosis

Diagnosis is based on symptoms, a history of ear infections, and otoscopic examination of the ear.

Treatment

Treatment with antibiotics may effectively control the infection. When it has persisted for a long time, however, destruction occurs in the middle ear and the mastoid process. These patients have marked loss of hearing, and often they are in danger of the infection spreading to the brain. Surgery usually is recommended to eradicate the disease and to prevent further complications. Often, a radical mastoidectomy is necessary to remove the diseased tissue.

Mastoiditis

Mastoiditis is an inflammation of the mastoid process that results from an acute or chronic otitis media.

Symptoms

Symptoms include pain and tenderness behind the ear, fever, malaise, headache, and symptoms of otitis media (see earlier discussion).

Diagnosis

Diagnosis is based on a patient's symptoms, palpation of the mastoid bone, and radiography. A computed tomographic (CT) scan or magnetic resonance imaging (MRI) also may be performed.

Treatment

Treatment of the otitis media (see earlier discussion) may eliminate the inflammatory process of the mastoid. If poor response is obtained, it may be necessary to remove the mastoid bone (mastoidectomy).

Chronic mastoiditis carries a less favorable prognosis. Chronic infection in the mastoid process leads to destruction of the tissue, causing hearing loss. The infection usually involves the middle ear because chronic otitis media frequently causes chronic mastoiditis. Often, radical mastoidectomy is necessary to remove the diseased tissue. Usually, the hearing is reduced markedly because of the necessity to remove important structures.

Otosclerosis

Otosclerosis is a common cause of hearing impairment among adults. It results from bony ankylosis of the stapes, which interferes with the vibration of the stapes and the transmission of sound to the inner ear. Fixation of the stapes occurs gradually over a period of many years.

Symptoms

The hearing loss, which is more common among women, usually becomes apparent to the patient in the second and third decades of life. Heredity is an impor-tant causative factor; most patients have a family history of the disease. The underlying cause is unknown.

The progressive loss of hearing is the most characteristic symptom. The patient notices this symptom when it begins to interfere with the ability to follow conversation. The patient has particular difficulty in hearing others when they speak in soft, low tones, but hearing is adequate when the sound is loud enough. Tinnitus (a ringing or buzzing in the ears) may appear as the loss of hearing progresses. Tinnitus, which can occur in any type of hearing loss, is especially noticeable at night, when the surroundings are quiet, and can be distressing to the patient.

Diagnosis

The diagnosis is made by an otologist after noting the family history, examining the ears, and testing the hearing. Although the hearing loss in otosclerosis is of the conductive type, with progression of the disease, often involvement of the cochlea supervenes, and the hearing loss becomes a mixed type.

Treatment

Although otosclerosis has no cure, the hearing loss can be corrected by surgery and the use of a hearing aid. The potential success of surgery, as well as the ability to wear an aid, depends greatly on the severity of the sensorineural involvement; the prognosis is best when the hearing loss is purely conductive.

In a procedure known as stapedectomy, which is usually performed under local anesthesia, surgeons remove the entire stapes and replace it with a prosthetic device composed of such substances as fat, Teflon, or a vein.

The surgery is carried out using fine instruments and an operating microscope designed specifically for surgery on the ear. Once the stapes is removed, the patient, if under local anesthesia, can hear. When surgery is completed, hearing is even better.

Trauma to the Tympanic Membrane

Perforation of the tympanic membrane (ruptured ear drum) may occur because of acute otitis media, severe head injuries that result in skull fractures, foreign objects that enter the external acoustic meatus, and extremely loud noises.

Symptoms

A patient may or may not experience sharp pain at the time of rupture. Hearing loss also may be noted.

Diagnosis

Diagnosis is based on a patient's symptoms (if any) and otoscopic examination of the tympanic membrane.

Treatment

Most injuries to the ear drum heal without need for medical intervention. A large rupture may result in a permanent opening in the membrane, however, and a tympanoplasty (surgical repair of the tympanic membrane) may be performed to close the opening. This surgery may restore hearing as well as decrease the risk of contamination of the middle ear by water. If an infection was the cause, treatment is instituted.

Meniere's Disease

The cause of Meniere's disease is unknown, and the pathologic changes responsible for the symptoms are not entirely clear.

Symptoms

This condition is characterized by severe vertigo, tinnitus, and progressive hearing loss. Nausea and vomiting often accompany the vertigo. It usually involves only one ear.

An attack may last from a few minutes to weeks and may occur with alarming suddenness. Often, patients become afraid to leave their homes, lest they have an attack in public. For some patients, continued employment becomes impossible.

Diagnosis

Diagnosis is based on a patient's history of symptoms. A CT scan or MRI may be performed to rule out other possible causes of the symptoms. A complete medical and allergy history is taken.

Treatment

Symptomatic treatment includes the use of a low-sodium diet to lessen edema. Allergy to certain substances may be implicated as the cause of the disorder. Treatment of the allergy or avoidance of the allergen is recommended. Antihistamines also may be of value. Bed rest is usually necessary during an acute attack. Patients may recover spontaneously from the disorder, or they may be so incapacitated that surgery is necessary. In one type of surgery, the labyrinth is destroyed by ultrasonic waves, thus relieving symptoms. Another type of surgery establishes permanent drainage of excessive endolymph from the inner ear into the subarachnoid space.

Motion Sickness

Motion sickness (sea sickness) is an inner ear disorder that results from constant movement, usually a repetitive or a spinning motion. The rocking of a boat (repetitive) or a carnival ride (spinning) are examples of movements that may result in motion sickness.

Symptoms

Symptoms include dizziness, nausea, and sometimes vomiting, which may persist for more than an hour after the motion stops.

Diagnosis

Diagnosis is based on a patient history of activity and symptoms.

Treatment

Nonprescription drugs available for this disorder have helped some people. Others may need to use a prescription drug, such as transdermal scopolamine, which is a patch that is applied behind the ear.

NURSING PROCESS —THE PATIENT WHO HAS A DISORDER OF THE MIDDLE OR INNER EAR

Assessment

A history of symptoms and the length of time they have been present and a complete medical and allergy history are obtained. The experienced examiner may use an otoscope to inspect the tympanic membrane and external acoustic meatus.

Vital signs are taken if the patient has a suspected or known infection.

Nursing Diagnosis

Depending on the type and severity of the disorder, one or more of the following may apply:

- Anxiety related to pain, loss or decrease in hearing
- Pain related to infection
- Hyperthermia related to an infectious process
- Impaired verbal communication related to a decrease in hearing
- Self-care deficit related to vertigo secondary to a middle or inner ear disorder
- Potential for injury related to vertigo secondary to a middle or inner ear disorder
- Knowledge deficit of treatment regimen, technique of instilling medication, prevention of future infections

Planning and Implementation

The major goals of the patient include a reduction in anxiety, relief of pain, reduction of fever, improved communication, absence of injury, improved ability to care for self, and an understanding of the treatment regimen and preventive measures.

The major goals of nursing management are to relieve pain, discomfort, and other symptoms of the disorder and control the infection (when present).

If surgery is planned, see the later discussion under

Nursing Process—The Patient Undergoing Ear Surgery.

Anxiety, Pain.   Middle ear infections often cause moderate to severe pain. Until pain is decreased or eliminated with either drug therapy or surgical intervention, analgesics may be ordered.

A patient with a hearing impairment may exhibit anxiety and concern over the inability to hear. The patient is encouraged to discuss the planned treatment and the anticipated results of treatment with the physician.

Hyperthermia.   Antibiotic therapy is started if an infectious process is present. An antipyretic agent may be necessary if the temperature is elevated.

Impaired Verbal Communication.   If a hearing loss or a decrease in hearing in both ears has occurred, a patient may have difficulty communicating with others, especially if the hearing loss is sudden. Speaking slowly, clearly, and in a slightly louder voice may enable the patient to hear. If a hearing aid is being used or a hearing impairment is present, see the earlier discussion under Nursing Process—The Patient Who Has a Hearing Impairment.

Self-Care Deficit, Potential for Injury.   Inner ear disorders can cause severe vertigo, and a patient may be unable to perform the activities of daily living. Assistance is necessary in many activities because any motion (even lying still) can produce severe vertigo. These patients may require as much care as immobilized patients.

When a patient is allowed out of bed, assistance must be given; falls are not uncommon in patients with inner ear disorders that result in severe attacks of vertigo.

Knowledge Deficit.   If medication is prescribed for the outpatient, the patient or family member is taught how to instill ear drops.

Depending on the original disorder and the physician's prescribed treatment or recommendations, the following may be included in a teaching plan:

1. Follow the medication schedule and other treatments as prescribed by the physician.
2. Complete the prescribed course of therapy. Do not stop using the medication even if symptoms disappear.
3. Do not insert anything into the ear canal unless told to do so by the physician.
4. Follow-up care is necessary to be sure the infection has been eradicated.
5. If symptoms become worse or recur, contact the physician immediately.
6. For patients with a perforated tympanic membrane: Avoid getting water in the ear, take special precautions

when bathing, use custom-molded ear plugs plus a bathing cap (when recommended by the physician) during swimming or bathing, avoid swimming (when recommended by the physician).

The patient with an inner ear disorder that results in vertigo is taught the medication schedule and the importance of avoiding injuries such as falls. If a low-sodium diet has been recommended, the patient is given a list of foods that contain moderate to high amounts of sodium. If an allergy is suspected as the cause, the patient is advised to follow the recommended drug schedule and to avoid known allergens.

Patients who receive a prescription for medication to control the symptoms of motion sickness must be taught how to use the drug. Transdermal products contain instruction sheets; the patient is advised to read and follow them carefully.

If a hearing aid has been recommended, the audiologist instructs the patient in its use.

Evaluation

- Anxiety is reduced
- Pain and discomfort are controlled
- Temperature remains normal; no evidence of infection
- Communicates effectively with others; is able to understand directions, suggestions
- Self-care needs are met
- Requests assistance with ambulatory activities
- Shows no evidence of injury
- Verbalizes understanding and importance of treatment regimen, preventive measures
- Verbalizes understanding of technique of instilling ear drops

SURGERY OF THE EAR on test!

Tympanoplasty.   This reconstructive surgical procedure has several variations and may be performed to close or reconstruct a perforated ear drum, as well as to repair or restructure one or more of the ossicles of the middle ear to restore continuity of the structures. A myringoplasty is one type of tympanoplasty.

Myringotomy.   A myringotomy makes a surgical opening in the ear drum to drain an infection of the middle ear. Small tubes may be left in place to provide continuous drainage until the infection is controlled.

Stapedectomy.   This procedure removes the stapes and replaces it with a prosthetic device composed of such substances as fat, Teflon, or a vein. A stapedectomy is performed for otosclerosis.

Mastoidectomy. Through a postaural (behind the ear) incision, the surgeon removes the infected mastoid cells. Hearing impairment usually does not occur.

Radical Mastoidectomy. In this procedure, the diseased mastoid cells are removed, as well as the incus, the malleus, and the eardrum. The middle ear and the mastoid become one cavity. The stapes is left in position to protect the entrance to the inner ear. The extent of the infection determines the amount of surgery, and the more extensive the surgery, the greater the hearing loss. This operation is uncommon today because of early diagnosis and treatment of ear infections.   *results in hearing loss*

NURSING PROCESS —THE PATIENT UNDERGOING EAR SURGERY

Preoperative Period

Assessment
A history of symptoms and a medical and allergy history are obtained from the patient or family. If a hearing loss is present, the amount of loss or the ability of the patient to hear conversation is determined.

Nursing Diagnosis
Depending on the diagnosis and surgical procedure, one or more of the following may apply:

- Anxiety related to surgery, concern over the possible negative results of surgery
- Impaired verbal communication related to hearing loss
- Pain related to an infectious process
- Potential for injury related to vertigo secondary to an inner ear disorder
- Knowledge deficit of preoperative preparations, postoperative care

Planning and Implementation
The major goals of the patient include a reduction of anxiety, effective preoperative communication, a reduction of pain, absence of injury, and a knowledge of preoperative preparations and postoperative care.

The major goals of preoperative nursing management are to prepare the patient for surgery, reduce anxiety, and reduce pain or discomfort (when applicable).

Ear surgeries may be performed under local anesthesia with sedation administered before and possibly during surgery. For more extensive surgeries, such as a mastoidectomy, or for an extremely apprehensive patient, general anesthesia may be required.

Anxiety. If a patient exhibits extreme anxiety and is scheduled to have the procedure performed under local anesthesia, the surgeon must be notified *immediately*. The extremely anxious patient may not be cooperative and may not remain still (even with sedation) during surgery.

Impaired Verbal Communication. If a hearing loss is present, preoperative explanations may be misunderstood. Time must be taken to slowly explain preoperative and postoperative care.

Pain. Pain during the preoperative period may require administration of an analgesic. The type and severity of pain is recorded on the patient's chart. If pain is not controlled, the surgeon is notified.

Potential for Injury. If vertigo is present, the patient requires assistance with all ambulatory activities before surgery.

Knowledge Deficit. Preoperative preparations and immediate postoperative care are explained to the patient. When applicable, the nurse reinforces the instructions or information given by the surgeon. Postoperative instructions are especially important; the patient will be sedated or coming out of anesthesia, and activity is often restricted for about 24 hours or more after surgery.

The patient also is told that after surgery hearing may be the same as or worse than before surgery. This fact does not indicate that surgery was a failure but usually is due to the presence of packing or drainage in the external acoustic meatus.

Evaluation
- Anxiety is reduced
- Patient understands preoperative and postoperative instructions
- Pain is reduced or eliminated
- Self-care needs met during the preoperative period
- Shows no evidence of injury
- Demonstrates understanding of preoperative preparation and postoperative instructions given by the surgeon

Postoperative Period

Assessment
Vital signs are obtained, and the patient's chart is reviewed for postoperative orders. It is essential that the surgeon's orders are followed since displacement of a prosthesis, infection, or other complications could occur because of inappropriate nursing actions.

Nursing Diagnosis

Depending on the type of surgery, one or more of the following may apply:

- Pain or discomfort related to surgery
- Anxiety related to the anticipated results of surgery
- Sensory and perceptual alterations (auditory) related to surgery, packing in the external acoustic meatus, drainage, and so on
- Potential for infection related to contamination of the operative area
- Potential for injury related to vertigo secondary to surgery
- Knowledge deficit of the postdischarge treatment regimen and restrictions

Planning and Implementation

The major goals of the patient include a reduction of anxiety, relief of pain, absence of injury and infection, improved auditory perception, and an understanding of the postdischarge treatment regimen and restrictions.

The major goals of postoperative nursing management are to reduce anxiety, relieve discomfort or pain, prevent infection, and review the physician's postoperative instructions.

Postoperative instructions vary. Information about whether the patient is allowed to turn and on which side (operated or unoperated) the patient can or cannot lie is given by the surgeon in the postoperative orders.

Occasionally, oozing may be noted around the packing in the external acoustic meatus. The nurse should notify the physician if excessive drainage or bleeding occurs. The packing is not changed or added to, as pressure from an additional dressing may dislodge a prosthesis or affect the results of the surgical procedure. If fever, headache, severe pain, excessive drainage, or extreme dizziness occurs, the physician is notified immediately.

After a myringotomy, the discharge from the ear is bloody and then purulent. The external portions of the ear may be wiped with a dry sterile applicator. Cotton plugs are not inserted into the ear because the pus must drain; however, if ordered, a loose cotton plug may be inserted into the end of the external ear canal to collect drainage. The cotton plug is changed when it is moist or as directed by the physician.

Pain.   Postoperative pain is relieved by the administration of the prescribed analgesic. An antiemetic may be ordered for dizziness and nausea.

Anxiety, Sensory and Perceptual Alterations.   Blood may collect in the middle ear and cause a temporary decrease in hearing, which alarms the patient and raises questions about whether the surgery was a success. To eliminate this concern, the patient is told of the possibility before surgery. Surgical packing inserted in the external acoustic meatus canal and edema also contribute to a temporary postoperative hearing deficit.

If a stapedectomy is performed, the patient, if under local anesthesia, hears once the stapes is removed. When surgery is completed, hearing may be decreased because of the presence of packing or drainage in the external acoustic meatus. This fact also is explained to the patient during the preoperative period.

Potential for Infection.   Strict adherence to aseptic technique is essential when changing a dressing or cleaning the skin of the pinna. Because the ear is so close to the brain, any infection may endanger the patient's life. Antibiotics may be ordered to help prevent infection. Patients are instructed to keep their hands away from the dressing or packing. The external ear and surrounding skin are kept meticulously clean and free from purulent drainage. Any rise in temperature, excessive drainage, or sudden onset of pain is reported to the physician.

Potential for Injury.   Vertigo, which is due to the temporary effects on the body-balancing function of the semicircular canals, may occur. When a patient is allowed out of bed, special measures are employed to avoid injury. Side rails and handrails are used, and the patient is helped out of bed. Vertigo is distressing. It must be explained that this symptom is not unusual after ear surgery and that it gradually subsides.

Knowledge Deficit.   A discharge teaching plan is based on the type of surgery and the individual preferences of the surgeon. The prescribed medical regimen and restrictions given by the physician are discussed with the patient or family member. One or more of the following may be included in a teaching plan:

1. Avoid blowing the nose because this action may dislodge the prosthesis, loosen the eardrum before healing has taken place, or may result in infectious matter being blown into the eustachian tube to the middle ear.
2. Avoid high altitudes or flying.
3. Do not lift heavy objects, strain when defecating, or bend over at the waist; these activities increase pressure in the middle ear.
4. Do not get water in the ear. Swimming, showering, and washing the hair are avoided.

5. When recommended by the physician, place an ear plug (a small piece of cotton) in the external acoustic meatus after the packing is removed. The cotton is gently placed in the outer ear canal and never pushed into the ear. Change the ear plug as directed by the physician.

6. Wash the hands thoroughly before cleaning the outer ear or changing the ear plug. Do not touch the dressings except when changing the ear plug.

7. Avoid exposure to people with infections, especially upper respiratory infections. Should a head cold occur, contact the physician immediately.

8. Notify the physician immediately if severe pain, excessive drainage (of any kind), a sudden loss of hearing, or fever should occur.

The restricted activities recommended by the physician must be adhered to until the physician states they may be resumed.

Evaluation

■ Pain, nausea, or other discomforts are controlled or absent
■ Anxiety is reduced
■ Verbalizes understanding of temporary decrease in hearing
■ Temperature is normal; no evidence of infection
■ Shows no evidence of injury; seeks assistance when getting out of bed
■ Verbalizes understanding of postoperative medical regimen and restrictions

General Nutritional Considerations

☐ A low-sodium diet may be prescribed for the patient with Meniere's disease. A list of the foods that are and are not allowed must be given to the patient.

☐ Meniere's disease may be caused by an allergy to certain foods. Once the offending allergens are known, the patient requires a list of foods that should be avoided.

General Pharmacologic Considerations

☐ Before any drug is instilled into the eyes or ears, the label *must* be checked. Any drug instilled into the eye must be labeled as "ophthalmic" or "for use in the eyes." Any drug instilled into the ear must be labeled as "otic" or "for use in the ears." The labels also must be checked for drugs stored on the eye or ear tray.

☐ The patient with glaucoma must avoid any drug that contains atropine. The patient is advised to check with a physician or pharmacist before using any nonprescription drug.

☐ The advantage of using long-acting eye drops, such as echothiophate iodide (Phospholine), in the treatment of glaucoma is that they need be instilled only once or twice per day, thereby increasing patient compliance.

☐ Sympathomimetics, such as epinephrine and dipivefrin (Propine), dilate the pupil, relax the ciliary muscle, and reduce the manufacture of aqueous humor. These drugs may be given along with a miotic drug in the treatment of glaucoma.

☐ Miotic drugs in ophthalmic form may be used to treat glaucoma. These drugs constrict the pupil and pull the iris away from the drainage channels.

☐ The β-adrenergic blocking agents timolol maleate (Timoptic), betaxolol HCl (Betoptic), and levobunolol HCl (Betagen Liquifilm) appear to lower IOP by decreasing the production of aqueous humor. These drugs do not change the size of the pupil or affect visual accommodation.

☐ The use of nonprescription eye drops may disguise a more serious eye condition. Approval of a physician for the use of these products (for tired eyes, itching of the eye, redness of the eye) should be obtained.

☐ External acoustic meatus disorders may be treated with antibiotics in the form of ointment or drops.

☐ The microorganisms responsible for middle ear infections may be resistant to some antibiotics. The patient should be encouraged to contact the physician if the infection does not appear to improve.

□ Treatment of Meniere's disease may include drugs used for motion sickness, such as dimenhydrinate (Dramamine). Various other drugs, such as antihistamines, diuretics, and sedatives, also may be used.

□ The drugs used for motion sickness may have undesirable adverse effects, such as dry mouth and drowsiness.

General Gerontologic Considerations

□ Visual and hearing changes can result in accidents and injuries to the elderly patient. It is most important that these patients be assisted, as needed, in the activities of daily living.

□ The safety of the elderly patient with visual impairment is essential. The room should be dimly lit at night, objects that may cause falls or other injuries (eg, chairs, footstools) are placed away from areas where the patient walks, and assistance is given whenever the patient is out of bed.

□ Activities such as reading, watching television, and engaging in hobbies or other forms of recreation may be curtailed because of visual impairment, resulting, possibly, in depression and withdrawal.

□ The elderly person with a hearing impairment may become disoriented and confused in strange surroundings. Frequent contact and reassurance may prevent confusion.

Suggested Readings

□ Boyd-Monk H, Steinmetz C. Nursing care of the eye. Norwalk, CT: Appleton & Lange, 1987. *(Additional coverage of subject matter)*

□ Boyd-Monk H. Eye trauma: a close-up on emergency care. RN 1989;52:22. *(Additional coverage and illustrations that reinforce subject matter)*

□ Carver J. Cataract care made plain. Am J Nurs 1987;87:626. *(Additional coverage of subject matter)*

□ Gruendemann BJ, Meeker MH. Alexander's care of the patient in surgery. 8th ed. St Louis: CV Mosby, 1987. *(In-depth coverage of subject matter)*

□ Hahn K. . . . About sensory loss. Nursing '89 1989;19:97. *(Additional coverage of subject matter)*

□ Norris RM. Common sense tips for blind patients. Am J Nurs 1989;89:360. *(Additional coverage of subject matter)*

□ Wieck L, King EM, Dyer M. Illustrated manual of nursing techniques. 3rd ed. Philadelphia: JB Lippincott, 1986. *(Additional and in-depth coverage of subject matter)*

The Gastrointestinal Tract and Accessory Structures

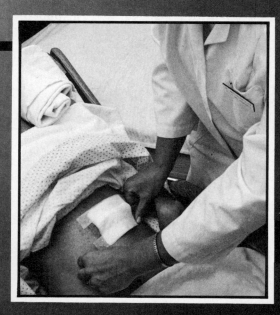

Unit 10

Chapter 42

Introduction to the Gastrointestinal Tract and Accessory Structures

On completion of this chapter the reader will:

- Be familiar with the basic anatomy and physiology of the gastrointestinal tract and accessory structures

- Know the basic principles of a physical assessment of the patient with a gastrointestinal disorder

- Discuss the common tests used for diagnosing gastrointestinal disorders

- Use the nursing process in preparing a patient for undergoing diagnostic testing for gastrointestinal disorders

The gastrointestinal (GI) tract may be arbitrarily divided into two sections: the upper GI tract and the lower GI tract. The upper GI tract begins at the mouth and ends at the jejunum. The lower GI tract begins at the ileum and ends at the anus. The accessory structures of the GI tract include the liver, gallbladder, peritoneum, and pancreas. Figure 42-1 is a diagram of the GI tract.

ANATOMY AND PHYSIOLOGY
Gastrointestinal Tract

Mouth. Food normally enters the GI tract by way of the mouth, where it is chewed (masticated) before swallowing. Food that contains starch undergoes partial digestion when mixed with the enzyme salivary amylase, which is secreted by the salivary glands.

Esophagus. The esophagus begins at the base of the pharynx and ends at the opening between the stomach and the esophagus. This muscular, tubular structure transports food to the stomach by the action of peristalsis.

Stomach. The opening between the stomach and the esophagus is called the *cardiac orifice*; that between the stomach and the duodenum is called the *pyloric orifice*. Both of these openings are controlled by sphincters that, when contracted, close the orifice. When the sphincters relax, the orifice opens, permitting the contents to flow to the next structure.

The stomach stores food and prepares it by mechanical and chemical action to pass in semiliquid form into the small intestine. Gastric juice that contains digestive enzymes is secreted continuously, but the amount of secretion increases when food is eaten. Gastric juice is acidic because it contains hydrochloric acid. The contractions of the stomach mix the food with the gastric juice and by peristalsis move the mixture of semiliquid food and digestive juice to the small intestine. The length of time required for the stomach to empty depends on the amount and the composition of the food eaten. For example, fats delay stomach emptying.

Small Intestine. The small intestine is divided into three portions: the *duodenum,* the *jejunum,* and the *ileum.* The greatest amount of digestion and absorption of nutrients takes place in the jejunum and ileum. Peristalsis moves the contents through the small intestine.

The duodenum, the first region extending from the pylorus to the jejunum, contains the openings for the common bile and pancreatic ducts. It is about 10 inches long. The jejunum, the second portion of the small intestine, is contiguous with the duodenum and the ileum. Most digestion, which begins in the mouth

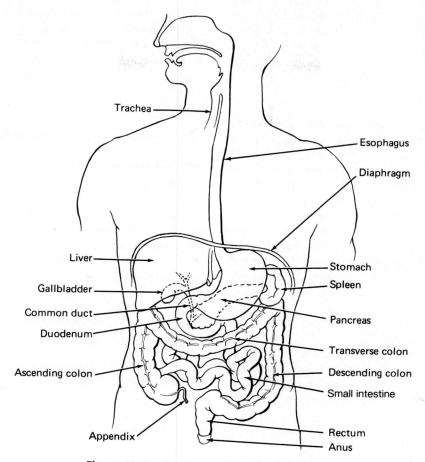

Figure 42–1. Diagram of the gastrointestinal tract.

and continues in the stomach, and absorption of food takes place in this portion of the small intestine. The ileum, the longest portion of the small intestine, ends at the beginning of the large intestine. The jejunum and ileum combined are about 23 feet long. Most of the absorption of nutrients occurs in the ileum.

Cecum. The cecum is a pouchlike structure at the beginning of the colon, or large intestine. The ileocecal valve between the end of the ileum and the cecum opens and closes to allow fecal matter to pass from the small to the large intestine. At this point, the fecal matter is liquid. The appendix is a narrow blind tube located at the tip of the cecum. It has no known function in humans.

Colon. The colon is divided into three parts—the ascending, transverse, and descending colon. Water is absorbed as the fecal stream is moved through the colon by peristalsis. By the time the fecal mass reaches the descending colon, it is more formed.

The material that moves through the large intestine is composed of food residues, microorganisms, digestive juices, and mucus that is secreted in the large intestine and aids in moving the feces toward the anus. Water normally is absorbed from the stool while it is in the colon.

Rectum. The rectum is a storage place for fecal matter. The fecal mass is stored here until defecation takes place. Distention of the rectum initiates the urge to empty its contents.

Anal Canal and Anus. The anal canal is the terminal structure of the rectum. The internal anal sphincter, which is controlled by the autonomic nervous system, normally is closed. Once the rectum becomes distended, the sphincter opens.

The external anal sphincter, which is controlled by the conscious mind, also normally is closed but opens to permit expulsion of the rectal contents (defecation).

Accessory Structures

Peritoneum. The peritoneum is a sac that lines the abdominal cavity. The walls of the digestive organs normally prevent the gastric and intestinal contents from escaping outside the lumen of the digestive tract. The intestine contains many microorganisms, and any perforation that allows material to seep out of the digestive tract is serious because the microorganisms will cause severe infection of surrounding tissues, primarily the peritoneum.

Liver.   The liver, the largest glandular organ in the body, normally weighs between 1 and 1.5 kg (2 and 3 lb). It is located in the right upper abdomen just under the right diaphragm, which separates it from the right lung. The liver has two major lobes, right and left, and two small lobes, the caudate and quadrate lobes, located on the undersurface. It is supported by intraabdominal pressure as well as by various attachments called *ligaments,* or *mesenteries.* These attachments connect the liver to the adjacent intestines, abdominal wall, and diaphragm. Unless it is abnormally enlarged, the liver usually is not felt when the abdomen is palpated.

The liver receives arterial blood from the hepatic artery, an indirect branch of the aorta. The portal vein transports blood from the intestinal tract to the liver. After it has traversed vascular pathways inside the liver, the blood is collected by the hepatic veins and transported to the inferior vena cava and then back to the heart.

Microscopically, the internal structure of the liver includes smaller ramifications of the hepatic artery, the hepatic and portal veins, the lymphatics, and the bile ducts. The cellular constituents of the liver are the hepatic parenchymal cells, which carry out most of the liver's metabolic functions, and the Kupffer, or reticuloendothelial, cells, which engage in the immunological, detoxifying, and blood-filtering actions of the liver.

The liver is involved in a multitude of vital, complex metabolic activities. Among the most important functions are the formation and excretion of bile; the use, transformation, and distribution of vitamins, proteins, fats, and carbohydrates; the storage of energy-yielding glycogen; the synthesis of factors needed for blood coagulation, including prothrombin and fibrinogen; the detoxification of endogenous and exogenous chemicals (including drugs), bacteria, and foreign elements that may be harmful; and the formation of antibodies and immunizing substances, including gamma-globulin.

Gallbladder.   The gallbladder is attached to the midportion of the undersurface of the liver. It normally has a thin wall, and a capacity of about 60 mL of bile. Bile formed in the liver enters the intrahepatic bile ducts and travels to the common hepatic duct. Then it usually passes into the cystic duct and is stored in the gallbladder. When required, the gallbladder empties its bile, which goes out of the cystic duct, into the common bile duct, and on into the duodenum. Stones can be found in any portion of the biliary system, but they are most frequently found in the gallbladder. Arteries, veins, and lymphatics are associated with all sections of the biliary tree and, along with the ducts themselves, are subject to considerable variation.

The liver forms up to 1 L/day of bile. On reaching the gallbladder, bile is altered by the absorption of water and minerals to form a more concentrated product. On reaching the intestine after gallbladder contraction (stimulated by ingested food, especially fats), bile functions in the absorption of fats, fat-soluble vitamins, iron, and calcium. Bile also activates the pancreas to release its digestive enzymes as well as an alkaline fluid that may neutralize stomach acids that reach the duodenum.

Pancreas.   The pancreas is a gland that has two major functions. As an endocrine organ, it produces the hormone insulin, which maintains the blood sugar level and is secreted directly into the bloodstream. As an exocrine organ, it produces a variety of protein-, fat-, and carbohydrate-digesting enzymes. These do not enter the bloodstream directly, but instead enter the ducts of the pancreas and eventually are released into the lumen of the duodenum, where they act directly on arriving food. By a complex interplay of chemical and nervous stimuli, the pancreas is activated by ingested foods to release its enzymes at the appropriate time for most efficient digestion.

ASSESSMENT OF A PATIENT WHO HAS A DISORDER OF THE GASTROINTESTINAL TRACT OR ACCESSORY STRUCTURES

Patients with GI disorders have a wide variety of health problems that involve disturbances in ingesting and digesting food, absorbing nutrients, and eliminating waste products from the GI tract.

Gastrointestinal problems may be caused by physical or emotional factors. Many GI disturbances cannot be neatly classified as emotional or physical in origin; these illnesses seem to stem from both psychological and physiologic malfunctions, which tend to interact.

Patient History

The extent of the patient history may be based on the chief complaint as well as an initial evaluation of the patient's general condition. The nurse should obtain a thorough patient history to identify the possible cause of the disorder as well as possible relations to other factors.

The following areas may be included in the patient history.

Symptoms. A complete history of all symptoms, the length of time the symptoms have been present, and what (if anything) appears to cause or be related to the symptoms should be noted. If pain is or has been present, the exact location should be determined.

History. A history of all past medical and surgical disorders and the treatment of each should be obtained. A family history should include the general health as well as illnesses of all family members (spouse, children, parents, and siblings). A work history, including the type of work and the physical location of employment, should be noted. The patient also should be questioned about any exposure to environmental toxic wastes or hazards or any known exposure to radiation or radioactive materials.

Ingestion, Digestion, and Elimination. This part of the history includes any problems associated with chewing and swallowing foods, any symptoms that occur during or after meals, and the color of the stool and the frequency and type of bowel movements.

Diet. A dietary history includes a list of foods that appear to cause any type of problem, such as nausea, vomiting, pain, or diarrhea. If the patient has had a sudden onset of nausea, vomiting, or diarrhea, it is important to know which foods were eaten and where in the past 24 hours. Any drastic changes in food intake with regard to the type or amount of food also are noted.

Allergy History. A complete allergy history should be obtained, including possible allergy to certain foods, as food allergies can result in various disorders of the GI tract.

Drug History. A list of all prescription and nonprescription drugs should be obtained, including the name of the drug, the dose, the frequency, and the reason for taking the drug.

Weight. The patient should be questioned regarding any weight gain or loss within the past year. If there has been a weight change, the patient should be asked if any method was used to gain or lose weight, or if weight loss was due to anorexia.

Physical Examination

Depending on the patient's symptoms and general physical condition, a complete or partial physical assessment may be performed. Physical appraisal also includes measurement of vital signs and weight.

General Appearance. The patient's general appearance should be evaluated with regard to evidence of pronounced weight loss, breathing pattern, emotional attitude, and mental status.

Skin. Using normal sunlight, the skin should be inspected for any abnormal color, such as jaundice. If the skin is jaundiced, the eyes should be checked to see if the sclerae are yellow. The skin of the face and abdomen should be inspected for other abnormalities, such as spider angiomas (red discolorations, actually a form of superficial skin tumor, consisting of blood vessels that assume a spider-shaped pattern), or scars.

Oral Cavity. The lips should be examined for sores, cracks, lesions, or other abnormalities. Using a tongue blade and a flashlight, the mouth should be examined for inflammation, sores, swellings, tumors, or other abnormalities. The teeth should be inspected for evidence of good or poor oral care, and the condition of the teeth and gums, the absence of teeth, and the presence of partial plates, bridges, or dentures should be noted. The patient should be questioned regarding the ability to chew food. If dentures are worn, the patient should be asked if they fit well and whether regular food can be eaten. If the patient can eat only soft foods, this should be noted on the Kardex.

Esophagus. Examination of the esophagus necessitates questioning the patient about the ability to swallow solid foods or liquids, any difficulty in swallowing, or pain or discomfort associated with swallowing. If the original complaint included regurgitation of food or burning in the chest or below the sternum, the patient should be questioned regarding any relief from or worsening of symptoms when position changes (eg, sitting upright or lying down) are made.

Stomach. The patient should be questioned regarding any pain in the area immediately below or to the left or right of the sternum. If pain or other symptoms appear to be related to the stomach, additional questions, such as those related to the type of foods eaten and when the symptoms occurred, should be asked.

Gallbladder. Gallbladder disorders can give rise to pain or discomfort in the area of the stomach or the gallbladder. The location of the pain or discomfort should be noted. The patient also should be questioned regarding when the pain occurs and if it appears related to meals or certain types of food.

Liver. The liver normally is not palpable. In certain disorders, the liver may be felt as extending below the right lower rib cage. Pain or discomfort in this area may be indicative of a liver disorder, but it also may indicate other GI disorders, such as gallbladder or intestinal disease. The experienced examiner may attempt to palpate the lower liver margin.

Pancreas. Diseases of the pancreas may produce a variety of symptoms. Pain in the midline above the umbilicus, pain in the middle of the back, and digestive disturbances may indicate a pancreatic disorder.

Abdomen. Using a stethoscope, the abdomen should be auscultated for the presence or absence of bowel sounds. The quality, pitch, and frequency of bowel sounds should be noted. The girth of the abdomen may be measured using a measuring tape placed at the iliac crest. The abdomen may then be palpated for areas of pain or tenderness and the presence of masses. The contour of the abdomen should be evaluated while the patient takes a deep breath. The exact location of any asymmetry should be noted.

Anus. The anal area should be examined for evidence of external hemorrhoids. The surrounding skin should be inspected for breaks, rash, inflammation, infection, and other abnormalities.

Diagnostic Tests

The diagnostic tests commonly used in disorders of the GI tract include radiographic studies, magnetic resonance imaging (MRI), computed tomographic (CT) scan, ultrasonography, endoscopy, nuclear imaging, biopsy, and laboratory tests.

Radiographic Studies. An radiograph of the abdomen may be ordered to note the approximate size of the liver or to detect the presence of air, fluid, tumors, or foreign objects in the abdominal cavity. A chest radiograph may be ordered to detect any upward displacement of the diaphragm or lungs by an abdominal disorder, such as fluid, tumors, or air.

Barium Swallow and Upper Gastrintestinal Series. Sometimes the terms *barium swallow* and *upper gastrointestinal series* are used interchangeably. A barium swallow is the fluoroscopic observation of the act of swallowing barium. An upper

GI series includes a barium swallow plus fluoroscopic or radiographic observation of the barium moving down the esophagus into the stomach. The barium normally leaves the patient's stomach about 6 hours after ingestion. Additional radiographs may be taken to check whether any barium remains in the stomach after this time. An upper GI series is used to identify abnormalities in the esophagus, such as tumors, strictures, or varices, peptic ulcer in the stomach or duodenum, gastric tumors, and hiatal hernia.

Small Bowel Series. This group of radiographs follows the movement of the swallowed barium through the small intestine, and may be used to identify disorders such as tumors, inflammation, and obstruction in the small bowel.

Barium Enema (Lower Gastrointestinal Series). Barium is given by enema in the radiology department. The patient is asked to retain the barium while films are taken. A barium enema is used to identify polyps, tumors, strictures, and other lesions of the colon.

A laxative and enemas usually are given by the nurse before the procedure, to cleanse the bowel of feces. The number of enemas, the type of solution, the times specified for their administration, and the type of laxative vary in different hospitals.

Oral Cholecystography (Gallbladder Series). Oral cholecystography is used to identify stones in the gallbladder or common bile duct and tumors or other obstructions of the gallbladder, as well as determine the ability of the gallbladder to concentrate and store dye. A radiopaque dye is taken orally in tablet form the evening before the examination, after which the patient is kept in a fasting state. After ingestion, the dye reaches the liver, is excreted into the bile, and passes into the gallbladder, making it radiographically visible. A fatty test meal may be given after initial radiographs are taken, to determine the ability of the gallbladder to empty. After eating the meal, the patient is returned to the radiology department for additional films.

Cholangiography. Cholangiography is essentially the same as oral cholecystography and is performed for the same reasons. The difference between these two tests is that instead of the dye being ingested in tablet form, it is given intravenously (IV cholangiography). It is either injected directly into the common bile duct or injected through a T tube immediately before radiographs are taken. IV cholangiography may be performed in the radiology department or may be used during surgery on the gallbladder, at which time the dye is injected directly into the common bile duct.

Postoperatively, the dye also may be injected into the T tube to determine patency of the biliary system.

Computed Tomography and Magnetic Resonance Imaging. A CT scan or MRI may be performed to detect lesions of the GI tract, and may be done before or after other radiographic studies, such as an upper GI series. These tests often are helpful in detecting metastatic lesions that might not be apparent on regular GI radiographs.

Ultrasonography (Ultrasound). In ultrasonography, high-frequency sound waves are passed through the body and then recorded. Organs such as the liver and pancreas may be outlined as the sound waves are bounced back off these structures.

Nuclear Imaging. In nuclear imaging, a radioactive isotope is injected intravenously or ingested orally, and a scanner is placed over the organ to be examined. The scanner picks up and records radioactive emission from the organ. A scan may be performed to detect lesions of the liver and pancreas, and demonstrates the size of the organ as well as defects or lesions such as tumors.

Biopsy. A biopsy may be performed during endoscopy to obtain a sample of the tissues of the GI tract. The liver also may be biopsied by means of a needle inserted through the chest wall. A local anesthetic is injected before insertion of the needle. The tissue sample is then examined by a pathologist.

Endoscopy. Endoscopy is the examination of organs through a flexible fiber-optic instrument passed through one of the body openings. This type of examination permits direct visualization of a section of the lining of the GI tract. A biopsy also may be performed at this time. Endoscopy may be performed to detect abnormalities such as inflammation, ulceration, and superficial lesions.

The following endoscopic procedures frequently are used in examination of the GI tract:

Esophagoscopy—Visualization of the esophagus
Gastroscopy—Visualization of the stomach
Endoscopic retrograde cholangiopancreatography—Radiographic and visual examination of the pancreatic ducts and radiographic examination of the hepatobiliary tree after insertion of an endoscope and injection of a dye
Sigmoidoscopy—Visualization of the sigmoid colon, the rectum, and the anus
Proctoscopy—Visualization of the rectum and the anus
Anoscopy—Visualization of the anus

The instruments used are named according to the procedures performed with them. All areas through which the scope passes are examined; therefore, sigmoidoscopy includes examination of the anus and the rectum as well as the sigmoid colon.

Laboratory Tests

Gastric Analysis. A nasogastric tube is inserted into the stomach for the purpose of obtaining a sample of gastric fluid for analysis, which is sent to the laboratory for examination. This test may be performed to diagnose gastric carcinoma and pernicious anemia, as well as determine the amount of fluid retained in the stomach in those with suspected or known obstruction of the pylorus or duodenum.

Stool Examination. One or more samples of stool may be sent to the laboratory and examined or tested for the presence of blood as well as ova and parasites. A culture and sensitivity test also may be performed on a stool sample.

Other Laboratory Tests. Depending on the suspected or known diagnosis, various blood and urine tests may be ordered. Examples of laboratory tests are a complete blood count; urinalysis; serum bilirubin, cholesterol, ammonia, protein electrophoresis, and enzymes, such as amylase and lipase; and prothrombin time.

NURSING PROCESS —THE PATIENT UNDERGOING DIAGNOSTIC TESTING FOR A GASTROINTESTINAL DISORDER

Assessment
A patient history should be obtained and may direct the examiner to the area or areas that require more detailed investigation and examination. Some radiopaque contrast media contains iodine. If the allergy history reveals a possible or known history of iodine allergy, the physician should be informed and the cover of the patient's chart labeled with this information.

Physical assessment of one or more areas of the GI tract should be performed when indicated by information obtained during the patient history. Vital signs should be and the patient weighed.

Nursing Diagnosis
Depending on the presenting symptoms, the condition of the patient, and other factors, nursing diagnoses in addition to the following may be necessary:

- Anxiety related to possible diagnosis, diagnostic tests
- Pain during or after a diagnostic procedure

■ Knowledge deficit of the diagnostic procedure, preparation for the procedure

Planning and Implementation

The major goals of the patient include reduction of anxiety, elimination of pain or discomfort, and an understanding of the purpose and preparation for a diagnostic test.

The major goal of nursing management is to prepare the patient for diagnostic testing.

Patient Preparation.   Proper preparation of the patient is essential. The procedure may need to be canceled or repeated because of failure to complete or properly carry out the required preparations. Because hospital and physician guidelines for patient preparation vary, the hospital procedural manual or the physician's orders should be consulted. The following are some possible measures that may be necessary to prepare the patient for diagnostic testing:

1. Fasting may be required for some laboratory tests, upper GI series, and cholecystography.
2. Enemas and laxatives may be ordered for colonoscopy, sigmoidoscopy, barium enema, and cholecystography. Enemas and laxatives may be given the night before and the morning of the test to remove gas and fecal material from the bowel, thus ensuring adequate visualization of the area being examined.
3. Special diets may be required for some diagnostic tests, for example a clear liquid diet for 24 hours before a colonoscopy or a high-fat meal after initial radiographs are taken of the gallbladder (oral cholecystography).
4. The radiopaque dye given for some studies may contain iodine. Patients who are scheduled for any study in which iodine is used should be carefully questioned regarding iodine allergy and allergy to seafood (which contains iodine). The hospital procedural manual should be consulted regarding those tests using iodine, in tablet or injectable form, as part of the diagnostic procedure. If the patient admits to an iodine allergy, or an iodine allergy is suspected, the physician should be notified, as the test may need to be canceled. All patients who take tablets that contain iodine before a diagnostic procedure should be observed for symptoms of iodine allergy (eg, nausea, vomiting, diarrhea, hypotension, and soreness or pain in the parotid glands). The appearance of these symptoms should be reported immediately.
5. Oral cholecystography requires that tablets that contain a radiopaque substance be administered the evening before the test.
6. A sedative may be given before some diagnostic procedures (eg, an endoscopic procedure). The sedative should be given at the exact time ordered so that the patient is relaxed and cooperative.

Postprocedure Management and Observations.   Nuclear imaging, CT scan, MRI, laboratory tests, plain film radiographic studies, ultrasonography, and cholecystography require no special postprocedure care.

Some tests require a series of radiographs at spaced intervals. When the patient returns to the unit from the radiology department, it is important to determine whether the test has been completed or further films are necessary. If additional films are necessary, the patient should be returned to the radiology department at the appropriate time.

After a liver biopsy, the patient should be instructed to lie on the right side for 2 or 3 hours. Vital signs should be monitored every 15 to 30 minutes, or as ordered, and the patient observed for signs of shock and internal bleeding.

Whenever an endoscopic procedure has been performed, with or without a biopsy, the patient should be observed for signs of possible perforation of the examined area. The vital signs should be monitored every 15 minutes for 2 to 4 hours and then hourly for 4 hours. Depending on the type of endoscopic procedure performed, the presence of any of the following signs and symptoms requires contacting the physician immediately: severe pain, vomiting of blood, bright red bleeding from the rectum, difficulty breathing, or a drop in blood pressure and a rise in pulse. If the endoscope was introduced through the mouth, fluids should be withheld until the gag and swallowing reflexes return.

If barium was introduced into the GI tract, provision should be made for its prompt elimination. Retained barium can become a hard mass that could cause intestinal obstruction or an impaction in the anus or rectum. A laxative or enema often is ordered after the procedure and fluids are encouraged. After barium has been given, it should be noted whether the barium has been passed and whether the patient is having regular bowel movements. The patient should be informed that the stool will appear light in color for a few days.

Anxiety, Fear.   Fear of the unknown often creates moderate to severe emotional responses. The general purpose and type of test and how it will be performed should be explained. For example, if the patient is scheduled for an upper GI series, the purpose of the test can be explained as a method of outlining and looking at the upper part of the GI tract.

Pain.   The discomforts associated with some of these tests are a long fasting period, the length of time required for the test, the awkward positions that must be assumed, and lying on a hard x-ray table. Elderly patients especially may experience difficulty during and after the test. Although it may not be possible to eliminate discomfort, the radiology department should be informed if the patient has a physical problem such as arthritis. Radiology personnel may be able to use pillows, blankets, or other measures to relieve the patient's discomfort.

Knowledge Deficit. Some diagnostic tests for GI disorders are performed on an outpatient basis. Also, some tests, such as a CT scan, MRI, and ultrasonography, require no special preparation other than a general explanation of the test. The procedure and the equipment to be used should be explained to the patient, and when applicable, the patient should be informed that the procedure is not painful.

One or more of the following points may be included in an explanation of a diagnostic test:

OUTPATIENTS

Date and time of the test and where to report for the test
When applicable, review of the preparations for the test
(which usually are given in printed form) to be sure the patient understands what is to be done before the examination
Importance of patient compliance to avoid cancellation or a repeat of the test

HOSPITALIZED PATIENTS

Explanation of preparations for the test
Review of each preparation (eg, enema or special diet) at the time it is carried out

Evaluation

■ Anxiety is reduced
■ Pain or discomfort is reduced or eliminated during and after the test
■ Patient and family demonstrate an understanding of the preparations required for the test

General Nutritional Considerations

☐ Diagnostic tests for the detection of disorders of the GI tract may require a special diet, such as a liquid or low-residue diet, before the test. The diet should be reviewed with the patient. The importance of following the recommended preparation should be stressed.

☐ Patients who are to undergo upper GI tract radiographic examinations, esophagoscopy, gastroscopy, or other studies that require fasting may experience hunger. The importance of fasting should be explained. An appetizing lunch should be available for the patient as soon as the tests are completed.

General Gerontologic Considerations

☐ Radiographic examinations can be tiring, especially for weak and aged patients. Besides fasting, they must assume various positions on the x-ray table while the series of films is being taken.

☐ Elderly patients may forget the instructions for a diagnostic test. Printed directions should be given to the outpatient and, when possible, reviewed with a family member.

Suggested Readings

☐ Alfaro R. Applying nursing diagnosis and nursing process: a step-by-step guide. 2nd ed. Philadelphia: JB Lippincott, 1990. *(Additional coverage of subject matter)*
☐ Alltop SA. Teaching for discharge: gastrostomy tubes. RN November 1988;51:42. *(Additional and in-depth coverage of subject matter)*
☐ Bates BA, Hoekelman RA. Guide to physical examination and history taking. 4th ed. Philadelphia: JB Lippincott, 1987. *(In-depth coverage of subject matter)*
☐ Becker KL, Stevens SA. Performing in-depth abdominal assessment. Nursing '88 June 1988;18:59. *(Additional coverage of subject matter)*
☐ Memmler RL, Wood DL. The human body in health and disease. 6th ed. Philadelphia: JB Lippincott, 1987. *(Additional coverage of subject matter)*
☐ Memmler RL, Wood DL. Structure and function of the human body. 4th ed. Philadelphia: JB Lippincott, 1987. *(Additional coverage of subject matter)*
☐ Smith CE. Assessing bowel sounds. Nursing '88 February 1988;18:42. *(Additional coverage of subject matter)*
☐ Smith CE. Assessing the liver. Nursing '85 July 1985;15:36. *(Additional coverage of subject matter)*

Chapter 43

Disorders of the Upper Gastrointestinal Tract

On completion of this chapter the reader will:

■ Use the nursing process in the management of the patient with anorexia, anorexia nervosa, bulimia, or obesity

■ Discuss the treatment of nausea and vomiting

■ Use the nursing process in the management of the patient with nausea and vomiting

■ Name and discuss the purpose of a gastrostomy and the various types of nasogastric tubes

■ Use the nursing process in the management of the patient with gastrointestinal intubation

■ Use the nursing process in the management of the patient with a gastrostomy

■ List and discuss the symptoms, diagnosis, and treatment of cancer of the oral cavity

■ Use the nursing process in the management of the patient having surgery for cancer of the oral cavity

■ List and discuss the symptoms, diagnosis, and treatment of esophageal diverticulum, hiatal hernia, and cancer of the esophagus

■ Use the nursing process in the medical and surgical management of the patient with an esophageal disorder

■ List and discuss the symptoms, diagnosis, and treatment of gastritis, peptic ulcer, stress ulcer, and cancer of the stomach

■ Use the nursing process in the medical and surgical management of the patient with a gastric disorder

EATING DISORDERS
Anorexia

Anorexia is a common problem related to the gastrointestinal (GI) tract. Although occasional short-lived periods of anorexia caused by emotional stress may be experienced by most people, prolonged periods of anorexia can have serious consequences. Anorexia may be related to the effects of a drug (eg, an appetite suppressant or a drug that causes anorexia as an adverse effect) or to such factors as emotional stress, fear, psychological problems, and terminal illnesses.

Treatment
Management of the patient with anorexia depends on the reason for the anorexia, if known. Short-term anorexia usually requires no medical intervention. Persistent anorexia may require a variety of approaches, such as a high-calorie diet, high-calorie interval feedings, tube feedings, total parenteral nutrition, and psychiatric treatment.

Anorexia Nervosa

A severe form of anorexia, anorexia nervosa is a psychiatric condition that occurs most commonly in women under age 30. When this disorder persists, it ultimately results in severe malnutrition and weight loss because the patient refuses to eat adequate amounts of food. People with anorexia nervosa have a bizarre preoccupation with eating, coupled with a morbid fear of being fat. Even though these patients may appear extremely emaciated, they see themselves as being fat. During discussions, they often express concern over their weight. Even when confronted with facts that prove that they are not fat, they refuse to believe that these facts are correct.

The cause of anorexia nervosa is unknown, although it is thought to occur because of conflicts with one or both parents, society's strong emphasis on being thin, some unexplained biologic factor, or other unknown elements.

Treatment
If weight loss and malnutrition are severe, the patient is admitted to a hospital. Treatment of anorexia nervosa includes the administration of fluids and electrolytes by a central or peripheral intravenous line or by a nasogastric tube. Some hospitals have opened special units for the treatment of this disorder. Treatment on a general hospital unit often is unsuccessful, as these patients require constant supervision and a low nurse/patient ratio.

If left untreated, or if treatment fails to correct the problem and the patient returns to poor eating habits, death may result from cardiac failure, electrolyte imbalances, or hypothermia.

Bulimia

Bulimia is the practice of binge eating followed by self-induced vomiting, starvation, or crash dieting, prolonged vigorous exercise, or the use of large doses of laxatives immediately after an eating binge. Although considered a separate disorder, bulimia may be seen in those with anorexia nervosa and is more common in women than in men.

In these patients, the consumption of a large amount of food (binge eating) usually occurs in private, the food often is high in calories and carbohydrates, and a large amount is consumed in 2 or fewer hours. Binge eating is terminated by the abdominal pain resulting from eating, by interruption (discovery by others), by sleep, or by self-induced vomiting.

After the binge, these patients become depressed over their behavior, and resort to measures aimed at getting rid of the food (eg, self-induced vomiting, fasting, or the use of laxatives).

Although some people practice bulimia occasionally, the condition becomes serious when the patient engages in this activity at frequent intervals. Frequent episodes can produce severe weight loss, and laxative use, starvation, and crash diets can result in electrolyte imbalances and dehydration.

Treatment

Management of bulimia includes psychotherapy, group therapy, behavior modification techniques, and the administration of antidepressants. Severe malnutrition is treated the same as for anorexia nervosa.

Obesity

Just as some people lose their appetites when they are under emotional stress, others overeat. Some people find that eating helps them to relax when they feel nervous and upset. Others, by overeating, may strive to make up for the lack of certain pleasures and satisfactions. Still others overeat because of habit. Some obese people alternate between stringent, nutritionally inadequate reducing diets and overeating. The exact reason why a person overeats is not always clear.

Treatment

With the increased emphasis on slimness, weight-reduction programs have been developed to help people with eating disorders. Although some programs follow good nutritional guidelines for the adjustment of eating habits, others advertise rapid weight reduction that requires strict adherence to an extremely low-calorie diet. Some people may be able to physically tolerate severe calorie restriction, but this method may be dangerous for others. In addition, some programs sell products, such as vitamin and mineral supplements

and foods, that are promoted as necessary when following their dietary program. Other diet plans sell all the food that is to be consumed by the person; still others use a diet plan combined with an exercise program.

People who want to lose weight through a commercial diet program should be encouraged to first discuss this approach to weight reduction with their physicians. Nonprescription diet aids also should be avoided, unless their use has been approved by the physician. Some nonprescription diet aids contain drugs that can raise the blood pressure and heart rate. Others use indigestible cellulose fiber to give the feeling of fullness. Still others use a combination of products (eg, vitamins, minerals, protein, and cellulose). Because hypertension as well as other medical disorders may accompany obesity, these products may not be safe for everyone.

The treatment of obesity is best conducted under the supervision of a physician. A weight-reduction diet usually is recommended, and the physician may prescribe an appetite suppressant for the first several weeks of the weight-reduction program.

Before a weight-reduction diet is prescribed, the patient should have a thorough physical examination. Diagnostic tests also may be ordered, if it is believed that the obesity may be due to a physical disorder, such as hypothyroidism.

If obesity cannot be corrected by conservative medical management and the patient is extremely overweight (morbid obesity) with accompanying problems that pose a threat to health, surgical intervention may be considered. The surgical procedures that may be used include the following.

Lipectomy. This procedure involves the surgical removal of fat from such areas as the breasts, hips, thighs, and abdomen. Suction lipectomy, or liposuction, is the removal of adipose tissue by suction through small incisions made in the skin. This procedure also has been used for cosmetic reasons and is not confined to the treatment of morbid obesity.

Jaw Wiring. Although the jaw may be wired for other reasons, such as fractures of or surgery on the mandible, this procedure may be used as a temporary measure to restrict food intake to fluids.

Gastric Stapling (Gastric Partitioning, Gastroplasty). This surgical procedure reduces food intake by stapling the stomach. In this procedure, staples are placed near the upper portion of the stomach (Fig. 43-1), leaving an open channel for the passage of food. If desired, the staples can be removed at a later date, but removal does require abdominal surgery.

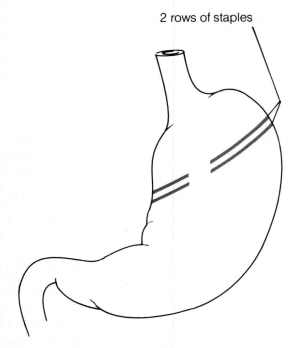

2 rows of staples

Figure 43–1. Gastric stapling procedure. A small channel remains for the passage of food.

Bypass Procedures. Several surgical bypass procedures have been used to correct morbid obesity. One, a gastric bypass, reduces food intake by making the stomach smaller, much like gastric stapling. Another uses the technique of bypassing a major portion of the small intestine, thereby reducing the amount of digested food that is absorbed.

The surgical approach for the correction of morbid obesity is not without dangers. Bypass procedures can result in malnutrition, vitamin deficiencies, and electrolyte imbalances. The skin of an obese person heals poorly, creating problems with the healing of the surgical incision. In addition, the obese person always poses a surgical risk, regardless of the type of surgery, and complications such as pulmonary embolus and pneumonia may occur.

NURSING PROCESS —THE PATIENT WHO HAS ANOREXIA, ANOREXIA NERVOSA, OR BULIMIA

Assessment

A complete medical and allergy history should be obtained from the patient or a family member. A dietary history, including a description of the patient's eating patterns, is most important. It should be remembered that the patient with any type of eating disorder may give an inaccurate or incomplete dietary history. The weight, height, and vital signs should be taken.

Nursing Diagnosis

Depending on the length of time the eating disorder has been present, as well as other factors, one or more of the following nursing diagnoses may apply:

■ Activity intolerance related to severe weight loss, electrolyte imbalance, decreased blood glucose levels, anemia
■ Altered nutrition: less than body requirements related to anorexia, self-induced vomiting, or laxative use
■ Potential fluid volume deficit related to self-induced vomiting, laxative use
■ Constipation related to decreased food and fluid intake, inactivity
■ Diarrhea related to decreased food intake, use of laxatives
■ Body image disturbance related to inaccurate perception of self as obese
■ Impaired skin integrity related to loss of subcutaneous fat and dry skin secondary to malnutrition
■ Impaired social interaction related to fear of discovery, mistrust, fear, and possibly unknown factors
■ Ineffective individual coping related to such factors as fear, mistrust, inappropriate use of defense mechanisms, unknown factors
■ Knowledge deficit of reasons for eating disorder, treatment regimen, dangers associated with eating disorder

Planning and Implementation

The major goals of the patient include increase in activity tolerance, improved nutritional intake, normal bowel elimination, correction of a fluid volume deficit, effective coping mechanisms, acceptance of (actual) body image, achievement of normal weight, prevention of skin breakdown, improved social interactions, and a knowledge of the treatment regimen.

The major goals of nursing management are to help these patients understand their eating problem and to teach them what may be done to gain weight.

The treatment of severe eating disorders often results in failure. Although positive short-term results may be attained, long-term results often are disappointing.

Nursing management of these patients can be frustrating for several reasons. It is difficult to understand why these patients continue in the firm belief that they are fat. In addition, they may appear to cooperate with their medical care, but once discharged from the hospital, they return in several months for treatment of the same problem. It also is difficult to see these patients die of a disorder that can be "cured" by something as simple as eating.

Activity Intolerance. The patient should be allowed time to complete the activities of daily living as well as rest between activities, as fatigue is a common problem. The patient may show disinterest in the activities of daily living and may need to be encouraged to take an interest in personal care and grooming.

Altered Nutrition, Potential Fluid Volume Deficit. A careful record of the food and fluid intake should be kept. Patients with anorexia nervosa may attempt to hide food while claiming that it has been eaten; patients with bulimia may offer excuses to go to the bathroom so that they can induce vomiting. Because of these activities, the intake and output record may be inaccurate. It should be remembered that questions asked about food that is eaten, water intake, and bowel movements may not always be answered truthfully.

When feeding measures such as the administration of intravenous fluids and nasogastric feedings are used, the patient should be under constant observation, as attempts may be made to remove the intravenous line or the nasogastric tube.

These patients should be closely observed for signs of electrolyte imbalance, dehydration, and cardiac, respiratory, and renal problems.

Constipation, Diarrhea. A record of bowel movements should be kept. Like the record of food and fluid intake, this, too, may be inaccurate. Constipation or diarrhea should be reported to the physician.

Body Image Disturbance. The nurse should listen to these patients and accept their comments about their weight. For most of these patients, individual or group psychotherapy sessions are necessary to restore a concept of their real self, that is, emaciated, not fat, bodies.

Impaired Skin Integrity. The skin, especially over bony prominences, should be inspected daily for signs of skin breakdown and decubitus ulcer formation. The patient should be encouraged to be out of bed as much as possible.

Impaired Social Interaction. Many of these patients are withdrawn and interact poorly with others. Attempts to encourage social interactions may or may not be successful. An attempt should be made to discover those activities that the patient likes and then provide situations in which the patient can interact with others.

Ineffective Individual Coping. These patients usually are totally preoccupied with their concept of being fat and how they can reduce their food intake, and ignore other problems or situations. They fear and mistrust others, and their thinking may be paranoid. Although extreme malnutrition may effect thinking, a psychiatric overlay is probably present. Psychotherapy, behavior modification, and social rehabilitation may be included in the therapeutic regimen.

The nurse should accept these patients, strive to gain their confidence, help them to work through their problems, and, above all, understand that this is an illness that must be treated.

The family and its structure often are strained. Family counseling, with or without the patient, is an important part of therapy.

Knowledge Deficit. The family often has a difficult time accepting and understanding eating disorders. Although there are many unanswered questions regarding these disorders, careful explanation of the possible causes and the short- and long-term treatment modalities may help the family to understand and deal with the situation. The patient, on the other hand, often is not willing to accept explanations regarding the possible causes or why treatment is necessary.

Evaluation

- Increased activity is tolerated
- Patient performs activities of daily living without assistance
- Patient increases food intake and gains weight
- Fluid or electrolyte imbalances are absent
- Elimination pattern is normal
- Patient begins to accept self as thin and not fat
- Skin remains intact
- Patient begins to socialize and interact with others
- Patient cooperates with treatment regimen
- Family demonstrates knowledge, understanding, and acceptance of eating disorder

NURSING PROCESS —THE OBESE PATIENT

Assessment

A complete medical and allergy history should be obtained from the patient or a family member. The dietary history should include the types of foods eaten, food preferences, previous attempts at weight loss, and previous enrollment in weight-loss programs. It may be important to determine the average amount and types of food eaten per day. The dietitian may be contacted to assess the patient's dietary habits, thus obtaining a more accurate account of the average daily calorie intake and eating profile.

Nursing Diagnosis

Depending on the individual patient, the degree of obesity, and other factors, one or more of the following nursing diagnoses may apply:

- Activity intolerance related to marked obesity
- Altered nutrition: more than body requirements because of depression, poor dietary habits, unknown factors
- Body image disturbance related to obesity
- Constipation related to dietary indiscretions, use of prescription or nonprescription weight-loss products or drugs
- Diarrhea related to dietary indiscretions, surgery, use of (some) weight-loss products
- Impaired social interaction related to morbid obesity, activity intolerance, disturbance in self-concept, other factors
- Knowledge deficit of treatment regimen, dangers associated with obesity

Planning and Implementation

The major goals of the patient include increase in activity tolerance, balanced nutritional intake, normal bowel elimination, effective coping mechanisms, attaining and maintaining normal weight, prevention of skin breakdown, improved social interactions, and a knowledge of the treatment regimen.

The major goals of nursing management are to help these patients understand their eating problem and to teach them what may be done to lose weight.

The obese patient must want to lose weight. When admitted to the hospital for a surgical procedure for obesity, planning should include short- as well as long-term weight-reduction and weight-maintenance goals. Before surgery, these patients should be evaluated by the physician with regard to their desire to follow a calorie-restricted diet after surgery.

If surgery is performed to reduce eating (and therefore calorie intake), postoperative management of these patients is the same as for those having gastric surgery (see Nursing Process—The Patient Undergoing Surgery for a Gastric Disorder later in this chapter).

Activity Intolerance. The person who is markedly obese often finds that any activity may result in shortness of breath, dizziness, and fatigue. Activities should be spaced so that the patient is able to complete them without undue discomfort. The extremely obese patient may require assistance with ambulation, grooming, and other activities.

Altered Nutrition. The obese patient requires instruction in maintaining a low-calorie diet. Depending on the medical history, type of surgery per-formed (if any), and other factors, a 600- to 800-calorie diet may be prescribed. A consultation with the dietitian helps the patient to understand the prescribed diet and how to read labels and compute calories.

Body Image Disturbance, Impaired Social Interactions. Some overweight patients accept their appearance, but others have difficulty dealing with their weight problem. Depression, lack of social activities, inability to participate in certain activities, and a low self-image often accompany obesity. Each patient should be approached differently. Often talking to someone who has lost weight, either by a physician-supervised diet or by a surgical procedure, gives emotional support and reinforces the desire to stick to a diet.

Constipation, Diarrhea. Intestinal bypass procedures often cause the patient to have frequent liquid stools, which may persist for many months after surgery. This condition poses additional short- and long-term problems with hydration, electrolyte imbalances, and vitamin deficiencies. Other patients may experience constipation caused by either a change in their eating habits or medications prescribed by the physician.

A record of bowel movements should be kept. Constipation or diarrhea should be reported to the physician.

Knowledge Deficit. A problem encountered with surgery for obesity is the need for these patients to readjust their eating habits, which is something they were not able to do before surgery. The nurse should work with the patient and family, the physician, and the dietitian in the dietary management of obesity. Patients who use a restricted-calorie diet to lose weight should thoroughly understand how to follow the diet. Fad diets should be discouraged, and the importance of eating a well-balanced, nutritious, low-calorie diet emphasized. The patient who requires surgery for morbid obesity requires intensive teaching regarding the dietary plan that will need to be followed after surgery.

Evaluation

- Increased activity is tolerated
- Patient demonstrates a strong desire to lose weight
- Patient adheres to a weight-reduction diet
- Patient socializes with others
- Elimination pattern is normal
- Patient demonstrates understanding of dietary management of obesity

NAUSEA AND VOMITING

Nausea and vomiting are common problems related to the GI system. If either continues long enough, weakness, weight loss, nutritional deficiency, dehydration, and electrolyte imbalances may result.

Some of the more common causes of nausea and vomiting include drugs, infections of the GI tract, intestinal obstruction, systemic infections, central nervous system lesions, food poisoning, emotional stress, and uremia.

Treatment

Sometimes the condition is short-lived and does not require medical intervention. In some instances, intravenous fluids, electrolyte replacement, and drug therapy may be necessary.

Elimination of the cause includes a variety of interventions ranging from stopping a drug to surgical intervention for intestinal obstruction. Symptomatic relief may be achieved by administering an antiemetic agent and intravenous fluid and electrolyte replacement, and by not allowing the patient to have anything by mouth until the cause can be eliminated. Serum electrolyte levels may be measured to determine the electrolyte status.

NURSING PROCESS —THE PATIENT WHO HAS NAUSEA AND VOMITING

Assessment

In addition to the assessments performed on the patient with a GI disorder (see Chapter 42), a complete medical, dietary, drug, and allergy history should be taken. A list of symptoms that occur before as well as along with the nausea and vomiting, the length of time the problem has been present, and the frequency, color, and amount vomited also are obtained. Because the cause may be unknown, a list of foods eaten in the past 24 hours and where the food was eaten also should be obtained.

The patient's general appearance should be noted and vital signs taken. The patient should be assessed for signs of a fluid volume deficit (see Chapter 12).

Nursing Diagnosis

Depending on the condition of the patient, one or more of the following nursing diagnoses may apply:

■ Anxiety related to symptoms, potential diagnosis
■ Altered nutrition: less than body requirements related to nausea and vomiting
■ Fluid volume deficit related to prolonged vomiting and decreased intake of oral fluids

Planning and Implementation

The major goals of the patient include reduction of anxiety, improved nutrition, and normal fluid intake.

The major goals of nursing management are eliminating the cause, if possible, and providing symptomatic relief. Antiemetics should be administered as ordered, and their effectiveness noted. If the drug fails to relieve symptoms, the physician should be informed.

Vital signs should be monitored every 4 hours. More frequent monitoring may be necessary if the patient is acutely ill or vomiting has been prolonged. Intravenous replacement fluids should be given as ordered.

Anxiety.   Some antiemetics also have a mild tranquilizing effect, thus helping to relieve some of the anxiety associated with the symptoms and discomfort. The patient should be observed at frequent intervals, and the emesis basin emptied and the bedding changed as needed. The room should be kept free from odors.

Altered Nutrition, Fluid Volume Deficit.   If vomiting is severe, intravenous fluids may be ordered. The patient should be observed for signs of electrolyte imbalances. Because a severe electrolyte depletion can be life-threatening, the physician should be contacted immediately if symptoms of an imbalance occur.

Once nausea has passed and oral fluids are tolerated, the patient should be given clear liquids hourly in small amounts. Other liquids that may be used are broth and carbonated beverages.

Dry, unsalted crackers and toast should be gradually added to the diet. If the nausea and vomiting remain controlled, the dietary intake should be gradually increased to include solid foods that are nonirritating to the stomach. Spicy foods, coffee, fried foods, and highly acidic foods should be avoided until all symptoms have disappeared and then added to the diet in small amounts. Meals should be small and served frequently, rather than as three large meals per day.

Intake and output should be measured, and the physician informed if urine output falls below 500 mL/day. Skin turgor and the oral mucous membranes should be assessed for signs of fluid volume deficit.

Evaluation

■ Anxiety is reduced
■ Oral fluid intake is increased
■ Patient is able to eat and retain small amounts of food

- Daily total of urine output is within normal range
- Serum electrolyte levels are within normal range
- Evidence of dehydration is absent; skin turgor is normal

GASTROINTESTINAL INTUBATION

Gastrointestinal intubation is the insertion of a tube into the stomach or intestine by way of the mouth or nose. The purposes of this procedure are as follows:

- To prevent and treat postoperative distention caused by gas or fluid, particularly after abdominal surgery
- To administer liquid feedings and medications
- To remove accumulated contents of the GI tract when there is obstruction in the tract
- To empty the stomach before emergency surgery or after the swallowing of poisons
- To withdraw specimens of gastric contents for diagnostic purposes
- To treat a disorder of the esophagus or stomach (eg, bleeding ulcer or esophageal varices)

Gastrointestinal decompression is the emptying or draining of the contents of the stomach or the intestines. If intestinal decompression is necessary, a special tube is used; it is longer, and has a device that facilitates its passage along the intestinal tract.

The contents of the GI tract are withdrawn by suction. When suction is continued for an extended period, a mechanical device is used that can be adjusted to continuously provide the amount of suction specified by the physician. Wall suction outlets also are used, and this type of suction eliminates excess equipment at the patient's bedside. If the withdrawal of gastric contents is to be carried out over a brief period, such as when specimens are obtained for diagnostic purposes, the suction is applied by attaching a syringe to the end of the tube and drawing back on the plunger.

Kinds of Tubes

There are several types of GI tubes. The type most commonly used for gastric decompression is the nasogastric (nose/stomach), or Levin, tube (Fig. 43-2). This tube has a single lumen, usually is plastic, and has holes in several locations near its tip to permit withdrawal of stomach contents.

Another type of nasogastric tube is the gastric sump tube (Salem, VENTROL). This tube has a double lumen and permits continuous suction, rather than the intermittent suction used with the Levin tube. The opening to the second lumen usually is a pale-colored

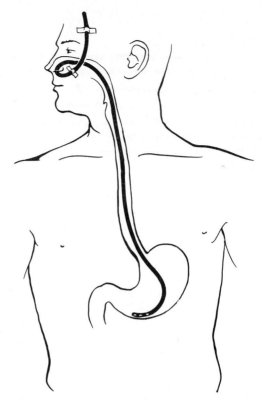

Figure 43–2. A nasogastric tube in place. The tube is used to aspirate gastric contents or to convey liquids to the stomach.

plastic, rather than the clear plastic of the main lumen. The second lumen is left open unless ordered otherwise; it allows a small amount of air to be drawn in when the nasogastric tube is connected to suction. This type of tube decreases the possibility of the stomach wall's adhering to and obstructing the tube openings.

The Miller-Abbott and the Cantor are nasoenteric (nose/bowel) tubes that can be used for intestinal intubation and decompression. They are longer than the nasogastric tube and contain devices that facilitate the passage of the tube along the intestinal tract. The Miller-Abbott tube has a double lumen (a tube within a tube; Fig. 43-3). One tube has a balloon at the tip; the other has holes near the tip. After the tube has passed through the pylorus, the balloon is inflated with mercury, water, or air and then propelled along the intestinal tract by peristalsis, carrying the rest of the tube with it. The weight of the mercury helps to propel the tube along the intestinal tract. The intestinal contents are sucked back through the holes.

Because the Miller-Abbott tube has two lumina, each with a separate opening, it is important to correctly identify each lumen. The end of the tube that remains outside the patient's body has an adapter on it. The

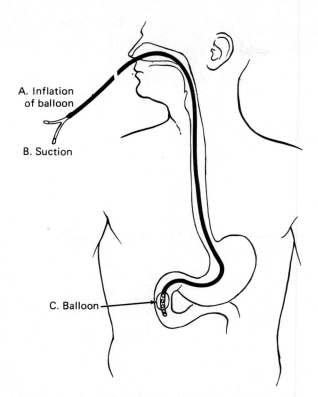

Figure 43–3. A Miller-Abbott tube in place. It is advanced through the intestines to the prescribed point. The Miller-Abbott tube has a double lumen. (*A*) Portion of the metal tip leading to the balloon. (*B*) Portion of the metal tip leading to the lumen that can be suctioned. (*C*) Balloon inflated with air.

adapter has two openings—one for suction and the other leading to the balloon. The latter is used by the physician to inflate the balloon, and should be labeled so that it is never connected to suction nor has irrigating solutions instilled into it.

The Cantor tube has just one lumen and a bag on the end, into which mercury is inserted (Fig. 43-4). The mercury is injected directly into the bag with a needle and syringe before the patient is intubated. The mercury remains in the bag because the needle does not make an opening large enough to permit the escape of the mercury. The bag is elongated when the tube is inserted, so that it can be passed more easily and with less discomfort to the patient. Because the Cantor tube has only one lumen, there is only one opening at the end outside the patient's body, and therefore no confusion can result about which opening to use for suction and which for irrigation.

The Harris tube is a single lumen tube weighted with mercury that is used for suction and irrigation. A Y tube may be attached to the end of the Harris tube, with one end connected to suction and the other clamped until it is used for irrigation. When the tube is irrigated, a clamp is placed over the suction tube.

NURSING PROCESS —THE PATIENT WHO HAS GASTROINTESTINAL INTUBATION

Assessment

In addition to the assessments performed on the patient with a GI disorder (see Chapter 42), the initial assessment should include a review of the patient's chart to determine the purpose of the GI tube. A flashlight should be used to inspect both nostrils to determine which nostril should be used for insertion of the tube, as some people have a deviated septum, with one side being more open than the other.

Vital signs should be taken. If the tube is being inserted for the administration of nasogastric feedings, the patient should be weighed.

Nursing Diagnosis

Depending on the patient's diagnosis and condition, the type of tube inserted, and the length of time the

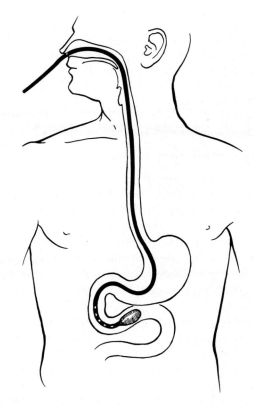

Figure 43–4. A Cantor tube in place. This intestinal tube ends in a bag that is filled with mercury to help it pass along the gastrointestinal tract to the point prescribed by the physician. Intestinal tubes are not taped in place until they have advanced fully. The holes for suctioning are behind the balloon.

tube is left in place, one or more of the following nursing diagnoses may apply:

- Anxiety related to anticipation of the procedure, discomfort of the procedure, diagnosis
- Fluid volume deficit related to continuous GI decompression
- Altered nutrition: less than body requirements related to inadequate oral intake of food and fluids
- Constipation related to liquid tube feedings, other factors (specify)
- Diarrhea related to liquid tube feedings, lack of bulk in the diet, other factors (specify)
- Impaired physical mobility related to connection of GI tube to suction apparatus
- Bathing/hygiene and dressing/grooming self-care deficits related to impaired physical mobility, diagnosis, discomfort
- Altered oral mucous membrane related to mouth breathing, restriction of oral fluids

Planning and Implementation

The major goals of the patient include reduction of anxiety, improved oral intake of food and fluids, normal bowel function, improved mobility, improved ability to carry out activities of daily living, and elimination of oral mucous membrane irritation.

The major goals of nursing management are keeping the patient as comfortable as possible and ensuring effective functioning of a GI decompression unit. When a nasogastric tube is used to provide nutrition, the goals of management also include meeting the patient's nutritional needs.

The patient's position should be changed and deep breathing encouraged every 2 hours. Vital signs should be monitored every 4 hours or as ordered. The temperature should be taken rectally, as mouth breathing may give an inaccurate reading.

When a GI tube is connected to suction, proper functioning of the unit must be maintained (see Chart 43-1).

Nasogastric Tube.
For insertion of the nasogastric tube, the patient usually is placed in a sitting position. Screening is important in preventing embarrassment because some gagging and expectoration are likely to occur. A large towel or plastic apron should be used to protect the gown and the bedding, and tissues made available for wiping the nose and the mouth. An emesis basin should be kept nearby. The patient should be instructed to relax as much as possible and to swallow when asked. A water-soluble lubricant is used to facilitate insertion. The patient usually is allowed to have a few sips of water through a straw while the tube is being passed. Swallowing water while the tube is being passed eases insertion of the tube.

Chart 43–1.   Checklist for Proper Functioning of Gastrointestinal Decompression Tube and Equipment

- ☐ Check tape on nose for secure anchoring and reapply as needed.
- ☐ Check entire external section of nasogastric tube for kinks, obstruction by mucus, or large blood clots.
- ☐ Check electrical function of machine: switch in "on" position, correct negative pressure setting, electrical cord firmly plugged into wall outlet. If nonelectric wall suction is used, check to be sure it is firmly seated in the wall outlet.
- ☐ Check drainage collection bottle for tight seal.
- ☐ Check glass or plastic connector between the nasogastric tube and machine tubing for tight fitting.
- ☐ Check for possible additional factors that may interfere with the function of the nasogastric tube or suction equipment: obstruction of the nasogastric tube lumen (which may require irrigation of the tube or slight withdrawal of the tube); coughing up of the tube; incorrect insertion of the tube; electrical cord problems; machine malfunction.*

---

* If electrical malfunction is suspected, a new machine sould be obtained. The machine in question should be inspected and repaired only by an electrician or a repair service representative.

After insertion of a tube for GI decompression, the tube is taped to the face to support the tube and to make the patient more comfortable. The tube is then attached to suction. After the desired amount of suction is achieved, it is important to maintain suction and note whether fluids are being drawn out of the GI tract by watching the flow through the adapter to the drainage bottle. Drainage dripping into the collection bottle also can be observed. If the suction does not seem to be operating satisfactorily, the equipment should be checked for proper functioning. Abdominal or gastric distention caused by failure of the suction can have serious consequences; for example, it may cause strain on the suture line in postoperative patients.

The physician may order irrigation of the tube to keep it patent. Before irrigating the tube, the following should be determined:

- Whether the physician has ordered the irrigations (they are not done routinely)
- How much solution is to be used, and how often the irrigation is to be done
- What solution is to be used
- Whether the procedure requires clean or aseptic technique

Harm can be done by improper irrigation. Injecting too much solution can cause distention, with strain on sutures. The irrigating solution should be injected with an Asepto syringe, or with a syringe that has been fitted with an adapter, so that it can be inserted tightly into the tube. After the fluid has been injected, it is aspirated with the syringe. The amount returned, as well as the amount injected, should be noted. The irrigating solution that is not aspirated should be suctioned into the drainage bottle. The amount of irrigating solution that is not removed immediately should be noted. At the end of the day, this amount should be totaled and then subtracted from the total amount of fluid in the drainage bottle.

When a nasogastric tube is used for the administration of tube feedings, the liquid usually is allowed to enter the tubing by gravity flow. In some instances, continuous feeding is given with a volumetric controlled pump mechanism. When intermittent feedings are ordered, 1 to 2 oz of water may be added before the feeding (depending on hospital policy) to ensure patency of the tube. After completion of the feeding, 1 to 2 oz of water also is added to clean the tube.

When GI decompression or nasogastric tube feeding is terminated, the tube is gently withdrawn. Nasogastric tubes can be withdrawn quickly, whereas intestinal tubes are first deflated—the water, air, or the mercury *must be removed before the tube is withdrawn*. Intestinal tubes are removed gradually, several inches at a time; some resistance to removal of the tube is felt, and removal is never forced.

A great deal of mucus usually is secreted because of the irritation caused by the tube. Tissues should be available to remove the excess secretions.

Intestinal Tube. After its insertion for intestinal decompression, the tube's course through the tract is followed by a series of radiographs and fluoroscopy. The physician orders the patient placed in various positions to facilitate passage of the tube through the pylorus and into the intestine. After the tube has passed through the pylorus, the physician may recommend that the patient walk about at the bedside to increase peristalsis and, therefore, help pass the tube along the intestinal tract. The specific time intervals and the desired positions are ordered by the physician in accordance with observations of the position of the tube by radiographic and fluoroscopic examinations.

The intestinal tube should never be taped to the patient's face or pinned to the bedding while it is being advanced through the intestinal tract because these fastenings would prevent the tube from being carried along the tract. The extra length of tubing is left coiled on the bed. When the tube has reached the desired location in the intestinal tract (for example, when it has passed to the point just above an obstruction), then it may be taped to the patient's face.

If peristalsis is not adequate to propel the tube (a condition that occurs in paralytic ileus), the weight of the mercury at the end of the Cantor tube helps it to pass through the intestines by gravity. With these exceptions, the management of a patient with an intestinal tube is essentially the same as for a patient with a nasogastric tube.

Anxiety. Passage of a nasogastric tube into the stomach is, for most patients, an unpleasant experience. Intestinal tubes that have a balloon on the end are especially uncomfortable to swallow. While the tube is in place, the patient is constantly aware of this foreign body that partially obstructs the nose and makes the nostril and throat feel irritated and sore. Most patients treated by intubation are permitted nothing by mouth. This restriction, plus the mouth breathing to which the patient often resorts, dries the oral mucous membranes.

Discomfort may be minimized by a brief explanation of the procedure and what is to be done as the tube is being passed. Most patients respond better if they know what to expect and what is expected of them.

Fluid Volume Deficit, Altered Nutrition. The large quantities of fluids lost during GI decompression must be replaced parenterally. A record of intake and output is necessary so that the need for parenteral fluids can be accurately determined. The total amount of fluid administered, as well as the amount of urine output and the amount of drainage obtained by GI decompression, should be recorded every 24 hours. The type of drainage should be noted and recorded, and specimens of any unusual drainage saved for the physician. The drainage bottle should be washed thoroughly each time it is emptied.

Whenever fluid is administered through a nasogastric tube, the placement of the tube should be determined *before* giving the feeding. If the nasogastric tube is in the trachea and not in the stomach, the fluid will enter the lungs.

One of two methods may be used to determine proper tube placement. The first is to insert a small amount of air (about 10 mL) into the tube with a bulb syringe while using a stethoscope placed over the stomach area to hear the bubbling of air. The second method is the aspiration of the tube. If the tube is in the stomach, liquid will appear in the syringe.

The patient is kept in semi-Fowler's position during and after the tube feeding. While the solution is flowing in by gravity, the patient should be continually observed for nausea, vomiting, and the regurgitation of the formula. After administration of the feeding, the nasogastric tube should be securely clamped.

The patient should be observed for signs of electrolyte imbalance (see Chapter 12). The physician may order periodic electrolyte determinations. In some instances, lost electrolytes will need to be replaced.

Constipation, Diarrhea.　Episodes of constipation or diarrhea should be brought to the attention of the physician. Patients who are receiving tube feedings may require a change in the formula to eliminate this problem.

Impaired Physical Mobility, Bathing/Hygiene and Dressing/Grooming Self-care Deficits.　Patients with GI decompression attached to suction require assistance with their activities of daily living. Some patient may be allowed out of bed for short intervals. If ordered, the nasogastric tube can be clamped and disconnected from suction.

Altered Oral Mucous Membrane.　Careful, frequent mouth care greatly lessens discomfort and helps to relieve the parched, dry feeling and to get rid of unpleasant tastes and odors. If the patient is able, the mouth may be rinsed with mouthwash. Cream or glycerin applied to the lips and the edge of the nostril helps to prevent dryness and cracking. A small amount of lubricant can be applied to the tube where it emerges from the nose, to prevent crusts of dried secretions from forming. Such crusts are irritating to the nostril.

The physician may allow the patient to suck on ice chips or order an analgesic throat lozenge if the patient's mouth and throat become sore. Mouth care should be given after the tube has been removed. Soreness of the throat may persist for several days.

Evaluation

- Anxiety is reduced
- Decompression apparatus functions correctly
- Comfort is maintained
- Normal fluid intake is attained and maintained
- Signs of dehydration are absent; urine output is normal
- Patient attains and maintains a normal nutritional balance
- Serum electrolyte levels are within normal limits
- Bowel elimination is normal
- Self-care needs are met
- Oral mucous membranes, lips, and nostril are normal in appearance

GASTROSTOMY

Gastrostomy, the creation of an artificial opening into the stomach, is performed to provide a method of administering fluids and (liquid) food. Cancer and stricture of the esophagus from swallowing chemicals are examples of conditions that cause obstruction of the esophagus and necessitate either a temporary or a permanent gastrostomy. Gastrostomy is a relatively minor procedure. It can be performed under local anesthesia if the patient is weak and debilitated.

NURSING PROCESS —THE PATIENT WHO HAS A GASTROSTOMY

Preoperative Period

Assessment
In addition to the assessments performed on the patient with a GI disorder (see Chapter 42), the patient's ability to understand the surgery and acceptance of the procedure are determined.

Nursing Diagnosis
Depending on the reason for the gastrostomy and the patient's physical and emotional condition, one or more of the following nursing diagnoses may apply. Additional diagnoses may be necessary if the patient has other problems, such as pain and difficulty breathing and swallowing.

- Anxiety related to surgery, diagnosis, need to use gastrostomy for nutrition
- Knowledge deficit of surgical procedure

Planning and Implementation
The major goals of the patient include reduction of anxiety and an understanding of the gastrostomy procedure.

The major goals of nursing management are to relieve apprehension and anxiety and explain the procedure to the patient and family.

In addition to normal preoperative preparations, the patient should be weighed. The abdominal skin area (eg, the probable site of the gastrostomy) should be prepared according to the surgeon's instructions. Shaving of the area usually is ordered. The patient's chart should be reviewed for potential problems (eg, severe malnutrition or diabetes mellitus) that may interfere with postoperative healing and skin integrity.

Anxiety.　The patient should be allowed time to talk about the impending surgery. Although anxiety may not be relieved, verbalization of concerns may make the patient understand the importance of the procedure.

Knowledge Deficit. The surgeon explains the purpose of and reason for the procedure. The patient and family should be allowed time to ask questions about the surgery as well as other points related to feeding by this method. They should be told that food in liquid form will go directly into the stomach.

Evaluation

- Anxiety is reduced
- Patient verbalizes understanding of the reason for and purpose of the procedure

Postoperative Period

Assessment
The patient's chart should be reviewed for the patient's condition during and immediately after surgery. Vital signs should be taken. The site and placement of the gastrostomy may be discovered from the chart and the stoma visually inspected.

Nursing Diagnosis
Depending on the reason for the procedure and the patient's original diagnosis and emotional acceptance of the gastrostomy, one or more of the following nursing diagnoses may apply. Additional diagnoses may be added under certain circumstances, such as a change in the patient's condition, inability of the patient to perform his or her own gastrostomy feedings, and lack of a support group after discharge from the hospital.

- Potential for infection related to surgery, skin breakdown, poor care of the stoma
- Altered nutrition: less than body requirements related to problems associated with gastrostomy (enteral) feeding
- Impaired skin integrity related to effect of gastric secretions on the skin
- Constipation caused by enteral feeding formula, other factors
- Diarrhea caused by enteral feeding formula, lack of bulk in the diet, other factors (specify)
- Ineffective individual coping related to inability to eat normally
- Body image disturbance related to change in obtaining nutrition (enteral feedings)
- Knowledge deficit of management of gastrostomy feedings

Planning and Implementation
The major goals of the patient include absence of infection, improved nutrition, absence of skin breakdown, normal bowel elimination, effective coping mechanisms, acceptance of changes in body image, and an ability to perform own gastrostomy feedings.

The major goals of nursing management are attaining and maintaining an optimal level of nutrition, preserving skin integrity, helping the patient adjust to the change in body image, and teaching the patient and family the technique of gastrostomy feeding and care.

Potential for Infection, Impaired Skin Integrity. When a gastrostomy is performed, a catheter is inserted into the opening and secured to the abdominal wall. The operative site should be inspected daily for signs of infection. Vital signs should be monitored, and any temperature elevation or other signs of infection, such as severe inflammation or purulent drainage around the tube site, should be reported to the physician.

To prevent the leakage of gastric contents, the end of the catheter should be clamped except for the time the patient is being fed. The leakage that may occur around the tube causes discomfort because gastric juices are irritating to the skin. Dressings should be applied to absorb any drainage that occurs around the tube and should be changed frequently. The skin should be washed often with mild soap and water to prevent excoriation. Ointments such as zinc oxide ointment may be applied to the skin to help prevent irritation. Any adhesive tape residue should be promptly removed, as this also may irritate the skin.

Altered Nutrition. The initial feedings through the tube usually consist of small amounts of tap water, which is gradually increased to larger amounts as tolerated. The amount of fluid and the frequency of administration are specified by the physician. When the patient is able to tolerate clear liquids, the feedings are begun. After sufficient healing, the gastrostomy tube may be removed and inserted only for feedings. About 300 to 500 mL is given at a time. Some patients feel uncomfortably full and even nauseated unless feedings are given in small amounts. It may be necessary to administer the feedings more frequently to deliver the total amount ordered.

Intake and output should be measured and recorded. The physician should be informed if there is any difficulty in administering the formula or liquids or if episodes of nausea should occur. The patient should be weighed daily to monitor the effectiveness of the prescribed feeding formula.

Constipation, Diarrhea.   Constipation or diarrhea may occur. Changes in bowel elimination should be reported to the physician, as a change in the formula or other measures may be necessary.

Ineffective Individual Coping.   It is hard for most patients to face the prospect of having a gastrostomy. Eating is one of the basic pleasures of life. Although nutrition can be maintained by gastrostomy, the patient is denied the physical satisfaction of taste and the emotional satisfaction of companionship during meals. In addition, a gastrostomy also indicates a serious or possibly terminal illness. Adjustment to the gastrostomy takes time, and the patient may, in the beginning, refuse to accept this change in body image.

Knowledge Deficit.   After discharge from the hospital, the patient or a family member will be responsible for managing the gastrostomy as well as preparing the feeding or prescribed formula. The physician may recommend that the patient's normal diet be converted to a form suitable for tube feeding by the use of a blender. This method is considered desirable if tube feedings must be continued for a long period because normal nutrition can be maintained.

The following points may be included in a teaching plan:

- Food or formula preparation, total daily fluid and calorie intake
- Insertion of the catheter, administration of the formula or blenderized food, care of the catheter and funnel or syringe after feeding
- Maintenance of weekly weight record

Evaluation

- Evidence of infection is absent; vital signs are normal
- Skin remains intact with no evidence of skin breakdown
- Patient achieves an adequate intake of nutrients
- Weight is maintained or gained
- Bowel elimination is normal
- Patient shows evidence of adjusting to gastrostomy
- Patient asks questions regarding care of gastrostomy and food or formula preparation
- Patient performs gastrostomy feeding with minimal supervision

CANCER OF THE ORAL CAVITY

The oral cavity includes the lips, any part of the mouth, and the pharynx. When they are detected early, many cancers of the oral cavity have a fairly good cure rate.

Smoking, the use of chewing tobacco, and the excessive use of alcohol have been linked to oral cancers. Cancer of the lips has been linked to pipe smoking and prolonged exposure to the wind and sun.

Symptoms

Early symptoms may be lacking in the early stages of oral malignancies. The first symptom the patient may notice is a lesion, lump, or other abnormality of the lips or mouth. Other symptoms, such as pain, soreness, and bleeding, may be seen later. When there is a lesion on the tongue, the patient may experience difficulty in chewing, swallowing, or tasting foods. Pain, numbness, and a loss of feeling also may occur. Dentists and oral hygienists examine the mouth for oral malignancies each time a patient is seen, and may be the first to notice a change in the tissues of the mouth.

Diagnosis

Diagnosis is made by visual examination and a biopsy of the lesion.

Treatment

Treatment depends on such factors as the location and type of tumor, the extent of involvement (or stage), and the patient's physical condition. Surgical excision of malignant tissue in the mouth may result in complete cure, provided that it is performed early.

Cancer of the lip may respond to excision of the lesion. Larger lesions may be treated with radiation therapy. A neck dissection may be performed if the cancer has spread to the lymph nodes.

Cancer of the tongue usually is treated with radiation and radical surgery, which involves removal of part of the tongue (hemiglossectomy). Cancer of the posterior third of the tongue is difficult to treat with radiation. A total glossectomy (removal of the tongue) may be performed, but the cure rate is low.

Cancer of the floor of the mouth, palate, and mandible may be treated with radiation therapy and chemotherapy. Radical surgery, which may involve removal of the jaw, part of the palate, and oral soft tissues, also is used; however, the cure rate is low and radical surgery is disfiguring.

In advanced cases, treatment is only palliative. Chemotherapy or radiation therapy may be used to relieve pain and temporarily decrease tumor size. Certain measures (eg, tracheostomy or gastrostomy) may be instituted to maintain an adequate airway or provide nutrition.

Nursing management of the patient receiving palliative treatment for an oral malignancy is the same as for any patient with cancer (see Chapter 19). Much of the material included in the management of a patient having surgery for oral cancer also applies to medical management. In addition, tumor invasion of adjacent blood vessels may result in sudden, severe hemorrhage. The management of this phenomenon is discussed in the section on planning and implementation during the postoperative period.

NURSING PROCESS —THE PATIENT UNDERGOING SURGERY FOR CANCER OF THE ORAL CAVITY

Preoperative Period

Assessment

In addition to the assessments performed on the patient with a GI disorder (see Chapter 42), a complete health history, including a drug, use of alcohol and tobacco, and allergy history, should be obtained from the patient or a family member. The patient should be questioned regarding symptoms, the length of time the symptoms have been noted, whether or not he or she is able to eat normally, and whether or not any weight has been lost and, if so, about how much. The lips and oral cavity should be examined visually for the presence of lesions or tissue changes.

The patient's understanding of the planned surgery also should be evaluated at the time of assessment.

Nursing Diagnosis

The nursing diagnoses depend on the type of surgery to be performed, and may include one or more of the following:

- Anxiety related to symptoms, diagnosis, planned treatment, possible disfigurement
- Pain caused by pressure of the lesion on adjacent nerves
- Impaired verbal communication related to involvement of the tongue or lips
- Altered nutrition: less than body requirements related to inability to chew and swallow
- Knowledge deficit of planned surgery, prognosis, disfigurement

Planning and Implementation

The major goals of the patient include reduction of anxiety, improved comfort, improved nutrition, ability to communicate needs to others, and an understanding of the planned surgery.

The major goal of nursing management is preparing the patient physically and emotionally for surgery.

Anxiety. The patient and family should be allowed time to talk about the planned surgery. Although it is difficult to eliminate anxiety, letting the patient ventilate feelings and talk about the surgery may provide some relief. If the patient is severely anxious, the physician should be informed, as a tranquilizer may be necessary.

Pain. Before surgery, the mouth or lips may be sensitive or painful. Depending on the degree of discomfort, topical or systemic analgesics may be ordered. Because oral tissues are sensitive, hot and cold liquids and spicy foods should be avoided during the preoperative period.

Impaired Verbal Communication. The patient may have difficulty speaking if the tongue or a large area of the lips are involved. Severe speech impairment may require the use of a pen and paper to communicate needs.

Altered Nutrition. If weight loss is severe and malnutrition is present, surgery may be delayed until the nutritional deficit is corrected. Intravenous fluids or parenteral nutrition may be necessary. If the patient is able to take oral fluids, a dietary consultation may be necessary to supply the patient with a diet that can be tolerated.

Intake and output records should be kept and the physician informed if the patient fails to take a sufficient amount of oral fluids or loses weight.

Knowledge Deficit. The patient and family should discuss the proposed surgery with the physician. Because surgery may be disfiguring and not offer a complete cure, or additional surgery may be necessary, the patient should fully understand the planned procedure. If the patient or family still do not seem to understand what will be done, the nurse should inform the physician, as further clarification is necessary.

The nurse is responsible for explaining the basic principles of postoperative nursing care (see Chapter 16).

Evaluation

- Anxiety is reduced
- Pain is controlled
- Patient is able to communicate effectively
- Weight is gained or remains stable
- Nutritional needs are met
- Patient demonstrates understanding of the surgical procedure, the structures involved, prognosis, and additional treatment modalities

Postoperative Period

Assessment

Immediately on the patient's return from surgery, vital signs should be taken, the patient's general condition evaluated, and the chart reviewed for information regarding the type and extent of surgery performed.

Assessment of the patient with an excision of an oral malignancy focuses on two major areas: maintenance of a patent airway and prompt detection of hemorrhage. Sometimes surgery is extensive and disfiguring, and may interfere with normal breathing and swallowing.

Nursing Diagnosis

Depending on the type and extent of surgery, one or more of the following nursing diagnoses may apply. Additional nursing diagnoses related to any surgical procedure also may be added (see Chapter 16).

- Anxiety related to the disfiguring results of surgery, airway obstruction, changes in body image
- Pain related to surgery
- Hyperthermia related to surgery, infection
- Potential for infection related to surgery
- Ineffective airway clearance due to edema of the surgical site, blood in the mouth, inability to cough and deep breathe
- Impaired verbal communication related to edema, removal of structures necessary for clear speech
- Ineffective individual coping related to disfigurement of surgery, diagnosis, prognosis
- Fluid volume deficit related to inability to take oral fluids
- Altered nutrition: less than body requirements related to inability to chew, eat, and swallow
- Altered oral mucous membrane related to surgery of the mouth
- Body image disturbance related to cosmetic changes secondary to surgery
- Social isolation related to impaired verbal communication, change in body image
- Impaired social interaction related to impaired verbal communication, change in body image
- Knowledge deficit of postdischarge care (eg, tube feedings and tracheostomy care)

Planning and Implementation

The major goals of the patient include reduction of anxiety, elimination of pain and discomfort, normal body temperature, absence of infection, maintenance of a patent airway, improved communication skills, acceptance of and coping with body image changes, attaining and maintaining a normal fluid and food intake, prevention of injury to oral mucous membranes, improved social interaction, movement through the grieving process, and an understanding of home care.

The major goals of nursing management depend on such factors as the type of surgery, the extent and site of the tumor, and the prognosis. The primary goals are to ensure a patent airway, identify compli-

cations such as hemorrhage and infection, help the patient cope with the physical change, and prepare the patient for home care management.

Hemorrhage. Large blood vessels, such as the carotid arteries, are near the oral cavity. Serious hemorrhage ("carotid blowout") and death may result when an artery is invaded by cancer and becomes ulcerated, or when necrosis follows radiotherapy. The physician should advise the nurse which patients are most likely to develop hemorrhage. Massive hemorrhage from the carotid artery has a poor prognosis, since the bleeding is difficult to stop.

If hemorrhage should occur, direct digital pressure should be applied over the bleeding point until the physician arrives. Another nurse should be asked to report the emergency so that the nurse who first applies digital pressure can remain with the patient and continue to apply pressure until further treatment is instituted by a physician. The physician may order a narcotic to relieve the patient's apprehension and transfusions to replace lost blood. Ligation of the bleeding vessel usually is necessary. After the bleeding is controlled, the patient is likely to be exhausted, and apprehensive lest it recur. Frequent observation and monitoring of vital signs are important in detecting further bleeding.

Pain. Analgesics should be given for pain. Judgment is necessary in the administration of narcotics postoperatively because they can cause respiratory depression and depress the cough reflex.

Firm support of the patient's head and neck helps to ease pain during coughing. At first, the nurse provides this support for the patient; later, the patient is taught to do it. The hands should be placed gently but firmly on either side of the patient's head, supporting the head to prevent excessive movement when coughing.

Hyperthermia, Potential for Infection. Vital signs should be monitored as ordered; the temperature should be taken rectally.

Antibiotic therapy usually is instituted after surgery. The suture lines should be inspected daily for signs of infection. Any rise in temperature or evidence of possible infection should be brought to the physician's attention.

Ineffective Airway Clearance. Equipment for suctioning, administration of oxygen, and care of a tracheostomy should be kept at the patient's bedside during the immediate postoperative period. If the patient does not have a tracheostomy, a tracheostomy tray is kept at the bedside for emergency use, as respiratory distress or obstruction may necessitate an emergency tracheostomy.

On return from the operating room, the patient is positioned flat, either on the abdomen or on the side, with the head turned to the side to facilitate drainage from the mouth. Suction should be carried out as necessary to prevent aspiration of secretions or blood, which may result in atelectasis or pulmonary infections.

After the patient recovers from anesthesia, the head of the bed should be elevated. This position usually makes it easier for the patient to breathe deeply and cough up secretions, and controls edema in the operative area. The lungs should be auscultated daily for signs of pulmonary congestion and abnormal or absent breath sounds. To prevent pulmonary complications, coughing and deep breathing should be encouraged hourly.

Although the raising of some dark blood is to be expected in the immediate postoperative period, the sudden appearance of blood on the dressing, rapid pulse rate, a fall in blood pressure, respiratory distress, or the coughing up of bright red blood is serious and necessitates immediate medical attention.

Impaired Verbal Communication. Communication with others presents a real problem to patients who have had extensive oral surgery. The ability to tell others about discomfort, to express fears, to ask questions, or to call for help is impaired at the time when the patient most needs to communicate with others. A Magic Slate can be used to write questions or answers. Lifting the plastic cover erases the writing, and the slate is ready for reuse. Special care should be taken that the patient's call button is within easy reach at all times, and that the call light is answered promptly.

Ineffective Individual Coping. The patient's emotional response to radical oral surgery is a very real and often difficult problem. Extensive surgery of the mouth and adjacent structures is not only disfiguring, but also usually interferes with communication, eating, and the control of saliva. Although the extent of surgery is explained before the operation, many patients and their families are unable to understand, at that time, the full implications of this type of surgery. The first time family members see the patient after surgery and the first time the patient looks into a mirror can be traumatic experiences.

Before family members visit the patient during the immediate postoperative period, the nurse should inform them of the patient's physical condition. Although what is included in this explanation depends on the extent of surgery, a brief description of the dressings and communication problems is needed.

The nurse can give additional basic information before subsequent visits.

To prepare the patient for the emotional shock of looking into a mirror for the first time, the physician may briefly describe what has been done at the time of the first dressing change. This is followed by further explanations each time the dressing is changed. If at all possible, it is best to have the physician present when the patient looks into a mirror for the first time. If there appears to be difficulty accepting the surgery, or if the patient or family does not seem to understand what has been done, the nurse should discuss this with the physician as well as document this fact in the patient's chart. This approach also applies to any patient who has had radical and disfiguring surgery.

The nurse may reduce the patient's distress over changes resulting from surgery by performing the following aftercare:

1. Provide privacy during the first attempts to swallow and eat.
2. Minimize the problem of drooling. An ample supply of tissues should be provided, and the patient directed to tilt the head at intervals so that the saliva is directed back, where it can be swallowed. Sometimes a small catheter attached to low-pressure suction is used to remove excess saliva from the mouth.
3. Help the patient to pay extra attention to personal cleanliness and grooming. Clean bedclothes, hair neatly combed, and attention to appearance (as soon as the physician permits) all help the patient feel more presentable.

When there is a marked change in body image, the patient usually goes through a grieving process, which may be evidenced by such actions as avoiding contact with others and refusing to talk about the surgery or changes in appearance. The patient should be allowed time to accept and adjust to these changes in body image.

Altered Nutrition, Fluid Volume Deficit. Parenteral fluids are ordered after surgery. Because the patient may be unable to swallow, nutrition and fluids also may be supplied by feedings through a nasogastric tube. Certain types of oral surgery may necessitate a temporary or permanent gastrostomy.

If the patient can swallow, the physician may order small amounts of liquid and a gradual progression from liquids to soft foods as tolerated. The patient should be carefully observed when first attempting to swallow small amounts of liquid. If there is coughing and difficulty in swallowing, the liquid should be suctioned from the mouth immediately. Further oral feedings should not be given without checking with the physician. Some patients have had such extensive surgery that they continue to require tube feedings through either a nasogastric tube or a gastrostomy tube.

Altered Oral Mucous Membrane.   Old blood and mucus collect in the mouth during the postoperative period. Unless the mouth is kept scrupulously clean, infection is likely to occur, and unpleasant odors and an offensive taste in the mouth are distressing to the patient and visitors. Cleansing should be done frequently, and precautions taken to prevent trauma or infection. Sterile technique is used in some hospitals; clean technique is used in others because the mouth normally harbors bacteria and cannot be kept sterile.

The mouth should be gently irrigated to keep it clean. The frequency of irrigations and the type of solution used are ordered by the physician. Normal saline solution or hydrogen peroxide and water are commonly used. The patient's head should be turned to the side to allow the solution to run in gently and flow out into an emesis basin. A soft catheter is useful for this purpose because it does not cause trauma. The mouth should not be irrigated until the patient regains consciousness after surgery because of the danger of the patient's aspirating the irrigation solution. Precautions should be taken to keep the dressings and the patient's bed and gown from getting wet during irrigations. The emesis basin should be placed in position to catch the return. Irrigations can be frightening. Only a small amount of solution should be allowed to run into the oral cavity, and this should be drained out before additional irrigating solution is used. Plastic material can be used to protect dressings and bed linen.

Once healing has begun and the patient takes oral food and fluids, mouth care should be given after each meal.

Social Isolation, Impaired Social Interaction, Body Image Disurbance.   Many patients want to be alone after surgery because they are self-conscious about their appearance. In the beginning, they may want to see only close family members. As healing takes place and they have begun to emotionally accept their diagnosis and surgery, they may be more willing to see visitors. Some patients continue to avoid social interaction with others after discharge from the hospital.

Knowledge Deficit.   The type and extent of patient teaching depend on the surgery performed. If nasogastric or gastrostomy feedings are to be continued after discharge from the hospital, the patient or a family member should be taught this technique. The patient should participate in nasogastric or gastros-

tomy feedings while hospitalized, if possible. The importance of a balanced diet by means of nasogastric or tube feedings should be emphasized.

If a permanent tracheostomy is necessary, tracheostomy care and suction techniques should be taught to the patient and family.

The available support system should be evaluated. Some patients require home nursing care, and they should be informed of the agencies in the area that supply such care. Financial obligations may be overwhelming; therefore, the social worker may need to discuss financial arrangements with the family.

Evaluation

- Pain is reduced
- Anxiety is reduced
- Evidence of infection, hemorrhage, or other complications from surgery is absent
- Airway is clear; lungs are clear to auscultation
- Patient coughs and deep breathes effectively
- Patient communicates effectively and socializes with others
- Patient shows evidence of coping with physical changes
- Patient is able to talk about surgery, diagnosis, and home care
- Adequate food and fluid intake is maintained
- Oral mucous membranes show normal healing pattern
- Patient demonstrates understanding of principles and techniques of home care

DISORDERS OF THE ESOPHAGUS

Treatment of an esophageal disorder may be medical or surgical. With the exception of cancer of the esophagus, failure of relief from medical intervention may necessitate surgery. Patients with esophageal cancer may or may not be candidates for surgery, depending on the extent of the tumor.

Esophageal Diverticulum

A diverticulum is a sac, or pouch, that results from a congenital or acquired weakness in one or more layers of the wall of an organ or structure. An esophageal diverticulum may be found at the junction of the pharynx and the esophagus or in the middle or lower portion of the esophagus.

Symptoms

The patient may experience difficulty or pain when swallowing, belching, a foul breath odor (caused by the decomposition of food trapped in the diverticulum), a gurgling sound high in the chest area, and coughing (caused by irritation and compression of the trachea).

Diagnosis

Diagnosis is made by a review of the patient's symptoms and by a barium swallow.

Treatment

For mild symptoms, treatment usually includes a bland diet. Small meals should be eaten four to six times per day. Antacids and cholinergic blocking drugs may be prescribed to relieve symptoms. Sleeping with the head of the bed elevated, avoiding lying down for at least 2 hours after meals, losing weight, and avoiding coffee, alcohol, tobacco, and spicy foods also may relieve symptoms. Drugs such as cimetidine (Tagamet), famotidine (Pepcid), and ranitidine (Zantac) may be prescribed. Patients with more severe symptoms may require surgical excision of the diverticulum.

Surgical repair of a diverticulum of the lower esophagus usually is performed by means of a thoracic (chest) approach. The surgical approach for an esophageal diverticulum at the junction of the pharynx and esophagus usually is above the clavicle (collar bone).

Hiatal Hernia   women

A hiatal, or diaphragmatic, hernia is a protrusion of part of the stomach into the esophagus. It is caused by a defect in the diaphragm wall at the point where the esophagus passes through the diaphragm. This condition may result from a congenital weakness in the diaphragm or from trauma. Factors that increase intraabdominal pressure, such as multiple pregnancies or obesity, contribute to the development of a hiatal hernia. The loss of muscle strength and tone that occurs with aging also is a contributing factor. The condition is common in older age-groups, particularly in women.

There are two types of hiatal hernia: the paraesophageal type (Fig. 43-5), which is a rolling up of the fundus and greater curvatures of the stomach through the diaphragm, and the sliding type, in which the junction of the stomach and the esophagus and part of the stomach slide up through the weakened portion of the diaphragm.

Symptoms

Symptoms include heartburn, belching, and a feeling of substernal or epigastric pressure after eating. These symptoms are more severe when the patient lies down.

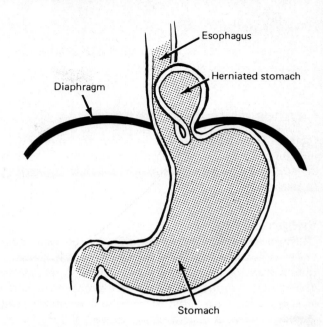

Figure 43-5. Hiatal hernia—paraesophageal type. The herniated portion of the stomach protrudes through the diaphragm into the chest cavity.

Diagnosis

The diagnosis is suggested by the history and confirmed by radiographic studies.

Treatment

Most patients can be managed medically by following a weight-reduction program, maintaining a bland diet, and taking antacids and drugs such as cimetidine (Tagamet), famotidine (Pepcid), and ranitidine (Zantac). Elevating the head of the bed on 3- or 4-inch blocks prevents stomach acid from refluxing and chemically attacking the esophageal mucosa. Patients with reflux esophagitis secondary to hiatal hernia may bleed acutely, especially in the more uncommon paraesophageal type. They also may have melena or hematemesis. Sometimes occult bleeding for long periods produces a typical iron deficiency anemia. Patients who do not respond to a rigid medical regimen are treated surgically.

Surgical treatment involves restoring the stomach or other protruding organs in the abdominal cavity to their proper position and repairing the defect in the wall. The thoracic cavity is entered, so that postoperative care is similar to that for any patient who has had chest surgery (see Chapter 23). Some repairs may be done with an abdominal, rather than a thoracic, approach, in which case nursing management is similar to that for any patient who has had general abdominal surgery. Continuous gastric suction usually is ordered postoperatively to prevent distention of the stomach and avoid pressure on the surgical repair.

Esophageal Varices

Esophageal varices is due to cirrhosis of the liver, which is discussed in Chapter 46.

Cancer of the Esophagus

Cancer of the esophagus is more common in men than in women, and usually occurs in the fourth or fifth decade of life. The tumor usually is a squamous cell carcinoma.

Symptoms

Symptoms usually develop slowly. By the time difficulty in swallowing (dysphagia) is noticeable, the cancer may have extended and invaded surrounding tissues and lymphatics. In the beginning, symptoms may be mild, with vague feelings of discomfort and difficulty in swallowing some foods. As the disease progresses, solid foods become almost impossible to swallow, and the patient resorts to liquids. Weight loss accompanies progressive dysphagia. Pain is a late symptom.

Diagnosis

Diagnosis is made by a barium swallow and esophagoscopy.

Treatment

Treatment mainly depends on the extent of the lesion and evidence of metastasis. When surgery is considered, the type of surgery depends on the site of the tumor as well as other factors. For tumors of the lower third of the esophagus, the esophagus is resected and the remaining two thirds are anastomosed to the stomach. Lesions of the upper two thirds of the esophagus are resected and the esophagus replaced with a section of jejunum or colon.

Patients who are not candidates for surgery are treated with palliative measures. Esophageal dilatation may be used to enlarge the area obstructed by a tumor, or a prosthesis (stent placement) may be inserted at the site of the tumor to widen the area narrowed by tumor growth. A prosthesis also may be inserted when a fistula has formed at the tumor site. Endoscopic laser therapy may be used to destroy some of the tumor in those with inoperable cancer.

If the patient is too ill to withstand surgery, a gastrostomy may be performed, which permits food to be introduced directly into the stomach through an opening in the patient's abdomen. If the patient's nutritional status improves sufficiently to permit surgery, the gastrostomy opening is closed.

NURSING PROCESS —THE PATIENT UNDERGOING MEDICAL TREATMENT FOR AN ESOPHAGEAL DISORDER

Assessment

In addition to the assessments performed on the patient with a GI disorder (see Chapter 42), a history of symptoms and a medical, drug, and allergy history should be obtained during the initial assessment. Vital signs should be taken and the patient weighed.

Nursing Diagnosis

Depending on the symptoms and the potential or actual medical diagnosis and treatment, one or more of the following nursing diagnoses may apply:

- Anxiety related to symptoms, diagnosis, treatment modalities
- Pain related to a tumor, reflux of gastric juices
- Altered nutrition: less than body requirements related to dysphagia
- Altered nutrition: more than body requirements related to an eating disorder and obesity
- Knowledge deficit of treatment regimen

Planning and Implementation

The two main problems associated with an esophageal disorder are nutrition and discomfort. The patient may experience pain or discomfort on swallowing, be unable or find it difficult to swallow, or experience mild to severe distress after eating.

The major goals of the patient include relief of pain or discomfort, reduction of anxiety, improved nutrition, and an understanding of the treatment regimen.

The major goals of nursing management are to improve nutrition, relieve pain or discomfort, and reduce anxiety associated with the symptoms.

Anxiety.   Being unable to eat or experiencing difficulty eating may create anxiety. In addition, the possible diagnosis of a serious or even terminal disorder and the planned treatment modalities may cause emotional distress. The patient should be allowed time to ask questions about the diagnosis and treatment.

Altered Nutrition.   Depending on the type of esophageal disorder and the patient's physical makeup, it may be necessary for the patient to gain or lose weight. If weight gain or loss is part of the treatment regimen, a bland weight-reduction or bland weight-gain diet may be ordered.

The nutritional needs of the patient with inoperable cancer of the esophagus are met with nasogastric or gastrostomy tube feedings or total parenteral nutrition.

Pain. Pain is a late symptom of cancer of the esophagus. In many instances, surgery is not possible because the tumor has metastasized. Pain is controlled with narcotics. Many patients with pain or discomfort associated with other esophageal disorders find relief with conservative treatment, such as antacid therapy and maintenance of a bland diet. Response to treatment should be noted and the physician informed if the patient fails to respond to these measures.

Knowledge Deficit. The prescribed treatment should be explained to the patient. The importance of adhering to the physician's recommendations should be stressed. When a special diet is ordered, the diet should be reviewed with the patient. A consultation with the dietitian may be necessary. The following points may be included in a teaching plan for patients with an esophageal diverticulum or hiatal hernia:

1. Avoid the use of alcohol, tobacco, and very hot, cold, or spicy foods. Bland foods are better tolerated.
2. Eat four to six small meals per day rather than three regular meals.
3. Remain upright for at least 2 hours after a meal.
4. Avoid strenuous physical activities and constipation. Some sports activities also may need to be avoided, especially if participation results in a return of symptoms.
5. Sleep with the head of the bed elevated on 3- to 4-inch blocks.
6. Follow the drug regimen prescribed by the physician. If symptoms worsen, do not increase the dose without contacting the physician.
7. Avoid overuse of nonprescription drugs such as antacids.
8. Contact the physician if symptoms worsen, steady weight loss is noted, or other symptoms occur.
9. Frequent rinsing of the mouth helps to relieve unpleasant taste and odor.
10. Maintain the diet (bland, weight reduction, weight gain) recommended by the physician.

The following points may be included in a teaching plan for patients with an inoperable esophageal tumor:

1. Eat four to six small meals per day rather than three regular meals.
2. Eat foods that are easy to swallow. A soft diet is better tolerated.
3. Take the prescribed medications as ordered.
4. Weigh yourself weekly.

5. Keep all physician, clinic, or radiation treatment appointments.
6. Notify the physician if the pain worsens, swallowing of soft foods becomes impossible, weight is lost, temperature rises, chest pain occurs, or any other new symptoms appear.

Evaluation

■ Anxiety is reduced
■ Pain or discomfort is reduced or eliminated
■ Nutrition is improved
■ Patient gains or loses (specify) weight
■ Patient demonstrates understanding of treatment regimen

NURSING PROCESS —THE PATIENT UNDERGOING SURGERY FOR AN ESOPHAGEAL DISORDER

Assessment

In addition to the assessments performed on the patient with a GI disorder (see Chapter 42), a history of symptoms and a medical, drug, and allergy history should be obtained during the initial assessment. Vital signs should be taken and the patient weighed.

Nursing Diagnosis

Depending on the surgical approach used, one or more of the following nursing diagnoses may apply. Nursing diagnoses related to those having chest surgery (see Chapter 23) may need to be added.

■ Pain related to surgery, tumor metastasis
■ Altered nutrition: less than body requirements related to dysphagia
■ Potential for infection related to surgery
■ Knowledge deficit of home management

Planning and Implementation

The major goals of the patient include reduction in anxiety, relief of pain, improved nutrition, absence of infection, patent airway, and an understanding of home care.

The major goals of nursing management are to attain and maintain an adequate nutritional intake, relieve pain, and provide information regarding home care.

Vital signs should be monitored as ordered. If the surgical approach is above the collar bone, a dressing will be applied to the left or right side of the neck. A drain also may be inserted in the surgical wound. The patient should be observed for difficulty in breathing and swallowing as well as for excessive or purulent drainage on the surgical dressing. If any of these problems should occur, the surgeon should be contacted immediately. If a thoracic approach has been used, management is essentially the same as that for any patient who has had chest surgery (see Chapter 23). Pain is controlled with analgesics.

The drainage from the nasogastric tube should be carefully observed for any evidence of bleeding. Although a small amount of blood may drain through the tube when the patient first returns from the operating room, the drainage should promptly return to the yellow-green color of normal gastric secretions.

The patient may be allowed to take a few steps and sit in a chair the day after surgery, to stimulate deep breathing and improve circulation. Closed-chest drainage and drainage from the nasogastric tube are continued even when the patient is out of bed. Special care is required to see that the tubing is long enough to permit the patient to move a step or two toward a chair. Some patients are fed through a temporary gastrostomy for 4 to 7 days postoperatively. In these patients, the gastrostomy tube, rather than a nasogastric tube, is used to decompress the stomach.

Nutrition and Fluids. Several days after the surgery the patient is permitted small amounts of water at frequent intervals. The patient should be closely observed for regurgitation of the ingested fluid and for such symptoms as dyspnea and fever, which may indicate seepage of the fluid through the operative area to the mediastinum. Sitting up during and just after the ingestion of water helps to prevent regurgitation.

The patient gradually progresses to swallowing other liquids, soft foods, and, finally, a normal diet. If the stomach has been drawn up into the thoracic cavity, the patient may have a feeling of pressure in the chest and dyspnea after eating. These symptoms can be minimized by frequent, small meals and by not allowing the patient to lie down for several hours after eating.

Many patients with cancer of the esophagus become emaciated because of their inability to swallow and because they regurgitate food. Patients with other esophageal disorders also may have difficulty eating and have lost weight.

Preoperative preparation may involve improving nutrition and restoring water and electrolyte balances. The patient receives parenteral fluids as they are required and, if able to swallow liquids, is given a high-calorie, high-protein liquid diet. After surgery, the patient is given intravenous feedings and nothing by mouth for several days to allow the tissues to heal.

Knowledge Deficit. The following points may be included in a teaching plan for patients who have had esophageal surgery:

1. Chew food thoroughly before swallowing and avoid swallowing large pieces of food.
2. Follow the diet plan recommended by the physician.
3. Take all medications with a full glass of water unless directed otherwise.
4. Contact the physician immediately if difficulty is experienced in swallowing or administering tube feedings or if weight loss occurs.

If gastrostomy or nasogastric tube feedings are to be continued at home, the patient or family needs to be instructed in food preparation and administration.

Evaluation

- Anxiety is reduced
- Pain or discomfort is controlled or eliminated
- Patient demonstrates an understanding of treatment modalities (diet, medication, administration of tube feedings)
- Adequate nutritional intake is achieved
- Patient demonstrates an understanding of food preparation and administration by means of a nasogastric or gastrostomy tube

GASTRIC DISORDERS
Gastritis

Gastritis, or inflammation of the lining of the stomach (gastric mucosa), may be acute or chronic. The causes of acute gastritis include dietary indiscretions, certain drugs, ingestion of poisons, toxic chemicals, or corrosive substances, bacterial or viral infections, and food allergies. Chronic gastritis may be seen in patients with cancer of the stomach, gastric ulcer, alcoholism, or pernicious anemia.

Symptoms
Symptoms may vary, but usually the person complains of epigastric fullness and pressure, anorexia, nausea, and vomiting. When gastritis is due to a bacterial or viral infection, vomiting, diarrhea, fever, and abdominal pain may be present. Drugs, poisons, toxic substances, and corrosives can cause gastric bleeding in addition to some of the symptoms previously mentioned. Chronic gastritis may give rise to symptoms similar to those of acute gastritis or it be asymptomatic (without symptoms).

Diagnosis
Diagnosis is made by patient history, gastroscopy, and upper GI series. Other laboratory and diagnostic tests

may be performed to rule out disorders that produce symptoms similar to those of gastritis.

Treatment

Treatment depends on the symptoms experienced by the patient. Nothing is given by mouth until symptoms subside. This is followed by clear liquids as tolerated. Intravenous fluids may be necessary to correct dehydration and electrolyte imbalances if vomiting or diarrhea is severe. Drugs to control nausea, vomiting, and diarrhea may be ordered. Ingestion of poisons, toxic chemicals, or corrosive substances requires emergency treatment; for example, the patient who has swallowed a chemical that is acid in nature is given an alkali to neutralize the substance. Further treatment is based on the damage caused by the chemical.

Chronic gastritis usually is treated with a bland diet, antacid therapy, and avoidance of foods or substances that may aggravate the condition.

Peptic Ulcer

A peptic ulcer is a circumscribed loss of tissue in an area of the GI tract that is in contact with hydrochloric acid and pepsin. Most peptic ulcers occur in the duodenum (duodenal ulcers) (Fig. 43-6); however, they may occur at the lower end of the esophagus, in the stomach (gastric ulcer), or in the jejunum after the patient has had a surgical anastomosis between the stomach and the jejunum.

Peptic ulcer is common in adults. Much has been written about the relation of peptic ulcer to the stress of modern life; sometimes it is assumed that peptic ulcer occurs chiefly in those who do competitive work in an industrial society. Actually, peptic ulcer occurs widely throughout the world and in all societies, ranging from the primitive to the highly industrialized. Men are affected more frequently than women. The highest incidence occurs during middle life, but the condition can occur at any age. The immediate cause of peptic ulcer is the digestive action of acidic gastric juice and pepsin on the mucosa. The underlying cause is unclear.

Symptoms

Symptoms are largely due to the irritation of the ulcer by gastric acid. Pain, which may be described as "burning" or "gnawing," occurs in the epigastric region, and has a definite relation to eating. It usually occurs 1 to several hours after meals, and may be relieved by the ingestion of protein foods, such as milk. Sometimes the pain is accompanied by nausea, and the patient may find that vomiting relieves it. Patients who secrete a large amount of acid may experience pain during the night, which disturbs their sleep. Back pain

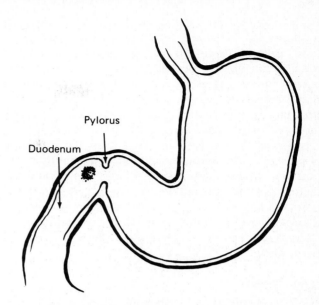

Figure 43-6. A peptic ulcer in the duodenum.

may indicate irritation of the pancreas by the ulcer. About 20% of patients may have bleeding as the first sign of the ulcer; hematemesis or melena also may occur. Protracted vomiting secondary to scarring and resultant obstruction also is seen as the first symptom in those who have ignored earlier symptoms.

Diagnosis

The diagnosis is suggested by the history and confirmed in most patients by an upper GI series or gastroscopy. Duodenal ulcers are benign, but gastric ulcers may be benign or malignant. To differentiate between benign and malignant ulcers, radiographic studies, gastric analysis, gastric washing for cytologic examination, and gastroscopy may be performed. Failure of radiographic examination and gastroscopy to show significant healing usually is reason to operate for suspicion of malignancy.

Complications

Complications of a peptic ulcer are common, and their symptoms may be responsible for the patient's seeking medical care.

Hemorrhage, which may be mild to life-threatening, is the most frequent complication of peptic ulcer. Bleeding occurs when a blood vessel is eroded by the ulcer. If the vessel is large, massive hemorrhage results. If the vessel is small, gradual blood loss occurs, and may be detected by examination of the stool for occult blood. Continuous bleeding may be noted only when the loss of blood has been sufficient to cause faintness, weakness, and dizziness.

Another complication of peptic ulcer is obstruction.

Edema, spasm, inflammation, and scar tissue surrounding the ulcer may interfere with the passage of food, causing retention of food in the stomach for longer than normal periods. Obstruction commonly occurs in the pyloric region. The formation of scar tissue results in pyloric stenosis. Physical examination, radiography of the GI tract, gastroscopy, and aspiration of the stomach contents help to determine the location and severity of the obstruction. If obstruction is present, large amounts of food and secretions are obtained when a nasogastric tube is passed and the contents of the stomach withdrawn by gentle suction.

Sometimes the ulcer penetrates the tissues so deeply that perforation occurs, allowing the contents of the GI tract to seep into the abdominal cavity, resulting in peritonitis.

Treatment

Medical treatment of peptic ulcer is designed to provide the optimal conditions for healing the lesion. Objectives of therapy are the neutralization of acid so that it does not further irritate the ulcer, and the reduction of hypermotility and gastric secretions.

Dietary management of the patient with a peptic ulcer varies. Bland diets and modified regular diets are recommended. Modification of a regular diet usually entails the omission of highly seasoned or spicy foods, alcoholic beverages, fried foods, coffee, cola beverages, or any food or drug (eg, aspirin) that causes gastric distress.

Drug therapy includes antacids to neutralize hydrochloric acid produced by the stomach. These preparations are not absorbed from the GI tract, and therefore do not produce alkalosis, even when given in large doses. Cholinergic blocking agents, such as tincture of belladonna and atropine, may be given to decrease gastric motility and acid secretion. These drugs are contraindicated if partial obstruction is present because they further decrease the motility of an atonic stomach and add to the obstructive symptoms. Cimetidine (Tagamet), famotidine (Pepcid), nizatidine (Axid), and ranitidine (Zantac) are histamine H_2-receptor antagonists used in the treatment of duodenal ulcers. Administration of these agents decreases the production of hydrochloric acid, allowing the ulcer to heal.

The long-term management of peptic ulcer includes avoiding fatigue and stress. Foods that might cause irritation and excess secretion of hydrochloric acid are avoided. Patients are advised to avoid smoking, alcoholic beverages, coffee, and tea, and to take medications as they are ordered. Peptic ulcer tends to recur, and each recurrence brings the possibility of complications.

When complications occur, treatment may be of an emergency nature. Treatment of hemorrhage includes complete rest and blood transfusions. Nothing is given by mouth, and intravenous fluids are administered until the bleeding has stopped. Every effort is made to control the bleeding without immediate surgical intervention because patients who undergo surgery need supportive treatment beforehand, such as transfusions to replace lost blood. When bleeding cannot be controlled by these measures, surgery may be necessary to ligate the bleeding vessel. Sometimes a subtotal gastrectomy is necessary to control bleeding or prevent future episodes of bleeding.

Obstruction caused by edema and inflammation often subsides when the patient has careful medical treatment for the ulcer. Gastric intubation and decompression are used to remove food and secretions. Nutrition may be maintained by intravenous therapy, total parenteral nutrition, nasogastric feedings, or a clear liquid diet. The choice of therapy depends on the severity of the obstruction and the anticipated length of therapy. Severe obstruction or persistent symptoms usually necessitate surgical intervention (ie, vagotomy and antrectomy).

Perforation is an emergency condition. Treatment includes immediate surgical closure of the perforation so that no further leakage can occur, suction during surgery to remove the gastric contents from the peritoneal cavity, and the administration of large doses of antibiotics. The longer the perforation goes untreated, the less likely is the patient's recovery.

Stress Ulcer

The term stress ulcer is used to describe a duodenal or gastric ulcer that occurs as a result of an extremely stressful condition, such as extensive third-degree burns, overwhelming infections, severe trauma, and prolonged shock.

Symptoms

Symptoms are essentially the same as for a peptic ulcer.

Diagnosis

Diagnosis is made by confirmation of GI bleeding, patient history, and endoscopic examination.

Treatment

Treatment includes antacid therapy and the administration of drugs such as cimetidine. If the patient is unable to take the antacid orally, it is administered through a nasogastric tube. Transfusions may be necessary to counteract blood loss. Ice water irrigation by means of a nasogastric tube also has been used to control episodes of bleeding. Endoscopic laser therapy may be applied to the bleeding areas.

Cancer of the Stomach

Heredity and chronic inflammation of the stomach appear to be causative factors in cancer of the stomach.

Symptoms

Early symptoms may be vague. As the tumor enlarges, symptoms include a prolonged feeling of fullness after eating, anorexia, weight loss, and anemia. The stool usually contains occult blood. Pain is a late symptom. Cancer of the stomach often metastasizes to the liver.

Diagnosis

Diagnosis is made by fluoroscopy, barium swallow, and gastroscopy. A gastric analysis may show the absence of free hydrochloric acid.

Treatment

The treatment of cancer of the stomach is partial (subtotal) or total gastrectomy. The type and extent of surgery usually depend on the location of the tumor, the symptoms, and whether metastasis has occurred. Depending on the location and the size of the tumor, it may be possible to perform a subtotal, rather than a total, gastrectomy, thus preserving a more normal digestive function. Even though surgery may not achieve a complete cure, it may still be performed to control bleeding or relieve obstruction at the cardiac or pyloric junction.

Chemotherapy, using drugs such as 5-fluorouracil (5-FU) or doxorubicin, and palliative radiation therapy also may be used.

NURSING PROCESS —THE PATIENT UNDERGOING MEDICAL TREATMENT FOR A GASTRIC DISORDER

Assessment

In addition to the assessments performed on the patient with a GI disorder (see Chapter 42), a complete medical, drug, and allergy history as well as a thorough history of symptoms should be obtained from the patient or family. Each symptom should be explored in depth. For example, if pain occurs, it is important to determine its type, location, and duration.

A dietary history also is important. Questions that may be relevant pertain to foods that cause distress, the amount of food eaten at each meal, if food relieves pain, and use of spicy foods, alcohol, tobacco, and coffee.

Vital signs and weight should be obtained.

Nursing Diagnosis

Depending on the tentative or actual diagnosis, symptoms, and treatment used, one or more of the following nursing diagnoses may apply:

- Anxiety and fear related to symptoms, diagnostic procedures, treatment modalities, tentative or actual diagnosis
- Pain related to inflammation or erosion of the gastric mucosa
- Diarrhea related to the laxative effect of blood in the GI tract
- Constipation related to medications
- Fluid volume deficit related to excessive vomiting or diarrhea
- Altered nutrition: less than body requirements related to symptoms (pain, vomiting, diarrhea)
- Self-care deficits (total or partial) related to treatment modalities (nasogastric tube, intravenous lines)
- Activity intolerance related to anemia, treatment modalities
- Knowledge deficit of treatment regimen

Planning and Implementation

The major goals of the patient include reduction of anxiety, relief of pain, normal bowel elimination, adequate nutrition and fluid intake, ability to carry out own activities of daily living, increased activity tolerance, and an understanding of the treatment regimen.

The major goals of nursing intervention are to relieve pain, reduce fear and anxiety, improve nutrition, improve the patient's understanding of the treatment modalities prescribed by the physician, and recognize complications associated with the disorder.

Vital signs should be monitored every 4 to 8 hours or as ordered. The patient should be weighed weekly, but more frequent weights may be necessary if parenteral, nasogastric, or gastrostomy tube feedings are given or if the patient has a history of marked weight loss.

The patient should be observed for symptoms that may indicate one of the following complications of the disorder:

1. *Hemorrhage.* The patient may have hematemesis or pass tarry stools. Blood that is vomited may appear either bright red or as dark material that resembles coffee grounds. If blood loss is severe, the symptoms of hemorrhage are acute: pallor, rapid and weak pulse, thirst, faintness, sweating, and collapse. When bleeding occurs high in the GI tract, the stools appear black and sticky. Bleeding near the anus, such as that which may occur with hemorrhoids, appears as bright red blood mixed with stool.
2. *Obstruction.* Symptoms vary with the degree of obstruction, ranging from a feeling of fullness, distention,

and nausea after eating to nausea, vomiting, pain, and abdominal distention caused by severe obstruction.

3. *Perforation.* The symptoms of perforation and ensuing peritonitis usually are dramatic. The patient experiences sudden, excruciating pain in the abdomen and sweats profusely; the face becomes ashen and drawn. The body temperature at this time may be normal or subnormal. The abdomen becomes rigid, extremely painful, and tender, and the patient resists having it touched. The patient may lie with knees flexed to lessen the pain. Breathing is rapid and shallow. After 1 or 2 hours, the patient's face may become flushed, and the body temperature rises. The abdomen becomes very distended and less rigid. Respirations become even more rapid and shallow, and the pulse becomes rapid and weak. Unless treatment is given promptly, the patient may die.

When a complication occurs, the patient should be kept as quiet as possible, and only the most essential aspects of personal hygiene should be carried out until the patient's condition has stabilized. The patient usually is aware that a serious complication has occurred and is frightened. The patient should be assured that measures are being promptly taken to treat the problem. The importance of resting quietly in bed should be emphasized. Sedatives are given as ordered by the physician to control restlessness. If hemorrhage or emesis has occurred, an effort should be made to prevent the patient from seeing the amount of blood or emesis lost. Soiled linen and utensils should be removed from the area as soon as possible.

Anxiety. The symptoms associated with some gastric disorders (eg, epigastric distress and intolerance to certain foods) and the potential or actual diagnosis may cause anxiety. The patient should be allowed to ask questions, and treatments and diagnostic tests should be fully explained.

Pain. Pain can be relieved or minimized by the administration of the prescribed medications. If drugs such as antacids, histamine H_2-receptor antagonists, and cholinergic blocking agents are prescribed, complete pain relief may not be immediate, but should begin to lessen in a few days. Patients who have cancer and are receiving analgesics for pain should be monitored for the effect of the prescribed analgesic.

If drug therapy fails to reduce or relieve pain, the physician should be notified. Any sudden onset of severe abdominal pain should immediately be brought to the physician's attention, as a life-threatening situation such as hemorrhage, obstruction, or perforation may be present.

Diarrhea, Constipation. Each stool passed should be examined for color and consistency. A sudden occurrence of tarry stools should be brought to the physician's attention and the patient closely observed for signs of hemorrhage and shock.

Constipation, which may be a side effect of drug therapy, should be reported to the physician, as an enema may be necessary.

Fluid Volume Deficit, Altered Nutrition. Intake and output should be measured. The physician should be notified if any of the following occurs: (1) excessive fluid loss because of vomiting or diarrhea, (2) decreased oral intake, or (3) epigastric distress, pain, or regurgitation resulting from nasogastric or gastrostomy feedings.

Self-Care, Activity Intolerance. Situations such as blood loss and chemotherapy produce varying degrees of fatigue. Certain treatments also may limit the patient's ability to attend to personal care. In these patients, nursing care should be given in a way that minimizes exertion and fatigue.

Knowledge Deficit. Successful treatment of some gastric disorders depends on a thorough understanding of the disorder and adherence to the prescribed therapeutic regimen. During patient teaching, the nurse should be alert for clues that may indicate indifference, misunderstanding, or other factors that may alter the patient's desire or ability to comply. The role of drugs in the treatment of the disorder should be discussed with the patient.

Depending on the prescribed or recommended treatment regimen, the following points can be included in a teaching plan:

- The importance of adhering to the prescribed diet or taking the prescribed medications
- The medication schedule
- The adverse effects that may occur with each medication, and what to do if these should occur
- Avoidance of foods that cause pain or discomfort, and beverages such as coffee, colas, and alcohol
- Drugs (aspirin, baking soda, laxatives) to be avoided or taken only with physician approval
- The importance of maintaining a well-balanced diet and eating meals at regular times
- The importance of rest and the reduction or avoidance of stressful situations
- Symptoms of complications, and what to do if these should occur
- The importance of continued medical supervision

Those with terminal cancer of the stomach require a specialized teaching program. The nurse should evaluate the patient's support system, since physical care may need to be carried out in whole or in part by a family member. Depending on the home situation, the patient or family may require instruction in gastrostomy or nasogastric tube feedings, meal planning and interval feedings, administration of analgesics, and specific aspects of personal care, such as bathing and skin care. See the Nursing Process in Chapters 15 and 19 for planning and management of these patients.

Evaluation

- Anxiety is reduced
- Pain is controlled or eliminated
- Bowel elimination is normal
- Evidence of complications is absent
- Vital signs are stable
- Fluid intake and urine output are normal
- Patient eats small, frequent meals; maintains weight
- Self-care needs are met (when applicable); patient performs most or all self-care activities
- Increased activity is tolerated
- Patient demonstrates an understanding of medical regimen (eg, diet, drugs, and rest), treatment modalities, adverse drug effects, and symptoms of complications
- Patient and family are able to perform nasogastric or gastrostomy feedings with minimal or no assistance
- Patient verbalizes acceptance of the prescribed medical regimen

NURSING PROCESS —THE PATIENT UNDERGOING SURGERY FOR A GASTRIC DISORDER

The following types of surgery may be performed on the stomach and adjacent structures:

Gastrectomy—Removal of the entire stomach with the continuity of the GI tract restored by joining the jejunum and the esophagus

Subtotal gastrectomy—Removal of part of the stomach (usually two thirds to three fourths). The remaining stomach is joined (anastomosed) to the jejunum or duodenum.

Vagotomy—Severing of the vagus nerve to reduce gastric acid secretion by cells in the stomach

Antrectomy—Removal of the lower portion of the stomach (the antrum) as well as a section of the pylorus. When the remaining stomach is joined to the duodenum (gastroduodenostomy), the procedure is called a Billroth I. When the remaining stomach is joined to the jejunum (gastrojejunostomy), the procedure is called a Billroth II.

Pylorectomy—Removal of the pylorus

Pyloroplasty—Repair or reconstruction of the pylorus

Preoperative Period

Assessment

Assessment is essentially the same as for the patient undergoing medical treatment for a gastric disorder. In addition, the nurse should assess the patient's understanding of diagnostic tests, the scheduled surgery, and the preparations for surgery.

Nursing Diagnosis

Depending on the patient's symptoms and information obtained during assessment, one or more of the following nursing diagnoses may apply:

- Anxiety related to diagnostic tests, diagnosis, surgery
- Altered nutrition: less than body requirements related to anorexia, nausea, vomiting, other factors (specify)
- Fluid volume deficit related to vomiting, diarrhea
- Pain related to inflammation or erosion of the gastric mucosa
- Knowledge deficit of preoperative preparations

Planning and Implementation

The major goals of the patient include reduction of anxiety, improved preoperative nutrition and fluid intake, reduction of pain, and an understanding of the preparations for surgery.

The major goals of nursing management include preparing the patient physically and mentally for diagnostic tests and surgery, relieving pain or discomfort, and attaining and maintaining an adequate nutritional, fluid, and electrolyte balance.

Anxiety.   The patient should be encouraged to talk and to ask questions about the surgery or preoperative diagnostic tests. The preparations for surgery should be explained; however, it may be best to explain some preparations, such as the insertion of a nasogastric tube, immediately before the procedure. If surgery is an emergency, the nurse may reduce fear and anxiety by briefly explaining the necessity for immediate surgery and offering reassurance.

Altered Nutrition, Fluid Volume Deficit.   Intake and output should be measured. Intravenous fluids may be administered if the patient is unable to take oral food and fluids.

Pain.   Pain during the preoperative period may require the administration of analgesics. Sudden, severe pain, with or without symptoms of complications such as hemorrhage or perforation, requires immediate notification of the physician, as immediate surgery may be necessary.

Knowledge Deficit.   All diagnostic tests, preoperative preparations, and the surgical procedure should be fully explained to the patient and family. The nurse is responsible for explaining the basic principles of postoperative nursing care (see Chapter 16).

Evaluation

- Anxiety is reduced
- Nutrition and fluid needs are met
- Pain is controlled
- Patient and family demonstrate an understanding of the surgery and the postoperative period

Postoperative Period

Assessment

When the patient returns from surgery, vital signs should be taken and the patient's chart reviewed for such information as the type of surgery performed and the patient's progress during and immediately after surgery. The surgical dressing should be checked for drainage, and tubes or catheters checked for placement, patency, and type of drainage. The general condition of the patient should be determined to provide baseline information.

Nursing Diagnosis

Depending on the type of surgery performed and complications during and immediately after surgery, one or more of the following nursing diagnoses may apply:

- Hyperthermia related to infection
- Pain resulting from surgery or a complication of surgery
- Fluid volume deficit related to taking nothing by mouth, GI intubation and suction
- Altered nutrition: less than body requirements related to surgery, taking nothing by mouth
- Potential for infection related to surgery
- Ineffective airway clearance related to pain, concomitant medical problems (eg, asthma or chronic obstructive pulmonary disease), failure to cough and deep breathe
- Knowledge deficit of postdischarge home care management

Planning and Implementation

The major goals of the patient include normal body temperature, reduction of pain, absence of infection, normal food and fluid intake, patent airway, and an understanding of home care management.

The major goals of nursing management are to relieve pain, prevent complications, help patient attain and maintain an adequate nutrition and fluid intake, and review with the patient the prescribed regimen to be followed after discharge.

When the patient returns from the operating room, a nasogastric tube usually is in place and con-nected to suction. After recovering from anesthesia, the patient should be placed in low Fowler's position.

Vital signs should be monitored as ordered. The dressing should be checked for bleeding or drainage. The function and type of drainage from the nasogastric tube should be noted. Early ambulation usually is ordered, to prevent venous stasis. Additional nursing measures that apply to any postoperative patient (see Chapter 16) are included in a plan of management.

If a total gastrectomy has been performed, the patient must receive vitamin B_{12} injections for the rest of his or her life. Once the entire stomach has been removed, the intrinsic factor necessary for absorption of vitamin B_{12} is no longer produced. Therapy usually is not necessary for 1 or 2 years after surgery, since the body uses very small amounts of this vitamin and body stores often are sufficient for several years.

Complications.   The patient should be closely observed for potential complications of surgery, such as shock, hemorrhage, perforation or leakage at the site of anastomosis, cardiovascular and pulmonary problems, dumping syndrome, paralytic ileus, and wound evisceration. Any of the following may indicate a complication of surgery:

- Change in the vital signs
- Severe pain, even though an analgesic has been given; pain in an area other than the operative site (eg, legs, head, or chest)
- Abdominal distention or rigidity
- Failure to pass flatus or stool for 48 hours after surgery
- Extreme restlessness
- Profuse diaphoresis
- Excessive bloody drainage from the nasogastric tube, surgical drains, or surgical dressing
- Difficulty breathing, increased respiratory rate, cyanosis
- Separation of the surgical wound edges
- Unusual odor to drainage

The dumping syndrome occurs when the patient begins to take solid food. After a meal, the patient experiences weakness, dizziness, sweating, palpitations, abdominal cramps, and diarrhea. These symptoms may be due to the rapid emptying of large amounts of food and fluid through the gastroenterostomy into the jejunum. (Food normally would pass through the entire stomach and the duodenum before reaching the jejunum.) The presence of this hypertonic solution in the gut draws fluid from the circulating blood volume into the intestine, reducing the effective blood volume and producing a syncopelike syndrome. As the syndrome progresses, there may be a rapid elevation of the glucose level followed by increased insulin secretion, which in turn causes hypoglycemia. The precise cause of the dumping syndrome is not fully understood. If this syndrome occurs, the physician should be notified, as a diet change may be necessary. Patients who experience the dumping syndrome usually are given small, frequent, low-carbohydrate, high-protein, moderate-fat meals. The patient also should be instructed to lie flat after eating.

Hypoglycemia after a meal (postprandial hypoglycemia) is considered a variant of the dumping syndrome. As in the dumping syndrome, there is gastric emptying of a large amount of food and fluid high in carbohydrates. This sudden appearance of carbohydrates in the jejunum stimulates the pancreas to secrete excessive amounts of insulin. A secondary hypoglycemia then follows within about 2 hours after a meal. The symptoms include weakness, light-headedness, sweating, and palpitations. If these symptoms should occur, the physician should be notified, as a diet change may be necessary. Treatment is similar to that for the dumping syndrome, with greater emphasis placed on the avoidance of high-carbohydrate meals.

Pain.   Narcotic analgesics should be administered as ordered. The patient's response to the analgesic effect of the drug should be noted. If the drug fails to relieve pain, or a sudden onset of severe pain or pain in an area other than the operative site is noted, the physician should be notified.

Fluid Volume Deficit.   Intake and output should be measured and intravenous fluids given at the rate and volume ordered. The patient should be observed for signs of fluid and electrolyte imbalance (see Chapter 12), which may occur because of continuous gastric suction. As soon as the nasogastric tube is removed, the physician usually orders the patient started on sips of water.

Altered Nutrition.   Bowel sounds should be auscultated every 4 to 8 hours. The patient usually is given nothing by mouth until peristalsis returns. Once oral fluids are ordered, sips of water and then a clear liquid diet are prescribed. If the patient is able to tolerate this diet, a soft and then a regular diet are ordered. A soft bland diet may be prescribed for 1 or 2 weeks after surgery. Because the stomach is now smaller, the patient may note that only a small amount of food can be taken at one time. Four to six small meals may be better tolerated.

Potential for Infection.   Aseptic technique should be used for dressing changes and the dressing rein-forced as needed. When dressing changes are allowed, the wound should be inspected each time the dressing is changed for approximation of wound edges, excessive drainage, and signs of infection.

An antibiotic usually is ordered during the postoperative period, and should be given as directed to maintain adequate blood levels of the drug.

Ineffective Airway Clearance.   The patient should be turned and deep breathing, coughing, and leg movement encouraged every 2 hours. The incision should be supported when the patient coughs and deep breathes.

The lungs should be auscultated every 4 to 8 hours, or more frequently if the patient appears to have respiratory distress. Any change in the respiratory rate or pattern, cyanosis, or abnormal breath sounds should be reported to the physician.

Knowledge Deficit.   Postoperative teaching depends on many factors, such as the preoperative diagnosis, the type and extent of surgery, and the physician's orders. The following points may be included in a patient teaching plan:

■ Follow the diet (eg, foods to eat or avoid) recommended by the physician.
■ Begin by eating small meals (this may avoid the dumping syndrome), and drink fluids between meals rather than with meals.
■ Take planned rest periods during the day and rest particularly after meals.
■ Try to avoid stressful situations.
■ Take medications exactly as prescribed. Follow the directions on the container, paying particular attention to when the drug should be taken (eg, before, after, or with food or meals).
■ Weigh yourself weekly. Report any significant weight loss to the physician.
■ Periodic follow-up office visits are necessary.

Evaluation

■ Evidence of postoperative complications is absent
■ Pain and discomfort are controlled or eliminated
■ Evidence of a fluid volume deficit or electrolyte imbalance is absent
■ Patient is able to take fluids and food by mouth
■ Evidence of infection is absent
■ Patient coughs, deep breathes, and performs leg exercises; ambulates as ordered
■ Respirations are normal; lungs are clear to auscultation
■ Patient demonstrates an understanding of postdischarge diet plan, drug regimen, periodic follow-up office visits
■ Patient verbalizes importance of avoiding stressful situations

General Nutritional Considerations

☐ Inadequate intake of foods by the patient and problems in absorption of nutrients can result in severe emaciation.

☐ Neutralization of gastric acid (hydrochloric acid) by dietary measures may be part of the treatment of gastric and duodenal ulcers. The dietary method used varies, and may be based on physician preference, location of the ulcer, and the individual patient. The diet prescribed may vary from a bland to a modified regular diet.

☐ Foods to be avoided by patients on a bland diet include fried foods, canned soups, raw vegetables, gas-forming vegetables, pork, meat gravies, smoked meats, raw fruits (except bananas and orange juice), whole-grain breads and cereals, coffee, tea, alcoholic and carbonated beverages, pastries, candy, nuts, raisins, and spicy and highly seasoned foods.

☐ Weight-reduction diets should be well balanced and nutritious. Unless directed otherwise by the physician, the patient should be encouraged to lose weight at a slow, steady rate rather than to crash-diet to lose a large amount of weight in a short period.

☐ Patients who have surgery for morbid obesity require extensive dietary instruction as well as modification of their eating patterns.

General Pharmacologic Considerations

☐ Histamine H_2 antagonists used in the treatment of peptic ulcer and esophageal diverticulum inhibit the action of histamine at H_2 receptors of the parietal (hydrochloric acid–secreting) cells of the stomach. An excess of hydrochloric acid usually is present in patients who have peptic ulcers. These agents decrease healing time and reduce the incidence of surgical intervention for the management of peptic ulcer.

☐ Cholinergic blocking agents usually are given 30 minutes before meals, to suppress the increased acid secretion that follows food ingestion; they also may be administered at bedtime.

☐ Cholinergic blocking agents may be given to patients with a peptic ulcer to decrease gastric motility and secretions. These drugs may cause a variety of adverse effects, most notably dry mouth, urine retention, and blurred vision. When combined with sedatives, these products may cause drowsiness; the patient should be cautioned about engaging in any activity that requires alertness (eg, driving a car). These drugs are contraindicated in patients with glaucoma or prostatic enlargement.

☐ Antacids are used to neutralize gastric hydrochloric acid. These drugs may be given two to four times per day or as frequently as every 1 or 2 hours. The antacid may be ordered left at the patient's bedside for self-administration.

☐ If the patient is to be responsible for taking the prescribed antacid, the nurse should (1) demonstrate how to measure the drug in a medicine glass, (2) explain the importance of antacids in the treatment of peptic ulcer, (3) explain the time of day the drug is to be taken (eg, every hour, every 2 hours on the even hour), (4) be sure that the patient has a clock or watch, (5) periodically check the supply of the drug and measuring cups, and (6) periodically check to see if the patient is taking the medication.

☐ In some patients the use of antacids causes constipation or diarrhea.

☐ Patients with intestinal bypass surgery for morbid obesity require vitamin and mineral supplements as well as antidiarrheal medication after surgery.

☐ Although sodium bicarbonate (baking soda) is an antacid, it is readily absorbed from the GI tract and in large doses may produce alkalosis. Its use should be avoided by patients for whom antacids have been prescribed in the treatment of gastric disorders.

General Gerontologic Considerations

☐ Severe and prolonged episodes of vomiting can be especially serious for elderly patients whose nutritional and fluid intake may be marginal; more profound electrolyte imbalances and severe dehydration can result.

☐ Anorexia, which may have many causes, is not uncommon in the elderly. To avoid malnutrition, elderly patients with anorexia should be given four to six small, well-balanced meals per day. The ability of the patient to chew certain foods (because of the lack of teeth or ill-fitting dentures) and the patient's food preferences should be taken into consideration when planning a diet.

☐ Most patients with hiatal hernia are in the older age-group. A patient is not considered a candidate for surgery unless symptoms are severe and not manageable by more conservative means.

Suggested Readings

☐ Alfaro R. Applying nursing diagnosis and nursing process: a step-by-step guide. 2nd ed. Philadelphia: JB Lippincott, 1990. *(Additional coverage of subject matter)*

☐ Brunner LS, Suddarth DS. The Lippincott manual of nursing practice. 4th ed. Philadelphia: JB Lippincott, 1986. *(Additional and in-depth coverage of subject matter)*

☐ Burtis G, Davis J, Martin S. Applied nutrition and diet therapy. Philadelphia: WB Saunders, 1988. *(Additional coverage of subject matter)*

☐ Caine RM, Buffalino PM (eds). Nursing care planning guides for adults. Baltimore: Williams & Wilkins, 1987. *(Additional coverage of subject matter)*

☐ Caldwell L. Nutrition education for the patient: The handout manual. Philadelphia: JB Lippincott, 1984. *(Additional coverage of subject matter)*

☐ Carroll P. Safe suctioning. Nursing '89 December 1989;19:48. *(Additional coverage of subject matter)*

☐ Dudek SG. Nutrition handbook for nursing practice. Philadelphia: JB Lippincott, 1987. *(Additional coverage of subject matter)*

☐ Feickert DM. Gastric surgery: your crucial pre- and postop role. RN January 1987;50:24. *(Closely related to subject matter)*

☐ Irwin M. Managing leaking gastrostomy sites. Am J Nurs March 1988;88:359. *(Additional coverage of subject matter)*

☐ Johnson BS. Psychiatric mental health nursing: adaption and growth. 2nd ed. Philadelphia: JB Lippincott, 1989. *(Additional coverage of subject matter)*

☐ Kozier B, Erb G. Techniques in clinical nursing: a nursing process approach. 2nd ed. Menlo Park, CA: Addison-Wesley, 1987. *(Additional coverage of subject matter)*

☐ McConnell EA. Clinical considerations in perioperative nursing: preventive aspects of care. Philadelphia: JB Lippincott, 1987. *(Additional and in-depth coverage of subject matter)*

☐ Tilkian SM, Conover MB, Tilkian AG. Clinical implications of laboratory tests. 4th ed. St Louis: CV Mosby, 1987. *(Additional coverage of subject matter)*

Chapter 44

Disorders of the Lower Gastrointestinal Tract

On completion of this chapter the reader will:

- Discuss the symptoms, diagnosis, and treatment of constipation and diarrhea

- Use the nursing process in the management of the patient with constipation or diarrhea

- Discuss the symptoms, diagnosis, complications, and treatment of inflammatory bowel disease

- Use the nursing process in the nursing management of the patient with an inflammatory bowel disease

- Discuss the symptoms, diagnosis, and treatment of appendicitis and peritonitis

- Use the nursing process in the nursing management of the patient with peritonitis

- Use the nursing process in the nursing management of the patient with a paralytic ileus

- Discuss the symptoms, diagnosis, and treatment of diverticular disorders

- Use the nursing process in the nursing management of the patient with a diverticular disorder

- Discuss the types, symptoms, diagnosis, and treatment of hernias

- Use the nursing process in the nursing management of the patient having surgical repair of a hernia

- Discuss the symptoms, diagnosis, and treatment of cancer of the colon and rectum

- Discuss the symptoms, diagnosis, and treatment of anorectal disorders

- Use the nursing process in the medical and surgical nursing management of the patient with an anorectal disorder

ALTERATIONS IN BOWEL ELIMINATION

The material that moves down the large intestine is composed of food residues, microorganisms, digestive juices, and mucus that is secreted in the large intestine and aids in moving the feces toward the anus. Water normally is absorbed from the stool while it is in the large colon. When feces are propelled rapidly through the tract, less water is absorbed, and the stool is softer, or even liquid. When feces are retained in the sigmoid because of spasm, or in the rectum because of inattention to the defecation reflex, too much water is absorbed, and the stool becomes hard and dry. People differ greatly in bowel habits. Some people normally have bowel movements every other day, whereas others have two or three movements a day. In differentiating normal from abnormal function, the consistency of stools is more reliable than their frequency.

Constipation

Constipation may result from emotional stress or from poor diet or bowel habits. Other causes of constipation include certain drugs, the chronic use of laxatives, lack of exercise, inadequate fluid intake, and certain diseases and disorders (eg, multiple sclerosis, paraplegia, diabetes mellitus, and tumor of the colon).

Some patients are not actually constipated but defecate less frequently than what is considered normal. Too much emphasis on the importance of a daily bowel movement can lead to a dependence on laxatives. Instead of a normal movement (for some patients) every other day, a loose stool is produced because of the use of a laxative. This often is followed by no bowel movement the next day, which leads to the administration of another dose of a laxative. Patients need to be assured that daily evacuation is not necessary, provided the stool is not hard and dry, and that avoiding laxatives usually allows the bowel to function normally again.

Symptoms

Stools are hard and dry, and occur infrequently. Defecation often is difficult. Diarrhea also may be present because a hard, dry stool in the lower colon and rectum stimulates nerve endings, which in turn increases peristalsis. The increase in peristalsis produces a watery stool that bypasses the impacted stool.

Diagnosis

Diagnosis is made by patient history, examination of the stool, and, possibly, a rectal examination. Laboratory and diagnostic tests may be performed to rule out an underlying cause.

Treatment

When constipation is related to diet, stress, or other nondisease entity, the major emphasis is helping the patient to maintain habits that foster normal elimination. A diet that includes plenty of raw fruits and vegetables and whole-grain bread and cereal, a high fluid intake, and regular periods of rest and exercise are important. Allowing sufficient time for evacuation at a definite time each day also is helpful in restoring normal function. The program of therapy is designed to help the patient return to normal patterns of elimination with the least possible use of enemas and laxatives.

When constipation is due to an underlying disorder, it is necessary to determine if treatment of the disorder plus dietary management will correct the situation, or if the constipation should be treated separately. Depending on the underlying disorder, treatment may include the administration of enemas or laxatives (in oral or suppository form). Although frequent administration of products or drugs to produce a bowel movement may themselves produce constipation because of a loss of intestinal tone and a diminishing of the defecation reflex, their short-term use may be necessary. Long-term use may be necessary for patients with neurologic disorders that permanently diminish or abolish the defecation reflex, such as paraplegia and multiple sclerosis.

NURSING PROCESS —THE PATIENT WHO HAS CONSTIPATION

Assessment
Some people are overly concerned about their bowel elimination pattern, and may not realize that people differ greatly in their bowel habits. In discussing the subject with the patient, it may be helpful to determine the patient's definition of constipation, as well as bowel elimination pattern; the frequency of bowel movements and their appearance, color, and consistency; dietary habits; fluid intake; and amount of exercise.

In addition to the assessments performed on the patient with a gastrointestinal (GI) disorder (see Chapter 42), a complete patient history should be obtained as well as a drug history, including the use of laxatives or enemas. Assessment of the patient may need to include examination of the anal area while looking for fissures, redness, and hemorrhoids. The abdomen should be palpated for distention and masses, and auscultated for bowel sounds.

Nursing Diagnosis
Depending on the probable cause, one or more of the following nursing diagnoses may apply:

- Constipation related to dietary habits, decreased fluid intake, underlying disease, or other factors (specify, if known)
- Anxiety related to possible diagnosis, treatment modalities, scheduled diagnostic tests, inability to have a bowel movement, abdominal discomfort
- Knowledge deficit of methods that may be used to attain normal bowel function

Planning and Implementation
The major goals of the patient include reduction in anxiety, normal bowel function, and an understanding of the methods used to attain normal bowel function.

The major goals of nursing management include the restoration of normal bowel elimination; reduction of anxiety, pain, or discomfort; and effective teaching regarding the prevention of constipation.

Anxiety. Diagnostic studies should be explained, and the patient assured that once bowel movements return to normal, discomfort will probably be reduced or eliminated.

Knowledge Deficit. Many older patients are overly concerned with their frequency of bowel movements. The definition of constipation should be discussed with the patient and misinformation clarified. Included in the discussion and teaching plan is the importance of diet, fluids, exercise, and avoiding the use of laxatives and enemas. The patient also should be warned not to strain to have a bowel movement, as this can promote the formation of hemorrhoids or make them worse. Straining also results in the Valsalva maneuver, which increases arterial blood pressure and decreases the flow of blood to the heart, which can be dangerous in cardiac as well as other disorders.

The frequency of bowel movements and their appearance should be recorded. Patients with constipation caused by an improper diet or inadequate fluid intake should receive instruction in the methods that may be used to prevent future episodes of constipation. A diet high in fiber, the addition of bran to cereal or juice, exercise, and drinking eight or more full glasses of liquid per day should be recommended. The patient should be given a list of high-fiber foods.

Elderly patients may need to be frequently reminded to drink fluids throughout the waking hours. If fluid intake appear inadequate, intake and output should be measured. If the patient fails to take sufficient fluids, the physician should be informed of the problem.

Evaluation

■ Normal bowel elimination pattern is established
■ Anxiety and discomfort are reduced or eliminated
■ Patient drinks adequate amount of fluid (eight or more glasses daily)
■ Patient eats the prescribed diet
■ Patient verbalizes understanding of areas covered in the patient-teaching plan

Diarrhea

Temporary diarrhea may be due to many factors, such as bacterial or viral infections that affect the intestine, diverticulitis, food poisoning, uremia, stress, a diet high in roughage, food that is highly spiced or seasoned, ulcerative colitis, irritable colon, intestinal obstruction, and food allergies. Diarrhea also may be caused by the overuse of laxatives, or it may be an adverse effect of drugs. Constipation may result in episodes of diarrhea because of the increase in peristalsis as the bowel attempts to empty itself of the hardened fecal mass.

Diarrhea is due to an increase in peristalsis, which rapidly moves the products of digestion through the GI tract. A decreased amount of water is absorbed in the large intestine, and the stool becomes either soft or liquid. Three major problems that may occur with severe or prolonged diarrhea include electrolyte imbalances, dehydration, and vitamin deficiencies. When diarrhea is due to a disease that causes malabsorption, a nutritional deficiency may occur. Prolonged diarrhea can cause excoriation of the skin around the anus.

Symptoms

Stools are loose and watery stools, and occur frequently.

Diagnosis

Diagnosis is based on patient history as well as examination of the stool. Stool samples may be ordered to determine the causative microorganism or to check for blood or parasites in the stool.

Treatment

Mild diarrhea or diarrhea of short duration, such as that caused by a dietary change, usually does not require treatment. When diarrhea persists, when the stools are frequent and large, or when the person is very young or elderly or has another illness, medical treatment is required.

Before treatment is instituted, the physician determines the seriousness of the problem, the possible or known cause, and what medical management is necessary to correct the disorder as well as the problems created by frequent bowel movements. Treatment may include one or more of the following:

■ An antidiarrheal agent, such as diphenoxylate hydrochloride with atropine sulfate (Lomotil), loperamide hydrochloride (Imodium), opium tincture deodorized, or camphorated tincture of opium (Paregoric), or a combination product such as Kaopectate (kaolin and pectin)
■ Fluid and electrolyte replacement by either the oral or the intravenous route
■ Dietary adjustments, which may include eliminating foods that may cause diarrhea or, when diarrhea is severe, not allowing the patient to take anything by mouth or allowing clear liquids as tolerated. If clear liquids are tolerated, the patient may be advanced to a soft bland diet followed by other foods as tolerated.
■ Total parenteral nutrition if diarrhea is severe and prolonged, and if the introduction of oral fluid and food results in another episode of diarrhea

When diarrhea is due to an infectious process, the patient may be placed in isolation.

NURSING PROCESS —THE PATIENT WHO HAS DIARRHEA

Assessment

In addition to the assessments performed on the patient with a GI disorder (see Chapter 42), a complete patient history should be obtained as well as a dietary and drug history, including the use of laxatives or enemas. Because diarrhea can occur if there is an impacted fecal mass, the patient should be asked about the occurrence of periodic episodes of constipation.

To help determine the possible cause of the diarrhea, the following information should be obtained:

■ Relation of start of diarrhea to taking a new drug, eating, bouts of constipation, or other occurrence
■ Description of the frequency, character, and color of the stools
■ When bowel movements occur (eg, immediately after eating, at any time, or without warning)
■ If excessive flatus, pain, or cramping is present, and if it is related to the passage of stool or occurs at any time

Depending on the severity of the diarrhea and the length of time it has been present, assessment of the patient may include examination of the anal area for redness or other tissue changes. The abdomen should be palpated for distention and masses, and auscultated for bowel sounds. The patient should be checked for signs of dehydration and electrolyte imbalance. Vital signs should be taken to provide baseline data.

Nursing Diagnosis

Depending on the probable cause, one or more of the following nursing diagnoses may apply:

- Diarrhea related to infection or inflammation of the bowel, constipation, tumor of the bowel, diet, other factors (specify, if known)
- Pain (cramping) related to excessive peristalsis
- Anxiety related to frequent bowel movements, odors, other factors (specify)
- Fluid volume deficit related to frequent passage of stools, inadequate fluid intake
- Altered nutrition: less than body requirements related to rapid passage of stool through the entire GI tract, anorexia
- Impaired skin integrity related to the passage of frequent, loose stools
- Potential for infection related to infectious process of the lower GI tract

Planning and Implementation

The major goals of the patient include reduction of anxiety and discomfort, normal bowel function, correction of fluid deficit, and maintenance of skin integrity.

The major goals of nursing management include the restoration of normal bowel elimination, reduction or elimination of pain or discomfort, reduction of anxiety, prevention of a fluid and electrolyte deficit, maintenance of skin integrity, and prevention of the spread of infection.

If the patient has severe diarrhea, vital signs should be monitored every 2 to 4 hours; more frequent assessments may be necessary if the patient is extremely ill. When diarrhea is severe, the patient should be kept on bed rest.

Although cramping may occur when diarrhea is severe, the sudden onset of acute abdominal pain or a rise in temperature may indicate a perforation of the bowel, and the physician should be contacted immediately. Any appearance of blood or excessive mucus in the stool should be reported to the physician.

Anxiety. If the stools have a foul odor, a room deodorizer should be used. A bedpan or commode should be kept at the patient's bedside and emptied after each use.

Fluid Volume Deficit, Altered Nutrition. When diarrhea is severe, the patient should be closely observed for signs of dehydration and electrolyte imbalances, especially hypokalemia and hyponatremia (see Chapter 12). Intake and output should be measured, and the physician notified if urine output decreases or falls below 500 mL/24 hr.

Fluids should be offered at frequent intervals. Intravenous administration of fluids may be necessary if the patient becomes dehydrated. A bland diet may be prescribed and the patient encouraged to eat. Patients who have had prolonged episodes of diarrhea may require total parenteral nutrition or nasogastric feedings.

Impaired Skin Integrity. After each bowel movement, the patient's anal area should be washed with soap and water, rinsed with clear water, and thoroughly dried. An ointment, such as vitamins A and D ointment, may be applied if the skin appears reddened. If skin breakdown occurs, the physician should be notified, since infection may easily occur because of contamination of the area. The bedding should be changed as needed and disposable pads placed under the patient's buttocks to prevent soiling of bed linen.

Potential for Infection. Good hand washing technique is imperative when caring for the patient with diarrhea to prevent transfer of microorganisms to oneself and other patients.

Evaluation

- Normal bowel elimination pattern is established
- Anxiety and discomfort are reduced or eliminated
- Normal fluid and electrolyte balance is maintained
- Nutritional needs are met; patient eats the prescribed diet
- Skin integrity is maintained
- Evidence of infection transmission is absent

INFLAMMATORY BOWEL DISEASE

Crohn's Disease (Regional Enteritis)

Most prevalent in young adults, Crohn's disease usually affects the terminal portion of the ileum. Distribution of the disease often is patchy, with the intestinal wall becoming thick and edematous. The exact cause is unknown.

Symptoms

Symptoms include abdominal pain, distention, and tenderness; diarrhea; fever; and leukocytosis. As Crohn's disease progresses, there may be weight loss, dehydration, and electrolyte imbalance. Onset usually is insidious, and the course of the disease variable. Some patients have a gradual increase in symptoms, whereas others have acute exacerbations alternating with remissions. The condition sometimes subsides spontaneously. Intestinal obstruction, perforation, or abscesses may occur, and fistulas may form between the loops of the intestine.

Diagnosis

Diagnosis is made by the symptoms, barium enema, and sigmoidoscopy or colonoscopy. Laboratory tests may show leukocytosis and, in advanced cases, electrolyte imbalances due to diarrhea. Stool samples may contain occult blood.

Complications

The complications associated with Crohn's disease include intestinal obstruction, fistula formation between the small intestine and the bladder, intraabdominal fistulas, and perforation.

Treatment

Treatment is supportive. Rest, relief of emotional stress, and diet modification may be prescribed. The dietary approach may vary, but a low-residue, high-calorie, high-protein diet often is prescribed. Parenteral therapy with fluids, electrolytes, and whole blood may be necessary to correct anemia and restore the fluid and electrolyte balance.

Drug therapy may include supplementary vitamins, iron, antidiarrheal drugs, tranquilizers, and corticosteroids. None of these treatments is curative.

Surgical treatment, usually reserved for complications such as intestinal obstruction or perforation, is made more difficult because the disease tends to be widely scattered. An attempt may be made to divert the flow of the intestinal contents from the diseased area by joining the proximal healthy portion of the ileum with the colon (ileocolostomy). The diseased portion of the ileum may later be removed; if the patient progresses satisfactorily, this may not be necessary. Irrespective of the type of treatment used, recurrence of the disease is common.

Ulcerative Colitis

In ulcerative colitis, the mucosa of the colon becomes hyperemic, thickened, and edematous. Sometimes the ulceration is so extensive that large areas of the colon are denuded of mucosa.

Ulcerative colitis is most common in young and middle-aged adults, but it can occur at any age. Although the exact cause is obscure, some believe that ulcerative colitis is a disease of multiple causative factors, including infection, allergy, autoimmunity, and emotional stress. The term *idiopathic* (no known cause) is used to describe ulcerative colitis.

Symptoms

Onset may be abrupt or gradual. The patient experiences severe diarrhea (12 or more bowel movements per day) and expels blood and mucus along with fecal matter. Weight loss, fever, severe electrolyte imbalance, dehydration, anemia, and cachexia may follow. Diarrhea often is accompanied by cramps, and the patient may experience anorexia, nausea, vomiting, and extreme weakness. The urge to defecate may come so suddenly and with such urgency that the patient is incontinent of feces. Some patients have particular problems with incontinence while they are asleep; they are unaware that defecation has taken place until they awaken.

Ulcerative colitis may continue in a fairly mild form for years, or it may run a rapid, fulminating course, and cause death from hemorrhage, peritonitis, or profound debility. Some patients have sudden, dramatic recoveries and may remain free of the disease for years.

Diagnosis

Diagnosis is made by the patient history and physical examination. Radiographic studies such as a barium enema as well as proctoscopy, sigmoidoscopy, and stool examination are performed. A careful search is made for other conditions that could be responsible for the symptoms, such as cancer, amebic dysentery, or diverticulitis. Laxatives are contraindicated in the preparation of these patients for a barium enema unless they are specifically ordered by the physician. This is especially so if the disease is acute. If the diagnosis can be made by sigmoidoscopy, the physician may postpone other studies until the more acute phase is passed, and order gentle tap-water enemas the morning of the examination.

Laboratory tests such as serum electrolyte level determination, complete blood count, and stool examination for occult blood may be ordered, to determine the effect of fluid, electrolyte, and blood loss, and other changes brought about by severe diarrhea.

Complications

Complications of ulcerative colitis include hemorrhage and perforation of the bowel. If the disorder has persisted for an extended period of time or symptoms are severe, weight loss, dehydration, electrolyte imbalance, and anemia may be seen.

Treatment

Medical treatment is supportive, and designed to provide rest for the bowel, opportunity for healing, and correction of anemia and malnutrition. Some patients can be managed medically and helped into remission. Others may require a total colectomy and permanent ileostomy when medical treatment fails or an acute complication such as perforation or severe hemorrhage occurs.

The patient may be prescribed a bland diet. Any substances that might further irritate the bowel, such as raw fruits and vegetables or highly seasoned foods, are eliminated. The patient is encouraged to eat as nourishing a diet as possible. Protein foods, such as meat and eggs, are important.

Blood transfusions and iron may be given to correct anemia. Parenteral fluids and electrolytes also may be needed. Because frequent bowel movements can interfere with absorption of nutrients, supplementary vitamins may be prescribed.

A variety of drugs may be given. Although they do not cure the disease, they may lessen symptoms and promote healing of the diseased intestine. Sedatives and tranquilizers often help the patient to relax and rest. Drugs that slow peristalsis, such as atropine or tincture of belladonna, or drugs that coat and soothe the mucosa, such as kaolin and pectin, may be ordered. Antispasmodics should be given with great caution because they may be precipitating factors in producing toxic megacolon—a marked dilatation of the colon that may lead to perforation and death. Any sudden onset of abdominal distention in a patient with acute ulcerative colitis is an ominous sign that should be reported at once.

Corticosteroids, administered either as an oral preparation or as an enema, may be given if the disease does not respond to other measures. A dramatic relief of symptoms often follows their use. In the acutely ill patient with severe diarrhea, fever, and abdominal pain, these drugs may be given intravenously until they can be taken orally. To maintain a remission, the patient may remain on the drug for weeks or months, with as low a dose as possible prescribed. The use of these potent drugs is not without hazard. They may mask the symptoms of peritonitis or produce adverse reactions, such as moon face and edema. Although they are potentially dangerous, corticosteroids have helped many patients with this disease to live longer and more comfortably and have helped some to recover who might otherwise have succumbed to the disease. They have played a major role in reducing the operative mortality of elective colectomy by decreasing patient risk and debilitation before surgery.

Sulfasalazine (Azulfidine), a sulfonamide, also may be used in the long-term management of ulcerative colitis. Psychotherapy may be helpful when it is largely of a supportive nature. As symptoms improve, the patient may be helped to recognize some of the emotional problems related to the illness.

Surgery may be necessary when the disease does not respond to other treatment or when complications occur (eg, perforation of the colon or hemorrhage). Surgical treatment of severe, intractable ulcerative colitis usually includes total colectomy (removal of the entire colon and rectum) and a permanent ileostomy.

Management of the patient with an ileostomy is discussed in Chapter 45.

NURSING PROCESS —THE PATIENT WHO HAS INFLAMMATORY BOWEL DISEASE

Assessment
In addition to the assessments performed on the patient with a GI disorder (see Chapter 42), a thorough patient history should be obtained, including a medical, drug, and diet history. At this time it is important to obtain information about the symptoms, the average number of stools passed each day, and a description of the stools. It also is important to know whether blood and mucus were present. The patient should be asked about weight loss, the drugs prescribed for the disorder (if any), and whether any foods increase the frequency of bowel movements or cause abdominal pain or discomfort.

Vital signs should be taken and the patient weighed.

Nursing Diagnosis
Depending on the severity of the disorder and the length of time present, one or more of the following nursing diagnoses may apply:

- Anxiety related to symptoms, diagnosis, treatment
- Diarrhea related to inflammation of the bowel
- Pain related to abdominal distention, inflammation of the bowel, increased peristalsis
- Altered nutrition: less than body requirements related to rapid passage of food through the bowel, anorexia
- Ineffective individual coping related to symptoms, diagnosis, treatment modalities
- Fluid volume deficit related to diarrhea, anorexia, rapid passage of food through the bowel
- Activity intolerance related to fatigue, anemia
- Potential impaired skin integrity (around anus) related to diarrhea
- Knowledge deficit of treatment regimen

Planning and Implementation
The major goals of the patient include reduction in anxiety, normal bowel elimination, relief of pain, improved nutrition and fluid intake, improved activity tolerance, prevention of skin breakdown, ability to cope with the disorder, and an understanding of the treatment regimen.

The major goals of nursing management are to attain normal bowel elimination, reduce anxiety, relieve discomfort or pain, correct fluid and electrolyte balance, improve nutrition, and help these patients cope with their disorder.

Vital signs should be monitored at 2- to 4-hour intervals. More frequent assessments may be necessary if the patient develops signs of complications, passes large volumes of watery, bloody stools, or experiences a rise in temperature and pulse and a drop in blood pressure.

The patient should be continually assessed for response to treatment. The nurse should know the action, indications for use, and adverse effects of the drugs administered to interpret and evaluate the patient's response to therapy. Thus, if an antidiarrheal agent is ordered, and the patient continues to have the same number of stools after several days of drug therapy, this fact should be documented in the patient's chart as well as reported to the physician.

Anxiety. Supportive care, both physical and emotional, can do a great deal to lessen symptoms and assist the patient in overcoming the disease. Any illness that is associated with fecal incontinence or frequent and urgent bowel movements is physically and emotionally distressing to the patient. The importance of not soiling oneself is stressed from earliest childhood, and finding that the bedding or clothing is soiled can cause the patient a profound sense of anxiety and embarrassment. Soiled bedding and clothing should be changed immediately and a room deodorizer used if needed.

The patient also should be given time to discuss and ask questions about the illness, the proposed treatments, and the possibility of surgery.

Diarrhea. The character, color, amount, and frequency of stools should be noted and recorded. Any increase in the frequency or amount of blood in the stool or the development of abdominal distention, pain, or tenderness requires prompt notification of the physician.

The abdomen should be inspected at frequent intervals for signs of distention or rigidity, especially if the patient is acutely ill.

Pain. The type of pain as well as its location, severity, and pattern of occurrence should be documented. Drugs may be prescribed to slow peristalsis and thus decrease pain. The patient's response to medication should be observed and recorded. Any sudden onset of more severe pain accompanied by other symptoms, such as abdominal rigidity, should be immediately reported to the physician.

Altered Nutrition. Helping the patient to maintain an adequate diet and fluid intake is essential. Small portions of food that the patient enjoys should be served in an environment that is clean and odor-free. The quantity and type of food the patient eats are noted. Some physicians advocate greater flexibility in the diet prescription for the patient who is not acutely ill, advising restriction only of those foods that are known to increase symptoms. The rationale behind this approach to diet therapy is that there is no clear evidence that certain categories of food worsen the condition.

Ineffective Individual Coping. Some patients appear to be both emotionally and physically ill. Some may show excessive dependence on the nurse or family members; others display apathy or constantly criticize whatever is done for them. These emotional responses may indicate that the patient is having difficulty coping with the diagnosis, symptoms, and proposed treatment modalities.

The period of acute illness is not the time to expect the patient to overcome emotional problems—even those that seem extreme, or those that present difficulties in relations with the medical team or family. Later, when the patient has improved physically, the combined efforts of the physician, the nurse, and the family may help the patient to deal more effectively with the diagnosis.

Fluid Volume Deficit. Intake and output should be measured, and the patient observed for signs of dehydration and electrolyte imbalances (see Chapter 12). If dehydration or electrolyte imbalances occur, intravenous fluids and electrolyte replacement may be necessary.

Activity Intolerance. Anemia, weight loss, and nutritional deficits are some of the causes of fatigue. The patient should be allowed to perform activities of daily living, when able, at a pace that does not produce fatigue.

Because rest in bed is important during the acute phases of the illness, it is continued until the severe symptoms subside and the patient begins to gain weight and feel stronger. The patient on bed rest may need assistance with self-care activities.

Potential for Impaired Skin Integrity. The patient should be helped to minimize soiling by keeping a clean bedpan or commode within easy reach and available if needed in a hurry. The patient should be assisted in cleaning the anal area and washing the hands after each bowel movement. If the patient is acutely ill, these tasks are performed by the nurse.

Skin care is important not only for aesthetic reasons but also because the skin around the rectum can easily become excoriated. Application of a protective ointment after the area has been cleaned may help to prevent irritation. If incontinence cannot be controlled (eg, if the patient defecates while sleeping), the use of perineal pads and disposable pads under the buttocks helps to control the extent of soiling and makes the area easier to clean.

Knowledge Deficit. Teaching the patient and family is an important aspect of managing inflammatory bowel disorders. The family will require a great deal of assistance from the physician and the nurse in understanding the patient's illness and their role in helping the patient to achieve normal bowel elimination.

DIET. The importance of maintaining the prescribed diet should be emphasized. A sample menu may be given as well as a list of foods that are either included in the diet or to be avoided.

DRUG THERAPY. Drug therapy should be reviewed with the patient, and the purpose, dose, and adverse drug effects explained. It is important to emphasize that although the drugs (when taken as directed) cannot cure the disorder, they often can control symptoms. If bowel movements become more frequent while the patient is taking the prescribed drugs, the physician should be immediately contacted, since this development may represent an adverse drug effect or a worsening of the disorder.

Sulfasalazine (Azulfidine) may cause oligospermia (reduction in the sperm count). Men who want to father children should be advised of this fact by the physician. Because this drug is a sulfonamide, the patient must drink six to eight glasses of water per day.

REST. Taking rest periods throughout the day is important. Once symptoms have subsided, the physician will allow activity to be resumed at a gradual pace.

PROBLEMS. The physician should be promptly notified if symptoms return or if extreme fatigue, severe abdominal pain, blood in the stool, adverse drug effects, or weight loss occurs.

FOLLOW-UP CARE. Periodic evaluation is necessary to determine the effectiveness of therapy.

Evaluation

■ Anxiety is reduced
■ Frequency of liquid stools decreases; stools become more formed
■ Pain is reduced or eliminated
■ Evidence of abdominal distention is absent; bowel sounds are normal
■ Patient takes oral fluids in adequate amounts; evidence of dehydration or electrolyte imbalances is absent

■ Patient tolerates small interval feedings; patient maintains or gains weight
■ Patient demonstrates ability to cope with the disorder and its treatment
■ Patient is able to increase activity tolerance
■ Evidence of skin breakdown is absent
■ Patient demonstrates an understanding of treatment modalities, including medications, diet, rest periods

ACUTE ABDOMINAL INFLAMMATORY DISORDERS
Appendicitis

Appendicitis is a common surgical emergency. The appendix—a narrow, blind tube located at the tip of the cecum—may become inflamed. Although the cause for inflammation is not clear, it is believed that obstruction occurs, making it difficult or impossible for the contents of the appendix to empty normally. Because the intestinal contents are laden with bacteria, an injury to the tissues in contact with the contents often results in an infection. A hard mass of feces, called a *fecalith*, may obstruct and mechanically irritate the appendix. Inflammation and infection may quickly follow. The pressure from the fecalith and the edema of tissues that occurs during the inflammation may interfere with the blood supply, making the tissues more vulnerable to infection and sometimes leading to gangrene and perforation. Perforation is a serious complication that may be followed by peritonitis.

Symptoms

Appendicitis can occur at any age but seems to be more common in adolescents and young adults. An attack of severe abdominal pain is the most frequent symptom of appendicitis. At first, the pain is generalized throughout the abdomen or around the umbilicus. Later, the pain typically occurs in the right lower quadrant of the abdomen. *McBurney's point*, midway between the umbilicus and the right iliac crest, usually is the site of the severest pain. Often the pain is worse when manual pressure over McBurney's point is suddenly released. This is called *rebound tenderness*. Slight or moderate fever and moderate leukocytosis usually are present. Nausea and vomiting also may be present.

Diagnosis

The physician performs a physical examination, noting especially the location of the abdominal pain and tenderness. A white blood cell count is taken, and additional tests and examinations may be ordered as necessary, to rule out other conditions that might be causing the same symptoms.

Treatment

The appendix is surgically removed (appendectomy), resulting in complete cure. The appendix has no known function within the body, and its removal causes no change in body function. Parenteral fluids may be administered before and after surgery. On the day after surgery, the patient may be permitted food and fluids as tolerated and usually is allowed out of bed. Convalescence may be rapid, but depends on the patient's age and general physical condition. A healthy young adult usually is able to return to regular activities within 2 to 4 weeks but is advised to avoid heavy lifting or unusual exertion for several months.

For nursing management of the patient undergoing appendectomy, see Chapter 16.

Peritonitis

In peritonitis, the peritoneum, a serous sac lining the abdominal cavity, becomes inflamed. The intestines, normally filled with bacteria, are among the organs enclosed in the peritoneum. Any break in the continuity of the intestines that causes a leakage of intestinal contents can lead to inflammation and infection of the peritoneum. Peritonitis may be caused by perforation of a peptic ulcer, the bowel, or the appendix; trauma, such as gunshot or knife wounds; ruptured ectopic pregnancy; or infection introduced during peritoneal dialysis. The infection may be widespread within the peritoneum (generalized peritonitis), or it may be localized, and lead to the formation of an abscess.

Symptoms

Symptoms include severe abdominal pain and tenderness, nausea, and vomiting. Fever may be absent initially, but the temperature rises as the infection becomes established. The patient avoids movement of the abdomen when breathing because such movement increases pain. The knees may be drawn up toward the abdomen because this position seems to lessen the pain. The pulse rate usually is elevated, and respirations are rapid and shallow.

Paralytic ileus typically accompanies peritonitis. The abdomen is rigid and boardlike. As the condition progresses, the abdomen becomes somewhat softer and distended with the gas and the intestinal contents that cannot pass normally through the tract. Marked leukocytosis usually is present.

If the infection is uncontrolled, severe weakness, a rapid and thready pulse, a markedly distended abdomen, and a drop in body temperature are seen. The patient is moribund, and death follows.

Diagnosis

Diagnosis is made by symptoms, a history of a disorder or event that may lead to peritonitis, and physical examination. The most severe pain and tenderness usually occur over the area of the greatest peritoneal inflammation. The location of the pain helps the physician to determine the possible cause. A white blood cell count and differential and radiographs of the abdomen are other important aids in diagnosis.

Treatment

The early diagnosis and treatment of such conditions as appendicitis have decreased the incidence of peritonitis. Strict surgical asepsis and the use of antibiotics before performing surgery on the intestines have reduced the number of patients who develop peritonitis as a complication of surgery.

Preventing further leakage of intestinal contents into the peritoneal cavity is an important measure in treatment. For example, if the duodenum has perforated as a result of peptic ulcer, the area of perforation is closed surgically so that no further escape of the intestinal contents can take place.

Gastrointestinal decompression is used to drain the accumulated gas and the intestinal contents. The replacement of fluids and electrolytes also is important, as water and electrolytes are being lost in vomitus and in drainage from GI intubation.

Large doses of antibiotics are given to combat infection. Analgesics such as meperidine (Demerol) often are necessary to relieve pain and promote rest. After successful intensive medical or surgical treatment, symptoms subside.

NURSING PROCESS —THE PATIENT WHO HAS PERITONITIS

Assessment

In addition to the assessments performed on the patient with a GI disorder (see Chapter 42), the initial assessment consists of documenting vital signs and all symptoms. Depending on the situation, a review of the patient's past and present medical, drug, and allergy histories can be made from the patient's chart or, if the patient is newly admitted to the hospital, obtained from the family.

Nursing Diagnosis

Depending on the severity of the disorder, one or more of the following nursing diagnoses may apply. Additional diagnoses may be necessary if the patient does not respond to treatment or if surgery is performed.

- Pain related to irritation and inflammation of the peritoneum, edema and distention of the bowel
- Hyperthermia related to the infectious and inflammatory process

- Fluid volume deficit related to inability to take oral fluids, GI decompression
- Altered oral mucous membrane related to hyperthermia, nasogastric intubation, restriction of oral fluids, surgery
- Impaired tissue integrity related to surgical incision, drains, infection

Planning and Implementation

The major goals of the patient include relief of pain, normal body temperature, correction of a fluid volume deficit, elimination of oral mucosa irritation, and healing of tissues.

The major goals of nursing management are to relieve pain, protect the patient from injury, and detect further complications, such as shock, electrolyte imbalances, and dehydration.

The patient with peritonitis is very ill and requires detailed assessment, care, and observation. Symptoms often change rapidly, and assessments, conducted at frequent intervals, should consist of the following:

- Inspection and palpation of the abdomen for signs of distention and rigidity
- Evaluation of pain with a description of the location, type, and intensity
- Measurement of vital signs
- Measurement of fluid intake
- Measurement of output—urine, nasogastric or GI decompression tube, drains (if any)
- Observation for signs of fluid or electrolyte imbalance

Intravenous fluids should be started immediately and continued until the patient is able to take oral fluids. Antibiotic therapy also should be started immediately. An antipyretic agent such as aspirin or acetaminophen may be used to reduce fever.

Any change detected during ongoing assessments or the development of any new problem should be reported to the physician immediately.

Pain. The patient with peritonitis requires *gentleness*, as every movement causes added pain. If the patient must be moved from the bed, the nurse will require assistance in moving the patient as gently and smoothly as possible. Precautions should be taken to avoid placing any accidental pressure on the abdomen.

Because shock may occur at any time, narcotic analgesics, even in low doses, should be administered with care. The blood pressure should be taken before administration, and the drug withheld if the systolic pressure is 100 or lower or if there have been recent decreases in the blood pressure determinations. After administration, the patient should be closely observed for a drop in blood pressure or re-

spiratory depression. If these occur, the physician should be contacted immediately, as a narcotic antagonist may be necessary to reverse the depressant effects of the narcotic.

The patient may become disoriented because of severe pain, narcotic administration, dehydration, or overwhelming infection. Side rails on the bed should be raised to prevent injury. If the patient is extremely confused and pulls at the surgical dressing, intravenous line, or nasogastric or GI tube, an order for wrist restraints may be obtained.

Altered Oral Mucous Membrane. Mouth care is important. The inability to take anything by mouth, the presence of a GI tube, and fever make the patient's mouth feel dry and cause an unpleasant taste and odor. If the patient is cooperative, oral rinses should be offered. If the patient is unable to use an oral rinse, the mouth should be cleaned with moist cotton swabs.

Impaired Tissue Integrity. If surgery is performed, drains may be inserted during surgery, and retention sutures used to support the surgical incision and decrease the possibility of wound separation. The surgical dressing and dressings over the drains should be checked at frequent intervals, and the amount and color or type of drainage recorded. During dressing changes, the incision and the entrance and exit points of the retention sutures should be inspected for signs of inflammation, abscess formation, drainage or exudate, retarded wound healing, and wound separation.

Evaluation

- Pain is controlled
- Temperature is normal
- Abdomen is less distended; peristalsis returns to normal
- Fluid volume deficit is corrected; serum electrolyte levels are normal
- Evidence of injury is absent
- Oral mucous membranes are normal in appearance
- Evidence of wound separation is absent; surgical wound appears normal

INTESTINAL OBSTRUCTION

Intestinal obstruction, which blocks the normal flow through the intestine, can be paralytic or mechanical. *Paralytic obstruction* occurs when there is an absence of normal nerve stimulation to muscle fibers of the intestine. *Mechanical obstruction* occurs when the intestinal lumen becomes obstructed.

Paralytic Obstruction

In paralytic ileus, peristalsis is absent. Peristalsis normally is absent for 12 to 36 hours after abdominal surgery (functional paralytic ileus), but this absence also may be seen with other types of surgery.

Most commonly, paralytic ileus is a complication of abdominal surgery seen after normal peristalsis is expected. It also may be seen in other disorders such as peritonitis and severe hypokalemia.

Symptoms

The patient complains of severe abdominal pain. The abdomen is distended, and bowel sounds are absent. Nausea and vomiting may occur, and, in some instances, there is a reverse peristalsis and the patient vomits fecal material.

Diagnosis is made by auscultation and palpation of the abdomen and by radiographs of the abdomen.

Treatment

The patient is given nothing by mouth, and a nasogastric tube is inserted and connected to suction. Neostigmine may be administered to restore normal peristalsis. Fluid and electrolyte imbalances are treated.

NURSING PROCESS —THE PATIENT WHO HAS A PARALYTIC ILEUS

Assessment

In addition to the assessments performed on the patient with a GI disorder (see Chapter 42), complete medical, drug, and allergy histories are obtained. It is important to document all symptoms and obtain detailed information about each. For example, if vomiting has occurred, information regarding the onset, amount, and color of the vomitus should be obtained.

Physical assessment includes examination of the abdomen for distention and tenderness and auscultation of the abdomen for bowel sounds. The girth of the abdomen should be measured to provide a data base; a measuring tape is placed under the hips at the iliac crest and the measurement is taken when the patient exhales. Vital signs should be taken.

Nursing Diagnosis

Depending on the severity of symptoms and the patient's general condition, one or more of the following nursing diagnoses may apply:

■ Pain related to bowel inflammation and distention
■ Anxiety related to symptoms, treatment modalities

■ Altered nutrition: less than body requirements related to vomiting
■ Fluid volume deficit related to vomiting, inability to take oral fluids

Planning and Implementation

The major goals of the patient include relief of pain, reduction in anxiety, improved nutrition, and correction of fluid volume deficit.

The major goals of nursing management are to relieve pain, reduce anxiety, restore normal peristalsis, improve nutrition, and correct and maintain fluid and electrolyte balance.

Vital signs should be taken and bowel sounds auscultated at frequent intervals. The abdomen should be measured every 4 to 8 hours for any increase or decrease in size. The function of the nasogastric tube should be checked at frequent intervals and the color and amount of drainage noted.

Pain, Anxiety.   Narcotic analgesics usually are ordered to control pain, which often is severe. The blood pressure and pulse rate should be measured before administration, and the drug withheld if symptoms of shock or a recent marked decrease in blood pressure has occurred. About 30 to 45 minutes after administration, the patient should be assessed for relief of pain. The relief of severe pain and discomfort also helps to reduce anxiety.

Altered Nutrition, Fluid Volume Deficit.   Intravenous fluids should be administered until peristalsis returns. Once peristalsis returns and the nasogastric tube is removed, clear fluids may be ordered given in small amounts and at frequent intervals. When the patient begins to pass flatus and tolerates clear liquids, a soft diet usually is ordered.

Serum electrolyte levels may be measured to monitor the electrolyte status. The patient also should be observed for signs of dehydration and electrolyte imbalance (see Chapter 12). Intake and output should be measured, and the physician notified if output falls below 500 mL/day.

Evaluation

■ Peristalsis returns; bowel sounds are normal
■ Pain is reduced or eliminated
■ Patient is able to take clear liquids and then solid food
■ Evidence of fluid deficit or electrolyte imbalance is absent
■ Anxiety is reduced
■ Nutritional needs are met

Mechanical Obstruction

Mechanical obstruction can be partial or complete. An example of partial mechanical obstruction is a tumor of the bowel; an example of complete obstruction is a volvulus.

Etiology

Adhesions. Adhesions are one of the most common causes of mechanical intestinal obstruction. Most instances of adhesions that cause an obstruction are the result of abdominal surgery. Adhesions also may form after inflammatory disorders, such as peritonitis.

Tumors. Benign tumors may obstruct the bowel lumen, but malignant tumors are one of the most common cause of intestinal obstruction, particularly in older people. The malignant or benign tumor gradually enlarges until it completely obstructs the bowel.

Hernia. A strangulated hernia is another cause of mechanical intestinal obstruction, and is described in the section on hernias, under incisional hernia.

Volvulus. A volvulus is a twisting or kinking of a portion of the intestines (Fig. 44-1). Complete obstruction usually occurs.

Intussusception. In this disorder, part of the intestine folds (or invaginates) into an adjacent part of the intestine.

Symptoms

Symptoms of severe intestinal obstruction may arise suddenly in a previously healthy person. When the bowel is obstructed, the portion proximal to the obstruction becomes distended with intestinal contents, whereas the portion distal to the obstruction is empty. If obstruction is complete, no gas or feces are expelled

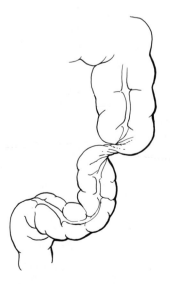

Figure 44–1. Volvulus of the colon. The twisting can cause complete obstruction.

rectally. One or two bowel movements may occur soon after the intestine has been obstructed because the material already past the obstruction is being expelled. Peristalsis becomes forceful in the proximal portion as the body attempts to propel the material beyond the point of the obstruction. These forceful peristaltic waves cause severe intermittent cramps.

When an obstruction occurs high in the GI tract, the patient usually vomits whatever contents are in the stomach and small intestine. On the other hand, if the obstruction is low—for example in the colon—vomiting usually does not occur.

The patient becomes dehydrated, is unable to take oral fluids, and loses water and electrolytes through vomiting. Failure of the mucosa to reabsorb the secretions that are poured into the intestine contributes to water and electrolyte imbalances.

Increasing pressure on the bowel due to severe distention and edema often impairs circulation and leads to gangrene of a portion of the bowel. Perforation of the gangrenous bowel (which results from pressure against weakened tissue) causes the intestinal contents to seep into the peritoneal cavity, resulting in peritonitis. Intestinal obstruction is extremely dangerous and may prove fatal if prompt treatment is not instituted.

The chief symptoms of cancer of the colon are a change in bowel habits, blood in the stool, and anemia. Changes in bowel habits may be noted while an obstruction is partial. There also may be alternating constipation and diarrhea. Diarrhea results from forceful peristalsis, which is the body's way of pushing the intestinal contents through the narrowed lumen of the bowel. If the patient receives prompt diagnosis and treatment, complete obstruction may be averted.

Diagnosis

Diagnosis is based on a thorough patient history and physical examination. Radiographic examination of the GI tract usually is necessary.

Treatment

Mechanical obstruction most frequently is treated surgically. The obstruction may be relieved by a temporary colostomy. After the patient's condition has improved as a result of relief of the obstruction and supportive therapy, more extensive surgery may be undertaken. Sometimes, because of the location and extent of a malignant process, a permanent colostomy is necessary.

These patients may be acutely ill. GI decompression, intravenous fluids, and antibiotics may be used before surgery to help improve their condition, so that surgery is less traumatic and recovery more rapid.

Gastrointestinal decompression is performed by passing a long tube, such as the Miller-Abbott tube, into the intestine. Large amounts of accumulated secretions and gas are drawn out through the tube by gentle suction, relieving distention and vomiting. Intravenous fluids with electrolytes are administered to correct fluid and electrolyte imbalances. Antibiotics may be ordered to treat infection.

Treatment of cancer of the colon is primarily surgical. Sometimes a combination of surgery, chemotherapy, and radiation therapy is used. Depending on the location of the tumor and the presence or absence of metastasis, it may be possible to completely remove the malignant tissue of the affected section of bowel and restore the normal continuity of the GI tract by joining the remaining portions of the intestine. If this treatment is not possible because of the size of the tumor, metastasis, or the patient's general condition, a permanent colostomy may be performed to relieve the obstruction. Sometimes a temporary colostomy is done to relieve obstruction, and more radical surgery, to remove the malignant growth and reestablish the continuity of the bowel, is performed when the patient's physical condition has improved.

Nursing management depends on treatment. If general abdominal surgery is performed, see Chapter 16. Management of the patient with a colostomy is discussed in Chapter 45.

DIVERTICULAR DISORDERS

Diverticula are sacs or pouches caused by herniation of the mucosa through a weakened portion of the muscular coat of the intestine or other structure. Diverticula are common in the esophagus and the colon, and are especially likely to occur in the sigmoid colon.

The cause of diverticula is unknown. It is believed that some diverticula are congenital, although most are thought to be due to weakness in the muscular coat associated with aging. Diverticula are most prevalent in people over age 50.

Diverticulosis

Diverticulosis is the presence of multiple diverticula.

Symptoms
Diverticulosis is almost always asymptomatic.

Diagnosis
Diverticulosis may not be discovered until GI radiographs are taken for some other condition or at autopsy. Sigmoidoscopy, colonoscopy, and barium enema studies may be performed to confirm the diagnosis.

Treatment
Diverticula noted during routine examination require no treatment if they do not cause symptoms. Avoiding foods that contain seeds of any kind is recommended. A high-fiber diet as well as bran added to cereal or juice may be recommended. Constipation should be avoided. Any appearance of blood in the stool or sudden pain and fever require seeking immediate medical attention.

Diverticulitis

Diverticulitis is inflammation or infection of the diverticula. The contents of the GI tract (eg, food and bacteria) may become trapped in these pouches, leading to irritation and infection of the diverticula.

Symptoms
Constipation, diarrhea, flatulence, pain and tenderness in the left lower quadrant, fever, leukocytosis, and rectal bleeding may occur. Intestinal obstruction, abscess formation, hemorrhage, or a perforation leading to peritonitis occasionally results from the inflammatory process.

Diagnosis
Diagnosis is based on symptoms and radiographic examination (see section on diverticulosis). Diverticulitis with resultant stricture formation may be difficult to differentiate from carcinoma except at surgery.

Treatment
Diverticulitis often responds to medical treatment. During an acute episode with pain and local tenderness, the patient may be maintained on intravenous fluids for several days with no oral intake. As the inflammation subsides under antibiotic therapy, oral fluids and food are prescribed. If the condition does not respond to medical treatment, or if complications such as perforation, intestinal obstruction, or severe bleeding occur, surgery may necessary. The portion of colon that contains the diverticula is removed, and the continuity of the bowel reestablished by joining the remaining portions of the colon. Depending on the location and extent of the disease and whether there is intestinal obstruction, a temporary colostomy may be necessary. The continuity of the bowel is restored in a later operation, and the colostomy is closed.

If treatment involves abdominal surgery, see Chapter 16. If a colostomy is performed, see Chapter 45.

Meckel's Diverticulum

In Meckel's diverticulum, a congenital disorder, a blind tube, like the appendix, opens into the distal ileum near the ileocecal valve.

Symptoms

There may be no symptoms, and like diverticulosis, diagnosis may not be made until radiographs are taken for another disorder. If symptoms do occur, they are the result of inflammation of the diverticulum. Pain in the right lower quadrant or umbilical pain, as well as the passage of stools containing dark red blood, may be seen.

Diagnosis

Diagnosis is made by radiography, examination of the stool for blood, and patient history.

Treatment

Treatment consists of surgical excision of the diverticulum. For nursing management, see Chapter 16.

NURSING PROCESS —THE PATIENT WHO HAS A DIVERTICULAR DISORDER

Assessment

In addition to the assessments performed on the patient with a GI disorder (see Chapter 42), a history of symptoms, diet, drug use, and allergies should be obtained. Important points to be covered in the history are questions regarding pain, bowel elimination, and diet habits.

Physical examination should include palpation of the abdomen for pain, tenderness, and masses. Vital signs should be taken.

Nursing Diagnosis

Depending on the diagnosis and symptoms, one or more of the following nursing diagnoses may apply:

■ Constipation related to low fiber intake, narrowing of the colon secondary to an inflammatory process
■ Diarrhea related to inflammatory process
■ Pain related to inflammation and infection
■ Knowledge deficit of treatment regimen

Planning and Implementation

In most instances, diverticula are treated medically.

The major goals of the patient include normal bowel elimination, reduction of pain or discomfort, and an understanding of the prescribed treatment regimen.

The major goals of nursing management are to relieve pain or discomfort and to restore normal bowel elimination.

Knowledge Deficit. The major focus of medical management is patient teaching. In most instances, pain or discomfort can be relieved and a normal bowel elimination pattern can be established with medical management and patient compliance. When a special diet is recommended, a dietary consult or a list of foods to eat or avoid is necessary.

The following points should be included in a teaching plan:

1. Follow the diet recommended by the physician. This will probably reduce pain and discomfort.
2. Bran adds bulk to the diet. Unprocessed bran can be sprinkled over cereal or added to fruit juice.
3. Avoid the use of laxatives or enemas except when recommended by the physician.
4. Avoid constipation. A regular evacuation schedule should be followed. Do not suppress the urge to defecate.
5. Drink at least 8 to 10 large glasses of fluids each day.
6. Take prescribed medications as directed, even if symptoms improve.
7. Exercise is especially important if work involves long periods of sitting.
8. If severe pain or blood in the stool occurs, see a physician immediately.

Evaluation

■ Patient demonstrates understanding of type of diet to be followed, medication schedule, and other prescribed or recommended treatment modalities
■ Bowel elimination pattern is normal

HERNIA

Although the term *hernia* may be used in relation to the protrusion of any organ from the cavity that normally confines it, it most commonly is used to describe the protrusion of intestines through a defect in the abdominal wall. Sometimes laypeople use the word *rupture* to describe this condition. When a hernia occurs, a lump or swelling appears on the abdomen beneath the skin. The swelling may be large or small, depending on how much of the intestine has protruded. Because hernia is common and may cause no symptoms other than a swelling, its potential seriousness often may be underestimated.

Types

The most common types of abdominal hernia are *inguinal* (Fig. 44-2), *umbilical, femoral,* and *incisional*. Certain points on the abdominal wall are weaker than others and more vulnerable to the development of a hernia. These points are the inguinal ring, the point on the abdominal wall where the inguinal canal begins; the femoral ring, at the abdominal opening of the femoral canal; and the umbilicus.

Inguinal Hernia. There are two types of inguinal hernia: direct and indirect. A direct inguinal hernia

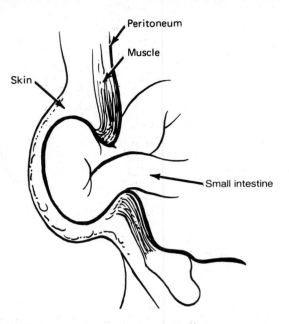

Figure 44–2. Inguinal hernia, demonstrating how the small intestine can become caught in the herniated sac.

extends into the floor of the inguinal canal, whereas an indirect inguinal hernia extends down into the inguinal canal.

Umbilical Hernia. An umbilical hernia usually occurs because the umbilical orifice fails to close shortly after birth. It is evidenced by a protrusion of the umbilicus. Obesity and prolonged abdominal distention also can result in an umbilical hernia.

Femoral Hernia. A femoral hernia occurs where the femoral artery passes into the femoral canal, below the inguinal ligament.

Incisional Hernia. An incisional hernia occurs through the scar of a surgical incision when healing has been impaired. Incisional hernias often can be avoided by careful surgical technique, with particular emphasis on the prevention of wound infection. Obese or aged patients and those who suffer from malnutrition are especially prone to the development of an incisional hernia.

If the protruding structures can be replaced in the abdominal cavity, the hernia is said to be *reducible.* Placing the patient in a supine position and applying manual pressure over the area may reduce the hernia. An *irreducible* hernia is one that cannot be replaced in the abdominal cavity. Edema of the protruding structures and constriction of the opening through which they have emerged make it impossible for them to return to the abdominal cavity. This condition is called *incarceration.* If the process continues without treatment, the blood supply to the trapped segment of

bowel can be cut off, leading to gangrene. This condition is called *strangulated hernia.*

Causes and Incidence

Congenital defects account for a large proportion of hernias, including those that appear after childhood. The hernia may be apparent in infancy, or it may appear in young adulthood in response to increased intraabdominal pressure, such as that which occurs during heavy lifting, sneezing, coughing, or pregnancy. Obesity and the weakening of muscles may be responsible for the development of hernia in later middle life and old age.

Inguinal hernias are the most common type. They are more prevalent in men than in women, whereas umbilical and femoral hernias are more frequent in women.

Symptoms

A hernia may cause no symptoms other than the appearance of a swelling on the abdomen when the patient coughs, stands, or lifts something heavy. Sometimes the swelling is painful, but the pain disappears when the hernia is reduced. Incarcerated hernias cause severe pain, and if not treated, they may become strangulated. The symptoms of strangulated hernia are discussed under the section on complications.

Diagnosis

Diagnosis usually is made by physical examination. Occasionally radiographs of the GI tract are ordered.

Complications

When a hernia first occurs, the defect in the abdominal wall usually is small. As the hernia persists and the organs continue to protrude, the defect grows larger, making surgical repair more difficult. The hernia may become incarcerated or even strangulated. *Strangulation is an acute emergency.* The patient suffers extreme abdominal pain, and the severe pressure on the loop of intestine protruding outside the abdominal cavity causes intestinal obstruction. Unless surgery is performed promptly, this section of the intestine will lose its blood supply and become gangrenous. The gangrenous part of the intestine must be excised, with anastomosis of the remaining portions of the intestine.

When a hernia is neglected for many years, the tissues in the area weaken, and postoperative healing may be impaired. Obese people who have put off surgical repair of their hernias for a prolonged period are especially prone to recurrence of the hernia, despite surgical repair. The physician usually advises the obese patient to lose weight before the surgery, to lessen the possibility of recurrence.

Treatment

The only recommended treatment for a hernia is a *herniorrhaphy*—surgical repair of the hernia. The protruding structures are replaced in the abdominal cavity, and the defect in the abdominal wall is repaired. Herniorrhaphy may be performed under local, spinal, or general anesthesia. Some patients, either because they are unwilling to have surgery or because they are not candidates for surgery, may wear a truss, which is an apparatus with a pad fitted to lie over the hernia and prevent protrusion of the bowel through the defect.

NURSING PROCESS —THE PATIENT UNDERGOING SURGICAL REPAIR OF A HERNIA

Assessment

Complete medical, drug, and allergy histories should be obtained. It is important to determine the length of time the hernia has been present, and if any activity, such as heavy lifting, produced the first signs of a hernia.

Nursing Diagnosis

Depending on the type of hernia and surgery performed, one or more of the following nursing diagnoses may apply:

- Pain related to surgery
- Potential for infection related to surgery
- Knowledge deficit of postdischarge home care

Planning and Implementation

The major goals of the patient include reduction of pain, absence of infection, and an understanding of postdischarge home care.

The major goals of nursing management are to relieve pain, prevent postoperative complications, and inform the patient of the measures necessary to prevent a recurrence of the disorder.

Preoperative preparations may be limited to routine preparations for surgery, as the current trend is to admit patients for this as well as other types of surgery on the morning of surgery.

After surgery, walking about and breathing deeply are important in preventing postoperative complications. The patient should be encouraged to move, provided no strain is placed on the operative area. Some patients are afraid to move or walk lest the hernia reappear. If the height of the bed is adjustable, it should be in the lowest position before the patient gets up, to avoid strain. If the bed is not adjustable, a footstool will help the patient to step easily from the high bed to the floor.

Coughing after surgery should be discouraged. The patient should be shown how to splint the incision with a hand if coughing or sneezing does occur.

Fluids and Nutrition. Most patients are able to tolerate food and fluids the evening of or the morning after surgery. Some patients, either because of the type and extent of the necessary surgery or because of the existence of such complications as strangulation, are permitted nothing by mouth for several days after the operation. These patients usually receive parenteral fluids until oral fluids are permitted. Intake and output should be measured.

Altered Urinary Elimination. Most patients are permitted out of bed on the day of or the day after the operation. If there is difficulty voiding, the male patient may be permitted to stand at the bedside, with assistance, while he uses the urinal. If permitted, the female patient may use a bedside commode.

Pain. Analgesics usually are given for 2 or 3 days after surgery. Some male patients develop pain and swelling of the scrotum due to inflammation and edema after repair of an inguinal hernia. Ice bags may be ordered for relief of the pain and swelling, and the scrotum may be supported with a suspensory.

Potential for Infection. Every effort should be made to prevent conditions that might impair healing and lead to a recurrence of the hernia. Strict aseptic technique is important in preventing infection. The wound should be inspected during each dressing change for signs of infection and wound separation.

Knowledge Deficit. Discharge teaching should include instructions to avoid strenuous exertion and heavy lifting until the physician determines that such activities can be safely undertaken. Many factors influence the extent to which the patient's activities must be restricted: the location and size of the defect repaired, the condition of the patient's tissues, the patient's age, and whether the patient is obese are examples. Patients who perform heavy physical labor may have to change occupations; those whose work is sedentary or light usually can return to full employment within a few weeks. Healthy young adults who have had an uncomplicated hernia repaired are likely to have few restrictions on activity.

The teaching plan also should cover the importance of drinking six or more glasses of liquids per day, eating a well-balanced diet, and avoiding constipation or straining to have a bowel movement.

Evaluation

■ Evidence of a fluid volume deficit is absent
■ Patient voids within 12 hours after surgery
■ Pain is controlled
■ Evidence of infection or wound separation is absent
■ Patient demonstrates understanding of home care and restriction of activities

CANCER OF THE COLON AND RECTUM

Cancer of the colon and rectum (colorectal cancer) is one of the most common types of cancer (Fig. 44-3). The incidence of colorectal cancer rises with age. Most malignant tumors arise from the lining of the intestine, and are adenocarcinomas. They may be found anywhere from the cecum to the rectum.

Polyps in the colon may be malignant or benign. When discovered during endoscopic examination, they are removed, and examined for malignant changes. In familial (occurring frequently in a family) polyposis, hundreds of polyps are present in the intestine.

Symptoms

Symptoms depend on the site and size of the tumor. The chief symptoms of cancer of the colon are a change in bowel habits, blood in the stool, and anemia. Other symptoms include abdominal pain and weight loss. A tumor of the cecum or rectum may give earlier warning signs, such as lower abdominal pain and cramps, bright red blood in the stool, and constipation alternating with diarrhea. If colorectal cancer goes undetected and untreated, it can cause a bowel obstruction.

Many times polyps in the intestine give no symptoms, and are discovered during endoscopic examination.

Diagnosis

A patient history plus diagnostic studies such as barium enema, sigmoidoscopy, colonoscopy, proctosigmoidoscopy, and examination of the stool for occult blood are performed. Laboratory tests include a complete blood count to detect anemia. Other laboratory tests, such as carcinogenic embryonic antigen, also may be ordered.

Physical examination may include palpation of the abdomen for masses, and digital examination of the rectum.

Treatment

Treatment of cancer of the colon is primarily surgical. Sometimes a combination of surgery, radiation therapy, and chemotherapy is used. Depending on the lo-

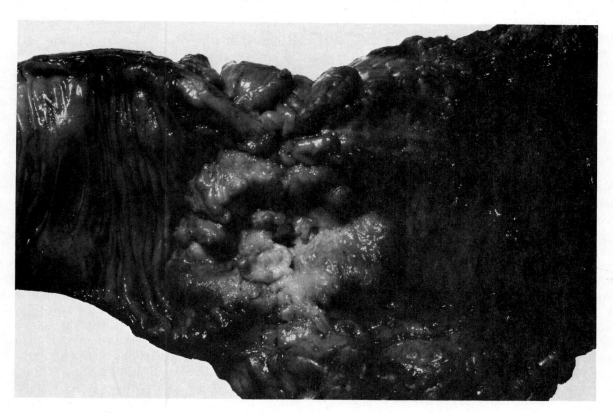

Figure 44-3.   Carcinoma of the transverse colon. (Courtesy of P. S. Milley, MD)

cation of the tumor and the time when treatment is instituted, it may be possible to completely remove the malignant tissue of the affected section of bowel and restore normal continuity of the GI tract by joining the remaining portions of the intestine. If this approach to treatment is not possible because of metastasis, the size of the tumor, or the patient's general condition, a temporary or a permanent colostomy may be performed to relieve the obstruction caused by the tumor.

Cancer of the rectum requires an abdominoperineal resection. Treatment of intestinal polyps includes removal of the polyps and examination of the removed tissue for malignant changes. Even if the polyp is benign, the patient should undergo periodic examination of the colon (eg, radiography and endoscopic examination) for recurrence. Familial polyposis necessitates removal of the entire colon, as this benign disorder almost always undergoes malignant changes if left untreated.

Management of the patient with a colostomy is discussed in Chapter 45.

ANORECTAL DISORDERS

Hemorrhoids

Hemorrhoids are varicose veins of the anus and the rectum. They may occur outside the anal sphincter (external hemorrhoids) or inside the sphincter (internal hemorrhoids; Fig. 44-4). The external and internal sphincters keep the orifice closed except during defecation. External hemorrhoids appear as small, reddish-blue lumps at the edge of the anus. Pregnancy, intraabdominal tumors, chronic constipation, and hereditary factors may foster the development of hemorrhoids.

Symptoms

External hemorrhoids may cause few symptoms, or they may produce pain, itching, and soreness of the anal area.

Thrombosed external hemorrhoids are painful lumps that appear near the anus. One or two such swellings may appear and disappear spontaneously within a few days. Pain and swelling are caused by clotted blood within the vein. Thrombosed external hemorrhoids seldom cause bleeding, but they may enlarge and become more numerous, causing pain and itching. Because the pain is especially severe while having a bowel movement, the person may put off defecation as long as possible. Constipation results or, if already present, is aggravated. Constipation and straining at stool make the hemorrhoids worse.

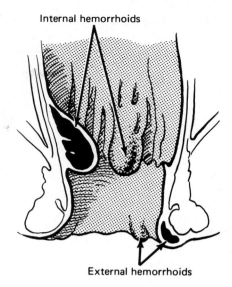

Figure 44–4. Internal and external hemorrhoids.

Internal hemorrhoids may cause bleeding but are less likely to cause pain, unless they protrude through the anus. The amount of bleeding varies from an occasional drop or two of blood on toilet tissue or underwear to chronic loss of blood, leading to anemia. Internal hemorrhoids usually protrude each time the patient defecates but retract after defecation. As the masses grow larger, they remain outside the sphincter, and often cause chronic discharge of blood and mucus.

Diagnosis

Diagnosis of external hemorrhoids is made by visual examination of the anus. Unless internal hemorrhoids protrude through the anus, the physician uses an anoscope or proctoscope to see them. Because the symptoms may be similar to those of cancer, a thorough examination of the anal and rectal areas is necessary. The patient who experiences rectal bleeding may have hemorrhoids or cancer or both.

Anyone who experiences pain, bleeding, or swelling in the anal area should be examined promptly, so that the cause of the condition can be determined.

Treatment

A small external hemorrhoid may disappear without treatment, or it may be relieved by warm sitz baths. The physician may recommend the application of an ointment that contains a local anesthetic, for the relief of discomfort. The correction of constipation is important both in relieving the condition and in preventing its recurrence. A stool softener may be ordered. Surgical excision of the dilated veins (hemorrhoidectomy) may be required.

Anorectal Abscess

An anorectal abscess is an infection in or around the anus.

Symptoms

Symptoms include pain, swelling, and redness in the affected area. Fever and abdominal pain may be seen if the abscess has extended into deeper tissues.

Diagnosis

Diagnosis is based on symptoms as well as visual examination of the area.

Treatment

Analgesics and sitz baths may be prescribed to relieve symptoms. An incision and drainage to remove the infected material also may be necessary. If a fistula has formed, deeper excision and removal of the fistulous tract are necessary.

Anal Fissure

An anal fissure (fissure in ano) is an ulcer in the anal canal.

Symptoms

Severe pain and bleeding on defecation are the most common symptoms.

Diagnosis

Diagnosis is established by visual examination with an anoscope.

Treatment

Treatment includes anesthetic suppositories, sitz baths, analgesics, and the prevention of constipation. Surgical excision of the area may be necessary.

Anal Fistula

An anal fistula (fistula in ano) is a tract leading from the anus into the anal canal.

Symptoms

Symptoms include pain on defecation and the leakage of pus and stool from the anus.

Diagnosis

Diagnosis is made by visual examination with an anoscope.

Treatment

Surgical excision of the fistulous tract often is necessary.

Pilonidal Sinus

Pilonidal means "a nest of hair." The words *sinus* and *cyst* are both used to describe the condition. The condition typically occurs after puberty, when the hair in the anogenital region becomes thick and stiff. The skin deep in the cleft in the sacrococcygeal region becomes macerated. People who have a deep cleft in this region and those who are hirsute (hairy) are predisposed to the condition. Inadequate personal hygiene, obesity, and trauma to the area contribute to the development of a pilonidal sinus. Stiff hairs in the sacrococcygeal region irritate and pierce the soft, macerated skin, becoming imbedded in it. The hairs then cause inflammation of the tissues. Infection readily follows because the break in the skin permits the entrance of microorganisms. Several channels lead from the sinus to the skin; their openings on the skin are called *pilonidal openings*. Hair may protrude from them.

Symptoms

The patient may be unaware that a pilonidal sinus is present until it becomes infected. Then, pain and swelling at the base of the spine and purulent drainage on clothing may be noted.

Diagnosis

Diagnosis is made by inspection of the affected area.

Treatment

Surgery usually is necessary. The sinus and all its connecting channels are laid open, and purulent material and hair are removed to encourage healing with normal, healthy tissue.

NURSING PROCESS —THE PATIENT WHO HAS AN ANORECTAL DISORDER

Assessment

A complete patient history, including drug and allergy histories, should be taken. Because bleeding often is seen in rectal disorders, the patient should be asked to describe the bleeding as well as all symptoms associated with the disorder. It also is important to determine if there is a history of constipation or alternating diarrhea and constipation, and if any prescription or nonprescription drugs were used to treat the problem. A diet history should be taken, with particular attention to the type of foods (especially fiber) included in the diet.

Nursing Diagnosis

Depending on the type of treatment, one or more of the following nursing diagnoses may apply:

Medical Treatment
■ Pain related to inflammation, swelling, infection, impairment of tissue integrity
■ Constipation related to diet habits, lack of exercise, inadequate fluid intake, pain on defecation
■ Knowledge deficit of medical treatment regimen

Surgical Treatment
■ Pain related to surgery
■ Anxiety related to surgery, postoperative pain and discomfort
■ Altered patterns of urinary elimination related to surgery
■ Constipation related to postoperative pain or discomfort
■ Knowledge deficit of home care regimen

Planning and Implementation

Medical Treatment

The major goals of the patient include relief of pain and discomfort, normal bowel elimination, and an understanding of the medical treatment regimen.

The major goals of nursing management are to relieve pain and discomfort, restore a normal bowel elimination pattern, reduce inflammation and infection, and promote adherence to the prescribed or recommended treatment modalities.

Treatments should be explained to the patient, with emphasis placed on the importance of adhering to the prescribed regimen, to relieve or eliminate symptoms.

If constipation is part of the clinical picture, the diet recommendations of the physician should be reviewed with the patient. In some instances, it is necessary to provide a list of foods high in fiber. The importance of exercise and increased fluid intake is emphasized. The patient should be cautioned against the prolonged use laxatives.

Surgical Treatment

The major goals of the patient include relief of pain, reduction of anxiety, normal bowel elimination pattern, and an understanding of postdischarge home care.

The major goals of nursing management are to relieve pain, establish a normal bowel and urinary elimination pattern, and promote adherence to the physician's recommendations for home care.

Preoperative preparations may be limited to routine preparations for surgery, as the current trend is to admit patients for this as well as other types of surgery on the morning of surgery. The operative area should be shaved and vital signs taken.

Postoperative management includes monitoring of vital signs and checking the rectal area for excessive bleeding. The temperature should be taken orally. The rectal area should be kept clean, and any external dressings changed or reinforced as needed. When sitz baths are prescribed, the patient should be assisted into the tub. The perineal area should be thoroughly dried after the bath.

Pain. Pain, which may be severe for the first 24 hours after surgery, is controlled with narcotic analgesics. Anxiety produced by pain can be reduced by promptly administering an analgesic as well as encouraging the patient to assume a position that provides the most comfort. When the patient is allowed out of bed and into a chair, sitting on a foam ring reduces pressure on the operative area.

If a rectal pack has been inserted during surgery, it is removed several days after surgery. Thirty minutes to 1 hour before removal of a rectal pack, the patient should be given a narcotic analgesic because removal of the packing is extremely painful. After the pack is removed, the patient should be checked hourly for several hours for evidence of rectal bleeding. The patient also may require a narcotic analgesic once or twice after removal of the pack.

If infection was present, wet dressings may be ordered, to relieve edema and promote drainage of the infected area.

Altered Patterns of Urinary Elimination, Constipation. Many patients have difficulty voiding after rectal surgery; thus it is important to check voiding for several days after surgery. The male patient may be assisted to a standing position to void.

The first bowel movement after surgery is painful. A stool softener may be ordered, to relieve some of the discomfort. Sitz baths are used to increase circulation to the rectal area, thereby reducing congestion and swelling, relieve pain, encourage voiding, and reduce pain on defecation.

Knowledge Deficit. The physician's home care instructions should be reviewed with the patient. The patient should be encouraged to keep the perineal area as clean as possible by using cotton wipes or commercially available wipes after each bowel movement. Constipation should be avoided by means of exercising, eating foods that contain fiber, and drinking extra fluids.

Evaluation

■ Pain is reduced or eliminated
■ Anxiety is reduced
■ Normal bowel and urinary elimination patterns are established
■ Patient demonstrates an understanding of the prescribed drug and dietary regimen, sitz baths, importance of keeping the area clean and dry

General Nutritional Considerations

☐ Dietary management of diverticulosis includes avoiding seeds of any kind. The physician also may recommend avoiding rice and nuts.

☐ Unprocessed bran must be kept refrigerated to prevent spoilage.

☐ Constipation may be relieved by adding high-fiber foods to the diet. Bran, fresh and cooked fruits and vegetables, and whole-grain cereals are excellent sources of fiber.

☐ When fiber is to be added to the diet, the patient should be advised to read the content labels of products, especially the percentage of content. Many products advertised as containing fiber may not have a high-fiber content.

General Pharmacologic Considerations

☐ Stool softeners, such as docusate calcium (Surfak), may be used in patients who should avoid straining at stool. Mineral oil also may be ordered; however, consistent use of mineral oil has two disadvantages: (1) it prevents the absorption of fat-soluble vitamins (A, D, E, K) and (2) with overuse and overdose, it has a tendency to leak past the rectal sphincter, which may slow healing of anal tissue. Patients should be advised to check with their physicians about the type of laxative to be used in rectal disorders.

☐ The nurse should discourage the overuse of laxatives to relieve chronic constipation.

General Gerontologic Considerations

☐ Constipation is a common problem in the elderly, and often is due to poor diet habits, lack of exercise, and decreased fluid intake.

☐ Elderly patients with constipation should be seen by a physician, since cancer of the colon may be responsible for the change in bowel habits.

☐ The frequent use of laxatives should be discouraged, especially when the patient is older. An attempt should be made to correct constipation by increasing fluid intake, eating foods high in bulk, and exercising.

Suggested Readings

☐ Caldwell L. Nutrition education for the patient: the handout manual. Philadelphia: JB Lippincott, 1984. *(Additional coverage of subject matter)*

☐ Cerrato PL. Fast action for a tube-fed patient's diarrhea. RN March 1988;51:89. *(Additional coverage of subject matter)*

☐ Cerrato PL. Is America really constipated? RN May 1989;52:81. *(Closely related to subject matter)*

☐ McConnell E. Meeting the challenge of intestinal obstruction. Nursing '87 July 1987;17:34. *(Additional coverage of subject matter)*

☐ Mertes JE. Action stat! GI bleeding. Nursing '89 August 1989;19:37. *(Additional coverage of subject matter)*

☐ Patras AZ, Paice JA, Lanigan K. Managing GI bleeding: it takes a two-tract mind. Nursing '88 April 1988;18:68. *(Additional coverage of subject matter)*

Chapter 45

The Patient Who Has an Ileostomy or Colostomy

On completion of this chapter the reader will:

- Describe the various types of ostomy procedures

- Discuss the preoperative preparations of ostomy surgery

- List the complications associated with an ileostomy or colostomy

- Use the nursing process in the management of the patient with an ileostomy

- Describe the two types of continent ileostomies

- Use the nursing process in the management of the patient with a continent ileostomy

- Describe the various methods of ostomy irrigation

- Discuss the major points of ostomy care and management

- Use the nursing process in the management of the patient with a colostomy

The term *ostomy*, as used here, is the creation of an opening of the bowel onto the skin. There are two main types: *ileostomy*, in which the ileum is opened onto the skin, and *colostomy*, in which the colon is opened onto the skin. Fecal material drains through these openings, which are called *stomas*.

The patient need not be disabled but must learn to manage and control a change in a body function. Teaching the patient to achieve this control is an important nursing role. Equally important is the nurse's role in supporting the patient during the preoperative and postoperative experience so that he or she is helped to accept the stoma.

An ostomy may be temporary or permanent. In some cases, the surgeon is not able to determine the extent of surgery required beforehand. Regardless of whether the ostomy is temporary or permanent, the patient requires assistance in learning to manage it.

Each patient requires a plan of care adapted to individual needs. A plan of care must consider the patient's preparation for surgery, recovery from surgery, and learning to live with an ostomy.

PREPARATION FOR SURGERY

Preoperatively, the physician explains the surgery required and why surgery is necessary. The patient is given an explanation of the type of ostomy that will be created, where the stoma will be placed, and what is involved in the care of the ostomy. The amount and detail of the explanation given by the physician during the preoperative period depends on the physician's evaluation of the patient's acceptance of the surgery as well as other factors. When the patient is acutely ill, preoperative explanations can be given only to the family.

Antibiotics such as neomycin sulfate may be used in preparing the patient for surgery, to decrease the number of bacteria in the bowel and thus lessen the possibility of infection.

Additional preparations for surgery include blood transfusions to replace blood lost by way of the gastrointestinal (GI) tract and improvement of the nutritional status.

Once the patient is scheduled for ostomy surgery, the nurse should discuss with the physician the possibility of preoperative or postoperative visits by a member of the local ostomy group. Some physicians approve of a visit before surgery; others believe that such visits are best made after surgery.

A visit from a person who has successfully mastered the care of a stoma and who has resumed work and family life can convey to the patient that it is possible to be well groomed, attractive, and successful despite an ostomy. It is helpful to give the ostomy group member who arranges visits the following information: type of visit (preoperative, postoperative, or both); the patient's age, occupation, sex, physical handicaps (if any), and language barrier (if any); and any other information significant to rehabilitation. The group's chairman of visiting arrangements will try to select a visitor with a background similar to that of the patient. Depending on the time of the visit (preoperative or postoperative), the visitor may bring literature to be left with the patient.

In some instances, the patient may be given instruction about the ostomy and ostomy equipment and the general principles of care before surgery. This makes some patients more receptive to teaching during the postoperative recovery period. Some physicians believe that this helps the patient to accept the ostomy; others believe that preoperative teaching that includes these facts creates unnecessary stress and anxiety.

The management of a patient with an ostomy should be patient-centered and living-oriented. It begins when the patient seeks care, and continues throughout the therapeutic phase and the period of recovery after discharge. The *ostomate* (one who has had ostomy surgery) continues to need medical and nursing care after hospitalization until there is security and competence in the management of the ostomy.

ILEOSTOMY

Surgery may be necessary when a disorder of the ileum does not respond to other treatment, or when complications occur (eg, perforation of the colon). The surgical treatment of severe, intractable ulcerative colitis usually includes total colectomy (removal of the entire colon and rectum) and a permanent ileostomy (opening of the ileum onto the abdomen for the passage of fecal matter).

An ileostomy is a surgically formed opening into the ileum for the drainage of fecal matter. A loop of ileum is brought out on the lower right quadrant of the abdomen slightly below the umbilicus, near the outer border of the rectus muscle, and a stoma is formed. The stoma is "matured" at the time of surgery by everting the bowel and suturing the cut end of the ileum to the skin. The rationale for maturing the stoma is that it provides a seal at the base of the stoma. This technique promotes healing and provides a smooth peristomal area, thus permitting the application of the permanent appliance much sooner than is permissible in the nonmatured stoma.

NURSING PROCESS
—THE PATIENT WHO
HAS AN ILEOSTOMY
Preoperative Period
Assessment
Complete medical, diet, and drug histories should be obtained. The patient's general physical and emotional status should be evaluated. Depending on

the patient's condition, a physical assessment also may be performed (see Chapter 42).

Nursing Diagnosis
Depending on the patient's physical condition, one or more of the following nursing diagnoses may apply. Nursing diagnoses related to problems such as nutrition or fluid volume deficit also may apply.

■ Anxiety related to surgery, change in body image and normal bowel elimination, other factors (specify)
■ Ineffective individual coping related to change in body image
■ Knowledge deficit of preoperative preparations

Planning and Implementation
The major goals of the patient include reduction of anxiety, beginning acceptance of an ostomy, and an understanding of the preoperative preparations.

The major goals of nursing management include reduction of anxiety and preparation of the patient physically and emotionally for the surgical procedure.

If the patient has been taking a steroid before admission, this drug must be given during the preoperative, intraoperative, and postoperative periods. An antibiotic such as neomycin sulfate may be used in preparing the bowel for surgery.

Preparations for surgery include insertion of an nasogastric tube, maintenance of a low-residue diet up until the evening of surgery, and those preparations that are routine for any general surgery.

Anxiety, Ineffective Individual Coping. Most patients know several days or weeks before surgery what the procedure entails and the physical changes that will occur as a result of surgery. Some patients may have had inflammatory bowel disease for a long period of time, and are ready to accept an ileostomy. Others experience difficulty in accepting this change.

A visit by a member of the local ostomy group may help to relieve some anxiety and concern. But the patient still needs time to talk with the family and members of the medical staff about the impending surgery.

The degree of anxiety and the manner and extent of the ability or inability to cope vary with each patient. The nurse should listen and look for clues, determine the patient's immediate needs, and develop a plan to meet those needs.

Knowledge Deficit. The nurse is responsible for explaining preoperative procedures such as shaving the operative site and the administration of antibiotics. The physician's explanation of the surgery also may be reinforced as needed. The patient or a family member may have questions regarding the surgical procedure or the ostomy. Depending on the questions raised, the nurse may further instruct the patient or refer the questions to the physician. Additional preoperative teaching includes the importance of coughing, deep breathing, and leg exercises.

Evaluation

- Anxiety is reduced
- Patient openly discusses and asks questions about the surgery
- Patient demonstrates understanding of and rationale for the operative procedure and preoperative preparations

Postoperative Period

Assessment

When the patient returns from the recovery room, immediate assessments should include vital signs and an evaluation of the patient's general status. The chart should be reviewed for information regarding the type of surgery and any problems encountered during or immediately after surgery. Information such as the type of collection appliance, special drains, packing, or tubes also should be obtained. All immediate postoperative findings should be recorded to provide a data base.

The surgical dressing and stoma should be inspected. A temporary ostomy appliance usually is placed over the stoma. Additional dressings may cover the surgical site. A rectal pack usually is used, and removed in 5 to 7 days.

Vital signs should be taken; the temperature should be taken orally.

Nursing Diagnosis

Depending on the postoperative condition of the patient, one or more of the following nursing diagnoses may apply. Diagnoses pertaining to general surgery may be added (see Chapter 16).

- Anxiety related to results of surgery, change in bowel elimination, care of the stoma, other factors (specify)
- Pain related to surgery
- Potential for infection related to fecal contamination of the surgical wound
- Ineffective airway clearance related to failure to cough and deep breathe
- Body image disturbance related to change in bowel elimination
- Ineffective individual coping related to changes in body image
- Impaired skin integrity related to effect of fecal material and adhesives on the skin

- Altered sexuality patterns related to change in body part
- Knowledge deficit of ostomy care, postdischarge treatment regimen

Planning and Implementation

The major goals of the patient include reduction in anxiety, relief of pain, absence of infection, maintenance of a patent airway, coping with the change in body image, maintenance of skin integrity, normal social interactions, resumption of previous sexual activity, learning ostomy care, and an understanding of the postdischarge treatment regimen.

The major goals of nursing management are to physically and emotionally help the patient through the postoperative period, prevent complications, and develop and use an effective teaching plan for the patient and family.

The use of a nasogastric tube connected to suction and the administration of parenteral fluids are usual in the immediate postoperative period. Within several days, these treatments usually are discontinued, and oral feedings of easily digested foods are ordered. A low-residue diet may be ordered once solid food can be taken.

The nasogastric tube should be irrigated as ordered. The abdomen should be checked for distention and auscultated for bowel sounds. Nausea and vomiting, which may indicate intestinal obstruction, should be reported to the physician immediately.

Before the rectal packing is removed, the patient usually is given an analgesic, as this procedure may cause considerable pain. After the packing is removed, the physician inspects the area for signs of infection or failure of the area to heal. Irrigations may be ordered, to promote healing. The nurse should continue to observe the rectal area for signs of inflammation or infection until healing is complete.

Complications.   Postoperative complications include intestinal obstruction, loss of blood supply to the stoma, stenosis of the stoma, and prolapse or excessive protrusion of the stoma.

Intestinal obstruction is a serious complication. It may be due to a twisted, strangulated, or incarcerated bowel, an internal hernia, or a bolus of poorly chewed, inadequately digested, stringy, pasty, or fibrous food. Spare or absent flow of fecal material from the stoma signifies an obstruction. The physician should be notified immediately if obstruction is suspected. When obstruction is caused food, the physician may attempt to correct the problem by irrigating the stoma. If the bowel is twisted or strangulated, surgical intervention may be necessary.

If the stoma steadily increases in size or becomes cyanotic, the physician should be notified immediately, as these symptoms may indicate obstruction or a loss of blood supply to the stoma or section of ileum. A temporary postoperative appliance with a larger disk opening than that of the appliance currently used should be applied until the patient can be seen by the physician.

Prolapse or protrusion of the ileostomy is fairly common. If it is of moderate degree (1 or 2 inches), no treatment may be required. A severe prolapse of the stoma is a serious complication. Edema may occur, and may lead to obstruction resulting from restriction of blood supply; necrosis may result if the prolapse is not promptly and skillfully managed. If there is a sudden prolapse of the stoma, the permanent appliance should be removed immediately, a temporary appliance applied, and the physician notified. Once prolapse of the stoma has occurred, recurrence is more likely.

Stenosis, tightening, and narrowing of the stoma may eventually require surgical revision. The surgeon may manually dilate the stoma daily for a while to prevent further difficulty. The surgeon also may instruct the patient to perform this maneuver after discharge from the hospital.

If the patient has been receiving a corticosteroid preparation before surgery, the dose of the drug may be tapered *slowly* over a period of time and the drug then discontinued. The patient should be closely monitored for signs and symptoms of adrenal insufficiency (eg, weakness, lethargy, drop in blood pressure, nausea, vomiting).

Anxiety.   Moving about in bed, coughing, and early ambulation may be made more difficult by the patient's fear of soiling clothing and bedding. The dressing or disposable plastic ileostomy pouch should be securely applied, so that the patient is more willing to move about. It is important to explain to the patient that some soiling is inevitable in the immediate postoperative period and that the changing of dressings and even of bedding is both expected and accepted. Soiled bedding, dressings, and gown should be changed promptly.

Pain.   Deep breathing, coughing, turning, and leg exercises are carried out as for other surgical patients. Medication for relief of pain and discomfort should be given as required. Nursing care should be planned to provide the patient with adequate time to rest. Some surgeons advocate the use of elastic bandages or antiembolism stockings on both legs to prevent thrombophlebitis until the patient can ambulate. If these are used, they should be removed and reapplied at least once during each 8-hour period.

Fluid and Electrolyte Balance.   Intake and output should be measured. The physician also may order measurement of the drainage from the stoma.

Electrolyte imbalance that is the result of a large output of fluid through the ileum is a particular problem for the patient with an ileostomy. The patient should be observed for weakness, trembling, and confusion, especially when the ileal output is profuse. Because administration of intravenous fluids for fluid and electrolyte replacement may be necessary, these symptoms should be immediately reported to the physician.

Potential for Infection.   Vital signs should be taken as ordered, and the temperature taken orally. The proximity of the stoma to the surgical incision makes it especially difficult to avoid fecal contamination of the incision. The temporary plastic pouch, which can be fitted snugly around the stoma, helps to prevent fecal drainage from seeping into the surgical incision. Dressings should be securely applied over the incision to protect it from fecal drainage.

Because of edema, the stoma is larger immediately after surgery than it will be later. The size of the stoma changes considerably during the initial postoperative period. The temporary appliance is especially useful because fresh appliances can be cut to fit the stoma as often as necessary. After healing has occurred and the stoma has reached its permanent size and shape, a permanent appliance is fitted.

Ineffective Airway Clearance.   The patient should be encouraged to cough, deep breathe, and move the extremities every 2 hours while awake. The patient should be shown how to splint the incision when coughing and deep breathing, and assistance should be given as needed until the patient is able to perform these activities without help. The lungs should be auscultated daily, and any abnormal findings reported to the physician.

Bowel Elimination.   The patient with an ileostomy cannot control bowel elimination or establish a regular evacuation pattern. An ilesotomy appliance must be worn continuously. The disposable bag should be changed or the permanent appliance emptied when the bag is about half full. If leakage occurs, the temporary appliance should be changed. The permanent appliance may require reapplication of the disk or other measures to reaffix the appliance to the skin.

The appliance should be changed or emptied at a time when the bowel is relatively quiet. For many patients this time is early in the morning, before eating, or 2 or 3 hours after mealtime.

Impaired Skin Integrity. The area around the stoma should be thoroughly cleaned each time the temporary appliance or the disk of the permanent appliance is changed. It is imperative that meticulous care be given to the area around the stoma to prevent excoriation and skin breakdown. Ileal discharge contains digestive enzymes and acids that undermine the skin; the resulting excoriation may take weeks to heal. Skin problems must be detected early so that they can be treated as soon as they occur.

It is especially important to protect the area around the stoma from ileal drainage while caring for the skin by placing a tissue cuff around the stoma or using a receptacle such as a small paper cup to collect the drainage.

Body Image Disturbance, Ineffective Individual Coping. The patient needs time to adjust to the stoma and change in bowel elimination. Most patients go through various stages of grieving and experience shock, depression, anger, and denial. The patient may at first refuse to look at the stoma when the appliance is changed, but she or he should be encouraged to look at the stoma and to help with such tasks as changing the appliance and skin care.

Odors. The room should be kept as free from odors as possible. Room deodorizers and frequent emptying of the ileostomy appliance help to control odor.

Altered Sexuality Patterns. The patient may or may not discuss concerns over relations with his or her sexual partner. Many times this problem is discussed

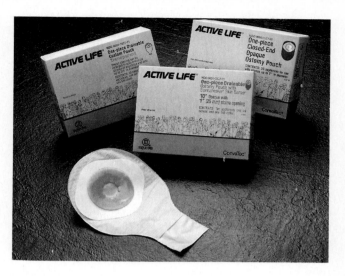

Figure 45-2. Various types and sizes of pouches are available for collection of drainage from an ostomy. (Courtesy of Convatec, Princeton, NJ)

with the physician during postoperative office visits. Local ostomy groups also can provide support and understanding in this matter.

Knowledge Deficit. The patient and family should be taught in logical steps and at a pace that allows the patient to learn each step before the next one is introduced.

The following nursing diagnosis topics may be included in a patient teaching program.

DIET. Follow the diet recommended by the physician. Foods that cause gas are best eliminated from the diet. An extra intake of fluids is especially important in warm weather.

PERMANENT ILEOSTOMY APPLIANCE. The three basic features of the permanent appliance are as follows:

- A disk (faceplate) that surrounds the stoma and usually adheres to the body (Fig. 45-1)
- A pouch for collecting the feces
- Accessories such as a belt, belt attachments, spout closures, bands, and clips

Considerations for choosing a permanent appliance involve the disk and its design (Fig. 45-2). The location and characteristics of the stoma and the characteristics of abdominal contour and texture must be analyzed for each person. The material and size of the disk depend on individual specifications and patient preferences. If there is no fitting problem, pouch size may be the deciding factor in choosing the appliance. Various types are used with respect to odor permeability. This may be the decisive factor for some patients. Allergy to rubber or other materials also may be a factor.

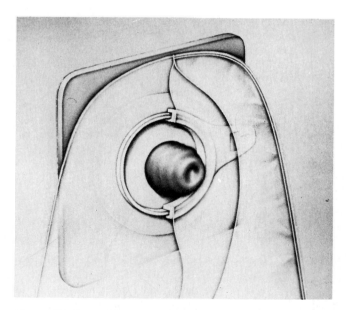

Figure 45-1. A disk surrounds the stoma, adheres to the body, and provides a surface for attachment of the collection appliance. (Courtesy of Convatec, Princeton, NJ)

Depending on the type of appliance chosen, a belt may be used to hold the appliance in place when adhesive is not used. The belt also provides pressure for a good bond when adhesive is used. It may be used to support the weight of the appliance and filled pouch and thus to prevent the disk from being pulled away from the abdomen by the weight of the liquid fecal material. It provides the new ostomate with the assurance that the appliance will not fall off.

Foam rubber, gauze, or flannel padding can be used under a belt that cuts into the flesh. Care should be taken to avoid upward or downward pull on the stoma. The belt should be placed at the level of the stoma, or double belts can be used to equalize pull on the top and bottom of the disk.

The permanent appliance may be secured with adhesive, a karaya gum ring, or a double-faced adhesive disk.

1. *Adhesive* (cement) is used to hold the appliance on the body and must be applied to a clean, dry surface (Fig. 45-3). It also protects the skin around the stoma. The adhesive is applied according to the manufacturer's instructions on the container. Finding the right adhesive is a trial-and-error procedure. The skin should be tested for sensitivity before an adhesive is used because sensitivity is common.

   Adhesive can be rolled off the skin and appliance after several days of wearing. If it does not roll off, a small amount of solvent applied to a gauze pad can be used to gently rub off traces of adhesive. The area should be wiped off with water after solvent has been used.

2. *Solvent* is a highly inflammable hydrocarbon. It also is irritating, and therefore should be applied sparingly between the body and the bag, using a medicine dropper. *Excessive* rubbing will irritate skin. *Carbon tetrachloride should never be used* in place of ileostomy solvent; it is the most toxic of all commonly used solvents.

3. *Karaya gum powder* and *karaya gum rings* protect the skin while permitting healing underneath; they also serve as adherents for the ostomy appliance. Karaya gum powder becomes gelatinous when brought in contact with moisture, and can be used in place of an adhesive. It can be resealed by applying pressure. Rings of karaya gum also are available commercially. One manufacturer supplies ostomy drainage bags with the karaya gum ring already attached. These rings can be cut, pulled, or pushed into any shape desired, and therefore can be used as a protection at the base of the stoma to correct the problems created by an ill-fitting appliance.

APPLICATION OF THE PERMANENT APPLIANCE.   There are several types of permanent appliances.

1. *Adhesive type.* Prepare the skin by cleansing with soap and water. Pat dry. Apply any agent (eg, tincture of benzoin) recommended by the physician. Dust on karaya powder or apply an adhesive. If tincture of benzoin is used, it should be tacky and dry before the appliance is applied. If the temporary bag does not have the exact size opening that is required, measure the stoma and add ⅛-inch clearance around the stoma to allow for size change. A karaya ring can be placed around the base of the stoma before applying the bag. Secure the end of the bag with a clamp.

2. *Karaya gum ring with adhesive facing.* Prepare the skin as recommended by the physician or manufacturer. Peel off the protective backing from the adhesive facing and align carefully to guide it over the stoma evenly. The karaya gum ring should fit snugly around the stoma. The end of the collection bag is secured.

3. *Karaya gum ring.* Prepare the skin as recommended by the physician or manufacturer. Remove the protective covering from the karaya ring and guide it over the stoma. Secure the end of the bag with a clamp. The karaya ring can fit snugly around the base of the stoma without injuring the stoma. Care should be taken not to use hard surface rings close to the stoma, to avoid injury to the stoma.

CHANGING THE APPLIANCE.   The important factors in changing the appliance are *time* and *frequency*. The appliance should be changed immediately when there is a burning or itching sensation underneath the disk or pain around the stoma. This should be done regardless of whether the appliance has been

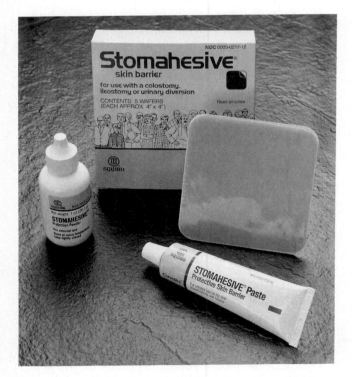

Figure 45–3. Adhesive may be used to hold an appliance in place. (Courtesy of Convatec, Princeton, NJ)

on for 1 hour or for several days. The stoma and skin should be carefully examined to determine the cause of the difficulty. Excoriation of the skin is to be avoided at all costs. Resorting to the use of a temporary appliance may be advisable until the cause is identified and eliminated. The most frequent cause of irritation is leakage of fecal drainage or a reaction to the solvent or adhesive. Stinging, tingling, or itching may be experienced immediately after an appliance change; these sensations quickly subside. If a sensation is prolonged or intensified, the appliance should be removed.

The appliance should be changed at a time when the bowel is relatively quiet (Fig. 45-4). At first, discharge from the stoma occurs frequently. As the bowel adjusts to its new state, the activity lessens. The bowel usually is most active after eating and relatively quiet at other times.

Most surgeons advocate changing the appliance ring when needed, that is, when the ring becomes separated from the skin. Too frequent changes are considered inadvisable because in removing the appliance, one also may remove the protective layers of epithelium and cause the skin to become raw and excoriated. The two-piece appliances permit inspection of the stoma by removing only the pouch while the disk remains cemented to the body.

DILATING THE STOMA. The physician may instruct the patient in how to dilate the stoma. To dilate the stoma, a finger cot is placed on the index or little finger and thoroughly lubricated; the finger is then gently inserted into the stoma for a few minutes. The fingernail should be cut short to prevent injury to the bowel.

CONTROL OF ODORS. Odor is an individual matter. There are two kinds of odor: that which is present when the ileostomy pouch is emptied and that which occasionally clings to the person. *Thorough* cleansing of the pouch is an absolute necessity for removing odors. Leakage, the pouch itself, too infrequent changing of the pouch, and certain foods may cause odors. Many types of deodorants and deodorizers are on the market. One method of controlling odor is to place deodorant tablets or liquids directly in the pouch. To deter the development of odor in warm weather, a plastic bag can be slipped over the appliance. Two pouches can be used alternately; while one is cleaned and dried, the other is worn.

To control odor at its source, a restricted diet of tea, toast, and marmalade and the addition of one food at a time may be tried. Foods that contain condiments, fish, eggs, onions, and cheese should be omitted, since they frequently cause odors that linger. Restriction of diet should be undertaken only with medical supervision. Some medications, especially antibiotics and antituberculosis drugs, cause particularly strong odors that cling to the appliance. Using an old pouch or disposable pouches while these medications are taken is helpful.

Intestinal gas can be caused by swallowing air. Sighing, chewing, gulping down food, and breathing with the mouth open all contribute to the formation of intestinal gas. Eating slowly and chewing food well with the mouth closed help to lessen the amount of gas that is formed.

Some foods, such as cabbage, onions, pork, beans, and peppers, produce intestinal gas, and should be avoided. Some people, however, find that they can add small amounts of these foods to their diet.

Evaluation

- Anxiety is reduced
- Pain is controlled during the postoperative period
- Evidence of dehydration is absent
- Evidence of complications during the postoperative period is absent
- Serum electrolyte levels are within normal range
- Evidence of wound infection is absent; vital signs are normal
- Patient coughs and deep breathes; lungs are clear to auscultation
- Patient begins to accept and cope with the change in body image
- Skin remains intact with no evidence of changes such as excoriation or rash; stoma is normal in size and color
- Odors are controlled or eliminated
- Patient accepts visits by the local ostomy group and openly discusses personal feelings and problems with the visiting ostomate, physician, or nurse
- Patient takes part in or is totally responsible for care of the stoma, skin, and appliance
- Patient demonstrates an understanding of application of the appliance, appliance care, changing the appliance, dietary measures, and control of odors

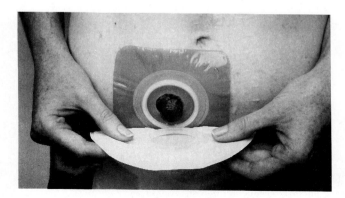

Figure 45–4. The ostomy appliance is changed when the bowel is relatively quiet. (Courtesy of Convatec, Princeton, NJ)

CONTINENT ILEOSTOMY (KOCK POUCH)

Whereas the conventional ileostomy involves the creation of a stoma from the distal portion of the ileum, the continent ileostomy is the creation of an internal reservoir for the storage of GI effluent (discharged fecal material or, in this case, liquid feces), thus eliminating the need for an external fecal collection bag.

After resection of the diseased portion of the ileum, a reservoir is formed by using a portion of the terminal ileum. A nipple valve is created by intussusception of the distal ileal segment into the reservoir. A permanent external stoma is formed and anchored to the abdominal wall (Fig. 45-5).

During surgery, a catheter is inserted through the nipple valve and sutured in place so that the end of the catheter protrudes from the external stoma. The reservoir stores GI effluent for several hours, until it is removed by means of a catheter.

ILEOANAL RESERVOIR

The *ileoanal reservoir* (also called the *ileoanal anastomosis*) (Fig. 45-6) usually is performed in two stages. In the first part of this two-stage procedure, a colectomy is done and a temporary ileostomy created. A distal part of the ileum is used to form a pouch or reservoir. The pouch is opened at one end, and the edges sutured to the anus. The second stage is done 2 or 3 months later. At this time, the surgeon closes the temporary ileostomy and reunites the two sections of ileum. This establishes a normal flow of fecal material through the ileum to the reservoir. The fecal material, which is stored in the reservoir, is then expelled from the anus.

This procedure, as well as the continent ileostomy, may be performed on selected patients with chronic ulcerative colitis or familial or multiple polyposis. Patients with conventional ileostomies also may be candidates for either one of these procedures.

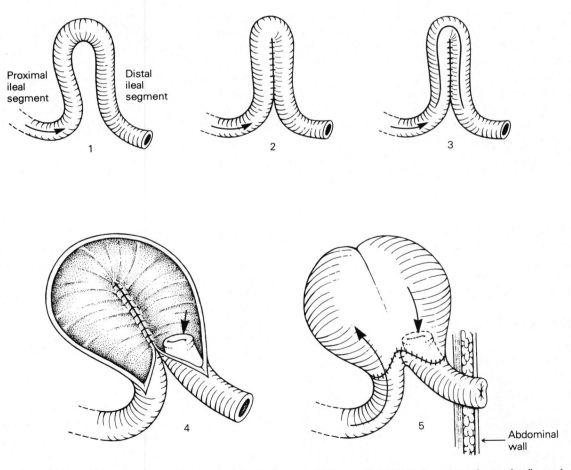

Figure 45–5.   The pouch ileostomy. (*1*) A loop of ileum is (*2*) sutured together (the arrow shows the flow of gastrointestinal effluent); (*3*) an incision is made on one surface, and (*4*) the ileum is opened. A nipple valve (*arrow*) is created by intussusception of the distal ileal segment; (*5*) a reservoir pouch is created by folding down and suturing the edges. The arrow shows the flow of gastrointestinal effluent, and the dotted lines show the internal nipple valve. The distal segment is brought through the abdominal wall to create an external stoma.

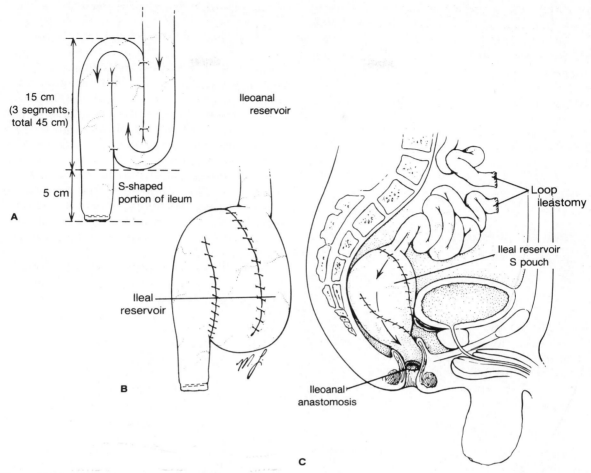

Figure 45–6. Ileoanal anastomosis. (*A*) A 50-cm portion of the distal ileum is aligned in an S shape. (*E*) The bowel is opened along the antimesenteric surface, and adjacent walls are anastomosed to create a reservoir. (*F*) A mucosal proctectomy precedes anastomosis of the ileal reservoir. A temporary loop ileostomy diverts effluent discharge for several months. (Brunner LS, Suddarth DS. Textbook of medical–surgical nursing. Philadelphia: JB Lippincott. 6th ed. 1988:818)

NURSING PROCESS —THE PATIENT WHO HAS A CONTINENT ILEOSTOMY OR ILEOANAL RESERVOIR

Preoperative Period

Assessment
The preoperative assessment of a patient having either procedure is essentially the same as for the patient with an ileostomy.

Nursing Diagnosis
Depending on the person, the procedure, and other factors, one or more of the following nursing diagnoses may apply:

- Anxiety related to surgery, change in normal bowel elimination, other factors
- Knowledge deficit of preoperative preparations

Planning and Implementation
The major goals of the patient include reduction in anxiety and an understanding of preoperative preparations.

The major goals of nursing management include the reduction of anxiety and preparation of the patient physically and emotionally for surgery. Additional preparations and patient teaching usually are the same as for the patient having an ileostomy.

Anxiety. The physician explains the procedure to the patient. With physician approval, a visit by a member of a local ostomy group who has had the same procedure may help to dispel any doubts and reduce anxiety.

Knowledge Deficit. Preoperative procedures as well as some of the aspects of the postoperative period, such as the presence of drains or catheters, are explained. The patient and family should be allowed time to ask questions and discuss the surgery. At this time the nurse may find it necessary to further explain the procedure to the patient or refer questions to the physician.

Evaluation

■ Anxiety is reduced
■ Patient openly discusses and asks questions about the surgery
■ Patient demonstrates an understanding of preoperative preparations and the surgical procedure

Postoperative Period

Assessment

In addition to routine postoperative assessments, the following observations should be made.

Continent Ileostomy. The abdominal dressing should be checked for drainage. The placement and patency of the ileal reservoir catheter, which is sutured into place and may be connected to suction, and the color and amount of drainage should be noted. The size and color of the stoma should be observed.

Ileoanal Reservoir. If the first stage of this procedure has been performed, the patient will have a temporary ileostomy and construction of an ileal reservoir. The observations are the same as for an ileostomy. In addition, the anal area should be inspected for drainage. There also may be a drain or drainage tube in the presacral area. If the second stage has been performed, the ileostomy has been closed and the ileum anastomosed to the anal reservoir, which was constructed during the first stage. The anal area and the operative sites should be inspected for drainage.

Nursing Diagnosis

Depending on the condition of the patient and the type or stage of the procedure, one or more of the following nursing diagnoses may apply. Diagnoses pertaining to general surgery (see Chapter 16) or an ileostomy (see earlier section) may be added.

■ Anxiety related to results of surgery, other factors (specify)
■ Fluid volume deficit related to passage of liquid stools, absence of large colon
■ Impaired skin integrity related to effect of fecal material and adhesives on the skin, frequent bowel movements (ileoanal reservoir, second stage), other factors (specify)

■ Knowledge deficit of management of continent ileostomy, care of stoma (Kock pouch, first-stage ileoanal reservoir), postdischarge home care

Planning and Implementation

The major goals of the patient include reduction of anxiety, correction of fluid volume deficit, maintenance of skin integrity, management of the continent ileostomy or ileostomy stoma, establishment of bowel continency, and an understanding of postdischarge home care.

The major goals of nursing management are to physically and emotionally help the patient through the postoperative period, prevent complications, help the patient establish bowel continency, and develop and use an effective teaching plan for the patient and family.

General postoperative management is the same as for the patient with an ileostomy, including observation for complications.

Continent Ileostomy. The stomal catheter usually is connected to low, intermittent suction that allows for continuous emptying of the pouch, thereby preventing tension on suture lines during the healing process. The ileal catheter should be checked frequently for signs of obstruction, that is, lack of fecal drainage or the patient's complaint of a feeling of fullness in the area of the ileal pouch. The physician may order either routine irrigations of the ileal catheter with small amounts of normal saline solution or irrigations only if the catheter appears to be obstructed. The perineal area is packed with gauze during surgery and reinforced, as needed, during the postoperative period. The packing is removed by the physician about a week after surgery. One hour before the packing is removed, the patient is given an analgesic because this procedure is painful.

The ileal output should be carefully monitored during the entire postoperative period. When GI function resumes, the amount of ileal drainage usually is high. If excessive fluid and electrolyte loss continues, parenteral fluid and electrolyte replacement is necessary. When ileal drainage stabilizes, the physician removes the ileal catheter. The patient is then taught to intubate (ie, insert a catheter into) the stoma.

The materials necessary for stoma intubation include a catheter, water-soluble lubricant, a basin, tissues, irrigating solution, an irrigating syringe, and gauze dressings. The patient sits on the side of the bed, and all necessary equipment is placed within reach. The catheter is lubricated and gently inserted into the stoma. Resistance will be felt when the catheter tip reaches the nipple valve (about 2 inches). A gentle thrust should push the catheter through the nipple and into the ileal pouch. Fecal material will then begin to drain through the catheter into the collecting basin. When drainage stops, the catheter is removed, washed, and thoroughly rinsed.

Initially, stoma intubations may be necessary every 2 to 4 hours. As the capacity of the reservoir increases (usually in about 6 months), the procedure may be performed three or four times daily.

Ileoanal Reservoir. After the first-stage ileoanal reservoir surgery, there is a mucous discharge from the anus. After the second stage, fecal material is discharged from the anus. The patient initially is unable to (consciously) control the frequent watery discharge. Later, as edema subsides and the anal sphincter is strengthened, control is attained. Disposable pads can be placed under the buttocks and changed as needed.

Anxiety. Although the patient may have had an explanation of the immediate postoperative discharge of fecal material from the ileostomy (Kock pouch, first-stage ileoanal reservoir), mucus from the anus (first-stage ileoanal reservoir), or fecal material from the anus (second-stage ileoanal reservoir), there still may be concern over the immediate results of surgery. It is important to review preoperative explanations as well as reassure the patient that this type of drainage is to be expected.

Fluid Volume Deficit. Electrolyte imbalance caused by the large output of fluid through the ileum is a particular problem for the patient with an ileostomy or ileoanal anastomosis. Intravenous fluids should be given until the patient is able to take oral liquids. Intake and output should be recorded, and the fecal discharge from the ileostomy measured. The patient with a second-stage ileoanal reservoir also requires measurement of fecal drainage.

The patient should be monitored for signs of dehydration and electrolyte imbalances, since there may be a copious amount of drainage from the reservoir.

Impaired Skin Integrity. Patients with a first-stage ileoanal reservoir initially experience an almost continuous mucous discharge from the anus. Those with a second-stage ileoanal reservoir initially experience a frequent discharge of fecal material. Severe excoriation of the skin around the anal area can occur after either stage. The perianal area should be inspected daily for redness and signs of skin breakdown. The area should be cleansed with warm water after each bowel movement or removal of mucus. The physician may order a protective cream or oint-

ment, such as A and D ointment (Desitin), applied to the area.

The patients who has a Kock pouch has a dressing around the stoma, which protects the skin from irritation. The dressing should be changed whenever mucus and secretions are apparent. Later, as drainage decreases, dressing changes may be required only every 6 to 8 hours.

Patients who have Kock pouches or a first-stage ileoanal reservoir may develop the same skin complications as patients who have ileostomies.

Knowledge Deficit. Some patients are discharged in a short period of time, and some aspects of the teaching plan may need to be covered on an outpatient basis.

Patients should be encouraged to contact their local ostomy group and talk to its members, especially someone who has had the same procedure. Ostomates often are able to help one another more than those who do not have the same problem.

The following material may be included in a patient-teaching plan, in addition to the information given to the patient with an ileostomy.

KOCK POUCH. The catheter is removed from the stoma about 10 to 14 days after surgery. After this time the Kock pouch needs to be drained periodically. The procedure for drainage is as follows:

1. A lubricated catheter is inserted about 2 inches into the stoma.
2. The end of the catheter is placed in a drainage basin held below the level of the stoma or the toilet bowl. Fecal material as well as gas may be expelled.
3. When drainage ceases, the catheter is removed. The area around the stoma is gently washed with warm water and patted dry.
4. An absorbent pad or dressing is placed over the stoma.
5. Initially, it usually is necessary to drain the pouch every 2 or 3 hours. Later, the interval between drainages is slowly lengthened.

ILEOANAL RESERVOIR. Performing perineal exercises four to six times per day helps to establish anal sphincter control. The anus is tightened (in the same manner as when trying to prevent having a bowel movement) for a count of 10 and then relaxed. Increasing sphincter control helps to enlarge the reservoir, and thus increase its capacity. These exercises should be performed daily for the rest of the patient's life.

Protective ointments or creams are applied as recommended by the physician. Because skin breakdown can be a problem, the anal area should be inspected daily by using a mirror. The physician should be contacted if the anal area becomes sore or skin changes (eg, sores, bleeding) are apparent. A thin sanitary shield or disposable, lined underpants can be used to prevent soiling by fecal drainage until anal sphincter control is achieved.

Evaluation

The following evaluations may be added to those for the ileostomy patient.

- Patient understands that fecal drainage normally is frequent during the early postoperative period
- Evidence of dehydration is absent; serum electrolyte levels are normal despite increased fecal drainage
- Skin of the perianal area appears normal
- Patient demonstrates an understanding of draining the Kock pouch
- Patient is able to perform perineal exercises to establish control over the anal sphincter (ileoanal reservoir)

COLOSTOMY

A colostomy is an artificial opening of the large bowel brought out to the abdomen and made into a stoma. The presence of a cancerous lesion, an ulcerative inflammatory process, multiple polyposis, or traumatic injury to the bowel are indications for a colostomy.

Types

A colostomy may be described in a number of ways, depending on its purpose, duration, and location. It may be temporary or permanent. If described by location, it may be ascending, transverse, or descending. It may have a single loop or a double loop (double-barrel). It may be described in terms of its therapeutic effect on the patient, that is, either curative or palliative.

Double-Barrel and Single-Barrel Colostomies

A double-barrel colostomy consists of two stomas, one of which connects with either the proximal or the distal portion of the bowel (Fig. 45-7). The portion of the bowel that leads from the small intestine to the stoma, through which the feces pass to the outside, is called the *proximal portion*, and its opening is called the *proximal opening*, or *loop*, of the colostomy. The *distal portion* of the bowel leads from the stoma to the anus. Because fecal drainage has been diverted, the distal portion of the bowel does not pass feces by way of the anus. Mucus often collects in this portion of bowel. Sometimes the double-barrel colostomy is a temporary procedure, and after disease or injury in the distal portion has been treated, the continuity of the bowel is restored.

When a double-barrel colostomy is performed, the stomas may be matured at surgery; that is, each stoma is everted and sutured down, and thus is open. If the stoma is not matured at surgery, a loop of bowel is brought out onto the abdomen. Sometimes a glass or plastic rod is placed between the underside of the loop and the skin to hold the exposed bowel loop in position. About 24 to 72 hours after the operation, the loop of bowel is opened by cutting or cautery to form the stoma. In this way, the initial healing of the incision takes place without danger of contamination. The latter procedure is not physically painful because the bowel is not sensitive to pain. The opening of the

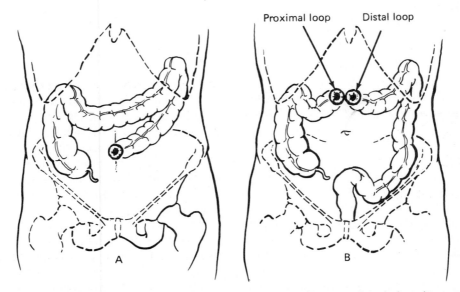

Figure 45–7. Single- and double-barrel colostomy. (A) One type of single-barrel colostomy. The distal portion of the bowel has been removed, and the colostomy is permanent. (B) One type of double-barrel colostomy, showing proximal and distal loops. This type of colostomy may or may not be permanent.

colostomy usually is carried out at the patient's bedside or in a treatment room. The bed should be well protected, and a temporary ostomy pouch, rather than a basin, used to receive the initial flow of liquid feces. The initial gush of fecal material from the stoma can be upsetting, even when the patient has been told what to expect. The patient should be prepared for the pungent odor of the cauterized tissue, which disappears shortly.

A transverse double-barrel colostomy often is temporary, and usually performed to rest a portion of the bowel, a procedure that may be necessary in the treatment of a disorder such as acute diverticulitis. The interval before the continuity of the bowel is reestablished may be 16 months or longer. When the diseased portion of the bowel is removed or healed, the bowel is reconnected by anastomosis.

A single-barreled colostomy consists of one opening through which fecal matter is passed (Fig. 45-7). The opening is that of the proximal portion of the bowel. The distal portion of the bowel usually is surgically removed, and the colostomy is permanent.

Abdominoperineal Resection

Abdominoperineal resection is performed when a tumor is in the lower sigmoid or rectal area. The colon is cut above the tumor area and brought through the abdominal wall to form a single colostomy stoma. A perineal incision is then made, and the tumor and structures below the tumor (sigmoid colon, rectum, and anus) are removed. A temporary drain is left in the perineal area.

Complications

Complications include a prolapse of the stoma, skin irritation, fecal impaction, stoma retraction, and a loss of blood supply to the stoma. If the latter occurs, the stoma may become gangrenous.

NURSING PROCESS —THE PATIENT WHO HAS A COLOSTOMY

Preoperative Period

The nursing process for the preoperative period is the same as for the patient having an ileostomy. A colostomy may be performed because the patient has cancer of the colon or rectum, which may make the patient more anxious about the procedure.

With physician approval, a visit by a member of a local ostomy group may be made during the preoperative period.

Postoperative Period

Assessment

After the patient returns from surgery, vital signs should be taken, the dressing should be checked, and the functions of the nasogastric tube and intravenous line should be monitored. If an abdominoperineal resection was performed, the drain left in the perineal space should be checked for placement and drainage. The patient's chart should be reviewed for the type of colostomy and the location of the stoma. The physician should be asked to identify the distal and proximal stomas of a double-barrel colostomy if a diagram has not been provided on the operative sheet or physician's progress notes.

Nursing Diagnosis

Depending on the type of colostomy, the condition of the patient, and the postoperative diagnosis, one or more of the following nursing diagnoses may apply:

- Anxiety related to results of surgery, change in bowel elimination, care of the stoma, other factors (specify)
- Pain related to surgery
- Potential for infection related to surgery
- Ineffective airway clearance related to failure to cough and deep breathe
- Body image disturbance related to change in manner of bowel elimination
- Ineffective individual coping related to changes in body image
- Impaired skin integrity related to effect of fecal material and adhesives on the skin
- Social isolation related to odor, accident (leakage, soiling of clothes)
- Altered sexuality patterns related to change in body part
- Knowledge deficit of colostomy management, postdischarge home care

Planning and Implementation

The major goals of the patient include reduction in anxiety, relief of pain, absence of infection, maintenance of a patent airway, coping with the change in body image, maintenance of skin integrity, normal social interactions, resumption of previous sexual activity, learning ostomy care, and an understanding of the postdischarge treatment regimen.

The major goals of nursing management are to reduce anxiety, relieve pain, maintain fluid and electrolyte balance, prevent infection, identify as well as prevent complications associated with this procedure, and physically and emotionally help the patient to care for the colostomy.

Perineal Wound Care. If an abdominoperineal resection has been performed, the perineal area should be checked for hemorrhage or excessive or purulent drainage.

A drain or pack usually is inserted at the time of surgery and removed in about 1 week. The physician may order irrigation of the perineal wound. Because irrigation is painful, an analgesic is given 30 to 45 minutes before the irrigation procedure.

About 10 days after surgery, sitz baths may be ordered, to promote further healing of the area, which fills in with granulation tissue. When the patient is allowed to sit in a chair, a foam ring may be used to reduce the discomfort associated with sitting.

Anxiety.
Anxiety may be reduced by relieving pain and instituting comfort measures such as position changes or back care.

The patient should be allowed time to talk and ask questions about the surgery and the care of the colostomy. Patients may become anxious because no one appears interested or concerned about their problem or takes the time to listen. Questions go unanswered or are answered as briefly as possible. Showing a caring and concerned manner often helps these patients through this emotional time, allows them to slowly accept the changes in their body image, and conveys an interest in their problems.

Pain, Potential for Infection.
Vital signs should be monitored every 4 hours or as ordered. The temperature should be taken orally. A sudden elevation in temperature, a temperature over 38.3°C (101°F), or an increase in pain and abdominal tenderness should be reported to the physician immediately.

Antibiotics usually are ordered during the postoperative period, and should be given at the time intervals ordered, to maintain adequate antibiotic blood levels. Narcotic analgesics normally are required for several days after surgery.

The surgical dressing should be checked frequently during the early postoperative period. The size and color of the stoma should be observed (see Chapter 16).

Fluid and Electrolyte Imbalances.
Intake and output should be measured. Intravenous fluids are given until the patient begins to take fluids orally. Serum electrolyte levels should be monitored, and the patient observed for signs of dehydration and electrolyte imbalance (see Chapter 12). An indwelling catheter may have been inserted before surgery to relieve pressure on the abdominal contents as well as prevent urine retention during the first few days after surgery. A marked decrease in urine output or a urine output of less than 500 mL/day should be reported to the physician immediately.

Ineffective Airway Clearance.
The patient should be encouraged to cough, deep breathe, and move the extremities every 2 hours while awake. The patient should be shown how to splint the incision when coughing and deep breathing; assistance should be given as needed until the patient can perform these activities without help. The lungs should be auscultated daily, and any abnormal findings reported to the physician.

Bowel Elimination.
The colostomy appliance should be checked frequently and changed as needed. The approximate amount of fecal material as well as its color and consistency should be recorded.

The content of the large bowel is liquid in the ascending colon, semiliquid to pasty in the transverse colon, semisolid in the descending colon, and solid in the sigmoid colon. The type and control of fecal evacuation, therefore, is based on the location of the stoma and the function of that portion of the bowel.

ASCENDING COLOSTOMY.   Because the fecal material is liquid, this type of colostomy requires a carefully applied temporary appliance or an ileostomy-type permanent pouch. Initially, the stoma constantly exudes soft to liquid feces. Frequent emptying of the plastic pouch day and night is necessary to keep the patient as clean as possible, to control odors, to maintain the seal of the ostomy pouch, to prevent excoriation of the skin around the stoma, and to protect against soiling bedding and clothing.

TRANSVERSE COLOSTOMY.   This type of colostomy is more manageable when irrigated daily to reduce the number of movements and to help eliminate odor. The use of a temporary ostomy bag protects the skin and prevents contamination of the surgical wound.

DESCENDING AND SIGMOID COLOSTOMIES.   Descending and sigmoid colostomies are easier to manage because the content of the bowel is semisolid to solid. Scheduled daily irrigation to establish regularity will help the patient to achieve control more rapidly. When control is obtained on a once-a-day basis, every-other-day irrigations may be recommended by the physician.

DOUBLE-BARREL COLOSTOMY.   When a double-barrel colostomy is irrigated, it is important to distinguish between the proximal and the distal loops. Irrigation may be ordered for both the proximal and distal portions of the bowel or for only the proximal portion.

Methods of Colostomy Management.
The three usual methods of colostomy management are irrigation by standard method, irrigation by bulb syringe, and nonirrigation.

Irrigations usually are begun on the fourth or fifth postoperative day. The day before the first irrigation, the irrigation procedure and equipment should be described or shown to the patient (Fig. 45-8).

It is essential that the patient be assisted with the irrigation procedure because the effectiveness of the irrigation is the basis for establishing control. It can be easily and simply taught, so that most patients can begin to do their own irrigation after it has been demonstrated once or more times by the nurse (Figs. 45-9 and 45-10).

The most widely advocated method for irrigation is the standard method, which consists of a daily scheduled irrigation with 500 to 1,500 mL of water. Equipment includes a receptacle for the irrigating solution, tubing, a catheter, and an irrigation sleeve or sheath for the fecal return. Several types of equipment are available commercially. After irrigation, the patient may be free of fecal spillage for 1 to 3 days.

Once the equipment is assembled, the irrigation solution prepared, and the air removed from the tubing, the patient is seated on a toilet seat or on a

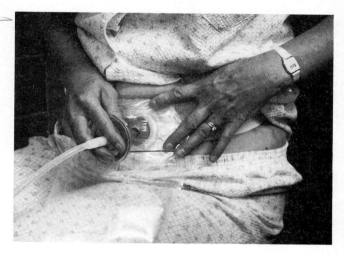

Figure 45–9. Patients must be instructed in the techniques of colostomy irrigation before discharge from the hospital. (Courtesy of Convatec, Princeton, NJ)

chair in front of a toilet with the irrigation sheath directed into the toilet bowl. The bottom of the bag containing the irrigating solution is hung at about shoulder height. The catheter is lubricated and then inserted into the stomal opening. The irrigation catheter should be inserted *slowly* and *gently* 2 or 3 inches by gentle rotation of the catheter. Difficulty in inserting the catheter may be due to a hard piece of stool, stool impacted in the catheter, or a fold of tissue. The catheter must *never* be forced into the stoma. If there is difficulty inserting the catheter, it can be removed, the irrigation clamp released, and water allowed to flow as the catheter is reinserted. Once the catheter is in place, it can be advanced 2 to

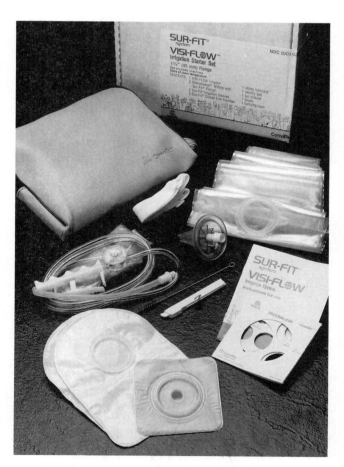

Figure 45–8. An irrigation starter set provides the new ostomate with materials necessary for colostomy irrigation. (Courtesy of Convatec, Princeton, NJ)

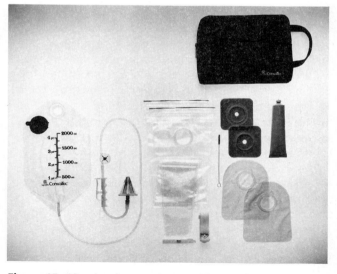

Figure 45–10. A colostomy irrigation kit. (Courtesy of Convatec, Princeton, NJ)

6 inches, as desired. The catheter only needs to be introduced far enough for water to be retained in the bowel.

The water should be allowed to enter the bowel slowly and gently because too rapid an instillation of fluid results in painful cramping and an ineffective irrigation. If water returns as it is being introduced, the tubing should be clamped until the return flow ceases.

After irrigation, the catheter is removed and the return flow permitted to drain into the irrigation sleeve. The patient may remain on the toilet seat, or may close off the edge of the sleeve and walk about to help stimulate an evacuation.

Return usually is completed in 20 to 30 minutes, but the time varies from person to person, and even in the same person. The patient will learn to determine when the irrigation is sufficiently effective and the bowel is clean of feces; the signal may be a spurt of gas or simply a sensation that the patient has learned to recognize. A clue to the effectiveness of the irrigation can be obtained by observing the return. If the return is watery and slightly colored, and contains no stool, the bowel is probably clean. If the return is heavy with stool, the bowel is probably not clean, and an additional instillation of irrigating fluid may be necessary. Patients should be discouraged from using more than 2 quarts of water at a time because of the possibility of water intoxication.

If the patient has a double-barrel colostomy, the proximal portion is irrigated in the same manner as for a single-stoma colostomy. Irrigation of the distal portion must be done with the patient sitting on a toilet or a bedpan, as the irrigation fluid will leave by way of the anus. A small amount of mucus usually is expelled along with the irrigating fluid. During the immediate postoperative period, necrotic tissue also may be expelled.

Cramping during irrigation is a problem for some patients. A slight cramp may simply be a signal that the bowel is ready to empty. Cramping also may be caused by water that is too cold or introduced too rapidly, or by failure to release air from the tubing before inserting the fluid. If cramping occurs, the tubing is clamped and the patient instructed to take a few deep breaths. When the cramp is gone, the clamp is released and the irrigation continued.

The water may fail to return if the catheter is inserted too far and the water remains in the bowel temporarily, or if it is trapped behind a hard stool. To encourage the prompt return of fluid material, one or several of the following measures may be used: gently massaging the lower abdomen, tightening the abdominal muscles, taking several deep breaths and relaxing, gently twisting the body (at the waist) from side to side, standing up, or sitting more erect. If these measures are not effective and the patient is uncomfortable or distressed, the physician should be notified.

After the irrigation is completed, the irrigation sheath is removed, rinsed in cool water to reduce odor, and discarded (if disposable) or cleaned in warm, soapy water (if reusable).

Another method of irrigation uses a bulb syringe and a short catheter. The equipment consists of the syringe, a container for solution, and an emesis basin or a plastic sheath or an apron. This method calls for several instillations of 250 to 500 mL of solution at a time. Some patients perform two instillations a day. Some patients have found this method effective for permitting freedom of spillage for 24 or more hours. It may be used as an alternate choice when the standard method cannot be used.

With the nonirrigation or natural method, the patient may use a variety of devices to stimulate an evacuation. Prune or orange juice on arising or before bedtime, liquid breakfast, coffee, mild exercises, a mild laxative (if approved by the physician), and lemon juice in warm water are a few measures that have been effective. The patient usually does not know when the evacuation will occur.

Another method used by nonirrigators is the insertion of a suppository, such as glycerin or bisacodyl (Dulcolax), into the stoma. It may take 7 or more days of daily use before a regular evacuation pattern is established. Initially, the movements may occur three or four times daily. Each day the movements become fewer and fewer, until the patient has one or two movements a day. Some patients use a suppository in addition to irrigation. The patient should not use suppositories unless their use is approved or recommended by the physician.

Stoma. The stoma may be covered with a gauze pad or a temporary postoperative ostomy bag. If a gauze pad is worn, a small amount of lubricating jelly should be applied over the area that comes into contact with the stoma, to prevent irritation. An adhesive drainable bag or a karaya seal drainable bag is recommended for those patients who continue to have drainage problems between irrigations.

Body Image Disturbance, Ineffective Individual Coping. As with the patient with an ileostomy, time is needed to adjust to the changes in body image. If a colostomy was performed because of a malignant tumor, the patient faces additional concerns over the future. The patient may have to cope not only with learning to care for and irrigate a colostomy, but also with weeks or months of radiation therapy and chemotherapy.

These patients should be allowed to go through the various stages of grieving. They need someone to talk to, to listen, to understand, and to care. The nurse should extend every effort to help the patient cope with the illness, face the future, and accept what must be done to maintain optimal physical and emotional wellness.

Social Isolation. The room should be kept as free from odors as possible. Room deodorizers may help to reduce odors.

Altered Sexuality Patterns. Although most patients discuss problems associated with sexuality with the physician, some find it easier to talk to the nurse or a member of a local ostomy group. Questions regarding sexual relations most often arise after the patient is discharged from the hospital and begins to resume a normal life-style. Discussions with the physician or an ostomy group member may help the patient to resume normal sexual activity.

Impaired Skin Integrity. Skin care for the colostomy patient is the same as for the ileostomy patient. The skin around the stoma should be thoroughly cleaned each time the appliance is changed. Excess powder, ointment, or karaya gum should be removed, and the skin wiped with a soft cloth moistened with warm water and a mild soap.

Knowledge Deficit. The patient should understand how to care for the colostomy, including the irrigation procedure, skin and stoma care, and applying and removing the appliance. The physician may show the patient how and when to dilate the stoma with a finger covered with a finger cot or a disposable plastic glove. If this is to be started immediately, the patient should be supervised in this procedure before discharge from the hospital.

A dietary consult may be needed to discuss foods to be avoided as well as to provide a well-balanced menu.

The following points may be included in a patient-teaching plan:

1. Changes in the size and color of the stoma vary with activity and emotional status. Anger or extreme annoyance may cause the stoma to turn red or purple. Small beads of blood may ooze from the surface. Fright may cause the stoma to blanch. These are normal reactions and are insignificant in that the tissues will revert to their normal state when the cause (eg, activity, emotional reactions) is alleviated.

2. A regular diet can be eaten, but gas-forming foods should be avoided.

3. In most cases, increasing the amount of bulk foods in the diet, drinking extra water, and eating laxative-type foods corrects constipation.

4. If diarrhea occurs, it may be related to diet. Eliminating food items that result in diarrhea may help to control the problem. If diarrhea persists for more than 2 days, the physician should be contacted.

5. Eating slowly with the mouth closed and chewing food well will lessen the amount of gas that is caused chiefly by swallowing air rather than by processes of digestion.

6. With the exception of tightly fitted clothing, no adjustment needs to be made in the type of clothing worn. Patients who require a firm support (eg, those who wear girdles, have back problems, or wear braces) may find a stoma shield helpful in preventing undue pressure on or irritation of the stoma.

7. Weekly weights should be obtained. The physician should be contacted if there is a sudden weight loss.

8. Irrigations should be done at about the same time each day. The best time to irrigate is after a meal, since food in the digestive tract stimulates peristalsis and defecation.

9. The physician may recommend that the schedule for irrigations gradually progress to every other day, every third day, or even twice a week. If constipation occurs, the physician should be contacted regarding a change in the irrigation schedule.

10. Travel or activities outside the home need not be restricted. Sets that contain all the materials needed for irrigation and changes of the colostomy bag are available (see Fig. 45-10). The necessary items also may be assembled individually and placed in a waterproof container.

Evaluation

- Anxiety is reduced
- Pain is reduced or eliminated
- Evidence of infection is absent; temperature is normal and lungs are clear on auscultation
- Evidence of dehydration or electrolyte imbalances is absent
- Patient drinks an adequate amount of fluid
- Patient maintains the prescribed diet; weight remains stable or shows a gain
- Patient verbalizes concerns and discusses them freely with the family and medical team
- Patient begins to accept the change in body image
- Skin around the stoma and perineal area appears normal with no evidence of skin breakdown
- Odors are controlled
- Leakage around the stoma and appliance is minimal
- Patient discusses fears and concerns regarding sexual activity and expresses desire to talk to others about this problem
- Patient participates in or assumes responsibility for irrigation of the colostomy, skin care, and application of an appliance
- Patient verbalizes an understanding of dietary measures to control or prevent constipation, diarrhea, excessive gas, and odors

General Nutritional Considerations

☐ The diet of the ostomy patient may have to be adjusted if excessive flatulence (gas) with or without cramping occurs. The colostomy patient may find it necessary to avoid foods that cause constipation or diarrhea.

☐ The formation of gas can be lessened or eliminated by eating slowly and chewing food well. Foods that cause gas, such as onions, cabbage, and beans, should be avoided or eaten in limited amounts.

☐ Ostomates who have a persistent problem with gas or odor, or who have severe constipation or diarrhea may need to eliminate almost all food from their diet and start a new diet with tea, toast, and marmalade. Then one food at a time is added to determine which foods may be causing the problem. A diet change such as this should not be attempted without the physician's approval.

☐ Fish, eggs, onions, and cheese are examples of foods that may cause lingering odors; it may be necessary to eliminate such foods from the diet.

☐ The colostomy patient usually can avoid constipation by increasing the daily fluid intake, eating laxative-type foods such as bran cereal, and drinking prune juice.

General Pharmacologic Considerations

☐ Patients who are scheduled for bowel surgery may receive an antibiotic that is capable of reducing the number of bacteria in the colon. A reduction in the number of bacteria lessens the chance of postoperative bowel or peritoneal infection. Examples of drugs used for this purpose are neomycin sulfate and kanamycin (Kantrex). When used for this purpose, the drug is given orally.

☐ Some drugs, such as antibiotics, impart a lingering odor to the ostomy appliance. The patient who is taking these drugs should be warned of the odor and encouraged to use a disposable pouch until the course of drug therapy is completed. A list of drugs that are capable of imparting an odor to an ostomy appliance can be obtained from an ostomy club or ostomy appliance manufacturers.

☐ Deodorizers for ostomy appliances include tablets that are taken orally and tablets or liquids that are placed directly in the pouch.

☐ Antidiarrheal drugs should not be used by the patient who has a colostomy unless the physician approves; overuse can result in fecal impaction. Use of laxatives also should be discussed with the physician.

General Gerontologic Considerations

☐ When teaching ostomy care to the elderly, the material is best presented in brief sessions, allowing the patient to master one task before another is presented. Illustrations and written directions may be necessary.

☐ A family member should be taught colostomy care in case the patient is temporarily unable to assume responsibility for this task.

☐ Difficulty in changing the appliance, skin care, irrigation of the (colostomy) stoma, and care of the permanent appliance may be encountered by the elderly ostomate because of chronic disorders such as poor vision and arthritis. These patients may require daily supervision by a family member.

☐ If it is believed that the elderly patient will be permanently unable to assume care for an ostomy, arrangements for daily care will have to be made. Depending on the situation, a family member, visiting nurse, or a home health care nurse will have to assume this responsibility. In some instances, transfer to a skilled nursing facility or nursing home that accepts ostomates may be necessary.

Suggested Readings

☐ Alfaro R. Applying nursing diagnosis and nursing process: a step-by-step guide. 2nd ed. Philadelphia: JB Lippincott, 1990. *(Additional coverage of subject matter)*

☐ Benedict P, Haddad A. Postop teaching for the colostomy patient. RN March 1989;52:85. *(Additional coverage of subject matter)*

☐ Burtis G, Davis J, Martin S. Applied nutrition and diet therapy. Philadelphia: WB Saunders, 1988. *(Additional coverage of subject matter)*

☐ Caldwell L. Nutrition education for the patient: the handout manual. Philadelphia: JB Lippincott, 1984. *(Additional coverage of subject matter)*

☐ Caine RM, Buffalino PM (eds). Nursing care planning guides for adults. Baltimore: Williams & Wilkins, 1987. *(Additional coverage of subject matter)*

☐ Dalton-Loehner D, Connor PA. Beyond ileostomy: surgery for a normal life. RN July 1989;52:29. *(Additional coverage and drawings that reinforce subject matter)*

☐ Dudek SG. Nutrition handbook for nursing practice. Philadelphia: JB Lippincott, 1987. *(Additional coverage of subject matter)*

☐ Kozier B, Erb G. Techniques in clinical nursing: a nursing process approach. 2nd ed. Menlo Park, CA: Addison-Wesley, 1987. *(Additional coverage of subject matter)*

☐ Neufeldt J. Helping the I.B.D. patient cope with the unpredictable. Nursing '87 August 1987;17:47. *(Additional coverage of subject matter)*

☐ Taylor MC, Lillis C, LeMone P. Fundamentals of nursing: the art and science of nursing care. Philadelphia: JB Lippincott, 1989. *(Additional coverage of subject matter)*

☐ Timby B. Clinical nursing procedures. Philadelphia: JB Lippincott, 1989. *(Additional coverage of subject matter)*

☐ Zastocki DK, Rovinski CA. Home care: patient and family instructions. Philadelphia: WB Saunders, 1989. *(Additional coverage of subject matter)*

Chapter 46

Disorders of the Liver, Gallbladder, and Pancreas

On completion of this chapter the reader will:

- Discuss the symptoms, diagnosis, and treatment for cirrhosis

- Discuss the modes of transmission, symptoms, diagnosis, treatment, and complications of hepatitis

- Discuss the symptoms, diagnosis, and treatment of tumors of the liver

- Use the nursing process in the medical management of the patient with a disorder of the liver

- Use the nursing process in the surgical management of the patient with a disorder of the liver

- Discuss the symptoms, diagnosis, and treatment of acute and chronic cholecystitis

- Use the nursing process in the medical management of the patient with a gallbladder disorder

- Use the nursing process in the surgical management of the patient with a gallbladder disorder

- Discuss the symptoms, diagnosis, and treatment of acute and chronic pancreatitis

- Use the nursing process in the management of the patient with pancreatitis

- Discuss the symptoms, diagnosis, and treatment of carcinoma of the pancreas
- Use the nursing process in the management of the patient having pancreatic surgery

HEPATIC DISORDERS
Jaundice (Icterus)

Jaundice is a greenish yellow discoloration of tissue caused by an abnormally high concentration of the pigment bilirubin in the blood. Total bilirubin concentration normally is about 0.1 to 1.0 mg/dL of blood. If serum bilirubin levels reach 3 mg/dL or higher, jaundice is visible, notably on the skin, mucous membrane of the mouth, and especially the sclera.

Jaundice occurs in a multitude of diseases that directly or indirectly affect the liver. It is probably the most common sign of liver disorder. A knowledge of bile formation and excretion is important to the understanding of jaundice.

When red blood cells are old or injured, they are picked up by the spleen and bone marrow, where they are broken down by reticuloendothelial cells. Hemoglobin released from these red blood cells is then reduced to the compound known as *unconjugated,* or *indirect,* bilirubin. This type of bilirubin is then carried by the blood to the liver, where further chemical processes transform it into *conjugated,* or *direct,* bilirubin. These two forms of bilirubin are distinct, can be differentiated chemically, and are important in the clinical discrimination between different diseases that produce jaundice.

The conjugated bilirubin formed by the liver enters the bile ducts, reaches the intestine, and is transformed into urobilinogen. Some of the urobilinogen is then changed into urobilin, the brown pigment of stool. Urobilinogen enters the bloodstream and is carried back to the liver where it is changed into bilirubin for reexcretion in the bile. Another portion of urobilinogen is carried from the intestine to the kidney and is excreted in the urine.

In diseases that cause jaundice, the laboratory determination of the type of pigment in the blood, urine, and stool contributes to a more accurate diagnosis and permits the most appropriate therapy.

There are three forms of jaundice: (1) hemolytic jaundice, caused by the overabundance of breakdown products of blood; (2) hepatocellular jaundice, caused by internal liver disease that prevents normal transformation of bile by the liver cells; and (3) obstructive jaundice, caused by the inability of normally formed liver bile to be passed into the intestine because of blockage in the bile ducts. Jaundice is both a sign and a symptom; it is not a separate disease.

Cirrhosis

In cirrhosis, liver damage is followed by scarring, with development of excessive fibrous connective tissue. This occurs as the liver attempts to repair itself, and leads to considerable anatomical distortion, including partial or complete occlusion of blood channels within the liver. There are several types of hepatic cirrhosis, depending on cause, pathology, and clinical manifestations. They are as follows:

1. *Laennec's (portal, alcoholic, nutritional, or toxic) cirrhosis* is associated with a heavy, chronic alcohol intake, usually coincident with poor nutrition (Fig. 46-1). It also can follow chronic poisoning with certain chemicals, such as carbon tetrachloride, a cleaning agent. Laennec's cirrhosis is most often seen in people between the ages of 45 and 65 who have a history of alcoholism.
2. *Postnecrotic (posthepatitic) cirrhosis* follows varies types of hepatitis.
3. *Biliary (primary, secondary) cirrhosis* may have an unknown cause or be the result of chronic obstruction or infection of the bile ducts.

Symptoms

General manifestations of liver damage occur. There are disorders of protein, fat, carbohydrate, and vitamin metabolism as well as defects of blood coagulation, fluid and electrolyte balance, and ability to combat infections and toxins.

Clinically, findings in advanced cirrhosis include poor nutrition with tissue wasting; poor hemostasis (stopping of bleeding) and easy bleeding; vitamin deficiencies; water retention; sodium deficiency; weight loss; weakness; mental dullness; anorexia, nausea, and vomiting; intraabdominal fluid (ascites); hypoglycemia; and low blood proteins (hypoproteinemia). The skin is thin, with dilated veins especially noted over the abdomen. Nosebleeds (epistaxis), jaundice, ecchymosis, scant body hair, palmar erythema (bright pink palms), and cutaneous spider angiomata (tiny, spiderlike skin vessels of the face and chest) also can occur. Testicular atrophy often is seen, and is probably due to the inability of the damaged liver to metabolize

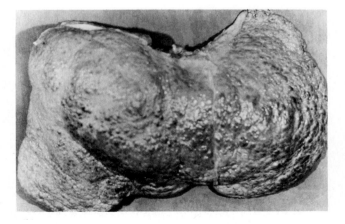

Figure 46-1. Top view of liver showing typical nodularity (hobnail liver) of alcoholic cirrhosis. (Photograph by Paul S. Milley, MD)

estrogenic factors produced by such organs as the adrenal gland.

In postnecrotic cirrhosis, the symptoms basically are the same as those seen in Laennec's cirrhosis. The earliest symptoms of biliary cirrhosis are jaundice, pruritus (itching of the skin), dark urine, and clay-colored stools. These symptoms usually are followed by diarrhea, weight loss, and bleeding tendencies. The liver is almost always enlarged.

Diagnosis

Diagnosis is made by patient history, physical examination, and diagnostic studies. Diagnostic studies include liver biopsy, ultrasound examination of the liver, computed tomographic (CT) scan, magnetic resonance imaging (MRI), and radioisotope liver scan. Laboratory tests include a complete blood count, serum enzyme studies, bleeding and coagulation tests, and serum albumin and globulin level determinations.

Treatment

No specific cure for hepatic cirrhosis exists. The principal aim of therapy is to prevent further deterioration by abolishing underlying causes and to preserve optimal liver function.

Treatment is aimed at relieving symptoms associated with the disorder. The physician may order a diet high in carbohydrates, proteins, and vitamins. If a high blood level of ammonia is present and impending liver coma is suspected, proteins (which are ammonia precursors) are omitted. If improvement occurs, proteins are slowly added to the diet. Because of the anorexia that accompanies severe cirrhosis, it is better to offer the patient frequent, small, semisolid or liquid meals rather than three full meals a day. Nausea and vomiting may necessitate parenteral feedings. Vitamin B complex, vitamin K, vitamin C, and iron may be prescribed. Intravenous albumin may be given in severe hypoproteinemia, and blood transfusions may be necessary for anemia. Because of the tendency toward salt and water retention (which can lead to edema, circulatory congestion, and heart failure), the intake of these substances is carefully regulated and often restricted. Antacids may be given to relieve gastric distress,

If treatment begins in the early phases, when signs and symptoms are few and mild, satisfactory recuperation is frequent and long-term prognosis is good. Rescuing patients with advanced disease who are jaundiced and hypoproteinemic and have ascites and other manifestations of severe liver damage is considerably more difficult.

Complications

Hepatic coma, bleeding esophageal varices, infection, and ascites are complications of advanced cirrhosis.

Hepatic Coma. Coma may occur in any form of hepatic failure. The patient becomes lethargic, drowsy, confused, irritable, and, eventually, stuporous, drifting into coma. If the patient has a history of alcoholism, delirium tremens may occur early in the development of hepatic coma. Increased serum ammonia levels seem to be related to the development or aggravation of hepatic coma, but are not the absolute cause. Therapy to reduce ammonia levels seems to reverse the comatose state in some people. Ammonia formed in the intestine by bacterial action on ingested proteins normally is detoxified in the liver by conversion to urea, which is then excreted by the kidneys. A failing liver, as in advanced cirrhosis, can no longer break down ammonia and, therefore, allows it to accumulate in the blood. Also, with portal venous obstruction, ammonia-rich intestinal blood may be diverted from the liver, further reducing detoxification.

Therapy of coma includes reduction of protein intake to zero, avoidance of drugs and stress, and removal of residual protein or blood (if there has been recent hemorrhage) from the intestine by laxatives and enemas. An antibiotic such as neomycin or kanamycin (Kantrex) may be ordered. Because these drugs are poorly absorbed from the gastrointestinal (GI) tract, their use reduces the number of microorganisms in the bowel, thereby lessening the production of ammonia by the intestinal flora. Cleansing enemas may be ordered, to reduce the fecal bacterial substrate in the colon. Careful medical support of the comatose patient involves maintenance of fluid and electrolyte balance with parenteral nutrition. Multivitamins often are added to infusions.

Portal Hypertension and Bleeding Esophageal Varices. The most important factor secondary to hepatic scarring in Laennec's cirrhosis is portal hypertension. In the scarred cirrhotic liver, the intrahepatic veins may be squeezed shut, so that blood backs up into the portal vein and on into diverting channels around the esophagus and stomach. These engorged collateral vessels are called *esophageal,* or *gastric, varices.* This buildup of pressure in the portal system is called *portal hypertension.*

The gastric and esophageal veins distend and may bleed. Subsequent bleeding into the stomach and esophagus often is rapid, and may result in massive hematemesis. The bleeding is aggravated by clotting disorders common to liver damage.

The most life-threatening complication is hemorrhage from esophageal varices. Patients with cirrhosis of the liver have a high incidence of duodenal ulcers, which may be another cause of GI bleeding.

Portal hypertension can be relieved by surgically draining blood from the portal vein into an adjacent systemic vein. Because less blood will now go through the portal system, the pressure drops, and there is less chance that a collateral vessel will burst, with resultant hemorrhage. The portal vein lies just next to the inferior vena cava. A connection can be made surgically between these vessels, so that portal blood is released into the vena cava, reducing hypertension. This is called a *portacaval shunt.* A similar beneficial effect is sometimes achieved by connecting the splenic vein (a tributary of the portal vein) to the renal vein (a tributary of the vena cava). This is called a *splenorenal shunt* (see Fig. 46-2). These procedures are major surgeries. If done electively or prophylactically to prevent future hemorrhage, the patient should be in the best possible condition before surgery.

Infection. Infection is due to a decrease in natural resistance as liver function is reduced. Antibiotics are administered as needed.

Ascites. Ascites is a collection of fluid in the peritoneal cavity. This complication results from portal hypertension (see earlier discussion).

The increased fluid retention manifested as ascitic intraabdominal fluid and tissue edema fluid involves several factors and relations that are not entirely clear. Overproduction of the hormone aldosterone by the adrenal glands probably occurs in cirrhosis. This hormone causes sodium and water retention combined with potassium excretion. This, in addition to associated protein deficiency and factors that affect kidney function, allows abnormal fluid collection. An abdominal paracentesis may need to be performed to remove ascitic fluid.

The rapid removal of abdominal fluid by paracentesis is achieved by carefully introducing a needle through the abdominal wall and allowing the fluid to drain. This may quickly relieve the severe discomfort of distention and difficulty in breathing secondary to pressure of a large volume of abdominal fluid on the diaphragm and lungs.

Only a few liters of fluid are removed at one time, since removal of large quantities of fluid at once can cause drastic shifts between the vascular and extravascular compartments with resultant circulatory collapse (shock). Shock can occur shortly after the tap because of the acute fluid, mineral, and protein shifts that act to replace the lost ascitic fluid. Other complications of paracentesis include perforation of the intestine or bladder, resulting in peritonitis, and leakage of fluid from the needle site. To avoid perforation of the bladder, it is important to have the patient void before the procedure is done. Vital signs should be monitored before and for several hours after this procedure. Any changes in vital signs, abdominal pain, or fever should be reported immediately.

Additional treatment includes diuretics and a so-

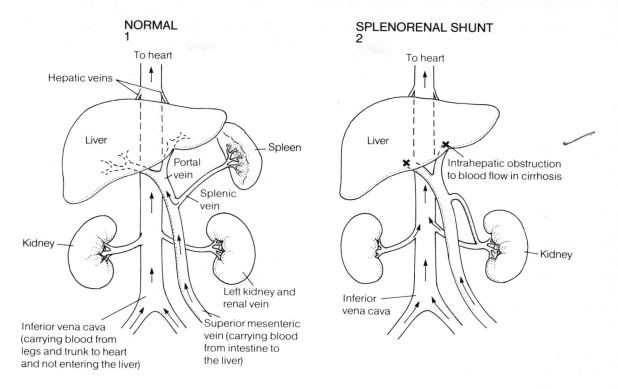

NORMAL
1

SPLENORENAL SHUNT
2

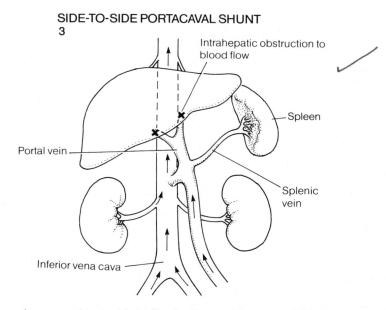

SIDE-TO-SIDE PORTACAVAL SHUNT
3

Figure 46–2. (*1*) Normal anatomy showing blood flow back to the heart. Note that the major veins pass through the liver. (*2*) Splenorenal shunt. The spleen has been removed and the splenic vein connected to the left renal vein. Now some portal blood can flow into the inferior vena cava by thus passing the liver. (*3*) Side-to-side portacaval shunt. The side of the portal vein is anastomosed to the side of the inferior vena cava. Now blood can flow from the portal circulation into the systemic circulation if there is significant intrahepatic obstruction.

dium-restricted diet. The potassium-sparing diuretic spironolactone may be used, as this drug specifically antagonizes aldosterone, reversing the effects of this hormone so that sodium and water are excreted, potassium is retained, and the amount of ascites reduced.

A surgical procedure called a continuous peritoneal jugular shunt (LeVeen shunt) redirects the fluid from the peritoneal cavity to the systemic circulation. This surgery involves the insertion of perforated tubing into the peritoneal cavity. The tubing is fitted with a one-way pressure-sensitive valve. The other end of the tubing is attached to the valve and threaded into the jugular vein and the superior vena cava. Peritonitis, blockage of the tubing, and electrolyte imbalances are some of the complications associated with this procedure.

Hepatitis

Viral Hepatitis

Pathology. Hepatitis is an infectious, contagious disease of the liver caused by a virus. The infection may cause simultaneous damage to the intestine and other organs, but the most significant damage is to liver cells, which may become necrotic and die. In fatal cases, liver parenchymal damage is severe. Internal damage to the liver may prevent normal bile secretion or excretion, causing jaundice in addition to the metabolic dysfunction of parenchymal injury.

Etiology. Although similar in nature, the following forms of hepatitis are slightly different clinical diseases with respect to such factors as incubation period and mode of transmission:

Hepatitis A—Caused by the hepatitis A virus; also known as infectious hepatitis or epidemic hepatitis
Hepatitis B—Caused by the hepatitis B virus; also known as serum hepatitis
Hepatitis C—A newly discovered virus that probably causes most of what was originally called non-A, non-B hepatitis
Hepatitis D—Also called delta hepatitis, appears to accompany hepatitis B in some patients, making the infection more severe
Hepatitis E—Resembles hepatitis A and is transmitted in the same manner

Modes of Transmission. *Hepatitis A* and *hepatitis E* are transmitted from person to person by contact with the virus in the feces and saliva of infected people. Transmission also may occur by means of water and food contaminated with the virus. In the hospital, contaminated rectal thermometers, bedpans, and linen may harbor the virus, which in turn contaminates the hands. Diseased food handlers, cooks, or waiters may create an epidemic, especially in the armed services, schools, restaurants, supermarkets, and similar close community conditions. The hepatitis A virus also may be found in the blood of infected people.

Hepatitis B is primarily transmitted by transfusions of blood or plasma and by needles, syringes, or surgical or dental equipment contaminated with the blood of people who have the disease. It also may be transmitted by sexual contact with carriers or with those who have the disease, since it may be found in the vaginal secretions, semen, and saliva of infected people.

Hepatitis C is transmitted by blood and probably sexual contact. This form of hepatitis apparently increases the risk of liver cancer.

Hepatitis D is apparently transmitted by contaminated blood and needles and by sexual contact.

Incubation Period. The incubation period for hepatitis A is about 3 to 5 weeks; for hepatitis B, about 2 to 5 months. The incubation period for other forms is variable, but averages about 7 weeks.

Symptoms. In some instances, the signs and symptoms of the various forms of hepatitis are indistinguishable, whereas at other times there may be a somewhat different set of symptoms. The signs and symptoms for the three phases of hepatitis are as follows:

Preicteric phase—Nausea; vomiting; anorexia; fever (which may be low- or high-grade); malaise (which may be severe); arthralgia; headache (which may be severe); right upper quadrant discomfort; enlargement of the spleen, liver, and lymph nodes; weight loss; rash; and urticaria
Icteric phase—Jaundice, pruritus, clay-colored or light stools, dark urine, fatigue (which may be extreme), anorexia, and right upper quadrant discomfort. Symptoms of the preicteric phase may continue
Posticteric phase—Liver enlargement may still be seen, and malaise and fatigue may continue even though other symptoms of the disease have disappeared

The patient with hepatitis may not experience all the symptoms listed above, and the severity of any one symptom may vary. Even though the symptoms are divided into prejaundice, jaundice, and postjaundice phases, all patients with hepatitis do not have jaundice.

Diagnosis. Diagnosis is based on the patient's symptoms and history (eg, blood transfusions, dental work, surgery, or contact with an infected person). Laboratory tests may include tests for hepatitis antibodies and radioimmunoassays.

Prognosis. A small number of patients with hepatitis proceed to hepatic coma and death. Most recover, but they can never donate blood. There also are a small number of patients who suffer from chronic active hepatitis, which usually progresses to cirrhosis and death unless corticosteroid treatment slows the active and inflammatory processes. Some researchers believe that some patients with hepatitis C develop mild to severe chronic liver disease that may lead to cirrhosis.

Prevention. For hepatitis A, immune globulin (gamma-globulin) may be given before or after exposure, but immune globulin is not indicated for patients who have clinical manifestations of hepatitis A. When an outbreak of hepatitis A occurs or when food handlers are diagnosed as having hepatitis A, the local health department may institute administration of immune globulin to all possible contacts. Thorough hand washing, good personnel hygiene, and environmental sanitation measures such as proper sewage disposal and a safe water supply also prevent the spread of the disease.

The spread of hepatitis B can be prevented by the administration of hepatitis B vaccine to those at risk for contracting the disease. Persons at risk include all medical and dental personnel and those exposed to blood or blood products. Administration of hepatitis B immune globulin is recommended for those who are exposed to hepatitis B and not protected by the hepatitis B vaccine.

A blood test to detect hepatitis C in donated blood as well as to diagnose this form of hepatitis is currently being developed.

Treatment. Treatment is symptomatic and includes bed rest, a well-balanced diet given as small, interval feedings, and intravenous administration of fluids if the patient is extremely ill or has a low oral intake of fluids. Vomiting may be treated with antiemetics, but it usually is advisable to avoid the use of any drug until the liver has recovered. Multivitamin therapy may be necessary if the patient eats poorly.

Nonviral Hepatitis

Exposure to solutions that contain carbon tetrachloride, insecticides, and a variety of other drugs and chemicals can cause severe liver damage. The degree of damage, signs, and symptoms vary with the extent of exposure to the toxic agent as well as associated damage to kidneys and other organs. The clinical picture may evolve gradually or abruptly and may be indistinguishable from viral hepatitis. A history of exposure, elevated white blood cell count, acute onset of jaundice, and hepatic failure with a rapidly enlarging, tender liver are more indicative of toxic hepatitis. Management is similar to that for viral hepatitis.

Prevention. Prophylaxis requires the education of children, parents, industrial workers, and others by nurses, physicians, and public health–minded people. The public should be advised to read labels carefully and to observe precautions when using cleaning solutions, insecticides, and other chemicals; to provide adequate ventilation when using volatile chemicals; to keep chemicals away from children; and to take no medicines unless specifically prescribed by the physician.

Tumors of the Liver

Tumors of the liver may be malignant or benign. Malignant tumors may be primary (classified as hepatomas) or secondary (metastatic tumors). Hepatomas are rare but appear to have a higher incidence in people with cirrhosis, especially those with the postnecrotic form. The most common malignant tumor of the liver is a metastatic lesion from the breast, lung, or GI tract. Among the causes of benign tumors of the liver are tuberculosis and fungal and parasitic infections. Oral contraceptives and anabolic steroids also have been implicated in the development of benign hepatic lesions.

Symptoms

The symptoms of a hepatoma may be vague and can be confused with those of cirrhosis. Once the tumor is sufficiently large, the patient may complain of pain in the right upper quadrant and a sudden onset of abdominal distention (due to ascites).

Diagnosis

Diagnosis is made by needle biopsy of the liver, liver scan, ultrasound examination, CT scan, MRI, and laboratory studies that indicate changes in liver function.

In patients with cancer, metastatic lesions may be suspected when tests show changes in liver function. These lesions also may be diagnosed during surgery for the primary lesion. Benign tumors may have few symptoms until the tumor causes liver enlargement, followed by signs of changes in liver function.

Treatment

If the tumor is confined to a single lobe of the liver, a hepatic lobectomy may be attempted for the removal of primary malignant or benign tumors. Metastatic tumors usually are considered inoperable because they often are scattered throughout the liver.

NURSING PROCESS —THE PATIENT WHO HAS A LIVER DISORDER

Assessment

A complete patient history, including all symptoms and diet and drug histories, should be obtained from the patient or family. Depending on the potential diagnosis as well as information given during the patient history, in-depth questioning may be necessary to obtain information that may help the physician establish or confirm a diagnosis. Contributing factors such as exposure to toxic chemicals, a history of hepatitis, or long-term alcohol abuse also may be revealed in the patient history.

A physical assessment should be performed (see Chapter 42) with special attention to the size of the abdomen and the presence or absence of jaundice and other symptoms of liver disease. A general evaluation of the patient's physical and mental condition should be made at this time.

Nursing Diagnosis

Depending on the condition of the patient, the diagnosis, and other factors, one or more of the following nursing diagnoses may apply:

- Anxiety related to symptoms (eg, hematemesis and tarry stools), diagnosis, other factors (specify)
- Pain related to ascites, liver enlargement, discomfort associated with pruritus
- Activity intolerance related to ascites, anemia, fatigue, other symptoms (specify)
- Potential for infection related to decreased antibody production
- Altered nutrition: less than body requirements related to anorexia, use of alcohol as a source of food, chronic gastritis, other symptoms (specify)
- Diarrhea related to the presence of blood in the GI tract and fats in the stool secondary to liver dysfunction
- Fluid volume excess related to peripheral edema, ascites, sodium retention.
- Impaired skin integrity related to jaundice, pruritus, edema
- Potential for injury related to mental changes (eg, confusion and disorientation), impairment of clotting factors secondary to liver dysfunction
- Altered thought processes related to increased serum ammonia levels and liver failure
- Knowledge deficit of postdischarge medical management

Planning and Implementation

The major goals of the patient include reduction of anxiety, relief of pain and discomfort, improved activity tolerance, absence of infection, improved nutrition, normal bowel elimination, reduction of fluid volume, prevention of skin breakdown, absence of injury, improved thought processes, and an understanding of postdischarge medical management.

The major goals of nursing management are to improve the nutritional status, recognize and prevent complications, reduce pain and discomfort, and protect the patient from injury.

The patient should be weighed daily. If ascites is present, the abdomen should be measured daily or as ordered. Measurements should be taken in the same manner each time to ensure accuracy.

Daily observations and assessments should include weight; intake and output; vital signs every 2 to 4 hours or as ordered; the number, color, and consistency of bowel movements; measurement of ab-dominal girth; and evaluation of the patient's mental status. Changes in any of these indicators should be reported to the physician. New symptoms or problems also should be noted and recorded. Diarrhea, especially black, tarry stools, should be reported immediately, as this may indicate bleeding in the GI tract.

Laboratory and diagnostic studies and the physician's progress notes provide an understanding of the patient's response (or lack of response) to therapy and should be reviewed daily.

ESOPHAGEAL VARICES. Patients who have severe cirrhosis with portal hypertension may bleed from esophageal varices. When bleeding occurs, a Sengstaken-Blakemore esophageal-gastric balloon tube may be inserted by the physician into the esophagus in an attempt to stop the bleeding. The use of this three-lumen tube can be hazardous and requires constant supervision. The tube has three separate openings: one inflates the esophageal balloon, one inflates the gastric balloon, and one aspirates the stomach (Fig. 46-3). The distended, bleeding varices are in the lower esophagus and upper stomach. As the physician inflates the gastric balloon, it is gently pulled up. Constant application of the balloon to the upper stomach wall squeezes any bleeding vessels shut. Similarly, as the physician inflates the esophageal balloon, it expands against the esophageal wall, and ruptured bleeding varices are pressed closed. Through the tube opening into the stomach, clots can be removed by irrigation to reduce protein by-products of digested blood, which can lead to ammonia production and, possibly, hepatic coma.

Because patients who have this tube in place require continuous care and observation, they usually are placed in the intensive care unit. As the patient's condition stabilizes, the physician may order the tube deflated in 24 to 48 hours. The tube is kept in place, so that rapid reinflation can be carried out if bleeding should recur. During this period, the patient is observed for melena, further hematemesis, fall in blood pressure, fall in hematocrit, and tachycardia, which indicate further bleeding. If bleeding occurs or is uncontrolled, an emergency shunt or ligation operation may be necessary. With this tube in place, the patient may be restless, apprehensive, and uncomfortable.

HEPATIC COMA. The patient with a liver disorder may go into hepatic coma. Management of a semicomatose or fully unresponsive patient involves observation of vital signs, frequent turning to avoid skin breakdown, mouth care, endotracheal suction to prevent aspiration pneumonia, use of side rails, frequent observation to prevent falling, and similar commonsense measures. When reversal of the pathological process is impossible, hepatic coma is a

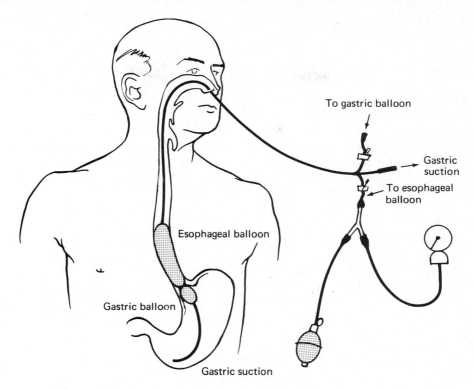

Figure 46-3. A Sengstaken-Blakemore tube in place. The clamp on the tube that leads to the esophageal balloon is kept tightly closed to maintain the inflated balloon at the prescribed pressure. The clamp is loosened to check the pressure with the manometer. The gastric suction tube is attached to continuous suction to keep the patient's stomach empty and to prevent vomiting, which would dislodge the esophageal balloon. Irrigations of the gastric suction tube may be ordered to prevent clogging with blood.

terminal state. In other instances, medical and nursing measures succeed, and the patient recovers from coma.

Anxiety, Alteration in Thought Processes. The patient may experience anxiety for any number of reasons, including a progressive decrease in liver function, which can result in mental changes. In patients with cirrhosis and a history of alcohol abuse, anxiety may be an early warning sign of alcohol withdrawal (see Chapter 11). Any change in the patient's mental status should be carefully evaluated, as changes may be indicative of a serious complication. Mental changes also necessitate more frequent observation of the patient, as falls and other injuries can occur if the patient becomes confused or disoriented.

Pain, Impaired Skin Integrity. The patient with ascites or an enlarged liver should be assisted to assume a position of comfort. Position changes should be made every 2 hours or more often if needed. Because muscle wasting and weight loss may be present, skin care should be given to bony prominences each time the patient's position is changed.

The use of tape or soap should be avoided when-

ever possible, to prevent trauma to the skin. When the use of soap is necessary, it should be used sparingly, the skin thoroughly rinsed and dried, and a protective lotion or cream applied.

Pruritus. Pruritus may be an extremely uncomfortable, difficult-to-control feature of obstructive jaundice. Itching may be relieved by some types of lotions or sponge bathing with tepid water. Starch or oatmeal baths or antipruritic ointments also may be tried. Relief is only temporary, and several methods may have to be tried before some relief is obtained.

If the patient scratches while asleep, he or she may wear light cotton gloves at night. The patient's fingernails should be kept short and clean to reduce the possibility of breaking the skin. If itching is severe, the physician should be consulted. Tranquilizers or sedatives such as barbiturates usually are avoided, because most of these drugs are detoxified by the liver and their use is contraindicated in liver disease.

Bleeding. Because of decreased production of clotting factors by the liver, patients with a liver disorder may have bleeding tendencies, such as rectal bleeding, tarry stool, hematuria, bleeding gums, and ecchymosis from minor skin trauma. In some instances, hemorrhage can occur.

The patient should be observed for bleeding, and procedures should be performed in a way that lessens the likelihood of bleeding. Bleeding, when it occurs, usually arises from the GI tract. Each stool and all vomitus should be inspected for signs of bleeding, and if found, this should be reported to the physician immediately. Intramuscular injections and intravenous fluids should be given with small-gauge needles (when possible), and the injection site firmly pressed and observed for hematoma formation. After an intravenous catheter or needle is removed, immediate and prolonged pressure should be applied to prevent seepage, which allows hematomas to form, making the vein unusable. These patients may require frequent blood tests or intravenous therapy, hence every effort is made to preserve the integrity of the veins.

Potential for Infection. Patients with severe liver disease should be protected from other patients with infection and from visitors with colds or other contagious diseases. Vital signs should be monitored, and a rise in temperature should be reported to the physician.

Activity Intolerance. The patient with a liver disorder usually is placed on bed rest, and encouraged to deep breathe and move the extremities every 1 or 2 hours. If ascites or liver enlargement is present, semi-Fowler's position may lessen discomfort and make breathing easier.

Depending on symptoms, the patient may require partial or complete assistance with all activities of daily living or ambulatory activities (when allowed).

Altered Nutrition. Sustained, adequate nutrition is important in the therapy of patients with a liver disorder. Food intake should be recorded. If the patient eats poorly, a dietary consult may be obtained in an attempt to provide foods that are preferred but remain within the confines of the prescribed diet. The physician should be informed if the patient continues to eat poorly.

Fluid Volume Excess. Intake and output should be measured. If the patient is seriously ill, urine output may be measured on an hourly basis. Diuretics and a salt-restricted diet may be used to reduce the fluid volume excess.

Knowledge Deficit. Discharge teaching depends on the type and cause of the liver disorder and the physician's prescribed or recommended home care.

The following points may be included in a teaching plan:

- Follow the diet recommended by the physician.
- Avoid situations that could further damage the liver, for example drinking alcohol or inhaling certain toxic chemicals.
- Take frequent rest periods, especially if fatigue occurs during activity.
- Avoid exposure to infection.
- Follow the physician's recommendations regarding care of the skin.
- Avoid the use of nonprescription drugs (especially aspirin and products that contain aspirin) unless they have been approved by the physician.
- Contact the physician immediately if the following should occur: vomiting of blood, tarry stools, extreme fatigue, yellowing of the skin, light-colored stools.

If the patient requires a special diet (eg, a low-sodium diet to prevent edema and ascites), a consultation with the dietitian may be necessary.

Evaluation

- Anxiety is reduced
- Patient increases nutrition intake; eats the prescribed diet
- Evidence of bleeding or infection is absent
- Activity tolerance is increased
- Skin remains intact without evidence of infection or breakdown
- Patient appears mentally clear and more comfortable
- Patient understands dietary restrictions or prescribed special diet
- Patient demonstrates an understanding of the importance of avoiding infection, taking special care of the skin, avoiding the use of nonprescription drugs, and rest

NURSING PROCESS —THE PATIENT UNDERGOING SURGERY FOR A LIVER DISORDER

Assessment
See Chapter 43, Nursing Process for the Patient Who Has a Gastric Disorder, for general preoperative nursing management.

Postoperative assessments include vital signs and checking the function of drains and tubes (chest and nasogastric). The patient should be continually observed for complications (eg, hemorrhage, shock, infection, electrolyte imbalances, and hepatic coma). In addition, those with cirrhosis may exhibit signs of alcohol withdrawal.

Nursing Diagnosis

Depending on the type of surgery, one or more of the following nursing diagnoses may apply. If chest tubes have been inserted, additional nursing diagnoses pertaining to chest surgery are added (see Chapter 23).

- Pain due to incision high in the abdomen, chest tubes
- Hyperthermia related to infection
- Potential for infection related to surgery
- Ineffective airway clearance related to incisional pain, chest tubes, failure to cough and deep breathe
- Self-care deficits related to pain and discomfort of surgery
- Knowledge deficit of postdischarge treatment regimen, home care

Planning and Implementation

The major goals of the patient include relief of pain, normal body temperature, absence of infection, patent airway, improved ability to care for self, and an understanding of the continued treatment regimen and home care.

The major goals of nursing management are relief of pain, early detection and prevention of complications, maintenance of an adequate respiratory status, maintenance of adequate nutrition and fluid intake, and teaching the patient and family the essentials of postoperative home care.

After recovering from anesthesia, the patient is placed in low sitting position. If chest tubes have been inserted, the collection bottles should be positioned to ensure proper removal of air and fluid from the chest. The function and drainage of all tubes and drains should be noted.

Vital signs should be monitored as ordered. The dressing should be checked for bleeding or drainage. Additional nursing measures that apply to any postoperative patient (see Chapter 16) or the patient with chest tubes (see Chapter 23) are included in a plan of nursing management.

The patient should be assisted with all activities of daily living as long as necessary.

Pain. Narcotic analgesics may be ordered; however, patients with chronic liver disease are given lower than normal doses, since the liver is unable to effectively metabolize central nervous system depressants (which includes narcotics) as well as many other types of drugs.

The patient's response to the analgesic effect of the drug should be noted. If the drug fails to relieve pain or a sudden onset of severe pain is noted, the physician should be informed.

Fluids. Intake and output should be measured. Intravenous fluids should be given at the rate and volume ordered, and the patient observed for signs of fluid and electrolyte imbalance.

If the patient has a history of cirrhosis, the ankles should be checked for edema and the abdomen measured daily. Diuretics may be ordered to relieve or prevent ascites, and salt-poor albumin given to treat hypoproteinemia.

Nutrition. Bowel sounds should be auscultated every 4 to 8 hours. Patients normally are not given anything by mouth until peristalsis returns. Ice chips (if allowed) may relieve a dry mouth. Nutrition should be supplied intravenously until clear liquids are started, after removal of the nasogastric tube. Initially, liquids should be given in small amounts until the patient appears able to tolerate oral fluids.

Potential for Infection. Aseptic technique should be used for dressing changes, and the dressing reinforced as needed. Because patients with liver disease are susceptible to infection, the wound should be closely inspected each time the dressing is changed for appearance, approximation of wound edges, excessive drainage, and signs of infection. Antibiotics usually are ordered during the postoperative period. Any sudden rise in the patient's temperature should be reported to the physician.

Ineffective Airway Clearance. The patient should be turned and deep breathing, coughing, and leg movement encouraged every 2 hours. When applicable, the area of chest tube insertion should be supported when the patient coughs and deep breathes.

The head of the bed should be elevated to improve respiratory function. The lungs should be auscultated every 4 to 8 hours and at more frequent intervals if the patient appears to have respiratory distress. Arterial blood gas analysis may be ordered. Any signs of respiratory distress should be reported to the physician immediately.

Knowledge Deficit. Postoperative teaching depends on the diagnosis, the type and extent of surgery, and the physician's orders. It may be necessary to reinforce the physician's recommendations and explanations of future treatment modalities. If the patient has a malignant tumor of the liver, further treatment and prognosis are explained by the physician and reinforced by the nurse.

The following points may be included in a patient-teaching plan.

1. Follow the diet recommended by the physician.
2. Take planned rest periods during the day, and avoid heavy lifting.

3. Take medications exactly as prescribed. Follow the directions on the container, particularly with regard to taking the drug before, after, or with food or meals.
4. Weight should be measured weekly or as recommended by the physician. Report any significant weight gain or loss to the physician.
5. Contact the physician if any of the following occur: significant weight gain or increase in the size of the abdomen, fever, nausea, vomiting, vomiting of blood (bright red, coffeeground), tarry stools, difficulty in concentrating, jaundice, swelling of the ankles.
6. Periodic follow-up office visits are necessary.

Evaluation

- Pain and discomfort are controlled or eliminated
- Evidence of fluid volume deficit or electrolyte imbalances is absent
- Patient is able to take fluids and food by mouth
- Evidence of infection is absent; surgical wound appears normal
- Patient coughs, deep breathes, and performs leg exercises; ambulates as allowed
- Respirations are normal; lungs are clear to auscultation
- Self-care needs are met
- Patient demonstrates an understanding of postdischarge diet plan, drug regimen, incision care, periodic follow-up office visits

DISORDERS OF THE GALLBLADDER

Cholecystitis is inflammation and possibly infection of the gallbladder; cholelithiasis is stones within the gallbladder. Gallstones represent the most common ab-

normality of the biliary system (Fig. 46-4). Incidence increases progressively with aging. Gallstones occur more frequently in women than in men, particularly in women with a history of pregnancies, diabetes, and obesity. The cause of cholelithiasis has not definitely been established, but bile stasis and infection have been implicated. Hemolytic anemias associated with excessive bilirubin formation are associated with the development of pigment stones; hypercholesterolemia is associated with the accumulation of cholesterol-type stones.

Cholelithiasis and cholecystitis are intimately related, and the two conditions almost always coexist.

Chronic Cholecystitis

Chronic cholecystitis is seldom present without cholelithiasis.

Symptoms

Symptoms are probably caused by transient blockage of the outflow of bile due to stones or spasms of the ductal system. After a meal containing fried, greasy, spicy, or fatty foods, the patient may experience belching, nausea, and right upper abdominal discomfort, with pain or cramps.

In simple, uncomplicated colic of chronic cholecystitis with stones, there is no jaundice, fever, chills, liver damage, leukocytosis, or evidence of peritonitis on abdominal examination. Many patients with stones in the gallbladder never have symptoms of the disorder.

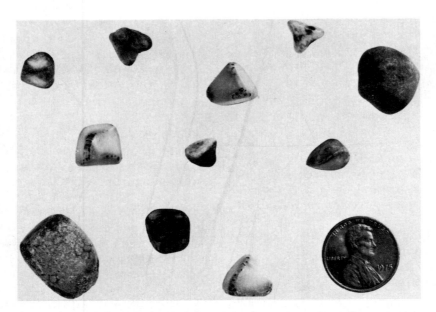

Figure 46–4. Gallstones. The one-cent piece is for comparison. Note that the stones are of different colors, sizes, and shapes. (Photograph by D. Atkinson)

Diagnosis

In addition to suggestive symptoms, definitive demonstration of cholelithiasis is obtained by means of cholecystography (gallbladder series), ultrasonography, and radionuclide imaging. Percutaneous transhepatic cholangiography may be performed to distinguish jaundice caused by liver disease from that of jaundice related to gallbladder disease.

Treatment

Because of the distress associated with this condition, removal of the gallbladder (cholecystectomy) usually is advised. Even in mild cases, because of the possibility of future distress and the complications of acute cholecystitis, cholecystectomy is advised by many surgeons who prefer to operate electively rather than in an emergency situation.

Medical management of cholecystitis includes a low-fat diet. Patients who are a surgical risk and have radiolucent stones may be given the drug chenodiol (Chenix) in an attempt to dissolve the gallstones. This drug is only moderately successful. The success rate is greatest when the stones are small. Because the drug can be hepatotoxic, frequent monitoring of liver function is necessary.

Lithotripsy may be used for selected patients. This nonsurgical procedure uses shock waves passed through water. The patient is given an anesthetic and immersed in a water bath. The lithotriptor generates shock waves directed at the gallbladder area. The stones fragment, and may be removed by endoscopy, which involves the passage of an endoscope through the mouth and down the GI tract to the common bile duct. Another method for removing the stones fragmented by lithotripsy is the insertion of a tube percutaneously into the common bile duct, followed by infusion of a solvent.

Acute Cholecystitis

Acute cholecystitis is a progression of chronic cholecystitis in which a stone completely blocks the flow of bile from the gallbladder. If the stone impacted in the cystic duct does not dislodge spontaneously, the walls of the distended gallbladder may become gangrenous, causing rupture and subsequent peritonitis.

Symptoms

Patients with acute cholecystitis usually are very sick with fever, vomiting, severe abdominal pain, and tenderness over the liver. The gallbladder may be so swollen that it becomes palpable; the white blood cell count is elevated; slight jaundice due to associated hepatic inflammation may be seen.

Severe pain is called *biliary colic*. The pain may radiate to the back and shoulders and is probably caused by a gallstone partly or completely obstructing the bile duct or the outlet of the gallbladder.

Diagnosis

Diagnosis is based on symptoms as well as the same studies performed for chronic cholecystitis.

Treatment

Medical management, including antibiotics, parenteral fluids, and nasogastric suction, fails to relieve a significant number of patients. In these cases, surgery consisting of either cholecystectomy or cholecystostomy (opening of the gallbladder, removal of stones, and placement of a tube for bile drainage to the exterior) may be lifesaving. If medical therapy is elected and is successful, cholecystectomy is carried out 2 or 3 months after inflammation has subsided.

NURSING PROCESS —MEDICAL MANAGEMENT OF THE PATIENT WHO HAS A GALLBLADDER DISORDER

Assessment

Patients admitted with the diagnosis of a gallbladder disorder should be questioned about symptoms, if any, experienced before admission. A description of symptoms should include the type and location of pain or discomfort and whether specific foods appeared to cause pain, discomfort, or other problems, such as nausea, vomiting, or abdominal cramping. Examination of the skin and sclera for jaundice, as well as palpation of the abdomen for tenderness, should be performed.

Nursing Diagnosis

Depending on the severity of symptoms, one or more of the following nursing diagnoses may apply. Additional diagnoses may apply if symptoms such as nausea, vomiting, or jaundice are severe.

- Anxiety related to symptoms, diagnosis
- Pain related to inflammation or presence of stones in the gallbladder
- Knowledge deficit of prescribed treatment regimen

Planning and Implementation

The major goals of the patient include reduction of anxiety, relief of pain, and an understanding of the prescribed treatment regimen.

The major goals of nursing management include relief of anxiety and discomfort and review of the treatment modalities with the patient and family.

During an attack of biliary colic, therapy usually involves rest, a bland liquid diet, and sedation. If vomiting occurs, nasogastric suction and parenteral fluids may be ordered.

If lithotripsy or some other method is used to remove the stones, the patient should be closely observed after the procedure for an increase in pain, shock, and signs of internal bleeding.

Anxiety. All diagnostic studies and treatment modalities should be fully explained. If lithotripsy or some other procedure is scheduled, the patient should be allowed time to ask questions about the procedure, with the nurse clarifying the explanations given by the physician.

Pain. A narcotic analgesic such as meperidine (Demerol) may be given to relieve severe pain. Narcotic analgesics also can cause spasm of portions of the common bile duct and the sphincter of Oddi, resulting in an increase in, rather than a relief of, pain. The patient's response to the administration of a narcotic analgesic should be carefully evaluated.

When pain is caused by certain types of foods, especially those high in fat, these foods should be omitted from the diet to decrease or eliminate symptoms.

Knowledge Deficit. Medical management should be explained to the patient. A consultation with a dietitian should be scheduled, and a complete list of foods that are to be avoided should be supplied. The patient also should be instructed to read the labels of all food products to determine their fat content.

When applicable, drug therapy should be explained, and the importance of taking the medication exactly as prescribed emphasized. The patient should be informed that the medication must be continued, even if symptoms disappear, and that frequent monitoring of the effect of drug therapy is necessary.

The importance of contacting the physician immediately if severe pain, jaundice, or a fever occur should be emphasized.

Evaluation

- Anxiety is reduced
- Pain is controlled
- Patient demonstrates an understanding of nonsurgical procedure to break up stones
- Evidence of complications after the procedure is absent
- Patient demonstrates an understanding of the recommended diet, medication schedule, and symptoms that necessitate examination by a physician

NURSING PROCESS —SURGICAL MANAGEMENT OF THE PATIENT WHO HAS A GALLBLADDER DISORDER

Assessment

Preoperative assessments are the same as for the patient with a medical disorder of the gallbladder. Preoperative preparations and nursing management are basically the same as for any surgery that requires a general anesthetic (see Chapter 16). A nasogastric tube usually is inserted the night before or the morning of surgery.

When the patient returns from surgery, vital signs should be taken and the chart reviewed for essential information, such as the insertion of drains or a T tube and the type of surgery performed. Types of gallbladder surgery include a cholecystectomy (removal of the gallbladder), choledochotomy (opening into the common bile duct), and a cholecystostomy (opening and drainage of the gallbladder). The nursing management of each is essentially the same.

Nursing Diagnosis

Depending on the patient's age and preoperative condition, one or more of the following nursing diagnoses may apply:

- Pain related to surgery
- Potential for infection related to surgery
- Impaired skin integrity related to bile drainage from T tube or drains
- Knowledge deficit of postdischarge treatment regimen, home care

Planning and Implementation

The major goals of the patient include relief of pain, absence of infection, prevention of skin breakdown, and an understanding of the postdischarge treatment regimen and home care.

The major goals of nursing intervention are to relieve pain, prevent complications, and provide the patient with an understanding of home care. Some of the complications associated with biliary surgery are thrombophlebitis, pulmonary embolus, peritonitis, and wound infection.

If a T tube has been inserted, it should be connected to straight gravity drainage unless ordered otherwise. The collection bag or bottle should be placed *below* the level of the operative site to prevent reflux of bile back into the duct. The collection receptacle must have a vent opening to prevent pressure buildup that would hinder bile drainage. Bile drainage should be measured every 8 hours. If more than 500 mL of drainage is collected within 24 hours, this should be reported to the physician. The drainage tube usually is left open, and should not be clamped without a physician's order. Kinking or occlusion of the tube should be avoided.

T tube cholangiography (in which dye is introduced into the tube and a radiograph is taken) may be done before removal of the T tube to ensure that there is no residual obstruction.

Nursing Care Plan 46-1 is an example of nursing management of the patient with a cholecystectomy.

Pain.   Medication for relief of pain should be administered frequently, so that the patient can rest and perform postoperative breathing and leg exercises, but not so frequently that activity is diminished and respirations become shallow or depressed. A sudden increase in pain or abdominal tenderness, or pain in other areas, such as the chest or legs, requires immediate medical attention.

Fluids.   Intravenous fluids should be administered at the rate ordered, and the patient observed for signs of electrolyte imbalance and dehydration (see Chapter 12). Intake and output, including output from the T tube and nasogastric tube, should be measured.

If a nasogastric tube has been inserted, it usually is removed in 24 to 48 hours, and liquid feedings are ordered with gradual progression to a general diet.

Potential for Infection.   Vital signs should be monitored every 4 hours or as ordered. The surgical wound should be inspected at the time of each dressing change. Any sudden rise in temperature or signs of wound infection should be brought to the physician's attention.

Respiratory Function.   After surgery, emphasis should be placed on deep breathing and coughing. Because the incision is high on the abdomen, these patients find full expansion of the chest more painful than those with a lower incision. The patient *must* be encouraged to cough and deep breathe every 1 or 2 hours. The incision should be supported with the hand or a pillow. The lungs should be auscultated daily.

Leg exercises should be encouraged hourly while awake. If the patient is unable to do so because of age or other problems, passive range-of-motion exercises should be performed.

Impaired Skin Integrity.   One or two drains may be placed in the area of the excised gallbladder to remove blood and bile that may accumulate after surgery. If the dressing is excessively stained with blood or bile, the physician should immediately be in-

formed. A T tube also may be used to drain bile from the common bile duct (Fig. 46-5). The skin around the area should be kept clean, as the bile may be irritating to the skin. If excessive drainage occurs around the T tube, this may be an indication that the tube is partly or completely obstructed. The skin and sclera should be inspected daily for jaundice, as this also may indicate obstruction of the T tube or other problem of the biliary system, such as edema of the common bile duct.

Knowledge Deficit.   The patient may be discharged with drains or a T tube in place and will require instructions in the care of the incision, drains, or T tube, as well as how to change the dressing. If a special diet or diet restrictions are recommended, written instructions regarding the foods that may be eaten or are to be avoided should be given. If drugs are prescribed, the dose and possible adverse effects should be explained.

The patient should be instructed to contact the physician if any of the following occur: fever, yellowing of the skin, severe pain in the abdomen or around the incision, dark urine, clay-colored stools, or pain the chest or legs.

Evaluation

- Pain is controlled
- Patient takes sufficient fluids orally
- Respiratory rate is normal; lungs are clear to auscultation
- Skin around incision appears normal
- Patient demonstrates understanding of drug therapy, incision care, care of drains or T tube, diet

DISORDERS OF THE PANCREAS
Acute Pancreatitis

Pancreatitis is an inflammatory disease characterized by the destruction of pancreatic tissue as well as functional capability. Its exact cause is unknown. It may be acute and mild, or it may occur abruptly with an often fatal course. Later, it may occur as a chronic disease, with a long history of relapse and recurrent attacks.

Pancreatitis has been noted to develop in people with a history of biliary tract disease, high alcohol intake, and hyperparathyroidism. Many people who have no other illness, however, also develop pancreatitis.

Symptoms
The most common complaint is severe middle-upper abdominal pain, which may radiate to both sides and straight through to the back. Nausea and vomiting usually are present. If inflammation is severe, with

Nursing Care Plan 46–1
Postoperative Management of the Patient Who Has a Cholecystectomy

Potential Problem and Potential Nursing Diagnosis	Nursing Intervention	Outcome Criteria
Pain (Incisional) *Pain related to surgery, immobility, improper positioning*	Administer analgesics as ordered; support incision during coughing and deep breathing; exercise care when repositioning patient; provide comfort measures such as a pillow for back support and pillow between the knees when on side, and adequate support of the head and shoulders when supine; place bed in low semi-Fowler's position when supine	Pain controlled
Thrombophlebitis	Encourage leg exercises q 2 hr; change position q 2 hr; check legs for signs of thrombophlebitis q 4 hr; notify physician immediately if fever, leg or calf pain, tenderness, swelling, or redness occurs	No evidence of thrombophlebitis
Skin Breakdown Due to Bile Drainage from Incision or Drains or Around T Tube (if one is inserted) *Impaired skin integrity related to surgery, secretions*	Check dressing q 2–4 hr and change or reinforce as needed; use nonallergenic tape or Montgomery straps to secure dressing; inspect skin around incision and drains at time of each dressing change; notify physician if skin breakdown is noted; connect T tube to gravity drainage (unless ordered otherwise); do not apply ointment or skin protectant unless use is approved by the physician	Skin integrity maintained
Wound Infection *Potential for infection related to surgery*	Use aseptic technique in changing dressing; inspect wound for drainage at each dressing change and note type and amount of any drainage present; monitor vital signs q 4 hr; notify physician of temperature elevation or purulent drainage from incision, drains, or T tube, or increased incisional pain	Wound clean and dry with no evidence of infection
Pneumonia *Ineffective airway clearance related to pain, tracheobronchial secretions*	Have patient cough and breathe deeply q 2 hr; change position q 2 hr; auscultate breath sounds q 2–4 hr; support incision during coughing, deep breathing; plan coughing and deep-breathing exercises when effect of analgesics is greatest; place patient in semi-Fowler's position when supine to encourage deep breathing at more frequent intervals; ambulate as soon as patient is allowed out of bed	Chest clear; normal breath sounds and respiratory rate
Paralytic Ileus	Auscultate bowel sounds q 4 hr; keep NPO until physician orders oral fluids; start oral fluids (when ordered) slowly with sips of water; encourage ambulation (as ordered); plan ambulation 45 to 60 min after administration of analgesic; notify physician if bowel sounds (when present) suddenly cease or abdominal distention is apparent	Normal bowel sounds 24 hr or more after surgery

Continued

Nursing Care Plan 46-1
Postoperative Management of the Patient Who Has a Cholecystectomy Continued

Potential Problem and Potential Nursing Diagnosis	Nursing Intervention	Outcome Criteria
Electrolyte Imbalance/Dehydration	Measure intake and output (including T tube and nasogastric drainage) q 8 hr; administer IVs at prescribed rate; notify physician if T tube or nasogastric drainage excessive or urine output decreased; observe for signs of electrolyte imbalance (especially sodium and potassium)	Hydration maintained; serum electrolytes normal

NPO, nothing by mouth.

necrosis and hemorrhage of the gland, peritonitis, severe fluid and electrolyte imbalance, and shock may ensue. In severe cases, fatty tissue around the pancreas is digested by lipase, a fat-digesting enzyme. Calcium binds with the released fatty acids. In rare cases, this reduces the level of circulating calcium to a dangerous degree, resulting in tetany and convulsions. Also, in the more advanced circumstances of hemorrhagic pancreatitis, released blood may discolor the skin of the lateral abdominal wall.

Diagnosis
Various radiographic and laboratory tests may be carried out in the diagnosis of pancreatitis, including the

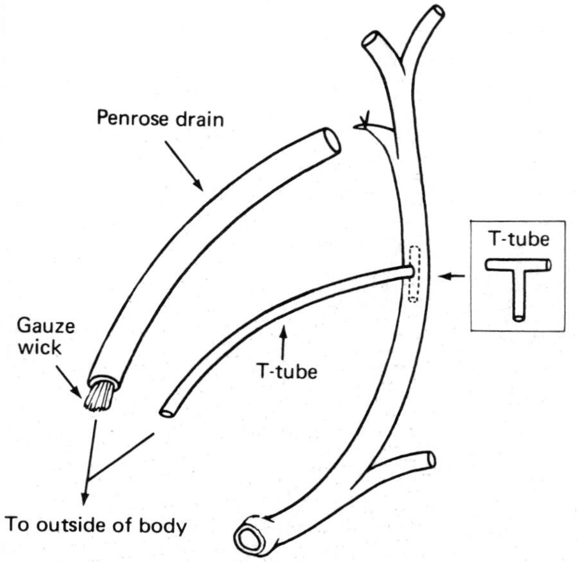

Figure 46-5. After cholecystectomy, the Penrose drain helps to remove exudate from the area formerly occupied by the gallbladder. The T tube diverts bile to the outside.

measurement of serum amylase and lipase levels. Elevated levels of these two enzymes, which are normal secretions of the pancreas, are found in most patients with significant pancreatitis.

Treatment
Measures are taken to relieve pain, reduce pancreatic secretion, and restore fluid and electrolyte losses. The patient usually is given nothing by mouth, and a nasogastric tube is inserted and connected to suction. This relieves nausea, distention, and vomiting, and reduces stimulation of the pancreas by gastric contents that enter the duodenum. Atropine or other anticholinergic drugs may be used to reduce the activity of the vagus nerve, which stimulates the pancreas.

Improvement usually occurs in about a week. The diet initially prescribed is extremely bland, with slow progress to a low-fat diet. Alcohol, coffee, tea, and other irritants or rich foods are withheld. Because prolonged use of narcotics may lead to addiction, care and thought in their prescription and administration are essential.

There is no direct surgical therapy for acute pancreatitis. If a pancreatic abscess is suspected, it must be drained surgically. If acute cholecystitis or obstruction of the common duct is thought to be a coincident or inciting factor, drainage and simple stone removal may be necessary.

Chronic Pancreatitis
Chronic pancreatitis is the reappearance of intermittent attacks of pancreatic inflammation after an initial episode. With chronicity, there may be partial to complete loss of function as pancreatic tissue is progressively destroyed.

Symptoms

With the development of chronic recurrent pancreatitis, stones and strictures may obstruct the pancreatic ducts. Areas of pancreatic breakdown may disrupt and form *pseudocysts*, fluid-filled pouches that bud from the diseased pancreas. The cysts cause symptoms by putting pressure on adjacent organs or by rupturing. With the development of chronic pancreatitis, pain, weight loss, digestive disturbances, diabetes, malnutrition, and steatorrhea (excessive fat in the stool) occur, in addition to the usual signs and symptoms of acute pancreatitis. These problems are caused by the progressive loss of exocrine and endocrine actions of the gland.

Diagnosis

Computed tomographic scans, MRI, ultrasonography, and endoscopic retrograde studies of the pancreas may be used in diagnosis. A glucose tolerance test may be used to evaluate function of the pancreatic cells that produce insulin. This test also may detect early diabetes mellitus, which results from decreased function of insulin-producing cells of the pancreas.

Treatment

Treatment depends on the cause and whether obstruction of the pancreatic duct is present. If pancreatic duct obstruction is not yet present, abstinence from alcohol, maintenance of a bland, fat-free diet, and correction of associated biliary tract disease or hyperparathyroidism may give good results. If there is scarring, with stricture and stenosis of portions of the pancreatic duct, various surgical measures can be performed to attempt reconstitution of the duct.

Chronic pain may be relieved by severing the nerve fibers that supply the pancreas, as well as by removing part or all of the pancreas. The insulin and digestive enzyme deficiencies seen with advanced pancreatic destruction may be treated with insulin and with exocrine enzyme replacement with pancreatin or pancrelipase, both of which help to absorb and digest fats, proteins, and carbohydrates.

NURSING PROCESS —THE PATIENT WHO HAS PANCREATITIS

Assessment

Initial assessment should include a history of symptoms experienced before admission as well as a complete medical history. It is important to obtain a description of the pain with respect to location and type. Physical examination should include an immediate evaluation of vital signs because shock often is an outstanding symptom of acute pancreatitis. A description of the patient's general appearance and palpation of the abdomen—especially the epigastric area—for pain, tenderness, distention, or rigidity should be included in the patient assessment. If weight loss has occurred, the patient should be weighed.

Stool (to test for steatorrhea) and urine (to test for glucose and ketones) specimens should be obtained and saved for laboratory examination.

Nursing Diagnosis

Depending on the severity of the disorder, the presenting symptoms, and whether the disorder is acute or chronic, one or more of the following nursing diagnoses may apply:

- Pain related to inflammation of the pancreas
- Fluid volume deficit related to vomiting
- Altered nutrition: less than body requirements related to nausea, vomiting, pain
- Diarrhea related to steatorrhea
- Knowledge deficit of treatment regimen

Planning and Implementation

The major goals of the patient include relief of pain, absence of fluid volume deficit, improved nutrition, normal bowel elimination, and an understanding of the treatment regimen.

The major goals of nursing management are to relieve symptoms, improve the fluid and nutritional status, and review the prescribed treatment modalities with the patient and family.

Most patients with acute pancreatitis are severely ill. The nurse should anticipate emergency treatment of these patients by obtaining the necessary equipment as soon as the patient is admitted to the hospital unit. Emergency treatment measures include the insertion of a nasogastric tube to decrease abdominal distention and discomfort, and the administration of intravenous fluids.

Ongoing assessments should be concerned with the patient's response to treatment, that is, a comparison of the current symptoms with those experienced before and at the time of admission. In addition, there should be continued monitoring of vital signs, as well as close observation for early signs of fluid and electrolyte imbalances and impending shock. Any sudden change in the patient's general condition, vital signs, or symptoms (eg, pain or abdominal distention) should be reported to the physician immediately.

Pain. Because severe pain is the outstanding symptom of acute pancreatitis, nursing intervention involves relief of pain by careful administration of prescribed analgesics and by other measures, such as changes of position. Failure of an analgesic to relieve pain should be reported to the physician.

Altered Nutrition, Fluid Volume Deficit. Intravenous fluids should be given to treat dehydration and electrolyte imbalances. In patients with acute pancreatitis, an intravenous line also may be used to treat or prevent shock.

During an acute attack, the patient should be given nothing by mouth, and insertion of a nasogastric tube usually is ordered. Both of these measures decrease pancreatic secretions. The patient should receive mouth care. The nasal passage may feel dry and sore from the tube; a small amount of water-soluble lubricant applied to the nares may relieve this discomfort. The gastric secretions removed by nasogastric suction should be measured every 8 hours or as ordered by the physician. The color, consistency, and amount should be recorded on the patient's chart.

The physician may order removal of the nasogastric tube and initiation of oral fluids once the acute stage has passed. Clear liquids in small amount usually are given first, followed by a progression to a soft, low-fat diet. An evaluation and recording of the patient's food intake is necessary. The physician may order daily to weekly weighings.

The patient's urine should be checked one to four times a day for the presence of glucose and ketones as a method of detecting a decrease in insulin production by the pancreas. The presence of glucose should be brought to the physician's attention. If diabetes mellitus has resulted from destruction of insulin-producing cells, the patient may require the administration of insulin.

Respiratory Function. The patient should be encouraged to cough and deep breathe hourly. The bed should be kept in semi-Fowler's position to decrease pressure on the diaphragm caused by abdominal distention.

Anticholinergic drugs given to decrease pancreatic and gastric secretions also reduce respiratory secretions, which in turn may result in pulmonary infection. The lungs should be auscultated daily. A rise in temperature, an increase in the respiratory rate, chest pain, or a change in the color of respiratory secretions should be reported to the physician.

Diarrhea. A description of all stools as well as a record of the number of stools passed each day should be recorded on the patient's chart. Severe diarrhea should be brought to the attention of the physician and the patient observed for signs of dehydration and electrolyte imbalance.

Knowledge Deficit. Most patients with acute pancreatitis are extremely ill and usually require a prolonged recovery period. Patient teaching should reinforce the treatment modalities prescribed or recommended by the physician.

A low-fat diet usually is recommended, and the patient should be given a list of foods to avoid. Four or more small meals per day instead of three large meals may be recommended. The importance of avoiding distention of the stomach by large meals should be emphasized.

The medication schedule should be reviewed with the patient. If alcohol abuse was known to be the cause of acute or chronic pancreatitis, the patient should be strongly encouraged to avoid *all* alcoholic beverages.

If insulin administration is necessary because of diabetes mellitus, see Chapter 48.

Evaluation

- Pain is reduced, controlled, or eliminated
- Nausea and vomiting are controlled
- Weight stabilizes or shows a gain
- Patient eats the prescribed diet
- Patient coughs and deep breathes at regular intervals
- Lungs are clear to auscultation
- Vital signs are normal
- Bowel elimination is normal
- Patient demonstrates an understanding of treatment modalities (diet, medications)
- Patient verbalizes importance of and desire to abstain from alcoholic beverages

Carcinoma of the Pancreas

Carcinoma of the pancreas may occur in the head, body, or tail of the gland. Most tumors involve the head of the pancreas. Early diagnosis may be difficult because symptoms may not be apparent until the disease is far advanced.

Symptoms

The most common symptoms of carcinoma of the head of the pancreas include pain, jaundice, severe anorexia, and sudden weight loss. Pain or jaundice usually is the first symptom that prompts the patient to seek medical attention. The first symptom of carcinoma of the body or tail of the pancreas most often is pain, which may be described as a boring pain in the midback. Marked weight loss also may be present.

Diagnosis

Physical examination, laboratory studies, CT scan, and radiographic examinations may establish a diagnosis in some patients. A pancreatic needle biopsy may be performed. Surgical exploration usually is necessary to rule out the possibility of a liver or gallbladder disorder as well as to remove or resect the tumor.

Treatment

Resection of tumors of the head of the pancreas is possible in some cases. Depending on the findings at the time of surgery, the surgeon may perform a *Whipple procedure* or attempt to relieve the obstruction causing jaundice by rerouting pancreatic and biliary drainage. There are various surgical techniques for the latter procedure.

The Whipple procedure has a high mortality and may be performed when there is no evidence of metastasis. The procedure consists of a subtotal gastrectomy, resection of the head of the pancreas and duodenum, and anastomosis of the bile and pancreatic ducts to the jejunum. The operation may be performed in one or two stages.

For inoperable tumors, radiation therapy or chemotherapy with fluorouracil (5-FU) or mitomycin (Mutamycin) may be tried. This form of treatment is palliative and does not cure the disease. The prognosis for patients with carcinoma of the pancreas is poor despite treatment with surgery, chemotherapy, or radiation therapy. Most succumb within 3 to 12 months after the onset of symptoms.

Nursing management for those treated medically is the same as for any patient with a malignant disorder (see Chapter 19).

NURSING PROCESS —THE PATIENT UNDERGOING PANCREATIC SURGERY

Preoperative Period

Assessment

On admission, some patients are acutely ill, whereas others may only experience symptoms such as jaundice, pruritus, and abdominal discomfort. Initial assessment should consist of evaluating the patient's general physical condition as well as obtaining a history of all symptoms that were present before admission. Questions about the onset of symptoms, weight loss, bleeding tendencies, and the type of pain or abdominal discomfort should be asked. Physical assessment should include checking for jaundice, visual examination of the stools and urine, and palpation of the abdomen for tenderness and distention. A urine sample should be obtained and tested for the presence of glucose. Vital signs and weight should be taken. The nutritional status of the patient should be assessed.

Nursing Diagnosis

Depending on the symptoms and condition of the patient, one or more of the following nursing diagnoses may apply. Additional nursing diagnoses may apply if the patient is dehydrated or has a nutritional deficit.

■ Anxiety related to symptoms, diagnosis, surgery
■ Knowledge deficit of preoperative preparations, postoperative care

Planning and Implementation

The major goals of the patient include reduction in anxiety and an understanding of preoperative preparations and postoperative management.

The major goals of nursing management are to relieve pain and discomfort and prepare the patient physically and emotionally for surgery.

Anxiety. The physician explains the tentative diagnosis and possible surgical procedure. Depending on the situation, the prognosis and future treatment modalities also are explained.

The patient and family should be allowed time to discuss and consider all aspects of surgery and the anticipated results. Because of the poor prognosis, some patients may refuse surgery and choose chemotherapy. The nurse should listen to the patient, answer questions as best as possible, and refer any problems or questions regarding the decision to the physician.

Nutrition and Fluids. Some patients may be poor candidates for immediate surgery because of severe anorexia and weight loss. Intravenous fluids, total parenteral nutrition, or a special diet may be ordered preoperatively to improve the patient's nutritional status as well as correct any fluid or electrolyte imbalances.

Knowledge Deficit. Before surgery, a nasogastric tube and indwelling urethral catheter usually are inserted. The insertion of these as well as other preoperative preparations should be explained to the patient. Other explanations include the routine postoperative assessments or treatments, such as monitoring vital signs and administering intravenous fluids.

Evaluation

■ Anxiety is reduced
■ Patient demonstrates an understanding of explanations given by the physician, and preoperative preparations

Postoperative Period

Assessment

Immediate postoperative assessments include vital signs and a review of the chart for the type and extent of surgery. The surgical dressing as well as all drains and tubes should be checked for patency, and the amount and color of drainage should be noted at this time as well as throughout the entire postoperative course.

Nursing Diagnosis

Depending on the type and extent of the surgery, one or more of the following nursing diagnoses may apply. Additional nursing diagnoses pertaining to routine care of any surgical patient may be added.

- Pain related to surgery, metastasis of the tumor
- Ineffective airway clearance related to pain and large upper abdominal surgical incision, prolonged period of anesthesia
- Potential for infection related to lowered resistance
- Impaired skin integrity related to terminal stage of the disease, pruritus, lack of movement, other factors (specify)
- Knowledge deficit of home care management, treatment modalities

Planning and Implementation

The major goals of the patient include relief of pain, maintenance of a patent airway, absence of infection, prevention of skin breakdown, and an understanding of home care management and treatment modalities.

The major goals of nursing management are to relieve pain and discomfort, improve the patient's nutritional status, recognize and prevent complications, and provide an understanding of home care and management.

Some of the complications associated with this surgery include diabetes mellitus, bleeding tendencies due to a vitamin K deficiency, and liver and kidney failure.

Patients who undergo palliative surgery for the relief of jaundice should be managed essentially the same as those having general surgery. Ongoing assessments include evaluation of the patient's general physical condition and a record of any increase in symptoms such as jaundice, pruritus, and pain. If jaundice was present, the color of the skin, stools, and urine should return to near normal color if the biliary obstruction was relieved.

Patients undergoing the Whipple procedure or one of its variations require more intensive nursing management. In addition to nursing management of the patient having general surgery or biliary or hepatic surgery, the patient should be closely observed for complications related to extensive surgery in this area (eg, shock, pancreatic abscess, and hemorrhage).

Jaundice. The skin and sclera should be inspected daily for signs of jaundice. The color of the urine and stools should be noted. Laboratory values, such as serum bilirubin, should be monitored.

Hyperglycemia, Hypoglycemia. Because of tumor infiltration of the pancreatic cells that produce insulin, diabetes mellitus may occur after surgery or may have been present before surgery. Hyperglycemia also may be seen. The urine should be tested every 4 hours for the presence of glucose and ketones. The physician may order daily blood glucose tests.

Bleeding. A vitamin K deficiency may require the administration of vitamin K. The patient should be closely observed for signs of bleeding. Easy bruising, blood in the urine or stool, or bleeding from the incision, drains, or tubes are signs of a bleeding tendency.

Pain. Opiates usually are avoided, but other narcotic analgesics may be prescribed. Lower than normal doses may be ordered if there is evidence of liver failure.

Pain should be carefully evaluated. If pain occurs in an area other than the surgical area, the physician should be contacted.

Fluids. Intake and output should be measured. If there is a decrease in urine output or kidney failure is suspected, the output may be measured hourly. Intravenous fluids should be administered until the patient is able to take oral fluids.

Ineffective Airway Clearance. If the Whipple procedure was performed, mechanical ventilation usually is necessary until the patient is fully awake and can breathe effectively without the use of the ventilator, and arterial blood gas analyses are normal.

When the ventilator is removed, the patient should be encouraged to cough, deep breathe, and perform leg exercises hourly. The lungs should be auscultated at frequent intervals if the patient appears to have difficulty breathing or has other respiratory difficulties, such as purulent sputum.

Potential for Infection. Antibiotics are ordered. The incision should be inspected for signs of infection at the time of each dressing change. Vital signs should be monitored, and the physician informed of a rise in the patient's temperature.

Nutrition.   Once the patient is allowed to take oral fluids, a diet high in proteins, carbohydrates, and vitamins usually is ordered. The patient should be encouraged to eat. Failure to meet nutritional needs may necessitate the administration of parenteral nutrition.

Because diabetes mellitus can occur, insulin administration may be necessary. A record of the amount of food eaten at each meal as well as urine and blood glucose determinations are necessary to monitor insulin therapy.

If extensive surgery was performed, the pancreatic cells that produce digestive enzymes may have been removed. Pancreatic digestive enzymes, which are taken with meals, are then ordered.

Impaired Skin Integrity.   The patient's position should be changed every 2 hours, and bony prominences inspected for signs of skin breakdown or irritation.

Knowledge Deficit.   The patient and family require extensive teaching regarding home care. Areas covered in the teaching plan depend on the patient's condition, problems associated with surgery, and future treatment modalities.

The following areas may be covered in a teaching plan:

- Medication schedule: oral medications, insulin administration
- How to check the urine for glucose and ketones
- Recommended diet
- Symptoms to report to the physician: jaundice, dark urine, bleeding tendencies, vomiting, tarry stools, increased pain, swelling of the extremities, abdominal enlargement, decreased urine output, weight loss
- Schedule for radiation therapy or chemotherapy
- Importance of drinking fluids, eating adequate diet
- Care of the skin (including the skin around the incision)

Evaluation

- Pain is controlled
- Evidence of dehydration or electrolyte imbalances is absent
- Vital signs are normal
- Evidence of serious postoperative complications is absent
- Respiratory function is normal; lungs are clear to auscultation; patient practices coughing and deep breathing on own
- Nutritional intake is adequate
- Skin appears normal; evidence of breakdown is absent
- Patient demonstrates an understanding of skin care, medication schedule, insulin administration, checking urine for glucose and ketones, importance of drinking fluids and eating the recommended diet
- Patient is able to discuss what problems require notification of the physician

General Nutritional Considerations

☐ Patients with hepatic cirrhosis need to maintain a well-balanced diet. The physician may order a low-fat diet because of the inability of the liver to manufacture bile, which is necessary for the digestion of fats.

☐ Patients with cirrhosis accompanied by edema and ascites may be placed on a low-salt diet. Because salt makes food more palatable, its restriction poses a challenge to find other seasonings that the patient enjoys and is permitted to have.

☐ If hepatic coma is present or impending, protein may be omitted from the diet.

☐ Patients with hepatic cirrhosis usually have poor appetites, and may require frequent, small feedings rather than three regular meals.

☐ Patients with cholelithiasis may require a low-fat diet. Foods such as eggs, pork products, rich dressings, cheese, cream, and whole milk are eliminated from the diet. It also may be necessary to avoid greasy, fried, and spicy foods and foods high in cholesterol. Special diets are seldom necessary once the gallbladder is removed.

General Pharmacologic Considerations

☐ When chenodiol (Chenix) is prescribed to dissolve gallstones, about 2 years of therapy with the drug are necessary.

☐ Barbiturates, narcotics, and any drug detoxified by the liver are *contraindicated* or *used with caution* in patients with liver disease.

☐ To reduce ascites and edema in the patient with cirrhosis, a diuretic may be ordered. One diuretic that is particularly useful is spironolactone, which antagonizes aldosterone. Reversing the effects of aldosterone increases water and sodium excretion, whereas potassium is retained.

☐ Patients with acute pancreatitis have severe pain that may necessitate the use of narcotic analgesics. Because the pain may persist for some time, care should be taken to avoid addiction.

☐ Patients with carcinoma of the head of the pancreas usually require vitamin K before surgery, to correct a prothrombin deficiency.

General Gerontologic Considerations

☐ Although hepatitis A commonly is found in younger people, elderly patients may develop hepatitis through contact with people who have the disease, such as waiters and supermarket employees.

☐ Elderly people may recover more slowly from surgery on the gallbladder. They also are more prone to develop postoperative complications, such as pneumonia and thrombophlebitis, because of an inability to move about in bed, adequately perform deep-breathing exercises, and ambulate shortly after surgery.

Suggested Readings

☐ Bates BA, Hoekelman RA. Guide to physical examination and history taking. 4th ed. Philadelphia: JB Lippincott, 1987. *(In-depth coverage of subject matter)*

☐ Bowers AC, Thompson JM. Clinical manual of health assessment. 3rd ed. St Louis: CV Mosby, 1988. *(In-depth coverage of subject matter)*

☐ Carpenito LJ. Handbook of nursing diagnosis 1989–1990. Philadelphia: JB Lippincott, 1990. *(In-depth coverage of subject matter)*

☐ Fuller J, Schaller-Ayers J. Health assessment: a nursing approach. Philadelphia: JB Lippincott, 1990. *(Additional coverage of subject matter)*

☐ Gahart BL. Intravenous medications: a handbook for nurses and other allied health personnel. St Louis: CV Mosby, 1989. *(Additional coverage of subject matter)*

☐ Malseed R, Girton SE. Pharmacology: drug therapy and nursing considerations. 3rd ed. Philadelphia: JB Lippincott, 1990. *(Additional and in-depth coverage of subject matter)*

☐ Munn NE. When the bile duct is blocked. RN January 1989;52:50. *(Additional coverage of subject matter)*

☐ Timby B. Clinical nursing procedures. Philadelphia: JB Lippincott, 1989. *(Additional coverage of subject matter)*

■ Introduction to the Endocrine System
■ Disorders of the Endocrine System

The Endocrine System

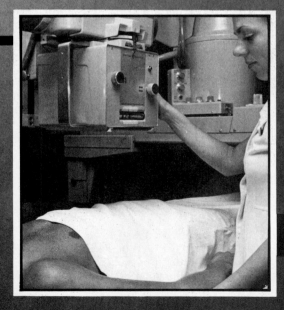

Unit 11

Chapter 47

Introduction to the Endocrine System

On completion of this chapter the reader will:

- Be familiar with the basic anatomy and physiology of the endocrine system

- Discuss the common tests used for diagnosing endocrine disorders

- Use the nursing process in preparing a patient for tests used in the diagnosis of endocrine disorders

Endocrine glands secrete their hormones directly into the bloodstream. Most disorders of the endocrine system are the result of overproduction or underproduction of the hormones that the glands secrete, causing a disturbance in the delicate balance that hormones normally maintain and often resulting in a widespread chain of pathological events within the body (Fig. 47-1).

Pituitary Gland

The pituitary gland (or hypophysis) lies within the sella turcica (Turk's saddle) of the sphenoid bone, and is connected by means of a stalk to the hypothalamus. The pituitary is divided into three lobes: anterior, intermediate, and posterior.

Many of the endocrine glands respond to stimulation from the pituitary (Fig. 47-2). If endocrine gland production is increased, the pituitary stimulating factor is decreased as a counterregulatory mechanism. This slows down the gland's activity. For example, an increase in the production of thyroid hormones results in a decrease in the amount of thyroid-stimulating hormone (thyrotropin or TSH) produced by the pituitary gland. Conversely, a decrease in the gland's output is countered by increased pituitary stimulation. This is called a *feedback mechanism*.

The middle or intermediate lobe (pars intermedia) secretes melanocyte, a hormone responsible for skin pigmentation. Only the hormones of the anterior and posterior lobes are discussed in this chapter.

The hormones of the anterior pituitary gland are as follows:

Growth hormone (also called somatotrophic hormone)—Stimulates the growth of bones, muscles and other organs
Adrenocorticotrophic hormone—Controls the growth, development, and function of the cortex of the adrenal glands
Thyroid-stimulating hormone (also called thyrotrophic hormone)—Controls the secretory activity of the thyroid gland
Follicle-stimulating hormone—Stimulates the development of eggs in the ovaries and sperm in the testicles
Luteinizing hormone—Causes ovulation in the female and the secretion of sex hormones in both sexes
Prolactin (also called lactogenic hormone)—Stimulates the production of breast milk in the female, but has no known function in the male.

The hormones of the posterior pituitary are as follows:

Antidiuretic hormone (also called vasopressin)—Controls the excretion of water by the kidneys by affecting the reabsorption of water from the kidney tubules
Oxytocin—Causes contraction of the uterus at term and the ejection of milk from the breasts

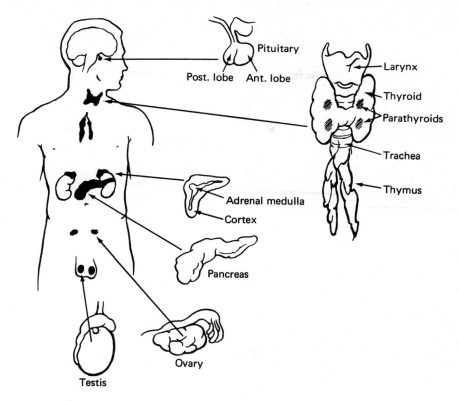

Figure 47–1. Location of hormone-producing glands in the body.

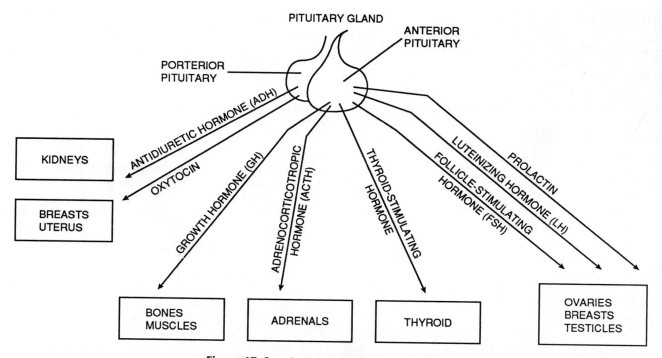

Figure 47–2. The hormones of the pituitary gland.

Thyroid Gland

The thyroid gland is located in the neck anterior to the trachea. It is divided into two lateral lobes that are connected by a band of tissue called the isthmus.

The thyroid has the ability to concentrate iodine in the manufacture of the thyroid hormones that help to regulate the production and use of energy for the body's dynamic processes. The important active hormones of the thyroid gland are tetraiodothyronine (thyroxine, or T_4) and triiodothyronine (T_3). Iodine is contained in these hormones. Another hormone produced by the thyroid is calcitonin, which is important in calcium metabolism.

Parathyroid Glands

The parathyroid glands are tiny bean-shaped bodies that normally are embedded in the lateral lobes of the thyroid. They usually number four, but there may be more. The upper parathyroid is found posteriorly at the junction of the upper and middle third of the thyroid. The lower parathyroids are more variable in location, but normally lie among the branches of the inferior thyroid artery. They secrete the parathyroid hormone—parathormone—that regulates the concentration of calcium and phosphorus in the blood and influences the passage of calcium and phosphorus among bloodstream, bones, and urine.

Thymus Gland

The thymus gland is located in the upper part of the chest above or near the heart. The known function of the thymus is the development of T lymphocytes, a type of white blood cell that is involved in immunity.

This gland is large during childhood but usually shrinks by the time the person reaches adulthood. Disorders of the gland are rare.

Adrenal Glands

The adrenal glands are located above the kidneys. The outer portion of the gland is called the cortex and the inner portion, the medulla. The adrenal *cortex* manufactures and secretes glucocorticoids, mineralocorticoids, and small amounts of sex hormones. Collectively, these hormones are called *corticosteroids*. The adrenal *medulla* produces two neurohormones: epinephrine and norepinephrine.

Glucocorticoids and mineralocorticoids are essential to life, and influence many organs and structures of the body. Glucocorticoids affect body metabolism, suppress inflammation, and help the body to with-

stand stress. Mineralocorticoids are concerned with the maintenance of water and electrolyte (sodium, potassium, chlorides) balances.

Pancreas

The pancreas lies below the stomach with the head of the gland close to the duodenum. In addition to the secretion of digestive enzymes (see Chapter 42), the pancreas secretes insulin, a hormone necessary for the metabolism of glucose.

The insulin-secreting cells of the pancreas, called the islets of Langerhans, are scattered throughout the pancreas.

Ovaries and Testicles

The sex glands, or the ovaries of the female and the testicles of the male, are important in the development of secondary sex characteristics, the manufacture of hormones, and the development of the egg (female) and sperm (male).

The hormone produced by the testicles is testosterone, which is concerned with the development and maintenance of secondary male sex characteristics such as facial hair and a deep voice. The hormones produced by the ovaries are the estrogens and progesterone. The functions and roles of these hormones are discussed in Chapter 49.

ASSESSMENT OF THE PATIENT WHO HAS AN ENDOCRINE DISORDER
Patient History

The symptoms of some endocrine disorders may be vague or indicative of many other physical or mental disorders. Examples are fatigue, personality changes, inability to sleep, and frequent urination. At other times symptoms may be dramatic, such as a change in the level of consciousness or sudden weight loss.

The patient history, including the medical history, becomes important in the diagnosis of many endocrine disorders. Some endocrine disorders are inherited or have a tendency to occur in families; therefore, a complete family history also is essential. Diet, drug, and allergy histories also are obtained.

Physical Examination

The physical examination may be generalized or focus on a specific area, depending on the tentative or actual physician's diagnosis.

General assessment includes height, weight, vital signs, and general physical appearance.

Specific areas of assessment include the following:

Skin, Nails, and Hair. The skin is inspected for excessive oiliness, dryness, ecchymosis (bleeding into skin or mucous membrane, producing blue-black discolorations), excessive or lack of pigmentation, excessive hair or loss of hair, and skin breaks that appear to be healing poorly. The nails are inspected for shape, color, and quality. It should be noted if the nails are thin, thick, or brittle.

Eyes. The eyes are examined for exophthalmos (abnormal bulging or protrusion of the eyes) and puffiness around the eyes.

Face and Neck. The patient's facial expression and general features are noted. The neck is inspected for enlargement in the thyroid. The experienced examiner may gently palpate the thyroid gland.

Cardiovascular System. The pulse rate and rhythm are noted, and the extremities are examined for edema and changes in color.

Respiratory System. The lungs are auscultated and abnormal sounds noted.

Neurologic System. The extremities are examined for the presence of tremors. Any loss of motor function or any decrease in sensitivity to pain or touch in the extremities is noted.

Mental and Emotional Status. The ability of the patient to respond to questions is recorded. The patient's attitude (eg, dull, apathetic, or extremely nervous) is evaluated.

LABORATORY AND DIAGNOSTIC TESTS

The type and extent of laboratory and diagnostic testing depends on the physician's tentative diagnosis. In some instances, the patient history may establish the scope of diagnostic testing.

Hormone Levels. The level of certain hormones may be used to evaluate the functioning of an endocrine gland. Examples of these tests include blood cortisol levels (morning and evening), antidiuretic hormone levels (blood), blood testosterone levels, and total thyroxine (blood).

General or Routine Laboratory Tests. Routine tests (eg, a complete blood count, SMA 12, blood glucose, and urinalysis) may be performed in conjunction with more specific tests to obtain a general profile of the patient's status as well as to rule out other disorders.

Radiography, Computed Tomographic Scan, Magnetic Resonance Imaging. These diagnostic studies may be performed in certain instances, such as a suspected pituitary tumor. General radiographs, such as a radiograph of the chest or abdomen, may be taken to detect tumors as well as to determine organ size and placement.

Radionuclide Studies. A radioactive iodine uptake test (RAI, ^{131}I uptake) may be performed to determine thyroid function.

Scans. By using radioactive materials, certain endocrine organs can be visualized or their activity determined. Examples of scans include thyroid scan, adrenergic tumor scan (^{131}MIGB), and parathyroid scan.

Radioimmunoassay. A T_4 determination by radioimmunoassay may be ordered, to evaluate thyroid function. Venous blood samples are required for radioimmunoassay tests.

NURSING PROCESS —THE PATIENT UNDERGOING TESTING FOR AN ENDOCRINE DISORDER

Assessment

A complete history, including allergy, drug, and family histories, should be obtained. Because some endocrine disorders may be accompanied by vague symptoms, the examiner may find it necessary to explore each symptom in detail.

Some thyroid function tests require the use of iodine. If an allergy history reveals a possible or known iodine allergy, the physician should be informed and the cover of the patient's chart labeled. It also is important to determine if within the past 3 months the patient has had any test that used iodine (eg, intravenous pyelography or gallbladder series). If so, the physician should be informed before the test is carried out.

An examination of one or more body areas should be performed when indicated by information obtained during the patient history. Vital signs should be taken and the patient weighed.

Nursing Diagnosis

Depending on the presenting symptoms, the condition of the patient, and other factors, the following nursing diagnoses may apply. Additional diagnoses may be necessary.

■ Anxiety related to possible diagnosis, diagnostic tests
■ Knowledge deficit of the diagnostic test (preparation, patient's responsibility)

Planning and Implementation

The major goals of the patient include reduction of anxiety, an understanding of the test, and responsibility and preparation for the test.

The major goal of nursing management is to prepare the patient for the diagnostic tests.

Patient Preparation.   Proper preparation of the patient is essential. The hospital procedure manual or the physician's orders should be consulted for the required preparation for each diagnostic procedure. Fasting may be required for some of these tests. The patient's participation in the test should be fully explained; for example, the patient may be required to save all voided urine. Some tests, such as a computed tomographic scan, require no special preparation other than a general explanation.

Anxiety.   The general purpose of the test, the type of test, and how it will be performed should be explained. The patient and family should be encouraged to ask any questions they may have about the test. The patient also should be encouraged to discuss the results of tests with the physician.

Evaluation

■ Anxiety is reduced or eliminated
■ Patient and family demonstrate an understanding of the preparations required for the test

General Nutritional Considerations

☐ Some health foods, especially sea salt and kelp, are high in iodine. A diet history should include the use of any type of health food or health food supplements.

General Pharmacologic Considerations

☐ When a patient is scheduled for thyroid tests, it is necessary to obtain an accurate drug history. If the patient has recently taken a drug that contains iodine or has had radiographic contrast studies that used iodine, the test results may be inaccurate. Other drugs (eg, salicylates and corticosteroids) also may affect the results of thyroid tests. All drugs taken by the patient should be entered on the laboratory request slip.

General Gerontologic Considerations

☐ Elderly patients may forget the instructions for a diagnostic test. Printed directions should be given to outpatients and, when possible, reviewed with a family member. This is especially important if test preparations are complicated.

Suggested Readings

☐ Bates BA, Hoekelman RA. Guide to physical examination and history taking. 4th ed. Philadelphia: JB Lippincott, 1987. *(In-depth coverage of subject matter)*
☐ Fischbach FT. A manual of laboratory diagnostic tests. 3rd ed. Philadelphia: JB Lippincott, 1988. *(Additional coverage of subject matter)*
☐ Memmler RL, Wood DL. Structure and function of the human body. 4th ed. Philadelphia: JB Lippincott, 1987. *(Additional coverage of subject matter)*
☐ Memmler RL, Wood DL. The human body in health and disease. 6th ed. Philadelphia: JB Lippincott, 1987. *(Additional coverage of subject matter)*
☐ Porth CM. Pathophysiology: concepts of altered health states. 3rd ed. Philadelphia: JB Lippincott, 1990. *(In-depth, high-level coverage of subject matter)*
☐ Wallach JB. Interpretation of diagnostic tests: a handbook synopsis of laboratory medicine. Boston: Little, Brown, 1986. *(In-depth, high-level coverage of subject matter)*

Chapter 48
Disorders of the Endocrine System

On completion of this chapter the reader will:

■ Discuss the symptoms, diagnosis, and treatment of acromegaly, Simmond's disease, diabetes insipidus, and syndrome of inappropriate antidiuretic hormone secretion

■ Use the nursing process in the management of the patient with a pituitary disorder

■ Discuss the symptoms, diagnosis, and treatment of hyperthyroidism, hypothyroidism, thyroid tumors, goiters, and thyroiditis

■ Use the nursing process in the management of the patient receiving medical treatment for a thyroid disorder

■ Use the nursing process in the management of the patient undergoing thyroid surgery

■ Discuss the symptoms, diagnosis, and treatment of hyperparathyroidism and hypoparathyroidism

■ Use the nursing process in the management of the patient with hypoparathyroidism

■ Discuss the symptoms, diagnosis, and treatment of adrenal insufficiency and acute adrenal crisis

■ Use the nursing process in the management of the patient with adrenal insufficiency

■ Discuss the symptoms, diagnosis, and treatment of pheochromocytoma and Cushing's syndrome

■ Use the nursing process in the management of the patient with Cushing's syndrome

■ Use the nursing process in the management of the patient having an adrenalectomy

■ Discuss the types, cause, pathology, symptoms, diagnosis, treatment, and complications of diabetes mellitus

■ Use the nursing process in the management of the patient with diabetes mellitus

DISORDERS OF THE PITUITARY GLAND (HYPOPHYSIS)
Acromegaly

Hyperplasia or tumors of the anterior pituitary can result in an overproduction of growth hormone. When there is an excess of this hormone in a young person, before the ends of the long bones are fully united (epiphyseal union), gigantism results. Overproduction of growth hormone during adulthood brings about acromegaly.

Symptoms
Acromegaly results in coarse features, huge lower jaw, thick lips, bulging forehead, bulbous nose, and large hands and feet. When the overgrowth is due to a tumor, headaches caused by pressure on the sella turcica are common. Partial blindness may result from pressure on the optic nerve. The heart, liver, and spleen may enlarge. Despite enlarged tissues, muscle weakness is common, and hypertrophied joints may become painful and stiff. Men often become impotent, and women may have amenorrhea, increased facial hair, and deepened voices.

Diagnosis
Diagnosis is made by symptoms as well as by skull radiographs, magnetic resonance imaging (MRI), and computed tomographic (CT) scans.

Treatment
Acromegaly is sometimes treated by surgical removal of the pituitary gland. Radiation and consequent destruction of the pituitary also may be used. Even if the disease is arrested successfully, physical changes are irreversible.

Simmonds' Disease

Simmonds' disease, or panhypopituitarism, is a rare disorder that results from the destruction of the pituitary gland by events such as postpartum emboli, surgery, tumor, or tuberculosis.

Symptoms
The gonads and the genitalia atrophy gradually. Because of an impairment of pituitary stimulus, the thyroid and adrenals fail to secrete adequate amounts of their hormones. Symptoms of hypothyroidism and adrenocortical insufficiency (Addison's disease) are apparent. The patient ages prematurely and may become extremely cachectic.

Diagnosis
Diagnosis is based on symptoms as well as on laboratory tests for hormone levels, such as thyroid, corticosteroid, and male and female hormones.

Treatment

Treatment includes the administration of substitute hormones of the glands that depend on the pituitary for stimulation.

Diabetes Insipidus

The hormone vasopressin, also called antidiuretic hormone (ADH), regulates the reabsorption of water in the kidney tubules.

Symptoms

In this rare disorder, secretion of ADH is reduced, leading to an outpouring of water through the kidneys. The urine is so copious that the patient does not have an unbroken night's sleep. Some 15 to 20 liters of urine may be passed in a 24-hour period. The urine is dilute, with a specific gravity of 1.002 or less. The excretion of urine cannot be controlled by limiting the intake of fluids. Thirst is excessive and constant. The need for drinking and emptying the bladder embarrasses the patient and limits activities. The patient is weak and anorectic and loses weight.

Diagnosis

Diagnosis is based on symptoms as well as on the fluid deprivation test. In the fluid deprivation test, fluids are withheld for 8 to 12 hours, and urine specific gravity and osmolarity are determined at the beginning and end of the test. Failure to concentrate urine during the time of fluid deprivation is characteristic of this disorder.

Treatment

Treatment is the administration of vasopressin subcutaneously or by nasal spray. The objective is to reduce the patient's urine output to 2 or 3 L/24 hr.

Syndrome of Inappropriate Antidiuretic Hormone Secretion

The syndrome of inappropriate antidiuretic hormone (SIADH) can be caused by lung tumors, central nervous system disorders, and some drugs. This disorder is characterized by an inability to excrete dilute urine.

Symptoms

Symptoms include severe hyponatremia, excessive thirst, headache, muscle cramps, water retention, and anorexia. As the condition becomes more severe, nausea, vomiting, muscular twitching, and changes in the level of consciousness occur.

Diagnosis

Diagnosis is based on symptoms, a history of those disorders capable of causing SIADH, and laboratory tests such as a serum sodium.

Treatment

When possible, treatment is aimed at eliminating the underlying cause. Diuretics help correct water retention. Severe hyponatremia is treated with the intravenous administration of a hypertonic sodium chloride solution.

NURSING PROCESS —THE PATIENT WHO HAS A PITUITARY DISORDER

Assessment

A complete history of the patient's symptoms, a medical history, and a drug history should be obtained. Depending on the symptoms, a physical examination related to the presenting symptoms may be performed. For example, if the patient complains of frequent urination and passage of large amounts of urine, he or she should be examined for signs of dehydration. Because a pituitary disorder may affect the function of one or more endocrine glands, the patient's general appearance should be noted, and a general appraisal of the endocrine system should be performed (see Chapter 47). Vital signs and weight should be obtained.

Nursing Diagnosis

Depending on the possible diagnosis and the patient's symptoms, one or more of the following may apply. If the patient has total impairment of pituitary function, nursing diagnoses relevant to decreased function of the thyroid and adrenal glands also apply.

- Anxiety related to symptoms, diagnosis
- Body image disturbance related to changes in physical appearance (acromegaly, panhypopituitarism)
- Fluid volume deficit related to large urine output (diabetes insipidus)
- Fluid volume excess related to water retention (SIADH)
- Chronic pain related to effect of disorder on the musculoskeletal system (acromegaly)
- Altered nutrition: less than body requirements secondary to pituitary disorder (panhypopituitarism, diabetes insipidus)
- Total or partial self-care deficit (if partial, specify areas) related to weakness and fatigue secondary to pituitary disorder

- Sexual dysfunction related to inadequate stimulation of the gonads by the pituitary (acromegaly, panhypopituitarism)
- Knowledge deficit of treatment modalities, home care management

Planning and Implementation

The major goals of the patient may include a reduction in anxiety, correction of a fluid volume excess or deficit, relief of pain, acceptance of body image changes, improved nutrition, improved ability to attend to self-care needs, frank discussion of problems associated with sexual dysfunction, and understanding treatment modalities and home care.

The major goals of nursing management are to relieve symptoms (when possible); to assist in correcting hormonal, electrolyte, and fluid imbalances; and to assist the patient in understanding the disorder. If treatment requires surgery (removal of the pituitary or hypophysectomy), see Chapter 38.

The patient with a pituitary disorder may be extremely ill, or he or she may experience only mild symptoms of the disorder. Nursing management depends largely on the disorder, the symptoms, and the patient's needs as identified through assessment.

Anxiety, Body Image Disturbance.   The patient must be allowed time to discuss the disorder. Symptoms, such as frequent urination or changes in body image, may be disturbing. In some instances, the nurse can assure the patient that symptoms will be controlled with treatment. The nurse must be alert to the patient's emotional status and discuss these problems with the physician. Changes in appearance, especially changes that are drastic and permanent, may require psychiatric counseling.

Fluid Volume Deficit or Excess.   Intake and output is carefully measured. When the urine output is excessive, as seen in diabetes insipidus, the physician may order measurement of the urinary output at 15- to 30-minute intervals. Sufficient fluids should be provided, and the patient should be weighed daily to identify weight gain or loss and should be observed for signs of fluid volume excess or deficit (see Chapter 12). If the patient has diabetes insipidus and is unable to take oral fluids to meet an excessive fluid volume loss, intravenous fluids may be necessary.

Diuretics may be ordered to increase the urinary output in those patients with a fluid volume excess. Sudden or steady weight gain or loss should be brought to the attention of the physician.

Chronic Pain.   Pain should be evaluated carefully. The physician may order a mild analgesic, such as aspirin, acetaminophen, or ibuprofen, for relief of pain.

Altered Nutrition.   The patient should be weighed daily to weekly, depending on the degree of anorexia. Four to six small meals per day may be better tolerated than three regular meals. The patient should be encouraged to eat; failure to eat or a steady weight loss should be brought to the attention of the physician.

Self-Care Deficit.   Extreme fatigue or muscle weakness may interfere with the patient's ability to attend to daily needs. The ability to perform self-care activities should be evaluated during the initial assessment, and the amount of assistance needed should be included in the nursing care plan.

Sexual Dysfunction.   A decrease in pituitary stimulation of the gonads may result in sexual dysfunction or amenorrhea (cessation of menstruation). In most instances, any sexual dysfunction should be discussed during a visit to an outpatient clinic or physician's office. Referral to a sex therapist may be made by the physician.

Knowledge Deficit.   If treatment requires drug therapy, the patient needs extensive information about the medication schedule and the adverse effects of each drug, especially if many different medications are prescribed. The importance of adhering to the medication schedule and not omitting a dose should be emphasized. If desmopressin acetate (DDAVP) or lypressin (Diapid) nasal spray is prescribed for treatment of diabetes insipidus, the patient should be taught the technique of instillation.

The following are additional points that may be included in the teaching plan:

- The importance of maintaining adequate nutrition and fluid intake
- Weekly weigh taking (or as recommended by the physician) and the importance of notifying the physician of any marked weight loss or gain
- Importance of clinic or office appointments
- Avoiding undue fatigue and resting between activities

Evaluation

- Anxiety is reduced
- Pain or discomfort is controlled or eliminated
- Fluid volume excess or deficit is corrected
- Serum electrolytes are normal
- Patient shows evidence of accepting changes in physical appearance
- Weight remains stable; patient eats prescribed diet
- Self-care needs are met

- Patient openly discusses sexual dysfunction with appropriate individuals
- Patient demonstrates knowledge of treatment regimen, importance of continued medical supervision

DISORDERS OF THE THYROID GLAND
Hyperthyroidism

In hyperthyroidism (also called Graves' disease, thyrotoxicosis, Basedow's disease, and exophthalmic goiter), the patient's metabolic rate increases because of an excessive secretion of thyroid hormones. The cause of hyperthyroidism is unknown. The disorder is more common in women than in men.

Symptoms

Symptoms vary from mild to severe. Patients with well-developed hyperthyroidism are characteristically restless, highly excitable, and constantly agitated. Fine tremors of the hands and clumsiness caused by tremors may be seen. Diarrhea also may be present. The symptoms of hyperthyroidism and hypothryroidism are compared in Table 48-1.

Some patients exhibit bulging of the eyes (exophthalmos) that gives them a permanently startled expression (Fig. 48-1). Usually, there is visible swelling of the neck caused by the enlarged thyroid gland.

Diagnosis

In addition to the patient history and symptoms identified during the physical examination, the physician may use one or more tests to confirm the diagnosis. Examples of tests include protein-bound iodine (PBI), serum T_3 and T_4 determination, thyroid ultrasonogra-phy, thyroid scanning, and radioactive iodine uptake test (RAI, RAIU).

Treatment

The treatment for hyperthyroidism may be medical or surgical.

MEDICAL TREATMENT. The antithyroid drugs propyl-thiouracil and methimazole (Tapazole) block the production of thyroid hormone and may be prescribed as medical treatment for hyperthyroidism. Iodine (as strong iodine solution) also may be given along with an antithyroid drug. The effects of antithyroid therapy usually do not become evident until the excess thyroid hormone stored in the thyroid gland has been secreted into the bloodstream. This process may take several weeks or more.

Radioactive iodine (^{131}I) may be given to a patient with hyperthyroidism to destroy hyperplastic thyroid tissue by radiation. The thyroid is quick to remove iodine, including radioactive iodine, from the bloodstream. The usual therapeutic dose of radioactive iodine does not seriously affect other tissues of the body. Antithyroid drugs may be given for 6 months or more prior to the administration of radioactive iodine.

If no remission of symptoms occurs, a second and perhaps third dose may be given. Possible transient symptoms following use of ^{131}I are nausea, vomiting, malaise, and fever, and the gland may feel tender. These reactions are rare. A more common unfortunate result of treatment is hypothyroidism (discussed next). Because this complication may not occur until long after the administration of ^{131}I, patients must remain under medical supervision for many years.

About 6 to 8 weeks after the initial dose of ^{131}I, the patient often notices some remission of symptoms. The long time required before the patient notices im-

---

Table 48–1.   Symptoms of Thyroid Dysfunction   *Study this!*

Body System or Function	Hypothyroidism	Hyperthyroidism
Metabolism	Decreased, with symptoms of anorexia, intolerance to cold, low body temperature, weight gain despite anorexia	Increased, with symptoms of increased appetite, intolerance to heat, elevated body temperature, weight loss despite increased appetite
Cardiovascular system	Bradycardia, moderate hypotension	Tachycardia, moderate hypertension
Central nervous system	Lethargy, sleepiness	Nervousness, anxiety, insomnia, tremors
Skin and skin structures	Pale, cool, dry, face appears puffy; hair coarse; nails thick and hard	Flushed, warm, moist
Ovarian function	Heavy menses, may be unable to conceive, loss of fetus also possible	Irregular or scant menses
Testicular function	Low sperm count	

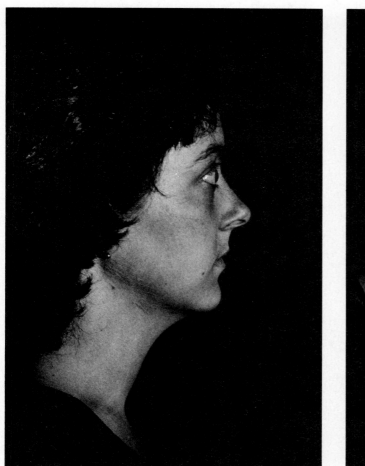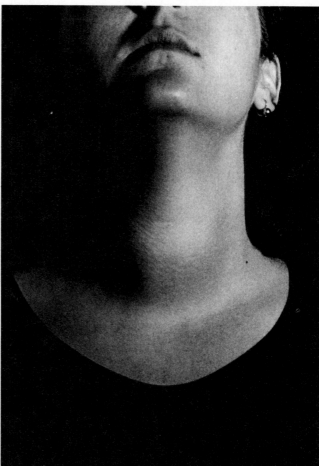

Figure 48–1. Thyroid enlargement with exophthalmos. (Photograph by D. Atkinson)

provement is one of the disadvantages of this treatment.

SURGICAL TREATMENT. Subtotal thyroidectomy is an effective treatment for hyperthyroidism. Total thyroidectomy may be performed if a malignancy is present.

Hypothyroidism

Hypothyroidism is a disorder that occurs when the thyroid gland fails to secrete an adequate amount of thyroid hormones. As a result, the rates of all metabolic processes slow (see Table 48-1). Severe hypothyroidism is called *myxedema*. This disorder may originate within the thyroid (primary hypothyroidism) or within the pituitary, in which case insufficient thyroid stimulating hormone (TSH) is produced. Regardless of the cause of the disorder, the symptoms are similar.

Symptoms

Symptoms of hypothyroidism are opposite in many respects to those of hyperthyroidism. The metabolic rate and both physical and mental activity are slowed. The patient feels lethargic and lacking in energy, dozes frequently during the day, is forgetful, and has chronic headaches. The face takes on a masklike unemotional expression, yet the patient is often irritable. The tongue may be enlarged and the lips swollen, and there may be edema of the eyelids. The temperature and pulse are decreased, and there is an intolerance to cold. The patient gains weight easily. The skin is dry, and hair characteristically is coarse and sparse, tending to fall out. Menstrual disorders are frequent. Constipation may be severe. The voice of the myxedema patient is low-pitched, slow, and hoarse. Hearing may be impaired. There may be numbness or tingling in the arms or legs, unrelieved by change of position.

Hypothyroidism may lead to enlargement of the heart caused by pericardial effusion and an increased tendency toward atherosclerosis and heart strain. Anemia also may be present. A problem in the early recognition of hypothyroidism is that many of the symptoms are nonspecific and may not be sufficiently dramatic to bring the patient to the physician. This condition can go untreated for years.

Diagnosis

A physical examination and patient history may reveal one or more of the general signs of hypothyroidism. Laboratory tests, such as one or more of those performed for the diagnosis of hyperthyroidism, may be ordered.

Treatment

Hypothyroidism is treated by replacement therapy. The patient is prescribed thyroid hormone in the form of desiccated thyroid extract, or with one of the synthetic products, such as levothyroxine sodium (Synthroid) or liothyronine sodium (Cytomel). These drugs are taken orally. Patients may be started on a low dose and the dose increased as needed.

The adverse effects of replacement therapy may include dyspnea, rapid pulse, palpitations, precordial pain, hyperactivity, insomnia, dizziness, and gastrointestinal disorders, in other words, signs of *hyper*thyroidism. Once replacement therapy has begun, a dramatic change may be seen in a few weeks.

Thyroid Tumors

Tumors of the thyroid may be malignant or benign. A follicular adenoma is the most common benign thyroid lesion, and papillary carcinoma is the most common malignant lesion.

An increased incidence of thyroid malignancies has been traced to the former use of radiation treatment for such problems as enlarged tonsils and facial acne during early childhood and the young adult years. It is recommended that individuals with a history of such treatment consult their physicians. External radiation of the head and neck areas for these problems is no longer used.

Symptoms

Symptoms may not be apparent, and the patient may be unaware of the lesion, which often is discovered during a routine physical examination. As the tumor enlarges, the patient may notice a swelling in the neck. Benign tumors may cause symptoms of hyperthyroidism in some patients.

Diagnosis

Diagnosis is confirmed by biopsy of the lesion. Thyroid cancer is suspected when there is a firm palpable area of the gland and when the RAI shows poor concentration in the suspicious area.

Treatment

Treatment of benign lesions depends on the symptoms. If the patient has no symptoms of hyperthyroidism, treatment is usually not needed. The lesion should be examined yearly, and if the enlargement results in symptoms such as difficulty swallowing or a noticeable swelling in the neck, surgical removal of the lesion may be considered.

Although treatment of malignant lesions varies, a thyroidectomy (total or subtotal) usually is performed. A modified or radical neck dissection may be necessary if there is metastasis.

After a thyroidectomy, replacement therapy (consisting of thyroid hormones) is given to supply those hormones no longer produced and to suppress pituitary TSH so that it no longer stimulates growth of any residual thyroid tissue. ^{131}I may be administered to destroy any remaining thyroid tissue as well as to treat lymph node metastasis, if present.

The cure rate of thyroid cancer depends on the type of tumor present. Papillary carcinoma, the most common thyroid carcinoma, does not grow rapidly, whereas undifferentiated cancer grows more rapidly and is more difficult to control. Because most thyroid cancers are papillary carcinomas, the physician often can convey optimism to the patient.

Endemic and Multinodular Goiters

The word *goiter* refers to an enlargement of the thyroid gland. *Endemic goiter* (also called simple or colloid goiter) is an enlargement of the thyroid, usually without symptoms of thyroid dysfunction. *Nodular goiters* contain one or more areas of *hyperplasia* (overgrowth of cells). This type of goiter appears to develop for essentially the same reasons as an endemic goiter. A goiter may be caused by a deficiency of iodine in the diet, by the inability of the thyroid to use iodine, by relative iodine deficiency caused by increasing body demands for thyroid hormones, or by goitrogens. *Goitrogens* are substances, primarily foods and drugs, that are capable of causing a goiter in some individuals. Foods labeled as goitrogens include turnips, carrots, seafood, and soybeans. Drugs known to be goitrogenic include iodine, propylthiouracil, salicylates, and sulfonamides.

Symptoms

The thyroid gland enlarges, and there is often a sense of fullness in the neck area. Eventually, continued gland enlargement can result in difficulty in swallowing and breathing when the thyroid presses on the trachea and esophagus. The gland is visible as a swelling in the neck when the thyroid has enlarged sufficiently. Nodular goiters also produce enlargement, but the gland has an irregular surface on palpation.

Diagnosis

Diagnosis is made by a thyroid scan, patient history, and physical examination. Tests of thyroid function, such as a serum T_4, also may be performed.

Treatment

Treatment depends on the cause of the goiter. If the diet has been deficient in iodine, foods high in iodine are recommended. Potassium iodide to supplement iodine intake may be ordered. In some instances, a thyroidectomy is recommended, especially when the gland is grossly enlarged. If the cause is related to goitrogenic foods, these are excluded from the diet or their intake is markedly reduced. Drugs that are potentially goitrogenic are avoided, when possible.

Thyroiditis

Thyroiditis, or inflammation of the thyroid gland, may be acute, subacute, or chronic. Acute thyroiditis appears to be the result of a bacterial infection of the gland. Subacute thyroiditis may follow a viral infection. There are two types of chronic thyroiditis: Hashimoto's thyroiditis and Riedel's thyroiditis. The latter is rare. Hashimoto's thyroiditis is thought to be an autoimmune disorder.

Symptoms

Symptoms of acute thyroiditis include fever, malaise, and tenderness and swelling of the thyroid gland. Subacute thyroiditis may produce symptoms of a swollen, painful gland, chills, fever, and malaise. Hashimoto's thyroiditis may be manifested by enlargement of the thyroid and symptoms of hypothyroidism.

Diagnosis

Diagnosis may be based on symptoms. In acute thyroiditis, laboratory tests may show an elevated white blood cell count and normal thyroid function. Subacute thyroiditis may show an elevation in some thyroid tests, such as the T_3 and T_4. Radioactive uptake studies and a needle biopsy also may be performed.

The diagnosis of Hashimoto's thyroiditis is based on the patient's symptoms, physical examination, and thyroid function studies.

Treatment

Acute thyroiditis requires administration of an antibiotic. The treatment of subacute thyroiditis is symptomatic and includes prescribing analgesics for pain and discomfort. A corticosteroid preparation also may be prescribed to reduce inflammation.

The treatment of Hashimoto's thyroiditis includes thyroid hormone replacement therapy. Surgery may be required if the gland becomes excessively large.

NURSING PROCESS —THE PATIENT UNDERGOING MEDICAL TREATMENT FOR A THYROID DISORDER

Assessment

Initial assessment includes a medical, drug, and allergy history as well as the patient's description of all symptoms. Physical examination includes checking vital signs and weight and looking for any overt symptoms of the disorder, such as tremors of the hands, nervousness, puffiness around the eyes, or swelling in the neck. The experienced examiner may palpate the thyroid for enlargement or other abnormal findings. The thyroid gland must be carefully palpated; excessive manipulation should be avoided because it can stimulate a sudden release of thyroid hormones.

Nursing Diagnosis

The following diagnoses are related to a disorder of the thyroid, namely hyposecretion, hypersecretion, or enlargement. Depending on the type of thyroid disorder and the symptoms, one or more may apply.

- Anxiety related to hypersecretion of thyroid hormones
- Self-care deficit: bathing, grooming related to fatigue secondary to hypothyroidism
- Activity intolerance and fatigue secondary to hyposecretion of thyroid hormones
- Diarrhea related to hypersecretion of thyroid hormones
- Constipation related to hyposecretion of thyroid hormones, inactivity
- Altered nutrition: less than body requirements related to hyperthyroidism
- Altered nutrition: more than body requirements related to hypothyroidism
- Ineffective individual coping related to symptoms, changes in physical appearance
- Knowledge deficit of treatment regimen

Planning and Implementation

The major goals of the patient may include a reduction in anxiety, improved ability to care for self, an increase in activity tolerance, normal bowel elimination, improved ability to cope with symptoms or changes in physical appearance, and understanding the treatment regimen.

The major goals of nursing management are to decrease the symptoms associated with the disorder, make the patient more comfortable, and instruct the patient in the medical management of the disorder.

Anxiety. The patient is assured that medical management may reduce or eliminate symptoms.

Certain conditions, such as room temperature, may upset the patient and increase anxiety. Providing cool liquids, reducing noise, reducing room temperature, and frequently changing bedding and gown if the patient is diaphoretic may help reduce some of the anxiety associated with hyperthyroidism. On the other hand, the hypothyroid patient may require a warmer room, warm liquids, and extra blankets at night. When possible, comfort should be maintained and situations causing anxiety should be reduced or eliminated.

Self-Care Deficit, Activity Intolerance, Fatigue. Acutely ill patients, such as those with myxedema (severe hypothyroidism) or thyroiditis, may require assistance with their activities of daily living (ADL). Depending on the severity of the disease, the hypothyroid patient may experience varying degrees of fatigue and may require some assistance with self-care activities. To reduce fatigue, tasks should be spaced so that the patient has time to rest between activities.

The hyperthyroid patient also may have difficulty attending to personal needs and require assistance. Marked nervousness and tremors may interfere with his or her ability to carry out activities such as shaving, bathing, and grooming.

Altered Nutrition. The hypothyroid patient may require a calorie-restricted diet, especially if an appreciable amount of weight has been gained. If the patient is hyperthyroid, the physician may order a high caloric diet, which may be better tolerated when given as four to six meals per day. If profuse diaphoresis or diarrhea is present, the patient should be placed on intake and output and fluids should be encouraged.

The patient should be weighed weekly, and any significant weight gain or loss should be brought to the attention of the physician.

Diarrhea, Constipation. The hyperthyroid patient may experience diarrhea caused by hypermotility of the gastrointestinal tract, whereas the hypothyroid patient may be constipated. A record of bowel movements should be kept, and problems with elimination should be brought to the attention of the physician. Diarrhea may require the administration of an antidiarrheal drug and constipation the administration of a laxative or enema.

Ineffective Individual Coping. The patient may be distressed over symptoms such as fatigue, nervousness, or a change in appearance. The nurse must help the patient understand that the disorder may be responsible for some of these symptoms and that once therapy is instituted, symptoms may disappear after a time. It should be noted that certain symptoms, such as exophthalmos, are permanent.

Knowledge Deficit. Because the symptoms of hyperthyroidism and hypothyroidism may affect the patient's learning and retention ability, the treatment regimen must be carefully explained. The dose of the medications and possible adverse drug effects that may occur during therapy should be discussed. If a special diet has been recommended, a dietary consultation should be obtained and sample diets given.

The patient should be instructed to obtain weekly weights. It is important for the patient to keep a record of symptoms and weight because the dose of the prescribed medication may require adjustment, depending on the relief or nonrelief of symptoms.

The importance of avoiding stressful situations, maintaining good nutrition, and receiving continuous medical supervision should be emphasized. The patient also should be instructed to notify the physician if symptoms become worse or adverse drug effects occur.

Evaluation

■ Anxiety is reduced
■ Patient eats a well-balanced diet
■ Weight remains stable
■ Bowel elimination is normal
■ Patient shows evidence of being able to cope with symptoms of the disorder
■ Patient demonstrates understanding of the medical regimen

NURSING PROCESS —THE PATIENT UNDERGOING THYROID SURGERY

Preoperative Period

Assessment

A complete medical, drug, and allergy history should be obtained. To decrease bleeding during surgery, patients scheduled for a thyroidectomy may have a short course of treatment with an antithyroid preparation for at least 2 weeks before surgery. If a preoperative medication was prescribed, it is important to determine if the patient completed the prescribed course of therapy.

A physical assessment (see Chapter 47) may be performed, but the thyroid gland should not be palpated because manipulation of the gland may release additional amounts of thyroid hormones.

Nursing Diagnosis

Depending on the reason for surgery, one or more of the following may apply.

- Anxiety related to surgery, diagnosis
- Fear related to possible diagnosis of cancer during or after surgery
- Knowledge deficit of preoperative preparations, postoperative management techniques

Planning and Implementation

The major goals of the patient may include a reduction in anxiety and fear and an understanding of preoperative preparations and postoperative management.

The major goal of nursing management is to prepare the patient physically and emotionally for surgery.

A suction machine and emergency tracheostomy tray should be obtained and placed at the bedside. Intravenous calcium should be obtained if the drug is not routinely stocked.

Anxiety, Fear, Knowledge Deficit.   Normal preoperative anxiety may be increased if the patient is hyperthyroid. Anxiety and fear also may be present if there is a tentative or actual diagnosis of cancer of the thyroid. The patient may need time to talk and ask questions about the surgery and about what further treatments may be necessary if a malignancy is found. Some questions may need to be referred to the surgeon.

In addition to the usual preparation of any patient undergoing surgery, these patients should be shown how to support the head when rising to a sitting position (Fig. 48-2). They also should be instructed in the technique and importance of deep breathing and leg exercises.

Evaluation

- Anxiety and fear is reduced
- Patient appears emotionally prepared for surgery
- Physical preparations for surgery are completed

Postoperative Period

Assessment

Complications associated with thyroid surgery include hemorrhage, airway obstruction, paralysis of

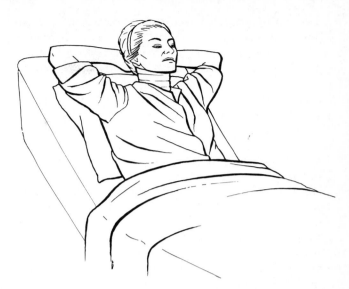

Figure 48–2.   After a thyroidectomy, the patient uses the hands to support the head while rising to a sitting position. This type of support helps avoid strain to the neck muscles and surgical incision.

the recurrent laryngeal nerve (responsible for speech), hypoparathyroidism, and hypothyroidism. The latter complication may not be apparent for several days or weeks after surgery.

On return from the operating room, vital signs should be taken. The patient's breathing should be assessed and the dressing inspected for bleeding or drainage. The patient should be asked to say a few words (such as his or her name) to check the voice for tone, pitch, and hoarseness. The extremities should be examined for tetany or spasm, the presence of which may indicate iatrogenic hypoparathyroidism (inadvertent removal of the parathyroid glands).

Nursing Diagnosis

Depending on the extent of surgery, the location and amount of gland removed, and possible complications, one or more of the following may apply.

- Pain related to surgical incision
- Ineffective airway clearance related to bleeding, edema, bulky surgical dressing
- Impaired verbal communication related to damage to edema around the recurrent laryngeal nerve
- Knowledge deficit of postdischarge treatment regimen

Planning and Implementation

The major goals of the patient may include relief of pain, a patent airway, absence of impaired verbal communication, and understanding the postdischarge treatment regimen.

The major goals of nursing management are to

maintain a patent airway and recognize complications.

An infrequent postoperative complication is tetany (muscular hypertonia with spasm and tremor), caused by a low concentration of calcium from the inadvertent removal of the parathyroid glands during the thyroidectomy. In this case, the patient complains of numbness, tingling of the extremities, and muscle cramps. Tetany also can cause laryngeal spasm. If these symptoms are present, the physician should be notified because treatment, which involves administration of intravenous calcium, must be instituted *immediately*. The treatment of permanent hypocalcemia is discussed in the next section.

Thyroid crisis or storm, now a rare complication of thyroid surgery, may occur within the first 12 hours after surgery. All the symptoms of hyperthyroidism are exaggerated. The patient's temperature may be as high as 41°C (106°F), the pulse is very rapid, and cardiac dysrhythmia are common. There may be persistent vomiting and extreme restlessness with delirium. The patient becomes exhausted and could die from cardiac failure. If these symptoms are present, the physician should be notified immediately. Emergency treatment includes intravenous sodium iodide, intravenous corticosteroids, oxygen, and cooling by the application of ice or a controlled thermoblanket.

Nursing Care Plan 48-1 is an example of postoperative nursing management of the patient with a thyroidectomy.

Pain. Analgesics are administered as ordered. Support of the head when the patient's position is changed may help relieve some pain in the area of the incision.

The patient usually returns from the recovery room in a supine position with the head slightly elevated. Following transfer to a hospital bed, the patient should be placed in a semi-Fowler's position. Pillows should be positioned under the head, neck, and shoulders to support these structures, to prevent excessive pulling on and possible separation of the suture line, and to reduce pain or discomfort in the area.

Ineffective Airway Clearance. During the early postoperative period, the patient should be observed for signs of respiratory obstruction. Edema or bleeding can compress the trachea, causing an inability to breathe. This serious problem must be treated within minutes by the insertion of an endotracheal tube or by a tracheostomy. A call light should be placed within easy reach, and the patient should be instructed to use it if he or she has difficulty breathing.

The surgical dressing should be inspected at frequent intervals for bleeding and drainage. Vital signs should be checked every 2 to 4 hours or as ordered. Attention should be given to the patient's complaints of a sense of fullness in or around the surgical incision because a small amount of blood in the incision can obstruct respirations.

Blood may not be evident on the front of the dressing, but it may ooze around to the back of the patient's neck. During the first 24 postoperative hours, a hand should passed behind the patient's neck to see whether it feels damp. When the patient is turned, the dressing and bed linen should be checked for blood. If the dressing becomes too tight, it should be loosened but not removed, and the surgeon should be contacted. Restlessness, apprehension, respiratory distress, increased pulse or temperature, decreased blood pressure, and cyanosis may occur and must be treated immediately by the physician.

Aspiration is a danger because there is depression of laryngeal and tracheal reflexes. When swallowing and coughing reflexes have returned, the patient should be encouraged to breathe deeply every 2 hours the first day. The lungs should be auscultated every 8 hours. Some surgeons prefer that only the deep-breathing exercises be performed during the immediate postoperative period because coughing places added strain on the incision and could precipitate bleeding. The postoperative orders should be checked to determine the surgeon's preference in this matter.

Impaired Verbal Communication. Infrequently, the recurrent laryngeal nerve is injured during surgery. The patient may be hoarse or unable to speak because of vocal cord paralysis. Respiratory obstruction also may occur. The patient should be asked to speak a few words every 2 to 4 hours. Although some hoarseness is to be expected, severe hoarseness or other voice changes should be reported to the physician. Talking should be kept to a minimum during the first 2 postoperative days. Humidification of the bedside area may be ordered.

Knowledge Deficit. Before discharge from the hospital, the patient should be instructed in the care of the surgical incision. Care should be taken to avoid excessive strain on the incision until it is healed. Because the incision is made in a crease of the neck, the healed scar is barely visible. If a patient seems concerned about it, clothing that covers the neck can be worn until the scar is almost invisible.

The symptoms of hypothyroidism, hyperthyroidism, and hypoparathyroidism should be discussed

Nursing Care Plan 48-1
Postoperative Management of the Patient Who Has a Thyroidectomy

Potential Problem and Potential Nursing Diagnosis	Nursing Intervention	Outcome Criteria
Respiratory Distress Due to Edema or Bleeding at the Operative Site *Ineffective airway clearance related to edema or bleeding near upper airway structures*	Keep tracheostomy tray and suction machine at bedside (or nurse's station); place call light within easy reach and instruct patient to use if respiratory difficulty occurs; vital signs q 1–4 hr or as ordered, with special attention to respiratory rate; instruct patient to use voice as little as possible during first few postoperative days; check surgical dressing and area behind neck for bleeding; support patient's head when moving or turning; place a small pillow under patient's head to prevent tension on the suture line; encourage deep-breathing exercises, but do not encourage voluntary coughing unless ordered by the physician; report signs of respiratory distress immediately	Patient maintains normal breathing pattern
Voice Loss Due to Edema or Laryngeal Nerve Damage	Voice check q 2–4 hr or as ordered; report any voice change immediately (some hoarseness is to be expected); keep talking to a minimum by asking questions that can be answered by yes or no	Voice normal; no difficulty in speaking
Hypocalcemic Tetany (Due to Accidental Removal of the Parathyroids)	Observe q 2 hr for signs of tetany (eg, apprehension, tingling of extremities and around the mouth, muscle twitching); have IV calcium immediately available; report symptoms of hypocalcemia immediately	If hypocalcemia occurs, it is detected and treated immediately
Thyroid Crisis (Storm)	Observe for sudden fever, marked tachycardia, cardiac arrhythmia, extreme restlessness, and delirium, and report immediately	If thyroid crisis occurs, it is detected and treated immediately

with the patient with instructions to immediately notify the physician if they occur.

If medication is prescribed, instructions should be given regarding the drug, dose, and adverse drug effects.

Evaluation

■ Pain is controlled
■ Incision remains intact; no evidence of wound separation, bleeding, or drainage
■ Respiration is normal; lungs are clear to auscultation
■ Patient deep breathes every 2 hours
■ Voice is normal; patient communicates effectively

■ Patient demonstrates understanding of wound care, medical regimen, symptoms requiring notification of the physician

DISORDERS OF THE PARATHYROID GLANDS
Hyperparathyroidism

In hyperparathyroidism, overproduction of parathyroid hormone (parathormone) results in increased urinary excretion of phosphorus and loss of calcium from the bones. The bones become demineralized as the calcium leaves and enters the bloodstream.

Symptoms

The excess serum calcium that has been taken from the tissues is lost in the urine. The large amounts of calcium and phosphorus passing through the kidneys may lead to the development of stones in the genitourinary (GU) tract, pyelonephritis, and uremia; thus, renal disease is a serious outcome. The amount of serum phosphorus is decreased. The shift of calcium from the bones to the blood leads to events that include muscle weakness, fatigue, apathy, nausea and vomiting, constipation, and cardiac dysrhythmia. Excessive blood calcium depresses the responsiveness of the peripheral nerves, accounting for the fatigue and muscle weakness. The muscles become hypotonic (loss of or decrease in muscle tone). Because the bones have lost calcium, there is skeletal tenderness and pain on bearing weight; the bones may become so demineralized that they break with little or no trauma (pathologic fractures).

Diagnosis

The diagnosis is made on the basis of elevated serum calcium and low serum phosphorus levels in the absence of other causes of hypercalcemia. A 3-day, low-calcium diet may be given, and the amount of calcium excreted in the urine measured to help establish the diagnosis and determine the severity of the disease. Other diagnostic studies may include skeletal radiographs (to detect loss of calcium from bones) and the immunoassay method of measuring parathyroid hormone levels.

Treatment

Treatment involves surgical removal of hypertrophied gland tissue or of an individual tumor.

Nursing management is similar to management of the patient with a thyroidectomy, as the surgical approach is similar. Also included is observation of the patient for the symptoms of hypoparathyroidism (discussed in the next section).

Hypoparathyroidism

The most common cause of hypoparathyroidism is trauma to the glands or inadvertent removal of these structures during a thyroidectomy. The idiopathic form of this disorder is rare. In hypoparathyroidism, calcium in the blood is decreased, phosphorus in the blood is increased, and both are decreased in the urine.

Symptoms

The main symptom of acute, sudden hypoparathyroidism is tetany. The patient may feel numbness and tingling in the fingers or toes or around the lips. A voluntary movement may be followed by an involuntary, jerking spasm. Muscle cramping may be present. Tonic (continuous contraction) flexion of an arm or a finger may occur. If the facial nerve (immediately in front of the ear) is tapped, the patient's mouth twitches, and the jaw tightens (positive Chvostek's sign). A spasm may occur in the larynx, causing the patient to become dyspneic, with long, crowing respirations as air tries to get past the constriction. Cyanosis may be present, and the patient may be in danger of asphyxia and cardiac dysrhythmia. Generalized convulsions may be seen.

Diagnosis

The diagnosis is made on the basis of low serum calcium and elevated serum phosphorus levels in the absence of other causes of hypocalcemia. Recognition of hypoparathyroid tetany—as might be seen after a thyroidectomy—usually is based on symptoms and decreased serum calcium levels.

Treatment

Severe hypoparathyroidism must be treated immediately. Intravenous calcium gluconate should be given intravenously. Endotracheal intubation and mechanical ventilation may be necessary if acute respiratory distress occurs. Bronchodilators also may be ordered.

Long-term treatment following trauma to or inadvertent removal of the parathyroids includes administration of vitamin D or vitamin D_2 (calciferol), which increases the blood level of calcium. The dosage is related to the degree of hypocalcemia, which is determined by frequent measurements of the blood calcium. The urine calcium levels also may be checked. A diet high in calcium and low in phosphorus is usually recommended.

NURSING PROCESS —THE PATIENT WHO HAS HYPOPARATHYROIDISM

Assessment

Patients having thyroid surgery should be observed for the development of hypoparathyroidism. If the patient has chronic hypoparathyroidism, a complete medical, drug, and allergy history should be obtained. The patient should be examined for symptoms of the disorder, primarily for the effect of a decreased serum calcium on the nervous system. The extremities should be examined for evidence of muscle spasm (tetany). If tetany is suspected, the area in front of the ear should be tapped to elicit a positive Chvostek's sign. The lungs should be auscultated because the patient may have dyspnea or other respiratory difficulty. Vital signs should be taken with particular attention to the cardiac rate and rhythm.

Nursing Diagnosis

Depending on the degree of hypoparathyroidism, one or more of the following may apply:

- Anxiety related to symptoms (muscle spasms, laryngospasm, etc.)
- Pain or discomfort related to muscle spasms
- Total or partial (specify areas) self-care deficit related to muscle contractions or cramping
- Knowledge deficit of postdischarge treatment modalities

Planning and Implementation

The major goals of the patient may include a reduction in anxiety, relief of pain, improvement in ability to care for self, and understanding treatment modalities.

The main goals of nursing management are to recognize and report symptoms of the disorder promptly and to assist in the elimination of symptoms associated with hypoparathyroidism.

Those with severe hypocalcemia require administration of an intravenous calcium salt. The patient should be closely observed during administration of the drug for adverse effects associated with calcium administration, namely flushing, cardiac dysrhythmia (usually a bradycardia), tingling in the extremities, and a metallic taste. Local tissue necrosis may occur if the intravenous fluid escapes into surrounding tissues. Serum calcium levels are drawn periodically to determine the effectiveness of therapy.

Anxiety, Pain, Discomfort. Prompt recognition and treatment usually relieve symptoms and thus relieve anxiety and pain or discomfort. The patient should be observed closely for the relief of the symptoms of hypocalcemia, and the physician should be kept informed of the patient's response to treatment.

Self-Care Deficit. Until hypocalcemia is corrected, the patient may require assistance with activities such as bathing and grooming. Because movement, noise, and other environmental disturbances can precipitate tetany, care should be taken to keep disturbances to a minimum until serum calcium levels approach normal and symptoms are relieved.

Respiratory Function. An emergency tracheostomy tray, mechanical ventilation, and endotracheal intubation equipment should be kept at the bedside if the patient has severe hypocalcemia. The patient should be closely observed at frequent intervals for respiratory distress, and the physician should be notified immediately if this problem occurs.

Knowledge Deficit. Those requiring lifetime treatment of the disorder need a careful review of the physician's prescribed medical regimen. Consultation with a dietitian may be necessary to provide the patient with a list of foods to include or avoid in the prescribed diet.

The patient must be given a list of the symptoms of hypercalcemia and hypocalcemia, either of which can occur if the dose of the prescribed drug is either too high or too low or if the drug is omitted. The patient should be reminded that the physician may need to periodically adjust the dose of the drug and therefore it is important to remember the symptoms associated with hypercalcemia and hypocalcemia. The need to contact the physician immediately if one or more of these symptoms occurs should be emphasized.

Because normal calcium levels depend on drug and diet therapy, the importance of these two aspects of treatment should be strongly emphasized.

DRUG THERAPY. The prescribed drugs must be taken at the dose and intervals prescribed. The dose of the drugs should not be increased, decreased, nor omitted, unless advised so by the physician. Increasing the dose can result in symptoms of hypercalcemia; decreasing or omitting the dose can result in a return of the original symptoms.

If unable to take the prescribed drug because of nausea and vomiting, or should severe diarrhea occur, the physician should be contacted immediately.

DIET. Adherence to the recommended diet is absolutely necessary. Food labels must be carefully read so that foods that are and are not a part of the diet can be included and avoided, respectively.

Evaluation

- Serum calcium levels are normal
- Symptoms are reduced or eliminated
- Anxiety is reduced
- Comfort is attained and maintained
- Self-care needs are met
- Respiratory function is normal
- Patient demonstrates understanding of treatment regimen
- Patient is able to list and discuss the symptoms of hypocalcemia and hypercalcemia

DISORDERS OF THE ADRENAL GLANDS
Adrenal Cortical Insufficiency

Primary adrenal cortical insufficiency, also called Addison's disease, results from destruction of the adrenal cortex. Disease, such as tuberculosis, can affect the adrenal cortex; in many instances, however, the cause of the disease is unknown. *Secondary* adrenal cortical insufficiency may be caused by surgical removal of both adrenal glands (bilateral adrenalectomy), hemorrhagic infarction of the glands, hypopituitarism (caused by pituitary failure or surgical removal of the pituitary), or suppression of adrenal function by the administration of corticosteroid drugs.

Those with secondary adrenal cortical insufficiency caused by bilateral adrenalectomy or surgical removal of the pituitary gland technically experience adrenal cortical insufficiency. When these surgeries are performed under a *controlled* situation, however, these patients do not actually experience true adrenal cortical insufficiency because during and after surgery corticosteroid drugs are administered to prevent adrenal cortical insufficiency.

Symptoms

Although there are some differences between the symptoms of primary and secondary adrenal cortical insufficiency, the symptoms basically are much alike.

A decrease in or absence of adrenal cortical hormones leads to the symptoms of adrenal cortical insufficiency, which include the following:

- An increase in the urinary excretion of sodium and retention of potassium, followed by dehydration and a reduction of blood plasma volume
- Weakness, fatigue
- Hypotension, hypothermia
- Postural hypotension, dizziness
- Potential for vascular collapse because of poor myocardial tonus, decreased cardiac output, and hypotension
- Weight loss, anemia, anorexia, gastrointestinal symptoms
- Nervousness, periods of depression
- Hypoglycemia caused by a deficiency of those hormones that facilitate the conversion of protein into glucose; episodes of hypoglycemia may develop 5 or 6 hours after eating; the early morning before breakfast is an especially dangerous time
- Abnormally dark pigmentation, especially of exposed areas of the skin and mucous membranes, and a decrease in hair growth (primary adrenal cortical insufficiency)

Those with primary adrenal cortical insufficiency (Addison's disease) usually experience symptoms of adrenal insufficiency over a period of time. Those with secondary adrenal cortical insufficiency also may develop symptoms over a period of several days to weeks, or they may suddenly develop symptoms.

Diagnosis

Diagnosis is based on symptoms as well as on laboratory and diagnostic tests. The pituitary gland secretes adrenocorticotropic hormone (ACTH), which stimulates the adrenal cortex to secrete its own hormones. A test used to diagnose Addison's disease is the determination of the adrenal cortical response to ACTH. The excretion of adrenal cortical hormones is measured after the administration of intravenous ACTH. Normal people have an increased excretion of 17-hydroxycorticosteroids (17-OH) and 17-ketosteroids, whereas patients with Addison's disease show little or no increase. Eosinophils in the patient's blood also are measured. The eosinophil count normally drops 60% to 90% after the ACTH is given, but there is less change in patients with Addison's disease.

Other laboratory tests show low serum sodium and high serum potassium levels. A glucose tolerance test may be done. In Addison's disease, the glucose in the bloodstream does not rise as high as normal, and it returns to its fasting level more quickly than it would under normal conditions.

Treatment

Those with secondary adrenal cortical insufficiency caused by bilateral adrenalectomy or removal of the pituitary must receive corticosteroids daily for the rest of their lives. If for some reason the person is not given or does not take the medication, acute adrenal crisis can develop (see next section). This also applies to patients on long-term corticosteroid therapy for treatment of disorders such as allergies, rheumatoid arthritis, and collagen diseases. If the drug is to be discontinued, the dose *must be tapered* over a period of time, until the patient is finally off the medication.

Addison's disease is treated by replacement of the missing hormones. Fludrocortisone (Florinef), a synthetic corticosteroid preparation that possesses glucocorticoid and mineralocorticoid properties, is often selected for corticosteroid replacement therapy.

Treatment for secondary adrenal cortical insufficiency caused by bilateral adrenalectomy or pituitary failure is the same as treatment for Addison's disease. Treatment of secondary adrenal cortical insufficiency caused by suppression of adrenal function resulting from discontinuation of corticosteroid therapy or hemorrhagic infarction of the gland is variable and depends on the ability of the adrenals to return to normal function.

Acute Adrenal Crisis (Addisonian Crisis)

Acute adrenal crisis occurs when there is a *sudden* failure of the adrenal glands. Because the hormones of the cortex of the adrenal glands are prominent in effecting the body's adaptive reactions to stress, patients with Addison's disease may develop acute adrenal crisis when they are faced with extreme stress. Even uncomplicated surgery, such as an appendectomy, requires more physiologic adaptive ability than a patient with Addison's disease usually possesses. Salt deprivation, infection, trauma, exposure to cold, overexertion—any abnormal stress—can cause adrenal crisis.

Symptoms

The crisis may start with anorexia, nausea, vomiting, diarrhea, abdominal pain, headache, intensification of hypotension, restlessness, or fever. Unless the dosage of the corticosteroid is increased to meet the demand, the patient progresses to acute adrenal crisis. The blood pressure becomes markedly decreased, and the patient is in adrenal shock.

Acute adrenal crisis also may occur when corticosteroid therapy is suddenly stopped. Normally, cessation of corticosteroid therapy is accomplished by tapering the dose over a period of days. However, omission of one or more doses or suddenly discontinuing therapy can also produce adrenal crisis.

Diagnosis

Diagnosis of acute adrenal crisis is based on symptoms and history.

Treatment

Adrenal (Addison's) crisis is an emergency; death may occur from hypotension and vasomotor collapse. Corticosteroids should be given intravenously in solutions of normal saline and glucose. Antibiotics may be ordered because of the patient's extremely low resistance to infection. Vital signs should be taken frequently. The patient should be kept warm and as quiet as possible until the emergency is over.

NURSING PROCESS —THE PATIENT WHO HAS ADRENAL CORTICAL INSUFFICIENCY

Assessment

Regardless of cause, assessment of the patient with known or suspected adrenal cortical insufficiency or adrenal crisis includes recognition of the symptoms.

When a patient with Addison's disease is admitted for treatment of this or another illness, a complete summary of the history of the disorder, including the onset of symptoms, symptoms experienced since the disorder was first diagnosed, and the dose of prescribed medications should be obtained. All observable symptoms, such as skin color changes, body weight, and mental status should be recorded. The patient should be assessed for symptoms of electrolyte imbalance, especially hyponatremia and dehydration (see Chapter 12). Vital signs should be taken and the patient weighed. The patient's ability to perform any type of activity, including ADL, should be evaluated.

Assessment of those with known or suspected secondary adrenal cortical insufficiency is the same as for those with Addison's disease.

Both primary and secondary adrenal cortical insufficiency may progress to adrenal crisis. Immediate recognition of symptoms is most important because this complication is a life-threatening situation.

Nursing Diagnosis

The extent of the nursing diagnosis depends on many factors, such as the cause and severity of adrenal insufficiency and the presenting symptoms.

■ Total or partial (specify areas) self-care deficit related to weakness, fatigue, other symptoms of the disorder (specify)

■ Potential for injury related to hypotension secondary to fluid or electrolyte imbalances

■ Fluid volume deficit related to inadequate fluid intake, fluid loss secondary to inadequate adrenal hormone secretion

■ Altered nutrition: less than body requirements related to anorexia, nausea

■ Knowledge deficit of postdischarge treatment regimen

Planning and Implementation

The major goals of the patient may include improvement in ability to care for self, correction of fluid and electrolyte imbalances, improved nutrition, acceptance of changes in body image, absence of injury, and understanding the postdischarge treatment regimen.

The major goals of nursing management are to assist in correcting fluid and electrolyte imbalances, improve nutrition, decrease or eliminate stressful situations that place the patient at risk for adrenal crisis, educate the patient in the therapeutic management of the disorder, and recognize the symptoms of adrenal crisis, should they occur.

Nursing management of the patient with primary or secondary adrenal cortical insufficiency is essentially the same because the major problem is a lack of adrenal cortical hormone. The patient developing secondary adrenal cortical insufficiency because of surgery (bilateral adrenalectomy, surgical removal of the pituitary) has a controlled deficiency that is corrected with hormone replacement therapy.

It must be remembered that *any* patient with adrenal cortical insufficiency is a potential candidate for acute adrenal crisis. *It is imperative that the patient be given the prescribed corticosteroid replacement because omission of the drug can result in adrenal crisis.*

Vital signs should be taken at frequent intervals. Ongoing assessment of any patient with adrenal cortical insufficiency must always include observing the patient for early signs of adrenal crisis (see previous section).

Hypoglycemia is frequently a problem in patients with Addison's disease. Hence, no patient with this disorder should receive insulin by error because administration of insulin would lower the blood glucose to a critically low level that could result in brain damage or even death.

Self-Care Deficit, Potential for Injury. Bed rest with or without bathroom privileges may be ordered. Because fatigue and weakness may be seen, the patient may require complete or partial assistance with bathing and grooming. To partially eliminate fatigue, rest periods should be provided between activities.

Because of hypotension and muscle weakness, the patient may be subject to falling. Side rails should be used, and the patient should be instructed to ask for assistance in getting out of bed. The importance of getting out of bed slowly should be emphasized. If dizziness occurs on sitting up, the patient should be told to lie down again. The blood pressure is taken if symptoms such as weakness or faintness indicate that the blood pressure may be lower than previous readings.

Fluid and Electrolyte Balance, Altered Nutrition. Because the adrenal glands are closely related to the regulation of body water and electrolytes, careful records of fluid intake and urinary output are necessary. The patient should be weighed daily, and the physician should be notified if signs of dehydration, hyponatremia, or progressive weight loss appear.

The patient should be encouraged to drink fluids and eat the prescribed diet to maintain fluid and electrolyte balance. Because of recurrent hypoglycemia, the patient may do better on five or six small meals per day than on three regular meals. The physician may order the salt intake increased if serum sodium levels are below normal. If tolerated, extra salt can be added to the food. If excessive perspiration occurs, fluid and salt intake may have to be increased.

The symptoms of hypoglycemia are hunger, headache, sweating, weakness, trembling, emotional instability, visual disturbances, and, finally, disorientation, coma, and convulsions. If these symptoms are noted, the physician should be contacted immediately. Hypoglycemia is treated by giving glucose, orally or intravenously. To prevent recurring episodes of hypoglycemia, the physician may order between-meal snacks of milk and crackers, which is preferable to candy and other rapidly absorbed sugars. If the patient's meal is delayed because of diagnostic tests or for other reasons, the fasting period should be kept to a minimum, and the patient should be kept in bed and quiet.

Knowledge Deficit. Teach the patient and family what the disease is and the importance of lifetime corticosteroid replacement. The importance of physician or clinic appointments for lifetime supervision and following the recommended diet should be stressed.

The following may be included in a teaching plan:

1. The body has limited ability to handle stress of any kind.
2. Medical attention must be sought for the readjustment of dosage whenever there is stress. Examples of stress include an infection, a car accident (even if not noticeably hurt), exposure to cold, a family crisis, or an excessive work load.
3. Exposure to infections must be avoided.
4. If an infection (sore throat, upper respiratory infection) or other type of illness should occur, the physician should be contacted immediately because an increase in the dose of the medication may be necessary.
5. Vomiting, diarrhea, or any other condition that prevents taking the medication orally or interferes with proper absorption of the drug requires parenteral administration of the corticosteroid preparation. (Usually, the physician instructs the patient on the procedures to follow if the medication cannot be taken orally).
6. *Corticosteroids must be taken every day for the rest of the patient's life.* If the prescribed drug is not taken, adrenal cortical insufficiency, which is serious and can be life-threatening, will occur.
7. Identification, such as a medical alert tag or bracelet stating that the wearer has adrenal cortical insufficiency, is strongly recommended. If an accident or other problem should occur, medical personnel must be made aware of the need for corticosteroids.
8. The diet recommended by the physician must be followed.
9. Excessive fatigue must be avoided.

Evaluation

■ Self-care needs are met
■ Vital signs are normal
■ Fluid balance improved; no evidence of electrolyte imbalance
■ Patient eats the prescribed diet
■ Weight remains stable
■ No evidence of injury; patient asks for assistance with daily activities
■ Patient demonstrates understanding of importance of corticosteroid therapy, diet recommendations, need for lifetime medical supervision, avoidance of stress and infections, and wearing of identification tag or bracelet

Pheochromocytoma

A pheochromocytoma is a tumor, usually of the adrenal medulla, which causes increased hyperfunction of the adrenal gland, producing an excessive secretion of the catecholamines epinephrine and norepinephrine. The tumor is usually benign.

Symptoms

Symptoms include hypertension (intermittent or, more frequently, persistent), tremor, nervousness, sweating, headache, nausea and vomiting, hyperglycemia, polyuria, and vertigo.

Diagnosis

Diagnosis is made by measuring the urinary excretion of catecholamines and their breakdown products, such as vanillylmandelic acid (VMA). A CT scan, MRI, ultrasonography, aortography, and retrograde pyelograms also may be performed.

Treatment

Treatment involves the surgical removal of the tumor by means of an adrenalectomy.

Cushing's Syndrome (Adrenal Cortical Hyperfunction)

Cushing's syndrome is the opposite of Addison's disease. An overproduction of adrenal cortical hormones may result from (1) overstimulation by the pituitary gland, with resultant hyperplasia of the adrenal cortex (Cushing's disease), (2) benign or malignant tumors of the adrenal cortex, and (3) prolonged administration of high doses of corticosteroid preparations. In a few patients, Cushing's syndrome also is caused by an extraadrenal carcinoma, which produces an ACTH-like substance that causes adrenal hyperfunction and hyperplasia.

Symptoms

In Cushing's syndrome, extensive protein depletion leads to muscle wasting and weakness. Carbohydrate tolerance is lowered, and diabetes mellitus may result. There is a redistribution of fat, leading eventually to the typical moon face and buffalo hump. The skin is thin, and the face is ruddy. There is a susceptibility to infection because of a depressed production of white blood cells. Symptoms of infection may be masked.

The blood vessels are extremely fragile, the patient bruises easily, and striae may form over extensive skin areas. Wounds may be slow to heal, and the bones become so demineralized that the patient may have backache, kyphosis, and collapse of the vertebra of the spine. Sodium and water are retained; the patient suffers peripheral edema and hypertension. There is often a change in mood, and depression may be seen. Occasionally a psychosis develops. In women, Cushing's syndrome usually produces masculinization, with hirsutism and amenorrhea. The physical changes that occur with Cushing's syndrome are referred to as a *cushingoid appearance.*

Diagnosis

Diagnosis is usually based on the changes in the patient's physical appearance as well as on laboratory studies. The urine may be examined for 17-OH and 17-ketosteroids that are almost always increased. Plasma and urinary cortisol (a major adrenocortical hormone) levels also may be ordered. Laboratory tests may show an increase in serum sodium, a decrease in serum potassium, and an increase in blood glucose levels.

Abdominal radiographs, CT scan, or MRI may show an adrenal mass, and an intravenous pyelogram may show changes in the renal shadow caused by an abnormally large adrenal gland.

Treatment

Treatment depends on whether the disease is caused by a tumor or by adrenal hyperplasia (increase in the number of cells), and is directed toward removing the cause of the disorder and lowering plasma cortisol levels.

Radiation therapy to or removal of the pituitary may be used if there is adrenal hyperplasia. A bilateral adrenalectomy may be preferred if both adrenals are involved.

If Cushing's syndrome is caused by exogenous administration of a corticosteroid preparation, the drug can be slowly withdrawn by tapering the dose over a period of days or weeks. In some instances, as in the treatment of a serious disorder such as leukemia, the syndrome is allowed to persist.

NURSING PROCESS —THE PATIENT WHO HAS CUSHING'S SYNDROME

Assessment

A complete medical history as well as a head-to-toe examination should be performed to obtain a complete list of external symptoms. The patient should be weighed, and vital signs should be taken.

Initial assessment also includes a complete medical history (onset, symptoms, treatment) and a drug and allergy history. If the patient is currently taking a corticosteroid preparation for the treatment of another medical disorder, the name of the drug and the dose is most important because therapy with these drugs must *never* be abruptly terminated.

Nursing Diagnosis

The extent of the nursing diagnoses depends on the severity of the disorder and the number of symptoms present.

- Activity intolerance related to muscle weakness and wasting
- Self-care deficit related to muscle weakness and wasting
- Potential for injury related to osteoporosis
- Potential for infection related to depressed production of white blood cells
- Impaired skin integrity related to edema, dry skin
- Body image disturbance related to Cushing's syndrome
- Altered thought processes related to Cushing's syndrome
- Knowledge deficit of postdischarge treatment regimen

Planning and Implementation

The major goals of the patient may include an increase in activity tolerance, absence of infection, improved ability to care for self, absence of injury, prevention of skin breakdown or injury, and understanding the postdischarge treatment regimen.

The major goals of nursing management are aimed at preventing problems associated with the disorder, such as infection and impaired skin integrity. Additional goals are individualized according to the severity of the disorder and the needs of the patient as identified during assessment.

Activity Intolerance, Self-Care Deficit, Potential for Injury. If the patient tires easily, frequent rest periods should be allowed between activities. The patient with long-standing Cushing's syndrome may have widespread osteoporosis accompanied by pain, which may limit the ability to carry out many ADLs. The patient must be protected from falls and other types of injuries and should be instructed to seek assistance in getting out of bed. Shoes are preferable to slippers to prevent falls or slipping on waxed floors. When muscle wasting or osteoporosis is severe, the patient may require complete care and assistance with all activities.

Potential for Infection. Exposure to infections (other patients, hospital personnel, visitors) should be avoided because of the patient's decreased resistance to infection. The nurse should be especially alert for minor signs, such as a slight sore throat or a rise in temperature, that may indicate the presence of a more severe infectious process.

Impaired Skin Integrity. The patient should be encouraged to change positions frequently. Skin over bony prominences should be inspected daily for signs of breakdown. Skin abrasions and the development of decubitus ulcers should be avoided because wound healing may be retarded. Great care should be exercised when performing tasks that may damage the skin, such as removing the tape when discontinuing an intravenous infusion.

Body Image Disturbance. If the cause of the disorder can be eliminated, some or most of the physical changes may disappear with time. If the patient expresses concern over this problem, suggestions, such as the wearing of loose clothing, can be offered.

Altered Thought Processes. When they occur, the personality changes that may be seen with this disorder should be discussed with patient and family. Understanding that mood swings are part of the disorder may help the patient and family cope with the problem. If behavior changes, especially depression, become severe, the patient should be observed at frequent intervals, and the problem should be discussed with the physician. Psychiatric referral may be necessary.

Knowledge Deficit. If a cushingnoid appearance is caused by corticosteroid therapy, and the dose is to be tapered over a period of time, the patient requires a detailed explanation of the tapering schedule. The directions are printed on the prescription container but should be reviewed with the patient. The nurse can suggest using a calendar to write the dosage for each day of the tapering schedule. The entire tapering schedule can also be written on a card and each day crossed off. *The importance of strict adherence to the tapering schedule should be emphasized.*

Depending on many factors, such as age and severity of the disorder, those with Cushing's syndrome may or may not be scheduled for an adrenalectomy or removal or irradiation of the pituitary. Until such time as further treatment is scheduled, the importance of continued medical supervision should be emphasized. The following points can be included in a teaching plan:

1. Avoid trauma to the skin, contact the physician if sores or cuts do not heal or become infected or if easy bruising occurs.
2. Follow the diet recommended by the physician and read food labels carefully.
3. Avoid exposure to infection.
4. Do not use nonprescription drugs unless use has been approved by the physician.
5. Weigh self weekly and report marked weight gain or edema to the physician.

Evaluation

- Patient is able to tolerate some increase in activity
- Vital signs are normal; no evidence of infection
- Self-care needs are met
- No evidence of injury
- Skin remains intact
- Patient openly discusses methods of disguising physical changes
- No evidence of depression or other personality changes
- Patient demonstrates understanding of medical regimen, importance of good skin care, and avoiding infection

NURSING PROCESS —THE PATIENT UNDERGOING AN ADRENALECTOMY

An adrenalectomy may be performed for Cushing's syndrome and pheochromocytoma. Certain malignancies of the breast and prostate are under the control of hormones manufactured by endocrine glands, notably the ovaries and testes. To control metastasis, removal of the ovaries or testes reduces the hormonal effect of these glands. In some instances, removal of the gonads is not sufficient, and removal of the adrenal glands, which also secrete male and female hormones, is considered.

Preoperative Period

Assessment

A complete medical history, including a drug and allergy history, should be obtained. Vital signs should be taken, and blood pressure should be obtained on both arms with the patient standing, sitting, and lying.

Nursing Diagnosis

Depending on the diagnosis and reason for surgery, one or more of the following may apply:

- Anxiety related to impending surgery
- Knowledge deficit of preoperative and postoperative period

Planning and Implementation

The major goals of the patient may include reducing anxiety and understanding the preoperative and postoperative periods.

The major goal of nursing management is to prepare the patient physically and emotionally for surgery. If the patient has a pheochromocytoma, vital signs should be checked at frequent intervals during the preoperative period.

Additional nursing management is the same as for the patient having general surgery (see Chapter 16).

Anxiety, Knowledge Deficit. Anxiety may be reduced by briefly explaining the surgery, the necessary preparations for surgery, such as the shaving preparation, preoperative medications, and intravenous line. A brief explanation of the postoperative period, including the monitoring of vital signs and leg, coughing, deep-breathing exercises also should be given.

The patient with a pheochromocytoma is usually kept on bed rest, and anxiety-provoking events should be reduced to a minimum. The patient requiring surgery to halt the progression of a metastatic disease may have anxiety as well as depression and may need time to talk about the surgery and the anticipated results of surgery.

Evaluation

- Anxiety is reduced
- Patient demonstrates understanding of preoperative preparations and postoperative care

Postoperative Period

Assessment

Upon return from surgery, vital signs should be checked, and routine postoperative tasks, such as checking for a patent airway, should be carried out. The surgical record should be reviewed because the nursing diagnoses and postoperative observations and management depends on whether one or both adrenal glands were removed.

The patient should be closely observed for potential acute adrenal crisis (see previous section on acute adrenal crisis). Surgical removal of both adrenal glands is a *controlled* situation; therefore, these patients should not experience true adrenal cortical insufficiency because corticosteroid replacement is begun during and after surgery. Because the patient is experiencing the stress of surgery, however, the dose of the corticosteroid may require adjustment during this period. If symptoms of adrenal insufficiency occur, the physician should be notified immediately because an adjustment in the dose of the corticosteroid preparation may be necessary. *It must be remembered that corticosteroid replacement is absolutely essential to life.* The patient may experience adrenal crisis if the corticosteroid is omitted or the amount is insufficient to meet the needs of the body.

Surgical removal of one adrenal gland may not require corticosteroid replacement therapy. Even with one gland remaining, however, the patient may be a candidate for adrenal crisis if, for some reason, the remaining adrenal gland cannot supply a sufficient amount of corticosteroid hormone. Thus, these patients also should be observed for impending adrenal cortical insufficiency.

Nursing Diagnosis

Depending on the extent of surgery and the possible development of adrenal cortical insufficiency, one or more of the following may apply. Nursing diagnoses that apply to any surgical patient also may be added.

- Pain related to surgical incision
- Potential for infection related to surgical incision
- Potential for injury because of postural hypotension, weakness, and dizziness secondary to adrenal cortical insufficiency
- Knowledge deficit of postdischarge treatment regimen

Planning and Implementation

The major goals of the patient may include relief of pain, absence of infection, absence of injury, maintaining a normal body temperature, and understanding the postdischarge treatment regimen.

The major goals of nursing management are to recognize and prevent complications, maintain comfort, and develop an effective teaching plan.

The bilateral adrenalectomy patient must receive a corticosteroid drug to replace the hormones that are no longer supplied by the adrenal glands. During the immediate postoperative period, as well as throughout the patient's life, the dose may need to be adjusted to meet the body's needs.

During and after surgery, a corticosteroid is administered by the parenteral route. Once solid food is tolerated, the drug is given by the oral route. Because adrenal cortical insufficiency can lead to adrenal crisis, which is a life-threatening event, it is imperative that the prescribed corticosteroid drug *never be omitted.*

The patient with a unilateral adrenalectomy usually does not require hormone replacement because the remaining adrenal gland most probably will supply a sufficient amount of adrenal hormones.

Complications.   In addition to the complications that may be seen in any patient receiving a general anesthetic, the patient should be observed for problems such as hemorrhage, atelectasis, and pneumothorax because the adrenals are located close to the diaphragm and the inferior vena cava.

Vital signs should be monitored at frequent intervals, and the patient should be closely observed for signs of adrenal cortical insufficiency, which may occur in the following situations:

- When the prescribed dose of a corticosteroid preparation is not sufficient to meet the patient's individual needs (bilateral adrenalectomy)
- When the remaining adrenal gland (unilateral adrenalectomy) does not produce a sufficient amount of hormone to meet the patient's needs
- When the prescribed dose of a corticosteroid preparation is not given

Pain, Respiratory Function.   Analgesics should be administered as ordered. The patient's position should be changed every 2 hours, and deep-breathing, coughing, and leg exercises should be encouraged. Depending on the surgical approach, the patient with a bilateral adrenalectomy may have difficulty turning on either side. Firm support when turning is necessary.

The large incisions require firm support when the patient deep breathes and coughs. The lungs should be auscultated daily. Abnormal findings or failure of the patient to cough and deep breathe should be reported to the physician.

Potential for Infection.   A change in vital signs, purulent drainage on the dressing, or pain not controlled with analgesics should be brought to the attention of the physician. Once dressing changes are ordered to be performed by the nurse, the incision should be inspected at the time of each dressing change. Excessive redness, swelling of the suture line, or purulent drainage from the incision should be brought to the attention of the physician.

Potential for Injury.   Once allowed out of bed, the patient should be assisted with ambulatory activities and observed for weakness and dizziness. Although these symptoms may not be uncommon for 48 to 72 hours after surgery, continued episodes may be early signs of adrenal cortical insufficiency and require notifying the physician.

Knowledge Deficit.   The patient with an adrenalectomy requires detailed instruction in postdischarge management. The following areas may be covered in a teaching plan:

- The function of the adrenal glands and why they are necessary to life (which gives the patient insight into the importance of adhering to the prescribed treatment regimen)
- Care of the surgical incision until healed
- Medication schedule
- Importance of strict adherence to lifetime medication schedule, obtaining adequate rest, eating a well-balanced diet, ongoing medical supervision, avoiding infections, avoiding stressful situations, carrying identification indicating surgical removal of the adrenal glands

- Symptoms of adrenal insufficiency and adrenal crisis
- Contacting the physician if any of the following should occur: unable to take corticosteroid orally, diarrhea, fever, signs of adrenal insufficiency or crisis, any type of illness or stress

The patient with a unilateral adrenalectomy should be instructed in the care of the incision until healed. The importance of continued follow-up care, the symptoms of adrenal insufficiency, and the importance of seeing the physician if any of these symptoms occur should be emphasized.

Evaluation

- Pain is controlled
- No evidence of infection
- Respiratory function normal; lungs clear to auscultation; patient coughs and deep breathes effectively
- No evidence of complications
- No evidence of injury
- Vital signs normal
- Skin remains intact; surgical incisions show evidence of healing without complications
- Patient verbalizes understanding of medication schedule, incision care, signs of adrenal insufficiency, diet, and events requiring contacting the physician

DISORDERS OF THE OVARIES AND TESTES

Disorders associated with the female and male reproductive systems are covered in Chapters 50 and 51, respectively.

Diabetes Mellitus

The pancreas is both an endocrine and exocrine gland. The exocrine activity of the pancreas is discussed in Chapter 42.

Diabetes mellitus is a metabolic disorder of the pancreas in which glucose intolerance results from varying degrees of insulin insufficiency. Although no age group is exempt, diabetes is most frequently seen in people between ages 40 and 60.

The two major groups of diabetes mellitus are as follows:

Type I—Insulin-dependent diabetes mellitus (IDDM). Former names of this type of diabetes mellitus include juvenile diabetes, juvenile-onset diabetes, and brittle diabetes.

Type II—Non–insulin-dependent diabetes mellitus (NIDDM). Former names of this type of diabetes mellitus include maturity-onset diabetes, adult-onset diabetes, and stable diabetes.

Etiology

The exact cause of diabetes mellitus is unknown, but certain risk factors may play a role in the development of this disorder. Individuals at risk for developing diabetes mellitus include those with a family history of diabetes, overweight individuals, mothers giving birth to large infants, and individuals with premature manifestations of arteriosclerosis. It appears that the development of diabetes mellitus may involve a combination of factors rather than a single factor such as family history or obesity.

Pathology and Symptoms

A normal person has a fasting blood glucose level of 80 to 120 mg/dL of venous blood. Within about 30 minutes after eating, some of the ingested carbohydrate is digested and absorbed into the blood. The blood glucose level rises to about 150 mg/dL. Two hours after eating, the blood glucose has returned to its fasting level. In the liver and in muscle, glucose is converted to glycogen and stored. As the body needs fuel, the liver changes glycogen back to glucose and releases it into the bloodstream, where it becomes available to muscle and other body tissues as fuel for energy. Insulin is an important link in this process; it promotes the storage of glycogen in the liver, aids in the use of glucose by the tissues, and influences the metabolism of fats and proteins.

Insulin is secreted into the bloodstream by the β cells of the islets of Langerhans in the pancreas. Diabetics have less insulin available than their metabolic processes require. Because of inadequate insulin production, the ability of the liver to convert glucose to glycogen and the use of glucose by the tissues are impaired.

In diabetes mellitus, the fasting blood glucose content may be normal or elevated, but after eating it may rise to high levels (exceeding 150 mg/dL of blood).

The condition of excess glucose in the blood is called *hyperglycemia*. Some of the additional glucose in the blood is excreted by the kidneys. Glucose usually is found in the urine when the level rises over 180 mg/dL in the blood. This is called the renal threshold for glucose. The presence of glucose in the urine is called *glycosuria*.

To eliminate glucose, water also must be excreted. Therefore, one of the symptoms of untreated diabetes is *polyuria* (excessive urine). The patient complains of needing to urinate frequently and of passing a large amount each time. Because so much water has been lost in the urine, thirst (*polydipsia*) occurs, but the amount that the patient drinks is often not enough to compensate for water loss, and dehydration occurs.

While the needed glucose is being wasted, the body's requirement for fuel continues. The patient feels hungry and eats more (*polyphagia*). Hunger and weakness increases and weight is lost. To meet the rising need for energy, additional amounts of fats and proteins are metabolized.

Normally, when fat is metabolized, ketone bodies are formed in the liver and transported to muscle and other tissue, where they serve as a source of energy. *Ketone bodies* are chemical intermediate products in the metabolism of fat. In the process of serving as a source of energy, ketone bodies are oxidized to carbon dioxide and water. As more fat is metabolized, more ketone bodies are formed. The ketone bodies are β-hydroxybutyric acid, acetoacetic acid, and acetone (note that two of them are acids). All three are toxic if they accumulate in the body, a condition called *ketoacidosis*.

If ketone bodies are produced faster than they can be oxidized in tissues, they accumulate in tissues and body fluids. Ketone bodies are buffered by the bicarbonate buffer system. Thus, *ketonemia* (an increase in ketones in the blood) causes a decrease of plasma sodium, potassium, and alkali reserve. The loss of sodium and potassium salts in the urine further contributes to the development of acidosis. The carbon dioxide combining power of the blood is reduced, and the alkali reserve of the body is lowered, leading to further electrolyte imbalance. Chloride, particularly, is lost in the vomiting that accompanies acidosis, and sodium, potassium, and calcium also are wasted. The increased diuresis causes dehydration, which leads to diminution of the circulating blood volume and fall of the blood pressure. Air hunger (Kussmaul breathing) is common in ketoacidosis. Acetone, which is volatile, can be detected on the breath by its characteristic odor. If treatment is not given, the outcome is circulatory collapse, renal shutdown, and death. This complex is known as *diabetic coma* (though severe ketoacidosis can be present without the patient's being comatose).

Anything that causes glycogen depletion in the liver and therefore increases the need for oxidation of fat (eg, insulin deprivation, infection, surgery, anesthesia, vomiting) may result in an excess of ketone bodies. Infection and surgery invite ketosis and diabetic coma because they increase the demand for insulin that the diabetic's pancreas cannot deliver.

The metabolic situation is further complicated by overactivity of the anterior pituitary, the thyroid, and the adrenal cortex. The secretory activities of these glands may stimulate the formation of glucose, reduce the use of glucose, and therefore elevate blood glucose levels. Although these hormonal interrelations as they affect carbohydrate metabolism are not yet fully understood, indications are that diabetes is not merely an uncomplicated disease of the islets of Langerhans.

Diagnosis

Although diabetes mellitus is a highly complex disease, a diagnostic test for its detection is extremely simple. Normally, urine contains no easily detectable glucose or ketones; in this disease there may be both. Because glucose is not adequately used by the body, it is excreted in urine. If fats are metabolized faster than the body can use the ketone bodies, they will also appear in the urine. The relative ease of these urinary tests helps to facilitate case-finding programs for the early detection of diabetes. Because glucose in the urine is not always an indication of diabetes mellitus and because not all diabetics excrete glucose in the urine, blood glucose and glucose tolerance tests may be necessary to establish the diagnosis.

Urine Tests

Examples of materials used for testing the urine for glucose are Tes-Tape, Clinitest, and Diastix. Ketostix strips test the urine for ketones and Keto-Diastix checks the urine for glucose and ketones.

When a voided specimen is to be tested, it is important to test the *second voided specimen* because the first specimen voided may contain urine collected in the bladder for 7 or 8 hours (as, for example, the first voided specimen in the morning). In testing urine for glucose, it is essential that the test reflect the presence of glucose and ketones *at the moment*—not for the past several hours. The first specimen should be saved in case a second voided specimen cannot be produced. The patient should be encouraged to drink water and, about 30 minutes later, asked to void again so the second specimen can be tested. This procedure is essential if the dosage of insulin is based on the results of urine testing. When a patient has an indwelling catheter, it is essential *not* to take a specimen for testing from the drainage bag, because this urine may have been collected over a 6- to 8-hour period.

Testing for ketones becomes especially important when the patient has a fever, is vomiting, or consistently has glucose in the urine. In these situations, the chances for formation of ketone bodies are the greatest.

Blood Tests

A fasting blood glucose, or sugar (FBS), requires a single specimen of blood taken in the morning following about 8 hours of fasting. The normal range is 80 to 120 mg/dL. A postprandial glucose requires a single sample of blood taken 2 hours after the patient has eaten a high-carbohydrate meal. About 140 to 160 mg/dL are considered within the normal range.

An oral glucose tolerance test (OGTT) may be performed to confirm the diagnosis. A diet high in carbo-

electrolytes are determined. If the patient is comatose, the physician may order a catheterized urine specimen to be obtained and a retention catheter left in place for future specimens.

The main goals of treatment are (1) reduction of the elevated blood glucose, (2) correction of fluid and electrolyte imbalances, and (3) clearing the urine and blood of ketone bodies. To accomplish these goals, insulin must be given, usually by the intravenous route. Insulin reduces the production of ketones by making carbohydrates available for oxidation by the tissues and by restoring the liver's supply of glycogen. Regular insulin, added to an intravenous solution, should be given for its rapid effect. The number of units of insulin (regular insulin, regular Iletin) added to a specific volume of normal saline, electrolyte solution, or other intravenous solution, and the rate of infusion are ordered by the physician.

Depending on the severity of the disorder, periodic monitoring of serum electrolytes and blood glucose levels may be ordered. Urine should be tested for glucose and ketones at prescribed intervals.

Hyperosmolar Hyperglycemic Nonketotic Coma

Manifested by hyperglycemia and hyperosmolarity, hyperosmolar hyperglycemic nonketotic coma (HHNC) often occurs as a result of an event such as an acute illness. HHNC is more common in older diabetics, but it also may be seen in the nondiabetic with severe burns, renal dialysis, or total parenteral nutrition.

Because of persistent hyperglycemia, fluid moves from the intracellular compartment to the extracellular compartment. Diuresis occurs, and there is a loss of sodium and potassium. Ketoacidosis is rarely present.

Symptoms
Symptoms include hypotension, mental changes, dehydration, and fever. Neurologic signs may include seizures and coma. Symptoms of hypokalemia and hyponatremia are usually present.

Diagnosis
Diagnosis is made by patient history and laboratory tests. Blood glucose levels may be exceedingly high and serum potassium and sodium levels low.

Treatment
Treatment includes the administration of insulin and correction of fluid and electrolyte imbalances. A central venous pressure line may be inserted to monitor fluid balance, and electrocardiographic monitoring

may used to detect early signs of dysrhythmia associated with hyperkalemia.

Hyperinsulinism (Hypoglycemia)

When there is too much insulin (hyperinsulinism) in the bloodstream in relation to the amount of available glucose—in other words, when the blood glucose level falls below about 60 mg/dL of blood—hypoglycemia results. This is sometimes referred to as an *insulin reaction*. Hypoglycemia is as much a medical emergency as is diabetic ketoacidosis.

Symptoms
The pattern of symptoms varies somewhat from patient to patient, depending on the degree of hypoglycemia, the patient's individual reaction, and sometimes the type of insulin taken.

Initial symptoms may include weakness, headache, nausea, drowsiness, nervousness, hunger, tremors, a feeling of malaise, and excessive perspiration. Some patients have characteristic personality changes. One may become negative; another, weepy. Confusion, aphasia, delirium, and vertigo may occur. If hypoglycemia is not corrected, symptoms may progress to difficulty with coordination, and the patient may have double vision. If still untreated, there may be convulsions, and the patient become unconscious; if the condition is neglected further, the patient may suffer permanent brain damage. Death has been known to occur from severe hypoglycemia.

Although symptoms vary, they have a tendency to be repeated in the same person whenever there is too much insulin and too little food. The sequence may be extremely rapid, with the patient convulsing or becoming unconscious before other symptoms are recognized.

When a diabetic is found unconscious, the patient may have diabetic ketoacidosis *or* hypoglycemia (hyperinsulinism). These conditions are direct opposites; in ketoacidosis the blood glucose is too high, in hypoglycemia it is too low. Although the physician makes the diagnosis and prescribes the treatment, nurses and patients should be familiar with the symptoms of both hypoinsulinism and hyperinsulinism so that these can be recognized in their early stages (Table 48-3).

Diagnosis
Diagnosis is based on symptoms, patient history, and blood glucose level. The patient history also is important in differentiating between diabetic ketoacidosis (DKA) and hyperinsulinism. If the patient has had insulin and has not eaten, it is most likely that hyperinsulinism is present. If the patient has eaten and has

Table 48–3. Symptoms of Hypoinsulinism and Hyperinsulinism

	Hypoinsulinism	*Hyperinsulinism*
History	Insufficient or omitted insulin	Excessive insulin
	Intercurrent infection	Unusual exercise
	Dietary indiscretion	Too little food
	Gastrointestinal upset	
Onset	Slow, hours to days	Sudden, minutes
Skin	Flushed, dry, hot	Pale, moist, cool
Behavior	Drowsy	Excited
Breath	Acetone	Normal
Respirations	Air hunger	Normal to rapid, shallow
Pulse	Rapid, weak	Normal or slow; full, bounding
Blood pressure	Low	Normal
Vomiting	Present	May be absent
Hunger	Absent	Often present
Thirst	Present	Absent
Urinary sugar	Large amounts	Absent in second specimen
Response to treatment	Slow	Rapid

(Adapted from Lilly Research Laboratories. Diabetes mellitus.)

not taken or received insulin, it is most likely DKA is present.

Treatment

The treatment for a hypoglycemic reaction is the administration of a quick-acting carbohydrate. If the patient is conscious and able to swallow, orange juice, candy, warm tea or coffee with sugar, a cola beverage, honey, or a dextrose solution should be given. If the patient is unconscious, dextrose should be given intravenously. Whenever there is a diabetic on the unit, there should always be some orange juice in the refrigerator and some intravenous dextrose available. In a severe reaction, the patient may need repeated feedings before the symptoms are relieved. The physician may order glucagon to increase the patient's alertness and to stimulate the liver to release some of its store of glycogen.

Vascular Disturbances

Diabetics are particularly prone to circulatory disturbances. The incidence of arteriosclerosis in diabetics is higher than in nondiabetics, and there are many vascular changes in diabetics, some of which are not seen in nondiabetics, and some of which become more severe when the metabolic aspects of the disease are poorly controlled. An almost consistent finding in dia-

betic patients is thickening of the walls of some capillaries, arterioles, and venules. Coronary artery disease and increased cholesterol levels also appear to have a higher incidence in diabetics.

Any part of the body can be affected by vascular disturbances, but nerves (diabetic neuropathy), the retina of the eye (diabetic retinopathy), kidneys, and legs are particularly likely to be affected. The lower extremities are especially vulnerable to changes brought about by decreased blood supply to the tissues. Because of lessened blood supply, cramps may occur; infection is not fought effectively and may lead to ulcer formation and eventually to gangrene (Fig. 48-3), which may necessitate amputation. Surgery is an added strain on the body, and the surgeon and internist must work together to regulate the patient's diabetes during the period of extra stress. Uncontrolled diabetes frequently retards wound healing.

Visual Problems

In diabetics, the retinal capillaries tend to develop multiple tiny aneurysms, accompanied by small points of hemorrhage and by exudates. These hemorrhages may be treated with laser therapy, which seals off the retinal blood vessel. The scarring resulting from repeated hemorrhages may eventually cause blindness.

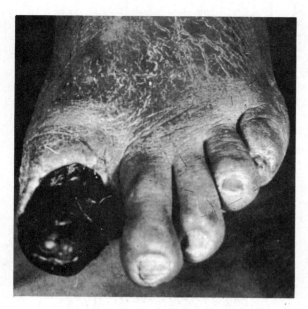

Figure 48–3. Gangrene of toe. (Dr. W. L. Lowrie, Detroit)

The incidence of cataracts also is higher in diabetic patients.

Neuropathy

Any nerve tissue can be affected. There may be facial paralysis, atony of the urinary bladder, diarrhea, or constipation. The legs are most frequently affected. The patient may experience itching and intense heat and can be burned without realizing it.

Other Problems

Insulin lipoatrophy, which is atrophy of subcutaneous fat, is common reaction to repeated insulin injections into the same area. It causes deep depressions of the skin and gives an undesirable cosmetic appearance. Lipohypertrophy, which is spongy, painless swelling occurring for the same reason as lipoatrophy, also is unsightly. Insulin is poorly absorbed when injected into such damaged tissue.

A risk associated with the oral hypoglycemic drugs is that some patients underestimate the seriousness of diabetes mellitus, fail to remain under medical supervision, or neglect diet, foot care, or urine testing. They may erroneously believe that the disorder can be ignored because taking a pill is so much simpler than the injections taken by others with the same diagnosis.

Poor regulation of carbohydrate metabolism, with the dangers of diabetic ketoacidosis on one hand and of hypoglycemia on the other, may be brought about by ignorance or carelessness on the part of the patient, by an infection, or by extreme emotional stress.

Noncompliance is another problem associated with the disorder. Some patients simply refuse to follow, for any number of reasons, their treatment regimen.

NURSING PROCESS —THE PATIENT WHO HAS DIABETES MELLITUS

Assessment
HISTORY. A complete medical, drug, and allergy history and a list of all symptoms should be obtained. The history should include information regarding the length of time diabetes has been present and a family history of diabetes. If the patient is a known diabetic, the prescribed treatment regimen should be recorded. It also is important to know if any complications associated with diabetes have occurred and the treatment instituted for each.

PHYSICAL EXAMINATION. The patient should be weighed, and a complete head-to-toe physical examination should be performed because diabetes affects many systems. The examiner should look for any changes that may be the result of diabetes, including the following:

Skin—Changes in the skin over insulin injection sites (if insulin is used as part of treatment), skin breaks that appear to be healing poorly, presence of ulcerations or evidence of infection

Cardiovascular—Vital signs, peripheral pulses, temperature of the extremities, inspection of the extremities for edema or changes in color

Eyes—Visual acuity should be determined and the patient questioned regarding any changes in vision

Neuromuscular—Examination for muscle atrophy, weakness, or loss of sensation

Nursing Diagnosis
The extent of the nursing diagnoses depends on factors such as whether the patient is a new diabetic, has had treatment for diabetes, or has not followed the prescribed medical regimen. The presence of complications may require additional diagnoses.

- Anxiety and fear related to diagnosis (new diabetic), complications of diabetes (if present)
- Potential impaired adjustment related to inability to accept diagnosis, treatment regimen
- Noncompliance to treatment regimen related to lack of knowledge, misunderstanding, or complexity of prescribed treatment program, other factors (specify)
- Altered health maintenance related to lack of knowledge, other factors
- Acute or chronic pain related to vascular complications
- Altered nutrition: more than body requirements re-

lated to failure to adhere to prescribed diet, decrease in exercise or activity pattern, change in insulin or oral hypoglycemic drug needs, other factors (specify)

■ Altered nutrition: less than body requirements related to failure to eat, change in exercise or activity pattern, change in insulin or oral hypoglycemic needs, other factors (specify)
■ Fluid volume deficit related to polyuria secondary to hyperglycemia
■ Impaired skin integrity related to susceptibility to infection, poor wound healing, hyperglycemia, pruritus secondary to vascular disturbances
■ Potential for infection related to depressed phagocytosis secondary to hyperglycemia
■ Potential for injury related to vascular complications, neuropathy, changes in visual acuity
■ Sexual dysfunction related to peripheral neuropathy
■ Knowledge deficit of prescribed treatment regimen

Planning and Implementation

The major goals of the patient may include a reduction of anxiety, adjustment to an acceptance of the diagnosis and treatment regimen, relief of pain and discomfort, adequate nutrition, correction of a fluid volume deficit, prevention of skin breakdown, absence of infection, absence of injury, ability to discuss sexual dysfunction with the appropriate individuals, and understanding of and compliance with the prescribed treatment regimen.

The major goals of nursing management are to attain a normal blood glucose, prevent complications, and develop an effective teaching program. Nursing management should be individualized and based on information obtained during assessment.

It is the nurse's responsibility to safeguard the hospitalized patient by ensuring the correct timing of insulin injection and meals. This is one medication that must always be given on time. If the patient is fasting for a blood glucose or glucose tolerance test, or does not eat for any other reason, a rapid-acting insulin should not be given until 15 to 30 minutes before the regular meal is served. Exact timing is most important with this type of insulin.

Diabetic Ketoacidosis. If the patient is comatose, the airway must be kept patent, and the oral cavity suctioned as necessary. Intravenous infusions are closely monitored, and vital signs taken at frequent intervals. It is especially important to note and keep the physician informed of the patient's response, or lack of response, to therapy.

Hyperinsulinism. The nurse should stay with the patient while administering treatment for hypoglycemia. The regulation of glucose metabolism is difficult for about 24 hours; therefore, the patient should be observed at frequent intervals for further episodes of hyperinsulinism.

The nurse may prevent hyperinsulinism in the hospitalized patient by doing the following:

■ Seeing that the meal is served within 30 minutes after regular insulin is administered
■ Informing the physician immediately if nausea, vomiting, or diarrhea occurs or if the patient refuses to eat
■ Seeing that the prescribed diet and between-meal or bedtime snacks are offered and eaten
■ Administering the correct type and dose of insulin at the prescribed times

Insulin Administration. Insulin may be administered in several ways. One method is the use of a needle and syringe. Use of the microfine needles has reduced the discomfort associated with an injection. Another method is the jet injection system, which uses pressure to deliver a fine stream of insulin below the skin. Another method uses a disposable needle and special syringe. The syringe uses a cartridge that is prefilled with a specific type of insulin (regular human insulin, isophane [NPH] insulin, or a mixture of isophane and regular insulin). The number of desired units are then selected by turning a dial and then locking the ring.

Another method of insulin delivery is the insulin pump, which is intended for a select group of individuals, such as the pregnant diabetic with early long-term complications and those with or candidates for renal transplantation. This system attempts to mimic the body's normal pancreatic function, uses only regular insulin, is battery-powered, and requires insertion of a needle into subcutaneous tissue. The needle is changed every 1 to 3 days. The amount of insulin injected can be adjusted according to blood glucose monitoring, which is usually done 4 to 8 times per day.

Anxiety and Fear. The new diabetic may experience varying degrees of anxiety and fear over events such as the diagnosis, ability to carry out the prescribed therapeutic regimen, or the need to give injections. On the other hand, disorders occurring as a complication of diabetes may cause severe anxiety or depression. Fear of needed treatment, such as an amputation necessary to treat advanced vascular disturbances, or fear of possible future complications also can cause emotional disturbances.

The newly diagnosed diabetic needs time to talk about the disorder, express concerns, and ask questions. An effective teaching program helps relieve some of the anxiety seen in the new diabetic as apprehension in those with complications associated with the disorder.

Potential Impaired Adjustment, Noncompliance, Altered Health Maintenance. The new diabetic may have difficulty accepting the diagnosis, and the apparent complexity of the therapeutic regimen can seem overwhelming. Before patients can be expected to learn to carry out treatment, they must accept the fact that they have diabetes, and then deal with their own feelings about having the disorder. The nurse has an important role in helping these patients gradually accept the diagnosis and begin to understand their feelings about it. Understanding diabetes may help patients work with physicians and other medical personnel in managing their diabetes.

Noncompliance is a problem with some diabetics. An occasional lapse in adherence to the prescribed diet occurs in most patients, as for example around holidays or other special occasions. This slip may not cause a problem if it is brief, not excessive, and there is an immediate return to the prescribed regimen. On the other hand, there are those who frequently stray from the prescribed regimen, take extra insulin to cover dietary indiscretions, fast for several days before follow-up blood glucose determinations, and engage in other dangerous behaviors.

While some patients can be convinced that failure to adhere to the prescribed treatment regimen is detrimental to their health, others continue to deviate from the prescribed regimen until a serious complication develops. The nurse must make every effort to stress the importance of adherence to the prescribed treatment during the initial teaching session as well as during follow-up office or clinic visits.

Pain. Some diabetics have mild to advanced peripheral vascular complications that may cause varying degrees of pain. Information regarding the type of pain the patient has should be obtained during the initial assessment and should form a database for future comparisons.

Vascular complications can be serious and even life-threatening. In some instances, the patient may require analgesics for relief of pain. The patient with vascular complications should be assessed at frequent intervals for the type and amount of pain, the relief of pain after administration of an analgesic, any changes in the appearance of the extremities, and any change in the quality of peripheral pulses, all of which should be reported to the physician.

Altered Nutrition. Various factors can change the patient's nutritional needs, and the diet or drug therapy (insulin, oral hypoglycemic) may require adjustment. Hypoglycemia and hyperglycemia must be avoided. The brittle diabetic—one who is difficult to keep normoglycemic—requires close supervision.

The hospitalized patient, especially the new or brittle diabetic, should be watched closely at the appropriate times after insulin administration (see Table 48-2 for onset and peak insulin levels) and after meals. The meal tray also should be checked to make sure that the patient has eaten all the food because the diet is calculated according to individual requirements as well as the insulin dose.

Fluid Volume Deficit. The new diabetic or the diabetic with DKA or HHNC may be dehydrated and may have one or more electrolyte imbalances. Intake and output should be measured, and the patient should be observed for signs of dehydration and electrolyte imbalances. When intravenous fluids are administered, the infusion rate should be closely monitored. Laboratory monitoring of electrolytes is usually necessary, and the nurse should keep the physician informed of the patient's response to treatment.

If the patient is able to take oral fluids, the patient should be encouraged to drink fluids and sufficient water should be kept at the bedside.

Impaired Skin Integrity, Potential for Infection. The diabetic is susceptible to infection, especially infection of the skin and subcutaneous tissues. Wounds, including surgical incisions, heal poorly, and minor infections or breaks in the skin may take a long time to heal.

The skin should be inspected daily and any breaks, changes in color or temperature, pruritus, infection, or evidence of poor healing should be brought to the attention of the physician. This is especially important when the diabetic has surgery, vascular complications, or is on prolonged bed rest.

The skin should be kept dry. The incontinent patient or the patient with profuse diaphoresis requires special attention. After bathing or care for incontinence, the skin should be patted dry. Special attention should be given to folds or creases in the skin and to the groin and axillary areas. Excessive use of powders should be avoided because perspiration cakes the material, and irritation may result. In addition, skin creases and folds are subject to fungal infections if not kept dry.

Potential for Injury. The diabetic with complications (peripheral neuropathy, retinal hemorrhages, cataracts) may have difficulty seeing or moving and is therefore subject to falls and other types of injuries. The patient should be instructed to ask for assistance when getting out of bed.

Diabetic neuropathy may result in a loss of sensation in the extremities. The patient may not feel intense heat and can be burned without realizing it. Bath and shower water should be checked before use, and heating or warming devices should be applied with care and checked at frequent intervals.

Sexual Dysfunction. Sexual problems occur more commonly in the male diabetic. If the patient indicates a problem with relations with the sexual partner, general questions may be asked to identify the problem. The information should then be discussed with the physician. Sexual counseling may be necessary in some cases.

Knowledge Deficit. One of the most important roles of the nurse is to work with members of the medical team in formulating and instituting a teaching plan. Some hospitals use a diabetic teaching team comprised of nurses and dietitians whose sole purpose is to teach patients. Individualized or group sessions may be used for teaching.

The extent of the teaching program depends on whether the patient has been a diabetic for a period of time or is a new diabetic. It must be remembered that even those who have had the disorder for years may have developed false ideas about their disorder as well as the treatment regimen.

Before teaching begins, the nurse should confer with the physician to determine the following:

- Type of diet to be prescribed
- Medication regimen (insulin or oral hypoglycemic agent)
- Materials to be used for insulin administration, such as needle and syringe, an insulin injection device such as NovolinPen, the Medi-Jector EZ (which uses pressure to inject a stream of insulin below the skin), or an insulin pump
- Materials (brand name) to be used for urine testing and whether urine is tested for glucose or glucose and ketones
- Frequency of urine testing
- Monitoring of blood glucose levels
- Additional information to be presented, such as skin care, signs of DKA or hyperinsulinism, and how to terminate hypoglycemia

Teaching is most effective when done in small steps, allowing the patient time to understand the material. Teaching should begin by explaining diabetes, what it is, why treatment is necessary, and the various methods of treatment. It should be stressed that treatment is highly individualized. The treatment of one person cannot be compared with that of another.

One of the easiest things to learn is urine testing. Once the patient understands how to perform this task, teaching can progress to the next step. Audiovisual materials (video tapes, booklets, drawings) enhance learning and should be used whenever possible. A chart showing the rotation of injection sites helps in selecting areas to be used for the injection of insulin.

Evaluation

Depending on the individual patient, one or more of the following may apply:.

- Anxiety is reduced
- Blood glucose levels are normal
- Patient demonstrates positive outlook and adjustment to diagnosis
- Patient verbalizes willingness to comply to the prescribed treatment regimen
- Discomfort is controlled or eliminated
- Electrolytes are within the normal range
- No evidence of dehydration
- Patient eats the prescribed diet
- Skin remains intact; no evidence of infection, skin breakdown
- No evidence of injury
- Patient openly discusses sexual problems with the appropriate individuals
- Patient demonstrates understanding of the information presented in teaching sessions
- Patient is able to test own urine, give own insulin injections

General Nutritional Considerations

☐ It is important to satisfy the need for food of the patient with a severely overactive thyroid. The patient with a less severe form of this disorder should also eat a high-calorie, high-carbohydrate diet.

☐ Before blood is drawn for some thyroid tests, the patient should not have ingested iodine or consumed large amounts of seafood for several weeks before the test is scheduled.

☐ The following foods are usually excluded from a diabetic diet: sugar, candy, honey, jam, jelly, marmalade, preserves, syrup, molasses, pie, cake, cookies, condensed milk, chewing gum, and soft drinks.

☐ The following foods are usually unrestricted in a diabetic diet: unsweetened gelatin, clear and fat-free broth, unsweetened pickles, cranberries, rhubarb, coffee, tea, and certain salads.

☐ Alcohol has a high caloric value. Any alcohol consumed is counted in the total diabetic diet. A large intake of alcohol is not advised because the high caloric value adds greatly to the amount of calories in the prescribed diet, thus reducing the permissible intake of foods necessary for adequate nutrition.

General Pharmacologic Considerations

☐ Substances containing iodine, such as some cough medicines and dyes administered for radiographs of the gallbladder, intravenous pyelograms, and bronchograms, cause errors in some thyroid tests.

☐ The adverse effects associated with the administration of a thyroid preparation are rare, but the patient may experience symptoms of overdose that are the same as the symptoms of hyperthyroidism.

☐ The most serious adverse effect of antithyroid drugs is agranulocytosis.

☐ The dose of an antithyroid preparation may need to be decreased or increased over a period of time until the optimal dose is attained. Certain situations such as severe illness and stress may require a change in dosage.

☐ Three properties of insulin—onset, peak, and duration—are of importance. *Onset* is when the insulin first begins to act in the body; *peak* is the time when insulin is exerting maximum action; and *duration* is the length of time the insulin remains in effect.

☐ Oral hypoglycemic agents are usually used to treat those who can be controlled on 40 or fewer units of insulin per day.

☐ The measurement of insulin *must* be accurate because patients may be sensitive to minute dose changes. The patient should be checked for signs of hypoglycemia after the insulin is given, at the expected onset, and again at the peak of action.

☐ Hospital policy dictates the actions to be taken when a patient taking insulin or an oral hypoglycemic agent experiences hypoglycemia. Most hospitals approve of the administration of oral glucose (fruit juice, Karo syrup and water, ginger ale, etc.) if the patient can *safely* swallow. The unconscious or semiconscious patient requires intravenous administration of 50% dextrose or glucagon.

☐ Oral hypoglycemic agents also must be given at the time of day ordered. The patient receiving these drugs also is observed for signs of hypoglycemia; however, the time when the reaction might occur is not predictable and could be from 30 to 60 minutes to many hours after the drug is given.

General Gerontologic Considerations

☐ Diabetes mellitus is especially prevalent among the elderly. Many older diabetics can learn to care for themselves if they are given sufficient time, instruction, and help in overcoming disabilities of age.

☐ Although it is useful for a family member to learn how to care for the elderly person with diabetes, excluding the patient from instruction and concentrating on teaching a family member should be avoided unless it is clear that the patient cannot assume responsibility for his or her own treatment.

☐ Some elderly patients experience difficulty in administering their insulin because of problems such as decreased visual acuity or arthritis. The nurse must evaluate the patient's ability to self-administer insulin before a teaching program is developed.

☐ A variety of aids (eg, a magnifier that fits over the syringe) are available for those experiencing difficulty in preparing insulin for injection.

☐ The elderly patient newly diagnosed as having diabetes mellitus may experience difficulty in conforming to the medical and dietary regimen required of the diabetic patient.

☐ The elderly patient often requires expanded instruction in the dietary regimen prescribed by the physician.

☐ The eating and sleeping habits of the elderly patient are often different from those of the young or middle-aged patient and must be taken into consideration when planning meals and selecting the proper type and dosage of insulin or oral hypoglycemic agent.

☐ During dietary instruction, the nurse or dietitian must discuss with the patient the ability to obtain certain types of foods, such as fresh vegetables, meat, and so on. Patients who live in areas where (for them) food shopping is limited to convenience-type foods may have their prescribed diets adjusted accordingly.

☐ The elderly patient taking an oral hypoglycemic agent requires the same detailed instruction for management of diabetes as the patient requiring insulin.

Suggested Readings

☐ Berkow R, Fletcher AJ, eds. Merck manual of diagnosis and therapy. 15th ed. Rahway, NJ: Merck and Co, 1987. *(In-depth coverage of subject matter)*

☐ Cerrato PL. What every diabetic patient needs to know. RN May 1987;50:73. *(Additional coverage of subject matter)*

☐ Fischbach FT. A manual of laboratory diagnostic tests. 3rd ed. Philadelphia: JB Lippincott, 1988. *(Additional coverage of subject matter)*

☐ Gavin JR. Diabetes and exercise. Am J Nurs February 1988;88:178. *(Additional coverage of subject matter)*

☐ Hernandez C. Surgery and diabetes: minimizing the risks. Am J Nurs June 1987;87:788. *(Additional coverage of subject matter)*

☐ Hughes B. Diabetes management: the time is right for tight glucose control. Nursing '87 May 1987;17:63. *(Additional coverage of subject matter)*

☐ Hurxthal K. Quick! Teach this patient about insulin. Am J Nurs August 1988;88:1097. *(Additional coverage of subject matter)*

☐ Huzar JG, Cerrato PL. The role of diet and drugs. RN April 1989;52:46. *(Additional coverage and illustrations that reinforce subject matter)*

☐ Huzar JG. Diabetes now: preventing acute complications. RN August 1989;52:34. *(Additional coverage of subject matter)*

☐ Karch AN, Boyd EH. Handbook of drugs and the nursing process. Philadelphia: JB Lippincott, 1988. *(In-depth coverage of subject matter)*

☐ Lockhart JS, Griffin CW. Action stat! Tetany. Nursing '88 August 1988; 18:33. *(Additional coverage of subject matter)*

☐ Lumley W. Controlling hypoglycemia and hyperglycemia. Nursing '88 October 1988;18:34. *(Additional coverage of subject matter)*

☐ Lumley WA. Reversing and recognizing insulin shock. Nursing '89 December 1989;19:34. *(Additional coverage of subject matter)*

☐ Luckmann J, Sorensen K. Medical–surgical nursing: a psychophysioloigic approach. 3rd ed. Philadelphia: WB Saunders, 1987. *(Additional and in-depth coverage of subject matter)*

☐ Mackowiak L, McCarthy R. Managing diabetes on "sick days." Am J Nurs July 1989;89:950. *(Additional coverage of subject matter)*

☐ Malseed R, Harrigan GS. Textbook of pharmacology and nursing care: using the nursing process. 2nd ed. Philadelphia: JB Lippincott, 1988. *(Additional and in-depth coverage of subject matter)*

☐ McFarland MB, Grant MM. Nursing implicationms of laboratory tests. 2nd ed. New York: John Wiley & Sons, 1988. *(Additional and in-depth coverage of subject matter)*

☐ Metheny NM. Fluid and electrolyte balance: nursing considerations. Philadelphia: JB Lippincott, 1987. *(Additional and in-depth coverage of subject matter)*

☐ Moore MC. Pocket guide to nutrition and diet therapy. St Louis: CV Mosby, 1988. *(Additional and in-depth coverage of subject matter)*

☐ Nath C, Murray S, Ponte C. Lessons in living with type II diabetes mellitus. Nursing '88 August 1988;18:45. *(Additional coverage of subject matter)*

☐ Orshan SA. The pill, the patient, and you. RN July 1988;51:49. *(Additional coverage of subject matter)*

☐ Robertson C. Coping with chronic complications. RN September 1989;52:34. *(Additional coverage of subject matter)*

☐ Robertson C. Diabetes now: the new challanges of insulin therapy. RN May 1989;52:34. *(Additional coverage of subject matter)*

☐ Robertson C. When the patient is also a diabetic. RN July 1987;50:33. *(Additional coverage of subject matter)*

☐ Sabo CE, Michael SR. Managing DKA and preventing recurrence. Nursing '89 February 1989;19:50. *(Additional coverage of subject matter)*

☐ Sarsany SL. Thyroid storm. RN July 1988;51:46. *(Additional coverage of subject matter)*

☐ Tomky D. A three-pronged approach to monitoring. RN March 1989;52:24. *(Additional coverage and illustrations that reinforce subject matter)*

☐ Tomly D. Tapping the full power of insulin pumps. RN June 1989;52:46. *(Additional coverage and illustrations that reinforce subject matter)*

☐ Wozniak L. Your teaching plan: the key to controlling type II diabetes. RN August 1988;51:29. *(Additional coverage and illustrations that reinforce subject matter)*

Disturbances of Sexual Structures or Reproductive Function

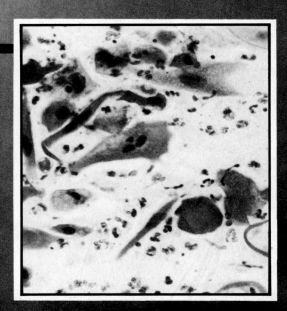

Unit 12

Chapter 49

Introduction to the Female and Male Reproductive Systems and Related Structures

On completion of this chapter the reader will:

- Be familiar with the basic anatomy and physiology of the female and male reproductive systems

- List and discuss the diagnostic tests used in the evaluation of the female and male reproductive systems

- Use the nursing process to prepare a patient for tests that diagnose disorders of the female or male reproductive system

ANATOMY AND PHYSIOLOGY OF THE FEMALE REPRODUCTIVE SYSTEM

The onset of puberty is characterized by breast development, redistribution of body fat, the growth of pubic and axillary hair, and the beginnings of menstruation. *Menarche*, which is the start of menstruation, usually occurs between ages 10 and 14.

The female reproductive system (Fig. 49-1) consists of two ovaries, two fallopian tubes, the uterus, and the vagina. The external female genitalia (Fig. 49-2) consist of the vaginal orifice (opening), the labia majora, the labia minora, and the clitoris. The two ovaries lie behind and slightly below the ends of the fallopian tubes. Each ovary contains thousands of ova (eggs).

The hormones of the anterior pituitary are shown in Figure 47-2 in Chapter 47. The influence of anterior pituitary hormones on the menstrual cycle is shown in Figure 49-3. Under the influence of the follicle-stimulating hormone (FSH) of the anterior pituitary, the ovarian follicle matures. With the release of a second pituitary hormone, the luteinizing hormone (LH), the mature follicle ruptures, discharging the ovum, which is drawn into the end of the fallopian tube. This process is called *ovulation* and occurs about every 28 days during the period between menarche and the menopause. After the ovum is released, the ruptured follicle is transformed into a small body filled with yellow fluid (*corpus luteum*).

Normally, the ovum meets a spermatozoon (sperm) in the fallopian tube and is fertilized. After fertilization, the ovum moves down to the uterus and implants itself in the endometrium, which is prepared to receive it. If fertilization does not occur, the ovum passes through the uterus and vagina and is expelled from the body.

Whether the ovum is fertilized or not, the endometrium, a highly vascular glandular tissue lining the inside of the uterus, prepares itself for a possible pregnancy during each menstrual cycle. The development of the uterine endometrium is governed by the hormone estrogen, produced by the maturing ovarian follicle. The follicle is under the influence of FSH. Estrogen production is, in turn, probably regulated by LH. After the follicle has ruptured, the corpus luteum produces another hormone, progesterone. This hormone stimulates a change in the endometrium, making it richer and thicker in preparation for a possible fertilized ovum. The pituitary production of FSH is inhibited at this point.

If the ovum is not fertilized, the prepared endometrium degenerates, and the menstrual flow begins about 2 weeks after ovulation. After menstruation, the endometrium again begins to grow thicker and more vascular. Because of these cyclical, hormone-dependent changes, the microscopic picture of the uterus is changing almost constantly. Thus, it is important that

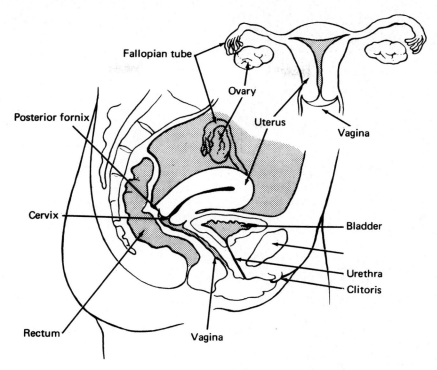

Figure 49-1. Anatomy of female reproductive organs.

each gynecologic specimen sent to the laboratory (eg, vaginal smears or scrapings obtained by curettage of the uterus) be marked with the date of the beginning of the patient's last menstrual period.

When conception occurs, the corpus luteum persists during early pregnancy. When conception does not occur, the corpus luteum degenerates and shrinks, and the thickened endometrium sheds its outer layers with bleeding. Menstrual flow usually lasts 4 to 5 days, with a normal loss of 30 to 180 mL of blood. Women who have a heavy menses may lose more blood.

PHYSIOLOGY OF THE BREAST

The breast is a complicated glandular organ that produces milk after pregnancy. Considerable space in the breast is devoted to a network of ducts that carry milk to the nipple. The area has an abundant supply of lymphatics and blood vessels. Axillary lymph nodes and the internal mammary lymph nodes drain the breasts.

The breast manufactures milk from elements in the blood. The transformation of amino acids and glucose in the blood into the proteins and lactose in milk is a chemical process not yet fully understood. To make 30 mL of milk, it has been estimated that the breast must process 12,000 mL of blood.

Although the most dramatic changes occur in the breast during preparation for its primary function, lactation, the mammary glands are a part of the female reproductive system, and, thus, they respond to the hormonal cycle associated with menstruation. Estrogen secreted by the ovaries brings about the growth and development of the duct systems and suppresses lactation. Progesterone secreted by the corpus luteum

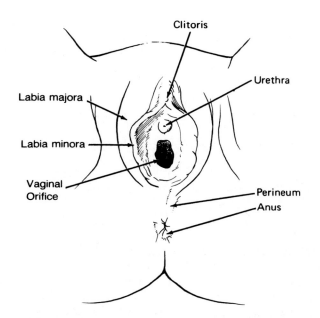

Figure 49-2. Diagram of female external genitalia.

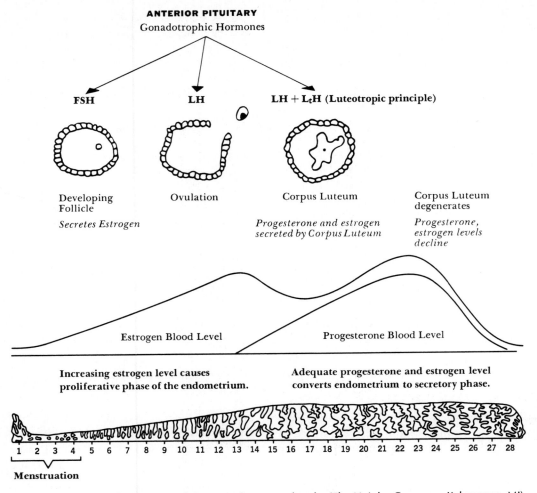

ANTERIOR PITUITARY
Gonadotrophic Hormones

FSH   **LH**   **LH + L$_t$H (Luteotropic principle)**

Developing   Ovulation   Corpus Luteum   Corpus Luteum
Follicle   degenerates

Secretes Estrogen   *Progesterone and estrogen*   *Progesterone,*
                                       secreted by Corpus Luteum   *estrogen levels*
                                                                       decline

Estrogen Blood Level   Progesterone Blood Level

Increasing estrogen level causes   **Adequate progesterone and estrogen level**
proliferative phase of the endometrium.   **converts endometrium to secretory phase.**

1 2 3 4 5 6 7 8 9 10 11 12 13 14 15 16 17 18 19 20 21 22 23 24 25 26 27 28

Menstruation

Figure 49–3.   Simplified version of the normal menstrual cycle. (The Upjohn Company, Kalamazoo, MI)

of the ovary stimulates lactation, as does the hormone prolactin.

ASSESSMENT OF THE PATIENT WHO HAS A DISORDER OF THE FEMALE REPRODUCTIVE SYSTEM AND RELATED STRUCTURES

Patient History

A thorough patient history is obtained and includes the following:

- A general health history
- A drug and allergy history
- Symptoms of present disorder and length of time present
- Pregnancy history: number of pregnancies, number of live births, number of stillborn births
- Abortion history (therapeutic, spontaneous, habitual)
- A family history of disorders that may be related to the patient's disorder, including a history of cancer

- Prior treatments (including drug therapy) or surgery for a gynecologic disorder (if any)
- Age of onset of menses (the menarche)
- Description of the menstrual pattern and flow, other symptoms associated with menstruation
- Age of menopause, symptoms associated with menopause (if applicable)

Physical Examination

Physical examination of the patient is performed almost always by a physician. Clinical nurse specialists may be assigned to perform certain examinations, such as examining the breasts and obtaining cervical smears. The nurse may be responsible for obtaining vital signs and the patient's weight as well as preparing the patient for examination.

Gynecologic Examination

The order in which the physician performs a pelvic examination varies. The physician usually begins the examination by observation of the external genitalia and adjacent structures. The vaginal wall and the cervix of the uterus are then visualized after insertion of a bivalve speculum. Next, the physician places one or two fingers of a gloved hand into the vagina. By palpation, the structures beyond the vaginal orifice are examined. The physician then performs the vaginal–abdominal examination. Without removing gloved fingers from the vagina, the fingers of the other hand are placed on the patient's lower abdomen. Between two hands, the position, the size, and the contour of the uterus, ovaries, and other pelvic structures can be palpated. At the end of the examination, the physician may place a gloved and lubricated index finger into the patient's rectum for palpation of the posterior surface of the uterus. The presence of hemorrhoids, fistulas, and fissures also can be noted.

Examination of the breasts also is performed at this time. The examiner notes breast size and symmetry and any unusual changes in the skin of the breasts and nipples. The breasts and the axilla are then palpated for masses, lymph nodes, tenderness, and any other abnormalities.

Laboratory and Diagnostic Tests

Cytologic Test for Cancer (Papanicolaou Test)

This test provides a means to examine cells that exfoliate (shed dead cells) for malignancy (Fig. 49-4). In gynecology, the Papanicolaou (Pap) test is used mainly to detect early cancer of the cervix, which is the most common form of malignancy of the reproductive tract. Physicians recommend that this test be taken every 6 to 12 months.

A sample of cells from the cervix is obtained by aspiration or scraping. In the most common method, a vaginal speculum is inserted, and a special applicator is used to scrape a sample of cells from the cervix. The applicator is then smeared on a special slide that is immediately placed in a fixing solution, labeled, and sent to the laboratory for examination by a pathologist. The findings are as follows:

Class 1—Absence of atypical or abnormal cells
Class 2—Atypical cells but no evidence of malignancy
Class 3—Suggestive of but not conclusive for a malignancy
Class 4—Strongly suggestive of a malignancy
Class 5—Conclusive for a malignancy

Dilatation and Curettage (D and C)

This procedure is performed under general anesthesia and involves the insertion of a weighted vaginal speculum followed by dilatation of the cervix and scraping of the endometrium. Samples of endometrial scrapings are labeled and sent to the laboratory for examination.

The diagnosis of endometrial carcinoma is best achieved by dilatation of the cervix and curettage of the uterus (D and C). Other uses of this procedure include the control of abnormal uterine bleeding and the removal of the products of pregnancy after an incomplete abortion.

Endometrial Smears and Biopsy

An endometrial smear and biopsy are used to determine the presence of carcinoma. Of the two, the en-

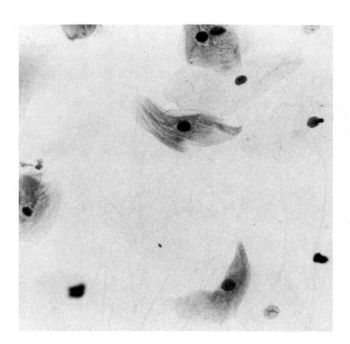
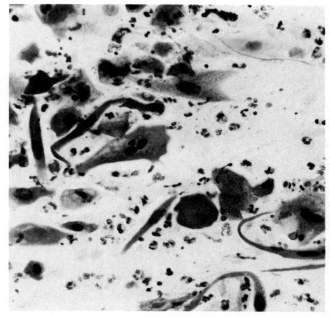

Figure 49-4. Papanicolaou smears from the vagina. (*Left*) Normal cells. (*Right*) Malignant cells. (Photograph by D. Atkinson)

dometrial biopsy is most accurate. It involves the insertion of a uterine sound followed by a special curet that obtains a tissue sample. Aspiration suction may be used to obtain an endometrial tissue sample. This procedure can be performed without anesthesia, but, if anesthesia is required, a paracervical block may be used.

An endometrial smear can be obtained by several methods. One method is to insert a malleable cannula in the uterine cavity. The cannula is attached to a syringe that is used to aspirate secretions. This procedure usually can be performed without anesthesia.

Cervical Biopsy

A cervical biopsy is usually performed as a follow-up when a cytologic test is positive or questionable. When the physician suspects cancer, a tiny piece of the cervix is obtained for microscopic examination. This procedure may be conducted in the physician's office or in a clinic. If the patient is still menstruating, the biopsy is usually scheduled for about 1 week after the cessation of the patient's monthly menstrual flow, when the cervix is least vascular.

Schiller's Test

When cancer is suspected or diagnosed, the physician may perform a Schiller's test. The cervix is painted with an iodine preparation, and biopsies are taken of all unstained tissues; cancerous tissues are among those that remain unstained.

Endoscopic Examinations

Endoscopic examinations are used to visualize areas of the female reproductive tract.

Culdoscopy.   Under local or general anesthesia, a culdoscope is inserted through an incision made in the posterior vaginal cul-de-sac to visualize the uterus, broad ligaments, and fallopian tubes. This procedure is performed to detect ectopic pregnancy but also may be used to visualize pelvic masses.

Laparoscopy.   This procedure is often performed under general anesthesia. A dilatation and curettage and pelvic examination usually are performed first. A needle is inserted into the peritoneal cavity through a small incision made in the abdomen about one-half inch below the umbilicus. The physician injects about 2 or 3 L of carbon dioxide or nitrous oxide gas into the peritoneal cavity to separate the intestines from the pelvic organs. The gas is removed at the end of the procedure.

This procedure may be performed to detect an ectopic pregnancy, for a tubal ligation (tying of the tubes to prevent pregnancy), to obtain a biopsy of the ovary,

and to detect pelvic abnormalities, such as tumors, endometriosis, and pelvic inflammatory disease.

Colposcopy.   This examination is used to visualize the cervix and vagina. A speculum is inserted into the vagina, and the surface areas are examined with a light and magnifying lens (colposcope). A cervical biopsy and Pap test also may be performed at this time.

Radiographic Examinations

Although not specific for disorders of the female reproductive system, radiographic examinations may be used in conjunction with other tests, including studies such as a barium x-ray, intravenous pyelogram (IVP), and flat plate (radiograph) of the abdomen. A computed tomographic (CT) scan or magnetic resonance imaging (MRI) also may be used to detect pelvic masses or other abnormalities of the female reproductive system.

Radiographic studies also may be performed if a breast lesion is thought to be malignant. The surgeon may order radiographic films of the lungs, spine, or other areas of the body to detect possible metastasis.

Hysterosalpingography (Hysterosalpingogram). Hysterosalpingography is a radiographic examination that visualizes the uterus and fallopian tubes. It is used to detect abnormalities, such as adhesions, as well as to determine fallopian tube patency, other tubal abnormalities, or congenital malformations of these structures.

With the patient in a lithotomy position, a cannula is inserted into the cervix and a contrast media injected. Fluoroscopic or radiographic films are then taken.

Mammography.   This radiographic technique is used to detect cysts or tumors of the breast, some of which may be so small as to be impossible to palpate. Mammography is used as a screening test for breast cancer. The frequency of a breast mammogram varies; the physician bases the need for screening intervals on factors such as a family history of breast cancer, early onset of menses, the patient's age, and exposure to radiation.

Xeroradiography.   Xeroradiography uses a low dose of radiation to produce a picture of breast tissue and may be used to detect abnormal breast lesions, such as breast cancer or breast abscess.

Breast Thermography

Like a mammogram, breast thermography is used to screen for breast cancer, but it also may indicate a breast abscess or fibrocystic breast disease. Infrared film and a camera are used to photograph the breasts. The special films detect the surface temperature of the skin of the breasts. Malignant lesions are more vascular and, therefore, appear as white areas ("hot spots") on the film.

Ultrasonography (Sonogram)

Ultrasound may be used to detect pelvic abnormalities, such as tumors, as well to detect pelvic organ size. A common use of ultrasound is to detect a single or multiple pregnancy, fetal abnormalities, fetal sex, and maternal abnormalities, such as an abnormal position of the placenta. Ultrasonography of breast tissue also may be used to detect malignant or benign breast lesions.

Breast Biopsy

A specimen of tissue from the breast for examination by a pathologist may be obtained in several ways. Incisional biopsy is performed in the operating room, where one or more sections of tissue are removed. A frozen section of the specimen is made and is examined microscopically by a pathologist while the patient remains anesthetized. If the tissue is negative (ie, benign), the remainder of the benign tissue is removed (if it had not been completely removed for biopsy), the incision closed, and the patient sent to the recovery room. If the tissue is positive (ie, malignant), the physician then performs the surgical procedure that offers the best chance of cure.

Some surgeons prefer an excisional biopsy, which is the removal of the entire lesion for detailed examination by a pathologist. Patients may be discharged from the hospital before the results of the biopsy are obtained, or they may remain hospitalized. If the lesion is malignant, the biopsy results and the proposed treatment are discussed with the patient. Unless the patient refuses the planned surgical treatment, a mastectomy is scheduled as soon as possible.

Aspiration biopsy, a procedure usually performed on an outpatient basis, uses a needle and syringe to obtain a sample of the suspicious tissue. A local anesthetic is first injected around the area, and a sample of tissue is removed. The tissue sample is examined by a pathologist.

Laboratory Tests

Various laboratory tests, such as a complete blood cell count (CBC), hemoglobin, and serum electrolytes, may be ordered to obtain a general survey of the patient. Culture and sensitivity tests of areas (eg, a vaginal smear) may be ordered if an infection is present.

Ovarian hormone activity may be evaluated by tests such as total urine estrogen and urine pregnanediol.

ANATOMY AND PHYSIOLOGY OF THE MALE REPRODUCTIVE SYSTEM

The male reproductive system consists of the testes, the epididymides (singular epididymis), vas deferens (or ductus deferens), seminal vesicles, prostate gland, and penis (Fig. 49-5). In the male, the lower urinary tract and reproductive system are so closely associated that disorders in this area frequently affect both systems. In the female, although close together, the systems are separated more.

During fetal life, the testes are formed near the lower pole of each kidney. During the latter half of the

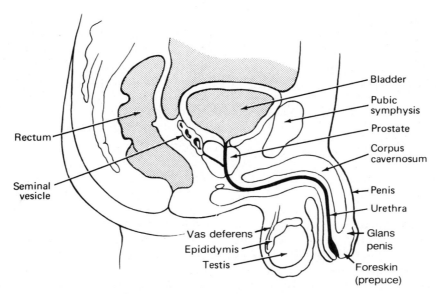

Figure 49–5. Male genitourinary tract.

eighth or early part of the ninth month of pregnancy, the testes descend into the lower abdominal cavity, through the inguinal ring, and into the scrotum.

The testes have a dual function: to form spermatozoa (sperm) and to manufacture the male sex hormone, testosterone, which is concerned with the development (at puberty) and maintenance of secondary male sex characteristics, such as muscle development, deep voice, and facial hair.

Sperm are manufactured in the testes, pass in tubules through the epididymides into the vas deferens, and are stored in the seminal vesicles. Sperm are discharged out of the body and into the urethra by rhythmic contraction of the muscles of the vas deferens and the penis during the sexual climax. At the time of ejaculation, seminal fluid (semen), which contains the spermatozoa, is released. The volume of the normal semen ejaculate is 2.5 to 3.5 mL, in which there are an average of 100 million spermatozoa.

The prostate is located just below the outlet (neck) of the urinary bladder and entirely encircles this section of the urethra. The prostate gland is an accessory sex organ that produces most of the alkaline seminal fluid. This fluid contains zinc, invert sugars, and other substances necessary for the nutrition of the sperm. Spermatozoa are rapidly immobilized in an acid environment. In human males, spermatozoa are produced continuously, even though they leave the body only periodically.

ASSESSMENT OF THE PATIENT WHO HAS A DISORDER OF THE MALE REPRODUCTIVE SYSTEM

Patient History

A thorough patient history is obtained and includes the following:

- A general health and family history
- A drug and allergy history
- Symptoms of present disorder and length of time present
- A family history of disorders that may be related to the patient's disorder, including a history of cancer
- Prior treatments (including drug therapy), diagnostic tests, or surgery for this disorder or any disorder related to the male reproductive system (if any)

Physical Examination

The physician examines the external genitalia, looking for abnormalities such as tumor growths and urethral discharge. The testes are palpated for tumors and the external scrotum examined. Using a gloved finger, a rectal examination is performed to examine the prostate for size as well as for evidence of a tumor.

Laboratory and Diagnostic Tests

Cystoscopy

In a cystoscopy, a cystoscope (an illuminated optical instrument) is inserted into the urethra to inspect the bladder and urethra. A cystoscopy may be performed for disorders of the male or female urinary tract. In the male, this procedure allows the physician direct view of the prostatic section of the urethra and, thus, an evaluation of prostatic size.

Radiographs

If a malignant process is suspected, radiographs may be ordered to determine possible metastasis of the tumor to areas such as the bones or lungs.

Biopsy

A biopsy of prostatic tissue may be obtained by the perineal approach or through the rectum. With a perineal approach, a local anesthetic is given, and a small incision is made in the perineal area. A needle is inserted through the incision and into the prostate. In the rectal approach, a needle is guided along a gloved finger and inserted through the rectal wall and into the prostate. The rectal approach usually does not require an anesthetic, although the procedure can produce pain at the moment the needle enters the gland.

A testicular biopsy may be obtained for evaluation of spermatozoa production. This procedure usually uses a local anesthetic and a needle to withdraw a small amount of tissue from the testis.

Laboratory Tests

Various laboratory tests, such as a CBC, hemoglobin, and serum electrolytes, may be ordered to obtain a general survey of the patient. Culture and sensitivity tests, such as a urethral smear, may be ordered if an infection is present or suspected.

Total urine estrogens require a 24-hour collection of urine. In testicular tumors, the total urine estrogens are elevated.

Infertility Studies

The causes of sterility in men can include general debility, hypopituitarism, hypothyroidism, obesity, infection, absence of a genital organ, undescended testicles (even when they are corrected), orchitis after mumps, radiation therapy to the testes, and mental stress. Conception can occur when the sperm count is low, but the chance that a sperm will contact an ovum is less than when the count is high.

Men who desire to father children may undergo tests for infertility (see Table 50-1 in Chapter 50). Fertility studies include a semen analysis to determine the sperm count, sperm viability, and the presence of abnormal sperm. Other laboratory tests for fertility may evaluate the plasma LH level in the blood. In the male, this hormone is necessary for the release of testosterone from the testes. A decrease in the blood level of this hormone may be responsible for decreased testosterone production and infertility.

NURSING PROCESS —THE PATIENT UNDERGOING DIAGNOSTIC EVALUATION OF THE REPRODUCTIVE SYSTEM

Assessment

A complete medical, drug, allergy, and family history is obtained. The patient is asked to list all symptoms that have been experienced and to describe the symptoms in detail. Vital signs and weight are obtained.

Nursing Diagnosis

Depending on the condition of the patient, possible diagnosis, and the diagnostic tests, one or more of the following may apply:

- Anxiety related to diagnostic test, knowledge deficit, possible diagnosis, other factors (specify)
- Pain related to diagnostic test or the existing disorder
- Knowledge deficit of diagnostic test, preparations, patient participation

Planning and Implementation

The major goals of the patient include reducing anxiety and pain (if present) and gaining knowledge of the diagnostic test, the preparations for the test, and what participation is required of the patient before, during, and after the test.

The major goals of nursing management include a reduction in patient anxiety, relief of pain, correct preparation of the patient for the diagnostic test, and observation of the patient after the diagnostic test (when required).

A female nurse should remain in the room the *entire* time that a female patient is being examined or a diagnostic test is being performed. All the needed equipment should be on hand.

Any tissue samples, cultures, or slides smeared with secretions taken from a male or female patient must be labeled with the type and source of the sample, the date, and the patient's name. Other pertinent data, for example, about the female patient's menstrual cycle, also may need to be added.

Anxiety. Some women dread having a gynecologic examination because they are embarrassed about being examined and they fear what the physician may find. When an apprehensive patient says that she is frightened or embarrassed, it may be helpful to ask what specifically makes her feel that way. The nurse can then do whatever is possible to alleviate these feelings and reduce anxiety. Encouraging the patient to breathe deeply may help lessen discomfort during the examination or test.

The male patient also may experience anxiety during a physical examination of the genitalia, especially if an infection or suspected disease is present.

Pain. Although the gynecologic examination is uncomfortable, the patient should not feel pain. Certain gynecologic or pelvic disorders, however, may cause varying degrees of pain or discomfort during and after a pelvic examination. The more relaxed the patient's lower abdominal muscles are, the better the physician can palpate the internal organs. Breathing deeply through the mouth may help to relax the abdominal muscles.

After an endometrial or cervical biopsy, the patient may have a cramped feeling that usually can be relieved by a mild analgesic recommended or prescribed by the physician. Severe pain after an examination or diagnostic test is brought immediately to the attention of the physician.

The male patient who has a digital (rectal) examination of the prostate may experience pain, which can be moderate to severe, during manipulation of the gland. The pain usually subsides quickly, but the physician may recommend a sitz bath to relieve the discomfort. After a prostatic biopsy, the physician may recommend or prescribe a mild analgesic.

Knowledge Deficit. The physician explains the purpose of the test and the basic procedure. The nurse may need to reinforce the physician's explanation.

Certain preparations for a specific test may be required but may vary according to hospital policy or physician preference.

1. Most tests require that the female patient not douche for 2 or 3 days before a test; irrigation of the vagina would remove the exfoliated cells or vaginal discharge that is to be examined.
2. The patient is asked to void before a test or pelvic or prostate examination because a full bladder may interfere with the procedure.
3. Some types of mammograms require that certain foods or substances, such as caffeine, be omitted from the diet for a specified length of time. These regulations usually are given by the department of radiology but may need to be clarified by the nurse.
4. If a general anesthetic is to be administered on a short-term admission basis, the physician gives the pa-

tient instructions about fasting from food and fluids. The nurse may need to review the instructions with the patient.

After a procedure, the physician may give the female patient such instructions as not to bathe or douche for a specified period or to avoid heavy lifting or straining. If a cervical or endometrial biopsy has been taken, the patient is instructed to call the physician or return to the clinic if bleeding is serious. If packing was inserted into the vagina, the patient is instructed not to remove it until the prescribed number of hours has passed (usually 24).

After some procedures, the physician may prescribe or recommend an analgesic for the relief of pain, cramping, or discomfort. The patient is instructed to notify the physician immediately if severe pain occurs.

An aspiration breast biopsy may produce redness and soreness in the area. The patient is instructed to notify the physician if drainage or bleeding from the biopsy site is more than slight, or if increased redness, pain, or fever occurs.

After an incisional biopsy of the prostate, the physician may instruct the patient to refrain from tub baths until the sutures are removed. If a female patient has a breast biopsy and is sent home, the physician instructs her to return to the office or clinic to have the sutures removed.

An antibiotic may be prescribed after a diagnostic test. Although it may be used to prevent an infection after a diagnostic procedure, in most instances, the antibiotic is used to treat an infectious disorder identified during the examination. The nurse should review the dosage schedule and adverse drug effects with the patient.

Evaluation

- Anxiety is reduced
- Pain is reduced or eliminated
- Demonstrates understanding of preparations for a diagnostic test or general anesthetic
- Demonstrates understanding of instructions given by the physician after a diagnostic test

Suggested Readings

☐ Bates BA, Hoekelman RA. Guide to physical examination and history taking. 4th ed. Philadelphia: JB Lippincott, 1987. *(In-depth coverage of subject matter)*

☐ Memmler RL, Wood DL. Structure and function of the human body. 4th ed. Philadelphia: JB Lippincott, 1987. *(Additional coverage of subject matter)*

Chapter 50

Disorders of the Female Reproductive System and Related Structures

On completion of this chapter the reader will:

- List and discuss the disorders of menstruation, providing the symptoms, diagnosis, and treatment of each
- Discuss the diagnosis and treatment of infertility
- List the types and treatment of abortion
- Discuss the symptoms, diagnosis, and treatment of ectopic pregnancy, menopause, and infectious or inflammatory disorders of the female reproductive system
- Use the nursing process in the management of a patient with an infectious or inflammatory disorder of the female reproductive system
- List and discuss the symptoms, diagnosis, and treatment of endometriosis
- Use the nursing process in the management of a patient with endometriosis
- List and discuss the symptoms, diagnosis, and treatment of vaginal fistulas, relaxed pelvic muscles, and uterine displacement
- Use the nursing process in the management of a patient who has medical or surgical treatment for a vaginal or uterine disorder
- List and discuss the symptoms, diagnosis, and treatment of malignant and benign tumors of the female reproductive system
- Use the nursing process in the management of a patient who has a vulvectomy or hysterectomy
- List and discuss the symptoms, diagnosis, and treatment of malignant and benign breast disorders
- Use the nursing process in the management of a patient who has a mastectomy

DISORDERS OF MENSTRUATION

Premenstrual Syndrome

Premenstrual syndrome, also known as premenstrual tension or PMS, is a group of symptoms that can occur in women 1 to 10 days before menstruation.

Symptoms

Symptoms include one or more of the following: weight gain, headache, nervousness, irritability, personality changes, depression, abdominal bloating, pain or tenderness of the breasts, breast enlargement, a craving for sweets, swelling of the ankles, feet, and hands, anxiety, and increased physical activity.

In some women, this syndrome occurs every month; in others it occurs less often. The symptoms of PMS may be mild and may not require treatment; or, the symptoms may be so severe and incapacitating that treatment is necessary.

Diagnosis

Diagnosis is based on the patient's description of symptoms. Additional diagnostic tests as well as a pelvic examination may be performed to rule out other abnormality of the female reproductive system.

Treatment

Treatment of PMS depends on the severity and type of symptoms experienced. Weight gain, edema, headache, and abdominal bloating may respond to a diet limited in salt; some patients may require diuretic therapy. Analgesics, such as acetaminophen (Tylenol) and ibuprofen (Advil), may be used. Large doses of aspirin should be avoided, especially if the woman has a history of a heavy menstrual flow. The use of drugs such as tranquilizers or antidepressants usually is avoided; in some women, however, the symptoms may be so severe that a short-term trial with these drugs may be necessary.

All patients with moderate to severe symptoms are advised to avoid self-treatment and to have an examination by a physician to rule out possible reproductive tract abnormality. Once the physician has determined that another disorder is not the cause, treatment can be instituted. The patient is encouraged to notify the physician if the symptoms have not lessened in intensity.

Dysmenorrhea

Dysmenorrhea is painful menstruation and may be primary or secondary. Primary dysmenorrhea usually is idiopathic, and no abnormality is found. Dysmenorrhea may be secondary to other abnormalities, such as endometriosis, displacement of the uterus, or narrowing of the cervical canal.

Symptoms

The main symptoms are pain and lower abdominal cramping. Mild pain may become more severe with fatigue, cold, and tension. Many patients with primary dysmenorrhea also experience PMS.

Diagnosis

Diagnosis is based on the patient's symptoms. Additional diagnostic tests as well as a pelvic examination may be performed if the disorder is believed to be caused by other abnormality.

Treatment

The patient with primary dysmenorrhea should consult a physician to uncover any possible abnormality. If none is found, symptomatic relief may be obtained with mild analgesics, such as acetaminophen, aspirin, or ibuprofen. Aspirin should be avoided in women with a heavy menstrual flow. On occasion, the physician may find it necessary to prescribe a mild narcotic analgesic, but prolonged use of these drugs is avoided because of their potential for addiction.

For some conditions, exercises may be suggested by the physician. If dysmenorrhea is related to retroversion of the uterus (ie, the uterus tilts backward), the knee–chest position may be prescribed. Surgery may sometimes be necessary, as with severe endometriosis, for example.

Amenorrhea and Oligomenorrhea

Amenorrhea is the absence of menstrual flow. *Oligomenorrhea* is infrequent menses. Amenorrhea occurs normally before menarche (onset of menstruation), during pregnancy, after menopause, and sometimes throughout lactation, if the new mother is breast-feeding her baby. Oligomenorrhea and amenorrhea may be caused by endocrine imbalance, endocrine gland tumors, wasting chronic disease (eg, tuberculosis or starvation), and psychogenic factors. Emotional reactions affect the menses in varying degrees.

Symptoms

An infrequent or total absence of menstrual flow is the primary symptom. Additional symptoms may be associated with an underlying disorder, such as pregnancy, a hormonal imbalance, or the beginning of menopause.

Diagnosis

A careful history of the menstrual pattern reveals whether the patient has amenorrhea or oligomenorrhea and the possible underlying cause. A pelvic examination and other diagnostic tests, such as pregnancy tests and blood and urine hormonal levels, may be used to determine the cause.

Treatment

The woman who misses menstrual periods should see a physician to determine the cause. Treatment includes correction of the underlying cause, such as the administration of female hormones or thyroid hormone (if the patient is hypothyroid). In some instances, for example with pregnancy or amenorrhea due to an emotional cause, no treatment is necessary.

Menorrhagia

Menorrhagia, which is excessive bleeding at the time of normal menstruation, may be caused by disorders such as endocrine imbalance, fibroid tumors, emotional upsets, abnormalities of blood coagulation, ovarian cysts, uterine polyps, and a variety of other pelvic abnormalities.

Symptoms

The symptom is primarily a heavy menstrual flow that may or may not be accompanied by cramping or severe pain.

Diagnosis

The symptoms of menorrhagia should bring the patient to a physician. Diagnosis is based on a description of the symptoms and the number of sanitary pads or tampons used compared to previous menstrual periods. Laboratory and diagnostic tests, such as hormone studies, dilatation and curettage (D and C) for examination of endometrial tissue, and an endometrial biopsy, may be performed to determine the cause.

Treatment

A dilatation and curettage may be performed in an attempt to stop the bleeding. Additional treatments depend on the underlying cause and include, for example, the administration of hormones or surgical removal of a fibroid tumor.

Unchecked menorrhagia can lead to anemia, which, if severe, also may require treatment.

Metrorrhagia

Metrorrhagia is vaginal bleeding at a time other than a menstrual period. It can be caused by the same abnormalities that cause menorrhagia or by abnormalities in the vagina or cervix, such as malignant or benign tumors or infection.

Symptoms

Symptoms may vary from a slight pink or brownish spotting to frank bleeding. Spotting also may occur in early pregnancy and sometimes is a warning symptom that abortion is imminent. Some women spot for a day or two midway between menstrual periods. This functional bleeding is thought to occur at the time of ovulation and may not be abnormal. Metrorrhagia always should be brought to a physician's attention, however, because it may be an early indication of cancer. The amount of blood is not important; however, the fact that it occurred when no bleeding was expected is important. Metrorrhagia may be difficult for the menopausal woman to identify if her menstrual cycle has become irregular.

Diagnosis

Diagnosis is based on patient history and additional tests to determine the underlying cause. Examples of diagnostic tests include a pregnancy test, cytologic examination of cervical smears, and urine and blood hormone levels.

Treatment

Treatment depends on the underlying cause; for example, surgery may be performed for cancer of the cervix. If all tests are negative, the physician may decide that no treatment is necessary.

INFERTILITY

High in the fundus of the uterus are two openings into the fallopian tubes, along which ova travel from the ovaries to the uterus and which sperm enter from the uterus. The tubes are about 4 inches long. After the ovum is released from the ovary (ovulation), movement of the cilia at the fimbriated end of the fallopian tube and muscular contractions of the tube itself draw the ovum down toward the uterus. Ovulation apparently occurs midway between menstrual periods, but can vary from month to month. Women are capable of becoming pregnant soon after ovulation. If the ovum is not fertilized, it degenerates and is shed.

For conception to occur, it is necessary for a spermatozoon to make its way, by movement of its taillike portion, up the entire length of the uterus and into the fallopian tube, to find an ovum and to insert its head into the ovum by piercing the outer coat (zona pellucida). Although the actual fertilization is by one spermatozoon, more than one sperm probably needs to be present to dissolve the zona pellucida sufficiently so that one can enter. It is likely that many spermatozoa find their way into the fallopian tubes. Usually, only one ovum is present as a result of ovulation.

Women may be infertile from systemic causes, or they may have problems that interfere with normal ovulation, such as endocrine disorders. A blockage in the fallopian tubes is a significant cause; gonorrheal,

streptococcal, or other infections can cause tubal strictures that prevent the ova from traveling down and the sperm cells from traveling up the tubes. Endometriosis is a common cause of infertility in women. Psychological factors sometimes help cause infertility.

Diagnosis

When a woman is unable to conceive after several years, she and her sexual partner should be examined by a physician. A complete physical examination is performed to rule out a possible systemic cause. Studies may be ordered to determine thyroid function, and urine may be examined for pituitary gland function. The man may be examined first because his examination can be made more readily.

Various tests may help determine the possible cause of infertility (Table 50-1).

Treatment

In some women, no physiologic defect can be found. If a systemic disorder such as endocrine imbalance or infection appears to be the cause of infertility, the physician treats the underlying disorder. Tubal strictures may be treated by surgery, though the operation is not always successful. Uterine displacement may be treated by surgery or by the use of a pessary and exercise. Other uterine conditions such as fibroids, polyps, or congenital malformations may be treated surgically.

Couples who wish to have a baby may be advised by their physician to have intercourse every other day from the 10th through the 16th day after the first day of the woman's menstrual period. Alternating days allows for an increase in the male sperm count. Couples must receive instructions about optimal times for sexual intercourse.

Newer techniques have helped some couples have children. One of these techniques is artificial insemination with either the male partner's or a donor's sperm. This technique introduces semen into the posterior vagina near the external cervical os (opening of the cervix). If a stricture of the cervical canal has occurred, a cannula may be inserted through the external cervical os and into the cervical canal and the semen inserted. The patient then lies quietly for about 30 to 45 minutes. The procedure may need to be repeated over a 2- to 4-month period. If it is not successful, the physician may advise waiting a year and attempting the procedure again.

Another technique is in vitro fertilization. An ovum is obtained usually with a laparoscopy and placed with sperm in an incubating dish for up to 18 hours to allow fertilization to take place. After another 48 to 72 hours, the fertilized ovum is removed and inserted into the uterine cavity by a cannula or catheter inserted through the cervix. The success rate varies. Failure may be due to many causes, including failure of

Table 50–1. Infertility Tests

Test	Description	Comment
Male		
Semen examination	The number, motility, and shape of sperm cells from a fresh semen collection are examined under microscope	Absence of sperm cells in *repeated* examinations suggests infertility A low sperm count decreases the possibility of conception
Testicular biopsy	Tissue is examined to see if sperm cells are being produced	If sperm are being produced but are not present in the semen, the problem may be an obstructive lesion
Female		
Rubin test ✓	Carbon dioxide is introduced through the uterus into the fallopian tubes and the peritoneal cavity to check for fallopian tube patency	In some instances, the gas may blow out the obstruction, resulting in fertility
Sims-Huhner (postcoital) ✓	Vaginal and cervical secretions are aspirated 6–12 hr after intercourse and examined microscopically	The interactions of the woman's secretions and the man's sperm can be observed
Hysterosalpingography	Radiographic study of the uterus and fallopian tubes with radiopaque dye	Bowel cleaning before the study is usually ordered
Endometrial biopsy	Microscopic examination of tissue shows whether the endometrium has been prepared for pregnancy	Frequently done premenstrually or on first day of period; also used to help diagnose cause of dysmenorrhea and amenorrhea
Culdoscopy	A lighted instrument inserted into the cul-de-sac allows visualization of the uterus, broad ligaments, and other abdominal structures	Performed to detect ectopic pregnancy and other pelvic abnormalities
Laparoscopy	A lighted instrument inserted through a small incision in the abdominal wall allows visualization similar to that possible with culdoscopy	Same as culdoscopy; also can be used to perform ovarian biopsy, (tubal) sterilization

the ovum to be fertilized or failure of the ovum to become attached to the uterine wall.

CONTRACEPTION

For people who wish to prevent pregnancy, several methods are available. Some methods have higher failure rates than others.

Rhythm Method

The rhythm method uses no drugs or mechanical barriers to prevent conception. Instead, sexual intercourse is avoided during the time that the women is able to conceive, that is, at the time of ovulation and for up to 72 hours after ovulation. The rhythm method requires keeping track of the menstrual cycle, noting the dates menstruation began and ended and the number of days between each cycle. This record must be kept for at least a year to determine the regularity of the cycle. This method also uses the basal body tem-

perature, which requires that the woman take her temperature when she first wakes up in the morning, before she drinks anything, smokes, or arises. Near ovulation, a slight drop in normal body temperature occurs followed by a slight rise within the first 24 hours after ovulation.

In addition to the basal body temperature, the woman also may check the cervical mucous with a kit such as the OvuSTICK Self-Test, which reportedly is able to determine the time of ovulation.

Oral Contraceptives

Oral contraceptives, which have the highest success rate of any single birth control method, are available as estrogen–progestin combinations or as progestin-only products. The decision to use a certain product and dosage rests with the physician and is based on many factors. The combination oral contraceptives inhibit ovulation by suppressing the follicle-stimulating hormone and luteinizing hormone and by affecting the cervical mucous so that sperm penetration through the cervical canal is inhibited. The progestin-only products, which have a slightly higher failure rate than the combination oral contraceptives, inhibit the release of luteinizing hormone and, thus, suppress ovulation.

An oral contraceptive is started on the fifth day of menstruation and is taken every day for 20 or 21 days (depending on the type used). Some of these products contain 21 hormone tablets and 7 inert tablets to ensure that the woman takes a tablet every day over the 28-day period. It is important that the pill is taken at the same time each day, preferably in the evening. The interval between doses must not exceed 24 hours.

The adverse effects associated with these drugs include nausea and vomiting, abdominal cramps, bloating, breakthrough bleeding and spotting, amenorrhea, rash, migraine headache, contact lens intolerance, weight gain, edema, and breast enlargement and tenderness. The more serious adverse effects include cerebral thrombosis, thrombophlebitis and thrombosis, pulmonary embolism, Raynaud's disease, hypertension, gallbladder disease, and liver tumors and other hepatic lesions. Patients should see a physician immediately should any adverse drug effect occur.

Mechanical and Chemical Methods

This group includes the intrauterine device (IUD), condom, diaphragm, cervical cap, vaginal sponge, aerosol foams, and gels or creams. Condoms also play a role in the prevention of sexually transmitted diseases (STDs).

The IUD is available in several shapes and is inserted through the cervix and into the uterine cavity by a physician. The IUD is thought to prevent pregnancy either by creating localized endometrial inflammation, thereby preventing attachment of the fertilized ovum to the endometrium, or, possibly, by being toxic to spermatozoa. While this method eliminates the need to take an oral contraceptive daily or to use another type of mechanical or chemical barrier, problems of excessive uterine bleeding, displacement of the IUD, and perforation of the uterus do occur.

Condoms are made of rubber or plastic and are applied over the erect penis before it enters the vagina. A small reservoir at the end of the condom collects the sperm; therefore, the condom must be removed while the penis is still erect to avoid spillage and possible invasion of sperm into the vagina. Some condoms also have a spermicide (a product capable of killing sperm) lubricant.

The diaphragm is a flexible round spring covered with a dome-shaped cap. A spermicide jelly or cream is applied into the concave part of the diaphragm before insertion. Diaphragms, which come in various sizes, must be fitted by a physician. Directions for insertion are given by the physician but also are supplied with the product. The cervical cap is similar to the diaphragm but smaller in size. A spermicide also is applied before insertion.

The vaginal sponge is made of urethane and is saturated with a spermicide. The vaginal sponge may be left in place up to 24 hours but must remain in place at least 6 hours after intercourse. A loop attached to the sponge allows it to be easily removed.

Various foams, gels, and creams that have spermicide activity are available. They are recommended for use with a diaphragm or cervical cap, although they may be used as a sole method of contraception. When used alone, their effectiveness is decreased.

Sterilization

A sterilization procedure may be performed on the male or female. Female sterilization involves ligation of the fallopian tubes (tubal ligation). This procedure does not affect the production of hormones by the ovary or the menstrual cycle. It may be performed in several ways, such as by a laparoscopy, a laparotomy (surgical opening of the abdomen), minilaparotomy (basically, a laparotomy with a smaller incision), or a colpotomy, which requires an incision in the vagina and use of a culdoscope to ligate the fallopian tubes. In the male, sterilization is accomplished by a vasectomy (see Chapter 51).

ABORTION

Abortion is the termination of a pregnancy before the fetus is viable. The term *abortion* is used to designate interruption of pregnancy before the fetus weighs more than 500 g (about 20 weeks of gestation). Between this time and a full-term delivery, the expulsion of the fetus is called a *premature birth*.

Spontaneous Abortion

About 10% of all pregnancies result in spontaneous abortion (*miscarriage* is the layman's term), usually before the 12th week. For people who associate the word *abortion* only with an intentional termination of pregnancy, the word *miscarriage* may be more acceptable. Abnormalities of the fertilized ovum or the placenta, inconsistent with life, are believed to be the most frequent causes of spontaneous abortion. Maternal disease, such as a severe acute infection, endocrine imbalance, or a chronic wasting disease, also may cause an abortion. Physical trauma rarely causes abortion.

The types of spontaneous abortion include the following:

1. *Threatened abortion*—Bleeding or spotting may indicate that abortion is imminent. Other symptoms include cramps or backache. The fetus may be lost, or the pregnancy may proceed normally.
2. *Incomplete abortion*—Some of the products of the pregnancy are expelled while some (usually a portion of the placenta) are retained. Incomplete separation of the placenta from the uterine wall causes hemorrhage.
3. *Complete abortion*—All the products of pregnancy (fetus, placenta, amniotic fluid) are expelled.

Symptoms

Abnormal uterine bleeding in any woman during the childbearing years may indicate an abortion in the early weeks of gestation—so early in pregnancy that she is unaware of being pregnant. Pain and bleeding are common symptoms. The pain may be so mild that it is disregarded, or it may be as severe as labor pains. Bleeding may range from spotting to hemorrhage.

Diagnosis

Diagnosis is based on symptoms. The physician also may perform a pelvic examination, including visualization of the cervix. A blood sample may be drawn for human chorionic gonadotropin. Below normal values may be found in threatened abortion.

Treatment

Threatened Abortion. If, in the physician's determination, the patient has symptoms of a threatened abortion, bed rest, a light diet, and warnings against any heavy lifting or straining, such as when having a bowel movement, are advised. The patient is told to save all formed vaginal discharges for the physician to examine. If the bleeding stops, the physician may allow her out of bed in several days, but only for quiet activity. If abdominal pain becomes severe or uterine bleeding increases, abortion may be imminent, and the patient usually is hospitalized.

All large clots and tissue are saved for the physician to examine. The patient should not use the toilet; instead, she should use the bedpan to avoid passing the fetus or the placenta unnoticed. If the patient begins to have cramps or bleeding, the physician is informed immediately.

Incomplete Abortion. An incomplete abortion is treated by a D and C. The patient may enter the hospital bleeding profusely. A type and cross-match for whole blood usually is performed, and an infusion of intravenous fluids, such as dextrose in water or saline,

is started. Sometimes a blood transfusion is necessary. Drugs such as oxytocin and ergonovine may be used to make the uterus contract and to control bleeding. If abortion is imminent or incomplete, bed rest prevents the increase of bleeding caused by activity.

Complete Abortion. A complete abortion may require no treatment, because the products of pregnancy (fetus, amniotic fluid, placenta) have been expelled. The patient is observed carefully for hemorrhage. If the patient does not require hospitalization, she is instructed to contact the physician immediately if frank bleeding occurs.

Habitual Abortion

Habitual abortions are those that occur repeatedly without apparent cause.

Treatment

If habitual abortion is due to an incompetent cervix (ie, a cervix that dilates during the third to six month of pregnancy, resulting in spontaneous abortion), a surgical procedure may be performed to prevent early dilatation of the cervix. The Shirodkar procedure places a pursestring (or drawstring) suture around the cervix that is left in place for the remainder of the pregnancy. Once labor begins, the suture is cut to allow the cervix to dilate. Delivery is often by cesarean section.

The patient with a Shirodkar procedure must inform anyone who gives her medical care at any time during pregnancy or at the start of labor that the suture is in place. Failure to remove the suture at the onset of labor can result in rupture of the uterus.

Other methods to treat patients with repeated abortions include bed rest from the beginning of pregnancy, the administration of progesterone, and correction or control of other medical disorders (if present), such as a thyroid deficiency and diabetes.

Therapeutic Abortion

The intentional termination of pregnancy by a physician, with the consent of the patient, is called a *therapeutic abortion.*

The methods of therapeutic abortion include the following:

■ Administration of an abortifacient (a drug used to induce abortion), including:
  □ Dinoprost tromethamine (prostaglandin $F_{2\alpha}$), which is injected into the amniotic sac (transabdominal intraamniotic instillation)

□ Dinoprostone (prostaglandin E₂), which is administered as a vaginal suppository

□ Carboprost tromethamine, which is administered intramuscularly

□ Sodium chloride 20% solution, which is injected into the amniotic sac

■ D and C

■ Dilatation and evacuation (by suction) of uterine contents

■ Hysterotomy or an opening into the uterus to remove uterine contents (fetus, placenta, amniotic fluid); this procedure requires an abdominal incision and may be selected when sterilization (tubal ligation) also is desired at the time of the therapeutic abortion

Patients who have a therapeutic abortion require the same consideration and care as those who have other types of abortions and may experience a variety of emotional reactions to the procedure and the loss of the fetus. If the procedure was recommended and consented to because pregnancy entailed a danger to the health of the mother, the patient may experience the same reactions as a woman whose pregnancy was terminated by a spontaneous, incomplete, or missed abortion. On the other hand, the women who has a therapeutic abortion because she wishes to terminate her pregnancy may experience a wide range of emotional reactions, including guilt about having the procedure, relief about the termination of pregnancy, or both positive and negative feelings.

Some women experience long-range emotional reactions after a therapeutic abortion. These reactions include guilt, depression, regret over having the procedure, and a sense of loss. The nurse must deal with each patient as an individual, recognizing that a variety of emotions may accompany the procedure and also may occur weeks or months after the procedure. Before a therapeutic abortion, some patients wish to vent their feelings, whereas others prefer not to discuss the situation. The nurse must respect each patient's feelings and reasons for the procedure as well as respect the privacy of those who prefer not to discuss the situation.

After a therapeutic abortion, the physician usually gives instructions to the patient. These instructions include not taking a tub bath, not douching, abstaining from sexual intercourse, and not using tampons for a specified number of days. Heavy lifting and straining also are avoided. The patient also is told to expect bleeding for about 5 to 7 days. A medication may be prescribed for bleeding. The patient also must have a follow-up visit after the procedure and is directed to contact the physician if excessive bleeding, pain, or temperature elevation should occur. Patients may desire information about birth control measures, especially when the patient is young or has limited knowledge of the various methods of contraception.

ECTOPIC PREGNANCY

[handwritten: painful sudden hemorrhage — Watch shock]

In an ectopic pregnancy, the fertilized ovum is implanted outside of the uterus. The fallopian tubes are the most common ectopic site, but implantation may occur elsewhere, such as in the abdominal cavity. The fetus starts to develop just as it would in the uterus. In most cases, the patient has all the classic signs of pregnancy. In addition, she may complain of spotting and pain in the lower abdomen.

[handwritten: Treat immediately]

Symptoms

Because the fallopian tube has so little room for expansion, the enlarging fetus and the placenta eventually rupture it. Symptoms of an ectopic pregnancy may begin as intermittent pain in the lower abdomen. If the pain is on the right side, it may mimic appendicitis. Some patients do not experience symptoms until rupture of the fallopian tube occurs. The patient then experiences a sudden, sharp pain and often is admitted to the hospital in severe shock from hemorrhage.

Diagnosis

Diagnosis is based on symptoms and patient history. If a patient does not know if she is pregnant, a pregnancy test may be done. A laparoscopy may be performed to confirm the diagnosis. An abdominal radiograph also may be done. If the patient is in shock, an exploratory laparotomy is scheduled immediately.

Treatment

If the patient is in shock, treatment is started immediately and the patient is prepared for emergency surgery. Treatment includes insertion of an intravenous line, administration of oxygen, and drawing blood for type and crossmatch. Blood transfusions may be given as soon as blood typing and crossmatching are done.

If the patient's condition is stable, depending on the site of the ectopic pregnancy and other factors, surgery is scheduled as soon as possible. The surgeon may make an opening in the fallopian tube (salpingostomy) to remove the products of pregnancy. Other surgical procedures include removal of the entire fallopian tube (salpingectomy) or removal of a small section of the fallopian tube followed by an anastomosis of the remaining sections of the tube. *[handwritten: Read]*

In the immediate postoperative period, careful and frequent observation of vital signs is imperative until they are well stabilized. The nature and the quantity of the vaginal discharge are noted, and perineal care is given as long as vaginal discharge occurs. Preoperative bleeding into the abdominal cavity may result in postoperative peritonitis. Sudden, severe abdominal pain, nausea, vomiting, chills, and fever are reported immediately to the physician. The rupture of a tubal pregnancy is a sudden and shocking event for the patient and family. After the operation, the patient needs time to assimilate the experience and to accept the fact that her pregnancy has been terminated.

MENOPAUSE

Menopause is the cessation of the menstrual cycle. *Climacteric* refers to the long period during which ovarian activity gradually ceases. The terms are often used interchangeably, and this period of time also is called the *change of life.* Menopause normally occurs between the ages of 45 and 55.

In menopause, ovulation gradually ceases and with it the menstrual cycle and the reproductive capacity. The change usually is not sudden and symptoms may persist for several years.

Symptoms

The menstrual pattern changes, and the menstrual flow may become scanty or sometimes unusually copious. The time between menstrual periods may remain the same or become irregular before the periods stop permanently. The uterus, vagina, and vulva decrease in size.

As ovarian function diminishes, so does the production of estrogen and progesterone. The resulting endocrine imbalance may lead to fatigue, nervousness, sweating, palpitation, severe headaches, and vasomotor disturbances (especially hot flashes). The vasomotor disturbances occur without warning and are characterized by perspiration, redness of the face and neck, and a feeling of warmth. They may be so mild and so transitory that they almost escape notice, or they may last as long as 2 minutes and occur frequently throughout the day. In some, they are disturbing enough to interfere with sleep. Because normal and abnormal changes may readily be confused, it is especially important for women to have regular gynecologic examinations during menopause.

Diagnosis

Diagnosis is based on the patient's history of symptoms and changes in the menstrual pattern. Additional diagnostic tests include a cytologic examination of a cervical smear (Papanicolaou or Pap smear), which also demonstrates a decrease in hormone production.

Treatment

Evidence suggests that administering estrogens to postmenopausal women increases the risk of endometrial cancer. This risk appears to apply to women who take estrogens in high doses for a prolonged period. Because of these findings, physicians usually prescribe estrogen therapy only for selected patients, such as those with moderately severe to severe symptoms.

Some physicians also believe that estrogen, in small doses, can help prevent osteoporosis and that the slight risk of endometrial cancer is outweighed by the seriousness of advanced osteoporosis.

The decision about administering estrogen is made for each patient on an individual basis. If estrogens are considered to be necessary, they are given in the lowest dose required to relieve symptoms and are discontinued as soon as possible. Some physicians use a cyclic pattern of administration: 3 weeks on estrogens followed by 1 week off. This method has been proposed as a way to reduce the risk of endometrial cancer.

The physician may find it necessary to treat some of the symptoms associated with menopause. Vaginal itching and drying may be prevented or reduced by drugs such as a cortisone cream or ointment. Headache may respond to a mild analgesic, such as aspirin, or acetaminophen. The vasomotor symptoms have no treatment except for the administration of estrogen, which can reduce or eliminate them.

INFECTIOUS OR INFLAMMATORY DISORDERS OF THE FEMALE REPRODUCTIVE SYSTEM

Vaginitis

The normal acidity of the vaginal secretion at maturity (pH 3.5 to 4.5) is a natural defense against infection. Nevertheless, a variety of pathogenic organisms can invade and infect the vagina, most commonly the protozoon *Trichomonas vaginalis*, the fungus *Candida albicans*, and certain bacterial species.

Trichomonal vaginitis (trichomoniasis) is an STD that may be found with other STDs (see Chapter 9). Monilial vaginitis, caused by the fungus *C. albicans* (candidiasis), is an infection common during pregnancy and after antibiotic treatment because antibiotics destroy the normal vaginal flora. It also is frequent in diabetics whose urine contains glucose (the monilial fungus is supported by carbohydrates), and occasionally this infection is seen after long-term corticosteroid therapy.

Symptoms

An abnormal vaginal discharge is a prominent symptom of a vaginal infection. In contrast to abnormal discharge, normal vaginal discharge has little odor and is colorless. Normal vaginal discharge changes in character and amount during the menstrual cycle, usually becoming more noticeable at ovulation and before menstruation. It varies from clear to cloudy.

Trichomonas vaginitis can cause a white, frothy,

highly irritating leukorrhea (a white or yellow-white vaginal discharge). Occasionally, the patient may be asymptomatic.

Symptoms of candidiasis include intense vaginal and perineal itching and a watery vaginal discharge that often contains cheesy particles. If the mouth of the urethra is affected, the patient may have urinary symptoms, such as burning on urination and the feeling that she has to void frequently. Also, some discomfort in the lower abdominal region may be felt.

Diagnosis

The patient must not douche before the examination; washing away the secretions prevents the physician from noting their characteristics and from taking an adequate smear. Diagnosis of vaginitis by infection with trichomonal or candidal organisms is based on the patient's symptoms and confirmed by microscopic examination of vaginal secretions.

Treatment

Vaginitis can be stubborn and discouraging. Vigorous early treatment may overcome its tendency to become chronic. At best, the patient can expect about 6 weeks of treatment before she is cured. At worst, vaginitis persists for years, recurring at the very moment when it appears to be cured. Patients with long-term vaginitis are understandably discouraged. They are tired of the malodorous discharge, of wearing perineal pads every day of the month, and of going to the physician for treatment.

The patient is often treated as an outpatient. After determining the cause of the infection, the physician may swab the infected area with a cleansing solution. The drug used to treat an infection with a *Trichomonas* organism is metronidazole (Flagyl), which may be given as a 1-day or a 7-day treatment. The dose for the 1-day treatment is 2 gm in a single or divided dose. The 7-day treatment dosage is 250 mg three times a day for 7 consecutive days. Usually, sexual partners are treated with the same dosage even though they do not have symptoms.

Clotrimazole (Mycelex-G) vaginal tablets and cream, nystatin (Mycostatin) oral and vaginal tablets, miconazole vaginal cream (Monistat 7) and suppositories (Monistat 3), and gentian violet tampons may be prescribed for the treatment of candidiasis. If the patient has diabetes, the elimination of glycosuria through control of the diabetes is an aspect of treatment.

Perineal Pruritus

Pruritus (itching) of the perineum can be caused by a deficiency of vitamin A (especially in older women who do not eat enough butter, milk, and yellow vegetables), an irritating vaginal discharge, glucose in the urine of those with uncontrolled diabetes mellitus (diabetic vulvovaginitis), uncleanliness, leukoplakia, urinary incontinence, and an inflammatory skin disease or local skin infection, such as moniliasis, scabies, and pediculosis pubis. Allergic reactions to fabric, soaps, or dye can produce or contribute to pruritus, which is a symptom, not a specific disease. It is seen in many genital conditions, both in the presence and in the absence of a vaginal discharge.

Symptoms

The primary symptoms are itching and inflammation of the vagina and vulva.

Diagnosis

Diagnosis is based on symptoms but also involves determining the possible cause. After examining the perineal area and questioning the patient, the physician may obtain vaginal smears for microscopic examination. Various tests to rule out possible causes may be performed, for example, a fasting blood sugar to rule out diabetes mellitus or a urinalysis to rule out a urinary tract infection.

Treatment

Treatment is directed at the underlying cause, such as controlling diabetes mellitus, improving the dietary intake of vitamin A, or treating an infection. Obese patients often suffer from pruritus because, as they walk, the skin surfaces rub against each other. In such cases, a light dusting with cornstarch may help to decrease friction. The physician may recommend cold or hot compresses or applications of a prescribed cream or ointment to help relieve the itching. The patient should be told to wear clothing that is light and nonrestrictive and to avoid tight-fitting undergarments and slacks.

Cervicitis

Cervicitis (inflammation of the cervix) may be caused by a number of infectious organisms. Streptococcal and staphylococcal infections are common, especially after childbirth when the organisms are able to enter cervical tissue through small lacerations. Gonorrhea is a frequent cause of cervicitis. Cervicitis also may be caused by a change in the pH of the cervical secretions, which are normally alkaline, pH 7.5 to 8.

Symptoms

Inflammation can cause erosion of cervical tissue, which may cause spotting or bleeding. Leukorrhea is the prominent symptom of cervicitis. Sexual intercourse may be painful (dyspareunia), or slight bleeding after sexual intercourse may occur. Early cervicitis may fail to show any symptoms. A severe cervicitis may cause a sensation of weight in the pelvis.

Diagnosis

Diagnosis is made by visual examination of the cervix during a pelvic examination. Smears may be taken to identify the causative microorganism.

Treatment

Unless acute cervicitis is treated promptly, it has a tendency to become chronic and difficult to cure. Examination of the cervix 6 weeks after giving birth, in addition to a regular gynecologic examination for all women, is important to discover the condition before it becomes chronic. Acute cervicitis may be treated with douches and local or systemic antibiotics. Chronic cervicitis may be treated with electrocautery. The procedure usually is performed on an outpatient basis 5 to 8 days after the end of the menstrual period. The patient is placed in a lithotomy position, a vaginal speculum is inserted, and the cervix is painted with an antiseptic. The eroded tissue is touched with a thin electrical rod that burns strips around the mouth of the cervix, destroying any cysts present. Usually no anesthesia is used because discomfort is minimal. If the cautery blade is inserted into the cervical canal, a momentary cramping sensation may be felt.

For a day or two after electrocautery, the patient should rest more than usual. No straining or heavy lifting should be done. If slight bleeding occurs, the physician may advise bed rest. Frank bleeding should bring the patient back to the physician. Cervical or vaginal packing or electric coagulation of the bleeding vessel may be necessary. A gray-green discharge may occur for about 3 weeks after cautery. The discharge is watery at first; then, as the burned tissues become necrotic, the discharge becomes malodorous. Slight bleeding may occur about the 11th day. The physician reexamines the cervix 2 to 4 weeks later. Dilatation is done if there is cervical stenosis. Sexual relations should not be resumed until the physician gives approval. Healing takes 6 to 8 weeks.

Severe chronic cervicitis may be treated by conization (removal of the diseased portion of the cervical mucosa). The procedure uses an instrument that simultaneously cuts tissue and coagulates the bleeding area. The procedure may be performed on an outpatient or short-term admission basis, and anesthesia may or may not be given.

As with cautery, about 6 to 8 weeks are required for healing. The follow-up visits (usually about every 2 weeks) to the physician are most important, so that the patency of the cervix can be checked. Successful treatment eliminates the distressing leukorrhea, may aid fertility, and eliminates the constant irritation.

Pelvic Inflammatory Disease

Pelvic inflammatory disease (PID) is an inflammatory disorder of the pelvic organs (except the uterus). Inflammation of the ovaries (oophoritis) or of the fallopian tubes (salpingitis), pus in the fallopian tubes (pyosalpinx), inflammation of the pelvic vascular system or of any of the pelvic supporting structures may be seen.

Infection may enter these structures through the vagina, the peritoneum, the lymphatics, or the bloodstream. The gonococcus is the most frequent cause, although other organisms, such as streptococci and staphylococci, also may cause PID.

Symptoms

Symptoms of PID include a malodorous discharge that is infectious and should be handled with care by both patient and nurse to prevent spread of infection. Backache, severe or aching abdominal and pelvic pain, a bearing-down feeling, fever, nausea and vomiting, menorrhagia, and dysmenorrhea may be seen. Pain may be felt during sexual intercourse or a pelvic examination. Severe infection may cause urinary symptoms or constipation.

Diagnosis

Diagnosis is based on symptoms as well as a gynecologic examination. A culture and sensitivity test of the vaginal discharge is obtained to identify the causative microorganism.

Treatment

The patient with acute PID may need to be hospitalized and kept in bed. Often the bed is adjusted to a semisitting position to facilitate pelvic drainage and to help prevent the extension of the infection upward. Antibiotics are administered. Intravenous fluids may be necessary if the patient is dehydrated.

One way to prevent PID is early medical attention to symptoms of infection in the genital or urinary tracts, such as a feeling of pressure in the pelvic area, burning on urination, and leukorrhea. Early treatment may prevent the infection from moving up the genital tract, resulting in complications such as peritonitis, abscess formation, and obstruction of the fallopian tubes. When early treatment of acute PID is delayed or inadequate, the infection may become chronic.

After discharge from the hospital, the patient should refrain from sexual intercourse as long as leukorrhea or any other abnormality exists; intercourse tends to extend the infection and also may infect the partner's genitourinary tract.

NURSING PROCESS —THE PATIENT WHO HAS AN INFECTIOUS OR INFLAMMATORY DISORDER OF THE FEMALE REPRODUCTIVE SYSTEM

Assessment

A complete medical, drug, and allergy history is obtained, and the patient is asked to describe all symptoms. Because the physician obtains a smear of vaginal secretions, the patient is instructed not to douche for 48 hours before being examined.

Nursing Diagnosis

Depending on the symptoms and severity of the disorder, one or more of the following may apply:

- Anxiety related to possible diagnosis, pelvic examination, discomfort, other factors (specify)
- Pain related to an infectious or inflammatory process
- Potential for infection transmission related to lack of knowledge of preventive measures, indifference
- Hyperthermia related to infectious or inflammatory process
- Knowledge deficit of treatment regimen, preventive measures, measures of preventing spread of infection to sexual partners

Planning and Implementation

The major goals of the patient include a reduction in anxiety, relief of pain or discomfort, prevention of transmission of infection to others, normal body temperature, and an understanding of the prescribed treatment regimen, preventive measures, and measures to prevent the spread of the infection to others.

The major goals of nursing management include a reduction of anxiety, relief of pain or discomfort, normal vital signs, and the preparation of an effective patient teaching plan.

If vaginal discharge occurs, the perineal pad is changed frequently and disposed of according to hospital policy for the handling of infectious material. The patient, as well as any auxiliary personnel who care for her, must thoroughly wash her' hands after changing the perineal pad. When discharge is copious, perineal care is given each time that the pad is changed and after the patient uses the bedpan. Amount, color, odor, and appearance of the discharge are recorded on the patient's chart.

Anxiety. Patients with this type of disorder often experience varying degrees of anxiety. Some may fear they have a malignancy, others may be concerned over the cause of the disorder. Tact and understanding, an explanation of diagnostic tests or physical examination, and thorough explanation of the treatment regimen may help relieve anxiety.

Pain. The physician may order a mild analgesic for pain. Severe pain may require short-term administration of a narcotic analgesic. Additional measures prescribed by the physician include bed rest and sitz baths.

Hyperthermia. Vital signs are monitored several times a day and more frequently if the temperature is elevated. An antipyuretic may be prescribed for fever. The physician is notified if the temperature remains elevated, if vaginal discharge increases, or if the patient complains of sudden, severe abdominal pain.

Pruritus. When pruritus is present, the physician may prescribe an ointment or cream to relieve discomfort. Pruritus also may be lessened by cleansing the perineal area frequently, especially if the vaginal discharge is copious. The patient is cautioned against scratching or rubbing the perineal area; a secondary infection may occur if the skin is broken. This symptom usually is relieved once the disorder is controlled.

Knowledge Deficit. Before discharge from the hospital, clinic, or physician's office, the patient must understand every detail of what she needs to do. In most instances, the treatment is performed by the patient at home.

Infectious disorders of the female reproductive tract may be spread to sexual partners. The importance of preventing the spread of infection is emphasized. Usually, the physician advises the patient to refrain from sexual intercourse until the infection is controlled. When intercourse can be resumed, the physician may suggest the male partner use a condom for a specified period of time to be sure the infection is completely eradicated and not retransmitted to the partner.

Although many medications supply directions and pictures for the use of vaginal products, the patient may still require instruction or a review of the package insert. Instructions about insertion or application of a suppository, tablet, or cream, the correct placement in the vagina, lying flat on the back while inserting the drug, how to hold an applicator, and any special instructions as they apply to a particular drug are reviewed with the patient.

If metronidazole (Flagyl) is prescribed, the patient is instructed not to drink alcoholic beverages. Doing so can cause a disulfiram (Antabuse) reaction, that is, nausea, vomiting, headache, and a hot, flushed feeling. At times this reaction can be serious.

Points for a teaching plan include the following:

1. Take the prescribed medication exactly as directed. Do not omit or skip a dose. Finish the prescribed course of therapy.
2. Follow the instructions of the physician about rest, warm baths, avoiding heavy lifting, and refraining from sexual intercourse. Do not resume sexual intercourse or physical activities such as heavy lifting until permitted to do so.
3. Wash the hands thoroughly before and after inserting or applying a medication, changing a perineal pad, or cleansing the perineal area.
4. Do not use tampons (except medicated tampons) because they may obstruct the flow of discharge. Do not resume the use of tampons until permitted to do so.
5. Lie flat for the prescribed period of time after inserting a vaginal medication.
6. Undergarments may be protected by wearing perineal pads or a disposable incontinence brief (eg, Attends).
7. Do not douche unless advised to do so by the physician.
8. Wear loose undergarments and thoroughly clean and dry the perineal area after voiding and having a bowel movement.
9. Contact the physician if the problem is not relieved, becomes worse, or abdominal pain, fever, or chills occur.

Evaluation

■ Anxiety is reduced
■ Pain or discomfort is relieved or eliminated
■ Vital signs are normal
■ Demonstrates understanding of treatment regimen, methods to prevent the spread of infection, activities to be avoided

ENDOMETRIOSIS

In this condition, tissue that histologically and functionally resembles that of the endometrium is found outside of the uterus, most frequently on the ovaries, commonly elsewhere in the pelvic cavity, and occasionally in the abdominal cavity. The ectopic tissue apparently responds to stimulation by estrogen and, perhaps, to progesterone. The tissue bleeds when the endometrium of the uterus does, and it shrivels after menopause and may regress during pregnancy.

Symptoms

Endometriosis is serious because the tissue bleeds into spaces that have no outlets. The free blood causes pain and adhesions. During menstruation, dysmenorrhea may be severe and bleeding copious. The fallopian tubes may be occluded, causing sterility. If endometrial tissue is enclosed in an ovarian cyst (called a *chocolate cyst*), the monthly bleeding has no outlet. Occasionally, the cyst ruptures, spilling old blood and endometrial cells into the pelvic or abdominal cavity. Menorrhagia, metrorrhagia, dyspareunia, and pain on defecation may occur.

Diagnosis

The diagnosis is based on the patient's symptoms as well as a pelvic examination. A laparoscopy confirms the diagnosis.

Treatment

This condition is relieved by natural or surgical menopause. Because this disease occurs during childbearing years, however, an artificially induced menopause raises many problems. Surgical treatment often is designed to remove the cysts and as much of the ectopic tissue as possible and to free the adhesions caused by bleeding, without destroying the childbearing function. Endometriosis that is widespread throughout the pelvic organs may necessitate extensive surgery, such as panhysterectomy (removal of the uterus, both fallopian tubes, and ovaries). Sterility and surgical menopause are results of this type of surgery.

One aspect of medical management is to administer hormones to keep the patient in a nonbleeding phase of her menstrual cycle for a prolonged time, such as 9 months. Sometimes this therapy controls the ectopic tissue so that the patient is then symptom-free for several years. Synthetic oral progestins prevent ovulation while the patient is taking the hormone, but pregnancy can occur when the drug is discontinued.

NURSING PROCESS —THE PATIENT WHO HAS ENDOMETRIOSIS

Assessment

A complete medical, drug, and allergy history is obtained. The patient is asked to describe all symptoms, including the length of time symptoms have been present, type and location of pain, number of days of menses, amount of menstrual flow, and regularity or irregularity of the menstrual cycle.

Nursing Diagnosis

Depending on the severity of symptoms, one or more of the following may apply:

■ Pain related to bleeding of ectopic endometrial tissue
■ Anxiety related to symptoms, sterility, other factors (specify)

■ Decisional conflict related to uncertainty of choice of treatment (surgical, medical)
■ Knowledge deficit of treatment regimen

Planning and Implementation

The major goals of the patient include relieving pain, reducing anxiety, choosing a therapy, and understanding the treatment regimen.

The major goals of nursing management include relieving pain and discomfort, reducing anxiety, encouraging patients about their treatment choice, and thoroughly explaining the treatment regimen.

Patients are treated for endometriosis on an outpatient basis, but they may be admitted to the hospital for diagnostic confirmation of their disorder or for surgery. If the patient is admitted for a panhysterectomy, see Nursing Process—The Patient Undergoing a Hysterectomy, later in this chapter.

Pain. The physician may recommend a mild analgesic, such as acetaminophen or ibuprofin (Advil), for the relief of pain. The use of aspirin is avoided; this drug has an effect on the clotting ability of the blood and is contraindicated with bleeding.

Other methods of reducing pain and discomfort include bed rest during the time of heavy menses and warm sitz baths.

Anxiety, Decisional Conflict. The patient may experience varying degrees of anxiety related to the symptoms experienced with each menstrual cycle, the inability to conceive, the proposed treatment regimen, and the possibility of having to make a choice between medical treatment and surgery.

The nurse must listen to the patient as she discusses her concerns and offer emotional support, especially if medical treatment does not provide complete relief. The nurse also must encourage the patient to be open and frank when discussing the treatment regimen with the physician and to ask questions as they arise.

Knowledge Deficit. The medical treatment regimen and the expected results are explained by the physician. The nurse must reinforce the physician's recommendations and emphasize the importance of adhering to the prescribed medication schedule for the best chance of success.

The importance of a regular gynecologic evaluation is stressed. The patient is told to contact the physician if pain increases, the menstrual flow is extremely heavy, or pregnancy occurs.

Evaluation

■ Pain is reduced
■ Anxiety is reduced

■ Begins to or does demonstrate an ability to reach a decision about treatment
■ Understands the prescribed treatment regimen

VAGINAL FISTULAS

Fistulas may be congenital or a result of obstetric or surgical injury; the most frequent cause in adults, however, is a breakdown of tissue due to cancer, irradiation for a pelvic malignancy, or damage to the tissues during a vaginal delivery of the fetus. The opening may be between a ureter and the vagina (*ureterovaginal fistula*), between the bladder and the vagina (*vesicovaginal fistula*, Fig. 50-1), or between the rectum and the vagina (*rectovaginal fistula*). Rectovaginal fistulas may be seen as a complication of ulcerative colitis.

Symptoms

Ureterovaginal and vesicovaginal fistulas cause urine to leak continuously from the vagina. The vaginal wall and the external genitalia become excoriated and often infected. The patient may not void at all through the urethra because urine does not accumulate in the bladder. Rectovaginal fistulas result in a discharge of fecal material and gas through the vagina.

Diagnosis

Diagnosis is made by physical examination of the vaginal wall after insertion of a speculum. A sterile probe may be inserted if the fistula is easily seen. A dye (usually methylene blue dye) also may be used to detect the exact location of the fistula. When a vesicovaginal fistula is suspected, the colored dye is injected into the bladder through a urethral catheter. A ureto-

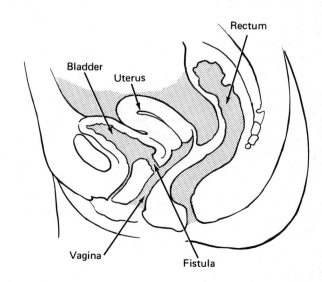

Figure 50-1. A fistula between the bladder and the vagina (vesicovaginal fistula).

vaginal fistula requires intravenous administration of the dye. A rectovaginal fistula may be located by looking for fecal drainage on the posterior vaginal wall. Intravenous pyelograms also may be performed to detect the flow of radiopaque dye through the lower genitourinary tract.

Treatment

Surgery is performed only when conditions are as close to optimal as possible—when inflammation and edema have disappeared. To attain this condition may take months of waiting.

The patient with a fistula usually is discouraged and uncomfortable. It is difficult for her to feel clean. She is always wet with urine or soiled by feces. The perineal area becomes raw and irritated. Good skin care is essential to prevent excoriation of the perineum and surrounding areas.

Sometimes the tissues are in such poor condition that surgical repair is not possible. When the fistula cannot be repaired, as in advanced cancer, frequent sitz baths and deodorizing douches help to control infection and odor and make the patient feel cleaner. A perineal pad or disposable incontinence brief, such as Attends, is needed.

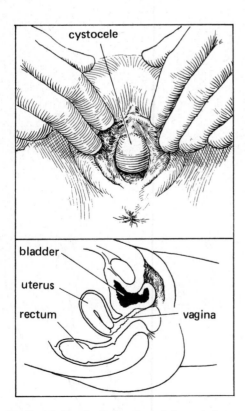

Figure 50–2. Cystocele. Relaxation of the anterior vaginal wall permits downward bulge of bladder on straining. (Brunner LS, Suddarth DS. Textbook of medical–surgical nursing. 5th ed. Philadelphia: JB Lippincott.)

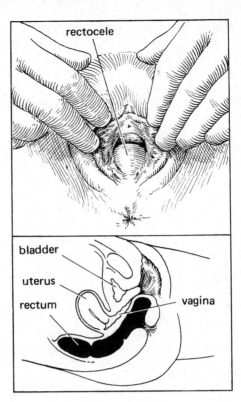

Figure 50–3. Rectocele. Relaxation of the posterior vaginal wall permits bulging of the rectum into the vagina on straining. (Brunner LS, Suddarth DS. Textbook of medical–surgical nursing. 5th ed. Philadelphia, JB Lippincott.)

RELAXED PELVIC MUSCLES

When the muscles and the fascia that support a structure relax, the structure sags. After unrepaired postpartum tears, childbirth, multiple births, or sometimes without apparent cause (perhaps from a slight congenital weakness), the floor of the pelvis relaxes, and the uterus, rectum, or bladder may herniate downward. The bulging of the bladder into the vagina is called a *cystocele* (Fig. 50-2), and it is the most common type of poor pelvic support. Herniation of the rectum into the vagina is called a *rectocele* (Fig. 50-3). Downward displacement of the uterus is called *prolapse*. A cystocele and a rectocele usually accompany uterine prolapse. The presence of the uterus low in the vaginal vault is a *first-degree prolapse; a second-degree prolapse* is the extension of the cervix beyond the vaginal os; and, when most or all of the uterus protrudes outside the vagina, a *third-degree* or *complete prolapse* (procidentia uteri) is present. The improved obstetric care available to many women before, during, and after delivery has greatly reduced the incidence of postpartum pelvic relaxation as a result of childbirth.

Symptoms

Symptoms of a uterine prolapse include backache, pelvic pain, fatigue, and a feeling that "something is dropping out," especially when lifting a heavy object, coughing, or with prolonged standing. A cystocele may cause difficulty in emptying the bladder, resulting in stagnation of the urine and possible cystitis (inflammation of the bladder). Stress incontinence may occur: a little urine seeps out every time the woman coughs, bears down, or strains. A rectocele can cause difficulty in evacuation, and constipation may result. In some instances, the patient may have to put her finger into the vagina and apply pressure to the posterior vaginal wall to reduce the herniation before she is able to evacuate the stool collected in the pocket.

Any tissue that protrudes below the vaginal orifice is subject to irritation from clothing or rubbing against the thighs in walking. This condition is seen especially in second- and third-degree uterine prolapse. Ulceration and infection frequently follow. These symptoms are annoying and may be incapacitating. They may preclude standing for long periods of time, walking with ease, lifting, and other activities that are difficult to avoid.

Diagnosis

Diagnosis is based on the symptoms and confirmed during a pelvic examination.

Treatment

The surgical repair of a cystocele is called *anterior colporrhaphy*. Repair of a rectocele is called *posterior colporrhaphy*. Repair of the tears (usually old obstetric tears) of the perineal floor is called *perineorrhaphy*. The operations are done by the vaginal route. A vaginal hysterectomy may be done to remove a completely prolapsed uterus.

UTERINE DISPLACEMENT

In some women, the uterus is abnormally placed. Displacement usually is congenital; sometimes backward displacement is due to childbearing. *Anteflexion* describes a uterus that is bent forward at an acute angle. In *retroflexion*, the uterus tilts backward, and the fundus is bent backward on the cervix (the opposite of anteflexion).

Symptoms

Displacement may be asymptomatic, or it may cause backache, dysmenorrhea, leukorrhea, easy fatigue, or, in the young patient, sterility. Anteflexion of the uterus also may cause urinary incontinence or retention.

Diagnosis

Diagnosis is made by pelvic examination.

Treatment

The condition may be treated by the insertion of a pessary and the assumption of the knee–chest position several times a day. If the displacement causes severe discomfort, or if the sterility possibly can be corrected, surgery may be performed to relocate and suture the uterus to a more natural position.

Because these conditions are most frequently found in older women, complicating diseases sometimes make surgery too great a risk. Under such circumstances, the displacement may be reduced by inserting a pessary, which repositions the uterus.

NURSING PROCESS —THE PATIENT UNDERGOING SURGERY FOR A VAGINAL OR UTERINE DISORDER

Preoperative Period

Assessment

A complete medical, allergy, and drug history is obtained. Although the diagnosis most likely has been established before admission to the hospital, a complete list of symptoms is obtained. Vital signs are taken, and the patient is weighed.

If the patient is admitted the morning of surgery, the physician may have prescribed neomycin or kanamycin to be taken before admission and may have recommended that the patient eat a low-residue diet 1 or 2 or more days before surgery. The nurse must check with the patient to be sure preadmission therapy has been completed.

Nursing Diagnosis

Depending on the patient and the type of surgery to be performed, one or both of the following may apply:

- Anxiety related to impending surgery
- Knowledge deficit of preoperative preparations, postoperative care, deep breathing and leg exercises

Planning and Implementation

The major goals of the patient include a reduction in anxiety and an understanding of care and exercises during the postoperative period.

The major goals of nursing management include preparing the patient physically and emotionally for surgery.

When surgery is performed for a rectovaginal fistula, both preoperatively and postoperatively the patient may be placed on oral neomycin or kanamycin (Kantrex) to clean the bowel of colon bacilli. A light, low-residue diet may be given before surgery to keep the stool soft.

An enema and a cleansing vaginal irrigation may be ordered for the morning of surgery. An indwelling catheter may be ordered to be inserted preoperatively to keep the bladder empty. If a catheter is not inserted before surgery, one usually is inserted in surgery.

Anxiety. Anxiety may be reduced by explaining preoperative preparations and postoperative nursing management.

Knowledge Deficit. Deep breathing and leg exercises are demonstrated, and, if time permits, the patient is allowed to practice the exercises under supervision. Preoperative preparations, such as a shaving of the operative area, enema, or catheter insertion, are explained as each procedure is carried out. Routine postoperative care is explained to the patient.

Evaluation

- Anxiety is reduced
- Demonstrates understanding of preoperative preparations and postoperative management
- Practices deep breathing and leg exercises before surgery

Postoperative Period

Assessment
On return from surgery, vital signs are taken and the chart reviewed for the type of surgery. The presence of drains, indwelling catheter, dressings, or vaginal packing is noted.

Nursing Diagnosis
Depending on the type and extent of surgery and the patient's general condition and age, one or more of the following may apply. Additional nursing diagnoses that pertain to patients who are having surgery may be necessary.

- Pain related to surgery
- Potential for infection related to surgery of a nonsterile area
- Impaired tissue integrity related to stress on the suture line secondary to failure of the bladder to remain empty during the healing phase
- Stress incontinence related to loss of tissue and muscle tone during the early postoperative period (after catheter removal)

- Urinary retention related to loss of bladder tone
- Knowledge deficit of postdischarge management

Planning and Implementation
The major goals of the patient include a relief of pain, absence of infection, a normal voiding pattern (after removal of the indwelling catheter), and an understanding of postdischarge management and home care.

The major goals of nursing management are to relieve pain and discomfort, establish a normal voiding pattern, and effectively teach postdischarge management.

After surgery, the patient who has had repair of a vaginal fistula may be kept on clear fluids for several days to inhibit bowel activity and graduated first to a light, low-residue diet and then to a general diet. The genitalia are cleansed gently, and warm perineal irrigations and perineal heat-lamp treatments may be ordered to promote healing and to lessen discomfort.

Deep breathing and leg exercises are encouraged every 2 hours during the immediate postoperative period. The patient is not encouraged to cough unless this is specifically ordered by physician.

The absence of urine in the vagina indicates healing of the fistula.

Pain. Analgesics are given as required. Pain that is not relieved by the analgesic, or sudden, severe abdominal pain, is reported immediately to the physician. If the patient has an indwelling catheter, the patency of the catheter is noted, as an obstructed catheter may be the source of sudden and severe abdominal pain.

Potential for Infection. Vital signs are monitored every 4 hours. During the immediate postoperative period, perineal care is given several times a day and always after the patient has urinated or defecated. The perineal area or the end of vaginal packing is inspected each time perineal care is given. Vaginal serosanguineous drainage is normal. The appearance of purulent drainage, chills, or a marked rise in body temperature is reported to the physician immediately.

Impaired Tissue Integrity. An indwelling catheter may have been inserted before or during surgery. The drainage is noted carefully. If the catheter becomes obstructed, and the bladder allowed to fill, the pressure of a full bladder on the operative site may break down the surgical repair and cause the fistula to reappear.

If a catheter has been inserted, it is attached to straight drainage while the patient is in bed. When the patient is ambulatory, the physician's orders are checked to determine whether the catheter is to be clamped or whether straight drainage is to be continued. Several days after surgery, clamping may be ordered to allow the bladder to fill and increase its muscle tone. It should be released every 4 hours, however, to prevent overdistention. No more than 150 mL should accumulate in the bladder until the catheter has been removed.

Every effort is made to prevent pelvic pressure and stress on the suture line. If sitz baths are given, a rubber or foam ring is placed in the bathtub. Until healing has taken place, the patient may be more comfortable sitting on a pillow placed over a rubber or foam ring. About the third or fourth postoperative day, the patient may be given a rectal suppository or an oral laxative to prevent strain when having a bowel movement.

If irrigations are ordered, they are done gently so that no pressure is applied to the suture line.

Stress Incontinence, Urinary Retention. After the catheter is removed (2 to 7 days after surgery), the patient is instructed to urinate at least every 4 hours, and the amount of each voiding is measured. Patients may have urinary frequency, which may or may not indicate adequate emptying of the bladder. Urinating in frequent, small amounts is reported to the physician. Catheterization for residual urine may be ordered.

After removal of the catheter, patients may experience urinary retention. If the patient has not voided within 4 to 6 hours after the catheter has been removed, the physician is notified. Reinsertion of an indwelling catheter or intermittent catheterization may be ordered.

Patients may experience stress incontinence because of edema around the surgical site. This usually disappears in a short period of time.

Knowledge Deficit. The physician's specific postdischarge orders are reviewed before developing a patient teaching plan. The physician may prescribe a mild analgesic for discomfort, a stool softener to prevent constipation and straining while having a bowel movement, and an antibiotic if infection occurred during the postoperative period. The physician also may recommend sitz baths, refraining from sexual intercourse for a specified period of time, and avoiding heavy lifting.

The physician also may recommend exercises to strengthen perineal muscles. Although the exercises vary somewhat, the usual routine is to tighten the perineal muscles for about 5 to 20 seconds and then relax. This procedure is repeated 10 or more times every 1 to 4 hours.

The patient is instructed to contact the physician if unable to void, if voiding is frequent and in small amounts, or if a purulent or bloody vaginal discharge is noted. Also, if the patient has had a repair of a vaginal fistula and urine or feces is leaking from the vagina, the physician must be contacted immediately.

Evaluation

- Pain is reduced
- No apparent infection; vital signs are normal
- Vaginal tissue appears intact; no evidence of leakage of urine or feces (after fistula repair)
- Voiding pattern is normal
- Demonstrates understanding of postdischarge management

NURSING PROCESS —MEDICAL MANAGEMENT OF THE PATIENT WHO HAS A VAGINAL OR UTERINE DISORDER

Assessment
A history of all symptoms and previous treatment (if any) and a complete medical, drug, and allergy history are obtained.

Nursing Diagnosis
Depending on the symptoms and the type of problem, one or more of the following may apply. If an infectious process also is present, see the earlier discussion under Nursing Process—The Patient Who Has an Infectious or Inflammatory Disorder of the Female Reproductive System.

- Anxiety related to symptoms, odor, other factors (specify)
- Chronic pain related to uterine displacement, vaginal or bladder infection
- Knowledge deficit of the prescribed or recommended treatment regimen

Planning and Implementation
The major goals of the patient include a reduction of anxiety, relief of pain, normal pattern of urine elimination, and an understanding of the treatment regimen.

The major goals of nursing management include a reduction of anxiety, improved comfort, and an effective patient teaching plan.

Anxiety. A large vaginal fistula causes the patient endless distress because of the odor and constant leakage of urine or fecal material. The nurse may help reduce anxiety due to odors by changing bedding and incontinent pads as they become soiled. At the same time, the patient also is offered soap and water for cleansing the perineum. If the patient is unable to perform this task, it must be done for her.

When performing these tasks, the nurse also may discuss ways to reduce odor at home.

Chronic Pain. Patients with chronic pain caused by uterine displacement usually find relief once a pessary has been inserted. A mild analgesic or warm sitz baths also may be recommended by the physician.

Knowledge Deficit. Although surgery offers the best treatment, all patients are not candidates for surgery. For many, medical treatment is supportive and emphasizes ways to eliminate odors and reduce the discomfort and problems associated with the disorder.

The following suggestions may be given to the patient who is experiencing difficulty with stress incontinence or the leakage of urine or feces.

1. Keep the perineal area as clean and dry as possible. Cleansing the area at frequent intervals throughout waking hours may be necessary.
2. Avoid the use of perfume or scented powders, lotions, or sprays. Mixing a perfumed scent with a fecal or urine odor may intensify the odor. In addition, powders may cake and cause irritation or a superficial skin infection. Perfumed sprays and powders also may irritate the area and increase discomfort. A thin dusting of plain cornstarch may be used but must be thoroughly washed off the skin when the area becomes wet with feces or urine.
3. Wear incontinence briefs day and night; they keep clothes from soiling and eliminate odors. The briefs may require frequent changing.
4. Avoid heavy lifting.
5. Use a commercial room deodorizer in the home.
6. Change clothes as they become soiled. After removing the soiled garment, soak it in warm soapy water and launder it as soon as possible.
7. Use plastic to cover such objects as mattresses and chairs to prevent soiling and lingering odors. The plastic must be washed with mild soapy water daily or more often if needed.
8. Contact the physician if any of the following occurs: increased discomfort, pain in the lower abdomen, fever, chills, or cloudy urine.

If the patient has a pessary inserted, it usually is removed, cleaned, and reinserted by the physician every 6 to 8 weeks. Some patients can be taught to perform these tasks. When removed, the pessary is thoroughly washed in water and dried. It is important to inspect the pessary to be sure that all secretions have been removed. A sterile lubricant is applied to the pessary before it is inserted.

When a pessary is in place, the patient should feel nothing. Discomfort may indicate that it has been inserted incorrectly, the pessary has moved, or that it is causing irritation. The appearance of leukorrhea may indicate an infection, in which case the patient should see the physician immediately. Assuming the knee–chest position for a few minutes once or twice a day helps to keep the pelvic organs and the pessary in good position.

Patients with uterine displacement or relaxed pelvic muscles are instructed to avoid heavy lifting and straining when having a bowel movement.

Evaluation

■ Anxiety is reduced
■ Comfort is maintained
■ Demonstrates understanding of methods to keep perineal area clean and dry and to eliminate odors
■ Demonstrates ability to remove, clean, and reinsert pessary
■ Discusses symptoms that require the notification of the physician
■ Lists situations to avoid

BENIGN TUMORS OF THE FEMALE REPRODUCTIVE SYSTEM
Tumors of the Uterus

Myomas (fibroids) that grow in the uterine wall are the most common tumor of the female pelvis (Fig. 50-4). The development of these tumors is believed to be stimulated by estrogen. They may be small or large, single or multiple. Growth usually is slow except during pregnancy.

Symptoms
Fibroid tumors can occur in various locations in the uterus: subserous (below the serous membrane), intramural (within the wall), and submucous (below the mucous membrane). The latter are most frequently associated with excessive menstrual bleeding. A benign tumor sometimes causes no symptoms, and the patient is unaware of its existence. When symptoms exist, menorrhagia is the most common. Also, the patient may have a feeling of pressure in the pelvic region, dysmenorrhea, anemia (from loss of blood), and malaise.

Diagnosis
Diagnosis is based on the patient's symptoms and pelvic examination. A Pap smear also may be done to rule out a malignancy. The diagnosis is not confirmed until the tumor has been removed and examined microscopically.

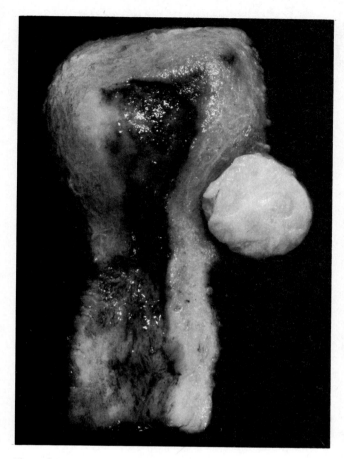

Figure 50–4. Fibroid tumor of the uterus. (Courtesy of P. S. Milley, MD)

Treatment

Treatment of benign uterine tumors is governed by a number of factors. An asymptomatic tumor in a woman who wishes to have children usually is watched closely by the physician, but it is not treated. The patient is reexamined every 3 to 6 months. A Pap smear is obtained every 6 to 12 months.

When the patient has had abnormal bleeding, she may be admitted to the hospital, and a D and C may be performed to determine the cause of bleeding, which may be a coexisting condition unrelated to the fibroid. Sometimes, a D and C is performed to control bleeding. Although it does not remove the tumor, it may make immediate, more extensive surgery unnecessary. Surgical removal of the tumor only (myomectomy) preserves the uterus and may be performed if a woman of childbearing years wishes to become pregnant in the future. A myomectomy is performed when the physician is certain that the tumor is benign. Future surgery may be required and is delayed, if possible, until the patient's family is complete. A hysterectomy is performed when the symptoms are severe and incapacitating, if the patient is past childbearing years, or a

future pregnancy is not wanted. Myomectomy or hysterectomy may be done by a vaginal or an abdominal approach.

Tumors of the Ovary

Ovarian cysts (benign tumors) are common. The types of ovarian cysts are listed in Table 50-2.

Symptoms

Ovarian cysts may or may not produce symptoms. Symptoms include pain, pressure in the lower abdomen, backache, and menstrual irregularities. Occasionally, the abdominal pain may be similar to the pain of appendicitis, ureteral stone, or other abdominal disorders.

Diagnosis

Diagnosis is based on the patient's symptoms as well as on palpation of the cyst by means of a pelvic examination. Surgery is the only means for confirming a diagnosis of a benign tumor.

Treatment

Occasionally, ovarian cysts require no treatment since they may rupture and not recur. If they persist, surgery is recommended. Surgery may involve complete removal of the ovary (oophorectomy), removal of the cyst (oophorocystectomy) leaving the ovary intact, or removal of the ovary and fallopian tube (salpingo-oophorectomy).

MALIGNANT TUMORS OF THE FEMALE REPRODUCTIVE SYSTEM

Cancer of the Vulva

This relatively rare malignancy usually occurs in women older than 60.

Symptoms

Pruritus is the most frequent early symptom. Later, a bloody discharge, enlarged nodules (as the adjacent lymph nodes become involved), ulceration and swelling of the vulva, and a visible mass may be seen; finally, severe pain is experienced. As the cancer ulcerates, a bloody, perhaps purulent, discharge from the vulva may be present.

Diagnosis

Diagnosis is confirmed by biopsy.

Treatment

Vulvectomy with removal of the inguinal lymph nodes (radical vulvectomy) is the treatment of choice. When

Table 50–2. Ovarian Cysts and Tumors

	Comments	*Treatment*
Ovarian Cysts		
Follicular cysts	Caused by retention of fluid, they often are asymptomatic and may disappear	Surgical excision may be required
Corpus luteum cysts	These cysts form when the corpus luteum fails to regress after the discharge of the ovum	Surgical excision of the corpus luteum is often necessary; the rest of the ovary usually can be saved
Ovarian Tumors		
Benign	May cause cessation of menstruation, hirsutism, atrophy of the breasts, sterility	Surgical removal of tumor, oophorectomy, may be performed
Serous		
Pseudomucinous		
Fibroma		
Cystic teratoma (dermoid)		
Malignant	May cause pressure on the bladder leading to frequency and urgency or pressure on the portal blood vessel leading to ascites; in the late stages, may cause weight loss, severe pain, and gastrointestinal symptoms	Surgery Deep radiation therapy Chemotherapy

the disease has spread to an inoperable stage, radiation therapy may be used. Exaggerated tissue reaction may cause the patient considerable discomfort.

Depending on the patient, the operation may be done in two stages: first the vulvectomy and later the groin dissection.

When cancer of the vulva is inoperable, wet dressings and perineal irrigations with a deodorizing solution may help to control the odor and the infection that usually occur in the ulcerating neoplasm. Narcotic analgesics usually are necessary in the terminal stage of the disease.

NURSING PROCESS —THE PATIENT UNDERGOING A VULVECTOMY

Preoperative Period

Assessment
A complete medical, drug, and allergy history is obtained. The patient is questioned about symptoms. Vital signs are taken, and the patient is weighed.

Nursing Diagnosis
Depending on the stage of the cancer, the age of the patient, and other factors, one or both of the following may apply:

■ Anxiety related to diagnosis, radical surgery
■ Knowledge deficit of surgery, preoperative preparations, postoperative management

Planning and Implementation
The major goals of the patient include a reduction in anxiety and an understanding of the surgery, preoperative preparations, and postoperative management.

The major goal of nursing management is to prepare the patient physically and emotionally for surgery.

Preoperative preparations include a shaving of the operative site, enemas, and insertion of an indwelling urethral catheter and intravenous line.

Anxiety. If the patient is older, many problems may be associated with the diagnosis and surgery, such as the care required after discharge from the hospital. The patient may live alone or have a spouse that is unable to care for her and manage the household after she is discharged from the hospital. Because of this and other types of problems, the patient may show great concern during the preoperative period.

The nurse must be willing to listen and to try to identify problems as they are made known. Once a problem is identified, steps can be taken to begin to solve it.

Knowledge Deficit. Preoperative preparations are explained before the procedure. The patient is taught and allowed to practice deep breathing and coughing.

Evaluation

■ Anxiety is reduced
■ Demonstrates understanding of preoperative preparations and postoperative coughing and deep-breathing exercises

Postoperative Period

Assessment

On return from surgery, vital signs are taken, and the patient's chart is reviewed for the extent of surgery. The surgical area is examined for the presence of drains, type of dressings, and whether or not drainage is on the dressing.

Nursing Diagnosis

Depending on the extent of surgery and other factors, such as the age and condition of the patient, one or more of the following may apply:

■ Anxiety related to diagnosis, radical surgery, change in body image
■ Pain related to surgery
■ Impaired skin integrity related to surgery, infection, maceration, wound drainage, other factors (specify)
■ Potential for infection related to surgery, proximity of surgical area to rectum
■ Self-care deficit: total to partial (specify areas) related to surgery, inability to move (pressure dressings on the perineal area, pain)
■ Body image disturbance related to removal of the vulva
■ Sexual dysfunction related to removal of vulva and adjacent structures
■ Knowledge deficit of postdischarge perineal care, treatment regimen

Planning and Implementation

The major goals of the patient include a reduction of anxiety, relief of pain, preservation of skin integrity, absence of infection, improved ability to care for self, acceptance of change in body image, return of adequate sexual function, and an understanding of postdischarge perineal care and treatment regimen.

The major goals of nursing management are to reduce anxiety, relieve pain, preserve skin integrity, prevent infection, give emotional support during the recovery phase, and develop a teaching plan that helps the patient care for the operative area.

An intravenous line is inserted before or during surgery, and intravenous fluids are prescribed until the patient is able to take oral fluids.

Because the urethra is involved in the operation, the patient returns from surgery with an indwelling urethral catheter. Intake and output are measured, and the physician is informed if the urinary output falls below 500 mL/day. The patency of the catheter is checked at frequent intervals; it is important to keep the bladder empty and prevent excessive tension on suture lines.

Deep breathing, coughing, and leg exercises are performed every 1 or 2 hours during the early postoperative period. The patient is assisted with passive leg movements until these exercises can be performed without assistance.

Anxiety.   Before and after surgery, the patient may express various concerns about the surgery, treatments, and prognosis. The nurse may help reduce anxiety by explaining all new treatments, even those as simple as applying a heat lamp. The patient's privacy must be ensured during activities such as perineal care, heat-lamp treatments, and sitz baths.

Once the patient begins to recover, she may provide indications that it is difficult to accept the change in body image and possible sexual dysfunction. The patient must be allowed time to talk and ask questions. Although some questions can only be answered by the physician, the nurse may offer suggestions, for example, about discussing concerns with her sexual partner and keeping the perineal area clean and as free as possible from odor. Showing the patient the healing tissues with the help of a mirror and encouraging participation in the changing of dressings may help the patient accept changes in body image.

Pain.   The patient usually is uncomfortable after a vulvectomy, and needs frequent administration of analgesics for at least a week or more. Placing the patient in a semirecumbent position may relieve some of the pressure on the sutures, which are probably taut. The patient must not remain in one position, even if a comfortable one is found. When on her side, the upper leg should be bent and supported with pillows to prevent pull on the operative area.

Impaired Skin Integrity.   The initial pressure dressing usually is held in place with a T-binder. After this dressing is removed, perineal care usually is ordered. Sterile technique is used when irrigating the area. Sterile saline, peroxide, or an antiseptic solution may be ordered for cleaning the surgical area. If drains were inserted, they are not disturbed. All drainage is noted and a description recorded.

After the sutures have been removed, warm sitz baths may be ordered. These also may help the patient to urinate after the indwelling urethral catheter has been removed.

Heat-lamp treatments may be ordered to dry the area after perineal care and also to improve circulation, which promotes healing.

Potential for Infection.   Antibiotics usually are ordered to prevent infection. Vital signs are monitored every 4 hours, and any temperature over 101°F (38.3°C) chills, cough, or chest pain is brought to the attention of the physician.

Straining at stool is avoided because the rectum is near the operative area. The patient is given enemas before surgery, and a low-residue diet often is prescribed during the postoperative period. After the patient has a bowel movement, the perineal area is gently and thoroughly cleansed to prevent contamination of the surgical site.

Once dressings are removed, the surgical area is inspected several times daily for signs of infection, such as purulent drainage from the incision. Any sign of infection is brought to the attention of the physician.

Self-Care Deficit.   In the beginning, the patient is unable to perform activities of daily living (ADL) because of pain as well as the dressings around the perineal area. Assistance with these activities is necessary. As healing occurs and dressings are removed, the patient may begin to participate in ADL. The patient's ability to assume responsibility for care is evaluated daily.

Knowledge Deficit.   The type of home management depends on many factors, such as physician's preference, patient's age, patient's acceptance of the surgery, and the healing of the surgical area. In most instances, a family member or health care giver needs to assume responsibility for aspects of home care. The nurse must evaluate the home situation and other problems that may have been identified about the availability of people to care for the patient during a relatively long recovery period. Problems with home care are discussed with the physician; referral to a home health care agency may be necessary.

One or more of the following may be prescribed by the physician: antibiotic therapy (which may continue for 6 or more months), a stool softener to prevent constipation, an ointment or cream to be applied to the operative area, and wound irrigations.

The following may be included in a patient teaching plan:

1. Avoid heavy lifting, straining to have a bowel movement, constipation, and sexual intercourse until approved by the physician.
2. Take, apply, or use the prescribed drugs exactly as ordered.

3. Rest at frequent intervals throughout the day; elevate the legs periodically; avoid sitting in one position for long periods.
4. Wear antiembolic stockings (if prescribed); remove and reapply two to three times daily.
5. Notify the physician if any of the following occur: chills, fever, pain, urinary frequency and urgency, drainage or bleeding in or from the operative site, swelling of the groin, legs, or ankles, adverse drug effects.

Evaluation

■ Anxiety is reduced
■ Pain is controlled
■ Operative site shows evidence of healing
■ Shows no evidence of infection
■ Self-care needs are met
■ Begins to assume responsibility for some or most of own needs: toileting, grooming, bathing
■ Openly discusses and asks questions about change in body image
■ Expresses desire to discuss relationship with sexual partner
■ Demonstrates understanding of treatment regimen, activities to avoid
■ Begins to assume responsibility for or participate in aspects of care of the surgical site

Cancer of the Vagina

Cancer of the vagina is rare and usually is seen in women older than 40. Studies have shown that a causal relationship may exist between the taking of diethylstilbestrol (DES) during early pregnancy and the development of vaginal carcinoma in the (young) female offspring. DES is no longer used to treat problems associated with pregnancy. All women who took this drug during a pregnancy should tell their daughters and advise them to have complete gynecologic examinations at regular intervals.

Symptoms

Abnormal vaginal bleeding usually is the predominant symptom. Dyspareunia also may occur.

Diagnosis

Diagnosis is made by visual examination of the vaginal canal and biopsy of the lesion.

Treatment

Cancer of the vagina is treated according to the extent of the tumor. Radiation therapy usually is the treatment of choice. Many complications, such as fistulas and bleeding, arise from the tumor itself and from radiation therapy. These complications are difficult to correct and control. Despite therapy, the prognosis is often poor.

Cancer of the Cervix

The most common malignancy of the female reproductive tract is cancer of the cervix. Only cancer of the breast exceeds it in frequency.

Theoretically, all cancer of the cervix begins in situ (in site, localized). It may take 10 to 15 years to become invasive. Regular Pap smears, therefore, are important for women of all ages.

Symptoms

The early stage has no symptoms. Even when the cancer has begun to invade the cervix, symptoms may still be absent. When symptoms do appear, bleeding and leukorrhea are most prominent.

At first, spotting occurs, especially after slight trauma, such as douching or intercourse. Later, if the condition is still untreated, the discharge continues, growing bloody and malodorous as the cancerous tissue becomes necrotic. Pain, symptoms of pressure on the bladder or bowel, and the generalized wasting of advanced cancer may be found.

Diagnosis

Routine inspection of the cervix, with Pap smears and biopsy of suspicious tissue, is imperative for early diagnosis. When cancer is suspected or diagnosed, the physician may perform a Schiller's test.

Treatment

Cure is possible if the disease is discovered before it has spread. When the cellular change is still confined to the mucosal layer of the cervix, it is called *carcinoma in situ*. Invasion of surrounding tissue may not occur for 5 years or more after the preinvasion period.

Treatment of cervical cancer usually depends on the stage of the tumor, which is determined by whether the tumor is localized (stages 0 or I) or has spread to other structures (stages II to IV), such as the vagina, pelvis, and bladder. Some physicians advocate radiation therapy or radium; others recommend surgery, such as a radical hysterectomy or radical pelvic surgery (pelvic extenteration). When radium is used, a rigid applicator that contains radium is placed near the cervix, left in place for a specified period of hours, and then removed.

Cancer of the Endometrium

Cancer of the lining of the uterus is more common in postmenopausal women. The risk of endometrial cancer increases when estrogens are taken for 5 or more years during and after menopause. When the lowest possible dose of estrogen is prescribed and therapy lasts for less than 5 years, the risk of this cancer appears to decrease.

Symptoms

Bleeding is the earliest and most common symptom. Before menopause, it may appear as menorrhagia. Because of the increased incidence in postmenopausal women, all vaginal bleeding must be investigated. Late symptoms include pain and signs of metastasis to other areas of the body.

Diagnosis

Microscopic examination of endometrial smears and of tissue removed by a D and C establishes the diagnosis. The D and C is dangerous because the scraping can spread the cancer cells. The endometrial smear is more accurate, less expensive, and does not require a surgical procedure.

Treatment

When the disease is diagnosed in its early stages, a hysterectomy is performed. Once metastasis has occurred, the physician may use radiation or radium implant. Chemotherapy with progestins, such as megestrol acetate (Megace) or medroxyprogesterone acetate (Depo-Provera), may be given as a palliative measure when the cancer is inoperable, recurrent, or metastatic.

HYSTERECTOMY

A hysterectomy may be performed for a variety of reasons, such as uncontrolled uterine bleeding, uterine fibroids, endometriosis, severe uterine prolapse, and malignancies of the uterus (cervix or endometrium).

The following are the types of procedures that remove the uterus:

Total hysterectomy—Removal of the entire uterus and cervix

Subtotal hysterectomy—Removal of the uterus only, with a stump of the cervix left intact

Radical hysterectomy—Removal of the uterus, cervix, ovaries, and fallopian tubes; part of the upper vagina and some pelvic lymph nodes also may be removed at this time

A hysterectomy may be performed with a vaginal or abdominal approach. The approach depends on many factors, such as the age and general condition of the patient. The vaginal approach may be used when the surgeon wishes to repair a cystocele or rectocele at the same time as the hysterectomy. This approach has fewer complications than the abdominal route and may be used to perform a total or subtotal hysterectomy.

An abdominal approach is required for conditions in which the abdominal organs need to be visualized directly, such as with endometriosis. This approach is always used for a radical hysterectomy, which is performed mostly for a malignant disorder of the cervix or endometrium. This approach also may be used for a total and subtotal hysterectomy.

NURSING PROCESS —THE PATIENT UNDERGOING A HYSTERECTOMY

Preoperative Period

Assessment
A complete medical, drug, and allergy history is obtained. The patient's records are reviewed for previous diagnostic and laboratory studies, as well as for the physician's diagnosis. Vital signs are taken, and the patient is weighed.

Nursing Diagnosis
Depending on the reason for surgery, the age and health of the patient, and other factors, one or both of the following may apply. Additional diagnoses may be necessary if the patient has problems such as anemia due to excessive bleeding that requires preoperative blood transfusions or concurrent medical problems such as diabetes mellitus.

■ Anxiety related to impending surgery, diagnosis
■ Knowledge deficit related to preparations for surgery, management after surgery, patient responsibilities after surgery

Planning and Implementation
The major goals of the patient include a reduction in anxiety and an understanding of preoperative preparations and postoperative management.

The major goals of nursing management are to prepare the patient physically and emotionally for surgery.

The preoperative preparations may vary, depending on the surgeon's preference and the planned surgical approach (abdominal or vaginal). If a vaginal hysterectomy is to be performed, the surgeon may order douches the night before or the morning of surgery. Either approach requires a shaving prep. Usually, an enema is ordered to be given the night before or the morning of surgery.

Preoperative preparation includes catheterization or the insertion of an indwelling catheter to minimize the chance of damaging the bladder. Surgeons may request the insertion of ureteral catheters by a urologist immediately before surgery. The purpose of these catheters is to help identify the ureters during abdominal surgery and prevent inadvertent cutting or tying of these structures. An intravenous line also may be inserted before surgery.

Surgeons may prescribe an antibiotic, usually one of the cephalosporins, such as cephradine (Velosef), cephalothin (Keflin), or cephapirin (Cefadyl), before a vaginal hysterectomy to prevent infection after surgery on a contaminated area. The drug is given both during and after surgery.

Anxiety. Because gynecologic tumors can be a threat to both life and reproductive power, the patient should receive as much emotional support as possible. The desire for children, the fear of cancer, the dread of mutilation, and of the loss of femininity are deeply felt emotions. Sterility, which results from removal of the uterus, often requires severe adjustment, especially if the patient is in her childbearing years.

Knowledge Deficit. The patient is given time to ask questions and to talk about the impending surgery. Routine preoperative preparations, such as shaving the area or inserting a catheter, are explained immediately before each task is performed. Preoperative teaching also includes demonstration and practice of deep breathing, coughing, and leg exercises.

Evaluation
■ Anxiety is reduced
■ Demonstrates understanding of preoperative preparations
■ Demonstrates understanding of postoperative deep breathing, coughing, and leg exercises

Postoperative Period

Assessment
On return from surgery, vital signs are taken, and the chart is reviewed for the operative approach and extent of surgery.

Nursing Diagnosis
Depending on the extent of surgery, intraoperative or postoperative diagnosis, the patient's age, and other factors, one or more of the following may apply:

■ Pain related to surgery
■ Anxiety related to pain, postsurgical diagnosis, other factors (specify)
■ Ineffective airway clearance related to failure to cough, deep breathe
■ Hyperthermia related to infection
■ Potential for infection related to surgery, failure to cough and deep breathe
■ Impaired skin integrity related to surgical incision
■ Constipation related to pain on defecation secondary to lower abdominal or vaginal surgery

■ Self-care deficit: complete to partial (specify areas) related to surgery, pain, discomfort
■ Body image disturbance related to loss of reproductive organs
■ Knowledge deficit of postdischarge management

Planning and Implementation

The major goals of the patient include relief of pain, reduction in anxiety, maintenance of a clear airway, absence of infection, presence of normal vital signs and normal bowel function, healing of the surgical wound, improvement in ability to carry out self care, acceptance of change in reproductive capacity, and an understanding of home care.

The major goals of nursing management are to relieve pain, reduce anxiety, prevent infection, identify complications associated with surgery, meet the patient's needs, and formulate and carry out an effective teaching plan.

Complications associated with the abdominal approach include infection, urinary retention, pulmonary embolus, paralytic ileus, hemorrhage, inadvertent ligation of a ureter, pneumonia, and thrombophlebitis. Complications are less common with the vaginal approach.

The management of the patient with a hysterectomy (Nursing Care Plan 50-1) is similar to that of the patient with general abdominal surgery. Vital signs are taken every 4 hours or as ordered. Intake and output are measured.

If ureteral catheters have not been inserted, it is extremely important that an accurate record of intake and output be kept. If ureteral catheters have been inserted, they are labeled as left and right. It is important to note if both catheters are draining urine. Output is measured from the indwelling urethral catheter as well as from each ureteral catheter.

Any complaints of back pain (which may be due to dilatation of the renal pelvis if a ureter is accidentally tied off) or severe abdominal pain (which may be due to urine leaking into the peritoneal cavity if a ureter was accidentally cut) are reported immediately.

Usually, the ureteral catheters are removed first. The drainage from the indwelling urethral catheter is monitored. A decrease or absence of urine output is immediately brought to the attention of the physician. Once the indwelling urethral catheter is removed, the urine output is measured after each voiding. Failure to void or voiding in frequent and small amounts is brought to the attention of the physician.

Antiembolic stockings may have been applied preoperatively or in surgery. These are removed and reapplied every 8 hours.

Pain.   The patient's pain is evaluated, and the prescribed analgesics are administered as ordered. The patient is helped to assume a position of comfort, and positions are changed at least every 2 hours. Pain in an area other than the surgical incision, such as the legs, chest, or back, must be carefully evaluated and then reported to the physician.

Anxiety.   Anxiety may be reduced by keeping the patient as comfortable as possible. If the patient is apparently comfortable but still seems to display anxiety, it may be necessary to spend time with her to try to determine the cause. The surgeon may have informed the patient that the lesion for which they performed the hysterectomy was found to be malignant. In this case, the patient may need someone to spend time with her as she discusses her concerns.

Anxiety also may occur in the younger patient who is concerned about the loss of reproductive function. Patients may believe that after a hysterectomy certain events occur, such as loss of libido, masculinization, premature aging, and severe depression or other mental disorders. The nurse must reassure the patient that these events have no connection with this type of surgery.

Ineffective Airway Clearance.   The patient is encouraged to cough and deep breathe every 2 hours. Support of the incision (abdominal approach) may be given to reduce the stress on the incision and, thus, reduce discomfort during these maneuvers.

The lungs are auscultated once or twice a day. Any abnormal breath sounds or chest pain is reported to the physician.

Hyperthermia, Potential for Infection.   A temperature higher than 101°F is brought to the attention of the physician. Antibiotics, which may have been started before surgery, usually are given during the postoperative period. Antibiotics may be administered by the intravenous or intramuscular route.

Impaired Skin Integrity.   If an abdominal approach was used, the dressing is checked for drainage. Abnormal or excessive drainage is reported to the physician. Once dressing changes are allowed, the incision is inspected for signs of wound separation and infection, such as purulent drainage, redness, and excessive pain in the incision. If any of these symptoms occur, the physician is notified.

Constipation.   Once peristalsis has returned and oral fluids are allowed, the patient is encouraged to drink water at frequent intervals. The physician may order a high-residue diet as well as a stool softener to prevent constipation and discomfort on defeca-

Nursing Care Plan 50–1

Postoperative Management of the Patient With a Total Abdominal Hysterectomy

Potential Problem and Potential Nursing Diagnosis	Nursing Intervention	Outcome Criteria
Pain/Discomfort *Altered comfort: pain: related to surgery, immobility, improper positioning*	Assess type of pain, location, onset, and duration; administer analgesics as ordered; change position q 2 hr; encourage active exercises; maintain correct body alignment; use pillows to support back and legs as needed	Patient reports decreased discomfort; pain adequately controlled with analgesics
Thrombophlebitis of the Veins in the Lower Extremities	Remove and reapply antiembolic stockings q 8 hr; encourage active leg exercises q 2–4 hr; assess lower extremities for color, warmth, pain, redness, blanching, or other changes in sensation q 4 hr; do not use pillows behind the knees or raise the foot gatch while patient is in a supine position; ambulate as ordered	No signs of thrombophlebitis in the lower extremities
Anuria Due to Accidental Ligation of One or Both Ureters During Surgery	Measure and record intake and output q 8 hr; report any decrease in urine output or alteration of the intake/output ratio to the physician immediately; carefully evaluate all abdominal pain (which could be due to the surgery or urine leaking into the abdominal cavity); report any increase in the severity of abdominal pain; check for back tenderness q 4 hr	Urinary output normal
Urinary Retention	Measure intake and output; palpate lower abdomen for distention q 4 hr; if patient is voiding in small amounts, measure urine each voiding (to detect retention with overflow); report any decrease in urine output to physician; encourage a liberal fluid intake; ambulate as ordered	Voiding in sufficient quantity
Abdominal Distention; Paralytic Ileus	Encourage ambulation; auscultate abdomen q 4 hr for bowel sounds; palpate abdomen q 4 hr for signs of rigidity; insert rectal tube if ordered; report signs of abdominal distention or rigidity or sudden absence of bowel sounds to physician immediately	Bowel sounds normal; abdomen soft; passes flatus
Vaginal Bleeding or Hemorrhage	Record number of perineal pads used; record color, amount, type of vaginal drainage; report excessive bleeding or passage of clots to physician immediately; monitor vital signs q 4 hr	Normal postoperative vaginal drainage; no change in vital signs

tion. Early ambulation encourages the passage of flatus (gas) and increases peristalsis.

Self-Care Deficit. Depending on the patient and the extent of surgery, the patient may be able to assume some self-care activities the morning after surgery. Assistance is given as needed until the patient is able to assume full responsibility for her own care.

Knowledge Deficit. The areas covered in a discharge teaching plan vary depending on the physician's recommendation or prescriptions, the age of the patient, the postoperative diagnosis, and other factors. If drugs have been prescribed, the dosage and adverse drug effects are reviewed with the patient.

The following areas may be included in a patient teaching plan:

1. Take the prescribed medications as ordered. Contact the physician if adverse drug effects occur.
2. Avoid heavy lifting, sexual intercourse, vigorous activity, douching, and the use of tampons until permitted by the physician.
3. Ambulate at intervals and avoid sitting in one position for a prolonged period of time.
4. Clean the incision as directed by the physician.
5. Contact the physician if any of the following occur: fever, redness, swelling, pain, or drainage of the incision, vaginal discharge that has a foul odor, bleeding from the vagina, pain in the chest, abdomen, or legs.
6. Avoid constipation and straining to have a bowel movement. Drink plenty of fluids. If constipation occurs, contact the physician.

Evaluation

- Pain is controlled
- Anxiety is reduced
- Coughs and deep breathes effectively; lungs are clear to auscultation
- Vital signs are normal
- Shows no evidence of infection
- Incision appears normal and is clean and dry with no evidence of drainage or wound separation
- Bowel elimination is normal
- Assumes responsibility for most or all of own care
- Talks openly about the surgery and its impact on reproductive function
- Demonstrates understanding of postdischarge management; asks questions about home care

Cancer of the Ovary

Malignant tumors of the ovary (see Table 50-2 and Fig. 50-5) are frequently far advanced and inoperable by

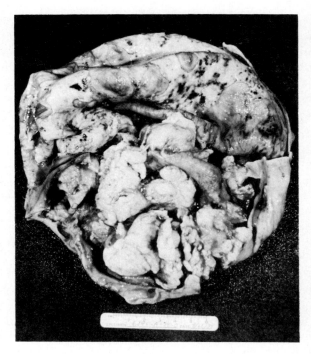

Figure 50–5. Gross appearance of a solid and cystic malignant tumor that has completely replaced an ovary. (Photograph by D. Atkinson)

the time they are diagnosed. It is believed that some of these tumors may arise from ovarian cysts. Many physicians feel that ovarian enlargement, found at the time of pelvic examination, requires surgical exploration.

Symptoms

In the beginning, symptoms such as lower abdominal discomfort are vague. As the tumor grows larger, urinary frequency and urgency may develop because of pressure on the bladder. Later, ascites, weight loss, severe pain, and gastrointestinal symptoms may occur.

Diagnosis

Diagnosis is made by surgical removal of the tumor with microscopic examination to confirm the diagnosis.

Treatment

Initially, exploratory surgery may have been performed for the diagnosis of a malignant or benign ovarian lesion. If the lesion was malignant, the ovary may be removed, but radical surgery is rarely performed. Treatment also includes deep radiation therapy followed by chemotherapy. Drugs used for chemotherapy include mitomycin (Mutamycin), doxorubicin (Adriamycin), and cyclophosphamide (Cytoxan). Usually, these drugs are given in combination.

Only a small percentage of patients with malignant tumors of the ovary survive 5 or more years despite intensive treatment. The emotional impact of the diagnosis requires support and understanding on the part of the nurse and other members of the health team. Many of these patients are young, the treatment is difficult, and the prognosis is poor.

DISORDERS OF THE BREAST

Both malignant and benign lesions of the breast are common in all age groups. The most common breast disorder is cystic disease. Benign tumors, such as fibroadenoma, are less common than cystic disease.

Symptoms

Pain. At times, breast pain is normal. It is not uncommon for the breasts to become enlarged and tender during the period immediately before menstruation. These physical changes are probably associated with the hormonal changes of the reproductive cycle and may be due to an increase in extracellular fluid tension; the mechanism, however, is not fully understood. Women with cystic disease also frequently experience fullness, tenderness, and some pain in their breasts immediately before they menstruate. Breast pain also may occur in breast abscess and as a late sign of a breast malignancy.

Masses. Changes in the breast are significant because they may be symptoms of a breast disorder. The most important reason to self-examine the breasts is to discover abnormal changes, such as a palpable mass (or lump), that may be a cyst or a benign or malignant tumor. Many disappear at the time of the menstrual period; only those that present postmenstrually are significant. Characteristically, malignant growths are painless in their early stages. The diagnosis can be made, but only if it is brought to the attention of the physician.

Nipple Discharge. A discharge that spots clothing or drips out without being elicited requires prompt medical attention. Cheesy and milky discharges usually are of no significance. Bloody, brown, or clear fluid discharges must be checked immediately.

Change in Appearance. A slight difference in the sizes of the two breasts may be normal; it also may indicate, however, a malignant or benign breast lesion.

A breast with an adhering mass near the surface may dimple the skin outside, or it may cause the nipple to retract. A deep-adhering tumor may fix the breast tissue to the underlying pectoral muscle. Firmness, redness, erosion, or edema may be seen. Redness (usually along with moderate to severe pain) may indicate a breast abscess.

Diagnosis

All women should have their breasts examined by a physician at least once a year. Women older than 30, those with cysts, and those who have a relative who has had cancer should be examined every 6 months. Women should go immediately to a physician when a lump or abnormality is discovered.

To discover carcinoma of the breast early enough so that its removal is life-saving, regular breast self-examination (BSE) is emphasized. The best protection against cancer is effective, early action. The technique for BSE is shown in Figure 50-6.

Many women are not aware of what they themselves can do to discover early disease. Some women have not been exposed to the idea of BSE; others have failed to attend to it.

It is essential to educate women about the need to protect themselves against death from breast cancer. Because so many emotional factors are involved, it is not enough to impart information. The educator must understand why women resist this knowledge and how they may be helped to overcome their apparent indifference. Apathy, fear, and the belief that cancer happens to other people lead to resistance to regular examinations of the breasts.

The knowledge that two thirds of all breast operations are for benign lesions is not necessarily reassuring. The patient knows that she may be in the other third. Those who have seen a close relative die of cancer of the breast may find BSE especially difficult.

Additional methods of early detection of breast lesions and ways to differentiate between a malignant and benign breast lesion, such as biopsy or mammogram, are discussed in Chapter 49.

Cystic Disease

Chronic cystic mastitis is not inflammatory (as the term *mastitis* would imply). In this benign disorder, normal breast tissue proliferates and forms many masses throughout the breasts. The masses become fibrotic and block the ducts, causing cysts to form.

Single or multiple breast cysts may develop. Some have a bluish color, prompting the name blue-domed cysts. Cysts usually are movable in the surrounding breast tissue. They are far less likely to adhere and to cause retraction than are malignant lesions.

Symptoms

Cystic disease of the breast may cause no symptoms other than lumps; or the breast may be tender or painful, especially before menstruation.

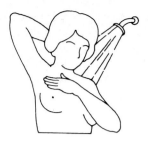

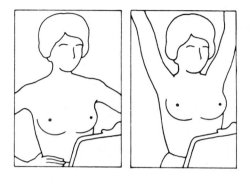

1. In the shower. Examine your breasts during bath or shower; hands glide easily over wet skin. With fingers flat, move them gently over every part of each breast. Check for any lump, hard knot, or thickening.

2. Before a mirror. Inspect your breasts with arms at your sides. Next, raise your arms high overhead. Look for any changes in contour of each breast—a swelling, dimpling of skin, or changes in the nipple. Then rest palms on hips and press down firmly to flex your chest muscles. Left and right breast will not match exactly—few women's breasts do. Regular inspection shows what is normal for you and will give you confidence in your examination.

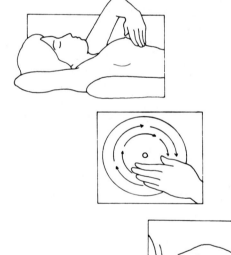

3. Lying down. To examine your right breast put a pillow or folded towel under your right shoulder. Place your right hand behind your head—this distributes breast tissue more evenly on the chest. With left hand, press gently in small circular motions around an imaginary clock face. Begin at outermost top of your right breast for 12 o'clock, then move to 1 o'clock, and so on around the circle back to 12. A ridge of firm tissue in the lower curve of each breast is normal. Then move in an inch, toward the nipple, keep circling to examine every part of your breast, including the nipple. This requires at least three more circles. Now slowly repeat the procedure on your left breast with a pillow under your left shoulder and your left hand behind your head. Notice how your breast structure feels. Finally, squeeze the nipple of each breast gently between your thumb and index finger. Any discharge, clear or bloody, should be reported to your physician immediately.

Figure 50-6. Self-examination of the breast. (Reprinted by permission of the American Cancer Society, Inc)

Diagnosis

Diagnosis is made by examination of the breasts by a physician.

Treatment

A well-fitted brassiere may be advised by the physician. During periods when the breasts are tender, the patient may feel more comfortable if she wears a brassiere during the night as well as the day. Multiple cystic disease sometimes is treated by partial mastectomy. The areola may be saved, and reconstructive surgery may be done with fat and fascia or a plastic insert to preserve the appearance of the breast (augmentation mammoplasty).

Malignancy in the breast seems to be somewhat more common in patients with cystic disease than in women with normal breasts. The physician usually recommends a BSE every month, examination of the breast by a physician every 6 months, and a mammogram every 1 or 2 years. The search for new breast masses is complicated by the already existing ones, but the woman who becomes familiar with her own breasts by periodic examination often can identify new growths.

Breast Abscess

Abscesses occur most frequently as a postpartum complication. Fissures and cracks in the nipple provide entry for microorganisms, especially staphylococci, which thrive in milk.

Symptoms

Symptoms include fever, chills, pain, redness, and swelling of an area of the breast. A purulent exudate may drain from the breast nipple.

Diagnosis

The physician bases the diagnosis on physical examination of the breast. If drainage from the nipple is found, culture and sensitivity tests may be ordered to identify the microorganism.

Treatment

The patient usually is hospitalized and may be placed on isolation precautions because the soiled dressings are highly infectious. Antibiotic therapy is started. A localized lesion may be incised, drained, and packed.

Montgomery straps may be applied so that the frequent removal of dressing tape does not irritate the skin. If warm soaks are ordered, zinc oxide may be applied to the surrounding skin to avoid maceration. The arm and shoulder are supported with pillows. The patient is instructed not to shave axillary hair on that side until healing is complete.

Benign Breast Tumors

A fibroadenoma is a benign tumor of the breast. Cystic breast disease may or may not be present.

Symptoms

The symptom of a benign breast tumor is a painless, nontender lump in the breast.

Diagnosis

Since an early malignant tumor also may have the same symptoms, diagnosis is based on microscopic examination of the lesion. Most surgeons advocate the immediate surgical removal of all breast lesions for microscopic examination.

Treatment

The entire tumor is removed at the time of a biopsy. Because it is not known if the lesion is malignant or benign until the tissue is examined under a microscope, the physician may, before surgery, discuss with the patient the prospects of finding a malignancy and the possible treatment. Depending on the patient and the physician, the discovery of a benign lesion only requires removal of the tumor. If the lesion is malignant, the surgeon may either proceed with a mastectomy or close the incision and discuss the possible treatments with the patient at a later time.

Malignant Lesions of the Breast

In women in the United States, the breast is the most common site of cancer (Fig. 50-7). When the disease is discovered and treated early, the 5-year level of cure for small lesions is about 80% or better.

A breast malignancy can occur at any age. The longer a woman lives, the greater chance she has of developing breast cancer. Though breast cancer primarily affects women, men, too, can develop breast cancer.

Symptoms

Although cysts and tumors start microscopically, they grow larger and sometimes cause physical changes in the breast before any discomfort or pain is felt.

The primary symptom of breast cancer is a mass felt in the breast. The lesion may or may not be painful, but it usually is painless in the early stages of the disease. Other symptoms include a bloody discharge from the nipple, a dimpling of the skin over the lesion, retraction of the breast nipple, and a difference in size between one breast and the other. The lesion may be

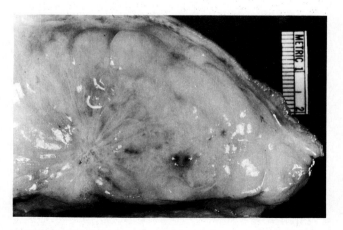

Figure 50–7. Typical cut surface of a primary scirrhous carcinoma of the breast. The center of the tumor is located toward the lower left-hand corner of the specimen. The radiating lines of infiltration extend into the surrounding breast fat. (Photograph by D. Atkinson)

fixed or movable, and lumps may be felt in the axilla. Many of these symptoms depend on several factors, such as the type and location of tumor cell and the length of time the tumor has been present.

Diagnosis

Because women have a better chance for cure when cancer is detected early, any lump or any change in the appearance of the breast that is noted during BSE is brought immediately to the attention of a physician. The earlier cancer is diagnosed, the less chance that it has spread.

Mammograms may be used to detect breast lesions. The radiologist can often differentiate between a benign and malignant lesion on radiograph. Diagnosis is confirmed by microscopic examination after removal of tissue by incisional, excisional, or aspiration biopsy (see Chapter 49).

Radiographs may be ordered if a breast lesion is thought to be malignant. The surgeon may order radiographs of the lungs, spine, or other areas of the body to detect areas of possible metastasis. These studies may be done before or after surgery, depending on the physician's findings and the patient's symptoms.

Treatment

If the lesion is found to be malignant, a mastectomy usually is performed immediately after the biopsy or is scheduled within the next few days. If the cancer is so far advanced that it has metastasized to other parts of the body, the removal of the breast does not cure the disease, and a mastectomy may or may not be done. In some instances, a simple mastectomy may be performed to remove a grossly enlarged, draining breast, thus making the patient more comfortable.

There is much controversy about which surgical procedure provides the most favorable prognosis. Various surgical interventions for malignant lesions of the breast are summarized here:

1. *Simple excision* (lumpectomy, tumorectomy)—Only the tumor is removed.
2. *Partial mastectomy*—The tumor and a small amount of breast tissue are removed.
3. *Simple mastectomy*—All breast tissue is removed. No lymph node dissection is undertaken.
4. *Subcutaneous mastectomy*—All breast tissue is removed, but the skin and nipple are left intact.
5. *Modified radical mastectomy*—The breast and the axillary lymph nodes are removed.
6. *Radical mastectomy*—The breast, axillary lymph nodes, and pectoral muscles are removed. In some instances, sternal lymph nodes (parasternal nodes) also are removed.

The main objective of surgery is to restore normal function to the shoulder and arm of the operative side. The surgical incision is planned so that skin grafting (if necessary) can be performed and so that the surgical scar is not visible when the patient wears normal clothing.

Normal function of the mammary gland depends on the action of several stimulating hormones. Changing the hormonal environment of the body may inhibit the growth of the primary tumor or metastatic tissue derived from the primary tumor elsewhere in the body. The hormonal environment of the body can be changed by ablation (removal) of an endocrine organ or by addition of exogenous sex hormones.

In premenopausal women with evidence of lymph node metastasis, a bilateral oophorectomy may be performed several weeks after the mastectomy. The rationale for this procedure is that some malignant breast tumors are thought to be hormone-dependent, that is, tumor growth is enhanced by the presence of the female hormone estrogen. When the source of the hormone—the ovaries—is removed, it is believed that tumor growth is slowed. Because the ovaries are removed to eliminate the source of estrogen from the body, no replacement estrogens are given to help relieve the distressing symptoms of a surgical menopause. The sudden lack of estrogen supply frequently causes more severe menopausal symptoms than those associated with natural menopause.

Some surgeons also advocate the removal of the adrenal glands (bilateral adrenalectomy) because the adrenal cortex also manufactures sex hormones. This surgery may be performed 1 or more months after the oophorectomy. Because the adrenals are removed, the patient is placed on lifetime corticosteroid therapy (see Chapter 48).

Additional treatment modalities depend on factors such as the presence or absence of metastasis, the type and stage of the tumor, the physician's preferences, the age of the patient, and, possibly, other factors. Depending on circumstances, additional treatment modalities include chemotherapy or chemotherapy plus radiation therapy.

Chemotherapy includes the following:

■ An antiestrogen drug, such as tamoxifen (Nolvadex), for postmenopausal women whose tumor is hormone-dependent as determined by a estradiol receptor (ERA) and a progesterone receptor assay (PRA), which is done on a tumor tissue sample

■ Androgen therapy for advanced breast cancer in postmenopausal women using testolactone (Teslac)

■ Using single or combined chemotherapy agents, such as cyclophosphamide (Cytoxan), doxorubicin (Adriamycin), fluorouracil (5-FU), methotrexate, and prednisone. Combined chemotherapy is most often used.

Radiation therapy may be given before or after surgery. If the surgeon finds that the axillary nodes contain cancer cells, a series of radiation treatments may be ordered prophylactically, even though the nodes have been removed. For palliative purposes, radiation therapy may be used to treat primary tumors, regional or distant metastases (especially to bone), or local tumor recurrence of the chest wall.

Patients may have reconstructive breast surgery at the time the mastectomy is performed or a few months to 1 or more years later. This type of surgery uses various techniques to reconstruct the breast and restore it to near normal size and shape. If this procedure is performed at the same time as or soon after a mastectomy, however, new tumor growth, if it does occur, is not detected easily and, therefore, goes unnoticed until a more advanced stage. For this reason, some surgeons prefer to wait 1 or more years before they perform reconstructive breast surgery.

Some women, despite treatment even in the early stages, develop metastatic cancer. Metastases often cause pain in the new site. Lymph nodes are most commonly involved in metastasis, with bone and pulmonary involvement following in order of frequency. Many organs and systems can be affected. When bone becomes involved, pathologic fracture (fracture after slight or no trauma) is possible. The patient is taught to take precautions against falling and to avoid bumps.

Treatment varies with the physician and specific type of metastasis and is aimed at providing the greatest period of palliation for the patient. Large doses of estrogen or testosterone sometimes alleviate the pain, weight loss, and malaise of metastatic cancer. Intramuscular androgen (testosterone) therapy is used especially when metastases are to bone. All forms of treatment carry the possibility of unpleasant effects and complications.

NURSING PROCESS —THE PATIENT UNDERGOING A MASTECTOMY
Preoperative Period

Assessment
A complete medical, drug, and allergy history is obtained. If possible, a family history of cancer (especially breast cancer) also is obtained. Vital signs are taken, and the patient is weighed.

The patient's records are reviewed for information about the location of the breast lesion, the diagnostic tests performed before admission (if any), and the information the physician has given the patient about the type and extent of surgery.

Nursing Diagnosis
The nursing diagnoses depend on factors such as the age of the patient, the planned extent of surgery, and what and how much the patient has been told by the physician.

■ Anxiety related to surgery, the diagnosis, other factors (specify)
■ Knowledge deficit of preoperative preparations, postoperative care, deep breathing and leg exercises

Planning and Implementation
The major goals of the patient include a reduction in anxiety and an understanding of routine postoperative care.

The major goal of nursing management is to prepare the patient physically and emotionally for surgery.

The preoperative area is shaved and an intravenous line may be inserted before the patient is transported to surgery. Other preoperative preparations depend on the physician's specific orders.

Some physicians refer the patient to support groups such as Reach to Recovery before surgery, whereas others prefer postoperative visits. A member of the group, who has had a mastectomy, visits the patient and answers questions about such matters as obtaining and wearing a breast prosthesis.

Anxiety. Opportunity must be provided for the patient to discuss her concerns and ask questions about the surgery. The patient who experiences extreme anxiety may be prescribed a tranquilizer before admission as well as during the preoperative period.

If the patient appears extremely nervous, the physician is informed. Patients with high levels of anxiety may require more anesthesia and thus run a greater risk of complications with anesthesia.

The nurse must also evaluate the patient's understanding of surgery. If, for any reason, the patient does not seem to understand the extent of surgery or the possible treatment modalities after surgery, it is noted in the patient's chart, and the physician is informed of the problem before surgery.

Knowledge Deficit. An explanation of the postoperative period is given to the patient and includes information about monitoring vital signs and administering intravenous fluids. Coughing, deep breathing, and leg exercises are demonstrated and practiced before surgery. Preoperative preparations, such as shaving the operative site or inserting an intravenous line, are explained.

Evaluation

■ Anxiety is reduced
■ Demonstrates understanding of preoperative preparations
■ Demonstrates understanding of postoperative management, including coughing, deep breathing, and leg exercises

- Demonstrates understanding of the type of surgery and potential postsurgical treatment modalities
- Openly discusses and asks questions about the surgery

Postoperative Period

Assessment

On return from surgery, baseline data include vital signs, inspection of the dressing, and checking the intravenous line. The patient's chart is reviewed for information about the type of mastectomy, presence of drains, problems that occurred during surgery (if any), and if skin grafting was necessary or any other surgical procedure was performed.

Drains are used to remove the serous fluid that collects under the skin, delaying healing and predisposing to infection. The physician may order the drainage tube attached to low-pressure suction or another drainage device.

A skin graft (often from the anterior thigh) may be required to close the resulting wound if a radical mastectomy has been performed. If so, a drain may be left in the axilla to clear fluid that may form under the graft. Pressure dressings are applied on both the donor and recipient graft sites.

Nursing Diagnosis

Nursing diagnoses depend on the patient and the extent of surgery (eg, simple lumpectomy, radical mastectomy). Nursing diagnoses that apply to any general surgery patient also may be added.

- Anxiety related to diagnosis, loss of breast, other factors (specify)
- Fear related to diagnosis, prognosis, planned treatment modalities
- Pain related to surgery
- Impaired skin integrity related to surgical incision, drains
- Impaired physical mobility (arm, operative side) related to surgery, pressure dressings
- Ineffective airway clearance related to failure to cough and deep breathe effectively secondary to pain and constriction of the surgical dressing
- Potential for infection related to surgery
- Ineffective individual coping related to loss of breast
- Dysfunctional grieving related to loss of breast
- Body image disturbance related to loss of breast
- Altered sexuality patterns related to mastectomy
- Bathing and hygiene and dressing and grooming self-care deficits related to partial immobility of upper extremity of operative side
- Knowledge deficit of postdischarge home care

Planning and Implementation

The major goals of the patient include a reduction in fear and anxiety, relief of pain, adequate healing of the surgical incision, improved mobility of the opera-

tive side, absence of infection, the development of family cohesiveness, ability to cope with and adapt to the diagnosis and results of surgery, improvement in ability to care for self, and an understanding of home care and future treatment modalities.

The major goals of nursing management are to reduce anxiety and fear, control pain, prevent infection, improve mobility on the operative side, emotionally support the patient and family, assist with or perform self-care needs, and prepare an effective patient teaching plan.

During the immediate postoperative period, vital signs are monitored every 30 to 60 minutes. The blood pressure and pulse, which are taken on the arm that did *not* undergo surgery, are monitored closely, as changes may indicate shock or hemorrhage.

Wounds may drain copiously. The color, amount, odor, and consistency of any drainage, whether from a drain or on the dressing, are noted and placed in the chart. The dressing is checked for drainage and oozing; any evidence of these is reported to the physician. The hand is used to feel under the patient's side; fluid seeping from the wound may not be visible on the front of the dressing but may flow underneath the patient. Immediately after surgery, the dressing is checked every 30 minutes for the first several hours. On the second and the third postoperative days, it is checked at least three times a day.

If skin grafting was necessary, the dressing that is applied is bulky to hold the skin flaps down and usually is left in place until about the fifth day after surgery. At that time, the dressing is changed by the surgeon.

COMPLICATIONS. Complications associated with a mastectomy include pneumonia, infection, damage to the brachial plexus (a network of nerves supplying the arm), hemorrhage, shock, and edema of the arm (operative side).

In some postmastectomy patients, lymphedema is disabling. Developing shortly after the operation or years later, lymphedema is most likely to occur when most or all of the lymph nodes are removed, leaving an insufficient amount of lymphatic tissue for proper lymph drainage of the arm. The cause is unknown. Radiation may aggravate lymphedema.

An air pressure machine may be used to treat lymphedema. It automatically fills the segments of the sleeve with air, exerting progressive cumulative pressure on the arm. The most distal portion of the sleeve fills first, then the next, and so on, forcing fluid past incompetent lymphatic valves toward the heart. After all the segments are filled, the air is released, and the cycle starts again. The machine is set about 5 mmHg below the diastolic blood pressure. This treatment must be used several times a day to be effective. Significant arm edema can be controlled in some cases with the use of an elastic sleeve or bandage. Obesity complicates the reduction of the edema, therefore, patients who are obese need help losing weight. Low-sodium diets and diuretics are sometimes prescribed.

Anxiety, Fear. Patients who have had a mastectomy immediately after an excisional biopsy frequently discover the diagnosis for themselves when they begin to recover from anesthesia. Unlike many other types of surgery, this operation makes the diagnosis evident to the patient. The physician and the family have no time to talk over how, if, and when to break the news. The patient, whose emotional and physical resources have been lowered by anesthesia, surgery, drugs, and suspense, needs a nurse to be there to help her at the time of the discovery.

During the postoperative period, the patient may have periods of anxiety; she may express fear and concern over the diagnosis and planned treatment modalities, such as radiation and chemotherapy. The patient must be allowed time to ask questions, express her concerns, and vent her feelings. If the patient seems extremely upset or fearful or unsure about future treatment, this problem is discussed with the physician.

Pain. Pain may be considerable, especially if a radical mastectomy has been performed. Narcotics are given liberally as ordered by the physician. Because the movement of the chest is painful and narcotics depress respirations, the patient is helped to take deep breaths after medication for pain has had its effect.

Respiratory Function. Because dressings tend to constrict the chest, the patient must be helped to cough deeply and take deep breaths every 2 hours. The hands or a pillow may be used to support the incision when the patient performs these maneuvers. The lungs are auscultated daily and abnormal findings reported to the physician.

Impaired Skin Integrity, Impaired Physical Mobility. When a radical mastectomy is performed, the incision is extensive, disturbing the integrity of a large area of skin and muscle. Immediately after the surgery, the upper arm on the affected side is protected from excessive motion, especially abduction (moving the arm away from the body). The arm on the operative side may be bandaged to the body, with the elbow bent at a right angle, especially if skin grafting has been done, as excessive motion might pull the skin graft free of its attachments. Whether the arm is bandaged or not, abduction of the arm on

the affected side is prevented. A pillow usually is placed under the arm (except with lumpectomy or simple mastectomy) to help support it and to elevate it above breast level. This practice helps to prevent lymphedema, which may develop after a radical mastectomy as a result of interference with the circulatory and lymphatic systems. The hands should be checked for signs of impaired circulation (eg, swelling, cyanosis, coldness, tingling). If such signs are noted, the surgeon is contacted.

The arm is inspected each day for evidence of lymphedema. If the patient is wearing a wedding ring after a left mastectomy, the ring and finger are inspected carefully each day. Any signs of swelling of the fingers or tightening of the ring require immediate removal of the ring. The patient with a left mastectomy with removal of axillary nodes should be discouraged from wearing her wedding ring on the left hand (it can be worn on the right).

Exercise of the arm on the operative side is ordered by the physician and may begin on the first or second postoperative day. With skin grafting, exercise is not instituted until the graft site has healed.

Exercises prevent shortening of muscles, contractures of joints, and loss of muscle tone. Active exercises are always more effective than passive ones. As soon as the physician has given permission, the patient starts a regular program that enables her to perform all normal activities. In those who do not have grafts, exercise of the operative side may begin by activities such as brushing the teeth, washing the face, and combing the hair. The first part of an exercise program may be opening and closing the hand, flexing and extending the fingers, and bending the wrist forward and backward. Squeezing a rubber or foam ball stimulates circulation and helps restore function. In some hospitals, no order is needed to commence these exercises, and they are started on the first postoperative day. The point of starting active exercises soon after surgery is psychologic as well as physiologic; it allows the patient to help in her own recovery.

When the drains are removed and the first dressing is changed, the surgeon may believe that the wound has healed sufficiently so that the patient can abduct her arm. The practice of raising the elbow away from the body can then be started. If fluid collects in the wound, exercises are delayed.

For the return of full function, the exercises must be practiced regularly. The removal of the pectoral muscle causes a temporary loss of strength but no loss of arm function. Although the arm on the operative side presents the most difficulty, exercises should be bilateral to avoid pain, postural change that results from inconsistent development, and consequent structural change.

Potential for Infection. Vital signs are monitored every 4 hours or as ordered. A temperature higher than 101°F, a cough, or a foul-smelling drainage may indicate an infection and must be reported to the physician immediately. Prophylactic antibiotic therapy may be prescribed during the postoperative period. Intramuscular or subcutaneous medications and intravenous fluid are never administered in the arm of the operative side. Blood samples for laboratory tests also are not obtained from this arm.

When dressing changes are allowed, the wound is inspected for pockets of swelling, redness, discharge, odor, and breaks in the suture line.

Ineffective Individual Coping. The emotional significance of a mastectomy varies from patient to patient. Effort should be made to help the patient look at the incision before she goes home. In addition to the incision, stab wounds for drains also may be present, and the overall appearance can greatly upset the patient, who may react with anger, tears, depression, or withdrawal. To help the patient, the nurse must anticipate and be sensitive to her reaction. Choosing the right time to encourage her to look at the incision requires an assessment of the patient's state of readiness.

The patient needs to know that, in time, redness, swelling, and irregularity of the incision will decrease, the scar will become less prominent, and tissues will become more normal in color. The healing period is 4 to 8 weeks for most patients.

Breast amputation is mutilating; it alters a woman's body. Particularly significant is the fact that it affects a part of her body intimately associated with sexual fulfillment and childbearing. Concern with appearance after surgery may be mitigated only partly by the use of prosthetic devices. The change in her body is one that the woman herself must learn to accept and cope with, regardless of what measures she may use to conceal the disfigurement from others.

These are deep and significant feelings that are not to be ignored. Nurses should help women to come to grips with these feelings by listening to them. Without prying, the nurse can help the woman to identify exactly what it is that troubles her. She can be encouraged to talk to her physician without feeling embarrassed, and she can be provided with the factual information she needs. The patient needs a great deal of support from all members of the health care team and her family.

The normal healing processes of grieving cannot be accelerated, and some patients need time, understanding, and artful listening before they are able to accept the changes in themselves and are ready to learn. As the patient's mourning and depression lessen, she becomes more aware of how the exercises are helping her and she becomes an active participant in the learning process.

Support from groups such as Reach to Recovery help many patients overcome anxiety and depression after surgery.

Self-Care Deficit. During the early postoperative period, the patient needs help with the activities that she cannot do for herself. As soon as possible, the patient is encouraged to be independent and to do as much as she can.

The way the nurse teaches exercises is important. The feelings and reactions of the patient provide the framework in which the nurse can teach. A perfect teaching plan can be a failure if the patient is not ready to learn or is so anxious that her perception is distorted. Because patients vary in their grief reactions, some may be too depressed to be able to participate in self-care activities.

The physician may order the patient out of bed for the first time on the operative night or the next day. Assistance is given until the patient appears able to ambulate without help. When assistance is necessary, the patient is supported on the *unaffected* side. Patients have a tendency to splint the operative site and to balance themselves by hunching that shoulder. Encourage the patient to keep the shoulder level and the muscles relaxed.

Knowledge Deficit. If no complications arise, most patients are discharged about 5 to 6 days after surgery. The patients need instructions in care of the surgical wound, mastectomy exercises, and other treatment modalities prescribed or recommended by the physician.

Some hospitals have group classes for postmastectomy patients. Exercising with other women who have the same difficulties can help a patient feel that she is not odd or clumsy and that she is among others who share a common problem and have common goals. A pamphlet that illustrates the exercises may help the patient practice them.

The following areas may be included in a patient teaching plan:

1. *Skin care*—Wash the area gently with a soft washcloth and soap. Complete healing of the wound takes considerable time and varies. It is not unusual to have some discomfort in the incision for several months. Do not apply creams or ointments to the incision unless approved by the physician.
2. *Prosthesis*—The physician determines when a breast prosthesis can be worn. There are several different types (Fig. 50-8). Some are made of foam rubber; others are inflated with air or filled with fluid. Sponge rubber is light and easily washable. Excessive heat and

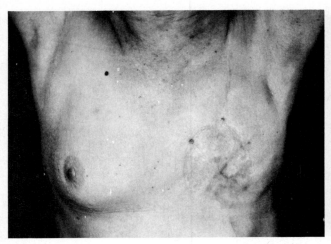 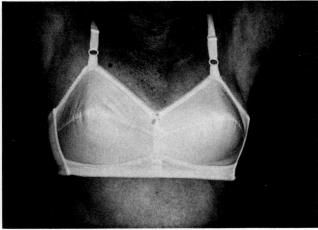

Figure 50–8. *(Left)* Radical mastectomy scar. The slight irregularity is typical. *(Right)* Same patient fitted with a prosthesis. (Photographs courtesy of Gordon F. Schwartz, MD, Professor of Surgery, Jefferson Medical College, Philadelphia)

careless handling should be avoided. If a rubber prosthesis is worn under a bathing suit, it can be squeezed dry unobtrusively with the forearm while drying the face with a towel. Prostheses that are filled with fluid assume natural contours like those of the other breast. These prostheses feel more like a normal breast and even assume body warmth.

Some surgical supply houses and department stores that sell breast prostheses have an experienced female prosthetist who can correctly fit the patient and give instructions for the care of the prosthesis. Some companies have excellent pamphlets prepared for post-mastectomy patients. (Be sure that the physician approves of the literature, the prosthesis, and the store before suggesting any of these resources to the patient. The addresses of several stores can be given to the patient. Some hospitals keep samples of different types of breast forms to show the patients).

3. *Swelling*—Slight and transitory swelling of the arm usually is relieved as soon as the arm regains function.
4. *Exercises*—Perform the exercises recommended by the physician. Postmastectomy exercises should continue, if possible, during radiation and chemotherapy treatments.
5. *Hand and arm care* (operative side)—Avoid injury, injections, having blood drawn, excessive heat, and exposure to the sun. A cream or lotion may be applied to the arm and hand several times a day.
6. *Notifying the physician*—The physician is contacted immediately if any of the following occur after dis-

charge or at any time in the future: fever, chills, drainage from incision, separation of incision, increased redness of and around the incision, sudden fatigue, sudden weight loss, loss of appetite, sudden swelling of the arm, pain in the opposite breast, infection of the arm or hand (eg, warmth, red streaks on the hand or arm, pain, fever).
7. *Follow-up*—Keep all physician or clinic appointments for follow-up care or further treatments.

Evaluation

- Anxiety and fear are reduced
- Pain is controlled
- Incision shows signs of a normal healing process
- Begins to use arm and hand of operative side
- Coughs and deep breathes effectively; lungs clear to auscultation
- No evidence of infection; vital signs normal
- Begins to demonstrate effective coping measures
- Openly discusses care of the incision; asks questions about home care
- Begins postmastectomy exercises
- Talks and asks questions about the surgery
- Looks at the incision
- Participates in daily care activities
- Demonstrates understanding of postdischarge home care
- Lists situations to avoid
- Discusses and asks questions about future treatment modalities

General Pharmacologic Considerations

☐ When gentian violet is prescribed, the patient is advised to wear a sanitary pad because the drug permanently stains clothing.

☐ Estrogen therapy can cause nausea and vomiting, pigmentation of the nipple and areola, and uterine bleeding. Stress incontinence may occur. Sodium may be retained, leading to excessive storage of intercellular fluid and edema. To help relieve this situation, diuretics and a low-sodium diet may be ordered.

Large doses of estrogen sometimes cause the mobilization of calcium into the bloodstream, damaging the kidney when it excretes the excess calcium.

☐ Patients who take oral contraceptive drugs may experience nausea, vomiting, and diarrhea. Taking the tablets with food may reduce the nausea. Breasts may become tender, and dizziness, weight gain, and stomach cramps may occur.

☐ Because synthetic hormones may cause thromboembolic phenomena, the patient is instructed to contact the physician should tenderness, pain, swelling, or redness occur in the legs. If vaginal bleeding should occur during hormonal therapy, the patient should contact the physician because the dose may need to be adjusted.

☐ When androgen therapy is prescribed, patients may have increased bone pain after the first few injections. As therapy continues, pain frequently lessens, some recalcification of bone occurs, and the patient has an increased appetite and gains weight. Androgen therapy may cause fluid retention, increased libido, and distressing symptoms of virilization, such as deeper voice and increased facial and body hair.

☐ Metastases of breast cancer to soft tissue and bone may respond to antineoplastic drugs. These drugs may cause bone marrow depression, granulocytopenia, anemia, nausea and vomiting, hypotension, dermatitis, malaise, diarrhea, and stomatitis.

General Gerontologic Considerations

☐ Older women may develop perineal pruritus. An effort is made to discover the cause of the pruritus; it may require asking questions about diet, type of clothing worn, presence of a vaginal discharge, and so on. The patient also may be tested for glucose in the blood and urine, and a pelvic examination may be performed to rule out other abnormalities, such as cervicitis, cystocele, rectocele, or cancer of the vulva, cervix, or uterus.

☐ When the elderly patient has a uterine prolapse, surgery may not be considered because of complicating disorders, such as cardiac or renal failure. A pessary may be inserted to return the uterus to its normal position in the pelvis.

☐ The elderly patient with a pessary is taught the importance of periodic removal and cleaning of the pessary. If the patient is unable to remove, clean, and reinsert the pessary, the importance of regular visits to a physician's office or a clinic is emphasized.

Suggested Readings

☐ Bates BA, Hoekelman RA. Guide to physical examination and history taking. 4th ed. Philadelphia: JB Lippincott, 1987. *(In-depth coverage of subject matter)*

☐ Bethea DC. Introductory maternity nursing. 5th ed. Philadelphia: JB Lippincott, 1988. *(In-depth coverage of subject matter)*

☐ Bowers AC, Thompson JM. Clinical manual of health assessment. 3rd ed. St Louis: CV Mosby, 1988. *(In-depth coverage of subject matter)*

☐ Brunner LS, Suddarth DS. The Lippincott manual of nursing practice. 4th ed. Philadelphia: JB Lippincott, 1986. *(Additional and in-depth coverage of subject matter)*

☐ Cerrato PL. Dietary help for PMS patients. RN January 1988;51:69. *(Additional coverage of subject matter)*

☐ Feather BL, Lanigan C. Looking good after your mastectomy. Am J Nurs August 1987;87:1048. *(Additional coverage of subject matter)*

☐ Fischbach FT. A manual of laboratory diagnostic tests. 3rd ed. Philadelphia: JB Lippincott, 1988. *(Additional coverage of subject matter)*

☐ Fox K. Ellen's going home: can she manage without you? Nursing '89 May 1989;19:80. *(Additional coverage of subject matter)*

☐ Kennedy BJ. I'm sorry, baby. Am J Nurs August 1988;88:1067. *(Additional coverage of subject matter)*

☐ Lewis LW, Timby BK. Fundamental skills and concepts in patient care. 4th ed. Philadelphia: JB Lippincott, 1988. *(Additional coverage of subject matter)*

☐ May KA, Mahlmeister LR. Comprehensive maternity care nursing. 2nd ed. Philadelphia: JB Lippincott, 1989. *(In-depth coverage of subject matter)*

☐ McKeon VA. Cruel myths and clinical facts about menopause. RN June 1989;52:52. *(Additional coverage of subject matter)*

☐ Nero F. When couples ask about infertility. RN November 1988;51:26. *(Additional and in-depth coverage of subject matter)*

☐ Rubin D. Gynecologic cancer: cervical, vulvar, and vaginal malignancies. RN May 1987;50:56. *(Additional coverage of subject matter)*

☐ Veatch RM, Fry ST. Case studies in nursing ethics. Philadelphia: JB Lippincott, 1987. *(In-depth coverage of the ethics of abortion)*

☐ Weiner SM. Clinical manual of maternity and gynecologic nursing. St Louis: CV Mosby, 1990. *(In-depth coverage of subject matter)*

Chapter 51

Disorders of the Male Reproductive System

On completion of this chapter the reader will:

■ Discuss the symptoms, diagnosis, and treatment of prostatitis, benign prostatic hypertrophy, and cancer of the prostate

■ Use the nursing process in the management of a patient who is having a prostatectomy

■ Discuss the purpose of a vasectomy and vasovasostomy

■ Discuss the symptoms, diagnosis, and treatment of cryptorchidism, epididymo-orchitis, spermatic cord torsion, hydrocele, and varicocele

■ Discuss the symptoms, diagnosis, and treatment of cancer of the testes

■ Use the nursing process in the management of a patient who is having surgery for cancer of the testes

■ Discuss the symptoms, diagnosis, and treatment of phimosis, paraphimosis, and cancer of the penis

■ Discuss the purpose of circumcision and rationale for this procedure in the adult

DISORDERS OF THE PROSTATE

Prostatitis

Prostatitis is an inflammation of the prostate gland due to situations such as infection, prostatic enlargement, and stricture (narrowing) of the urethra.

Symptoms
Symptoms vary depending on the cause and include perineal pain or discomfort, low back pain, fever, chills, and urinary urgency, frequency, pain, and burning. Nocturia (excessive urination during the night) may also be seen. Patients also may have no symptoms.

Diagnosis
Diagnosis is based on symptoms as well as a careful patient history. The physician usually examines the gland by inserting a finger in the rectum. In addition, the gland may be massaged to express prostatic fluid, which is then examined microscopically. A culture and sensitivity test may be performed on the prostatic fluid as well as on a voided urine specimen to determine if a bladder infection is also present.

Treatment
Antibiotics are given for 7 to 10 days. Patients with chronic prostatitis may be prescribed low doses of an antibiotic to be taken over a prolonged period of time.

The patient is instructed to rest as much as possible. A mild analgesic may be recommended or prescribed for pain or discomfort. Sitz baths taken 2 to 4 times a day for 15 to 20 minutes may be recommended. If a bladder infection is also present, treatment may include a sulfonamide or urinary antiinfective, such as nalidixic acid (NegGram), cinoxacin (Cinobac), or norfloxacin (Noroxin).

Additional recommendations by the physician may be to refrain from sexual intercourse until the disorder is under control, prevent constipation, take a stool softener, and avoid prolonged periods of sitting. Avoiding foods such as coffee, tea, alcoholic beverages, and spicy foods may also be recommended since these substances can irritate the bladder.

Benign Prostatic Hypertrophy

With advancing age and under the influence of male sex hormones, the periurethral glandular tissue undergoes hyperplasia (extra growth of normal tissue, increase in the number of cells), with gradual enlargement of the gland. This outward expansion is not of any clinical importance; inward encroachment of this tissue, however, which diminishes the diameter of the prostatic urethra, is of clinical significance.

707

Symptoms

The symptoms of benign prostatic hypertrophy (BPH) are all secondary to an increased difficulty in urinating. Symptoms appear gradually. At first the patient may notice that it takes more effort to void and decreasing force and narrowing of the urinary stream is seen. As the residual urine that remains in the bladder accumulates, the bladder fills more quickly, and the patient finds that the urge to void occurs more often. Urgency, to the point of incontinence, may occur. At night, the patient awakes for trips to the bathroom. It may be difficult to start the stream, and hematuria may be seen when it does start. Residual urine is a good culture medium for bacteria, and, if infection results, symptoms of cystitis are also present. The combination of hesitancy, narrowed stream, straining to void, frequency, urgency, and nocturia is known as *prostatism*.

Diagnosis

The physician performs a digital rectal examination, which demonstrates that the gland is enlarged and elastic. Cystoscopy reveals the extent of the infringement on the urethra and the effects on the bladder. Intravenous and retrograde pyelograms give information about the possible damage to the upper urinary tract due to urinary retention. Blood chemistry tests, such as serum creatinine, may be ordered to determine kidney function: prolonged obstruction at the bladder neck can result in renal damage. Measurement of significant quantities of residual urine (usually at least 60 mL) adds to the data that confirm the diagnosis.

Treatment

As BPH develops, the hyperplasia of the periurethral glands forms an adenoma that includes the bulk of the prostate. The adenoma thins and compresses the surrounding true capsule of the gland. Between the adenoma and capsule, a plane of cleavage can be developed easily by the surgeon. The aim of all surgical procedures for BPH is to remove the adenoma, leaving the true capsule behind. Subsequently, the patient urinates through this fossa. Healing, by reepithelialization, occurs over a 2- or 3-month period.

Benign prostatic hypertrophy with associated symptoms is treated by surgically removing part of the prostate gland. The four operative approaches used are suprapubic prostatectomy, retropubic prostatectomy, perineal prostatectomy, and transurethral resection of the prostate (TURP).

In open operations (retropubic, perineal, or suprapubic prostatectomy), the surgeon develops the cleavage plane between the adenoma and capsule by either finger or sharp dissection. The adenoma is removed along with the mucosa of the prostatic urethra. The transurethral method accomplishes the same objective except that the adenoma is removed piece by piece through an instrument (resectoscope) inserted into the urethra.

Transurethral prostatectomy is the easiest of the four operations for the patient because no external incision is made. It is performed most frequently on patients with complicating conditions, such as heart disease and advanced age, and those with minimal prostatic hypertrophy. If the patient is obese, the transurethral or perineal approach may be preferable to an abdominal one.

A newer procedure to establish patency of the prostatic urethra in patients with BPH is a transcystoscopic urethroplasty. In this procedure, a special catheter with an inflatable balloon is inserted into the prostatic urethra and dilated. This procedure is an alternative for patients who are poor surgical risks and can be performed under local anesthesia, but a general anesthetic may also be used. Usually, the patient is hospitalized for 3 or 4 days. Because the procedure is new, the time that the effects last are unknown; for those who are poor surgical risks, however, it may be an acceptable alternative, even if the procedure must be repeated.

Cancer of the Prostate

Prostatic carcinoma is most common in men older than 50. As the life expectancy increases, more people live to an age when incidence of this disease is highest.

Symptoms

At first, no symptoms occur, and none may occur for years. The disorder usually starts as a nodule in the posterior lobe of the gland that is farthest from the urethra. If the tumor grows large enough, it can obstruct urinary flow and cause frequency, nocturia, and dysuria (difficult or painful urination), which are also symptoms of other disorders, such as BPH or cystitis (inflammation of the bladder). BPH may also be present.

The malignancy is spread by the bloodstream and lymphatics to the pelvic lymph nodes and bone, particularly the lumbar vertebrae, pelvis, and hips. The first symptoms the patient notices may be back pain or pain down the leg due to metastasis to the nerve sheaths. A patient with these and other symptoms is often in the advanced stages of the disease.

Diagnosis

Diagnosis is made by rectal examination and the detection of a nodule on the gland. The physician may then order a series of tests, such as pelvic or spinal radiographs (to detect metastasis to the bone), a serum acid phosphatase (which is often elevated in prostatic cancer), bone scan, and magnetic resonance imaging (MRI). Intravenous pyelograms and other renal function studies may be ordered to detect kidney damage caused by longstanding urethral obstruction and urinary retention (if present).

The diagnosis is confirmed by a biopsy and microscopic examination of tissue removed from the gland, which may be obtained by needle biopsy, transurethral resection of the prostate, or during abdominal surgery for removal of the prostate. A perineal biopsy also may be performed.

If the tumor was not felt during the rectal examination before surgery, the diagnosis sometimes is made during or after surgery for BPH.

Treatment

Treatment depends on factors such as tumor size, presence or absence of metastasis, the age of the patient, and the patient's general health status.

If the nodule is localized, a radical perineal prostatectomy is performed. In contrast to a prostatectomy for benign disease, this surgery removes the entire prostate and its capsule and the seminal vesicles. The bladder neck is sutured to the membranous urethra over an indwelling urethral catheter, which is left in place for 10 to 14 days. Disadvantages of this surgery include virtually guaranteed impotence (versus a chance to be cured of cancer) and serious difficulty with urinary control in some patients.

The outlook for many patients with prostate cancer is relatively good. Men whose cancers are obviously incurable may experience prolonged palliation on conservative therapy. Manipulation of the patient's hormones may give surprising, if temporary, relief of symptoms. Where pain had been severe, it may be gone; where the bladder neck was obstructed, urine may flow freely. Many tumors progress under the influence of androgens and regress on estrogens. After the decrease in androgens by castration (bilateral orchiectomy) and treatment with estrogens, some patients with advanced prostate cancer are reasonably comfortable and well 5 years later. Because of fluid retention problems associated with estrogen therapy, the patient with congestive heart failure must be closely followed by the physician.

As androgens are decreased and estrogens are given, the patient's voice may become higher, hair and fat distribution may change, and breasts may become tender and enlarged; gastrointestinal disturbances also may occur. When estrogens are used in lower doses, the patient may not experience these feminizing changes.

One treatment regimen, using the antineoplastic agents cyclophosphamide (Cytoxan), doxorubicin (Adriamycin), and cisplatin (Platinol), has been successful in some instances. Another antineoplastic agent, estramustine (Emcyt), is a combination of estradiol (an estrogen) and nornitrogen mustard and may be used for palliative treatment.

Even after drug therapy, the tumor may obstruct the bladder neck, and a transurethral resection may be necessary to establish urinary drainage. Occasionally, permanent suprapubic drainage may have to be established.

In the late stage of the disease, severe pain may be treated by a chordotomy (severing of pain fibers in the spinal cord). Radiation therapy may give relief from painful metastases. Narcotics are usually necessary in the late and terminal stages of the disease when other methods fail to relieve pain.

NURSING PROCESS —THE PATIENT UNDERGOING A PROSTATECTOMY

Preoperative Period

Assessment

A complete medical, allergy, and drug history is obtained. The patient is questioned about symptoms and the length of time the symptoms have been present. In the patient history, it is important to note if the patient has had an acute, sudden episode of urinary retention.

Vital signs are taken, and the patient is weighed.

Nursing Diagnosis

Depending on the patient and the type of surgery to be performed, one or both of the following may apply:

- Anxiety related to surgery, inability to void
- Knowledge deficit of preoperative preparations, postoperative care, deep breathing and leg exercises

Planning and Implementation

The major goals of the patient include a reduction in anxiety and an understanding of the preoperative preparations and postoperative management.

The major goals of nursing management are to physically and emotionally prepare the patient for surgery.

Unless a patient has marked symptoms or is totally unable to void, a urethral catheter usually is not ordered to be inserted before surgery. In patients with sudden acute retention, a urethral catheter is inserted and connected to gravity drainage. If the amount of urine in the bladder is great, the physician may order gradual emptying of the bladder over a period of 1 or 2 hours. For this effect, a clamp is placed on the drainage tube and opened briefly for release of urine; it is then reapplied. Specific orders may require that the clamp be opened briefly every 15 minutes until the bladder is emptied. Rapid emptying of an extremely distended bladder can result in profound hematuria due to rupture of the numerous stretched mucosal blood vessels, diuresis with loss of large amounts of sodium in the urine, and moderate to severe hypotension.

If difficulty is encountered while inserting a urethral catheter, the procedure is terminated and the physician contacted.

Additional preparations for surgery include shaving the pubic area if abdominal surgery is performed and shaving the perineal area if the perineal approach is used. If a transurethral resection is to be done, shaving may or may not be ordered.

Anxiety. The patient is allowed time to ask questions about the surgery and to discuss any problems or concerns he may have. Most of these patients have already discussed any personal problems that relate to sexual dysfunction or ability to urinate with the urologist before surgery.

Knowledge Deficit. Preoperative preparations are explained before each task is performed. Deep breathing, coughing, and leg exercises are demonstrated as well as practiced before surgery. The routine postoperative monitoring of vital signs and intravenous fluids also is explained.

Evaluation

- Anxiety is reduced
- Demonstrates understanding of deep breathing, coughing, and leg exercises and postoperative management

Postoperative Period

Assessment

On return from surgery, vital signs are taken. The color of the urine is carefully noted and recorded to provide baseline information for later comparison. The surgical dressing is checked (except transurethral resection) for drainage of blood or urine.

Nursing Diagnosis

Depending on the surgical approach used, one or more of the following may apply:

- Pain related to surgery, bladder spasms
- Anxiety related to postoperative discomfort or pain, leakage of urine on dressings (except transurethral resection), poor control of urine after the catheter is removed, other factors (specify)

- Fluid volume deficit related to blood or fluid loss during surgery
- Potential for infection related to surgical procedure, drainage of urine on surgical dressing (except transurethral resection)
- Ineffective airway clearance related to failure to cough and deep breathe effectively
- Constipation related to anesthesia, surgery, other factors (specify)
- Bathing and hygiene and dressing and grooming self-care deficit related to surgery
- Knowledge deficit of home care management, additional treatment modalities

Planning and Implementation

The major goals of the patient include a reduction of pain and anxiety, correction of fluid volume deficit, prevention of infection, maintenance of clear airway, ability to perform self-care activities, and an understanding of home care and additional treatment modalities.

The major goals of nursing management are to reduce anxiety, control pain, assist the patient in maintaining a clear airway, provide assistance with self-care activities, correct a fluid volume deficit, and develop an effective teaching plan.

No matter which surgical approach is used, general principles of care are applicable to all postprostatectomy patients. An example of a nursing care plan developed for the postoperative management of a patient with a suprapubic prostatectomy is given in Nursing Care Plan 51-1.

When a patient returns to the room, one or more catheters are attached to gravity drainage. The catheters may be an indwelling urethral catheter and a catheter in the incision (cystostomy catheter). The urine output from each catheter is recorded separately. The urethral catheter usually has a balloon filled with 30 mL of fluid (usually normal saline). The balloon size of the cystostomy catheter may vary and usually is noted on the patient's operative record.

The patient may have a Penrose drain inserted into the tissues of the operative site (except transurethral resection). This drain, which does not enter the urinary tract, removes blood and urine that may have leaked into the area. The Penrose drain is removed by the physician when all drainage has ceased.

If the patient has had a radical perineal prostatectomy, one or more drains may be left in the incision. A large dressing usually is placed over the perineal area. The dressing may have a plastic facing since radical perineal prostatectomies tend to have copious drainage. This dressing may be reinforced but is normally changed by the physician.

BLEEDING. After a prostatectomy, hematuria generally is present; frank bleeding, however, is a serious emergency and a potential complication for several

Nursing Care Plan 51–1

Postoperative Management of the Patient With a Suprapubic Prostatectomy

Potential Problem	Nursing Management	Outcome Criteria
Hemorrhage/Shock	Check blood pressure, pulse, and respirations q 1–4 hr (as ordered); observe color of urinary drainage from catheters; report change in vital signs, increase in bleeding, formation of clots in the urine immediately (urine should be light pink to clear in 24 hr); check abdominal dressing q 2 hr, reinforce as needed and report an excessive drainage of urine or blood; check and maintain traction on urethral catheter (if traction is ordered)	No evidence of frank bleeding 24 hr after surgery; vital signs stable
Bladder Spasms	Maintain patency of catheters and irrigate as needed (if irrigation ordered); administer analgesic as ordered; instruct patient to avoid trying to urinate; observe for appearance of fresh bleeding when bladder spasms occur; increase oral fluid intake (if oral fluids allowed) unless contraindicated by other disorders such as congestive heart failure; check abdomen (gently) for bladder distention; note urinary output	Bladder spasms eliminated or controlled with analgesics
Pain/Discomfort *Altered comfort: pain: related to surgery*	Administer analgesics as ordered; change position q 2 hr; check patency of catheters; check catheter drainage tubing for clots q 2 hr	Normal postoperative pain; pain controlled with analgesics
Catheter Obstruction	Connect each catheter to a closed drainage system and label each drainage container; check catheters for patency q 1–4 hr; monitor rate of continuous irrigation (if one is used) q 1 hr	Catheters remain patent
Infection *Potential for infection related to surgery*	Monitor oral temperature q 4 hr (take temperature orally unless ordered otherwise; avoid rectal temperatures); use aseptic technique for dressing changes or reinforcement, irrigating catheters; maintain sterility of closed drainage system and change system if contamination occurs; encourage a liberal oral fluid intake (2,000 mL/day or more) when oral fluids are allowed; check urine for cloudiness q 4 hr; check surgical wound each time dressing is changed for signs of infection, purulent drainage	Temperature remains within normal range; urine clear no evidence of infection

days after surgery. The color of the urine and the presence of any clots must be noted. Bright red blood indicates an arterial bleeding source, whereas a deep red color suggests venous oozing. Clots can obstruct the catheter, causing bladder spasm, pain, and further bleeding. Therefore, the catheter must remain patent at all times. The bladder is gently palpated for fullness and tenderness. If these are present, the bladder could be distended with clots, and the physician is notified promptly.

To control arterial bleeding, the surgeon may apply traction to the urethral catheter to keep the balloon seated on the bladder neck and, thus, provide hemostasis. Taping the inflated catheter to the thigh is one method commonly used. Traction may be maintained for 6 hours; with any longer period of time, however, there is danger of damage to the bladder sphincter, which causes temporary incontinence. The physician may order the tension to be decreased gradually or may reapply more gentle traction overnight.

DRAINAGE AND IRRIGATION.   The physician may order straight drainage without irrigation. Overzealous irrigation may induce further bleeding and cause frequent and uncomfortable bladder spasms. The nurse follows the physician's instructions about *when* to irrigate and *how much* and *what kind* of solution to use. Normal saline or other irrigating solution may be ordered, especially if a large volume of solution is necessary, to prevent dilution of the blood as a result of absorption of the irrigating solution by the bladder mucosa.

In selected patients, continuous irrigation may be ordered. The continuous gentle flow of fluid helps to prevent clots from forming in the bladder and obstructing the catheters. The drip is regulated to maintain the drainage at a light pink. When continuous irrigation is ordered, the urethral catheter usually is used for inflow and the cystostomy tube for outflow. The danger of bleeding is increased if the irrigating fluid is continued when the outflow is obstructed by clots.

Pain.   Narcotic analgesics are given as ordered. Pain or severe discomfort may not be related to the surgical incision but to bladder spasms or an obstructed urethral catheter with consequent bladder distention.

It is important to distinguish between catheter obstruction and bladder spasm. Usually with catheter obstruction, discomfort is gradual and increasing, with diminished or absent urinary output. The bladder becomes distended and is tender on gentle palpation. The need for relief of the obstruction is urgent. If catheter irrigation is ordered, it is done gently. If patency is not achieved or if irrigation is not ordered, the physician is notified immediately.

When bladder spasm without catheter obstruction is present, the patient has a urinary output. Pain may be constant or intermittent. Some bladder spasms are extremely painful. Narcotics do not seem to lessen the spasms, but they help to decrease pain in the bladder and operative area.

Anxiety.   The patient may experience anxiety over symptoms present after surgery. When a catheter is

in the urethra, the patient has a sensation of having a full bladder even though the bladder is empty. If he tries to void around the catheter, the bladder muscles contract, causing painful spasms. The nurse must first check to be sure the catheter is draining and then explain to the patient that the bladder is kept empty by the catheter and that trying to void causes further irritation and pain. Explaining to the patient why he feels the need to urinate may help relieve concern over this problem. The explanation may need to be repeated, especially if the patient is older.

When the urethral catheter is removed, the time and amount of each voiding is recorded for several days. Occasionally, if urinary function does not progress satisfactorily, reinsertion of a urethral catheter may be necessary. Patients may experience dribbling after the urethral catheter is removed, and they become upset about losing control of their bladder function. If this problem occurs, the physician is notified.

After the cystostomy tube is removed, the suprapubic wound frequently leaks urine for a few days. A saturated dressing, the odor of urine, and wet bed clothes can be uncomfortable and embarrassing to the patient. A liberal fluid intake (when the patient's medical status permits) is encouraged, and the patient is assured that the dressings will be changed promptly.

Fluid Volume Deficit.   An intravenous line is inserted before surgery, and intravenous fluids and possibly whole blood are given during and after surgery to compensate for fluid and blood loss during surgery.

Once able to take oral fluids, the patient is encouraged to drink fluids at frequent intervals. A high fluid intake (if permitted) helps to decrease bladder mucosal irritation because fluid is constantly passing over the irritated area.

Potential for Infection.   Prophylactic antibiotics may be prescribed after surgery to prevent infection. Vital signs are taken every 4 hours or as ordered. A temperature higher than 101°F is brought to the attention of the physician. Only an oral or axillary temperature is taken unless the physician orders otherwise. Generally, the use of rectal tubes, rectal thermometers, and enemas is not resumed until at least a week or more after surgery to avoid perforation of the rectal mucosa.

The abdominal dressing is changed (unless the physician orders otherwise, then the dressings are reinforced) as frequently as necessary to keep the patient clean and dry. Care must be taken not to disturb any tissue drains placed by the surgeon.

Strict aseptic technique is essential to prevent wound infection. The wound is inspected at the time of each dressing change. Any sign of infection, such as purulent drainage, odor (other than a urine odor) to the drainage, redness, and swelling, is brought to the attention of the physician.

Ineffective Airway Clearance. The patient is encouraged to cough, deep breathe, and perform leg exercises every 2 hours. The lungs are auscultated daily, and abnormal breath sounds or failure of the patient to cough and deep breathe is reported to the physician.

Constipation. After this type of surgery, the patient is cautioned against straining to have a bowel movement because this can result in prostatic hemorrhage. The physician may order a stool softener or a mild laxative about the third day after surgery. Drinking extra fluids, ambulating, and a diet high in roughage help prevent constipation.

Self-Care Deficit. The patient requires assistance with bathing and grooming for the first day or two after surgery. After that time, most patients can assume responsibility for their self-care needs.

Knowledge Deficit. Most patients who have prostatic surgery are elderly, and surgery can be a severe physical and emotional strain. The patient may be concerned over loss of urinary control (which does not occur in all patients). The physician may recommend perineal exercises: the usual routine is to tighten the perineal muscles for about 5 to 20 seconds and then relax. This exercise is repeated 10 or more times every 1 to 4 hours. The physician also may recommend that the patient stop the urinary stream after starting to void, wait a few seconds, and then continue to void. These exercises are explained to the patient.

The following areas may be included in a patient teaching plan:

1. Avoid heavy lifting, strenuous exercise, straining, sexual activities, prolonged periods of sitting, spicy foods, and alcoholic beverages until they are permitted by the physician.
2. Drink plenty of fluids (unless the physician instructs otherwise).
3. Take the prescribed medication as directed on the container.
4. Avoid constipation. Do not use enemas if constipated. If constipation occurs, talk to the physician before using any laxatives. Constipation may be avoided by drinking fluids (including prune juice), eating a well-balanced diet that contains roughage, and walking.
5. If the physician recommends perineal exercises, perform them as directed.

6. Contact the physician if any of the following occur: burning or pain on urination, blood in the urine, pain in the perineal area, cloudy urine, different odor to the urine, fever, or chills.

Evaluation

- Pain and discomfort are relieved
- Anxiety is reduced
- Fluid volume deficit is corrected
- No evidence of infection; vital signs are normal; surgical wound appears normal
- Coughs, deep breathes, and performs leg exercises; lungs clear to auscultation
- Bowel elimination normal
- Urinary elimination normal
- No evidence of hemorrhage
- Self-care needs are met; assumes responsibility for own needs before discharge from hospital
- Demonstrates understanding of perineal exercises, medication schedule, activities to avoid, when to contact the physician
- Verbalizes importance of increasing fluid intake

VASECTOMY AND VASOVASOSTOMY

Vasectomy is a minor surgical procedure that involves the ligation of the vas deferens for the purpose of sterilization or for the treatment of chronic epididymitis.

The vas deferens transports sperm from the testes to the seminal vesicles. Interruption of this pathway results in sterility. Several weeks or more after surgery, the ejaculatory fluid should not contain sperm.

This surgical procedure, when performed for the purpose of sterilization, is often done in a physician's office or clinic. The patient is warned that the ejaculatory fluid contains sperm for a period of time after surgery and that contraceptives have to be used until ejaculation samples are found to be free of live sperm.

After surgery, the patient usually is instructed to wear a scrotal support. Ice packs may be recommended for swelling, and a mild analgesic for pain. The physician tells the patient when to return for follow-up examinations.

On occasion, the patient may complain of impotency, although the surgical procedure has no effect on erection or ejaculation. This problem is best discussed with the physician.

A vasovasostomy is a surgical attempt to reverse the effects of a vasectomy by restoring patency and continuity to the vas deferens. Microsurgical techniques have been successful in some instances. Because there is no guarantee that fertility can be restored by this procedure, it is most important that the patient fully understand the long-term ramifications of a vasectomy.

DISORDERS OF THE TESTES AND ADJACENT STRUCTURES

Cryptorchidism (Undescended Testicle)

Failure of the testicle to lie in the scrotum is known as *cryptorchidism* (or *undescended testicle*). At least one testis (plural, testes) must be in its normal position in the scrotum for the patient to have reproductive function. One or both testes may be undescended.

The undescended testis may lie in the inguinal canal, in the abdominal cavity, or, rarely, in the perineum or femoral canal. If undescended testes are not placed in the scrotum by age 5 or 6, the likelihood that they will produce sperm is diminished. Undescended testes have a significantly higher incidence of malignant degeneration whether or not they are placed in the scrotum, but the overall incidence of tumors of undescended testes is low. During childhood or at puberty, undescended testes occasionally find their way into the scrotum without treatment.

Symptoms
One or both testes are absent from the scrotal sac.

Diagnosis
The physician makes a diagnosis by physical examination. The inguinal area is palpated to determine if the testis is lying in the inguinal canal.

Treatment
Some physicians advocate a short (1-week) trial of hormone (androgen) therapy. If a response is not noted within 3 weeks, surgery may be performed (orchiopexy). Other physicians think that surgery should be performed in all patients with undescended testes, preferably before puberty. After orchiopexy (also called *orchidopexy*), the patient may have three incisions: inner thigh, scrotal, and inguinal. The surgeon makes an inguinal incision and locates the testis and then moves it downward into the scrotal sac. The testes is held in the scrotum on tension to a taped rubber band or other device attached to a suture through the lower pole of the testis and to the skin of the upper thigh. The suture usually is removed in 5 to 7 days. Often an associated congenital hernia is present, and it is repaired at the time of orchiopexy. The patient can move his leg, but undue pressure should not be placed on the traction. The nurse should inspect the traction, which is outside the dressings, several times a day to make sure that the suture taped to the leg is taut and provides the necessary pull.

Epididymo-Orchitis

Infection and inflammation of the testis and epididymis usually occur simultaneously. The most common cause is infection that ascends from the vas deferens and its surrounding lymphatics because of prostatitis. A less common cause of acute epididymitis is untreated gonorrhea.

Symptoms
The symptoms are chills, fever, scrotal pain, and tenderness. The scrotal skin may be erythematous and tense. A markedly swollen testis and epididymis are usually present.

Diagnosis
Diagnosis is based on physical examination and patient history.

Treatment
Elevation of the scrotum with a four-tail bandage or adhesive taped across the upper thighs (Bellevue bridge) relieves the pain by lessening the weight of the testes. Strict bed rest usually is ordered during the early stage. An ice bag may be ordered to help relieve pain and is placed under the tender scrotum, not on top of it or leaning against it. The cold bag should not be kept constantly next to the skin because it may damage tissue. On 60 minutes, off 30 minutes is one routine that may be prescribed. Heat is not applied to the scrotal area because spermatozoa are damaged by heat that is even a few degrees above body temperature. (The normal temperature of the scrotum is lower than that of the rest of the body.) As with any infection, copious fluid intake is encouraged. Antibiotics may be prescribed.

Orchitis without epididymal involvement is most often caused by mumps that occur after puberty. This viral orchitis may result in testicular atrophy and sterility. For this reason, men who have not had mumps as children and who are exposed to it are advised to receive immediate medical attention. Immunization against mumps has helped reduce the incidence of viral orchitis and sterility in males.

Bilateral epididymitis frequently leads to permanent azoospermia (absence of sperm), especially when the infection recurs frequently, or when it becomes chronic. Vasectomy (removal of a section of the vas deferens) prevents recurrent attacks but causes sterility if it is performed bilaterally.

Torsion of the Spermatic Cord

This condition occurs in prepubescent boys and in men whose spermatic cords are (congenitally) unsupported in the tunica vaginalis (a membrane surrounding the testes) and move freely. Torsion may follow severe exercise, but it also may occur during sleep or after such a simple maneuver as crossing the legs.

Symptoms

Symptoms include a sudden, sharp testicular pain and local swelling. The pain may be so severe that nausea, vomiting, chills, and fever occur. The testis is extremely tender, and the usually posterior epididymis may be located anteriorly. In contrast to inflammatory conditions, elevation of the scrotum increases the pain by increasing the degree of twist.

Diagnosis

Diagnosis is based on the patient's symptoms and a physical examination.

Treatment

Treatment consists of immediate surgery to prevent atrophy of the spermatic cord and to preserve fertility. The torsion is reduced, excess tunica vaginalis is excised, and the testis is anchored with sutures in the scrotum. A similar prophylactic procedure may be performed on the opposite side.

Hydrocele

Normally, a small amount of fluid is in the space between the testis and the tunica vaginalis. A large accumulation of fluid in that space is known as *hydrocele*. This common cause of scrotal enlargement may be due to an infection, commonly epididymitis or orchitis, or trauma; most occur without known cause. When the accumulation of fluid is slow (chronic hydrocele), it usually is painless, even when the scrotum becomes large.

Symptoms

A hydrocele causes few symptoms in most instances except for its weight and unsightly bulk. Acute hydrocele is accompanied by both pain and swelling and may follow trauma or local infection.

Diagnosis

Diagnosis is made by examination and transillumination (passing a light through an organ or cavity) of the scrotum.

Treatment

Treatment, if indicated, consists of surgical excision of the sac. The fluid may be aspirated as a temporary measure; fluid reaccumulates, however, and the danger of introducing infection arises. After surgery, the patient has a drain and a pressure dressing. A scrotal support is required for weeks afterward.

Varicocele

This condition usually occurs on the left side of the scrotum and consists of dilatation and tortuous clumping of tributaries of the spermatic vein.

Symptoms

Swelling and pain are the major symptoms. Rarely does a varicocele per se cause enough symptoms to warrant surgery. In certain instances of infertility, correction of a varicocele has resulted in significant improvement in the semen specimens. The reason for this effect is unknown.

Diagnosis

Diagnosis is made by physical examination and palpation of the scrotum.

Treatment

Surgery involves an inguinal exploration of the spermatic cord with ligature and division of the major spermatic vein tributaries in this region.

Cancer of the Testes

Cancer of the testes is more common in young men. Testicular tumors tend to metastasize early.

Symptoms

Unless discovered early, the first symptoms may be related to tumor metastasis and include abdominal pain, general weakness, and aching in the testes. Gradual or sudden swelling of the scrotum or a lump felt on palpation should always receive prompt medical attention.

Diagnosis

The diagnosis is made when the patient or physician discovers a hard, nontender nodule of the testis. Because biopsy risks spilling the highly malignant tumor cells, surgery is recommended immediately. Laboratory and diagnostic tests that confirm the possibility of a malignant process include α-fetoprotein, levels may be increased; C-reactive protein, only indicates an active, widespread malignancy process; total urine estrogens, may be elevated if a testicular tumor is present; human chorionic gonadotropin, may be elevated; and intravenous pyelogram, to detect lymph node enlargement that may displace the ureters.

Treatment

Treatment of testicular tumors includes radiation, surgery, and chemotherapy. Surgery involves the removal of the testis and ligation of the spermatic cord. Radical lymph node dissection of the retroperitoneal lymph nodes may be performed at the same time. Not all physicians believe that radical lymph node dissection is necessary and prefer to use radiation of the lymph node channels after the patient has recovered from surgery.

A multiple antineoplastic drug regimen usually is instituted after surgery. One therapeutic regimen consists of administration of cisplatin (Platinol), cyclophosphamide (Cytoxan), vinblastine (Velban), bleomycin (Beloxane), and dactinomycin (Cosmegen) for induction (initial) therapy, followed by vinblastine and dactinomycin every 3 weeks for 1 year. Another treatment regimen uses cisplatin, vinblastine, and bleomycin given at intervals for 12 weeks. Plicamycin (Mithracin) also may be used when successful treatment by radiation or surgery is impossible. All of these drugs are given intravenously.

When the patient is young, he has many concerns, especially over sterility, as well as loss of libido and inability to engage in sexual activities. The type of treatment selected determines if any of these problems will occur. If only one testis is removed, sexual activity, the libido, and fertility are usually not affected. A gel-filled prosthesis can be implanted at the time of surgery or at a later date.

If radiation is used, the remaining testis is covered to preserve fertility. Usually, the libido and sexual activity are not impaired. After a radical lymph node dissection, sexual activity and the libido usually are not impaired, but the patient is most likely sterile.

The success of treatment depends on the type of testicular tumor and the extent of metastasis. Like tumors of the breast, testicular tumors can be identified early when the patient practices monthly self-examination of the scrotum.

NURSING PROCESS —THE PATIENT UNDERGOING SURGERY FOR CANCER OF THE TESTES

Preoperative Period

Assessment
A complete patient history, including a medical, drug, and allergy history, is taken. Information about symptoms and the length of time symptoms have been present is obtained. Vital signs are taken, and the patient is weighed. The patient's records are reviewed for the findings of all preoperative tests and studies as well as for any notations or comments made by the physician.

Nursing Diagnosis
Depending on the patient, one or more of the following may apply:

- Anxiety related to diagnosis, extensive surgery, prognosis
- Knowledge deficit of preoperative preparations, postoperative management

Planning and Implementation
The major goals of the patient include a reduction in anxiety and an understanding of preoperative preparations and postoperative management.

The major goal of nursing management is to prepare the patient physically and emotionally for surgery.

Depending on the planned extent of surgery, an intravenous line, nasogastric tube, and indwelling urethral catheter may be inserted before surgery.

Anxiety. Most patients with this type of cancer are young, usually are not acutely ill, and have many questions about the surgery and prognosis. The physician discusses the diagnosis, planned treatment modalities, and prognosis with the patient and family.

The patient may or may not wish to talk about the diagnosis and planned treatment modalities. If he does, the nurse must be willing to listen and offer encouragement. If the patient appears to be unclear about treatments or appears to be extremely anxious, the physician is informed before the patient goes to surgery.

Knowledge Deficit. Since a high level of anxiety may exist, it is important to explain all preoperative preparations, such as shaving the skin, enemas, and preoperative medications.

Although questions about the diagnosis, treatments, and prognosis must be answered by the physician, the nurse can answer questions about the preparations for surgery and general postoperative care.

Coughing, deep breathing, and leg exercises are taught, and the patient is given time to practice.

Evaluation
- Anxiety is reduced
- Openly discusses problems associated with the diagnosis, planned treatments, and surgery
- Demonstrates understanding of preoperative preparations

Postoperative Period

Assessment
On return from the operating room, vital signs are taken, and the patient's chart is reviewed for the extent of surgery (orchiectomy with or without radical lymph node dissection).

If a radical lymph node dissection was performed, there is a large abdominal incision and dressing. The surgical incision is checked for drainage. If drains have been inserted, the physician may order them connected to low suction. After an orchiectomy, the physician usually orders a scrotal support applied over the dressing.

Nursing Diagnosis
Depending on the extent of surgery, one or more of the following may apply. Additional diagnoses that apply to general surgery may be added.

- Pain related to surgery
- Potential for infection related to surgery
- Urinary retention related to scrotal swelling, extensive abdominal surgery (radical lymph node dissection)
- Self-care deficit: total to partial (specify areas) related to surgery
- Constipation related to painful defecation secondary to radical lymph node dissection, immobility
- Ineffective airway clearance related to failure to cough and deep breathe effectively secondary to long abdominal incision
- Body image disturbance related to loss of testis
- Knowledge deficit of home care management

Planning and Implementation
The major goals of the patient include a reduction of pain, absence of infection, normal pattern of urinary and bowel elimination, increased ability to care for self, acceptance of the results of surgery (loss of testis), a clear airway, and an understanding of home care management.

The major goals of nursing management are to relieve pain, prevent infection, assist with bathing and grooming, offer emotional support and understanding, and develop an effective patient teaching plan.

COMPLICATIONS. Complications depend on the extent of surgery and include hemorrhage, wound infection, pneumonia, and shock. Vital signs are monitored every 1 to 4 hours or as ordered. The intravenous line is checked at frequent intervals to recognize possible extravasation or infiltration of intravenous fluid. Any sudden or gradual decrease in the blood pressure or increase in the pulse rate is brought immediately to the attention of the physician.

Pain. Analgesics are administered as ordered. Pain must be evaluated as to location and intensity. Surgery may be extensive, and pain is often severe because of the long abdominal incision necessary for a radical lymph node dissection. If tissue supporting the kidneys was removed, the patient may be kept in a Trendelenburg position for a time after surgery to keep the kidneys in good position. In this position, it is difficult to eat, urinate, and defecate.

Potential for Infection. When dressing changes are permitted, the incisions are inspected for redness, tenderness, swelling, or drainage. If these occur, the physician is notified. Vital signs are monitored every 1 to 4 hours or as ordered. A temperature higher than 101°F is brought to the attention of the physician. Prophylactic antibiotics usually are given during the postoperative period.

Urinary Retention. Intake and output are measured until the patient is voiding in sufficient quantity. If an indwelling catheter was inserted, it is connected to gravity drainage unless another type of drainage system is ordered by the physician. Once the catheter is removed, the patient may still have scrotal swelling and difficulty urinating. The amount of each voiding is measured, and the frequency and amount are recorded on the patient's chart. If an indwelling catheter was not inserted, the patient's voiding pattern is monitored closely. Each time the patient urinates, the amount is measured until a sufficient quantity (usually 200 mL or more) is passed at the time of each voiding.

The physician is notified if the patient has difficulty voiding, if small amount are voided each time, or if voiding is frequent and in small amounts.

Self-Care Deficit. The patient is assisted with bathing and grooming until able to assume these responsibilities. Those who have a radical lymph node dissection may require complete care for several days.

Constipation. When oral fluids are allowed, the patient is encouraged to drink extra fluids. The physician may order a stool softener to reduce discomfort when defecating, which is more likely to occur if a radical lymph node dissection was performed. A record of bowel movements is kept. If constipation occurs, the physician is notified.

Respiratory Function. The patient is encouraged to cough and deep breathe, and his position is changed every 2 hours. Because of the length of the incision of a radical lymph node dissection, coughing usually is uncomfortable. The patient is encouraged to place a pillow on his abdomen and apply light but firm pressure while coughing.

The lungs are auscultated once or twice per day, especially if the patient has had a radical lymph node dissection and remains immobile for several days after surgery.

Body Image Disturbance. The patient may or may not discuss concerns about loss of a testis, possible loss of libido, or inability to engage in sexual activities. If the discussion does arise, he is encouraged to talk about his concerns with the physician.

Knowledge Deficit. The teaching plan depends on the type of surgery and the future treatment modalities.

When prescribed, the schedule for intravenous chemotherapy and radiation therapy is reviewed with the patient.

One or more of the following may be included in a patient teaching plan:

1. Drink plenty of fluids (unless the physician instructs otherwise) and eat a well-balanced diet. Avoid constipation.
2. Obtain adequate rest; avoid fatigue and heavy lifting.
3. Wash the incision with warm soap and water or care for the incision as instructed by the physician. Contact the physician if redness, drainage, pain, or swelling is seen.
4. Take the prescribed medication (if any) exactly as directed. Avoid nonprescription drugs unless their use is approved by the physician.
5. Perform self-examination of the remaining testicle every month.
6. Contact the physician if any of the following occur: fever, chills, adverse drug effects, weight loss, or anorexia.

Evaluation

- Pain is controlled
- Shows no evidence of infection; vital signs normal
- Pattern of urinary elimination is normal
- Self-care needs are met; assumes responsibility for all care before discharge
- Bowel elimination is normal
- Verbalizes intention of discussing body image change with physician and sexual partner
- Coughs and deep breathes effectively; lungs clear to auscultation
- Demonstrates understanding of planned treatment modalities, drug regimen, incision care, self-examination of the remaining testis, activities to avoid
- Lists symptoms that require the attention of the physician

DISORDERS OF THE PENIS
Phimosis and Paraphimosis

Phimosis is the constriction of the foreskin (prepuce), which results in the inability to retract the foreskin back over the end of the penis. *Paraphimosis* is the retraction of the foreskin behind the glans.

This condition occurs only in uncircumsized males.

Symptoms

No symptoms may be associated with phimosis other than the inability to retract the foreskin. When long-standing, the area beneath the foreskin may collect dried secretions. Chronic inflammation with possible scarring and formation of adhesions may be seen.

Pain and edema of the penis are the most prominent symptoms of paraphimosis. If the condition is allowed to continue, severe edema and urinary retention may be seen.

Diagnosis

Diagnosis is made by visual inspection.

Treatment

Circumcision is recommended for phimosis if scarring and adhesions make it impossible to retract and clean under the foreskin. If paraphimosis is present, the physician usually tries to return the foreskin to its normal position. If successful, the patient is instructed to clean the area under the foreskin daily. If the physician is unable to release the constriction and retract the foreskin or if the condition becomes chronic, circumcision is necessary.

Circumcision involves the removal of the foreskin and usually is performed under local anesthesia. Although sometimes performed on infants shortly after birth, circumcision may be necessary in the adult for conditions such as phimosis and paraphimosis. The area is covered with a nonadhering dressing and an analgesic is prescribed. Though rare, excessive bleeding may occur and requires immediate medical attention. Usually, additional sutures are needed to tie off the bleeding vessels.

Cancer of the Penis

The exact cause of this malignancy is unknown, but it is thought to be related to poor personal hygiene and phimosis. It is rare in circumcised males.

Symptoms

Growths that resemble warts or ulcers appear on the glans penis, the skin of the penis, or at the posterior border of the glans (corona glandis). Other symptoms include a foul-smelling discharge and bleeding from the tumor. Pain usually is a late symptom.

Diagnosis

Diagnosis is made by visual inspection of the growths and is confirmed by biopsy and microscopic examination.

Treatment

Depending on the stage of the malignancy, treatment includes excision of the tumor and, possibly, chemo- therapy and radiation therapy. When the tumor in- vades deeper tissues, it may be necessary to amputate part or all of the penis.

General Pharmacologic Considerations

☐ The patient with prostatic carcinoma may be treated with estrogens. Depend- ing on the dose used, the patient may or may not experience feminizing changes: enlargement and tenderness of the breasts, change in fat distribution in which the hips and thighs often increase in size, voice changes (rise in pitch). Because these changes may be distressing to the patient, they should be explained before therapy is begun.

☐ Chemotherapy for testicular cancer is often intensive because the tumor me- tastasizes rapidly. The patient often becomes acutely ill from the drugs, and hospitalization may be necessary during drug therapy.

General Gerontologic Considerations

☐ Regardless of the reason for admission to the hospital, all elderly male patients should be questioned about urinary tract problems.

☐ The elderly patient who is having prostatic surgery may have periods of con- fusion after surgery and may attempt to remove his urethral or suprapubic catheter. The urethral catheter usually has a 30-mL retention balloon. Acci- dental removal of the catheter without deflating the balloon may cause severe trauma to the urethra.

☐ Occasionally, urinary incontinence may occur after a prostatectomy. In some patients, it disappears with time; but, in others, dribbling of urine may persist, leading to depression and social withdrawal.

☐ Incontinence in elderly men may require the use of disposable waterproof pants that are worn under the clothing. Nighttime urinary leakage may be helped by wearing a sheath over the penis, which is connected to a closed drainage system. Patients may require an indwelling urethral catheter or a permanent cystostomy tube.

Suggested Readings

☐ Berkow R, Fletcher AJ, eds. Merck manual of diagnosis and therapy. 15th ed. Rahway, NJ: Merck and Co, 1987. *(In-depth coverage of subject matter)*

☐ Brunner LS, Suddarth DS. Textbook of medical–surgical nursing. 6th ed. Philadelphia: JB Lippincott, 1988. *(Additional and in-depth coverage of subject matter)*

☐ Casey MP. Testicular cancer: the worse disease at the worse time. RN February 1987:50:36. *(Additional coverage of subject matter)*

☐ Farrell J. Nursing care of the older person. Philadelphia: JB Lippincott, 1990. *(In-depth coverage of subject matter)*

☐ Gruendemann BJ, Meeker MH. Alexander's care of the patient in surgery. 8th ed. St Louis: CV Mosby, 1987. *(In-depth coverage of subject matter)*

☐ Jenkins B, Carbaugh C. Action stat! Testicular torsion. Nursing '89 July 1989;19:33. *(Additional coverage of subject matter)*

☐ Zastocki DK, Rovinski CA. Home care: patient and family instructions. Philadelphia: WB Saunders, 1989. *(Additional coverage of subject matter)*

The Urinary Tract

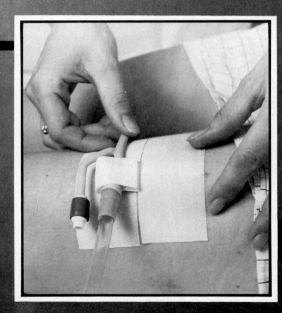

Unit 13

Chapter 52

Introduction to the Urinary Tract

On completion of this chapter the reader will:

- Be familiar with the basic anatomy and physiology of the urinary tract

- List and discuss the diagnostic tests used in the evaluation of the urinary tract

- Use the nursing process to prepare a patient for tests used to diagnose urinary tract disorders

ANATOMY AND PHYSIOLOGY

The urinary tract consists of the kidneys, ureter, bladder, and urethra (Fig. 52-1A).

Two kidneys lie posteriorly to the left and right of the midline of the body. The kidneys are enclosed in a thin, fibrous capsule and separated from the abdominal cavity anteriorly by the peritoneum. They are the main excretory organs of the body.

The blood supply to each kidney consists of a renal artery and renal vein. The renal artery arises from the aorta and the renal vein empties into the vena cava (see Fig. 52-1B).

Each kidney contains about 1 million nephrons, which are the smallest functioning unit of the kidney. The nephron consists of glomerulus, afferent arteriole, efferent venule, Bowman's capsule, distal and proximal convoluted tubules, Henle's loop, and the collecting tubule (see Fig. 52-1C).

The glomerulus (see Fig. 52-1D) consists of a tuft of blood vessel comprised of an afferent arteriole and an efferent venule. The removal of waste products, electrolytes, and water from the blood takes place in the glomerulus. The formed urine moves from the glomerulus into Bowman's capsule, flows out through the proximal and then distal tubules and into the collecting tubules, then into the renal pelvis, and is carried down the ureter to the bladder. Here, the urine is stored until the capacity of the bladder is reached, at which time the the urine is voided to the outside through the urethra.

The kidneys have at least three known functions: (1) they excrete excess water and the nitrogenous waste products of protein metabolism; (2) they play a significant role in maintaining the acid–base balance of the body and the equilibrium of plasma electrolytes; and (3) they produce enzymes, such as renin, which act on certain plasma constituents to form a compound that raises the blood pressure. The kidneys selectively filter more than 50 gallons of plasma daily. All but a quart or so of this volume is resorbed back into the circulation every 24 hours.

Any disorder that interferes with the process of filtering waste products, electrolytes, and water may be serious unless the situation can be corrected. These disorders include interference with the circulation of blood to the kidney, disease of the kidney itself, and obstruction anywhere in the urinary tract.

ASSESSMENT OF THE PATIENT WHO HAS A URINARY TRACT DISORDER

Patient History

The following may be included in the patient history: a history of all past and present symptoms, a general health history, drug and allergy history, history of this

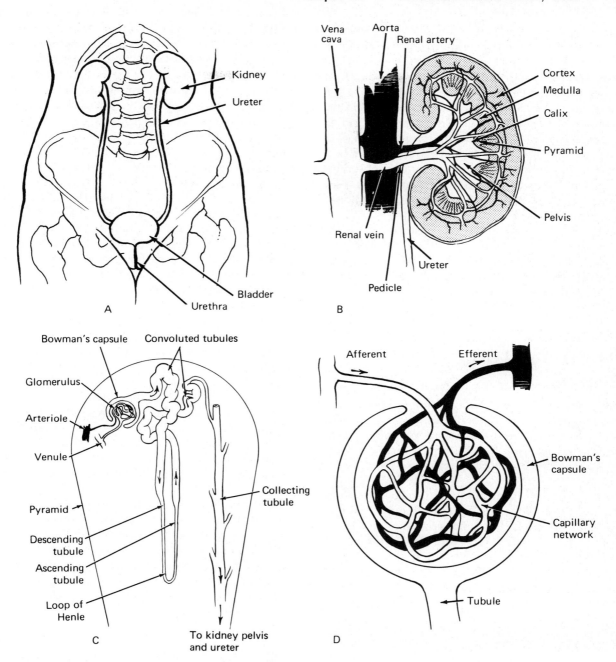

Figure 52–1. Structures of the urinary tract: (*A*) the urinary tract; (*B*) cross-section of kidney; (*C*) a nephron; (*D*) glomerulus.

or other disorders related to the urinary tract, and family history of illnesses. Depending on symptoms and other factors, an occupational or work history, history of exposure to toxic chemicals or gasses, and a history of childhood diseases also may be included in the health history.

It is most important that a complete history and description of the symptoms be obtained. If, for example, the patient has had to urinate frequently, it is important to know the average number of times the patient voided during the day as well as during the night. It also is important to determine whether pain accompanied urination and whether the urine was an abnormal color, for example, bloody, dark, pale, or cloudy.

Physical Examination

The physician usually performs an initial general physical examination, which includes abdominal palpation of the kidneys to determine if tenderness or pain is felt in either area of the kidney. In the obese patient, it is not always possible to palpate the kidneys. The physician also may look for costovertebral angle tenderness by striking one or more light blows with a fist to the area where the lower ribs meet the vertebrae.

The nurse obtains baseline data during the initial assessment. The function of the urinary tract is to eliminate metabolic products and electrolytes, and, because water is the vehicle for the movement of these substances, the initial assessment includes observing for signs of electrolyte and water imbalance (see Chapter 12). The patient's general physical appearance is evaluated for other symptoms, such as swelling around the eyes (periorbital edema), edema of the extremities, signs of cardiac failure, and mental changes, all of which may indicate the presence of certain urinary tract disorders. Vital signs and weight also are obtained at this time.

LABORATORY AND DIAGNOSTIC TESTS
Urinalysis

Much information about the condition of the kidneys, electrolyte balance, and overall health can be learned by studying the urine. Urinalysis is one of the most important diagnostic studies of the urinary tract. The characteristics of normal urine are listed in Table 52-1.

A red color of the urine may be caused by blood, but this cause must be proved by microscopic examination. Certain metabolic disturbances, ingested dyes, or foodstuffs may impart a red color that is not blood. Cloudiness of the urine may be due to phosphates (a normal finding), or to white cells (an abnormal finding), suggesting an infection or irritation of the tract.

Table 52–1. Characteristics of Normal Urine

Characteristic	Finding
Specific gravity	1.005–1.035
Color	Pale yellow to dark amber
Turbidity	Usually clear (cloudiness is not always abnormal)
pH	4.5–8.0
Protein	None to trace
Glucose	None to trace
Red blood cells	0–3 per high-power field
White blood cells	0–4 per high-power field
Casts	Rare per high-power field

Proteinuria (protein in the urine, which usually is albumin) may occasionally be normal, but more often it implies disease of the kidneys. Casts are molds of the renal tubules, and their size varies with the size of the portion of the nephron from which they originate. They may consist of red cells, white cells, or precipitated protein.

When infection is suspected, a urine specimen may be taken for culture. In men, it usually is sufficient to cleanse the glans penis with an antiseptic and have the patient void about 60 mL, which is discarded, and then void into a sterile specimen bottle. The bottle is capped so that it is not contaminated. In women, specimens for culture may be obtained by catheterization. Because of the danger of introducing infection into the urinary tract with a catheter, however, the sterile (or clean) catch procedure is used in many hospitals. The labia are held apart, and the area is cleansed. The patient voids into a sterile container after the initial 60 mL is discarded. To prevent the growth of bacteria in the urine, as well as its decomposition, the urine specimen is delivered immediately to the laboratory or promptly refrigerated until it can be taken to the laboratory.

Sometimes, a specimen of all urine excreted over a period of time, such as 24 hours, may be needed for examination of such constituents as tubercle bacilli or 17-ketosteroids. The patient voids immediately before the start of the time period, and this urine is discarded. The urine is then collected for the required length of time.

Depending on the test, the entire specimen may or may not need to be refrigerated to prevent bacteria growth. To prevent any part of the specimen from being lost or contaminated, the patient is instructed to use separate receptacles for voiding and defecation. If any urine is discarded by mistake or lost while defecating, the test is stopped; loss of even a small amount of urine invalidates the test.

Blood Chemistry

When the nephrons fail to remove waste products efficiently from the body, the blood chemistry is altered. Deterioration in renal function is manifested chemically by rises in the blood urea nitrogen (BUN) and creatinine values, both of which are protein breakdown products. A moderate decrease in function occurs, however, before these values rise. The normal BUN value is 8 to 20 mg/dL, and creatinine is 0.5 to 1.2 mg/dL.

Serum electrolyte values (Table 52-2) may give information about kidney function; the kidney is responsible for the regulation of electrolyte concentration in the extracellular fluid compartment. Blood calcium, phosphorus, and uric acid studies may be ordered

Table 52–2. Serum Values

	Normal Serum Value*	Changes in Pathology
Calcium	9–11 mg/dL	Lower in renal failure
Carbon dioxide-combining power	24–32 mEq/L	Higher in alkalosis
Potassium	3.6–5.0 mEq/L	Higher in renal failure
Proteins, total		
Albumin	3.5–5.5 g/dL	Lower in renal failure
Globulin	1.5–3.0 g/dL	
Sodium	135–145 mEq/L	Lower in renal failure
Blood urea nitrogen	8–20 mg/dL	Higher in renal failure

* May vary, depending on references consulted or laboratory methods used.

when the physician is evaluating metabolic causes for certain types of urinary calculi (stones).

Urine Concentration Test

Specific gravity shows the concentration of particles, such as electrolytes, in water. The specific gravity of distilled water is 1.000. Normally, the specific gravity of urine is responsive to the water and electrolyte balance in the body. On a hot day, a person who is perspiring profusely and taking little fluid has urine with a high specific gravity. Conversely, a person who has a high fluid intake and who is not losing excessive water from perspiration, diarrhea, or vomiting has copious urine with a low specific gravity.

When the kidneys are damaged, the ability to concentrate urine is impaired: the specific gravity remains relatively constant, no matter what the water needs of the body are or how much the patient drinks. To test the kidneys' capacity to adjust the specific gravity of urine, the patient is dehydrated. Fluids are restricted starting at 6 PM and are withheld until the test is complete. The patient voids at 10 PM, and the specimen is discarded. If the patient voids during the night, the specimen is saved and labeled with the time of voiding. The next-morning urine specimens are collected at 6 AM, 7 AM, and 8 AM. Each specimen is placed in a separate container and labeled with the time collected. A specific gravity of less than 1.020 on all specimens indicates renal disease.

Urine Protein

Urine protein (proteinuria) may be detected by dipping a test reagent stick in the urine and comparing color changes with the provided color chart. It also may be determined by collecting the urine for 24 hours in a container supplied by the laboratory. The exact start and end of the test is entered on the label. Normal values are 50 to 80 mg in 24 hours.

Creatinine Clearance Test

This test is used to determine kidney function and is not influenced by dietary intake. Creatinine, a substance that results from the breakdown of phosphocreatine present in muscle tissue, is excreted at a fairly constant rate by the kidney. For this test, a 24-hour urine specimen and a sample of blood are collected. First, the urine is collected for 24 hours. Immediately after the last specimen of urine, a sample of blood is drawn. Both urine and blood are sent to the laboratory. The normal creatinine clearance is 600 to 1800 mg in 24 hours, although normal values may vary from laboratory to laboratory. A decrease in the creatinine clearance indicates depressed renal function.

Intravenous Pyelogram

The intravenous pyelogram (IVP) is a radiographic study based on the ability of the kidneys to excrete a contrast (radiopaque) media in the urine. Injected intravenously, the contrast medium shows the outlines of the kidney pelvis, the ureters, and the bladder on radiographic film as the radiopaque material passes through the urinary tract.

The contrast medium usually contains iodine, to which the patient may be allergic. The physician may inject a minute amount of medium intravenously and observe the patient for 5 to 10 minutes to determine whether an allergy to iodine is present. New contrast media that do not contain iodine, called *nonionic contrast agents*, are available and produce fewer allergic reactions.

If the patient is undergoing extensive diagnostic testing, the physician probably will delay barium studies of the gastrointestinal tract until urologic studies are completed. It may take several days for barium to be removed from the gastrointestinal tract, and its presence can distort IVP findings. The physician's orders before an IVP usually include the following:

1. The patient should eat nothing by mouth for 12 hours before the pyelogram is scheduled. This fasting dehydrates the patient so that the urine (and, therefore, the contrast medium) is at maximum concentration.
2. The bowel should be cleansed, so that its contents do not interfere with visualization of kidneys on the film. Usually, a laxative is ordered the evening before and a rectal suppository or enema early on the morning of the pyelogram. Because poor cleansing of the intestinal tract may require that the test be repeated, it is important that the bowel preparation is effective.

Patients may have other conditions that make the usual preparation inadvisable. For example, in peptic ulcer or ulcerative colitis, because of the danger of gastrointestinal perforation, the bowel-cleansing procedure may be modified. To obtain additional information that helps the physician with diagnosis, additional films may be taken up to 24 hours later.

Cystoscopy and Retrograde Pyelograms

Cystoscopy is the visual examination of the inside of the bladder using a metal instrument (cystoscope). The cystoscope consists of a sheath with a light bulb for illumination at its tip. A telescope is inserted into the sheath for visualization. The cystoscope enables the physician to see a magnified view of the interior of the bladder. Inflow and outflow valves allow for irrigation. The size of the cystoscope is graded in the French (F) scale; usually, one that is 20 to 24 F is used in adults.

A retrograde pyelogram is the insertion of a radiopaque ureteral catheter into the pelvis of each kidney with a cystoscope. Radiopaque dye is injected, and radiographs are taken. Cystoscopy and retrograde pyelograms may be done for the following purposes.

Inspection.   Prostate, urethra, bladder, and ureteral orifices can be seen. Cystoscopy usually is performed with bleeding of the urinary tract because bleeding can be a symptom of cancer. A catheter may be threaded into each ureter to gather separate speci-

mens of urine from each kidney to indicate which one is affected by pus, cancer cells, tubercle bacilli, or other evidence of disease. To obtain a retrograde pyelogram, contrast medium (about 3 ml to 5 ml) can be injected into the catheters to outline the upper urinary tract. Retrograde pyelograms may be performed when visualization during an IVP has been inadequate.

Biopsy.   Specimens of tissue may be taken from the bladder or urethra through the cystoscope either with a biopsy forceps or by using the brush technique. In the latter, a biopsy brush is introduced through the cystoscope and into the ureter and renal pelvis. The brush is withdrawn, and the tissue samples are examined microscopically.

Treatment.   Tumors of the urethra or bladder can be treated by electrosurgery (fulguration), with electrodes passed through the cystoscope. Small stones and other foreign bodies sometimes can be removed through the cystoscope. Sometimes, larger stones are crushed and then removed. A narrowed ureteral orifice can be incised, ureters dilated, the kidney pelvis drained and irrigated, and radon seeds implanted around or into malignant tumors.

Cystourethrogram

In this test, contrast material is instilled into the bladder through a urethral catheter, and radiographs are taken. This test also may be performed if the patient is having retrograde pyelograms.

A voiding cystourethrogram is similar to a cystourethrogram except that the patient is instructed to void (the urine contains the contrast material), and a rapid series of radiographs are taken.

Arteriograms

Renal arteriograms are used to evaluate blood vessels to the kidneys and to delineate the nature of mass lesions. Using this radiographic study, the surgeon can obtain accurate information about the location and number of renal arteries, especially because multiple vessels to the kidney are not unusual. The percutaneous catheter technique is the method commonly used. A catheter is passed up the femoral artery into the aorta to the level of the renal vessels. At this point, contrast medium is injected. The dye first outlines the aorta in the area of the renal artery, then it enters the renal artery and the kidney, and radiographs are taken. The catheter may be manipulated into separate arteries individually.

Computed Tomographic Scanning

A computed tomographic (CT) scan may be performed to diagnose renal pathology. In this procedure, a contrast medium may be injected intravenously after the initial scan to enhance the images, especially when vascular tumors are suspected.

Ultrasonography

The size, shape, position, and the internal structures of the kidneys may be determined by using ultrasound. This test is not invasive, does not require the injection of a contrast medium, and does not require fasting. The structures of the kidney are not as clearly defined, however, as they are with other methods, such as a CT scan and the use of a contrast medium.

Needle Biopsy

A needle biopsy may be performed to obtain a sample of tissue from the kidney. Usually, this procedure is done under local anesthesia in the operating room. Before the procedure, the patient fasts for 6 to 8 hours, and a mild sedative may be given. An intravenous line is inserted before the patient is placed in a prone position with a sandbag under the abdomen. Radiographs (eg, IVP, retrograde pyelograms, flat plat of the abdomen [also called a KUB, or *k*idneys, *u*reters, and *b*ladder]) are used to determine placement of the needle. Once needle placement is determined, the patient is asked to take in a deep breath and hold it while the needle is inserted. The "swing" of the needle usually indicates that the needle is properly placed. Ultrasound and fluoroscopy also may be used to determine needle placement. Samples are removed, visually examined, and placed in a container with preservative. When the surgeon is satisfied that renal tissue has been obtained, the needle is withdrawn.

An open biopsy also may be obtained by a small incision in the flank. Many physician's prefer to attempt a needle biopsy first and, if tissue samples are not satisfactory, then perform an open biopsy.

General Radiographs

General radiographs (eg, a KUB) may be used to detect abnormal renal or bladder shadows as well as to visualize radiopaque stones in the urinary tract. A radiograph of the pelvis, chest, or other area may reveal metastatic bone lesions that are occurring as a result of renal or bladder tumors. CT scans or magnetic resonance imaging (MRI) may be used for this purpose and also to determine kidney size and the presence of abnormalities, such as tumors or cysts.

NURSING PROCESS —THE PATIENT UNDERGOING TESTS FOR A URINARY TRACT DISORDER

Assessment
A complete history of symptoms and a general medical, drug, and allergy history are obtained. It is important to determine if the patient is allergic to iodine or seafood (which contains iodine) because iodine is a component of some contrast (radiopaque) materials used in radiographs, such as an IVP. If an allergy is suspected or known, the patient's chart must be clearly labeled with this information, and the physician must be informed *before* any tests are performed.

Nursing Diagnosis
Depending on the patient or type of test, one or both of the following may apply:

- Anxiety related to diagnosis (actual, potential), diagnostic test
- Knowledge deficit of type of test, patient preparation and participation

Planning and Implementation
The major goals of the patient include a reduction in anxiety and an understanding of the preparations for diagnostic tests.

The major goals of nursing management are to reduce anxiety, correctly prepare the patient for diagnostic tests, and observe the patient after the tests.

Whenever a contrast medium that contains iodine is used, the nurse carefully observes the response of the patient and promptly reports to the physician any untoward effect, such as increasing anxiety, restlessness, wheezing, tachycardia, or signs of cardiovascular collapse. Oxygen, antihistamines, epinephrine, corticosteroids, and vasoconstrictor agents, such as metaraminol (Aramine), as well as resuscitation equipment should be readily available when a patient has a radiograph that uses a contrast medium with iodine.

After some tests, such as an IVP, cystoscopy, or retrograde pyelogram, the physician may order "push fluids" to overcome the dehydration and to flush any remaining dye from the urinary tract.

Underlying abnormality may be aggravated by instrumentation procedures, such as a cystoscopy. For example, significant prostatic obstruction may result in complete urinary retention. With a urinary infection, instrumentation may be followed by chills, fever, and possibly septicemia. The patient is observed for these symptoms, and they are promptly reported to the physician. The physician may order antibiotics administered after genitourinary instrumentation.

Many patients have a dull ache caused by distention of the renal pelvis with dye. The physician may order a hot bath or codeine to relieve pain.

After an arteriogram, the physician usually applies a pressure dressing to the femoral area. This dressing may be ordered to be left in place for several hours, and the pulses in the legs and feet are palpated for signs of interference with the circulation. The dressing is observed for bleeding: if bleeding occurs, the physician is contacted immediately.

If the patient has had a needle, brush, or open kidney biopsy, the urine is checked for hematuria. After a needle or open kidney biopsy, vital signs are taken every 15 to 30 minutes until stable. The physician is notified if hematuria persists or becomes worse, the blood pressure drops and the pulse rises, or the patient complains of pain in the back or abdomen. These events may indicate bleeding and require immediate examination by the physician.

Anxiety. Many patients experience anxiety—and sometimes fear—when scheduled for diagnostic tests that involve the insertion of an instrument or catheter. A thorough explanation of what to expect can relieve the patient's anxiety about the procedure.

The physician normally explains the test, what it involves, and why it is being done. The nurse may reinforce or reexplain the test to the patient. For example, if a cystoscopy is being performed, the nurse advises the patient that an urge to void is felt when the instrument is passed into the bladder and when the bladder is filled with fluid. This feeling is normal, and the patient is reminded not to push down or try to void because these actions may increase discomfort.

Knowledge Deficit. All preparations are fully explained to the patient before the test. In some instances, it may be necessary to inform the patient of what to expect; for example, a laxative that is given to empty the bowel before kidney radiographs may result in several loose stools and abdominal discomfort.

The patient is told that voiding is painful for about a day after a cystoscopy. Mild hematuria is not unusual. Discoloration of the urine may be expected if dyes were used, and the patient should be informed of this fact.

The collection of single or multiple urine specimens may require repeated explanations and reminders, especially if the patient is elderly. The patient is closely supervised when a 24-hour urine specimen is obtained; *all* urine excreted in that period must be placed in the appropriate collection container.

Outpatients should be instructed to return to the physician if frank bleeding, anuria, pain, or fever occurs.

Evaluation

- Anxiety is reduced
- Demonstrates understanding of and necessary participation for a diagnostic test

Suggested Readings

☐ Fischbach FT. A manual of laboratory diagnostic tests. 3rd ed. Philadelphia: JB Lippincott, 1988. *(Additional coverage of subject matter)*

☐ Kozier B, Erb G. Techniques in clinical nursing: a nursing process approach. 2nd ed. Menlo Park, CA: Addison–Wesley, 1987. *(Additional coverage of subject matter)*

☐ McConnell EA. Assessing the bladder. Nursing '85 November 1985;15:44. *(Additional coverage of subject matter)*

☐ Memmler RL, Wood DL. Structure and function of the human body. 4th ed. Philadelphia: JB Lippincott, 1987. *(Additional coverage of subject matter)*

☐ Porth CM. Pathophysiology: concepts of altered health states. 3rd ed. Philadelphia: JB Lippincott, 1990. *(In-depth, high-level coverage of subject matter)*

☐ Stark JL. A quick guide to urinary tract assessment. Nursing '88 July 1988;18:56. *(Additional coverage and illustrations that reinforce subject matter)*

Chapter 53

Disorders of the Urinary Tract

- Discuss general points of observation made during the management of a patient with a urinary tract disorder

- Use the nursing process in the management of a patient with an indwelling catheter and closed drainage system

- Use the nursing process in the management of an incontinent patient and a patient with urinary retention

- Discuss the symptoms, diagnosis, and treatment of infectious or inflammatory disorders of the lower and upper urinary tract

- Use the nursing process in the management of a patient with an infectious or inflammatory disorder of the lower or upper urinary tract

- Discuss the symptoms, diagnosis, and treatment of obstructive disorders of the urinary tract

- Use the nursing process in the management of a patient with urinary tract obstruction

- Use the nursing process in the management of a patient who is having ureteral surgery

- Discuss the symptoms, diagnosis, and treatment of a malignant kidney or bladder tumor

- Use the nursing process in the management of a patient who is having kidney surgery or a urinary diversion procedure

- Discuss the symptoms, diagnosis, and treatment of congenital disorders of the urinary tract

- Discuss the symptoms, diagnosis, and treatment of acute and chronic renal failure

- Use the nursing process in the management of a patient in renal failure

- Discuss hemodialysis, peritoneal dialysis, continuous ambulatory peritoneal dialysis, and renal transplantation

- Discuss the symptoms, diagnosis, and treatment of traumatic urinary tract injuries

GENERAL OBSERVATIONS

The kidneys are the major organ of excretion of water and waste products and regulate electrolyte and acid–base balance. These functions are essential to life. Observation of the patient with a urologic disorder must include specific tasks:

1. An accurate measurement of the intake and output is *most important* in patients with urologic disorders.
2. The patient is observed for edema, which may first become obvious as puffiness around the eyes (periorbital edema) or in the legs. Whenever edema is present, the patient is weighed every day to keep track of possible loss or gain of fluids.
3. The blood pressure, pulse, and respirations are monitored at intervals, depending on the patient's diagnosis and physical condition.
4. The patient is frequently assessed for signs of electrolyte, acid–base, and water imbalance, especially for those who are in renal failure.

Observation of the urine can reveal a great deal. The daily amount is an important indication of the adequacy of renal function. Less than 500 mL/day when the intake has been adequate means that the urinary tract is in serious trouble; the physician must be notified. Total intake and output measurements for the 24- or 8-hour period are checked to see if the figures are about equal. Any wide discrepancy is reported to the physician.

Color and content of the patient's urine should also be observed for sediment, clots, and shreds of material; odor, color, and degree of opacity are also noted. If the patient has any type of catheter, the urine is observed as it passes through the tube connected to the drainage system. This index is better than the old urine in the drainage receptacle.

Each day, the specific fluid-intake goal for each patient must be established. The amount of fluid that should be taken orally in a 24-hour period is calculated, and then a schedule of fluid intake is planned for the patient's waking hours. Three quarters or more of the total intake should be given during the day. As a general rule, fluids are encouraged to keep the urine dilute. Dilute urine does not crystallize and form calculi as easily as concentrated urine. In those with cystitis, burning on urination is less. An increase in urine output rids the kidney of noxious substances and removes products of inflammation.

When fluids are to be encouraged (often 3,500 to 4,000 mL), frequent, small offerings may be more palatable than large quantities presented less often, especially with geriatric patients. Often, the patient takes responsibility for drinking fluids. It is essential that the patient understand how much should be taken, how to keep track of the amount, and why fluids are important. The fluids available to the patient may take the form of ice water, certain fruit juices, gelatin, fruit flavored drinks, or (some) carbonated beverages.

All patients for whom fluids are encouraged are observed for a fluid volume excess (ie, edema, dyspnea, rales), especially those who are elderly and those with a heart ailment or potential renal failure.

In some urologic disorders, fluids may be limited (often 600 to 800 mL/day), such as when edema or renal failure is present. If the patient's body is unable to rid itself of water efficiently, damage results when large amounts of fluid are given. When the fluid intake is limited, the amount of oral fluids given over a 24-hour period is evenly distributed during the patient's waking hours. The patient should understand the reason for the restriction. Thirst may be a problem, especially in hot weather. Icechips, when allowed, need to be counted in total fluid intake. If fluid intake is provided by intravenous administration, the flow rate is calculated so that administration also is evenly spaced during the 24-hour period.

Records of intake and output must be accurate; otherwise, the physician bases treatment on incorrect information. Every person who works with the patient should understand and agree to the method of keeping records and the amount of fluid that the cups and glasses hold.

Blood pressure is another index of the course of illness. The patient's usual blood pressure and its value on admission are noted during the initial physical assessment and give a standard by which to judge readings. Blood pressure usually is taken every 4 hours for patients with nephritis, all those with active renal abnormality, and those with uremia. If the blood pressure is not stable, it is taken more frequently. If the patient seems sluggish or complains of headache, the blood pressure should be taken more frequently. A progressive rise in blood pressure is reported to the physician.

URINARY DRAINAGE

When urine does not leave the body normally, a catheter may need to be inserted to provide urinary drainage. A catheter may be inserted in the kidney (nephrostomy tube), ureter (ureteral catheter), or bladder to provide adequate drainage of urine.

If a patient has one or more catheters in place, it is imperative that the placement and function of each tube is understood. If this information is not immediately known, it may be found in the operative record or physician's progress notes. Each catheter should be labeled (label can be put on the drainage vessel or on the catheter itself with a tag or a loop of tape) so that all personnel can note and chart the material that comes from each catheter.

Types of Catheters

Catheters are sized according to the French system. The higher the number, the larger the diameter of the catheter. The several types of catheters (Fig. 53-1*A*) are suited for different purposes.

Drainage

A drainage catheter may be an indwelling urethral (Foley) catheter (see Fig. 53-1*B*) placed in the bladder, a retention catheter in the kidney pelvis (Figs. 53-2 and 53-3), a ureteral catheter, or one for drainage through a suprapubic wound that leads to the bladder (cystostomy tube).

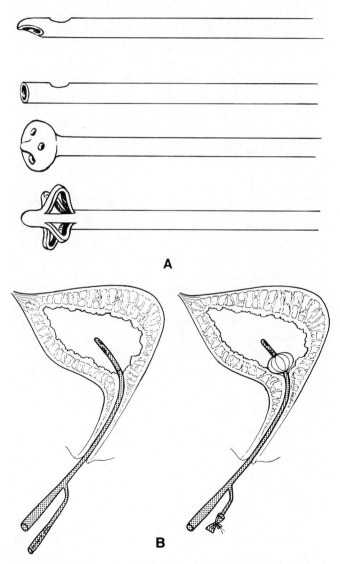

Figure 53–1. (*A*) Some catheter tips. (*Top to bottom*) Whistle-tip, hole-in-tip, de Pezzer mushroom, Malecot four-wing. (*B*) Foley catheter. (*Left*) The catheter is inserted into the bladder. (*Right*) The inflation of the bag prevents the catheter from leaving the bladder. The inner tube that leads to the balloon is tied.

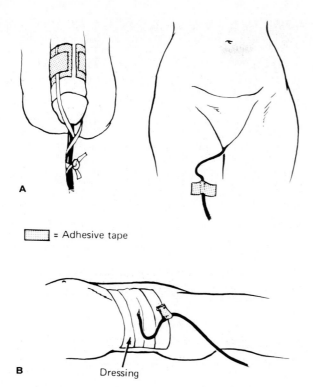

= Adhesive tape

B   Dressing

Figure 53–2. Indwelling catheters should be anchored securely to prevent pull on them. (**A**) Indwelling urethral catheter. (**B**) Catheter in the kidney pelvis.

Drainage. As soon as a catheter is inserted, it is connected to a closed sterile drainage system. If there is more than one catheter, *each* drainage system is labeled according to the source of the catheter, for example, "suprapubic" and "urethral," or "left ureter" and "right ureter." The intake and output record is set up with a separate column for each source of urine. Each drainage tube is secured to the bed linen with an anchoring device. Enough tubing is allowed between the anchoring device and the patient so that there is no pull on the catheter when the patient turns or moves, but not so much so that the tubing becomes tangled. A catheter must never be bent at right angles because this closes the lumen of the tubing. The *entire* length of the tubing is inspected—from insertion into the patient to the closed drainage system—for kinks. The kidney pelvis has a capacity of 5 to 8 mL. If a tube draining is blocked for a half-hour (eg, because a clot is stuck in the lumen, patient lying on the tube, tube kinked), urine backs up, perhaps strains the suture line, and increases pain for the patient. The end of the tube that drains the kidney pelvis is always handled with aseptic technique.

Splinting

A second type of catheter, one that is used solely for splinting, may be inserted after a plastic repair of the

ureter and may be kept in place for 1 or more weeks after surgery.

GENERAL PRINCIPLES OF CATHETERIZATION

The following general principles apply to the insertion and maintenance of urethral drainage catheters:

1. Aseptic technique is always used for insertion of a catheter and gloves are always worn.
2. The meatus is thoroughly cleansed before insertion of a catheter.
3. An adult urethra usually takes a size 18 to 24 F indwelling catheter; a smaller size may be used for intermittent (straight, single) catheterization.
4. When an indwelling catheter is inserted, the balloon should be tested before insertion of the catheter by filling the balloon with the solution in the prefilled syringe supplied with the catheterization tray. The solution is then withdrawn into the same syringe. The catheter is lubricated with a sterile water-soluble lubricant and inserted. The balloon is then inflated with the solution in the prefilled syringe.
5. Catheters are connected to a sterile closed drainage system.
6. Indwelling urethral catheters are changed according to the physician's orders or hospital policy.
7. An indwelling urethral catheter that accidentally becomes dislodged should never be reinserted but is replaced by a new sterile catheter.

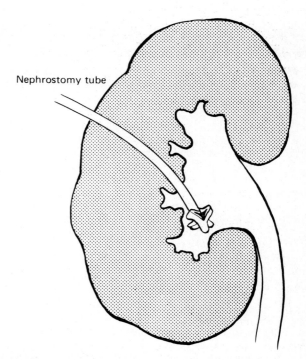

Nephrostomy tube

Figure 53–3. A nephrostomy tube with a Malecot four-wing tip draining the kidney pelvis.

NURSING PROCESS —THE PATIENT WHO HAS AN INDWELLING CATHETER AND CLOSED DRAINAGE SYSTEM

Assessment

In addition to the initial patient history and physical examination, the patient's chart is reviewed for the diagnosis, reason for insertion of a catheter, the type and size of catheter, the location of the catheter (eg, urethra, ureter, kidney pelvis, suprapubic cystostomy catheter), and the physician's orders about specific tasks, such as catheter irrigation or catheter changes.

Ongoing assessments are summarized in Charts 53-1 through 53-4.

Nursing Diagnosis

Depending on the type and location of the catheter and the patient's diagnosis, one or more of the following may apply. Additional nursing diagnoses that pertain to the patient's medical diagnosis also may be added.

- Anxiety related to feeling the urge to void (urethral catheter), inability to control voiding, diagnosis, proposed additional treatments, other factors (specify)
- Potential for infection related to contamination of the urinary tract, inflammation due to catheter placement
- Impaired tissue integrity (mucous membranes) related to infection, localized inflammation due to mechanical trauma of the catheter

---

Chart 53-1. Assessment and Management of the Patient Who Has an Indwelling Urethral Catheter

- ☐ Connect catheter to sterile closed gravity drainage system; empty drainage system q 8 hr and as needed.
- ☐ Anchor catheter with tape (see Fig. 53-2) to keep tension off catheter and avoid trauma to urethra and bladder neck; remove and reapply tape.
- ☐ Force fluids to 3000 mL/day unless contraindicated by other concurrent disorders (congestive heart failure, renal shutdown, increased intracranial pressure, etc.).
- ☐ Measure and record intake and output; note and record appearance of urine.
- ☐ Irrigate catheter (if ordered) using strict aseptic technique.
- ☐ Cleanse perineal and periurethral areas twice daily and as needed.
- ☐ Apply water-soluble bacteriostatic ointment to urinary meatus twice daily or as ordered.
- ☐ Visually inspect external section of catheter and drainage tubing for kinks, torsion, or obstruction q 2–4 hr (or more often if necessary).

Chart 53-2. Assessment and Management of the Patient Who Has an Indwelling Ureteral Catheter

- ☐ Connect ureteral catheter to a sterile closed gravity drainage system (unless ordered otherwise) with a sterile adapter; if two catheters were inserted, connect each to a separate drainage system and label each catheter and drainage system (left, right).
- ☐ Anchor catheter to thigh (or abdomen if catheter exists through a surgical incision); remove and reapply tape.
- ☐ Use strict aseptic technique for irrigation (if ordered); use *no more than* 5 mL of sterile irrigant each time.
- ☐ Measure and record output of *each* catheter q 8 hr or as ordered.
- ☐ Check for patency of catheter by visually noting urine output (urine dripping from end of ureteral catheter into drainage tubing adapter or upper section of drainage tubing).
- ☐ Report immediately any pain or discomfort in region of kidney (mid- to upper back) or failure of catheter to drain urine.
- ☐ Force fluids to 3000 mL daily unless contraindicated.

- Knowledge deficit of home care management (urethral, nephrostomy, cystostomy catheters)

Planning and Implementation

The major goals of the patient include a reduction of anxiety, an absence of infection, an absence of mucous membrane trauma, and an understanding of the care of the catheter at home.

The major goals of nursing management include a reduction in anxiety, prevention of infection, prevention of mucous membrane trauma, and the development of an effective teaching plan for the patient after discharge from the hospital.

Ongoing nursing management is summarized in Charts 53-1 through 53-4.

When a patient has a catheter (or tube) in any part of the urinary tract, the physician is informed if fever, chills, or sudden onset of pain in the area occurs or if the catheter fails to drain.

When caring for patients, catheters are checked frequently for patency and drainage of urine. Catheters that drain from the kidney pelvis or the ureter are checked every half-hour, and others at least every 2 hours. If a catheter is not draining, the nurse can do the following:

1. Check the entire length of the tubing from the patient to the closed drainage system for kinks, pressure, and other external compression of the tube that may be compressing the lumen.

Chart 53-3. Assessment and Management of the Patient Who Has a Cystostomy Tube

- ☐ Connect cystostomy tube to drainage system specified by the physician (closed gravity drainage, continuous bladder irrigation system).
- ☐ If other catheters (ureteral, urethral) also are inserted, label each catheter and drainage system.
- ☐ Change or reinforce dressing around catheter as needed.
- ☐ Visually inspect cystostomy tube for evidence of obstruction: kinks, blood clots, mucus plugs.
- ☐ Measure and record intake and output. Record outputs separately if more than one catheter has been inserted.
- ☐ If continuous bladder irrigation system is used, check container of irrigant at specified intervals; replace or refill as needed; record amount of irrigant added to system each time irrigant is replaced or refilled; subtract 8-hr total irrigant from 8-hr cystostomy tube drainage to obtain urinary output.
- ☐ Force fluids to 3000 mL daily unless contraindicated.

Chart 53-4. Assessment and Management of the Patient Who Has a Nephrostomy Tube

- ☐ Connect nephrostomy tube to sterile gravity drainage; label each drainage system if bilateral nephrostomy tubes are inserted.
- ☐ Measure and record output from each tube q 8 hr; note and record appearance of urine.
- ☐ Force fluids to 3000 mL daily unless contraindicated.
- ☐ Reinforce dressing around nephrostomy tube as needed; report excessive drainage immediately.
- ☐ Maintain security of tubes by anchoring to flank with tape or any other method approved by the physician.
- ☐ Check each tube for evidence of urinary output q 2–4 hr; report a decrease or absence of urinary drainage immediately.
- ☐ Nephrostomy tubes usually are *not* irrigated by nursing personnel.

---

2. Clamp the tube off near the patient and "milk" the remainder of tube toward the closed drainage system; feel for gravel (sediment made of phosphates and other mineral crystals); after milking, release the clamp and watch for urine.
3. Replace the tubing and closed drainage system (without removing the catheter that goes to the patient).
4. If urine still does not flow from the catheter, notify the physician immediately.

Nephrostomy tubes (catheters) that are positioned deep into the kidney pelvis through a flank incision can, at times, be replaced only by reopening the wound. It is extremely important that all catheters are anchored properly and protected from accidental dislodging from the surgical wound.

Ureteral catheters are smaller than other types of catheters used for urinary drainage and may become obstructed easily if blood or pus is in the urine. The physician may order irrigation of a ureteral catheter with 5 mL of sterile normal saline. The technique of irrigation is ordered by the physician. Irrigation may be performed by using a syringe and allowing the irrigant to flow in and be returned by gravity. Another method of irrigation is to instill the irrigant with a special ureteral syringe and adaptor or a syringe and blunt needle. The solution is slowly instilled and then withdrawn. Force must never be used. The physician is notified immediately if patency of the catheter cannot be established by the prescribed irrigation method.

Special adaptors are available to connect ureteral catheters to closed drainage systems. If a ureteral catheter is in each ureter, they are labeled "right" and "left."

CHANGING CATHETERS.   Indwelling urethral catheters are changed according to hospital policy or the physician's orders. Catheters such as nephrostomy or cystostomy catheters are inserted surgically and may be sutured in place. Ureteral catheters are inserted by a cystoscope and are never removed or changed except by a physician.

DRAINAGE AND IRRIGATION.   Drainage is usually accomplished by gravity, though suction may occasionally be used. When the end of the catheter is in the kidney pelvis, only gravity drainage is used. The physician orders the type and amount of suction.

Catheters are irrigated with sterile saline or distilled water, but only by a physician's order. Irrigation serves to keep the system of tubing open and not to rinse the cavity being drained. Because every irrigation carries with it the danger of infection, aseptic technique always is employed. If fluid is instilled and does not return, gentle aspiration with the irrigating syringe may be used, *except* in recent postoperative patients and those whose catheters enter the kidney pelvis. If there is no return after one aspiration, the procedure is stopped, and the tubing is reattached to the drainage system and observed. If nothing has returned after 30 minutes, the physician is notified. The amount of fluid that was instilled must be noted and subtracted from the total output.

The amount of fluid used for irrigation is ordered by the physician; a common amount for irrigating urethral tubing is 30 mL of sterile saline. No more than 5 mL at a time is used to irrigate tubing that goes into the ureters or kidney pelvis. Nephrostomy tubes are not usually irrigated by nursing personnel. Whenever a patient complains of pain during an irrigation, it should be stopped momentarily. Irrigations should be done *slowly* and *gently*.

If frequent irrigation is required, a closed system may be set up to decrease the chance of infection. Intermittent irrigation can be accomplished by releasing the clamp. When constant irrigation is ordered, a drip device is incorporated into the tubing, and a three-way Foley catheter (one tube admits fluid, one allows for drainage, and the third fills the balloon) may be used. Usually, the fluid is allowed to drip at a rate of 30 to 60 drops/min. A closed system such as this one is not used when the catheter is inserted into the kidney pelvis because of the danger of admitting too much fluid.

After a catheter is removed from a wound, the closure of the surgical fistula usually is rapid. If a wound catheter inadvertently slips out, the physician is notified immediately. When a catheter is removed by the physician, the site is observed. Urine may drain from it for a short time, but it should gradually stop. When a catheter has been removed from the urethra, the patient's voiding pattern is observed, and the time and amount of fluid are recorded.

Anxiety.   Some patients accept the insertion of a catheter into the urinary tract because it offers relief from pain and discomfort. Others find the procedure uncomfortable and are distressed by having a catheter inserted to provide drainage of urine. Normally, the insertion of a urethral catheter is not painful, but pain may be experienced if the urethra is inflamed or infected. The male patient with an enlarged prostate also may experience varying degrees of pain as the catheter is inserted into the prostatic urethra. To reduce anxiety, the patient must be told why the procedure is necessary, that discomfort usually is relieved in a short time, and that the urge to void may be noted. The patient is instructed not to bear down to void, since urine is being continually drained from the bladder and trying to do so may result in pain or discomfort.

Surgery is required for insertion of a catheter in the kidney or bladder (suprapubic approach). The surgical incision is checked for signs of inflammation and infection as well as for proper seating of the catheter. After removal of the catheter, urine usually seeps until the wound closes. To reduce anxiety associated with a constant leakage of urine, the dressing is changed frequently until the site of insertion remains dry.

Knowledge Deficit.   Patients who go home with catheters in place can be shown how to change them before discharge from the hospital. If the patient is unable to change the catheter, a family member or home health care personnel may be required to perform this task. The patient or family member also is taught the technique of connecting the catheter to a closed drainage system, to use aseptic technique when connecting and disconnecting the catheter from the drainage system, and how and when to empty and change the closed drainage system. The patient or family member is shown how to measure intake and output when this task is recommended by the physician.

The type of closed drainage system depends on the activity of the patient (eg, bed versus ambulatory). During the day, the ambulatory patient may use a drainage system that can be attached to the leg. When in bed, a drainage system attached to the bed frame and lower than the level of the bed is used. The importance of always keeping the drainage system below the level of the point of catheter insertion is stressed.

Where to obtain the necessary supplies (eg, catheter, equipment for insertion, closed drainage system) also is discussed with the patient and family.

The physician is consulted about the areas to be included in the teaching plan, such as the time interval between catheter changes or the type of irrigating solution. Usually, the following areas are included:

- How and when to change the catheter (if the catheter can be changed)
- Care of the skin around the catheter (nephrostomy, cystostomy); importance of and how to clean around the urethral meatus (urethral catheter)
- Application of dressings (if necessary)
- What to do if the catheter does not drain
- How to irrigate the catheter and the type of solution used
- When to notify the physician: if the catheter cannot be removed or reinserted (urethral catheter), fails to drain, or if fever, chills, or sudden pain occurs or the urine is bloody or extremely cloudy

Evaluation

- Anxiety is reduced
- No evidence of urinary tract infection
- Is free of trauma to the urethra, bladder, suprapubic or nephrostomy incision
- Demonstrates understanding of home management, catheter change, catheter care, irrigation procedure, what requires contacting the physician
- Asks questions about catheter care during the teaching sessions

URINARY INCONTINENCE

Ordinarily, the excretion of urine is controlled by two sphincters: the internal sphincter, which is close to the most dependent part of the bladder, and the external sphincter, which surrounds the urethra at a lower point. As the bladder fills, nerve endings are stimulated, giving the sensation of needing to void.

The anesthetized, unconscious, retarded, or elderly patient may not receive these stimuli, and, in many of these patients, the urinary sphincters relax involuntarily. Infection of the urinary system and accidental or surgical damage to either sphincter also can cause loss of control. The sphincters may not function adequately when local tissue has been damaged. Interference with the spinal nerves, such as that which occurs in tumors of the spinal cord, herniated disc, postoperative edema of the spinal cord, and spinal cord injuries, can interfere with the impulse conduction to the brain, resulting in a neurogenic bladder (a bladder that does not receive adequate nerve stimulation) and incontinence. Many paraplegic patients do not know when they void because they have lost all sensation in the lower parts of their bodies. A neurogenic bladder may be spastic, preventing the retention of urine, or it may be flaccid, preventing the complete expulsion of urine.

Symptoms

The symptoms may seem obvious, but it is important to determine if the patient is truly incontinent as the result of a specific disorder or if situations prevent the patient from voiding normally.

Diagnosis

Diagnosis is based on symptoms, but it is important to determine if incontinence is a temporary situation, as might be seen the first day after surgery, or if incontinence is due to a physical or mental disorder, such as paraplegia or Alzheimer's disease.

The physician may, in certain situations, perform tests, such as a urine culture and sensitivity, cystoscopy or cystourethrogram, to determine if incontinence is due to a treatable disorder.

Treatment

Treatment is aimed at correction of the physical disorder that is causing incontinence (when possible), correcting the situational problems that may be causing incontinence, or institution of a bladder training program.

NURSING PROCESS —THE INCONTINENT PATIENT

Assessment

A general health assessment is performed, and the patient's record is reviewed for the possible causes of incontinence. The patient's voiding pattern is evaluated. The patient is evaluated for possible situations that may cause incontinence, such as not being taken to the bathroom at regular intervals or not being able to reach the bedpan or urinal.

The patient's voiding pattern is noted and recorded over a period of at least 1 week.

Nursing Diagnosis

Depending on the possible cause and whether incontinence is temporary or permanent, one or more of the following may apply:

- Anxiety related to loss of voluntary control of urine, odors, other factors (specify)
- Total incontinence related to known (specify) or unknown factors
- Knowledge deficit of methods to reduce odor, prevent soiling, train the bladder to empty

Planning and Implementation

The major goals of the patient include reducing anxiety, being continent day and night, and understanding a bladder training program and ways to reduce soiling and prevent odors.

Some incontinent patients never achieve complete freedom from incontinency; others do. Success of a bladder training program depends not only on the degree of injury but also on the motivation of the patient and the amount of skillful help and encouragement received from the medical team.

Management of the incontinent patient is directed at establishing a voiding routine, when that is possible, and, when that is not possible, at finding the most convenient way to collect the urine and to keep it off the skin.

ESTABLISHING A SCHEDULE. The patient and the nurse working together may be able to set up a schedule so that voiding is regular and predictable. Such a program takes great patience by all concerned. If it is successful, it gives the patient freedom from constant odor, wetness, and the embarrassment of accidents at social gatherings or in the company of others. The first step is to observe and evaluate the patient's pattern of urination. If a pattern is observable, a bedpan or a commode should be made available (or the patient should be helped to the bathroom, if possible) just before it is believed the bladder will empty.

Fluid intake can be spaced to help to establish a regular time of voiding. Spacing fluids requires experimentation. If the patient limits fluids before going to bed or going out on a social occasion, it is essential that the fluid intake is adequate at other times of the day. A patient with a neurogenic bladder may not completely empty the bladder when voiding. Because of the danger of infection and stone formation, it is especially important that the patient drink sufficient fluids—at least 2,500 mL/day. Increasing intraabdominal pressure by gentle manual pressure just above the symphysis pubis may aid a patient with a neurogenic bladder to void.

Until a routine is well established, a record of the time and the amount voided is recorded. Such information can help the physician decide whether there is overflow with retention of residual urine and can help the patient begin to establish a voiding schedule.

REHABILITATION. An indwelling catheter may be used to prevent retention of urine and incontinence. Initially, it may be allowed to drain constantly, but, later, if the urologist determines that a reflex is present, a method of bladder training may be instituted. One method is to alternate clamping and unclamping of the catheter. The catheter is clamped for a specified length of time and then opened for a specified length of time. In the beginning, the catheter is unclamped for 5 to 15 minutes every 1 or 2 hours. In this time, the bladder is given a chance to hold urine and then to empty it, thus beginning to reestablish normal function. Gradually, the interval for releasing the catheter is lengthened to 3 or 4 hours, giving the bladder a chance to fill more completely. Patients can be taught to release the clamp on their own catheter at scheduled times. The retention catheter is changed once a week or as ordered by the physician.

The catheter later is removed entirely, and the patient is instructed to void every hour. Usually the patient is not able to retain the urine longer than 1 hour, and frequent voiding is necessary to prevent incontinence. Gradually, the interval is lengthened to 2, 3, or 4 hours. Because such frequent voiding would disturb the patient during the night, external drainage may be used on the male patient. A sheath (condom catheter, condom sheath) is placed over the penis and is connected by tubing to a drainage system or to a disposable urinary drainage bag. Women can wear absorbent pads and moistureproof pants.

The rehabilitation process takes a great deal of patience, and accidents do happen during the training period. When an accident occurs, the linen is changed promptly, and the patient is assured that accidents are to be expected during the retraining process. Patients should not be made to feel that the program has failed.

At first, many patients void in insufficient quantity, and they must be catheterized after voiding to remove residual urine. Patients should keep careful records of their fluid intake and output.

ODORS. Urea-splitting organisms, among them *Micrococcus ureae*, cause the urea in urine to react with water. An end product of this reaction is ammonia, which causes both the urine odor and skin damage. One way to protect skin is to avoid any contact with urine. When contact is unavoidable, an antiseptic such as methylbenzethonium chloride (Diaparene), which kills the ammonia-forming organism in urine, may be used. The antiseptic can (with the physician's approval) be applied to the skin of the incontinent ambulatory or bed patient. Light dusting with an absorbent powder, such as cornstarch, also helps to prevent ammonia dermatitis. The powder must be washed off, the skin thoroughly dried, and the powder reapplied four or more times a day.

If powder, an antiseptic, liners, and protective pads are used, odor or ammonia dermatitis should not be a problem; these measures should not be a substitute, however, for scrupulous cleanliness and the changing of padding as soon as it becomes wet. The buttocks and the genital area of the incontinent patient must be washed with soap and water several times a day. Unlike feces, urine on the skin is not visible. To prevent skin breakdown, the area actually must be free of urine; it is not sufficient that it appears to be clean. To avoid irritation, all soap and powders or ointments must be removed from the skin and the skin dried thoroughly. If an ammonia dermatitis is present, the affected area is kept clean, dry, and exposed to the air.

Total Incontinence. If it is not possible to establish a voiding routine and incontinence persists, the nurse and the patient together should devise a system of collecting the urine. The arrangement must be individualized, as not any one system works well for all patients. The objective is to provide for the urine an external reservoir that meets the following criteria:

- Protects the skin from contact with urine
- Is inexpensive to maintain
- Is convenient for the patient
- Can be worn under clothes
- Does not leak
- Is comfortable to wear

The male patient who is incontinent, bedridden, and unable to attend to his own needs can use a condom sheath during the day as well as at night; female patients can wear absorbent pads and moistureproof pants. Both male and female patients are provided with disposable absorbent pads that are placed under the buttocks. For ambulatory patients, various brands of protective pants that are available for men and women have a plastic outside layer and absorbent material inside. These pants can be pinned or snapped in place. Liners also are available and are worn next to the skin. Because they are nonabsorbent, the urine passes through them; because they dry quickly, they leave the skin dry and free of urine, even though the absorbent material is soaked.

Anxiety.   Anxiety may be reduced once the patient notes the effort, concern, and interest of the medical team. Discussing possible ways to establish normal bladder function actively involves the patient in a bladder rehabilitation program.

Patients are encouraged, when possible, to actively participate in a bladder training program by keeping a personal record of their fluid intake and time of voiding. Recommendations, such as drinking more fluids during the afternoon or drinking less in the evening, can be made once the patient's diary of fluid intake and voiding is reviewed.

Knowledge Deficit.   Many times, several methods need to be tried to establish a voiding program and effective control of urination. In some instances, control is never achieved, and incontinence continues.

A teaching plan is formulated to meet the patient's individual needs and includes one or more of the following:

1. Control odors by frequent cleansing of the perineum, changing clothes when they become soiled, wearing incontinence briefs (eg, Attends), and changing them when they become soiled. Electric room deodorizers may be used to control odors, but avoid the use of perfume or scented powders, lotions, or sprays. Mixing a perfumed scent with a urine odor may intensify the odor, irritate the skin, or cause a skin infection. Wash soiled garments as soon as possible in warm, soapy water. Use plastic to cover objects, such as a mattress and chairs, to prevent soiling and lingering odors. The plastic must be washed with mild soapy water daily or more often if needed.
2. Follow the recommendations of the physician about clamping and unclamping the catheter (when this method is prescribed).
3. Keep a record of fluid intake. Drink plenty of fluids during waking hours. Drink most of the required fluids in the morning and early afternoon hours, and decrease the intake toward evening.
4. Follow the recommended bladder training program. Time is often required to achieve success.
5. Contact the physician if any of the following occurs: increased discomfort, pain in the lower abdomen, fever, chills, or cloudy urine.

Evaluation

■ Anxiety is reduced
■ Actively participates in bladder training program by keeping own records
■ Urinary elimination pattern is normal or begins to show improvement
■ Patient and family openly discuss urinary elimination problem, ask questions, demonstrate willingness to adhere to bladder training program
■ Demonstrates understanding of importance of drinking fluids, adhering to bladder training program

URINARY RETENTION

Urinary retention may be defined as an inability to urinate and may be either acute or chronic. Chronic urinary retention may be seen in patients with disorders such as prostatic enlargement (males) and neurogenic bladder. Acute urinary retention may be seen in those with disorders such as complete urethral obstruction or after general anesthesia or the administration of certain drugs such as atropine or a phenothiazine.

The patient with acute urinary retention usually is not able to void. The patient with chronic urinary retention may or may not be able to void. If the patient with urinary retention is voiding (retention with overflow), the bladder is not being completely emptied. The urine retained in the bladder after the patient voids is called the *residual urine*. The amount of residual urine may vary from 1 oz to several hundred milliliters. Normally, a small amount of urine may remain in the bladder after voiding. When the amount exceeds 30 mL, it usually is considered a residual urine.

Symptoms

Symptoms of acute urinary retention are inability to void, which usually is accompanied by severe lower abdominal pain and discomfort. Chronic urinary retention may produce no symptoms, and the patient is unaware that the bladder is not emptying completely. If the amount of residual urine is large, the patient may void frequently in small amounts. Additional symptoms that may be seen in chronic urinary retention are signs of a bladder infection (eg, fever, chills, pain on urination) and dribbling of urine.

Diagnosis

Diagnosis of acute urinary retention is based on the patient's symptoms. Palpation of the bladder area reveals bladder distention. Diagnosis of chronic urinary retention also is based on the patient symptoms as well as catheterizing the patient for residual urine immediately after voiding.

Treatment

Treatment of acute urinary retention requires immediate drainage of urine from the bladder by catheterization. If a catheter cannot be inserted or if moderate to severe resistance is felt when inserting the catheter, force must not be used. Instead, the physician must be notified immediately; special urologic instrumentation may be necessary.

Chronic urinary retention may be treated in several ways. The first method is to remove the cause, when possible, such as surgery on the prostate gland. The insertion of an indwelling urethral catheter is another method that may be used on a temporary or permanent basis. To teach the patient ways to empty the bladder use Credé's maneuver or abdominal strain and Valsalva's maneuver.

For patients who do not respond to other methods or who have bladders that have lost all nervous system control either by disease or injury, intermittent catheterization may be necessary. Other possible treatment for patients who have lost nervous system control is to surgically insert a suprapubic cystostomy tube or use Credé's maneuver or abdominal strain and Valsalva's maneuver.

NURSING PROCESS —THE PATIENT WHO HAS URINARY RETENTION

Assessment

Patients with acute urinary retention are immediately treated for the disorder. Assessment may be limited to vital signs until the condition is relieved and the patient is able to give a medical history and a description of symptoms that lead to the acute episode.

Patients with chronic urinary retention require an investigation of symptoms, including the voiding frequency, the amount (eg, small, moderate) of urine passed each time, the presence of pain or discomfort in the lower abdomen, pain or discomfort on voiding, and difficulty in starting the urinary stream. The lower abdomen is gently palpated or percussed to determine if the bladder is enlarged and the possible degree of enlargement. Vital signs are taken, and the patient is weighed. A complete medical, drug, and allergy history also is obtained.

Nursing Diagnosis

Depending on whether the condition is acute or chronic, one or more of the following may apply:

- Pain related to severe, acute urinary retention
- Urinary retention related to urinary tract disorder (specify), neurogenic disorder or injury
- Anxiety related to inability to void, discomfort or pain secondary to acute or chronic urinary retention
- Knowledge deficit of ways to empty bladder

Planning and Implementation

The major goals of the patient with acute urinary retention include the relief of pain or discomfort, a reduction of anxiety, and a normal voiding pattern. The major goals of the patient with chronic urinary retention include a reduction of anxiety, relief of discomfort, a normal voiding pattern, and understanding ways to empty the bladder.

The major goals of nursing management are to reduce pain and anxiety and develop a teaching plan for patients with chronic urinary retention.

CHRONIC URINARY RETENTION. Patients with chronic urinary retention are monitored for intake and output. The time, amount, and color of each voiding is recorded. In some instances, this information is used to establish a voiding pattern, employ intermittent catheterization to empty the bladder, or use a manual maneuver to empty the bladder. The physician also may order catheterization for residual urine until 30 mL or less remains in the bladder.

If surgical insertion of a cystostomy tube is necessary, the patient requires the same postoperative care as any surgical patient or the patient with a catheter. The incision is inspected for leakage of urine around the catheter. Once a permanent fistula has formed, the size of the cystostomy tube may need to be increased or decreased to prevent leakage of urine or discomfort.

ACUTE URINARY RETENTION. If the patient is in acute urinary retention, the physician orders insertion of a urethral catheter. If the bladder is markedly distended, the physician may order gradual emptying of the bladder. About 300 to 500 mL is allowed to drain, and the catheter is clamped for the prescribed time (usually 15 to 30 minutes). Some believe that if too much urine is removed at a rapid rate, moderate to severe hypotension and bladder hemorrhage can occur.

After emptying of the bladder, the patient is monitored for intake and output. The time, amount, and color of each voiding is recorded. If the patient fails to void again in 6 to 8 hours or if the urine appears bloody, the physician is notified.

CREDÉ'S MANEUVER. Place hands on top of one another just below the umbilicus and press firmly down toward the lower abdomen. Repeat until no more urine is expelled.

ABDOMINAL STRAIN AND VALSALVA'S MANEUVER. Lean forward, contract the abdominal muscles, and bear down while holding the breath. Wait 1 minute and repeat until no more urine is expelled.

If intermittent catheterization is used, the patient or a family member is taught the procedure as well as given time to practice before discharge from the hospital. When an indwelling urethral catheter is used, the catheter must be changed at the time interval specified by the physician. Depending on the patient's home situation, the catheter may be changed by a family member or health care personnel who make home visits. If a family member assumes responsibility, demonstration of the procedure and time to practice the procedure under nursing supervision are required.

Patients who have a permanent cystostomy tube

develop a permanent fistula between the bladder and abdominal wall. The tube can often be changed by the patient or family member at the intervals prescribed by the physician. The procedure for changing the tube and time to practice the procedure must be taught to the patient or family member.

Anxiety, Pain.   Once the bladder has been emptied, the patient is probably less anxious and more comfortable. Pain is usually relieved after emptying of a distended bladder, but discomfort may remain for several hours. The physician may order an analgesic for discomfort.

Knowledge Deficit.   If the patient is to be taught one or more methods of emptying the bladder, the physician is consulted as to which methods are to be included in a patient and family teaching plan.

The following manual methods are performed in the sitting position (male and female). The physician must approve of their use.

Evaluation

- Pain is relieved
- Establishes a normal voiding pattern or uses an effective method for emptying the bladder
- Anxiety is reduced
- Demonstrates understanding of manual methods to empty the bladder and is able to effectively and correctly perform these maneuvers
- Demonstrates understanding of intermittent catheterization or changing the urethral or cystostomy catheter; patient or family is able to effectively and correctly perform the procedure

INFECTIOUS AND INFLAMMATORY DISORDERS OF THE LOWER URINARY TRACT

Cystitis

Cystitis is inflammation of the urinary bladder. Urine is normally sterile. Bacteria reach the bladder by way of infected kidneys, lymphatics, and the urethra. Because the urethra is short in women, ascending infections are more common in women than in men. Causes of cystitis include urologic instrumentation (eg, cystoscopy), fecal contamination, indwelling catheters, and sexual intercourse.

Cystitis is prevented from being even more common than it is by a natural resistance of the bladder lining, which helps to prevent an inflammatory process from taking hold as the result of occasional invasion of the bladder by bacteria.

Symptoms

The symptoms of cystitis include urgency (feeling a pressing need to void although the bladder is not full), frequency, dysuria (painful urination), perineal and suprapubic pain, and hematuria, especially at the termination of the stream (terminal hematuria). If bacteremia is present, the patient also may have chills and fever. Chronic cystitis causes similar symptoms, but usually they are less severe.

Diagnosis

The diagnosis is made by the patient's history, the total physical examination, and urinalysis, including microscopic examination of the urine and culture and sensitivity studies.

Treatment

Medical management includes locating and correcting contributing factors and antimicrobial therapy—usually with a sulfonamide drug. When there is a partial obstruction, no cure of cystitis is fully effective until adequate drainage or urine is restored by the removal of the obstruction. In some instances, treatment may be prolonged and may necessitate many visits to the physician.

Urethritis

Urethritis, or inflammation of the urethra, is seen more commonly in men than in women. Urethritis caused by microorganisms other than gonorrhea is called *nonspecific urethritis*. Gonorrhea, on the other hand, is a specific form of infection that can attack the mucous membrane of a normal urethra (see Chapter 9). In women, urethritis may accompany cystitis but also may be secondary to vaginal trichomonal or monilial infections.

The distal portion of the normal male urethra is not totally sterile. Bacteria normally present there cause no difficulty, however, unless these tissues are traumatized, usually after instrumentation such as catheterization or cystoscopic examination. Under such conditions, bacteria may gain a foothold to cause a nonspecific urethritis. Other causes of nonspecific urethritis in men include irritation during vigorous intercourse or vaginal intercourse with a female with a trichomonal or monilial infection.

Symptoms

The symptoms of infection of the urethra are discomfort on urination varying from a slight tickling sensation to burning or severe discomfort and urinary frequency. Fever is not common, and its appearance in men implies further extension of the infection to areas such as the prostate, testes, and epididymis.

Diagnosis

Diagnosis is based on the patient's history and symptoms. In men, a urethral smear is obtained for culture and sensitivity testing to identify the causative microorganisms.

Treatment

Treatment includes appropriate antibiotic therapy, liberal fluid intake, analgesics, warm Sitz baths, and improvement of the patient's resistance to infection by a good diet and plenty of rest. If urethritis is due to a sexually transmitted disease, it is treated with appropriate antibiotic therapy (see Chapter 9).

NURSING PROCESS —THE PATIENT WHO HAS AN INFECTIOUS OR INFLAMMATORY DISORDER OF THE LOWER URINARY TRACT

Assessment

A complete medical and drug history is obtained, and the patient is asked to describe the symptoms and when the symptoms began. A record of the patient's voiding history also is obtained, because lower urinary tract infection is associated with problems such as urinary incontinence or retention. Vital signs also are taken.

Nursing Diagnosis

Depending on the type and severity of the disorder one or more of the following may apply.

- Anxiety related to pain, discomfort, need to urinate frequently
- Altered comfort: pain related to urethral inflammation
- Knowledge deficit of treatment regimen, avoidance of future episodes of infection or inflammation

Planning and Implementation

The major goals of the patient may include a reduction in anxiety, relief of pain, and an understanding of methods that may be used in preventing future infection or inflammation of the lower urinary tract.

The major goals of nursing management may include a reduction of anxiety, relief of pain, and development of an effective teaching plan for ways to reduce or prevent future infection or inflammation of the lower urinary tract.

If a hospitalized patient exhibits cystitis or urethritis, fluids are forced, unless there is a specific order limiting fluids because of a coexistent medical disorder. The physician may prescribe antibiotic therapy and Sitz baths to relieve discomfort if the patient is ambulatory. Cranberry juice may be offered to the patient. This acidifies the urine and provides a less favorable climate for bacterial growth.

If the patient has an indwelling urethral catheter, gentleness is exercised when it becomes necessary to change catheters. Urethritis is commonly caused by irritation from indwelling catheters. Patients who have indwelling catheters should be washed more frequently, especially if the female patient is incontinent of feces. It is not sufficient to wash only around anus and buttocks; the meatus and labia also must be washed. When cleaning the anal area, wiping toward the urethra is avoided. If cotton pledgets are used, wipe from the urethral meatus to the anus in a single stroke and discard the pledget.

Anxiety and Pain. The patient is assured that symptoms will diminish once the infection/inflammation is under control, but it may take 3 or more days before relief is felt.

Knowldge Deficit. Most cases of cystitis and urethritis are treated on an outpatient basis. The following can be included in a patient teaching plan:

1. Take the prescribed medication as directed on the container. Do not stop taking the medication even though symptoms have disappeared. It is important that the entire course of therapy be completed.
2. Take warm tub baths if discomfort is severe.
3. Drink at least 8 large glasses of fluids per day. Include one or more glasses of cranberry juice in the daily fluid intake.
4. Fluids include water, cranberry juice, tea, coffee, carbonated beverages or any food (flavored gelatin, ice cream, and so forth) that is liquid at room temperature. Those on special diets (eg, low-sodium or diabetic diets) must check with the physician about drinking juices or beverages or eating goods that are liquid at room temperature. Some of these liquids either must be considered part of the daily dietary allowances or may not be allowed because they contain substances that must be eliminated from the diet. In some diets, a limited amount of certain liquids may be allowed.
5. Notify the physician if symptoms persist after the course of drug therapy is completed, if the symptoms become worse, or if fever or chills occur.
6. Follow the recommendations of the physician for preventing future episodes of infection or inflammation.

Evaluation

- Anxiety is reduced
- Pain is relieved
- Demonstrates understanding of drug regimen, importance of drinking fluids, measures to prevent future episodes

INFECTIOUS AND INFLAMMATORY DISORDERS OF THE UPPER URINARY TRACT

Pyelonephritis

Pyelonephritis means infection of the renal parenchyma and the lining of the collecting system. Pyelonephritis may be acute or chronic. Acute pyelonephritis is often associated with pregnancy and diabetes.

If the treatment of acute pyelonephritis is not permanently successful (eg, if the infection is recurrent, or if urinary stasis continues due to an obstruction), the disease may enter a chronic stage. The kidney shows irreversible degenerative changes and becomes small and atrophic, and the pelvic mucosa becomes pale and fibrotic. Many nephrons are destroyed. If enough nephrons are destroyed, the patient develops uremia.

Symptoms

In the acute form, the patient is clinically quite ill. Pain in the kidney, chills, fever, and malaise are usually seen. Frequency and burning on urination may be present if the bladder also is infected.

Although chronic pyelonephritis may be asymptomatic, the patient can have a low-grade fever, vague gastrointestinal complaints, and anemia. Acute attacks may occur; some patients develop hypertension due to renal ischemia. Sometimes stones form in the affected kidney.

Diagnosis

In the acute form, the urinalysis shows pyuria (pus cells in the urine). Diagnostic tests, such as cystoscopy and an intravenous or retrograde pyelogram, may be performed to determine if the infection has resulted in obstruction or damage to any of the structures of the urinary system.

Treatment

Treatment of acute pyelonephritis includes treating the symptoms (eg, fever, pain), antimicrobial therapy, and a liberal fluid intake.

No known substance can restore scarred kidney tissue. The aim of treatment for chronic pyelonephritis is to prevent further damage. Intensive therapy with antimicrobial agents is given. Any urinary tract obstruction is relieved. An effort is made to improve the patient's overall health. A nephrectomy may be performed if severe hypertension develops and if the other kidney can support life. The fight against chronic pyelonephritis is a long one. Prolonged medication and constant attention to general health habits may be a dull and discouraging routine for patients.

Tuberculosis

Since the advent of antitubercular drug therapy, tubercular infections of the urinary tract are less common than they used to be. Tuberculosis of the urinary tract usually occurs secondarily to lesions in the lungs. The upper pole of the kidney usually is involved first, and the disease may eventually involve the ureters, bladder, prostate, and scrotal contents.

Symptoms

Symptoms depend on the location of the infection. Fever, anorexia, and weight loss may be early symptoms of kidney involvement. Since these symptoms are nonspecific, they may be overlooked. As more involvement of the kidney and the lower urinary tract occurs, symptoms may intensify. Symptoms of lower urinary tract involvement include dysuria, polyuria, fever, urinary frequency, and pain.

Diagnosis

Diagnosis is based on the patient's symptoms as well as a culture of the urine for the mycobacterium (causative agent of tuberculosis). Special staining techniques (acid-fast stain) and microscopic examination of the urine also may identify the microorganism.

Treatment

If the renal tuberculosis does not respond to antitubercular drug therapy and is unilateral, a nephrectomy may be done. Rest is part of the treatment. Although the pulmonary lesion may no longer be active, in the early stage of treatment the urine contains the mycobacterium bacillus.

Acute Glomerulonephritis

The term *nephritis* refers to a group of noninfectious diseases characterized by widespread kidney damage. Glomerulonephritis is a type of nephritis characterized by inflammation of the glomeruli that occurs most frequently in children and young adults. It has been observed that symptoms of acute glomerulonephritis appear about 2 weeks after an upper respiratory infection, usually one that has been caused by group A streptococci infection. The exact relation between the respiratory infection and the nephritis is not clearly understood. The microorganisms are not present in the kidney when the symptoms of nephritis appear. The disease may represent an altered tissue reaction to infection, a result of host response rather than damage from infection.

Symptoms

Early symptoms may be so slight that the patient does not seek medical attention, although occasionally the onset is sudden. Symptoms include nausea, malaise, headache, generalized edema, facial puffiness especially around the eyes, and pain or tenderness over the kidney area. There may be cerebral and cardiac involvement.

In some instances, this disorder is discovered during a routine physical examination. More often, the patient or family notices that the person's face is pale and puffy and that slight ankle edema occurs in the evening. The appetite is poor, and nocturia may be present. Irritability and shortness of breath also may be seen. Visual disturbances, often due to papilledema or hemorrhage in the eye, and nosebleeds (epistaxis) may occur. As the condition progresses, the patient may develop hematuria, anemia, convulsions associated with hypertension, congestive heart failure, oliguria, and perhaps anuria.

Diagnosis

The diagnosis is based on the patient's symptoms. Laboratory findings include proteinuria, an elevated antistreptolysin-O titer (ASO titer) due to a recent streptococcal infection, decreased hemoglobin, elevated blood urea nitrogen (BUN) and serum creatinine, elevated serum potassium, and an elevated erythrocyte sedimentation rate (ESR). Gross or microscopic hematuria gives the urine a dark, smoky, or frankly bloody appearance.

Treatment

No specific treatment exists for acute glomerulonephritis. The therapy is guided by the symptoms and their underlying abnormality. The following regimen may be used:

1. *Bed rest*—While the blood pressure is elevated and edema is present, bed rest may continue for several weeks. When progressive ambulation is slowly started, daily urine specimens are usually collected, and blood pressure is taken daily or more often. Any increase in hematuria, proteinuria, or blood pressure is an indication for a return to bed rest.
2. *Hydration*—Fluids are given according to the patient's total daily urinary output and daily weight.
3. *Diet*—Sodium is restricted when edema is present. Carbohydrate intake is encouraged, especially when the protein intake is purposely limited. Vitamins may be added to the diet to improve the patient's general resistance. Iron may be needed to counteract anemia.
4. *Medication*—Antibiotics may be given to prevent a superimposed infection on the already inflamed kidney. Penicillin may be ordered to treat any remaining streptococci from the recent infection. Diuretics may be given to reduce edema, and antihypertensive agents may be given for severe hypertension.

In a seriously ill patient, a trial of corticosteroids may be given to attempt to alter the course of the disease. When the blood pressure climbs to high levels, antihypertensive drugs are usually given. The patient is not considered to be cured until the urine is free of albumin and red blood cells for 6 months. Return to full activity usually is not permitted until the urine is free of protein for 1 month.

Most patients with acute glomerulonephritis recover, usually completely. A few develop chronic glomerulonephritis. Subsequent infections with the same strain of hemolytic streptococci usually do not cause a second attack of acute glomerulonephritis. This is in sharp contrast with chronic glomerulonephritis, in which upper respiratory infections must be avoided to prevent exacerbations of the disease. Most patients survive the disease without sequelae, but death from uremia may follow delirium or convulsions, or the patient may die in congestive heart failure.

Chronic Glomerulonephritis

Chronic glomerulonephritis causes irreversible damage to the nephrons. Some disappear entirely. Bands of scar tissue contract the kidney and replace the functioning units. The cortex becomes distorted and shrunken. A small number of patients with chronic glomerulonephritis are known to have had acute glomerulonephritis, but most give no such history.

Symptoms

Some people experience no symptoms of this disorder until renal damage is severe. Others may have generalized edema, headache and hypertension, visual disturbances, nocturia, dyspnea, and proteinuria. Anemia, cardiac failure, and cerebral symptoms are not uncommon. The patient who develops anasarca (generalized edema) is said to be in the nephrotic stage. The generalized edema is due to the depletion of serum proteins, with loss of plasma osmotic pressure. These patients may remain markedly edematous for months or years. Quiescent periods occur between exacerbations. During this latent stage, the patient is relatively free of symptoms and feels well, but the urine contains protein.

The course of the disease is highly variable. The patient may live for years, with only occasional acute episodes or none at all; or the disease may be rapidly fatal due to renal failure (uremia).

Diagnosis

Diagnosis is based on the patient's symptoms and a general physical examination. Laboratory tests include examining the urine for protein, sediment, casts, and red and white blood cells. Other laboratory tests may be based on the severity of the disease and include serum electrolytes, complete blood cell (CBC) count, arterial blood pH, and albumin/globulin (A/G) ratio. Hyperkalemia, metabolic acidosis, hypermagnesemia, anemia, and hypoalbuminemia may be seen.

Chest radiograph and ECG may be performed to determine cardiac involvement. A percutaneous kidney biopsy also may be performed to confirm the diagnosis and to determine the severity of the disorder.

Treatment

Management is aimed at treating the patient's symptoms, such as hypertension, edema, and infections, with appropriate therapies. Patients are observed for any new signs of the disorder as well as any increase or decrease in the intensity of all present symptoms. Renal failure is always a possibility in patients with chronic glomerulonephritis; hence, it is important that symptoms be recognized early so that proper treatment can begin as soon as possible.

NURSING PROCESS —THE PATIENT WHO HAS AN INFECTIOUS OR INFLAMMATORY DISORDER OF THE UPPER URINARY TRACT

Assessment

A complete medical, drug, and allergy history is obtained from the patient or family member. A list of all symptoms is obtained and should include an in-depth description and onset of symptoms.

A general head-to-toe physical examination may be performed since these disorders may produce symptoms in many areas, such as the lungs, heart, and extremities. Laboratory and diagnostic tests are reviewed.

Vital signs are taken, and the patient is weighed.

Nursing Diagnosis

Depending on the symptoms and severity of the disorder, one or more of the following may apply:

- Hyperthermia related to infectious process
- Activity intolerance related to infectious process, chronic renal disease
- Anxiety related to disease process, knowledge deficit, diagnosis, other (specify)
- Colonic constipation related to enforced bed rest
- Pain related to inflammatory or infectious process (acute pyelonephritis or glomerulonephritis)
- Fatigue related to chronic disease state, effect of disorder on other body systems (cardiac, musculoskeletal)
- Potential for infection related to chronic disease state
- Self-care deficit: total or partial (specify areas) related to chronic fatigue

- Knowledge deficit of treatment regimen, home care management

Planning and Implementation

The major goals of the patient include a reduction of anxiety, increase in activity tolerance, normal body temperature, normal bowel elimination pattern, relief of pain and discomfort, absence of fatigue, absence of infection, increased ability to assume self-care activities, and an understanding of the treatment regimen and home care.

The major goals of nursing management are to relieve symptoms, achieve a normal bowel elimination pattern, meet the patient's physical and emotional needs, and prepare an effective postdischarge teaching plan.

Major nursing observations include the following:

- *Vital signs*
- *Intake and output*—Ratio of intake to output, color of urine, presence of blood, sediment, or cloudiness
- *Daily weights*—Sudden or slow increase or decrease
- *Signs of electrolyte or fluid imbalance* (especially hyperkalemia and hypermagnesemia)
- *Edema*—Face (especially around the eyes), extremities
- *Changes in cardiac and neurologic status*—Changes in blood pressure, pulse, respiratory rate; occurrence of dyspnea; auscultation of lungs for changes in breath sounds; observation for mental changes (confusion, disorientation, change in the level of consciousness)

The physician is notified if nursing observations reveal any change in the patient.

Anxiety. Patients may exhibit varying degrees of anxiety, depending on factors such as their degree of illness and what information has been given by the physician. Time must be allowed for the patient and family to talk about the illness and ask questions about treatments. Many times, a simple explanation of what a certain medication does helps them understand their treatment.

If the patient or family do not seem to understand the diagnosis, prescribed treatment regimen, or other facts about the disorder, this problem is brought to the attention of the physician.

Hyperthermia. Vital signs are monitored every 4 hours and more frequently if the patient is acutely ill. The physician is notified if the oral temperature is higher than 101°F, as an antipyretic may be ordered to reduce the temperature. The blood pressure is carefully watched. Any steady rise in the blood pressure is brought to the attention of the physician. If the patient is given antihypertensive medication, the response to therapy is noted. Failure of the drug to lower the blood pressure after several days is brought to the attention of the physician.

Colonic Constipation.   A record of bowel movements is kept, and the physician is informed if constipation occurs. A diet high in fiber or a stool softener may be ordered.

Pain.   Patients may experience moderate to severe pain. Pain is carefully evaluated and the location, onset, and description of pain are recorded. Analgesics, if ordered, are given. The physician is notified if the patient continues to have pain despite administration of an analgesic or if pain suddenly appears or becomes worse.

Potential for Infection.   Some patients should avoid exposure to people with infections, including other patients, hospital personnel, and visitors. The family is reminded that the patient must avoid exposure to infections. People should postpone a visit when they have any type of infection, such as an upper respiratory infection or sore throat.

Activity Intolerance.   Patients may be placed on complete bed rest but may be allowed to perform activities such as bathing and grooming. While some patients have few symptoms, others may note moderate to severe fatigue. The ability of the patient to perform activities of daily living is assessed on a daily basis. As response to treatment is noted, the patient may be able to assume some or all of bathing, grooming, and other personal needs.

When fatigue is present but patients are allowed to perform some of their own daily activities, these activities are spaced so that rest can be taken between activities.

Knowledge Deficit.   Some patients may be able to care for themselves; others require assistance with household management and personal activities. Patients' abilities to care for themselves at home or their available support systems are evaluated before they are discharged. If the patient lacks a support system, the physician is consulted; referral to a social agency or home health care agency may be necessary. If a special diet is prescribed, a dietary consultation may be necessary.

After a conference with the physician about the postdischarge treatment regimen and areas to be included in discharge teaching, the nurse can develop a patient teaching plan which includes the following general areas:

1. Follow the diet and fluid regimen recommended by the physician as outlined by the dietitian.
2. Take medication exactly as directed on the container label. Do not omit or discontinue any medication unless ordered to do so by the physician.
3. Monitor and record temperature and weight daily. (In

some instances, patients may be asked to monitor their blood pressure.)
4. Follow the physician's recommendations as to physical activity and exercise. Take frequent rest periods if fatigue occurs.
5. Contact the physician with any question about the medication, if symptoms become worse, or if fever, chills, blood in the urine, weight gain, swelling of the extremities or around the eyes, difficulty in breathing, difficulty in thinking, severe fatigue, excessive sleepiness, constipation, loss of appetite, or upper respiratory infection occurs.
6. Frequent follow-up visits and laboratory tests are necessary to monitor response to treatment.

Evaluation

- Able to tolerate increased activity
- Anxiety is reduced
- Vital signs are normal
- Bowel elimination is normal
- Pain and discomfort are relieved or absent
- Episodes of fatigue are decreased or absent
- No evidence of infection
- Able to assume some or all responsibility for own care
- Demonstrates understanding of treatment regimen, home care management, follow-up visits to the physician
- Asks pertinent questions about diet, medications, symptoms that require contacting the physician

OBSTRUCTIVE DISORDERS OF THE URINARY TRACT

An obstruction can occur anywhere in the urinary tract—from the kidney pelvis to the tip of the urethra. Obstruction may be caused by a tumor, a stone, a cyst, a kink in the ureter, stenosis or spasm of the ureter, or a diverticulum in the bladder wall that distends and blocks one or more of the three openings (two ureteral, one urethral) into the bladder. In older men, enlargement of the prostate gland is a common obstructing lesion (see Chapter 51). Urethral strictures may follow traumatic instrumentation and infection. Neurogenic dysfunction of the bladder that causes stasis of urine is essentially an obstructive condition.

When urine cannot pass freely by the obstruction, it backs up. For example, if an obstruction is at the end of the ureter where it opens into the bladder (ureteral orifice), the ureter becomes more and more distended because urine cannot flow into the bladder. The back pressure moves into the kidney pelvis, which also becomes distended. Next, the parenchyma of the kidney is squeezed between the pressure from the expanding pelvis and the internal pressure of the glomerulus and its continuous formation of urine. Likewise, the tiny blood vessels that supply the kidney tissue are being compressed, a dangerous condition because of the

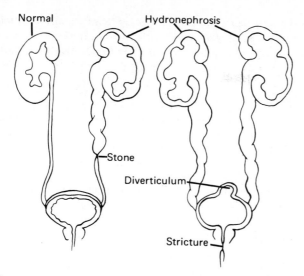

Figure 53–4. Hydronephrosis caused by blockage of the urinary tract. Dilatation occurs above the point of obstruction.

possibility of permanent kidney damage. When the kidney pelvis is swollen with backflow, the condition is called *hydronephrosis* (Fig. 53-4).

The lower the level in the tract at which obstruction occurs, the more slowly the kidney pelvis may become distended with the backflow of urine. When the obstruction of the urethra is partial, the bladder distends, and, finally, diverticuli (outpouchings) of the muscular wall may form. Urine becomes trapped in the diverticuli, stagnates, and becomes a culture medium for bacteria. For this reason, infection often occurs with an obstruction of the urinary tract. Control of infection

is extremely difficult until the underlying obstruction is corrected.

When the obstruction is minor and the pressure from backed-up urine develops slowly, symptoms may be few until the kidney pelvis and ureter become markedly enlarged. When the kidney pelvis becomes markedly distended, a mass may be palpated through the abdomen. Advanced hydronephrosis causes renal tenderness and pain. If a diverticulum of the bladder exists, the patient may be able to pass more urine after voiding and waiting a few minutes. The final quantity of urine comes from the diverticuli and may be malodorous.

The aim of treatment is to establish adequate drainage of urine. The first measure that the physician takes may be temporary, designed to permit free flow of urine, to relieve urinary retention, and to allow the enlarged kidney to heal until it is sufficiently healthy to withstand surgery to correct the obstruction.

Methods to relieve obstruction in the urinary tract depend on the location and cause of the obstruction.

Calculi (Stones, Lithiasis)

When the salts in urine precipitate instead of remaining in solution, they adhere and form stones (Fig. 53-5). Stones, most of which form in the kidney, can obstruct the urinary tract, so that obstruction with stasis of urine is frequently found. The exact conditions that cause salts to precipitate are not fully understood. Excessive excretion of calcium, such as

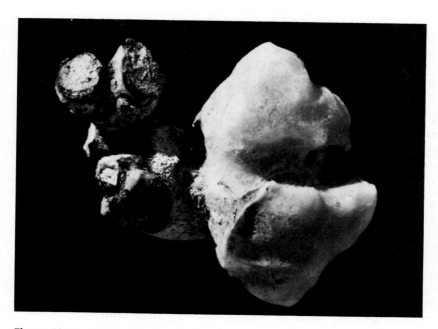

Figure 53–5. Kidney stones can be large. This stone was removed from the pelvis of the kidney. (Photograph by D. Atkinson)

occurs in patients with hyperparathyroid disease, appears to be one possible cause of stone formation.

Infection (particularly with *Proteus* species) and stones tend to coexist, but it may not always be clear which came first. Infection can make the urine alkaline, and the result may be the precipitation of calcium. On the other hand, when the pH of the urine becomes excessively acidic, cystine and uric acid may precipitate and cause stone formation. Patients with gout are likely to form uric acid stones. Osteoporosis (demineralization of bones) also may be a contributing factor.

Urinary stones may occur in patients who are relatively immobile or on long-term bed rest, such as those with fractures or paraplegia. When urine flow is sluggish and gravity drainage from the kidneys is poor, diffuse decalcification of bone may occur, and stones may form. This hazard of immobility may be prevented by nursing action, such as active range-of-motion exercises practiced several times every day and encouraging liberal ingestion of fluids (when both of these are allowed).

Symptoms

Small stones may pass right through and cause no symptoms; others are troublesome because they traumatize the walls of the urinary tract and irritate the lining, or because they obstruct the ureter or ureteral orifice, preventing urine flow and causing infection.

Renal Calculi.   Symptoms of a stone in the kidney include hematuria, symptoms of a urinary tract infection, abdominal pain, pain radiating to the genital area, and pain in the kidney area. Patients also may have no symptoms.

Ureteral Calculi.   One or more of the following symptoms may be seen if the patient has a stone in the ureter:

- Hematuria, gross or microscopic, as the stone traumatizes the walls of the urinary tract
- Pyuria (pus in the urine) due to infection behind the obstruction; the patient may experience chills and fever and can develop serious hypotension and other signs of a gram-negative septicemia
- Retention of urine or dysuria from blockage of the orifice between the bladder and urethra
- Flank pain
- Acute renal or ureteral colic (spasm accompanied by pain) due to violent contractions and spasms as the ureter tries to pass along a stone; the severity of pain is almost inversely proportional to the size of the calculus; smaller stones frequently travel more rapidly down the ureter, causing more forceful ureteral spasm and, therefore, greater pain

The colicky pain is characteristic. It is agonizingly severe, coming in waves that may start in the kidney or the ureter and radiate to the inguinal ring, the inner aspect of the thigh, or, in the male patient, to the testicle or the tip of the penis. In a female patient, the pain may go to the urinary meatus or the labia of the affected side. The patient may double up with pain and be unable to lie quietly in bed until it passes. The severity of the pain can cause nausea, vomiting, and shock.

Until the kidneys and the ureters are free of stones, the pain tends to recur. The violent spasm that causes pain may move a stone along, and, sometimes after an attack of pain, the patient may pass gravel or the offending stone itself. On the other hand, a spastic ureter may clamp down on a stone and hold it in place.

Bladder Calculi.   Symptoms of bladder calculi include hematuria, suprapubic pain, difficulty starting the urinary stream, symptoms of a bladder infection, and a feeling that the bladder is not completely empty.

Diagnosis

Diagnosis is based on patient symptoms, especially when the symptoms are typical of a stone in the urinary tract. Diagnostic tests for a ureteral calculi include an abdominal radiograph (KUB), intravenous pyelogram (IVP), and retrograde pyelogram, which locate the radiopaque stone. Kidney stones may be visualized by an IVP, KUB, and ultrasonography. Bladder stones may be detected by cystoscopy, KUB, IVP, and ultrasonography.

Blood chemistries for serum calcium and uric acid and a 24-hour urine record for calcium, uric acid, creatinine, and sodium also may be ordered.

Because stones may not be visible by radiography (radiolucent stones), the physician bases the diagnosis on the patient's symptoms and the appearance of the kidney, ureter, or bladder on radiograph. If a stone is present in an area (eg, in the ureter), an IVP probably shows the radiopaque dye stopping at a certain point in the ureter and an enlarged ureter above the obstruction and possibly an enlargement of the kidney and kidney pelvis.

Treatment

Most ureteral calculi are 1 cm or less in diameter and pass into the bladder spontaneously. Unless the bladder outlet is obstructed, such as with an enlarged prostate or urethral stricture, they may be voided spontaneously.

The patient may be observed for several days to see if the stone will pass spontaneously. The physician may order a large fluid intake to reduce the concentration of crystalloids in the urine and to foster the passage of stones. As soon as the acute pain subsides, the patient is encouraged to walk and drink, as ambulation and extra fluids may help pass the stone.

If the stone does not pass spontaneously and pain continues, if infection is above the stone, or if, in the opinion of the physician, spontaneous passage is unlikely, removal is necessary.

Renal Calculi.   For a stone in this area, the surgeon may perform one of the following procedures:

1. *Pyelolithotomy*—An incision is made into the renal pelvis, and the stone is removed. This procedure requires the same surgical approach (abdominal or flank incision) as a nephrectomy.
2. *Nephrolithotomy*—An incision is made into the parenchyma of the kidney to remove a stone in the calyx. This procedure also requires the same surgical approach as a nephrectomy.
3. *Nephrectomy*—The kidney is removed if the stone has permanently and severely damaged it so that kidney function is no longer possible. This operation is used when kidney damage has been unilateral, and the other kidney retains at least some healthy tissue.
4. *Percutaneous nephrostolithotomy* (or percutaneous ultrasonic lithotripsy)—Under general anesthesia, a nephrostomy tube is surgically inserted through a flank incision. Ultrasound waves are directed at the stone, which then breaks up into fragments that are irrigated, suctioned, or retrieved with a stone basket out through the nephrostomy tube.
5. *Extracorporeal shock wave lithotripsy*—The anesthetized patient is immersed in a special water-filled tank. Electrically generated shock waves from a machine called a lithotriptor are directed at the kidney stone, reducing the stone to fine gravel that passes out through the urinary tract. A newer lithotriptor does not use a water tank but instead uses a chair equipped with a water cushion through which the shock waves pass.

Surgery for kidney stones also includes correction of any anatomical obstructions that are thought to contribute to the development of stones. For example, a congenital ureteropelvic junction obstruction may require that the surgeon perform a pyeloplasty along with removal of calculi, or stones will reform.

Ureteral Calculi.   Stones in the ureter may be removed surgically. This procedure is called a *ureterolithotomy*. In one method, an abdominal or flank incision is made, depending on the location of the stone in the ureter. The ureter is identified, and a small incision is made in the ureter over the stone.

Occasionally, a stone in the lower portion of the ureter can be crushed or grasped and pulled out with a special catheter (stone basket) during cystoscopy. Snaring the stone is an extremely delicate procedure because of the constant danger of rupturing the ureter.

Usually, this cystoscopic procedure is performed under general anesthesia to avoid any sudden movement of the patient; and, if any complications are encountered, open surgery is begun at once. If the procedure is uncomplicated and successful, the patient has a ureteral catheter attached to a closed drainage system. The purpose of the catheter is to splint the ureter and to divert the urine past any possible tear in the ureteral wall. It is kept in place for 3 or more days. Sometimes after a cystoscopy, a ureteral catheter is left in place for 24 hours to dilate the ureter in the hope that the stone will pass through it or that it will be pulled into the bladder when the catheter is removed.

A newer therapy uses the laser to destroy stones, especially those in the lower half of the ureter. A fine wire, which is the laser, is inserted by means of a cystoscope into the ureter. Repeated bursts of the laser reduce the stone to a fine powder.

Bladder Calculi.   Bladder stones may be removed through the transurethral route, using a stone-crushing instrument (lithotrite). The procedure (*litholapaxy*) is suitable for small and soft stones. Larger, noncrushable stones must be removed through a surgical (suprapubic) incision.

When it has been possible to determine the chemical composition of stones that have been passed or removed, dietary treatment then may be attempted to adjust the pH of the urine to keep the urinary salts in solution. These diets, however, are not fully effective. Sometimes, the desired pH of the urine can be achieved by relatively minor changes in the diet. To acidify the urine, the physician may suggest elimination of citrus fruits, fruit juices other than cranberry, and carbonated beverages from the diet. To make the urine more alkaline, the physician may prescribe sodium bicarbonate. Uric acid stones may be prevented by a low-purine diet, and alkalinization of the urine by oral sodium bicarbonate. The physician may recommend the patient test for urinary acidity with litmus or nitrazine paper. Cystine stones may be prevented by a vigorous fluid intake and stringent alkalinization of the urine. Patients with gout and a history of stone formation may need to limit purine intake to prevent uric acid stones. Patients who have had stones of calcium may have to limit their intake of milk and milk products. Despite dietary changes and urine pH regulation, some patients continue to form calculi in the urinary tract.

Strictures

Strictures (narrowing) may be seen in the ureter and urethra. Because strictures are a form of obstruction, they are a danger to the upper urinary tract.

Strictures of the ureter are relatively rare but may be seen in patients with chronic ureteral stone formation that is accompanied by inflammation and infection. They also may be congenital. Strictures of the urethra may occur after infections such as untreated gonorrhea or chronic, long-standing, nonspecific urethritis.

Symptoms

The symptoms of a ureteral stricture are the same as a stone in the ureter. The symptoms of a urethral stricture include a slow stream of urine, hesitancy, burning, frequency, nocturia, and the retention of residual urine in the bladder, which may lead to bladder distention and infection. A voiding urethrogram aids in the diagnosis. If the patient is unable to void, a retrograde urethrogram may be performed.

Diagnosis

Diagnosis is based on the patient's symptoms as well as on cystoscopy, retrograde pyelograms, and IVP.

Treatment

Ureteral strictures may be treated by insertion of a ureteral catheter in an attempt to dilate the ureter. If obstruction persists, the physician may perform a ureteroplasty. This surgical procedure involves the removal of the narrowed section of ureter followed by reanastomosis of the ureter. A ureteral catheter is left in place until healing has occurred. Another approach is to insert a ureteral stent, which is a hollow tubular device that may be placed in the ureter with a cystoscope or nephrostomy tube or during surgery on the ureter (ureteroplasty). The purpose of the stent is to maintain the flow of urine through the ureter and into the bladder when the patient has a ureteral obstruction. Urethral strictures may be treated two ways.

Dilatation. This procedure uses specially designed instruments (eg, bougies, sounds, filiforms and followers) that are passed gently into the lumen of the urethra. Although done gently, the procedure is still painful.

Because forceful stretching of the urethra may cause bleeding and further stricture formation, the physician gently uses graduated instruments. He may start with only a 6 or 8 F instrument and gradually increase the size until a 24 or 26 F can be tolerated. Depending on the cause of the stricture and the patient's response to the therapy, the condition may subside after one or two treatments; usually, however, periodic dilatations are required indefinitely or until the condition is corrected surgically.

Urethroplasty. The urine is diverted from the urethra by way of a cystostomy tube or perineal urethrostomy tube attached to straight drainage until the urethra has been repaired. In one method of reconstructing the urethra, the constricted area is resected, and a mucosal graft (which may be taken from the bladder) is inserted to restore the continuity of the urethra. After surgery, the patient has a splinting catheter in the urethra that remains until healing has taken place. This operation may be performed in two stages: urinary diversion at the first operation and plastic repair at the second.

NURSING PROCESS —THE PATIENT WHO HAS URINARY TRACT OBSTRUCTION

Assessment

Many patients with a urinary tract obstruction are in moderate to severe pain; therefore, an accurate and complete history may need to be obtained, in part, from the family.

A complete medical, drug, and allergy history is obtained. A complete description of the symptoms, including the type and location of the pain as well as if the pain radiates to an area, is obtained. It also is important to determine if the patient is allergic to iodine or seafood, because iodine-containing radiopaque substances may be used to confirm the diagnosis and locate the obstruction.

Vital signs are taken, and a urine sample is obtained if the patient is able to void.

Nursing Diagnosis

Depending on the type and cause of the obstruction and the patient's symptoms, one or more of the following may apply:

- Anxiety related to pain, discomfort, need for immediate relief of symptoms, treatment measures
- Pain related to obstruction in urinary tract
- Potential for infection related to obstruction of urine flow secondary to a stone or stricture
- Hyperthermia related to urinary tract infection
- Knowledge deficit of proposed treatment, results expected, postdischarge treatment regimen

Planning and Implementation

The major goals of the patient include a reduction in anxiety, relief of pain and discomfort, absence of nausea and vomiting, absence of infection, normal body temperature, and an understanding of the treatment regimen and ways to prevent future stone formation.

The major goals of nursing management are to reduce anxiety, relieve or control pain, relieve nausea and vomiting, prevent infection, and develop an effective postdischarge teaching plan.

Intake and output are measured, and the color of the urine is noted. Any evidence of gross hematuria is reported immediately. The patient is encouraged to drink fluids (unless an order restricts fluid intake); fluids help pass stones and reduce the chance of infection or inflammation.

The physician may order all urine strained through gauze or wire mesh to retrieve a stone that may have been passed. If solid material is found, it is saved in a container until it is examined by the physician, who may have the material analyzed by the laboratory.

If the stone or stricture requires a nephrostomy, see the later discussion under Nursing Process—The Patient Undergoing Kidney Surgery. If a repair of the ureter is necessary, see the later discussion under Nursing Process—The Patient Undergoing Ureteral Surgery. Open surgery for bladder stones requires the same management as for the patient with a suprapubic prostatectomy (see Chapter 51).

CYSTOSCOPY. After a cystoscopy to dilate the ureter or remove a stone from the ureter, the urine is checked for hematuria, and vital signs are recorded hourly until stable. Any gross blood in the urine or bleeding from the urethral meatus is reported immediately to the physician.

LITHOTRIPSY. After the procedure, which is usually done under anesthesia, the patient may experience pain or discomfort in the back or flank. The area is inspected for ecchymosis, which is not uncommon, and the location of discoloration is recorded. The patient also may experience pain similar to the original pain (ureteral colic), which may be due to the gravel (small, broken pieces of stone) being passed down the ureter. An analgesic usually is ordered and must be given as needed.

Fluids are encouraged once the patient is awake and responding. Fluids are important to help excrete the gravel. If nausea and vomiting occur, the physician may order intravenous fluids to promote passage of the gravel.

PERCUTANEOUS NEPHROSTOLITHOTOMY. General anesthesia is administered. A nephrostomy tube was inserted during the procedure and connected to drainage. After the procedure, vital signs are taken at frequent intervals until stable. As soon as the patient is able to swallow, oral fluids are encouraged. A narcotic analgesic is ordered for pain. The physician may or may not order irrigation of the nephrostomy tube. If irrigations are ordered, they are done gently. Usually, 5 to 10 mL of irrigant is used for each instillation. A urethral and a ureteral catheter also may have been inserted and remain in place after the procedure. The output of *each* catheter is measured and recorded.

The incision area is checked for bleeding and placement of the catheter. If the catheter becomes dislodged, the physician is contacted immediately. All drainage tubes (nephrostomy, ureteral, urethral) are checked for urine drainage. The color of the urine is noted. The physician is contacted if one or more of the tubes fail to drain urine, the urine suddenly becomes more bloody (slight bleeding for 1 to 3 days is normal), the patient complains of severe flank pain, the urine appears cloudy or purulent, or the patient experiences chills and fever.

Anxiety, Pain. If the patient has moderate to severe pain, the physician usually orders a narcotic analgesic. In some instances, the pain is so severe that shock may develop. In this instance, the physician may order the analgesic given intravenously. The physician is notified if the analgesic fails to relieve at least some of the pain or if the pain becomes worse despite administration of an analgesic. The nurse assures the patient that every effort is being made to reduce symptoms. Once the patient has relief from pain, anxiety may be reduced.

Patients may find that walking or a certain position in the bed or chair relieves pain. The patient is encouraged to walk (if able to do so); it also may help pass the stone.

The physician explains the procedures that is to be used to remove the stone or correct the stricture. The nurse may find it necessary to reinforce the physician's explanation and to provide details about the procedure, such as a description of equipment, where the procedure is performed, and how long it takes.

Nausea and Vomiting. Patients may develop nausea with or without vomiting. If this symptom occurs, the physician is notified because an antiemetic may be necessary.

Hyperthermia, Potential for Infection. Prophylactic antibiotics usually are ordered before and after the stone has passed or been removed by an invasive or noninvasive procedure. Vital signs are monitored every 4 hours or as ordered. An elevation in temperature higher than 101°F orally is reported to the physician.

Knowledge Deficit. Patients who have a tendency to form stones should always ingest adequate fluids (minimum of 2,500 to 3,000 mL/day) to help prevent recurrence. The physician may order the patient to strain each voided urine for stones. The patient is taught how to strain urine and is told to bring any stone found to the physician for examination.

The following areas may be included in a teaching plan for a patient with stones in the urinary tract:

1. Follow the diet recommendations of the physician.
2. Take the prescribed or recommended medications as directed.
3. If symptoms return, see the physician immediately.
4. Drink plenty of fluids (at least 10 large glasses each day) and exercise regularly.
5. If a stone is passed and saved, take it to the physician.
6. Contact the physician if hematuria, burning, chills, fever, pain, or infection in any other part of the body occurs. (An infection in another part of the body may set up a secondary focus of infection in the urinary tract that can help to recreate stones).

The following may be included in a teaching plan for a patient with a urethral stricture:

1. When the physician recommends regular treatments for dilating the stricture, appointments for the procedure should be kept. Waiting until a reduction in the size of the urinary stream becomes severe or waiting for other symptoms of obstruction may result in future complications.
2. After a treatment, follow the recommendations of the physician.
3. Voiding is uncomfortable after the procedure (urethral stricture). Sitz baths may help relieve discomfort.
4. Drink extra fluids for several days after the procedure.
5. Slight bleeding may be noticed for 1 or 2 days after a treatment. If a great amount of blood appears or if bleeding persists, notify the physician immediately.

If surgery has been performed to correct a ureteral stricture, see the upcoming section, Nursing Process — The Patient Undergoing Ureteral Surgery.

Evaluation

■ Anxiety is reduced
■ Pain and discomfort are relieved or controlled
■ Nausea and vomiting are decreased or absent
■ No evidence of infection
■ Vital signs are normal
■ Demonstrates understanding of postdischarge treatment regimen, prevention of stone formation
■ Expresses willingness to adhere to treatment regimen and methods of stone prevention
■ Lists and discusses events that require contacting the physician

NURSING PROCESS —THE PATIENT UNDERGOING URETERAL SURGERY

Preoperative Period

Assessment

A complete medical, drug, and allergy history is obtained along with a full description of all symptoms, including the length of time present. Vital signs are

taken, and the patient is weighed. The patient's record is reviewed for previous diagnostic tests and diagnosis.

Ureteral surgery may be performed for ureteral strictures (congenital or acquired), cancer of the lower ureter, accidental ligation of the ureter during abdominal surgery (the highest incidence is seen in hysterectomies), and a stone impacted in the ureter that cannot be removed by other means.

Nursing Diagnosis

One or both of the following diagnoses may apply:

■ Anxiety related to surgery, symptoms, diagnosis, other factors (specify)
■ Knowledge deficit of preoperative preparations, postoperative management

Planning and Implementation

The major goals of the patient include a reduction in anxiety and an understanding of preoperative preparations, postoperative management, and home care.

The major goal of nursing management is to prepare the patient physically and emotionally for surgery.

Routine preoperative preparations include insertion of an intravenous line and shaving of the skin. The physician also may order insertion of a nasogastric tube and an indwelling urethral catheter.

Anxiety, Knowledge Deficit.   To reduce anxiety, all preoperative preparations are explained. The physician has explained the type of and reason for surgery. If the patient or family appear to be unclear about the procedure, the physician is informed.

Deep breathing, coughing, and leg exercises are demonstrated to the patient. If time permits, the patient is allowed to practice these maneuvers before surgery.

Evaluation

■ Anxiety is reduced
■ Demonstrates understanding of preoperative preparations, deep breathing, coughing, and leg exercises

Postoperative Period

Assessment

On return from surgery, vital signs are taken. The operative records are reviewed for the type of surgery, the surgical approach, the type and placement of catheters, and whether or not a stent was placed in the ureter. All catheters are connected to a closed drainage system or to the type of drainage ordered by the physician.

Nursing Diagnosis

Depending on the extent of surgery and the condition of the patient, one or more of the following may apply. Additional diagnoses that apply to any surgical patient also may be added.

- Pain related to surgery
- Potential for infection related to surgery
- Self-care deficit: total to partial (specify areas) related to surgery
- Knowledge deficit of home care management

Planning and Implementation

The major goals of the patient include a relief of pain, absence of infection, improved ability to care for self, and an understanding of home care management.

The majors goals of nursing management are to relieve pain, prevent infection, assist with self-care needs, and develop an effective discharge teaching plan.

The main complication associated with ureteral surgery is failure of the ureter to transport urine from the kidney to the bladder. Failure may be due to any number of reasons, such as blockage of the ureteral catheter or stent, inflammation of the ureter resulting in obstruction of the stent, or failure of the anastamosis. To detect this complication, measurement of the urinary output from the ureteral catheter is an important nursing task. Measurements may be ordered hourly, with the physician specifying the minimal amount to be expected.

Vital signs are monitored frequently during the first postoperative day and usually every 4 hours thereafter until stable. Coughing, deep breathing, and leg exercises are encouraged every 2 hours. The physician is contacted if signs of shock appear or if the patient complains of excessive abdominal pain, which may indicate leakage of urine into the peritoneal cavity.

Pain. Narcotic analgesics are usually required for the first few days after surgery. Each time the patient complains of pain, the type and location of pain are carefully evaluated.

Potential for Infection. Prophylactic antibiotic therapy may be started before or after surgery. The physician is notified if the patient experiences chills, fever, or if the urine is cloudy or foul-smelling.

Self-Care Deficit. Most patients are able to assume some responsibility for their care the day after surgery. If the patient has had a long-term urinary tract problem or is weak and debilitated, complete care by a member of the nursing team may be necessary until the patient is able to assume this responsibility.

Knowledge Deficit. Discharge planning depends on whether the catheters must remain in place for an extended period of time or whether they are removed before discharge. Depending on the physician's discharge orders, the patient needs instruction in the care of the urethral or ureteral catheters, the type and management of the drainage collection system, incision care, and a review of the prescribed diet and medication schedule.

The patient is told to contact the physician if urine fails to drain from the ureteral catheter, or if abdominal pain, fever, chills, or bloody or foul-smelling urine occurs.

Evaluation

- Pain is relieved
- No evidence of infection; vital signs are normal
- Assumes responsibility for own care
- Demonstrates understanding of incision care, diet, medication schedule, and drainage collection system
- Discusses and lists events that require contacting the physician

MALIGNANT DISORDERS OF THE URINARY TRACT
Tumors of the Kidney

A malignant hypernephroma (renal adenocarcinoma) is the most common tumor of the parenchyma of the adult kidney. Because the kidneys are deeply protected in the body, tumors can become quite large before they cause symptoms. These tumors are dangerous because they usually metastasize early but may present distressing symptoms only late in the course of the disease.

Symptoms

The symptoms of a malignant tumor include weight loss, malaise, unexplained fever, and episodes of hematuria. Hematuria may occur if the tumor invades the collecting system. It may be both intermittent and painless. Later, pain may be caused by expansion of the kidney or coliclike discomfort from the passage of blood clots. Sometimes, the first symptom occurs at a secondary, metastatic site.

Diagnosis

An abdominal mass found on a routine physical examination or on radiographic examination for other purposes may lead to the discovery.

Tests used for diagnosis include an IVP, cystoscopy with retrograde pyelograms, ultrasonography, magnetic resonance imaging (MRI), renal angiogram, and computed tomographic (CT) scan. Sequential urine samples may be obtained and checked for red blood cells as well as malignant cells.

Treatment

When a renal tumor is diagnosed, a complete removal of the kidney (nephrectomy) and its surrounding perinephric fat may be performed. When the tumor arises from the collecting system or in the ureter, a complete nephroureterectomy may be done. The kidney and ureter as well as a cuff of bladder tissue are removed because the recurrence rate in any stump of ureter left behind is high.

Surgery may be followed by radiation therapy either while the patient is still in the hospital or on an outpatient basis. If the unaffected kidney cannot adequately assume the function of excreting urine, or if extensive metastases are found, only palliative treatment can be given.

NURSING PROCESS —THE PATIENT UNDERGOING KIDNEY SURGERY

Preoperative Period

Assessment

A nephrectomy may be performed for disorders such as malignant tumors or large stones in the kidney pelvis that have resulted in a nonfunctioning kidney. An opening into the kidney (nephrostomy) may be performed to remove stones or provide urine drainage by means of a nephrostomy tube (catheter). A nephrostomy may be performed under local or general anesthesia.

A complete medical, drug, and allergy history is obtained from the patient or family. A list of symptoms, including the length of time present and an accurate description of each, is included in the patient history.

Vital signs are taken, and the patient is weighed. The patient's record is reviewed for previous diagnostic tests and diagnosis.

Nursing Diagnosis

Depending on the reason for surgery and the patient's symptoms, one or more of the following may apply:

- Anxiety related to the surgical procedure, diagnosis
- Pain related to infection, stone in the kidney, enlarged kidney, malignant tumor, other (specify)
- Knowledge deficit of preoperative preparations, postoperative management

Planning and Implementation

The major goals of the patient include a reduction of anxiety, relief of pain or discomfort, and an understanding of preoperative preparations and postoperative management.

The major goals of nursing management are to relieve pain and discomfort and prepare the patient physically and emotionally for surgery.

Anxiety.   The patient and family are given time to ask questions about the surgery and the events that occur before and after surgery. The nurse uses judgment as to which questions must be answered by the physician. All preoperative procedures are explained to the patient and family.

Pain.   If pain is present before surgery, the physician usually orders a narcotic or nonnarcotic analgesic, depending on the degree of pain. If pain is not relieved, the physician is notified.

Knowledge Deficit.   Preoperative preparations may include inserting a urethral catheter, shaving the preoperative area, and inserting a nasogastric tube and central venous pressure (CVP) or intravenous line.

The postoperative period requires deep breathing, coughing, and leg exercises, which are demonstrated to the patient. When possible, the patient is allowed to practice these maneuvers before surgery.

Evaluation

- Anxiety is reduced
- Pain is controlled or eliminated
- Demonstrates understanding of preoperative preparations
- Practices coughing, deep breathing, and leg exercises

Postoperative Period

Assessment

On return from surgery, vital signs are taken, and the patient's chart is reviewed for the type of surgery, type of drains inserted, the surgical approach, and the presence of catheters in the kidney, urethra, or ureter. The color of drainage from each catheter is noted and recorded for further comparison.

Nursing Diagnosis

Depending on the type of surgery and the surgical approach, one or more of the following may apply:

- Pain related to surgery
- Potential for infection related to surgery
- Hyperthermia related to infection

- Ineffective breathing pattern related to pain, immobility, pain on coughing and deep breathing
- Ineffective airway clearance related to inability to cough and deep breathe
- Self-care deficit: total to partial (specify areas) related to pain, other factors (specify)
- Knowledge deficit of future treatment regimens, home care management

Planning and Implementation

The major goals of the patient include a reduction of pain, absence of infection, normal body temperature, normal respiratory function, effective airway clearance, improved ability to care for self, and an understanding of home care management and treatment regimen.

The major goals of nursing management are to identify complications, relieve pain, prevent infection, maintain effective airway clearance and adequate respiratory function, and develop an effective patient teaching plan.

All catheters, which are ordered to be connected to a closed drainage system, are checked at frequent intervals to be sure each is draining urine. The closed drainage systems are always placed *below* the level of the bed. The color and amount of urine from *each* catheter is recorded. In some instances, the physician may order hourly measurements of urine. Any sudden decrease in urine output or presence of bleeding (a slight pink tinge to the drainage of a nephrostomy tube may be normal for several days after surgery) is reported immediately to the physician.

The blood pressure, pulse, and respiratory rate are monitored at frequent intervals for the first 24 to 48 hours after surgery. A decrease in blood pressure, rise in pulse, restlessness, or sudden onset of flank pain may indicate internal hemorrhage and requires contacting the physician immediately. If internal hemorrhage occurs at the site of the renal artery or vein ligation of a patient who has undergone nephrectomy, death can occur in a short time unless the patient is returned to surgery and the vessel is ligated.

Patients with a nephrostomy are not turned on the operative side because this position may compress the lumen of the nephrostomy tube. If the patient has had a nephrectomy, the physician may or may not allow the patient to be turned on the operative side.

Once a urethral catheter is removed, the patient's voiding pattern is evaluated. Each voiding is measured. Failure to void after the catheter is removed or voiding in frequent, small amounts accompanied by suprapubic discomfort may indicate urinary reten-

tion with overflow and must be brought to the attention of the physician.

Intravenous fluids are usually necessary until the patient is able to take oral fluids.

COMPLICATIONS. Potential complications associated with this surgery include internal hemorrhage, pneumonia, infection, paralytic ileus, and atelectasis.

Pain. Because of the large incision, which may be an abdominal or flank incision, and the position of the patient on the operating room table, the patient has moderately severe to severe pain the first few postoperative days. A narcotic analgesic is necessary.

Before an analgesic is administered, the type, location, and intensity of pain are determined. Pain in an area such as the chest, abdomen, or legs is reported immediately to the physician. If pain is in the surgical area, the catheter (if a nephrostomy has been performed) is checked for drainage. Failure of a nephrostomy tube to drain urine results in enlargement and stretching of the renal pelvis followed by severe pain.

Potential for Infection, Hyperthermia. Prophylactic antibiotic therapy usually is given after surgery. The temperature is monitored every 4 hours. A temperature higher than 101°F or the development of chills, purulent drainage from catheters, or redness, swelling, warmth, and drainage from the incision is reported immediately to the physician.

The surgical dressing is checked every 1 or 2 hours for the first 24 hours and every 3 or 4 hours thereafter. When dressing changes are allowed, aseptic technique is necessary, especially for the nephrostomy patient because the nephrostomy tract provides direct communication from the skin to the kidney.

Respiratory Function. The patient is encouraged to deep breathe, cough, and perform leg exercises every 2 hours. If a flank approach is used, the incision is close to the lower ribs; coughing and deep breathing are painful. Support of the incision must be given, and the patient is encouraged to take deep breaths slowly.

The lungs are auscultated daily, and abnormal breath sounds are brought to the attention of the physician.

Self-Care Deficit. Patients may be able to assume some of the responsibility for personal care the day after surgery. The ability of the patient to perform bathing and grooming activities is evaluated daily, and assistance is given as needed.

Knowledge Deficit. Patients who have had a nephrectomy usually have the drains (if any) removed before discharge. A dressing over the incision may or may not be required. If the physician orders a dressing applied and changed at home, the patient and family need to be taught how to change the dressing and are given a list of the necessary materials.

The following may be included in a patient teaching plan:

1. Change the dressing as ordered by the physician.
2. Drink plenty of fluids and follow the diet recommended by the physician.
3. Avoid exposure to infection.
4. Take the prescribed medication as directed on the container. Do not omit a dose.
5. Contact the physician immediately if pain, fever, or chills occur or if the urine becomes bloody, cloudy, or foul-smelling.

Patients who have a nephrostomy tube may have the tube left in place after discharge from the hospital. Because of the placement of the tube and dressing, the patient requires assistance to care for the area. The patient and family need to be shown how to change a dressing. The following may be included in a teaching plan for a nephrostomy patient:

1. Wash hands *thoroughly* before and after each dressing change.
2. Wash the site using the solution (soap and water, antiseptic solution) recommended by the physician.
3. Use nonallergic adhesive tape to keep the tube taped to the skin.
4. Wear the type of drainage bag recommended by the physician. Usually, the drainage bag can be strapped to the leg during the day. At night, the drainage system must be kept below the level of the bed.
5. Empty the drainage bag when it is one-half to two-thirds full.
6. When changing the bag, wipe the ends of the bag and nephrostomy tube with the solution recommended by the physician (alcohol or antiseptic).
7. Take the prescribed medication as directed on the container. Do not omit a dose.
8. Drink plenty of fluids and follow the diet recommended by the physician.
9. Contact the physician immediately if any of the following occur: the tube comes out; redness, swelling, or drainage around the tube occurs; fever, chills, or flank pain occurs; the urine becomes cloudy, bloody, or foul-smelling.

Evaluation

- Pain is controlled
- No evidence of infection; vital signs are normal
- Coughs and deep breathes effectively; lungs clear to auscultation
- Performs most or all of own care

- Demonstrates understanding of drug regimen
- Discusses importance of drinking extra fluids
- Demonstrates understanding of incision care, care of nephrostomy tube, drainage bags
- Able to list events that require contacting the physician

Malignant Tumors of the Bladder

Malignant tumors of the bladder are more common in men than women and are more frequent in the 50 and older age group. It is believed that industrial occupations that expose the worker to materials such as aniline dyes, paint, and rubber may increase the risk of bladder cancer.

Symptoms

The most common first symptom of a malignant tumor of the bladder is painless hematuria. Additional early symptoms include urinary tract infection (UTI) with symptoms such as fever, dysuria, urgency, and frequency.

Later symptoms are related to metastases and include pelvic pain, urinary retention (if the tumor blocks the bladder outlet), and urinary frequency due to occupation of bladder space by the tumor. If bleeding has been present for a period of time, the patient also may have symptoms of anemia due to blood loss (see Chapter 33).

Diagnosis

Diagnosis is made by cystoscopic examination and biopsy of the lesion. Additional tests include retrograde pyelograms, CT scan, radiographs of the pelvis (which may show a tumor shadow or bony metastases), and ultrasonography. Routine laboratory tests may be performed to determine kidney function and degree of anemia.

Treatment

Treatment varies according to the grade and stage of the tumor. Metastases usually have not occurred as long as the muscle wall of the bladder has not been penetrated by the tumor. Small, superficial tumors may be removed by cutting (resection) or coagulation (fulguration) with a transurethral resectoscope (the same instrument used in a transurethral resection of the prostate). Bladder tumors removed in this manner have a high incidence of recurrence. These patients must have a cystoscopic examination every 3 months for the first year, and every 6 months for the rest of their lives so that recurrence of the tumor or a new malignant growth can be discovered early.

Topical application of an antineoplastic drug may be used after resection and fulguration of a tumor. The drug, in liquid form, is injected into the bladder by means of a catheter. Fluid intake usually is limited before and during this procedure so that the drug remains in contact with the bladder mucosa for about 2 hours. The patient then voids and is given extra oral fluids to flush the drug from the bladder.

Surgical removal of the bladder (cystectomy) and a urinary diversion procedure are often necessary when the tumor has penetrated the muscle wall. When a cystectomy is performed, the bladder and lower third of both ureters are removed. If the tumor has extended through the bladder wall, the surgeon may perform a radical cystectomy. In the female, a radical cystectomy usually includes removal of the bladder, lower third of both ureters, uterus, fallopian tubes, ovaries, anterior vaginal wall, and urethra. In the male, a radical cystectomy usually includes removal of the bladder, lower third of both ureters, prostate, and seminal vesicles.

Although urinary diversion procedures are used for the treatment of bladder tumors, these procedures also may be used for extensive pelvic malignancies and severe traumatic injury to the bladder. The more common types of urinary diversion procedures include the following:

1. *Cystostomy*—In this procedure, a surgical opening is made into the bladder and a large catheter (cystostomy tube) is inserted. The catheter is connected to a closed drainage system. This procedure may be used when the tumor is considered inoperable, the patient is extremely debilitated and cannot withstand a radical cystectomy, the tumor does not obstruct the ureteral orifices, or the patient's condition is considered terminal. This procedure may be performed under local anesthesia.

2. *Nephrostomy*—Nephrostomy tubes are inserted in the pelvis of each kidney, brought through the skin and connected to a closed drainage system. This procedure may be used as a temporary measure until the patient can withstand radical surgery. A permanent nephrostomy is used if the bladder tumor obstructs the ureteral orifices and the patient is unable to withstand a radical cystectomy.

3. *Ileal conduit* (ileal loop)—A small segment of ileum is resected from the intestines, with its nerve and blood supply kept intact. The proximal end of the segment is closed, and the distal end is brought out as a stoma in the lower right quadrant (Fig. 53-6). The ureters are anasto-

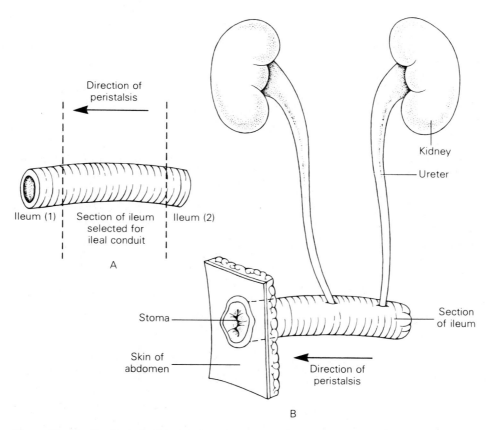

Figure 53–6.   The ileal conduit. (*A*) Once the section of ileum is removed, sections 1 and 2 are anastomosed to establish bowel continuity. (*B*) One end of the isolated segment of ileum is closed by suture, and the other end brought through the skin to create a stoma. The ureters are transplanted into the ileum. Peristalsis (*arrow*) aids in propelling urine from the ileal reservoir through the stoma.

mosed to this section of ileum. The ileal loop is no longer connected to the gastrointestinal tract.

4. *Continent ileal urinary reservoir* (Kock pouch; Fig. 53-7)—This procedure is similar to the continent ileostomy performed for bowel (ileum) disorders. The ureters are anastomosed to an isolated segment of ileum which has a one-way nipplelike valve (see Chapter 45). Urine is drained by periodic insertion of a catheter.

5. *Ureterosigmoidostomy*—The ureters are implanted in the sigmoid colon, which becomes the reservoir for urine. The patient voids and defecates through the rectum.

The advantage of attaching ureters to the bowel is that the patient need not adjust to caring for a continuously draining opening in the abdominal wall. No appliances are necessary, and no skin care surrounding the orifices is needed. The lower colon acts as a reservoir for urine, with the anal sphincter controlling the exit from the body of both urine and stool. The amount of urine that can be held is not as great as in the urinary bladder. The urine liquefies the stool, but some patients learn to regulate themselves so that they can continue with daily activities. The operation is not performed if disease of the large bowel, such as diverticulitis, is present or if the anal sphincter is incompetent because the main advantage, voluntary urinary control, would be lost.

The major disadvantage of ureterosigmoidostomy is that infection of the ureters and the kidney pelvis is frequent. The urinary tract is unprotected from the organisms that normally inhabit the lower bowel.

6. *Cutaneous ureterostomy*—This surgical procedure amputates the ureters from the bladder and brings the ends of the ureters to the surface of the skin. A cuff is formed at the end of each ureter and sutured to the skin. Urine drains from each ureter. The ends of the ureter that are sutured onto the skin resemble small stomas.

Each of the above procedures has advantages and disadvantages. The type of procedure used depends on many factors, such as the age and physical condition of the patient, the procedure that can produce the best results for the patient, and the extent of metastases.

NURSING PROCESS —THE PATIENT UNDERGOING A URINARY DIVERSION PROCEDURE

Preoperative Period

Assessment

Before surgery, the physician may order a complete physical examination to include cardiopulmonary and renal function studies as well as an evaluation of the patient's general health and nutritional status. Most of these studies may be performed on an outpatient basis. The type of surgery to be performed is based not only on the extent of the tumor but also on the patient's physical ability to withstand the surgery.

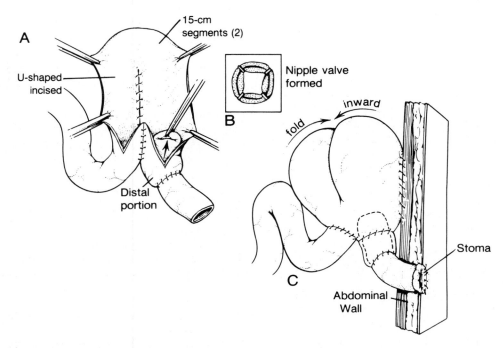

Figure 53–7. An ileal reservoir for the Kock pouch. (**A**) A 30-cm portion of the ileum is sutured together to form a U. It is then excised open, and the distal portion is pulled back into the ileum (similar to an intussusception). (**B**) A nipple valve is formed by suturing the pulled-back portion of the intestine to itself. (**C**) The top of the ileum is folded onto itself and a stoma is formed with the distal portion.

A complete medical, drug, and allergy history is obtained on admission. A list of all symptoms is obtained from the patient or family member. A general evaluation of the patient's physical and emotional status is made. Depending on the physical condition of the patient, a head-to-toe examination also may need to be performed. Vital signs are taken, and the patient is weighed.

Nursing Diagnosis

Depending on many factors, such as the type of surgery planned and the physical condition and age of the patient, one or both of the following may apply:

- Anxiety related to the diagnosis, planned surgery, concern over outcome of surgery, other factors (specify)
- Knowledge deficit of preparations for surgery

Planning and Implementation

The major goals of the patient include a reduction in anxiety and an understanding of the preparations for surgery.

The major goal of nursing management is to prepare the patient physically and emotionally for surgery.

Anxiety. The patient may display a variety of emotional responses before surgery. Some may appear depressed, while others show a mixture of anxiety and depression. The drastic change in the manner of excreting urine from the body, the diagnosis of cancer, the changes in body image are examples of situations that must be faced by the patient and family, especially if the patient has had several days or weeks to think about the surgery and what changes to lifestyle will occur.

By allowing these patients to talk about the surgery and the changes that will occur, extreme anxiety may be reduced. If the patient appears to have severe anxiety, the physician is contacted; a tranquilizer may be necessary 1 or more days before surgery.

Physicians may request that the patient or family be visited by a member of a local ostomy group to provide emotional support as well as information and reassurance that various types of assistance are available from agencies.

Knowledge Deficit. The physician explains the type of surgery to the patient and family and answers their questions. Often photographs or drawings may be used by the physician to show such information as the placement of the stoma and urostomy pouch.

Depending on the extent and type of surgery, preoperative preparations include insertion of a nasogastric tube, intravenous line, and CVP line; cleansing enemas; and a low-residue diet several days before surgery. Laxatives and enemas and a drug such as kanamycin (Kantrex) or neomycin may be ordered if a ureterosigmoidostomy is to be performed. These agents decrease the number of microorganisms in the bowel and, thus, lessen the possibility of infection as a complication of surgery on the bowel. Patients scheduled for an ileal conduit or continent ileal urinary diversion procedure also may have the bowel prepared in this manner.

All preoperative preparations are explained to the patient. The patient and family are given time to ask additional questions about the surgery, preparations for surgery, and management after surgery. The nurse must use discretion and refer certain questions to a physician.

Coughing, deep breathing, and leg exercises are demonstrated and, if possible, the patient is allowed to practice them before surgery.

Evaluation

- Anxiety is reduced
- Demonstrates understanding of the type and extent of surgery
- Understands reason for preoperative preparations
- Practices effective coughing, deep breathing, and leg exercises

Postoperative Period

Assessment

The patient's chart reveals the type and extent of surgery and the physician's orders, such as the connection of catheters or drains, intravenous fluids, and analgesics. Normal postoperative assessments, such as checking the vital signs, surgical dressing, and intravenous lines, are also carried out.

Nursing Diagnosis

Depending on the type of surgery and other factors, one or more of the following may apply. Additional diagnoses relating to any general surgery patient also may be added.

- Pain related to surgery
- Potential for infection related to surgery or type of urinary diversion
- Hyperthermia related to infection
- Diarrhea related to surgery (ureterosigmoidostomy)
- Anxiety related to difficulty in care for urinary diversion (stoma, drainage collection apparatus, catheterization of Kock pouch)
- Fluid volume deficit related to diarrhea (ureterosigmoidostomy)
- Body image disturbance related to loss of body function
- Ineffective individual coping related to loss of body function, diagnosis, prognosis

- Impaired tissue integrity related to stoma
- Self-care deficit: total to partial (specify areas) related to extensive surgery, degree of illness, or stage of disease
- Altered sexuality patterns related to anatomic disruption as a result of surgery, other factors (specify)
- Knowledge deficit of home care management, future treatment regimens, care of stoma or catheters

Planning and Implementation

The major goals of the patient include relief of pain, absence of infection, normal body temperature, absence or control of diarrhea, reduction in anxiety, correction of fluid volume deficit, increased ability to cope with the changes in body function, preservation of skin integrity, improved ability to care for self, and an understanding of the management of urinary function.

The major goals of nursing management are to relieve pain, prevent infection, reduce anxiety, recognize problems associated with the surgery, such as fluid volume deficit or impaired tissue integrity, and develop an effective teaching plan.

Position changes, coughing, deep breathing, and leg exercises are performed every 2 hours. The lungs are ausculated two to three times a day, depending on the patient's condition and ability to cough and deep breathe. Vital signs are monitored at frequent intervals immediately after surgery and then every 2 to 4 hours for the first few postoperative days. The patient's condition may require more frequent monitoring of vital signs.

CYSTOSTOMY. The patient returns from surgery with a catheter connected to a closed drainage system.

NEPHROSTOMY. The patient returns from surgery with a catheter (nephrostomy tube) inserted in both kidneys. Each catheter is connected to a separate drainage system.

ILEAL CONDUIT. The patient returns from surgery with a temporary drainage appliance, such as a disposable ileostomy or urostomy bag (Fig. 53-8), attached to the abdominal wall. Once the surgical area has healed and edema of the stoma subsides, the patient is fitted with a permanent ileal conduit appliance.

The physician may decide to insert a catheter into the conduit at times to check for residual urine (normally, the conduit is nearly empty because it does not have reservoir function as does the Kock pouch) or to provide for continued drainage if leakage occurs at one of the internal anastomoses.

The mucosa of the ileum produces mucus, which may plug the orifice and prevent the drainage of urine. The mucus may be removed with sterile gauze. The physician may dilate the stoma daily during the early postoperative period. Until the patient

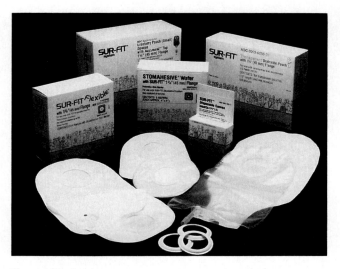

Figure 53–8. Various sizes and types of urostomy drainage pouches are available for the collection of urine after a urinary diversion procedure. (Photo courtesy of Convatec, Princeton, NJ)

is able to do this task, the nurse frequently checks the bag to see that the urine is draining adequately, empties it before it becomes full, and changes the temporary drainage bag as needed. Each time the patient's position is changed, the nurse and then the patient check to make sure that the drainage system is not impeded in any way.

CONTINENT ILEAL URINARY RESERVOIR (KOCK POUCH). The patient returns from surgery with a surgical dressing over the stoma and surgical incision. A urostomy drainage pouch placed over the stoma also may be used on a temporary basis in case urine leaks from the stoma during the healing phase.

The pouch must be emptied at routine intervals, usually every 2 or 3 hours, by insertion of a catheter into the stoma. The physician orders the type of catheter and the time intervals between draining of the reservoir.

URETEROSIGMOIDOSTOMY. At the end of the surgical procedure, a catheter is usually inserted in the rectum and taped to the buttocks. The catheter continuously drains urine from the sigmoid area and prevents a reflux (backflow) of urine into the ureters and kidney pelvis.

The rectal catheter usually is removed once peristalsis returns. At first the stool is liquid; as the bowel adjusts to being a reservoir, however, stools may become soft.

CUTANEOUS URETEROSTOMY. This procedure may be performed as a single or double ureterostomy. The single ureterostomy brings each ureter separately to the skin surface, resulting in two stomas that may be several inches or more apart. In a double ureterostomy, the two ureters are joined close together at the skin surface. This latter procedure also has variations.

Ureteral catheters usually are inserted at the time of surgery to keep the new stomas patent during the healing process. The catheters, labeled "left" and "right" denote the patient's left and right ureter and are connected to separate drainage systems.

After the catheters are removed, a collecting appliance is placed over each ureteral stoma, and urine drains through it to a drainage system that can be attached to the leg with straps once the patient is ambulatory. Care is taken that the straps are not too tight. The patient visits the bathroom at intervals during the day to release the stopper from the bottom of the bag, emptying it of urine. At night the bag is replaced by a closed drainage system kept below the level of the bed.

URINARY OUTPUT.   One of the most important postoperative nursing tasks is the measurement of urinary output. Accurate measurement is extremely important because complications of surgery can result in an interruption in the continuity of urinary tract drainage. Depending on the type of surgery, the urine output from each catheter or stoma is measured. If the patient has had a ureterosigmoidostomy, the output from the rectum or rectal catheter is measured.

The urine output from each drainage site or catheter is measured at the intervals ordered by the physician. During the early postoperative period, the urinary output may be measured hourly. The urine also is inspected for color (pale to concentrated), clarity (clear to cloudy), and presence of blood (eg, pink-tinged, which may be normal the first day or two after surgery, to grossly bloody). Concentrated urine or urine that is cloudy or bloody is reported immediately to the physician. If urinary drainage stops or decreases despite adequate oral or intravenous fluid intake, if the total urine output is less than 30 mL/hr, or if the patient complains of back pain, the physician is notified immediately.

NASOGASTRIC TUBE.   The patient may have had a nasogastric tube inserted before surgery. The tube usually remains in place for several days after surgery to prevent distention and pressure on the suture line due to the collection of gas in the bowel. The nasogastric tube is usually removed once peristalsis has returned.

Pain.   Narcotic analgesics may be necessary for 2 or more days postoperatively, depending on the extent of surgery. When the patient complains of pain, the type and location of the pain is determined. Pain in an área other than the operative site, for example in the legs or chest, is reported immediately to the physician.

Potential for Infection, Hyperthermia.   The temperature is monitored every 4 hours, and the blood pressure, pulse, and respiratory rate are monitored according to the physician's orders. The occurrence of fever, chills, back pain (over the kidney area), or cloudy, foul-smelling urine may indicate an infection in the urinary tract.

If the patient has a ureterosigmoidostomy, infection of the ureters and the kidney pelvis is a problem since the urinary tract is unprotected from the microorganisms that normally inhabit the lower bowel.

If the patient has an ileal conduit or Kock pouch, the nurse observes for and promptly reports any symptoms of peritonitis (eg, abdominal tenderness, fever, severe pain, distention) because the intestinal anastomosis can leak fecal material, or the ileal conduit may leak urine into the peritoneal cavity.

Diarrhea, Fluid Volume Deficit.   When the patient has had a ureterosigmoidostomy, the amount and color of drainage from the rectal catheter is checked every 1 or 2 hours. The anal and gluteal areas also are inspected at this time for signs of early skin breakdown. Patients are prone to fluid and electrolyte imbalances throughout the postoperative period (as well as for the rest of their lives) and, therefore, must be closely observed for signs of electrolyte losses (see Chapter 12). Frequent laboratory determinations of the patient's electrolyte status are usually necessary during the early postoperative period. All laboratory reports should be reviewed as soon as they are received, and abnormalities are reported to the physician promptly.

At first, urination (or the evacuation of urine from the rectum) is frequent. The patient also may leak urine mixed with stool and find it difficult to retain even small amounts of fluid in the rectum. The physician usually teaches the patient how to use special exercises to improve sphincter control. In time, the patient usually is able to differentiate between the presence of urine or stool in the rectum. Once good control is achieved, the patient is instructed to void (rectally) every 2 hours to prevent absorption of fluid and electrolytes through the rectal mucosa.

These patients usually are given a low-residue diet after surgery to minimize the formation of fecal material that would contaminate the operative area.

Anxiety.   Many of these patients develop a great deal of anxiety once they see the stomas. They become concerned about the (apparent) difficulty of tasks, such as dilating the stoma, caring for the stoma, or inserting a catheter for drainage of the Kock pouch. The nurse can help the patient overcome anxiety and feelings of insecurity by taking time during each procedure to explain what is being done. A few days after surgery, the patient or a family member can be asked to begin to help with these tasks. Ultimately, the patient or a family member can perform the necessary tasks, first under supervision and then alone.

Body Image Disturbance, Altered Sexuality Patterns, Ineffective Individual Coping.

The patient may worry about being able to function once discharged from the hospital. Acceptance of the urinary diversion, the equipment, and its care can be helped by giving the patient the responsibility for it in the early postoperative period.

Early ambulation (taking along the necessary equipment) demonstrates to patients that they can move about and are not chained to a collecting apparatus at the bedside. If they wish, patients should be allowed to discuss their fears and misgivings about the surgery and its effect.

There is no one easy way to help a patient cope with the physical changes that have occurred. Some patients quietly accept what has happened and try to deal with the problem as best they can. Others need someone to talk to—a nurse, a physician, or a therapist. What the nurse must do is recognize that the patient is having a problem dealing with the change in body image and then try to determine what can be done to help the patient.

Few patients openly discuss sexual dysfunction, although they may be concerned about it. Usually, female patients have no physiologic problem with sexual function, but the male patient may be impotent. Often, the male patient and physician have discussed this subject before surgery, and the patient is aware of the changes that probably will occur.

Impaired Tissue Integrity.

Each time a temporary drainage bag is changed, the skin around the stoma is inspected for signs of infection and skin breakdown. Excessive bleeding on the surface of the stoma, changes in the color of the stoma (eg, from a normal to a cyanotic color), or separation of the stoma edges from the surrounding skin is reported to the physician immediately.

Management of a patient with ureteral or ileal stomas is similar to that of a patient with a colostomy or an ileostomy (see Chapter 45). In both instances, the skin needs protection, the dressings should be changed promptly when they become soiled, and the appliances need care and cleansing. When the patient has a ureterosigmoidostomy, good skin care around the anal and gluteal areas is necessary to prevent skin breakdown.

If the patient has had a nephrostomy or cystostomy, the area around the catheter is inspected at the time of each dressing change. As for patients with a stoma, skin care is essential.

Self-Care Deficit.

The amount of assistance patients require with their daily activities after the first or second postoperative day depends on factors such as age, type of surgery performed, and physical condition of the patient. The ability of the patient to perform these activities is assessed daily, and the necessary assistance is given.

Knowledge Deficit.

During the postoperative period, the patient with an ileal conduit or cutaneous ureterostomy is measured for a permanent appliance. Then the patient is thoroughly instructed, along with another member of the family, in its application, cleaning, and care. Teaching is continued until the patient can leave the hospital, confident in the ability to manage care alone or with the help of family members or the public health nurse. A referral to the local ostomy association (with the physician's prior approval) is often beneficial. Members of these groups are able to share problems, encourage one another, and provide practical information about appliances, stoma and skin care, and the control of odors.

Many hospitals have an enterostomal therapist who works with and teaches the patient and family before and after surgery.

The material included in a patient teaching plan varies according to the type of surgery or the physician's specific discharge orders. For example, the patient with a ureterosigmoidostomy needs to be told of the signs of fluid and electrolyte imbalances; fluid and electrolytes removed by the kidney are reabsorbed by the sigmoid colon. This teaching is best accomplished by giving the patient a written or printed list of the symptoms that might occur, followed by a detailed explanation of the points covered.

The following may be included in a patient teaching plan:

1. *Urine output*—The output of urine from the catheter or stoma is continuous (with the exception of the Kock pouch). A urostomy pouch or closed drainage system (cystostomy or nephrostomy) is necessary at all times.

   During the day, a special type of closed drainage system may be worn strapped to the leg. The drainage system must always be kept below the level of the stoma or point of insertion of the nephrostomy or cyctostomy tubes. The tubing that connects the catheter or urostomy bag to the closed drainage system must be kept straight so that urine does not collect in a curve of the tube. Care is taken so that the tubing does not kink.

   Keeping the urine acidic helps to prevent urinary tract infections. Cranberry juice or vitamin C can be recommended (if the physician approves and in the dose recommended).

At night, a closed drainage system can be connected to certain types of urostomy pouches by a special adaptor. This connection prevents over-filling of the collection pouch during sleep. Patients with a nephrostomy or cyctostomy catheter also require connection to a closed drainage system at night. Whenever a catheter or special urostomy pouch is connected to a closed drainage system at night, the collection system must always be below the level of the bed.

2. *Fluids*—Drink plenty of fluids. Note the color of the urine. If the urine appears darker than usual, more fluids may be needed.

3. *Medications*—Take the medications as prescribed or recommended by the physician. Do not omit or stop taking the drugs. Do not take or use any nonprescription drugs without first checking with the physician.

4. *Color of urine*—Drinking fluids keeps the urine lighter in color. Some drugs and foods can affect the color of urine. Blood in the urine can also make the urine pink to red.

5. *Odors*—Cranberry juice, yogurt, or buttermilk helps control odors. Avoid foods that may impart an odor to the urine, such as asparagus or onions.

6. *Skin care*—Follow the recommendations of the physician or therapist in skin care. For all patients, the skin must be kept clean. When the adhesive wafer (to which the urostomy collection bag is attached) is changed, all remaining adhesive is removed before application of a new wafer. The skin is inspected closely at this time, and any problems are brought to the attention of the physician.

The skin around the stoma of a continent ileostomy or a nephrostomy or cystostomy tube is washed with soap and water, rinsed, and thoroughly dried. This task is necessary several times a day.

7. *Continent urostomy* (Kock pouch)—Drain four times a day or as directed by the physician. Follow the drainage schedule recommended by the physician.

8. *Care of the urinary collection pouch*—Wash thoroughly after changing, rinse with or soak in a solution of vinegar and water if crystals form in the pouch. Change the pouch as recommended by the physician or therapist.

9. *Contacting the physician*—Contact the physician if any of the following occurs: fever, chills, blood in the urine, failure of a stoma or catheter to drain urine, skin problems around the stoma, weight loss (more than 5 pounds), loss of appetite (more than a few days), inability to insert the catheter in the Kock pouch, pain in the flank (kidney area or lower abdomen), signs of fluid or electrolyte imbalance, or any unusual symptom or problem.

10. *Information for others*—Patients with a ureterosigmoidostomy must tell hospital personnel on readmission that they void rectally. They do not need laxatives, and enemas would force fecal material into the ureters.

Evaluation

- Pain is controlled or relieved
- No evidence of infection
- Vital signs are normal
- Anxiety is reduced
- Fluid volume deficit corrected (ureterosigmoidostomy)
- Demonstrates beginning to accept change in body image
- Demonstrates beginning of ability to cope with loss of body function, diagnosis, prognosis
- Skin remains intact; no evidence of skin breakdown
- Self-care needs are met
- Assumes most or all of responsibility for own personal care
- Discusses changes in sexuality patterns with appropriate people
- Demonstrates understanding of home care management, future treatment modalities, medication regimen
- Participates in or assumes all responsibility for care of stoma, care of skin, applying and changing urostomy bag, catheterizing continent ileostomy

CONGENITAL DISORDERS

Polycystic Disease

This disease is a congenital familial disorder. It is characterized by multiple bilateral kidney cysts and may not be diagnosed until mid life. As the cysts slowly enlarge, they squeeze the functioning kidney parenchyma between them until little functioning kidney tissue is left. The kidneys may become enormous and exert pressure on nearby abdominal and pelvic organs. Nephritis, calculi, infections, and hydronephrosis may result from and complicate the condition. Eventually, renal failure occurs.

Symptoms

The patient may have hematuria, pain, pyuria, anemia, and gastrointestinal symptoms from pressure caused by the expanding kidney. The patient usually is hypertensive.

Diagnosis

Diagnosis is based on the patient's symptoms, which often do not occur until renal function is poor. Intravenous and retrograde pyelograms and CT scan usually reveal the cystic structure and shape of the kidneys. Additional laboratory tests may be performed to determine the degree of remaining kidney function.

Treatment

Polycystic disease has no cure, and eventually uremia develops. Because the disease is often bilateral, the prognosis is poor. Dialysis is used to prevent uremia.

Horseshoe Kidneys

In this disorder, the kidney resembles a horseshoe because the two kidneys are joined by an island of additional kidney tissue. Each kidney may be about the same size or one may be smaller than the other. The amount of function in each kidney varies.

Symptoms

Unless renal failure occurs, symptoms are rare.

Diagnosis

The disorder may not be detected unless the patient has a diagnostic test that involves radiographs of the kidney area. If the kidney shadow is suspicious of a horseshoe kidney, intravenous and retrograde pyelograms may be ordered. Additional renal function tests usually are performed.

Treatment

No treatment is necessary unless renal failure is present.

Other Congenital Disorders

Hypospadias (in which the urinary meatus is on the underside of the penile shaft), epispadias (in which the urinary meatus is on the top of the penile shaft), exstrophy of the bladder (in which the bladder is everted, open, and lies on the outside of the abdomen), and many other congenital disorders are discovered at birth or shortly thereafter. These disorders are covered in pediatric nursing textbooks.

RENAL FAILURE

Renal failure, acute or chronic, is a serious inability of the kidneys to carry out the normal functions necessary to maintain fluid and electrolyte balance and eliminate the end products of metabolism from the body.

Uremia describes a toxic state characterized by a marked accumulation of urea and other nitrogenous wastes in the blood. Both acute and chronic renal failure may produce symptoms of uremia.

Acute Renal Failure

Causes of acute renal failure include thrombosis of the renal arteries; severe burns; severe, prolonged hypotensive episodes; blood transfusion reactions; severe infections; crushing injuries; and nephrotoxic drugs and chemicals.

Prevention.   Renal failure occurs more frequently when body fluid reserves are depleted. Nurses contribute to its prevention by planning with patients a system of oral fluid intake, particularly for those patients who may be too old, too weak, disinterested, or otherwise unable to reach for a glass of water.

Lowered cardiac output due to such conditions as cardiac dysrhythmias, shock, or accidental blood loss interferes with normal renal blood flow. Careful nursing observation of the patient and prompt reporting of hypotension helps the physician initiate a course of action that minimizes the threat of renal damage.

In a teaching role, the nurse can encourage patients with possible streptococcal infection to seek medical attention promptly to reduce the risk of glomerulonephritis, a disorder that can result in renal failure. Alerting the public to the importance of keeping drugs where they cannot be accidentally ingested is important because some drugs are toxic to the kidney and can damage it, also resulting in renal failure. Nurses and physicians, as well as ancillary personnel, must take utmost care to prevent the transfusion of incompatible blood.

Symptoms

Acute renal failure is usually characterized by a sudden decrease in urinary output (oliguria), usually less than 400 to 500 mL/24 hr. In some instances, urinary output may cease (anuria). The sudden decrease in urinary output is called the *oliguric phase* of acute renal failure and may last from a few hours to as long as 2 or more weeks. During this time, the BUN and serum creatinine rise as nitrogenous wastes accumulate in the blood.

The oliguric phase is followed by the *diuretic phase*—a period of increased urinary output. This phase of acute renal failure may last from a few days to a week or longer. At this time, the BUN and serum creatinine levels cease to rise and finally begin to fall. The diuretic phase is followed by the *recovery phase*, which begins to show signs of renal improvement. This phase usually lasts several months. Other symptoms of acute renal failure are variable and include anorexia, nausea, vomiting, diarrhea, pruritus, lethargy, hyperkalemia, hypertension, and edema. Some patients recover completely from acute renal failure, whereas others suffer loss of renal function.

Hypertension may be seen during the early phase of the disease. The skin and the appearance of the patient with acute renal failure may show changes similar to those seen in chronic renal failure. If treatment is begun early, however, the underlying cause corrected (when possible), and accumulated nitrogenous wastes removed by means of peritoneal dialysis or hemodialysis, the patient may show few of these or other symptoms of uremia.

Diagnosis

Diagnosis is based on symptoms, patient history, and laboratory tests. In acute renal failure, a sudden increase in the BUN and serum creatinine occurs early in the disease (oliguric phase). In the diuretic or second phase, the BUN and serum creatinine cease to rise and finally fall. Other electrolyte abnormalities of acute renal failure include acidosis and hyponatremia or hypernatremia. Hyperkalemia also may be seen early in the disease.

Treatment

If the primary cause can be removed or quickly remedied, such as in acute renal tubular necrosis (lower nephron nephrosis) or urinary tract obstruction, acute renal failure is reversible in a majority of patients, providing renal function was normal before the disease that caused renal failure. The treatment objective in acute renal failure is to keep the patient alive and free from complications during the 2 or 3 weeks required for regeneration of the damaged epithelium of the renal tubules. Kidney function may gradually return to normal over a period of several weeks.

The serum creatinine is monitored frequently, as this test is a better gauge of renal failure than the BUN. A progressive and steady rise indicates progressive renal dysfunction.

Treatment modalities for acute renal failure include dialysis (hemodialysis or peritoneal dialysis), correction of electrolyte and fluid imbalances, diuretics, correction of acidosis (if present), and the limiting of dietary proteins. Ion-exchange resins (eg, sodium polystyrene sulfonate [Kayexalate]) also may be used to remove excess potassium.

Chronic Renal Failure

Chronic renal failure is a slow, progressive decrease in kidney function. Causes of chronic renal failure include polycystic disease of the kidneys, urinary tract obstruction, renal calculi, glomerulonephritis, chronic pyelonephritis, renal tumors, and disseminated lupus erythematosus.

Symptoms

Chronic renal failure usually begins slowly. At first, the symptoms of (unsuspected) renal failure may be vague and nonspecific and include lethargy, headache, anorexia, and dry mouth. As the disease progresses, symptoms include pruritus, dry skin, metallic taste, uremic odor to the breath, diarrhea or constipation, edema, anemia, bleeding tendency, muscle cramps, and mental changes. Oliguria or anuria may be present; however, the volume of urinary output may be near normal even in later stages of the disease.

In chronic renal failure, usually the BUN and serum creatinine gradually rise because, as in acute renal failure, the kidney's ability to excrete nitrogenous wastes is impaired. The patient may be hyponatremic or hypernatremic depending on dietary intake and remaining renal function. Acidosis also may be present.

Hypertension usually occurs in most patients with chronic renal failure. The patient is often pale because of anemia, which is a common symptom of the disorder. The skin is often dry and scaly, and pruritus is common, especially when elevation of the BUN and serum creatinine is marked.

Halitosis generally is marked, and ulceration of the oral mucosa due to increased capillary fragility is common. The patient's breath and body may have an odor characteristic of urine.

Edema is often present in chronic renal failure and may result from failure of the kidneys to excrete water and sodium, as well as from congestive heart failure. Patients also may have edema around the eyes (periorbital edema).

Although people in chronic renal failure may remain mentally alert for a long time, mental processes are progressively slowed as electrolyte imbalances become marked and nitrogenous wastes accumulate. A loss of concentration and memory impairment may occur.

Anorexia is a common early symptom of chronic renal failure. Later in the disease, vomiting often becomes a serious problem because severe and prolonged episodes can cause further fluid and electrolyte imbalance.

Uremia.   The terminal stage of chronic renal failure is called *uremia*. Symptoms include oliguria or anuria, mental changes (confusion, disorientation), changes in the level of consciousness, uremic odor to the breath, elevated BUN and serum creatinine, acidosis, hyperkalemia, severe anemia, hypertension, anorexia, nausea, vomiting, hiccups, lethargy, diarrhea or constipation, hypocalcemia, muscular twitching, and convulsions.

Because the skin also serves as an excretory organ, *uremic frost*, which is a white film composed of waste products excreted by the skin instead of the failing kidneys, may be seen.

Another serious problem is ulceration and bleeding of the gastrointestinal tract. The mucous membranes of the mouth bleed, and blood may be found in the feces. These as well as other symptoms are typical of uremia and often signal the terminal stage of the disease.

Because of the availability of hemodialysis and peritoneal dialysis, many patients in chronic renal failure are kept out of the terminal stage of the disorder.

Diagnosis

Diagnosis is based on symptoms and a history of kidney disease as well as laboratory tests for kidney function. An intravenous pyelogram may be performed to determine kidney function (ability to absorb and excrete a radiopaque dye). In patients with severe renal failure, appearance of the dye in the kidneys may take 1 or more hours instead of a few minutes. A kidney biopsy also may be performed.

Treatment

Renal disorders such as glomerulonephritis, nephrosis, pyelonephritis, and polycystic kidneys progress to deterioration of the nephron, involving either the glomeruli or the tubules or both, and may finally result in chronic renal failure. The onset of oliguria or anuria is an ominous sign. Remissions can occur, however. One objective of treatment is to avoid conditions that increase the workload of the kidneys, through control of diet, activity, and obesity and avoidance of infection. Another is to treat the various symptoms of the uremia itself. The prognosis for the patient in chronic renal failure usually depends on the degree of renal failure (early versus terminal), the effect the disease has had on other body systems, and the success of the treatment instituted.

Treatment modalities include ion exchange resins, hemodialysis, peritoneal dialysis, administration of antihypertensive agents, limiting the dietary intake of protein, and treatment of electrolyte imbalances. Kidney transplantation may be considered for some patients with chronic renal failure.

NURSING PROCESS —THE PATIENT IN RENAL FAILURE

Assessment

Before conducting an initial interview and physical assessment, it may be of value to learn the cause (if known) and prognosis of the patient's renal disorder. This information might be obtained from the physician or from previous hospital admission records and may help the nurse decide what information should be obtained. Patients may be unable to give an accurate history because of the effect of renal failure on the thought process or because they are acutely ill. The nurse may find it necessary to obtain information from the family.

The following areas may be covered when obtaining a medical history:

- History of the illness, including when the problems were first noticed; symptoms and physical changes (eg, edema) are an essential part of the history

- History of other medical or surgical disorders and the treatment of each
- Problems or symptoms experienced at the present time; the nurse may find it necessary to ask questions related to renal failure, such as problems with bleeding (eg, after minor cuts or abrasions) or symptoms of nausea, vomiting, or diarrhea
- Drug history, including prescription and nonprescription drugs
- Allergy and dietary history

The physical assessment can include the following:

- General physical appearance
- Identification of areas of edema (if any)
- Skin: color, evidence of pruritus, uremic frost
- Condition of the oral mucosa
- Vital signs and weight
- Sample of urine (if possible) with a description of the color and amount obtained in one voiding
- Appraisal of the patient's thought processes

Nursing Diagnosis

The extent of the nursing diagnosis depends on the type and degree of renal failure and the general condition of the patient. Many of these diagnoses are related to the effect of renal failure on organs and systems.

- Activity intolerance related to anemia, weight loss, other symptoms (specify)
- Fatigue related to anemia, weight loss, other symptoms (specify)
- Altered nutrition: less than body requirements related to anorexia, nausea, vomiting
- Constipation related to fluid and electrolyte imbalances, immobility, other factors
- Diarrhea related to electrolyte imbalances, blood in the gastrointestinal tract, other factors
- Potential for infection related to altered immune response
- Sensory and perceptual alterations (specify type, such as visual, auditory, or tactile) related to acidosis, fluid and electrolyte imbalances
- Potential for injury related to sensory and perceptual alterations
- Self-care deficit: total or partial (specify areas) related to extreme fatigue, mental changes, severe anemia, other (specify)
- Potential impaired skin integrity related to immobility, dry skin, uremic frost
- Altered oral mucous membranes related to dry mouth, dehydration, decreased fluid intake, other factors (specify)
- Knowledge deficit of home care management, treatment regimen

Planning and Implementation

The major goals of the patient include increased ability to tolerate physical activities, decrease in fatigue, improved nutrition, improved comfort, normal bowel elimination, absence of infection, normal electrolyte and fluid balance, improved ability to care for self, maintenance of skin and oral mucous membrane integrity, and an understanding of home care management.

The major goals of nursing management are to improve comfort, improve nutrition, prevent infection, prevent injury, provide assistance with care, maintain skin and oral mucous membrane integrity, recognize complications, and develop an effective teaching plan.

OBSERVING FOR COMPLICATIONS.   Many complications, such as fluid and electrolyte imbalances, hemorrhage, cardiac and respiratory failure, infection, and severe hypertension, may be seen in renal failure. When the patient is acutely ill, the physician orders almost daily laboratory tests to determine the fluid, acid–base, and electrolyte status as well as to monitor renal function. Other complications may first be detected by ongoing physical assessments. Vital signs, daily weights, auscultation of the heart and lungs, measuring intake and output, checking the stools for signs of gastrointestinal bleeding, and observing for signs of electrolyte imbalance are examples of assessments and observations that may be performed. Any change that is noted is recorded as well as reported to the physician.

Activity Intolerance, Fatigue, Self-Care Deficit.   Patients may be in an early stage of chronic renal failure or the recovery phase of acute renal failure and are able to perform activities without undue fatigue. Others may be in a terminal phase of chronic renal failure and require complete care.

The nurse must evaluate the patient's ability to perform any activity, such as bathing, eating, or getting out of bed, on a daily basis and plan nursing management according to an evaluation of the patient's ability to carry out specific activities.

Patients must be allowed time to carry out their activities of daily living and must be given adequate periods of rest between activities. Assistance must always be given if the patient seems unable to complete a task.

Altered Nutrition.   Nausea, vomiting, anorexia, and mental changes may prevent the patient from eating adequately. The patient's food intake is monitored after every meal, and weight is measured daily. If the patient dislikes the diet (especially when a special diet is prescribed and favorite foods must be omitted), a dietary consult may be obtained. Although dietary restrictions need to be maintained, the dietitian may be able to include some of the patient's food preferences. Small, frequent meals may be better tolerated than three regular meals a day, especially if the patient experiences nausea.

If the patient still fails to eat, the physician may order total parenteral nutrition and daily vitamins to meet the patient's dietary needs.

Potential Impaired Skin Integrity.   Pruritus may be severe during the terminal stage of renal failure. The skin must be rinsed frequently with warm water and patted dry to remove the crystals collecting on the skin (uremic frost). Creams or lotions may be used to moisten the skin and reduce itching. The patient's position is changed every 2 hours, and bony prominences are inspected for early signs of skin breakdown. The physician is notified if signs of skin breakdown are present.

Constipation, Diarrhea.   Constipation or diarrhea may be present. Each stool is inspected for signs of gastrointestinal bleeding, and the physician is informed if bleeding is apparent or the patient develops diarrhea or constipation. If diarrhea is severe, the patient is observed for early signs of dehydration.

Potential for Infection.   If the patient's immune system has been affected by renal failure, it is most important that any type of infection be avoided. The patient is closely monitored for signs of infection, such as chills, fever, sore throat, and signs of a urinary tract or respiratory infection. The skin is inspected daily for evidence of breaks in the skin, due to scratching or other causes, or signs of a superficial or deep skin infection.

Aseptic technique must be maintained when performing invasive procedures, such as insertion of an intravenous line or indwelling urethral catheter. Hospital personnel and visitors with upper respiratory infections should avoid contact with the patient.

Urinary Output.   When renal function begins to markedly deteriorate, the urine output usually is less than 400 mL/day. Measurement of intake and output may be ordered hourly. The patient is closely observed for edema, rising blood pressure, and signs of congestive heart failure, which are indications that a fluid volume excess probably has occurred.

The physician is notified of these events, as fluid intake may be restricted and drug therapy with a diuretic or antihypertensive agent may be prescribed. The patient must be closely observed for the results of the prescribed therapy and for an intensification of symptoms.

Sensory and Perceptual Alterations, Potential for Injury.   Electrolyte imbalances as well as end-stage (or terminal) renal disease can result in various types of mental changes, such as confusion, disorientation, and hallucinations. Depending on the activities of the patient, restraints may be necessary to prevent injury by getting out of bed unassisted or by pulling out intravenous lines or a urethral catheter.

Altered Oral Mucous Membranes.   If the patient is eating, oral care is given after each meal. Frequent oral care may be necessary, especially if the patient is acutely ill. The mouth is inspected daily for ulcerations and inflammation. Glycerin or a water soluble lubricant may be applied to dry lips.

Knowledge Deficit.   The discharge teaching plan depends largely on the type and degree of renal failure, the patient's condition and prognosis, and the physician's discharge orders or recommendations. If medications are prescribed, the dose regimen and adverse drugs effects are reviewed with the patient. If a special diet is recommended, the dietitian reviews the prescribed diet with the patient and family.

The following general points may be included in a patient teaching plan:

1. Follow the diet recommended by the physician. Do not use salt substitutes (which often contain potassium) unless allowed by the physician.
2. Take the medication exactly as prescribed by the physician.
3. Measure and record fluid intake and urine output. Limit fluids as recommended by the physician.
4. Avoid exposure to those with any type of infection (eg, colds, sore throats, flu).
5. Monitor blood pressure and pulse.
6. Do not use any nonprescription drug unless use has been approved by the physician.
7. Keep skin clean and dry. Shower daily, pat dry skin, use lotions or creams for itching. Avoid scratching.
8. When laundering clothing and towels, use an extra rinse cycle to remove all detergent. Avoid the use of harsh detergents.
9. Weigh self daily. Keep a record of weight, and report any rapid weight gain or loss to the physician.
10. Take frequent rest periods; avoid heavy exercise.
11. If any of the following occurs, contact the physician immediately: inability to urinate, slow decrease in daily urine output, weight gain or loss (more than 5 pounds or amount recommended by physician), chills, fever, sore throat, cough, blood in the urine, easy bleeding or bruising, lethargy, extreme fatigue, persistent headache, nausea, vomiting, diarrhea.

Evaluation

■ Able to tolerate increased activity; episodes of fatigue are reduced
■ Eats prescribed diet; episodes of nausea and vomiting reduced or absent
■ Pruritus is decreased or absent; skin less dry and scaly
■ Bowel elimination is normal

■ No evidence of infection; vital signs are normal
■ Weight remains stable; no evidence of edema; urine intake and output ratio approaches or is normal
■ Is mentally clear
■ No evidence of injury
■ Assumes most or all responsibility for own care
■ Skin intact; no evidence of bruising, decubitus formation, excessive dryness
■ Oral mucous membranes normal; no evidence of stomatitis or ulcerations
■ Demonstrates understanding of home care management, medication regimen, diet, activities to avoid

SUBSTITUTES FOR KIDNEY FUNCTION

Hemodialysis

Hemodialysis is a process designed to bring blood into contact with a semipermeable membrane through which diffusion takes place. Diffusion means the spontaneous movement of solutes and solvent from areas of high concentration to areas of low concentration until a state of equilibrium is established. Substances that should be removed from the patient's blood, such as urea, creatinine, and dangerously high levels of potassium, are removed because they are all absent from the dialysate fluid (the bathing solution). They move from the patient's blood through the semipermeable membrane to the dialysate fluid. Hemodialysis also permits the replacement of substances that may be low in the blood and present in the dialysate, such as bicarbonate and calcium.

In many types of dialyzers, the basic components are a synthetic semipermeable membrane and dialysate fluid. The dialysate fluid is similar to the electrolyte composition of normal human plasma. The composition is ordered by the physician and changed as needed. The patient's blood is removed from an artery, pumped through the coil (semipermeable membrane), and returned to a vein. Water and ions are able to pass through the walls of the membrane, but protein and red blood cells cannot.

Blood samples are taken before and after dialysis and may measure BUN, creatinine, sodium, potassium, chlorides, carbon dioxide, and hematocrit. These are indicators of the efficiency of dialysis.

External Arteriovenous Shunt.   When a patient is to be dialyzed, cannulas (the shunt) are placed surgically in an extremity where blood vessels are available. This placement allows for repeated treatments without having to perform a cut-down for each dialysis. Between treatments, the cannula ends are connected by an external Teflon joint, and blood is shunted between the artery and the vein. To attach the patient to the hemodialysis unit, the joint is opened and the arterial cannula is attached to the inflow tubing of the coil; the venous cannula is attached to the outflow tubing. When the treatment is finished, the joint is reconnected and blood flows through the shunt. Two cannula clamps (or rubber-tipped hemostats) should be close by at all times for use in the event that the cannulas disconnect at the Teflon joint.

Internal Arteriovenous Shunt. Instead of an external shunt, some patients on permanent dialysis may have an arteriovenous fistula (internal shunt) formed by way of a surgical anastomosis of an artery and vein lying in close proximity. The vein enlarges and assumes the characteristics of an artery. Venipuncture is performed in a proximal site and is used for the outflow from the machine. A distal needle puncture is used for the inflow. When dialysis is completed, the needles are removed and pressure dressings applied for several hours. Blood pressures and blood samples should not be taken in the cannulated extremity.

Patient Preparation
The physician usually orders any preparations for dialysis. These preparations include weighing the patient, obtaining blood for laboratory tests, and measuring vital signs. Fasting is not necessary.

Nursing Management After Hemodialysis
Vital signs are taken as ordered. No intramuscular injections are given for 2 to 4 hours after dialysis because the administration of heparin during dialysis may cause bleeding at the injection site.

The patient is observed for the following:

- Bleeding (urine, gastrointestinal, at site of arteriovenous shunt, mouth) because of the administration of heparin; epistaxis and bleeding from the gums are not uncommon
- Cardiac dysrhythmias, which may result from potassium removal
- Hypotension, which may result from excess fluid removal
- Fever
- Thought processes; an unconscious patient may become aware and coherent during dialysis, or vice versa; restlessness frequently occurs; the physician is notified if the patient becomes extremely restless or if a decrease in the level of consciousness occurs
- Complications; headache, muscle cramps, nausea and vomiting, fever, diaphoresis, anxiety, or chest pain that occurs during or after hemodialysis may reflect serious complications

Daily care is given to the external shunt, and it is observed for patency. Fluid and dietary restrictions are regulated according to the degree of recovery of renal function and the patient's clinical condition. Chronic dialysis patients continue on fluid restrictions based on urinary output. The potassium and sodium contents of the diet may be restricted. A normal protein diet may be allowed, or the patient may be placed on a special diet that allows only certain types and amounts of proteins.

Peritoneal Dialysis
The simplicity of peritoneal dialysis and the availability of the equipment for this procedure are in sharp contrast to the complexity of the technique and equipment used in hemodialysis. The latter is limited to hospitals that have the equipment and the personnel trained to use it, or to those who have been trained in the use of the equipment at home. Peritoneal dialysis can be performed in any hospital or at home. It provides, however, only a fraction of the plasma clearance that hemodialysis can provide.

In peritoneal dialysis, a dialysate is made to flow into and out of the peritoneal cavity (Fig. 53-9). The peritoneum acts as the semipermeable membrane. The dialysate causes urea, electrolytes, and dialyzable poisons to pass across the peritoneum and into the dialysate solution.

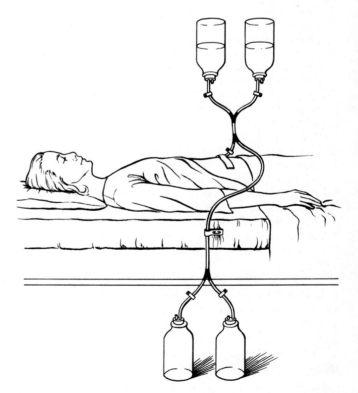

Figure 53–9. Peritoneal dialysis. After the solution flows into the patient, it is allowed to remain *in situ* for the time ordered by the physician. During this period, dialysis takes place. Then the clamps on the lower bottles are opened and the solution is drained off.

Patient Preparation

The purpose and general technique of the procedure is explained to the patient and family by the physician. The nurse may provide more details of the procedure, such as how long each cycle lasts and what nursing tasks are performed before, during, and after the procedure.

Laboratory tests such as BUN, serum creatinine, and serum electrolytes, are ordered to be drawn before the procedure. Vital signs are taken, and the patient is weighed. The patient is asked to void.

Technique of Administration

The physician makes a small incision in the midline of the abdomen. A catheter with many perforations is inserted so that the end lies free in the peritoneal cavity. The catheter is sutured in place, and a dressing is applied. Blood pressure, pulse, and respirations are recorded. Drugs (eg, heparin) may be ordered to be added to the dialysate solution before the bottles are attached to the administration tubing. The bottles of dialysate are set up and the administration tubing (inflow tube) is attached to the catheter in the patient. The outflow tubing leading to a closed drainage system is clamped off. The circuit run by the dialysate can be broken into three periods:

1. *Instillation period*—Two liters of dialysate should run into the peritoneal cavity by gravity in 10 to 15 minutes. If the drip is slow, the physician may need to reposition the catheter. When the bottles are empty but the tubing is still filled with dialysate to prevent entrance of air, the inflow tube is clamped. The nurse records instillation time, the volume and type of dialysate, plus any medications added.
2. *Equilibration period*—The solution is left in the abdomen for the length of time ordered by the physician (usually 15 to 45 minutes).
3. *Drainage period*—The outflow tube is unclamped, and the dialysate drains into a closed sterile drainage system. Gravity drainage facilitated by raising bed height or changing the patient's position should take no longer than 10 to 15 minutes. If it takes longer, the physician may need to irrigate the catheter to remove plugs or may need to reposition or replace the catheter.

The time of the start and finish of the drainage period and the appearance of the fluid removed is recorded. The removed drainage may be blood-tinged because of bleeding due to heparin or cloudy from protein loss. The difference between the volume instilled and the volume removed is recorded. The physician should be notified of excessive fluid retained or removed from the patient (about 500 mL).

The number of exchanges performed in peritoneal dialysis is ordered by the physician. When the final dialysis is completed, the physician removes the catheter, and a dry sterile dressing is applied. A purse string suture may be necessary. A bacteriologic culture may be obtained from the catheter tip as well as from the last dialysate drained. A postdialysis weight is obtained.

Observations During Peritoneal Dialysis

Blood pressure and pulse are taken frequently, usually at the end of each drainage period. A drop in blood pressure and increased pulse rate may occur when fluid removal is too rapid, especially when the dialysate has a high concentration of dextrose. If the patient is acutely ill, a bed scale is used for weight measurements. The physician may order that the patient be weighed as often as every 8 hours while the procedure is in progress.

Pain in the left shoulder may be due to diaphragmatic irritation caused by the high concentration of dextrose in the dialysate. Abdominal pain that occurs at the end of the drainage period may be relieved by the next instillation. Pain accompanied by marked abdominal distention warrants contacting the physician and delaying the next dialysis cycle until the physician has examined the patient.

The patient's position should be changed frequently; the patient can turn from side to side unless the physician orders otherwise. The patient who is undergoing peritoneal dialysis may eat and drink as permitted. The patient's mental state is observed, and any changes are reported to the physician.

Peritonitis (chemical or bacterial) is a major complication of peritoneal dialysis and may be evidenced by fever, nausea, vomiting, and severe abdominal pain, rigidity, or tenderness. If these symptoms occur during or after the procedure, the physician is notified.

Postprocedure Management

The physician may order specific observations after the procedure. Ongoing observations include the following:

- Vital signs (usually at 1- to 2-hour intervals for 24 or more hours)
- Checking the abdomen for tenderness, rigidity
- Measuring intake and output
- Observing for signs of fluid and electrolyte imbalances, peritonitis
- Weight

Daily laboratory tests to evaluate renal function and serum electrolyte levels usually are ordered. Daily weights are usually continued. A special diet high in carbohydrates but low in protein, potassium, and sodium usually is ordered. Drug therapy usually is continued after dialysis and includes drugs such as an antihypertensive agent, diuretic, a multivitamin preparation, and oral calcium. Dialysis may need to be repeated if renal function does not improve.

Continuous Ambulatory Peritoneal Dialysis

Continuous ambulatory peritoneal dialysis (CAPD) allows some patients with end-stage renal disease the freedom to carry on the activities of daily living while performing dialysis at home. Before the use of this technique, the patient who required dialysis had to rely on a machine for hemodialysis (at home or at a hospital hemodialysis center) or on admission to a hospital for peritoneal dialysis.

The technique of CAPD requires the insertion of an abdominal catheter into the peritoneal cavity. The catheter is connected to a flexible plastic bag that contains the dialysate. The dialysate solution (usually 2 L) is allowed to flow into the abdominal cavity by gravity. The flexible plastic bag is then rolled up and placed under the patient's clothing while the solution remains in contact with the peritoneum. Once the contact time is concluded, the plastic bag is unrolled and lowered below the abdomen to allow the fluid to drain. The solution and container are then discarded, and another container is added and allowed to infuse. This cycle (or exchange) is usually repeated four times a day.

The patient or a family member requires detailed instruction in the administration of CAPD; however, the technique is easier to learn than hemodialysis. A schedule for the exchange is developed by the physician, who takes into consideration the patient's daily activities. Patients on CAPD are usually allowed more fluids and have fewer dietary restrictions than those on hemodialysis, but restrictions may vary from patient to patient.

RENAL TRANSPLANTATION

Some patients with chronic, progressive end-stage renal disease may be candidates for a kidney transplant. Donors for a transplant may be selected from living relatives or from people who are brain dead, when permission has been granted to remove the kidneys (and possibly other organs) for transplantation.

Once people with end-stage renal disease are selected as candidates, their names are placed on a computerized recipient list, along with their tissue typing. When a kidney becomes available, a patient is scheduled for immediate transplantation of the organ.

Cyclosporine is often used to prevent the rejection of transplanted organs, including the kidney. It appears to have reduced the incidence of organ rejection. If transplantation is successful, the patient can lead a normal life.

TRAUMATIC INJURIES

Various types of injury can effect the urinary tract. Gunshot and stab wounds, crushing injuries, and forceful blows can result in tears, hemorrhage, or penetration of part of the urinary tract.

Injury to the urinary tract may be initially overlooked when the patient has incurred widespread, massive injuries. During treatment, an indwelling catheter usually is inserted, and hematuria or lack of urine output may be the first sign that a urinary tract injury has occurred. On the other hand, certain other types of injuries, such as stab or gunshot wounds, may be immediately identified as urinary tract injuries.

Symptoms

Symptoms vary according to the area affected and the type of injury. Anuria, hematuria, pain in the abdomen (which may indicate bleeding or leakage of urine into the abdominal cavity), pain in the bladder or kidney areas, and symptoms of shock may be indicators of urinary tract injury.

Diagnosis

Diagnosis may be based on the outward signs of injury (gunshot or knife entry wounds) and symptoms. Diagnostic tests usually are based on the possible type and site of injury and include abdominal radiographs, cystoscopy, and IVP. Exploratory surgery may be necessary to identify the exact type and extent of the injury.

Treatment

Treatment depends on the type, location, and extent of injury as well as on the condition of the patient. For example, a stab wound in the kidney area may require emergency exploratory surgery. Once the kidney is exposed, the physician needs to determine if the trauma to the kidney can be repaired or if the kidney must be removed immediately.

Examples of surgeries that may be performed for urinary tract trauma include cystostomy (temporary or permanent), nephrectomy, insertion of a nephrostomy tube, repair (reanastomosis) of the ureter, and cystectomy.

General Nutritional Considerations

☐ For patients in renal failure, dietary intervention becomes important and includes restrictions to alleviate symptoms of uremia. The type of diet or dietary restriction usually depends on the degree of severity of renal disease.

☐ The diet may be restricted in sodium, potassium, protein, and fluids. Restrictions depend on laboratory serum values, which show the kidneys' ability to eliminate specific waste products of metabolism.

☐ Salt substitutes, some of which contain potassium, may *not* be used unless approved by the physician (by specific name-brand product).

☐ The patient needs to be given detailed dietary instructions by the dietitian and at times by the nurse. Patients and families should be informed of the availability of foods and recipes made especially for those with dietary restrictions.

☐ When it is important to limit potassium intake, certain fruit juices, tea, coffee, and chocolate beverages, all of which have high potassium contents, are limited or omitted. Juices that are high in potassium include grapefruit, orange, prune, tangerine, and tomato. Juices that can be included in a 1,500-mg potassium-restricted diet include apple, cranberry, pear, peach, and pineapple.

☐ Patients with edema have severe restriction of their sodium intake. Salt substitutes that contain potassium for seasoning should not be used without the physician's approval.

General Pharmacologic Considerations

☐ Patients scheduled for intravenous or retrograde pyelography or arteriography should have an allergy history taken because the contrast media used in these studies contain iodine. The physician may first inject a small amount of the dye and wait before giving the remainder to be sure that the patient does not have a reaction to the dye. All patients who have these studies should be observed for signs of iodine sensitivity: tachycardia, restlessness, cardiovascular collapse.

☐ Sodium bicarbonate (baking soda), usually in tablet form, may be used to alkalize the urine of patients with kidney stones to try to prevent stone recurrence.

☐ Antibiotics and sulfonamides are drugs commonly used to treat urinary tract infections. Other drugs used are furan derivatives, nitrofurantoin microcrystals (Macrodantin) and nitrofurantoin (Furadantin), and acids, methenamine mandelate (Mandelamine) and nalidixic acid (NegGram). An azo dye, phenazopyridine (Pyridium), may be ordered for its soothing effect on bladder mucosa and is often used in conjunction with urinary antibiotics.

☐ Other drugs used in kidney disease include corticosteroids to control the inflammatory process of acute glomerulonephritis and diuretics to reduce edema in acute and chronic glomerulonephritis.

☐ Patients who receive drugs for urinary tract infections should be instructed to finish the course of therapy even though they may feel improved and be symptomfree after several days of therapy. A *completed* course of therapy is essential to be sure the infection is under control.

☐ Patients must be advised to follow the instructions of their physician about the medication and any instructions specific to that medication, such as drinking extra fluids.

☐ Drugs excreted from the body by the kidney are given with caution to the patient with renal disease. If the drug is deemed necessary, it may be given in lower than normal doses; the patient is closely observed for any changes in renal status if normal doses are necessary. The nurse should pay special attention to the patient's urinary output, as this method is a way to determine a change in renal status.

☐ Drugs that are toxic to the kidney (nephrotoxic) are not given to the patient with renal disease unless the patient's life is in danger and no other therapeutic agent is of value.

General Gerontologic Considerations

☐ Elderly patients often have slightly abnormal renal function tests. Mild abnormalities are due to the aging process and are usually of no clinical significance.

☐ The elderly patient may have some form of incontinence. In some, involuntary leakage of urine may occur when the patient coughs or sneezes, whereas others may be completely incontinent.

☐ Some elderly patients may be unable to follow the instructions of a bladder rehabilitation program; others may have involuntary relaxation of the bladder sphincter, making rehabilitation extremely difficult.

☐ Elderly patients with continence problems must not be treated like infants or scolded for their behavior (eg, bed wetting, soiling clothes). The nurse must make every effort to help rehabilitate the patient. If bladder rehabilitation is not successful, other methods to keep the patient clean, dry, and odorfree must be tried.

☐ If the elderly patient is incontinent, the perineal area is particularly susceptible to skin breakdown.

☐ Patients should not be made to feel isolated when they have a problem with urinary continence. Planned exercise and social activities should be a part of a bladder rehabilitation program.

☐ Elderly patients usually are not considered candidates for kidney transplants but may be able to use CAPD. Supervision of the procedure by a family member may be necessary. More frequent monitoring of the patient's progress is required when this technique is used.

Suggested Readings

☐ Baer C. Why does this patient have polyuria? Nursing '88 October 1988;18:94. *(Additional coverage of subject matter)*

☐ Baer C. Investigating dysuria. Nursing '89 May 1989;19:108. *(Additional coverage of subject matter)*

☐ Barkett PA. Action stat! Ruptured arteriovenous shunt. Nursing '87 October 1987;17:33. *(Additional coverage of subject matter)*

☐ Brady S. Getting the kinks out of a bladder drainage system. RN February 1988;51:39. *(Closely related to subject matter)*

☐ Bristoll SL, Fadden T, Fehring RJ, et al. The mythical danger of rapid urinary drainage. Am J Nurs March 1989;89:344. *(Additional coverage of subject matter)*

☐ Brogna L, Lakaszawski ML. The continent urostomy. Am J Nurs February 1986;86:160. *(Additional coverage and illustrations that reinforce subject matter)*

☐ Brunner LS, Suddarth DS. The Lippincott manual of nursing practice. 4th ed. Philadelphia: JB Lippincott, 1986. *(Additional and in-depth coverage of subject matter)*

☐ Caldwell L. Nutrition education for the patient: the handout manual. Philadelphia: JB Lippincott, 1984. *(Additional coverage of subject matter)*

☐ Farrell J. Nursing care of the older person. Philadelphia: JB Lippincott, 1990. *(In-depth coverage of subject matter)*

☐ Fischbach FT. A manual of laboratory diagnostic tests. 3rd ed. Philadelphia: JB Lippincott, 1988. *(Additional coverage of subject matter)*

☐ Ghiotto DL. A full range of care for nephrostomy patients. RN April 1988;51:72. *(Additional coverage of subject matter)*

☐ Hahn K. The many signs of renal failure. Nursing '87 August 1987;17:34. *(Additional coverage of subject matter)*

☐ Hahn K. Think twice about urinary incontinence. Nursing '88 January 1988;18:65. *(Additional coverage of subject matter)*

☐ Horne MM, Swearingen PL. Pocket guide to fluids and electrolytes. St Louis: CV Mosby, 1988. *(Additional coverage of subject matter)*

☐ Jaffe MS, Melson KA. Laboratory and diagostic cards: clinical implications and teaching. St Louis: CV Mosby, 1988. *(Additional coverage of subject matter)*

☐ Kidd PA. Action stat! Ruptured bladder. Nursing '89 January 1989;19:33. *(Additional coverage of subject matter)*

☐ Knezevich BA. Trauma nursing: principles and practice. Norwalk, CT: Appleton-Century-Crofts, 1986. *(Additional coverage of subject matter)*

☐ Long BC, Phipps WJ. Medical–surgical nursing: a nursing process approach. St Louis: CV Mosby, 1989. *(Additional and in-depth coverage of subject matter)*

☐ Luckmann J, Sorensen K. Medical–surgical nursing: a psychophysioloigic approach. 3rd ed. Philadelphia: WB Saunders, 1987. *(Additional and in-depth coverage of subject matter)*

☐ Malti J, Wellons D. CAPD: a dialysis breakthrough with its own burdens. Nursing '88 January 1988;18:46. *(Additional coverage of subject matter)*

☐ Moorhouse MF. Critical care plans. Philadelphia: FA Davis, 1987. *(Additional and in-depth coverage of subject matter)*

☐ Newman DK, Smith DA. Incontinence: the problem patients won't talk about. RN March 1989;52:42. *(Additional coverage of subject matter)*

☐ Preshlock K. Detecting the hidden UTI. RN January 1989;52:65. *(Additional coverage of subject matter)*

☐ Pritchard V. Geriatric infections: the urinary tract. RN May 1988;51:36. *(Additional coverage of subject matter)*

☐ Reilly NJ, Torosian LC. The new wave in lithotripsy: implications for nursing. RN March 1988;51:46. *(Additional coverage of subject matter)*

☐ Ruge C. Catheter related UTIs: what's the best way to prevent them? Nursing '87 December 1987;17:50. *(Additional coverage of subject matter)*

☐ Snyder TE. An exercise program for dialysis patients. Am J Nurs March 1989;89:362. *(Additional coverage of subject matter)*

☐ Strangio L. Believe it or not . . . peritoneal dialysis made easy. Nursing '88 January 1988;18:43. *(Additional coverage of subject matter)*

☐ Swearingen PL, Sommers MS, Miller K. Manual of critical care: applying nursing diagnosis to adult critical illness. St Louis: CV Mosby, 1988. *(Additional and in-depth coverage of subject matter)*

☐ Traines S. Ileal pull-through surgery. Nursing '87 November 1987;17:92. *(Additional coverage of subject matter)*

☐ Tucker SM, Canobbio MM, Paquette EV, Wells MF. Patient care standards: nursing process, diagnosis and outcome. St Louis: CV Mosby, 1988. *(Additional and in-depth coverage of subject matter)*

☐ Wieck L, King EM, Dyer M. Illustrated manual of nursing techniques. 3rd ed. Philadelphia: JB Lippincott, 1986. *(Additional and in-depth coverage of subject matter)*

☐ Zastocki DK, Rovinski CA. Home care: patient and family instructions. Philadelphia: WB Saunders, 1989. *(Additional coverage of subject matter)*

Orthopedic and Connective Tissue Disorders

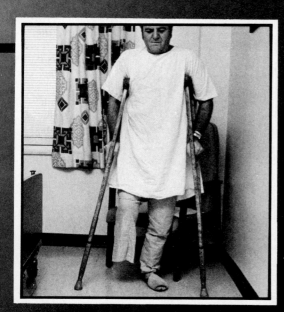

Unit 14

Chapter 54

Introduction to Orthopedic and Connective Tissue Disorders

On completion of this chapter the reader will:

■ Be familiar with the basic anatomy and physiology of the skeletal system

■ List and discuss the diagnostic tests used in the evaluation of orthopedic disorders

■ Describe the assessment of a patient with an orthopedic disorder

■ Use the nursing process in preparing a patient for tests used in the diagnosis of orthopedic disorders

ANATOMY AND PHYSIOLOGY

The musculoskeletal system consists of bones, muscles, joints, tendons, ligaments, cartilage, and bursae. These connective tissue structures are responsible for locomotion, the storage of calcium, the production of blood cells (in red bone marrow), and protection and support of many organs of the body, such as the lungs, heart, and brain.

Bones

The bones of the skeleton are classified as *short bones* (the bones in the fingers), *long bones* (the femur), *flat bones* (the sternum), and *irregular bones* (the vertebrae). There are two types of bone tissue: cancellous or cortical. *Cancellous* bone is spongy and has many spaces. *Cortical* bone is compact. Examples of these two types of bone tissue may be found in the long bones, such as the femur. Cancellous bone is found at the rounded, irregular ends (epiphysis) of the femur, and compact bone is found in the shaft (diaphysis).

Bone formation and resorption (breakdown) continues throughout life, although the greatest activity occurs during childhood. Bone cells that build bone are called *osteoblasts*. These cells manufacture a substance that is located between the cells. Calcium is then deposited, and the cells become hardened and are called *osteocytes*. Other cells contained in bones are called *osteoclasts*, which are responsible for resorption of bone.

There are two types of bone marrow: red marrow and yellow marrow. *Red bone marrow* is concerned with the manufacture of blood cells and hemoglobin. *Yellow bone marrow*, which consists primarily of fat cells and connective tissue, does not participate in the manufacture of blood cells. Red bone marrow is primarily found in the ribs, sternum, and iliac crest. Yellow bone marrow is found chiefly in the interior of the long bones.

Except for the joints, bones are covered by a layer of tissue called the *periosteum*. The inner layer of the periosteum contains the osteoblasts necessary for bone formation. The periosteum is rich in blood and lymph vessels and supplies the bone with nourishment.

Muscles

There are basically three kinds of muscles: skeletal, smooth, and cardiac. *Skeletal muscles* are voluntary muscles; that is, movement of the muscles is under the control of the conscious mind. The skeletal muscles are those that control movement and are attached to the bones of the skeleton. Examples of skeletal muscles are the biceps in the arms and the gastrocnemius in the calf of the leg. The movement of skeletal muscles normally is controlled by impulses that travel from efferent nerves of the brain and spinal cord.

Smooth muscles and *cardiac muscles* are involuntary muscles; their activity is not under the control of the conscious mind. Smooth muscles are found mainly in the walls of certain organs or cavities of the body, such as the stomach, intestine, blood vessels, and ureters. Cardiac muscle is found only in the heart.

Joints

A *joint* is the area of junction between two or more bones. Examples of joints are the knee, elbow, and ankle. Joints may be classified as *immovable joints* (synarthrosis), *slightly movable joints* (amphiarthrosis), and *freely movable joints* (diarthrosis or synovial joints). An example of an immovable joint is the suture line between the temporal and occipital bones of the skull. An example of a slightly movable joint is the joint between two vertebrae of the spine. An example of a freely movable joint is the knee.

Freely movable joints, which make up most of the joints of the skeleton, have a space between them. This space is filled with *synovial fluid*, which acts as a lubricant.

Tendons

Tendons are cordlike structures that attach muscles to the bony skeleton. A muscle has two or more attachments. One is called the *origin* and is more fixed. The other is called the *insertion* and is more movable. When a muscle contracts, both points of attachment are pulled, and the insertion is pulled closer to the origin. An example of this can be found in the biceps of the arm, which has two origin tendons, attached to the scapula, and one insertion tendon, attached to the radius. When the biceps contracts, the lower arm (with the insertion tendon) moves toward the upper arm (with the origin tendon).

Ligaments

Ligaments connect freely movable bones to other freely movable bones and consist of bands of fibrous tissue. Ligaments help protect the joints by stabilizing the joint surfaces and keeping them in proper alignment. In some instances, ligaments completely enclose a joint.

Cartilage

Cartilage is a firm, dense type of connective tissue that consists of cells embedded in a substance called the *matrix*. The matrix is firm and compact, thus enabling it to withstand pressure and torsion. *Articular cartilage* covers the surface of movable joints, such as the elbow, and acts as a protection for the surface of these joints. Examples of other types of cartilage include *costal cartilage*, which connects the ribs and sternum, *semilunar cartilage*, which is one of the cartilages of the knee joint, and *fibrous cartilage*, which is found between the vertebrae (intervertebral discs).

Bursae

A *bursa* is a small sac filled with synovial fluid and is found in connective tissue. Bursae reduce friction between areas such as tendon and bone and tendon and ligament. Inflammation of these sacs is called *bursitis*.

ASSESSMENT OF THE PATIENT WHO HAS AN ORTHOPEDIC OR CONNECTIVE TISSUE DISORDER

History

The original history depends on whether the patient has a chronic disorder or whether there has been a traumatic injury, such as a bone fracture. If the disorder is chronic, such as arthritis, a thorough medical, drug, and allergy history should be obtained. If the patient has been injured, information regarding when and how the injury occurred should be obtained. A medical history should be obtained as soon as possible because a medical disorder, such as diabetes mellitus, may also require the attention of medical personnel.

The medical history should include all past medical and surgical disorders and their treatment. A list of symptoms should be obtained that includes information about the onset, duration, location of discomfort or pain, whether any activity made the symptoms better or worse, whether any injury occurred, and any possible associated symptoms, such as muscle cramping or skin lesions. A family history—especially a history of these same symptoms—should be obtained, along with an occupational history.

Physical Assessment

The physical assessment also depends on the type and location of symptoms and whether an injury has occurred or whether this is a chronic disorder. A physical assessment for a chronic disorder may begin by taking vital signs and weighing the patient and then include the following observations of the affected area:

- Looking for and palpating for pain, tenderness, swelling, redness
- Assessing for the degree of movement, range of motion
- Assessing for stiffness
- Looking for abnormal size or alignment
- Testing for muscle strength
- Looking for muscle wasting

Depending on the symptoms, additional assessments may include looking for changes in gait, body posture, favoring one side over the other, and the patient's ability to bend and twist the trunk, head, and extremities. The patient's general appearance also should be noted.

A physical assessment for a traumatic injury should begin with taking vital signs. Assessment also depends on the type and area of injury, and may include the following:

- Looking for external bleeding
- Looking for broken skin, open wounds, superficial or embedded debris in or around the wound, protrusion of bone or other tissue from the wound
- Looking for injury beyond the original area
- Looking for incorrect alignment of the limb of the extremity of the injured part
- Assessing for pain (type and location)

Open wounds should not be touched, cleaned, nor disturbed and the injured extremity should not be moved until the patient has been examined by the physician.

Diagnostic Tests

Radiographs, Computed Tomographic Scans, and Magnetic Resonance Imaging

Radiographs, computed tomographic scans, or magnetic resonance imaging scans may be used to identify traumatic disorders, such as fractures and dislocations, and other bone disorders, such as malignant bone lesions, joint deformities, calcification, degenerative changes, osteoporosis, and joint disease.

Arthroscopy

Arthroscopy is the visual inspection of a joint by means of an instrument called an *arthroscope*. The most common use of arthroscopy is to visualize the knee joint, a common site of injury. After local or general anesthesia, the physician inserts a large-bore needle into the joint and injects sterile normal saline to distend the joint. The arthroscope is inserted, and the area is examined. Joint fluid may be removed and sent to the laboratory for examination.

Arthrocentesis

Arthrocentesis is the aspiration of synovial fluid from a joint. The patient is given local anesthesia for this procedure. The physician inserts a large needle into the joint and removes the fluid. Synovial fluid may be aspirated to relieve discomfort caused by an excessive accumulation of synovial fluid in the joint space or to inject a drug, such as a corticosteriod preparation. The removed synovial fluid may be sent to the laboratory for microscopic examination or for culture and sensitivity studies. Arthrocentesis may also be performed at the time of an arthrogram or arthroscopy.

Bone Scan

A *bone scan* uses the intravenous injection of a radioactive isotope, such as technetium polyphosphate, to detect the uptake of the radioactive substance by the bone. A bone scan may be ordered to detect metastatic bone lesions, fractures, and certain types of inflammatory bone disorders.

Biopsy

A biopsy of the bone may be taken to determine the structure of bone tissue or to obtain a sample of a bone lesion for microscopic examination. A bone biopsy most frequently is done for tumors of the bone.

Arthrogram

An *arthrogram* is a radiographic examination of a joint, usually the knee or shoulder. The physician injects a local anesthetic and then inserts a needle into the joint space. The synovial fluid present in the joint is aspirated and may be sent to the laboratory for analysis. Fluoroscopy may be used to verify correct placement of the needle. A contrast media is then injected, and radiographs are taken.

Laboratory Tests

Synovial Fluid Analysis

Synovial fluid may be examined to diagnose disorders such as traumatic arthritis, septic arthritis (which is caused by a microorganism), gout, rheumatic fever, and systemic lupus erythematosus.

Normally, synovial fluid is clear and nearly colorless. Laboratory examination of synovial fluid may include microscopic examination for blood cells, crystals, and formed debris that may be present in the joint space following an injury. If an infection is suspected, culture and sensitivity studies may be ordered. A chemical analysis for substances such as protein and glucose may also be performed.

Blood Tests

A routine blood test, which often is part of any complete physical examination, may be ordered to detect infection, inflammation, or anemia. Examples of routine blood tests are complete blood count, white blood cell and differential, and hemoglobin.

Examples of other blood tests that may be performed to diagnose various musculoskeletal disorders include the following:

- Alkaline phosphatase, which may be elevated in disorders such as bone tumors, Paget's disease, and healing fractures
- Serum calcium, which may be elevated in Paget's disease and rickets
- Serum phosphorus, which may be elevated in malignant bone tumors
- Serum uric acid, which usually is elevated in untreated or treated gout
- Antinuclear antibodies, which usually are elevated in lupus erythematosus

Urine Tests

Twenty-four–hour urine samples may be collected for determination of the levels of uric acid and calcium excretion. In gout, the 24-hour excretion of uric acid is elevated. Elevated calcium levels may be found in metastatic bone lesions and in those subject to prolonged periods of immobility.

NURSING PROCESS —THE PATIENT UNDERGOING TESTS FOR AN ORTHOPEDIC OR CONNECTIVE TISSUE DISORDER

Assessment

In the case of a traumatic injury, information regarding the injury should be obtained from the patient, family, or individual accompanying the patient. Vital signs should be taken at the time of admission to the hospital and at frequent intervals until the patient's condition is stabilized.

If the patient has a chronic disorder, a general medical, drug, and allergy history and a history of symptoms should be obtained.

Nursing Diagnosis

Depending on the symptoms and the condition of the patient, one or more of the following nursing diagnoses may apply:

- Pain related to injury or symptoms of disorder
- Anxiety related to possible diagnosis, pain or discomfort, knowledge deficit
- Knowledge deficit of diagnostic test

Planning and Implementation

The major goals of the patient may include relief or pain or discomfort, reduction in anxiety, and understanding of the diagnostic tests to be performed.

The major goals of nursing management are to relieve pain, reduce anxiety, and prepare the patient for and observe the patient after the diagnostic tests.

Pain. If the patient has severe pain as a result of an injury, the physician may order a narcotic analgesic. Patients with traumatic injuries should be closely observed after the administration of a narcotic analgesic for signs of shock. The physician may prescribe an analgesic for the patient with chronic pain or discomfort.

Knowledge Deficit. To reduce anxiety, the tests should be explained or described, and the patient should be allowed time to ask questions. The patient should be told how long the test or examination will take, where it will be done, and what preparations (if any) are necessary.

Some of these tests are performed on an outpatient basis. No special care is required after laboratory tests, general radiographs, or a bone scan. If the patient has had synovial fluid removed for laboratory examination, the area should be inspected for swelling and ecchymosis. If the patient has severe pain in the area before leaving the hospital or physician's office, the physician should be informed.

After an arthroscopy, the physician may order the application of ice and an analgesic for pain or discomfort. The area should be observed for swelling, redness, and drainage. The dressing should be changed or reinforced as needed.

After arthrocentesis or an arthrogram, a small dressing should be applied to the area. The area should be examined for redness, swelling, and drainage before the patient leaves the hospital or physician's office.

The physician often gives the patient special instructions after the procedure. The nurse should reinforce the physician's instructions.

Patients who have an arthroscopy may be admitted to the hospital on a short-term basis and discharged several hours after the procedure. The patient may remain in the hospital if the arthroscopy reveals a necessity to perform surgery or provide other treatment to the area.

Although the physician's instructions after an arthroscopy or arthrocentesis may vary, the patient usually is told to rest the extremity for several days. If the knee was examined or aspirated, weight bearing on the leg should be avoided for several days. The patient should be told to contact the physician if chills, fever, or increased pain, swelling, or redness of the area occur.

Evaluation

- Pain is relieved
- Anxiety is reduced
- Patient demonstrates understanding of the procedure
- Patient demonstrates understanding of home management after the procedure as well as symptoms that require contacting the physician

Suggested Readings

☐ Bates BA, Hoeckelman RA. Guide to physical examination and history taking. 4th ed. Philadelphia: JB Lippincott, 1987. *(In-depth coverage of subject matter)*

☐ Bowers AC, Thompson JM. Clinical manual of health assessment. 3rd ed. St Louis: CV Mosby, 1988. *(In-depth coverage of subject matter)*

☐ Doenges ME, Moorhouse MF. Nurse's pocket guide: nursing diagnoses with interventions. 2nd ed. Philadelphia: FA Davis, 1988. *(Additional coverage of subject matter)*

☐ Fischbach FT. A manual of laboratory diagnostic tests. 3rd ed. Philadelphia: JB Lippincott, 1988. *(Additional coverage of subject matter)*

☐ Fuller J, Schaller-Ayers J. Health assessment: a nursing approach. Philadelphia: JB Lippincott, 1990. *(Additional coverage of subject matter)*

☐ Long BC, Phipps WJ. Medical–surgical nursing: a nursing process approach. St Louis: CV Mosby, 1989. *(Additional and in-depth coverage of subject matter)*

☐ McFarland MB, Grant MM. Nursing implicationms of laboratory tests. 2nd ed. New York: John Wiley & Sons, 1988. *(Additional and in-depth coverage of subject matter)*

☐ Memmler RL, Wood DL. The human body in health and disease. 6th ed. Philadelphia: JB Lippincott, 1987. *(Additional coverage of subject matter)*

Chapter 55
Orthopedic and Connective Tissue Disorders

On completion of this chapter the reader will:

- Discuss the symptoms, diagnosis, and treatment of sprains and dislocations

- Use the nursing process in the management of a patient with a sprain or dislocation

- Discuss the types, symptoms, diagnosis, and treatment of fractures

- Discuss the principles of cast application

- Use the nursing process in the management of a patient with a cast

- Use the nursing process in the management of a patient in traction

- List and discuss the various types of orthopedic surgeries

- Use the nursing process in the management of a patient undergoing orthopedic surgery

- Discuss the symptoms, diagnosis, and treatment of rheumatic disorders

- Use the nursing process in the management of a patient with a rheumatic disorder

- Discuss the symptoms, diagnosis, and treatment of low back pain, osteoporosis, and bursitis

- Use the nursing process in the management of a patient having joint surgery

- Discuss the symptoms, diagnosis, and treatment of osteomyelitis, bone tumors, and Paget's disease

- Discuss amputation of the upper and lower extremities

- Use the nursing process in the management of a patient undergoing an amputation

- Discuss the symptoms, diagnosis, and treatment of disorders of the hands and feet

SPRAINS

Sprains are injuries to the ligaments surrounding a joint. Often sprains are caused by an accidental fall or a forceful twisting of the joint. Areas most subject to sprains are the wrist, elbow, knee, and ankle.

Symptoms
Sprains are accompanied by pain, swelling, and loss of motion. The skin over the area may become ecchymotic because of the rupture of nearby blood vessels.

Diagnosis
Diagnosis is made by examination of the affected part and symptoms. A radiograph may be taken to differentiate a sprain from a fracture.

Treatment
Treatment consists of the application of ice to the area to reduce swelling and relieve pain for the first 24 to 36 hours after the injury. Elevation of the part and application of an elastic bandage also may be recommended by the physician. Occasionally, the sprain may involve tearing of the ligaments surrounding the joint. Depending on the degree of injury, the physician may apply a light cast to the area. After 2 days, heat may be recommended to relieve discomfort.

DISLOCATIONS

Dislocations occur when the articular surfaces of a joint are no longer in contact. Dislocations are caused by trauma or, less frequently, by disease of the joint.

Symptoms
The symptoms of a dislocation are pain, malposition leading to an abnormal axis of the dependent bone, and loss of the function of the joint.

Diagnosis
Diagnosis is based on symptoms, physical examination of the affected area, and radiographs.

Treatment
The physician manipulates the joint until the parts are again in normal position, then immobilizes the joint, using an elastic bandage, cast, or splint, for several weeks to allow the joint capsule and surrounding ligaments to heal. A local or general anesthetic may be required for manipulation of the joint.

Some dislocations may require surgery, either to correct the dislocation or to repair damage caused by the injury. An example of a dislocation requiring surgery is a severe knee dislocation that has caused injury to the ligaments and blood vessels around the joint.

779

NURSING PROCESS —THE PATIENT WHO HAS A SPRAIN OR DISLOCATION

Assessment

Most patients with this type of injury are seen in the emergency department or physician's office. The nursing assessment should include a brief medical history (especially for patients with dislocations) and a visual examination of the affected area.

Nursing Diagnosis

Depending on the type of injury and age of the patient, one or more of the following nursing diagnoses may apply:

- Pain related to traumatic injury of the area
- Anxiety related to pain, other factors (specify)
- Knowledge deficit of home management

Planning and Implementation

The major goals of the patient may include reduction in pain, reduction in anxiety, and understanding of home care management.

The major goals of nursing management may include reduction in anxiety, relief of pain, and effective instruction in home care. After the correction of the dislocation, the nurse should watch for compression resulting from tight bandages or a tight cast.

Pain. The physician may recommend an analgesic such as aspirin or ibuprofen (Advil) for pain. In some instances, a narcotic analgesic may be prescribed.

Anxiety. Anxiety is usually reduced once the injury is diagnosed and treated and a drug given to relieve pain. The nurse should assure the patient that although there may be discomfort, following the physician's recommendations for treatment usually reduces or eliminate discomfort in a short period of time.

Knowledge Deficit. Patients with simple sprains and dislocations not requiring surgery are usually discharged from the emergency department. If the patient is to use an elastic bandage, the application of this type of bandage should be demonstrated to the patient. Those with a dislocation that was corrected by simple manipulation should be instructed to return to the physician for follow-up care and evaluation of treatment.

The following general areas may be included in a patient teaching plan:

1. Follow the physician's recommendations regarding care of the injured area.

2. Take the prescribed or recommended drugs.
3. Do not apply elastic bandages so tightly that circulation is impaired. When applying an elastic bandage, check the extremity below the bandage. If the extremity becomes cold, mottled, or blue, remove the bandage for a few minutes and then reapply it using less tension on the bandage.

For sprains, the patient should be instructed to elevate the extremity until swelling is no longer present, to avoid using the extremity until allowed by the physician, and to notify the physician if pain continues (after 2 or 3 days) or becomes worse.

For dislocations, the patient should be instructed to avoid using the extremity until the physician permits it and to apply the immobilization devices (slings, braces, and so forth) until told by the physician that they are no longer necessary. It is important to stress that the physician must be notified if pain is not relieved in 3 or 4 days or becomes worse, if the dislocation recurs, or if numbness, tingling, loss of feeling, or change in color of the extremity occur.

Evaluation

- Pain is reduced or controlled
- Anxiety is reduced
- Patient demonstrates understanding of home management, drug therapy, application of splint or bandage, and problems that require notifying the physician

FRACTURES

A fracture is a break in the continuity of a bone. The incidence of fractures is greater among people who have predisposing conditions that affect bone, such as osteoporosis and cancer. Poor coordination, diminished vision and hearing, frequency of dizziness and faintness, and general feebleness make falls and resultant fractures a common problem among the elderly. Other high-risk groups include those with diseases affecting locomotion, such as arthritis, Parkinson's disease, and multiple sclerosis. The fact that bone breakage in older people is more frequent across the neck of the femur is attributed partially to atrophy of bone. Some common types of fractures are shown in Figure 55-1.

The following is a simple classification of fractures:

Open (compound)—The bone breaks through the skin. Because there is an open wound, the danger of infection is greatly increased.
Closed (simple)—Any fracture that is not open is a closed fracture.
Displaced—The bone ends are separated at the fracture line.
Greenstick—The bone bends and splits, but it does not break clear through. This kind of fracture occurs primarily in children.

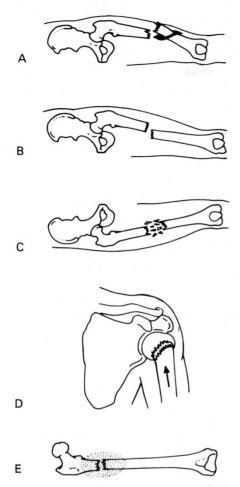

Figure 55–1. Types of fractures. (*A*) Open fracture. (*B*) Closed fracture. (*C*) Comminuted fracture. (*D*) Impacted fracture. (*E*) Pathologic fracture. (Brunner LS, Suddarth DS: Medical-Surgical Nursing. 4th ed., Philadelphia: JB Lippincott, 1980:1293. Courtesy of Ethicon, Inc)

Complete—The fracture line goes all the way through the bone.

Comminuted—The bone is splintered into many small fragments at the fracture site, with the bone ends separated and usually misaligned.

Impacted—One portion of the bone is driven into another.

Complicated—A fracture with injury to the surrounding tissues, such as blood vessels, nerves, muscles, tendons, joints, or internal organs.

Pathologic (spontaneous)—The bone breaks without sufficient trauma to crack a normal bone. This kind of fracture generally occurs in people with conditions such as osteoporosis (porous bones), cancer, certain types of malnutrition, and Cushing's syndrome, and as a complication of corticosteroid therapy.

For 10 to 40 minutes after a fracture occurs, the muscles surrounding the bone are flaccid, after which they go into spasm, often resulting in increased deformity and additional interference with the vascular and lymphatic circulations.

When there are bone fragments as a result of a fracture, the local periosteum and surrounding blood vessels are torn. The tissue surrounding the fracture shows inflammation, with swelling caused by hemorrhage and edema. The blood in the area clots, and a fibrin network forms between bone ends, which changes into granulation tissue. The osteoblasts, proliferating in the clot, increase the secretion of an enzyme that restores the alkaline pH, and the result is the deposition of calcium in the callus and the formation of true bone. At the stage of the consolidation of the clot (6 to 10 days after the injury), the healing mass is called a *callus*. The callus holds the ends of the bone together, but it cannot endure strain. Bone repair is a local process. About a year of healing should take place before bone regains its former structural strength, becomes well-consolidated and remolded, and possesses fat and marrow cells.

Symptoms

The symptoms of a fracture may vary, depending on the type and location of the fracture, and may include the following:

Pain—One of the most consistent symptoms of a fracture is pain. It may be severe, and it is increased by attempts to move the part and by pressure over the fracture.

Loss of function—Skeletal muscular function depends on an intact bone.

Deformity—A break may cause an extremity to bend backward or to assume another unusual shape.

False motion—Unnatural motion occurs at the site of the fracture.

Edema—Swelling usually is greatest directly over the fracture.

Spasm—Muscles near fractures involuntarily contract. Spasm, which accounts for some of the pain, may result in the shortening of a limb when a long bone is involved.

If sharp bone fragments tear through sufficient surrounding soft tissue, there will be bleeding and black and blue discoloration of the area. If a nerve is damaged, there may be paralysis.

Diagnosis

The diagnosis of a fracture almost always is made by one or more radiographs of the area. Different views may be needed to visualize the fracture. In some instances, a computed tomographic (CT) scan or magnetic resonance imaging (MRI) may be necessary.

Treatment

The aim of treatment is to help the body reestablish functional continuity of the bone. The method of treatment selected by the physician for a fracture depends on many factors, including the first aid given, the location and severity of the break, and the age and overall physical condition of the patient.

A fracture may be treated by one or more of the methods discussed in the following paragraphs.

Closed Reduction. In a *closed reduction*, the physician *reduces* the fracture (replaces the parts in their normal position) by external manipulation of the fragments, redirecting the bone to its normal position. The physician then immobilizes the area with a bandage, cast, or traction, and radiographs are taken to be sure the bone is correctly aligned. Depending on the site and type of fracture, the patient may be given a local (nerve block) or general anesthetic for this procedure.

Open Reduction. In an *open reduction,* which is performed in the operating room, the bone is surgically exposed and realigned. The operation usually is performed under general or spinal anesthesia. Radiographs are taken while the patient is still anesthetized so that any needed correction can be made. A cast or other method of immobilization usually is applied to the area. This procedure is used frequently for dealing with soft tissue, such as nerves or blood vessels, caught between the ends of the broken pieces of bone; for wide separation of the bone; for comminuted fractures; for fractures of the patella and other joints; for open fractures when debridement of the wound is necessary; and for *internal fixation* (using pins, nails, rods, wires, plates, or screws to immobilize and strengthen the bone) of fractures.

Cast Application. Some fractures do not require surgical or manual manipulation to realign the bone because the fractured bone still remains perfectly aligned. Casts hold the bone in place while it heals. Before the cast is applied, the patient may be given an analgesic or general anesthesia or local anesthesia (nerve block) to relieve pain.

Traction. Various types of traction can be used to maintain alignment and immobilization. The two most common types are skin traction and skeletal traction. *Skin traction* uses tapes or traction strips attached to the skin, usually by elastic bandages. The tapes or strips are connected to a traction apparatus that consists of ropes, pulleys, and weights. *Skeletal traction* uses a wire (Kirschner) or pin (Steinmann) inserted in the bone, with pull (traction) applied to the pin or wire. General anesthesia is required to insert these devices.

External Fixation. In external fixation, metal pins are inserted into the bone or bones from outside the skin surface, and a compression device is attached to the pins. Some complex or comminuted fractures may

require the use of an external fixator, such as a Hoffman device (Fig. 55-2), to stabilize and position the bone.

FRACTURE OF SPECIFIC SITES
Mandible

Fractures of the mandible (lower jaw) usually result from direct blows to the lower jaw or face. Teeth, especially the front teeth, also may be lost or broken. Lacerations in the mouth and of the tongue may be seen.

Symptoms
Pain, swelling, ecchymosis, bleeding in the mouth, and misalignment of the mandible may be seen.

Diagnosis
Diagnosis is based on radiographs and physical examination.

Treatment
Fractures of the mandible frequently are treated with wires that splint the lower jaw to the upper jaw. Broken or loose teeth are removed or repaired. Oral lacerations also may require suturing.

The nurse should be familiar with the wire loops

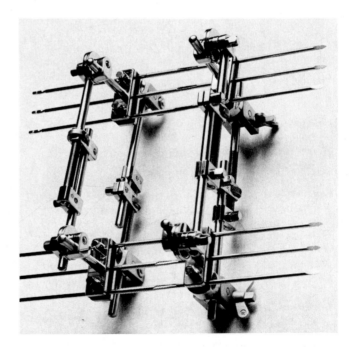

Figure 55–2. The external Hoffman fixator. The rods (which are horizontal in the photograph) are inserted through holes drilled in the bone. The external frames (which are vertical in the photograph) hold the rods in place and are adjustable. This device allows the surgeon to align and stabilize the fractured bone. (Photograph by D. Atkinson)

that can be unhooked. A pair of wire-cutting scissors is usually sent from surgery with the patient and should be taped to the head of the bed in plain view. These special scissors are used to cut the wires if the patient vomits. Cutting these wires is an emergency maneuver because vomitus is easily aspirated when the jaws are wired. All nursing personnel involved in the care of these patients should know how to cut these wires because this task must be performed quickly if the patient vomits. In addition, the patient should be instructed to use the call light if nausea occurs. A note also should be made on the Kardex about placement of the scissors (head of bed, bedside stand). Nursing personnel should check the patient's bedside stand one or more times per shift and especially after visiting hours to be sure the wire cutters are in their proper place.

Because the patient cannot chew, the diet should be liquid or, at best, semiliquid. The patient's mouth should be cleaned thoroughly after each meal and every 2 hours. The cheeks should be retracted with a tongue depressor and a flashlight used to see into the mouth. These fractures usually are compound. Complications include primary hemorrhage, asphyxia, and infection, which may lead to osteomyelitis.

Clavicle

The clavicle (collar bone) is a common fracture that often occurs from a fall (when the individual reaches out to break the fall) or a direct and forceful injury to the area. Dislocations of the clavicle also are common, and the bone may be both fractured and dislocated.

Symptoms

Pain, a droop in the shoulder of the injured side, inability to move the arm of the affected side, and muscle spasm of the affected area are the most common symptoms.

Diagnosis

Diagnosis is based on radiographs and physical examination.

Treatment

A fractured clavicle may be immobilized by a figure-of-eight bandage, a sling, or a clavicular strap, depending on which part of the clavicle is fractured and on the type of fracture. Some fractures may require open reduction.

Rib

One or more ribs may be fractured after a blow to the rib cage. Severe, crushing blows to the ribs may result

in injury to the lung, followed by blood in the thorax (hemothorax) and a collapse of the lung.

Symptoms

Severe pain in the chest, especially on inspiration, is the most common symptom. After more severe crushing injuries, acute respiratory distress and cyanosis is seen.

Diagnosis

Diagnosis is made by physical examination, history of trauma, and a chest radiograph.

Treatment

Broken ribs are uncomfortable because they must move when a person breathes. They usually heal without trouble. The patient should be observed for pulmonary complications (pneumonia, atelectasis) because of the tendency toward shallow respirations and suppression of the cough mechanism. Occasionally, the physician may support the injured rib cage with adhesive strapping, elastic bandage, or a rib belt. The disadvantage of limiting chest motion is the increased possibility of pulmonary complications.

Elbow and Upper and Lower Arm

Fractures of the upper and lower bones of the arm (humerus, radius, and ulna) range from simple hairline fractures without displacement of bone to complex injuries involving bone ends (eg, the head of the humerus), joints, tendons, and ligaments.

Symptoms

Pain, ecchymosis, inability to move the arm, and swelling are the usual symptoms of a less serious type of fracture. More serious fractures, such as a compound fracture after severe trauma, may produce additional symptoms, including bleeding, loss of feeling, and protrusion of bone through the skin.

Diagnosis

Diagnosis is based on radiographs and physical examination.

Treatment

Treatment depends on the type of fracture and the amount of displacement. Some fractures may require only application of a cast with or without closed reduction. Others may require open reduction and internal fixation, followed by application of a cast or even traction.

Wrist, Hand, and Finger

Fractures of the wrist or hand commonly occur from a fall. Some wrist fractures are actually fractures of the lower radius with or without fracture of the bones in the wrist (carpus and scaphoid). A fracture involving the lower radius with the distal end of the radius broken off and displaced is called *Colles' fracture.*

Fracture of a finger often results from blows, such as hitting the finger with or against a hard object, or catching the finger in a door.

Symptoms

Symptoms generally include pain and swelling after an injury to the area. In some instances, the wrist or finger is deformed in appearance.

Diagnosis

Diagnosis is based on radiographs and physical examination.

Treatment

Closed reduction may be attempted under either local (nerve block) or general anesthesia, followed by application of a cast. More severe injuries may require open reduction and internal fixation.

Fractures of the finger often require minimal treatment that includes the application of a splint to the finger. More severe fractures may require open reduction and internal fixation. A sling may be used to prevent edema of the hand (Fig. 55-3).

Spine

Fractures of the spine may be seen after severe injury, such as an automobile accident or serious fall. Osteo-porosis also may result in fracture of one or more vertebrae of the spine.

Symptoms

Symptoms usually include pain, tenderness over the area of fracture, neurologic deficits, and muscle spasm and sometimes even deformity of the spinal column.

Diagnosis

Diagnosis is based on symptoms, history of the injury, and radiograph examination.

Treatment

If there is injury to the spinal cord, immediate immobilization is necessary (see Chapter 38). Surgery, such as a laminectomy with spinal fusion or the insertion of stabilizing rods, may be necessary.

The patient with a fracture of the spine usually is placed in a position of hyperextension, which best reestablishes the normal position of the spinal column and exerts the least pressure on the spinal cord. Continuous hyperextension may be accomplished by applying a cast or by immobilizing the body with head traction and sandbags over a Gatch bed.

Traction for injury or fracture of the cervical spine may be accomplished by making small burr holes in the outer layers of the parietal bones on each side of the skull and inserting tongs, such as Crutchfield tongs, which then are connected to weights by means of rope and pulley attachments. Use of spring-loaded tongs does not require burr holes because these tongs are directly screwed into the skull after injection of a local anesthetic. Sometimes cervical traction is accomplished by leather or webbed straps on the head and under the chin and connected to ropes, pulleys, and weights to provide traction.

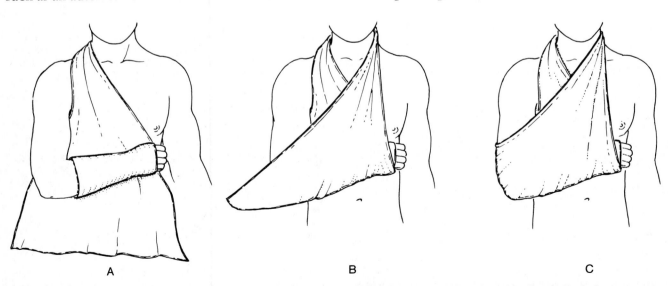

Figure 55–3.   Application of an arm sling. (*A*) The arm is positioned with the fingers higher than the elbow. (*B*) The entire arm is enclosed in the sling. (*C*) The flap is pinned snugly around the elbow.

Sandbags may be placed at the shoulders to help keep the patient in one position. If the physician allows it (usually requiring a written order), the patient may turn from side to side or the head of the bed may be raised. The patient must be turned without bending the spine. If the patient may be turned, a Stryker or a Foster frame facilitates care.

Simple, hairline fractures of the vertebrae that do not produce neurologic symptoms are usually treated conservatively with bed rest and a spinal brace.

Pelvis

The severity of a fracture of the pelvis may vary from minor fractures to severe or crushing injuries that result in the displacement of some of the bones of the pelvis.

Symptoms

Symptoms may vary from mild discomfort to serious internal hemorrhage and loss of function of one or both lower limbs. Tenderness over the area, ecchymosis, swelling, and symptoms of shock may be seen.

Crushing injuries may result in internal problems, including perforated bladder, severed nerves, and torn blood vessels, resulting in internal hemorrhage.

Diagnosis

Diagnosis is made by radiographic examination. Additional diagnostic tests may be performed if there has been a severe injury with possible damage to adjacent organs or structures.

Treatment

Treatment of small pelvic fractures is conservative. Sitz baths, bed rest, and analgesics for pain are usually prescribed. If the coccyx is fractured, defecation is often painful, and a stool softener may be ordered.

Treatment of more severe fractures may include pelvic traction, Buck's traction, a pelvic sling, a body cast (spica cast; Fig. 55-4), open reduction with internal fixation, or an external fixator (which uses the same principles as the fixator in Fig. 55-2).

Management of severe injuries often involves a multiple system approach because the bladder, intestines, arteries, veins, and nerves also may be damaged.

Femur

A fracture of the femur, or thigh bone, more commonly occurs in automobile accidents but may occur in falls from ladders or other high places or in gunshot wounds. Fractures of the femur often are accompanied by other injuries because they usually occur when there has been severe trauma accompanied by multiple injuries.

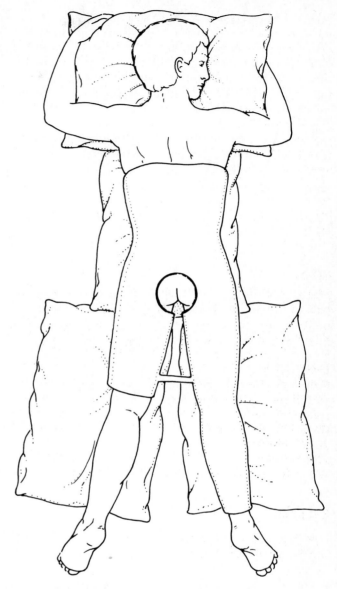

Figure 55-4. The wet spica cast is supported on pillows until it dries. When the patient lies on his abdomen, the feet are positioned over the edges of the pillows, which are placed such that they support the patient in good body alignment.

Symptoms

Severe pain, swelling, and ecchymosis may be seen. The patient usually is unable to move the hip or knee. If a compound fracture has occurred, an open wound or a protrusion of bone is seen. Dislocation of the knee or hip also may be seen.

Diagnosis

Diagnosis is based on radiographs and physical examination.

Treatment

Fractures of the femur are usually treated initially with some form of traction, including suspension traction with a Thomas splint or skin traction such as Russell traction (Fig. 55-5) or Buck's extension (Fig 55-6). Skin traction may be used initially to prevent deformities and soft tissue injury, which may be followed by the use of the Thomas splint with a Pearson attachment to keep the ends of the fracture separated in preparation for internal reduction and fixation. Balanced skeletal traction may be used if the fracture occurred in the lower two thirds of the femur. Attachment is made by use of a Steinmann pin or Kirschner wire. The Thomas splint with the Pearson attachment also is used with this type of traction. An external fixator also may be used in the treatment of femoral fractures.

Usually, internal reduction and fixation is done a week or more after the original injury.

Hip

Fracture of the hip is actually a fracture of the upper part of the femur (Fig. 55-7). This type of fracture is more frequent in older people with osteoporosis, and it is commonly a result of a fall or serious injury.

Symptoms
Symptoms include pain and a shortening of the leg, which is usually adducted (the extremity moves toward the midline), with the foot and leg externally rotated (turned outward).

Diagnosis
Diagnosis is based on radiographs and physical examination.

Treatment
Hip fractures may be treated with an internal fixation device, such as a nail or an *intramedullary rod* (a rod

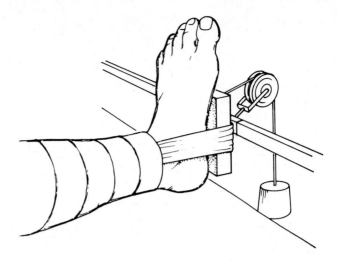

Figure 55–6. Buck's extension may be used for hip fractures until internal fixation (surgery) is performed. An elastic bandage is applied to anchor the moleskin straps applied to the skin. The strips may be applied in various ways, one of which is illustrated above.

inserted into the center of the bone with wires around the bone for stabilization), depending on the type and location of the fracture. Examples of internal fixation devices include the Jewett nail, the Richardson hip screw, the Moe intratrochanteric plate, and the Smith-Petersen nail.

Buck's extension or other forms of traction may be applied until surgery is performed. After surgery, the patient may be placed in a cast (hip spica) or in traction, or the limb may be left free.

The bone heals around the metallic device, which in the meantime holds the bone together. Thus, the bone is united immediately, and patients can be mobilized much earlier than with treatment by traction. Plates, bands, screws, and pins may be removed after the bone has healed, or they may be left permanently in place.

Knee

The kneecap (patella) may be fractured as a result of falls or blows. Because it is a joint, the knee is subject to various types of injuries to the ligaments and tendons and to fractures of the ends of the femur or tibia.

Symptoms
Symptoms include pain, swelling, ecchymosis, and inability or limited ability to bend or move the joint.

Diagnosis
Diagnosis is based on radiographs and physical examination. Arthroscopy may be used to determine the degree and extent of injury to ligaments and tendons.

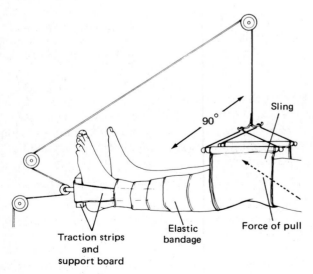

Figure 55–5. Russell traction, a form of skin traction, may be used for fractures of the hip and femur.

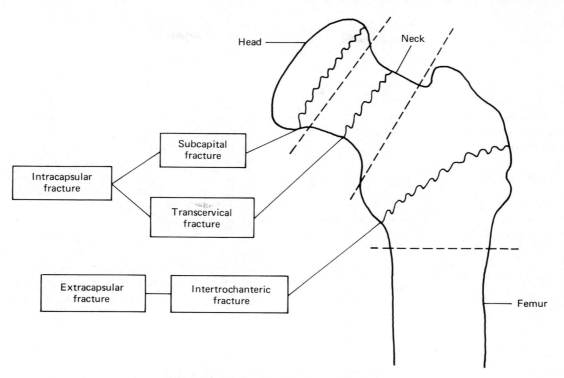

Figure 55–7. Types of fractures of the femur.

Treatment

A removable leg splint, which is fastened with Velcro straps, may be used to immobilize the leg in the treatment of a fractured patella. Arthroscopy may be performed to remove bone fragments. In some instances, open reduction and the insertion of wire sutures may be necessary. Removal of the patella may be necessary if there is extensive fragmentation of the patellar bone.

Skeletal traction may be used in the treatment of a knee injury if there is a fracture of the lower ends of the femur or tibia or both. Tears of the ligaments of the knee may be repaired by arthroscopy or by open surgery. Tears of the cruciate ligaments of the knee are a common athletic injury.

Lower Leg

Fractures of the two bones of the lower leg, the tibia and fibula, are most often the result of falls or forceful blows to the area. A fracture of the fibula by itself is rare; usually a fracture of the fibula is accompanied by a fracture of the tibia. Fractures of the tibia may or may not be accompanied by a fracture of the fibula.

Symptoms

Symptoms include pain, swelling, inability to put weight on the leg because of severe pain, ecchymosis, and possible deformity of the limb. Compound frac-

tures may result in bleeding and a protrusion of bone or bone fragments.

Diagnosis

Diagnosis is based on radiographs and physical examination.

Treatment

Closed reduction followed by the application of a cast may be used for simple fractures. If there are several fractures of the bone or a compound fracture (as may be seen in severe or crushing injuries), open reduction and internal fixation will be necessary. An external fixator also may be used.

Ankle

Because the ankle is a joint, it is subject to injury of the bones of the ankle, fracture of the ends of the tibia or fibula, and tearing of tendons and ligaments. Ligament tears often accompany ankle fractures.

Symptoms

Symptoms include pain, swelling, and severe pain when applying weight to the joint. Severe or crushing injuries may result in bone fragments in the joint or fragments protruding from the skin over the joint.

Diagnosis

Diagnosis is based on radiographs and physical examination.

Treatment

Depending on the severity and extent of injury, treatment may include the application of a splint or cast or open reduction and internal fixation with screws followed by the application of a cast.

Foot

Fractures of the foot may be seen alone or along with other fractures of the lower limb, such as the ankle, tibia, and fibula. Foot fractures may be caused by dropping heavy objects on the foot or by a trauma such as a fall or automobile accident.

Symptoms

Pain, swelling, ecchymosis, and an inability to put weight on the foot because of pain are the more common symptoms. Crushing foot injuries, like other crushing skeletal injuries, may result in the protrusion of bone or bone fragments through the skin.

Diagnosis

Diagnosis is based on radiographs and physical examination.

Treatment

Treatment depends on the bones involved and the extent and type of injury. A short leg cast may be used if the bones have not been displaced. Open reduction and internal fixation with pins may be necessary for some types of fractures.

Toe

Most toe fractures are the result of bumping into or hitting an object or dropping a heavy object on the toes when not wearing shoes.

Symptoms

Symptoms include pain, ecchymosis, swelling, and moderate to severe pain when walking.

Diagnosis

Diagnosis is made by physical examination. A radiograph is usually taken to rule out the presence of bone fragments.

Treatment

Treatment is conservative. Analgesics, elevation of the foot, and not wearing tight-fitting shoes until the fracture has healed are usually all that is necessary. If bone fragments are present, they may be removed surgically at a later date.

APPLICATION OF A CAST

Fractures, such as those of long bones, in which there is no impaction or misalignment of bone are immobilized by casts. Casts hold the bone in place while it heals and permit early ambulation when a leg is broken. The patient may be given a narcotic or general anesthetic before the cast is applied. Sometimes, a nerve block is performed, such as infiltrating the brachial plexus with a local anesthetic agent for closed reduction of a fracture of the arm.

When applying the cast, the physician positions the patient in a way that ensures the proper alignment of the part to be immobilized. An assistant holds the arm or leg exactly in place. A cast applied to an area that includes a joint usually is applied with the joint flexed to lessen stiffness.

The skin surface is cleaned and dried. The physician first applies a stockinette, which is made of knitted material and is longer than the anticipated length of the cast, onto the limb. Padding is then wrapped around the limb. The physician then wraps the wet cast material onto the limb. (The cast material is supplied in rolls of varying widths. There are different types of cast materials—some set in a few minutes, others take up to 24 hours to dry completely.) The edges of the cast are smoothed, and the stockinette is fastened to the outside of the cast (Fig. 55-8). Spica casts need special attention to the finishing area near the buttocks. After the cast has been applied, a second radiograph is taken to check bone alignment. Whenever a cast is removed or applied, a radiograph is taken.

The cast itself must be left uncovered so that water can evaporate from it. Many physicians prefer natural evaporation, but some order the use of a cast dryer to speed drying. Intense heat should never be used. Not only is there danger of burning the patient, but the heat dries the outside of the cast and leaves the inside wet, which later may become moldy. Intense heat also can crack the plaster.

Cast Windows.   A window cut in a cast over the area of discomfort permits visualization of that area of the skin. Some physicians cut a window or opening over the radial pulse in an arm cast to feel the pulse, which is one method of checking the circulation of the affected arm. The cast window can be observed for edema, which may cause the skin to protrude into the opening.

Bivalve Cast.   If a cast is put on an extremity before edema has developed fully, compression of the

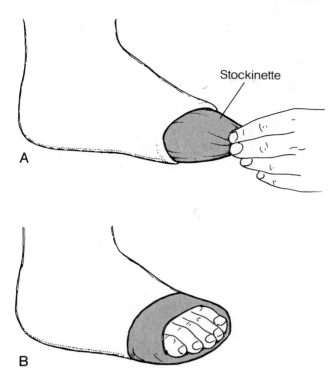

A

B

Figure 55–8. The edges of this cast are made smooth by (*A*) pulling out the stockinette and (*B*) fastening it to the outside of the cast.

Stockinette

tissues results because there will be no room for expansion inside the cast. To avoid this possibility, the physician may apply the cast and, as soon as it is dry, split it along both sides. The cast sides then are refitted on the patient's limb and bandaged in place. This kind of cast is called a *bivalve cast*. It also may be used for a patient who is being weaned from a cast, when a sharp radiograph is needed, or in the treatment of conditions such as arthritis, in which the method is a convenient one for splinting the part intermittently.

Cast Removal. Casts are removed by a mechanical cast cutter. Cast cutters are noisy and frightening, and the patient should be assured that the machine will not cut him or her.

When the cast is removed, continued support to the limb is necessary. An elastic bandage may be put on a leg or the arm may be kept in a sling.

The patient will have pains, aches, and stiffness, and the limb will feel surprisingly light without the cast. The skin will look mottled, and it may be covered with a yellow crust composed of exudate, oil, and dead skin. It may take a few days to remove this crust. Lotions and warm baths or soaks may be used to soften the skin and remove debris.

After removal of a cast, the patient's muscles are weak. Graded active exercise, directed by the physician or the physical therapist, helps the extremity to regain its normal strength and motion. Resistive exercises that are beyond the patient's capacity result in further limitation of motion. Exercises should be active, not passive, and progressively graded so that muscles and joints are coaxed rather than forced into full range and strength of motion.

NURSING PROCESS —THE PATIENT WHO HAS A CAST

Assessment

The patient's record should be reviewed for information regarding the type of injury, radiograph results, and treatment of the fracture. A medical, drug, and allergy history also should be obtained from the patient or family member.

After application of a cast, certain assessments are necessary, including the following:

- Check all cast edges for smoothness once the cast is dry.
- Check the extremities (fingers, toes, hand, foot) for *any* change in skin color or temperature.
- Look for drainage: observe the color, amount, or increase in the amount.
- Check the pulse of the extremity, if possible. Absence of a pulse must be reported *immediately*.

Nursing Diagnosis

Depending on the type of cast, the area of application, type of reduction, and other factors, one or more of the following nursing diagnoses may apply. Additional diagnoses may be necessary if the patient has multiple injuries.

- Pain and discomfort related to fracture, cast pressure, other factors (specify)
- Impaired physical mobility related to cast application, limited use of upper or lower limbs
- Anxiety related to traumatic injury, enforced inactivity, other factors (specify)
- Colonic constipation related to immobility
- Potential for infection (after open reduction) related to open wound, surgery
- Total or partial (specify areas) self-care deficit related to immobility, inability to use an extremity
- Impaired skin integrity related to immobility, cast pressure
- Knowledge deficit of home care maintenance, cast care

Planning and Implementation

The major goals of the patient may include reduction in pain and discomfort, improved physical mobility, reduction in anxiety, absence of infection, normal bowel elimination, improved ability to care for self, maintenance of skin integrity, and understanding of home care management and cast care.

The major goals of nursing management may include controlling pain and discomfort, helping the patient achieve physical mobility, reducing anxiety, preventing infection, meeting the patient's needs, maintaining skin integrity, and instructing the patient in management of the cast at home.

During the entire time that a cast is on a patient, the cast and adjacent areas should be inspected at regular intervals. During the first few days after application of a cast, these evaluations should be made every 2 to 4 hours. These observations are *extremely* important because serious complications result when casts become too tight and circulation is impaired or nerves compressed.

COLOR AND TEMPERATURE.   Color is a useful index of pressure. The skin showing at the ends of the cast should be the same color as that of the rest of the body; it should not be white or cyanotic. The blanching sign also is a useful color index. The nail of the big toe or of the thumb should be compressed briefly and then released. The blood should quickly rush back into the area once pressure is released.

The fingers and toes at the end of the cast should be as warm as those on the other side of the body. If they are not, the physician should be notified *immediately*. Compression of blood vessels and nerves by a cast can cause irreparable damage. The diminished supply of oxygen and food to the tissues may result in *necrosis* (death of tissue). Volkmann's contracture apparently results from pressure, perhaps on the radial artery. The cause is not entirely clear, but compression of vital structures in the arm plays a large role. The hand becomes swollen and blue, and the radial pulse is diminished or absent. Ultimately, atrophy and deformity of the hand result.

MOVEMENT.   Unless traction or another device has been applied to prevent movement, the patient should be able to move the fingers and toes free. If movement should be present but is not, the physician should be informed immediately.

The little toe has a tendency to get lost and be compressed inside a cast that covers most of the lower leg. If this occurs, the physician should be informed.

One of the benefits of motion is that it helps reduce edema in a nearby area. The patient should be reminded to move the fingers or toes at the end of a cast every few hours.

DRAINAGE AND ODOR.   If a cast is put on a patient after an open reduction and there is bleeding from the wound, it may take longer for the blood to seep through the plaster than it would to pass through an ordinary bandage. The physician may have cut a window over the operative site to permit drainage.

The patient may return from the operating room with a drain inserted inside the cast, in which case the drain may be removed in 24 hours through a cast window.

If there is no cast window and drainage on the cast surface is noted, it should be circled with a fiber-tipped or ballpoint pen, the time noted, and the physician notified. If the area enlarges beyond the marked boundaries, the bleeding is continuing and requires immediate attention by the physician.

The cast also should be checked for any unusual odor, which may (or may not) indicate an infection beneath the cast. Sometimes, the only indication that tissues inside the cast are undergoing necrosis is the odor emitted. The patient might not complain of any pain or discomfort *beneath* the cast because loss of sensation may develop in a pressure sore. When the pressure sore becomes necrotic, infection almost always results. If an odor is noted, the physician should be notified as soon as possible.

Vital signs should be monitored every 4 hours or as ordered. A rise in temperature or chills should be reported to the physician immediately because they may be early indications of an infection.

PERIPHERAL PULSES.   When possible, the pulses of the extremity with the cast should be checked every 4 to 8 hours. Absence of a pulse should be reported *immediately*.

PATIENT COMPLAINTS.   *Any* complaint the patient has should be thoroughly investigated, recorded, and brought to the attention of the physician.

Pain and Discomfort.   Although some pain at the fracture line is expected for the first few days, continued pain requires investigation. If the patient complains of any pain or discomfort above, below, or underneath the cast, the complaint should be thoroughly investigated before an analgesic is administered. The compression of a nerve or a blood vessel can lead to permanent damage and crippling.

The patient might push an object, such as a spoon or knitting needle, into the cast to relieve itching or discomfort under the cast. These objects may become lodged in the cast, or the skin under the cast may be injured by the foreign object. If this happens, the pain caused by the object may disappear in a few days as the wound becomes anesthetized. A hot spot will develop on the cast over the trouble area, and a stain will appear. This should be reported to the physician *immediately*.

Itching, especially during hot weather, can cause great discomfort. If itching is severe, the physician should be consulted.

Impaired Physical Mobility.   Most patients in lower extremity casts without traction can become mobile

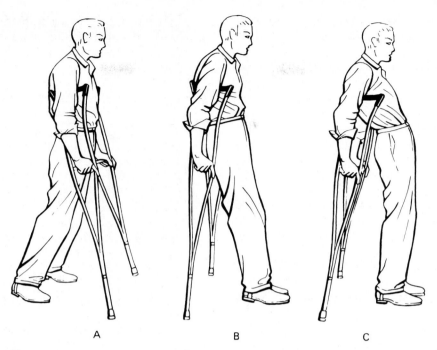

Figure 55–9.   Crutch walking using the swing-through gait. (*A*) He puts the crutches well in front of him. (*B*) The swing through. (*C*) The position in which he lands. He next puts the crutches in position (*A*).

in a short time. If the physician allows the use of crutches, the physical therapist should instruct the patient in their use. In Figure 55-9, both feet are on the floor. If the patient has a full leg cast, the extremity with the cast is bent at an angle, and only one foot is on the floor.

The patient in a body cast is completely immobile but should be turned every 2 hours. Two individuals are usually required for turning. After turning the patient, the exposed skin along the cast edges should be inspected.

EXERCISE.   The physician may prescribe physical therapy to establish a routine of daily exercises using the unaffected limbs. For example, the patient with a fracture of the left leg should exercise the left leg (if the cast does not completely immobilize the limb and hip) as well as the right leg and arms. For those whose activities are limited by the type or size of cast, coughing and deep-breathing exercises are necessary to prevent atelectasis and pneumonia.

Anxiety.   The physical discomfort of a cast, especially a body cast, can cause varying degrees of anxiety. Itching, the weight of the cast, imposed restrictions, immobility, and loss of income are some of the problems that can result in anxiety. The patient should be given the opportunity to discuss problems as they arise and, when possible, solutions should be recommended. Some problems, such as extreme itching or discomfort, require management by a physician. Other problems, such as loss of income, may require a referral to a social service worker.

Colonic Constipation.   Lack of mobility can result in constipation. The patient should be encouraged to drink extra fluids and to be as mobile as possible. The immobilized patient is more likely to develop constipation, which should be brought to the attention of the physician.

The patient in a body cast may have difficulty using the bedpan. To protect the cast from getting wet and soiled, the nurse can fit waterproof material around the edge of the cast opening and tape it to the cast. A consistently damp cast will become moldy and malodorous.

To place a patient in a spica cast on a bedpan, the space just behind the pan should be padded and the head of the bed slightly elevated. The legs should be supported with pillows to avoid strain on the cast. The anal area should be thoroughly cleaned and dried after the bedpan is removed.

Self-Care Deficit.   When an upper extremity is immobilized with a cast, implements for washing and grooming should be arranged so that the patient can perform as many of these activities as possible. Assistance always should be given as needed. The meal tray should be placed on a table or stand at the same level as the mattress so that the patient can eat. Food should be cut and liquids poured as needed.

Impaired Skin Integrity. While the patient wearing a cast is in bed, the injured limb should be kept elevated to prevent edema. Pillows may be used to elevate the limb, or the physician may order a special sling to provide greater elevation of the affected part.

During the drying period, the cast needs protection. A thumbprint applied to the cast while it is drying can leave an indentation that later may cause a pressure sore on the patient's skin. The cast should be supported with the palm of the hand rather than the fingertips.

Whenever the patient is turned or repositioned, the buttocks should be inspected, and any pieces of plaster that may have accumulated should be removed. The buttocks may be creased where the cast has pressed against the skin; these creases are lines of potential skin breakdown. Tincture of benzoin or an emollient may be applied to prevent skin breakdown. The physician should be notified if skin breakdown is apparent.

All edges of the cast—top and bottom—should be inspected several times a day for any place where it cuts into the skin. Although this is more likely to occur during the first 24 hours, it can happen at any time. In cases of pressure against the skin where there is no edema, the physician may split the cast and loosely pad the area with cotton. If there is edema around the edge of the cast, the physician should be notified at once. If edema causes pressure, the physician may bivalve the entire cast to release the pressure.

The physician may order a bivalve cast to be removed daily. The skin under the cast should be inspected for pressure areas or any signs of infection. Care should be taken not to pinch the skin when the cast is reapplied.

Knowledge Deficit. Some patients are discharged after application of the cast. Those requiring open reduction with or without internal fixation may be discharged several days to a week after surgery, and they may be sent home wearing a cast. Chart 55-1 is an example of a printed instruction sheet that gives directions for home care. The directions should be reviewed with the patient or family member.

The patient should be instructed to keep the cast dry and not allow water or other liquid to seep inside the cast. Although casts are durable, they do break. A particularly active patient may need to be told of this possibility.

If the patient with a fracture of the upper extremity is advised by the physician to wear a sling during the day, instructions for making and applying the sling must be given. The patient should be reminded to make sure that the knot does not rest exactly at the

---

Chart 55–1. Instructions for Home Care—Patients Who Have Casts

☐ Go to bed as soon as you get home. Stay in bed for the next 24 hr. You may get up to go to the bathroom.
☐ While you are in bed, keep the injured arm or leg elevated on a pillow. (Protect the pillow with plastic material as long as the cast is damp.) The hand or the foot should be the highest part of the body.
☐ Whenever you get out of bed, keep the injured arm in a sling. If your leg is injured, and you sit for longer than 15 min, elevate your leg on a chair or stool.
☐ Move your fingers (arm cast) or toes (leg cast) for several minutes every 30 min.
☐ If the cast feels tight, exercise the fingers or the toes and elevate the limb. If the tightness is not relieved, come to the hospital (emergency entrance). Immediately (day or night) report to the hospital or your doctor if you notice any of the following:
☐ Numbness of fingers or toes
☐ Swelling of fingers or toes
☐ Blueness of fingers or toes
☐ Severe pain in the limb
☐ A crack or break in your cast (if noticed at night, wait until morning to report to the hospital)

---

back of the neck but to the side. To prevent edema of the fingers, the sling should be adjusted so that the fingers are higher than the elbow. The patient should be advised to exercise the shoulder that bears the weight of the sling and the cast.

The physician also may give additional instructions to the patient, especially if an open reduction was required. These instructions should be reviewed with the patient.

Evaluation

■ Pain and discomfort are reduced
■ Physical mobility is improved
■ Anxiety is reduced
■ No evidence of infection; vital signs are normal
■ Bowel elimination is normal
■ Patient assumes some, most, or all of own care
■ Skin remains intact; no evidence of decubitus, nerve paralysis, loss of feeling
■ Patient demonstrates understanding of the care of the cast when at home

TRACTION

Traction is the pull provided by a series of weights, ropes, and pulleys that are connected to either a frame, to a wire or pin, or to straps applied to the skin of the patient. *Countertraction* is the force against the traction and is usually supplied by the weight of the patient's body. The application of traction is done by the physician. Maintenance of traction is absolutely necessary. Weights must hang free, ropes and pulleys must be free from interference, and splints and slings must be suspended without interference.

Several principles are involved in effective traction:

1. Traction must be continuous.
2. Countertraction must be applied.
3. The traction apparatus must be correctly maintained.

Various types of traction can be used to maintain alignment and immobilization. The two most common types are skin traction and skeletal traction. Skin traction uses pull-on tapes or traction strips attached to the skin, usually by elastic bandages. Examples of skin traction are Russell traction (see Fig. 55-5) and Buck's extension (see Fig. 55-6). *Skeletal traction* uses a wire (Kirschner) or pin (Steinmann) inserted in the bone, with traction applied to the pin or wire. The Thomas splint with the Pearson attachment is often used with the Kirschner wire or Steinmann pin to provide balanced skeletal traction.

NURSING PROCESS —THE PATIENT IN TRACTION

Assessment

Traction is usually set up by a physician. Once the traction apparatus is in place, the nurse should check all wires, pulleys, and weights to become familiar with each part of the traction apparatus.

The patient's chart should be reviewed for diagnosis, type of fracture, and prior treatments. Vital signs should be taken. The patient's general physical and mental condition should be evaluated to provide baseline data. Because the patient most likely will be in traction for several weeks or more, immobilization can lead to problems such as anxiety, confusion, disorientation, and anorexia.

If the patient had an open reduction with or without internal fixation, routine postoperative assessments should be carried out at the time of the initial assessment.

Nursing Diagnosis

Depending on the age and condition of the patient and whether other injuries are concurrently present, one or more of the following nursing diagnoses may apply:

- Anxiety related to immobilization, long period of treatment, discomfort, loss of income, other factors (specify)
- Pain or discomfort related to recent injury, surgery

- Impaired physical mobility related to traction
- Total or partial (specify areas) self-care deficit related to immobilization
- Colonic constipation related to immobility
- Impaired skin integrity related to immobilization
- Ineffective breathing pattern related to immobility
- Potential for infection related to initial injury, surgery (open reduction), insertion of Steinmann pin, Kirschner wire, or other device for balanced skeletal traction
- Knowledge deficit of treatment, traction device

Planning and Implementation

The major goals of the patient may include reduction in anxiety, relief of pain and discomfort, improved mobility, increased ability to care for self, absence of constipation, absence of skin breakdown and infection, and understanding of the treatment modalities.

The major goals of nursing management may include reduction in anxiety, relief of pain and discomfort, improvement in mobility, meeting the patient's self-care needs, prevention of constipation, prevention of infection and skin breakdown, and effective explanation of the purpose of traction.

The patient may remain in traction for many weeks, making nursing care a very important part of the return to optimal function. Because traction is used to realign and immobilize a fractured bone, it is imperative that correct principles of traction—that is, traction and countertraction—are maintained. All the ropes must be in the grooves of the pulleys (during movement a rope can jump its track). Ropes and pulleys must be checked several times a day to be sure they are functioning properly. *Weights never should be lifted, released, increased, or decreased unless there is a specific written order from the physician to do so.*

If suspension traction is working properly, the patient's leg will rise when the hips are lifted. If the leg does not rise, the ropes should be checked to make sure they are in the grooves of the pulleys, and the weights should be checked to make sure they are hanging free. If the leg still does not rise, notify the physician because the traction may require adjustment.

Nursing management of the patient in traction is summarized in Chart 55-2.

The patient in traction is more or less immobile in that he or she is confined to bed. This, then, prompts the institution of special points of nursing management to prevent the complications that arise from immobilization, including the following:

- Skin breakdown, decubitus formation
- Pneumonia and other respiratory problems
- Muscle atrophy, contractures, foot drop
- Urinary tract infection

Chart 55-2.   Nursing Management of the Patient in Traction

- □ Check traction alignment:
  - □ Weights, splints, and slings should hang free.
  - □ The body should be in alignment with the force of traction.
  - □ The head of the bed should be raised only to the prescribed height.
- □ Encourage motion and exercise in the *unaffected* limbs.
- □ Use a footboard to prevent footdrop.
- □ Use a trochanter roll for the unaffected leg.
- □ Encourage participation in daily care.
- □ Have the patient do deep-breathing exercises every 1 or 2 hr while awake.
- □ When giving care, use gentle movements and avoid excessive jarring of the bed.
- □ Give frequent skin care, with particular attention to bony prominences.
- □ Check for early signs of decubitus formation: blanched skin, reddened areas, pain or discomfort over pressure points.
- □ Keep bottom sheets taut and free of wrinkles.
- □ Use sheepskin pads, foam rubber supports, or an alternating pressure mattress at the first sign of skin breakdown (elderly patients may need these measures from the beginning).
- □ Be alert to signs of infection at sites of pin or wire insertion and operative site (if surgery was performed).
- □ Encourage intake of fluids unless specifically contraindicated by a physician's order.
- □ Keep all items within reach: bedside stand, call light, personal effects, etc.
- □ Make sure that traction is continuous and that weights are *never* released unless so ordered by the physician.
- □ Check for signs of circulatory impairment in all extremities but especially in the affected extremity:
  - □ Blanching or discoloration of the extremity
  - □ Coolness of skin when compared with the opposite extremity
  - □ Absence of peripheral pulses

- ■ Kidney stone formation
- ■ Thromboembolism, fat embolism (which may be seen after fractures of the long bones)
- ■ Heart failure, circulatory disturbances (especially in the elderly)
- ■ Constipation

Intake and output should be measured for the first several days and continued if fluid intake is low. Fluids must be encouraged because an increase in the fluid intake reduces the chance of kidney stone formation—a complication of prolonged bed rest and limited fluid intake. Fluids should be readily available by placement of the bedside stand close to the bed.

The extremities should be checked frequently to see that the affected hand or foot is warm and of normal color. Sensation should be normal when the foot or the hand is touched. There should be no numbness or tingling. If cyanosis, mottling, or coolness occur, if the patient complains of sudden numbness or tingling, or if a peripheral pulse cannot be obtained, the physician must be notified *immediately*.

Anxiety.   Many situations and events can create anxiety in the immobilized patient. Concerned nursing care and anticipation of the patient's needs may minimize the feeling of helplessness.

Diversion therapy is important for any patient confined for a long period of time. An occupational therapist can offer suggestions or plan therapy that is tailored to the patient's needs and preferences.

Because hospitalization is prolonged, the patient may encounter many types of problems. The nurse must allow time for these patients to discuss their problems and concerns and, when necessary, contact the appropriate individuals who may be able to solve or resolve the situation.

Pain or Discomfort.   Narcotic analgesics are often necessary for a period of time after placing the patient in traction. Gentleness is important because excessive movement causes pain. Linen changes are best done by two people, especially if the patient's movement is restricted.

Embolism and thromboembolism are complications of prolonged immobility. If the patient complains of pain or discomfort in the extremities or chest or if sudden neurologic symptoms occur, the physician should be notified immediately.

Sometimes, little annoyances cause great discomfort and anxiety. For example, if the patient complains of chilliness in the suspended arm or leg, and it is certain that there is no impairment of circulation, a small cover (flannel sheet or light blanket) may be placed over the extremity. The covering should be light and not interfere with the slings, splints, or ropes of the traction.

Impaired Physical Mobility, Self-Care Deficit.   Depending on the type and location of the fracture and the type of traction used, the patient may or may not be allowed certain movements—for example, turning, lifting the hips, or having the head of the bed raised. A trapeze may be suspended over the bed to help the patient lift the hips or turn. The amount of movement allowed should be ordered by the physician.

Exercises should be encouraged to prevent muscle atrophy. The physical therapist should direct the patient in those exercises performed on the affected extremity; the nurse must encourage use of the unaffected extremities. This can be done, in part, by having patients assist in their own care as often and as much as possible.

The ability of patients in traction to perform their care should be evaluated at least weekly. Although they should be encouraged to do as much as possible, whatever care cannot be performed must be done for them.

Range-of-motion (ROM) exercises may be ordered. The nurse or the physical therapist is responsible for performing these exercises on those incapable of self-exercise and for demonstrating and supervising the exercises of those not requiring physical assistance.

Colonic Constipation. A record of bowel movements should be kept, and the patient should be encouraged to drink extra fluids. A fracture pan (or orthopedic pan) rather than a regular bedpan usually is preferred because it eliminates elevation of the hips. A kidney (emesis) basin may be used for female patients if urination is difficult on a fracture pan. Stool softeners may be necessary because confinement to bed and the use of a bedpan encourage constipation.

A urinary tract infection or stone formation is a complication of prolonged immobilization. If the patient complains of difficulty in urinating, pain on urination, or sudden severe pain in the area of the kidney, back, or bladder, the physician should be notified.

Impaired Skin Integrity. The mattress on the traction bed should be firm and level. A bed board may be used under the mattress. Bottom sheets should be pulled taut, and all wrinkles eliminated. Bottom sheets may be changed from side to side or top to bottom. The latter maneuver is especially useful with accident victims who have incurred multiple injuries of the extremities and trunk.

The bony prominences (elbows, heels, sacrum, and so forth) should be checked for early signs of decubitus formation. The patient's elbows may become sore from rubbing the sheet. Long-sleeved gowns may help to protect them. The patient should be advised to use the overhead trapeze to lift and turn (when these movements are allowed) rather than the elbows.

Back care may offer a challenge, especially when movement is limited. Firm, downward pressure on the mattress near the part to be massaged gives room for the nurse's hand. Keeping the patient's skin soft and smooth is important because decubitus formation is a frequent complication, especially in the thin or elderly patient. Special attention should be given to the sacral area—a common early site of skin breakdown—which is not easily inspected when the patient cannot turn from side to side. Lamb's wool padding may be used to protect pressure areas. Lotion should be applied several times a day to those areas subject to skin breakdown. If early signs of skin breakdown are apparent, the physician should be consulted. An alternating pressure mattress or other type of mattress used to reduce pressure on bony prominences may be ordered.

Ineffective Breathing Pattern. The patient should be instructed to deep breathe and cough every 2 hours while awake because pneumonia and atelectasis are common complications of immobility. The lungs should be auscultated daily when vital signs are taken. Any sudden rise in temperature, chills, abnormal breathing sounds, or productive cough should be brought to the attention of the physician.

Potential for Infection. Systemic antibiotics are usually ordered after an open reduction or insertion of pins or wires for skeletal traction.

If skeletal traction or an external fixator is applied, the pin or wire sites should be inspected daily for signs of infection, namely redness, swelling, and purulent drainage. Although some swelling and slight redness may be normal, any increase should be reported. Serous drainage often is normal, but purulent drainage may indicate a serious infection in the underlying tissues and bone.

Knowledge Deficit. The array of bars, ropes, and pulleys may frighten the patient at first. Most fracture patients come to the hospital on an emergency basis, and they may be in traction before they have had time to recover from the shock of the experience. At first, simple and direct explanations should be given. Most important, these patients should be assured that their needs will be taken care of. It is important that the patient understand the purpose of the equipment, the approximate length of time that traction must be used, and the discomfort to be expected.

REMOVAL FROM TRACTION. When the patient is removed from traction, the physician orders the amount of movement to be allowed. Physical therapy also is ordered. The amount of movement allowed by the physician should be reviewed with the patient so there is complete understanding of what movement is permitted. The importance of adhering to any restrictions should be stressed.

If the limb has been in traction for a considerable time, it will at first feel stiff, and there also may be some atrophy of muscles, making the limb look thinner. These facts should be explained to the patient, and the patient should be reassured that the feeling of stiffness will disappear and that the muscles will gradually grow firm and strong again with therapeutic exercise.

Evaluation

- Anxiety is reduced
- Pain and discomfort are controlled
- Patient demonstrates improved physical mobility
- Patient is able to assume responsibility for most of own care
- Bowel elimination is normal
- Skin remains intact; no evidence of skin breakdown or decubitus formation
- Lungs are clear to auscultation; vital signs are normal; patient coughs and deep breathes every 2 hours
- No evidence of infection; pin or wire sites are clean
- Patient demonstrates understanding of treatment, traction device

ORTHOPEDIC SURGERY

Orthopedic surgery may be performed for many different reasons, including the following:

- To correct a deformity
- To remove a primary bone tumor
- To align bones that have been fractured (open reduction)
- To replace a joint
- To repair damage to tendons and ligaments
- To replace bone with a bone graft to stabilize or replace bone or aid in the healing of bone
- To stabilize a bone with rods, screws, nails, or wires (internal fixation)

NURSING PROCESS —THE PATIENT UNDERGOING ORTHOPEDIC SURGERY

Preoperative Period

Assessment
A complete medical, drug, and allergy history should be obtained from the patient or a family member. A general assessment of the patient's physical condition and mental status also should be made at the time of the initial interview. The patient's chart should be reviewed for the diagnosis, type of surgery to be performed, and any previous treatments, such as traction or drugs. If the disorder has been treated, it is important to know if any complications or problems occurred because of or during treatment.

Nursing Diagnosis
Depending on the diagnosis, type of surgery, age of the patient, and other factors, one or more of the following nursing diagnoses may apply:

- Anxiety related to surgery, diagnosis
- Pain related to traumatic injury
- Impaired physical mobility related to deformity, pain, injury, other factors (specify)
- Knowledge deficit of the preparations for surgery and postoperative management

Planning and Implementation
The major goals of the patient may include reduction in anxiety, relief of pain, and understanding of the preoperative preparations and postoperative management.

The major goals of nursing management may include reduction in anxiety, reduction in pain or discomfort, assistance with tasks requiring mobility, implementation of an effective preoperative teaching plan, and preparation of the patient physically and emotionally for surgery. The preoperative preparations may vary depending on the type of surgery to be performed and the physician's preference.

Anxiety, Knowledge Deficit. The physician discusses the type of and rationale for surgery and the results to be expected with the patient and family. In addition, postoperative management, such as the application of traction or physical therapy, also is discussed. The nurse may need to review the explanations given by the physician.

Many patients scheduled for orthopedic surgery have a deformity, injury, or pain and willingly accept the fact that surgery is necessary. These patients still have concerns about other matters, such as a prolonged period of inactivity, loss of income, and whether the surgery will be successful. These patients must be allowed time to talk about their concerns and, in some instances, the problem may need to be brought to the attention of the physician.

To reduce anxiety, all preoperative preparations should be explained to the patient. In addition, postoperative management, such as moving (as allowed), coughing, and deep breathing should be demonstrated, and the patient should be allowed to practice these maneuvers before surgery.

Pain. Some patients, such as those with a traumatic injury, may require analgesics for pain during the preoperative period.

Impaired Physical Mobility. The ambulatory patient (eg, the patient scheduled for a hip replacement because of arthritis), may require assistance in getting out of bed or walking. The patient should receive assistance with these activities because injuries can occur when the hip and lower extremities are affected by disorders such as severe and disabling arthritis.

Evaluation

■ Anxiety is reduced
■ Pain is controlled
■ Patient ambulates with assistance
■ Patient demonstrates understanding of preoperative preparations, postoperative management
■ Patient demonstrates understanding of physician's explanations of type of and reason for surgery and results expected

Postoperative Period

Assessment

When the patient returns from the operating room, vital signs should be taken, and the patient's chart should be reviewed for the type of surgery and for the condition of the patient during and immediately after surgery.

Nursing Diagnosis

Depending on the type of surgery, the condition of the patient, and other factors, one or more of the following nursing diagnoses may apply. Additional nursing diagnoses applying to general postoperative management or the patient in a cast or traction may be added.

■ Pain related to surgery
■ Hyperthermia related to infection
■ Potential for infection related to surgery
■ Impaired physical mobility related to surgical procedure, postoperative use of traction or other immobilizing devices (splints, casts, external fixator)
■ Anxiety related to pain, discomfort, immobilization, results of surgery, other factors (specify)
■ Colonic constipation related to immobility
■ Ineffective breathing pattern related to immobility
■ Impaired skin integrity related to immobility
■ Total or partial (specify areas) self-care deficit related to immobility, surgical procedure
■ Knowledge deficit of home care management

Planning and Implementation

The major goals of the patient may include relief of pain and discomfort, normal body temperature, absence of infection, improved physical mobility, reduction in anxiety, normal bowel elimination, maximum pulmonary function, absence of skin breakdown, improved ability to care for self, and understanding of home care management.

The major goals of nursing management may include relief of pain, prevention of infection, reduction in anxiety, attainment of normal bowel function and pulmonary function, prevention of skin breakdown and decubitus formation, assistance of the patient with activities of daily living, and preparation and implementation of an effective discharge teaching plan.

Vital signs should be monitored at frequent intervals. Shock and infection are two of the major complications of orthopedic surgery. Shock may occur after surgery because there is a tendency for bleeding during surgery. Severe pain that is not relieved also may cause shock. A decrease in blood pressure with a rise in pulse requires contacting the physician immediately.

A fat embolus is another possible complication after fracture of or surgery on the long bones. The symptoms of a fat embolus are the same as those of an embolus caused by a blood clot. In addition, petechial hemorrhages may be seen on the skin of the chest if the embolus is lodged in the lungs.

Nursing Care Plan 55-1 is an example of postoperative nursing management after surgery for a fractured hip.

Pain. Pain immediately after any type of orthopedic surgery can be severe. Narcotic analgesics should be given as ordered. Continued severe pain after the first several postoperative days requires investigation, as does pain in an area other than the operative area.

Hyperthermia, Potential for Infection. Infection is a serious complication of orthopedic surgery. The patient's temperature should be monitored every 4 hours, and elevations should be reported to the physician.

The surgical area may consist of pin or wire sites, a surgical incision, or a cast window over a surgical incision. These areas should be inspected every 2 to 4 hours for signs of infection. While pain is normally present, severe pain must be investigated and brought to the attention of the physician. Any signs of infection—elevated temperature, increase in pain, or wound drainage that has an odor or appearance of infection—must be reported immediately because intensive antibiotic therapy may be necessary.

Impaired Physical Mobility. Depending on the type of surgery, varying degrees of immobility may be present. The patient requires assistance moving in bed, and gentleness should be used when supporting, raising, or adjusting the patient's position.

Unless the physician orders otherwise, active or passive exercises should be performed on the unoperated extremities to prevent muscle atrophy. Patients able to do so should be shown how to perform these exercises.

As healing progresses, the patient may be allowed to become more mobile, and physical therapy should be instituted to improve use of the operated extremity.

Nursing Care Plan 55–1

Postoperative Management of the Patient With a Fractured Hip

Potential Problem and Potential Nursing Diagnosis	Nursing Intervention	Outcome Criteria
Pain/Discomfort *Pain related to tissue trauma*	Administer analgesics as ordered; change position q 2 hr or more frequently; exercise care when repositioning patient; encourage active exercises	Pain controlled; discomfort decreased or absent
Skin Breakdown *Impaired skin integrity related to immobility*	Reposition q 2 hr; keep skin clean and dry; massage skin over bony prominences q 4 hr; use sheep skin padding or other devices to protect bony prominences or place patient on an alternating pressure mattress; keep bed linen taut and free from wrinkles	No evidence of skin breakdown
Venous Stasis Resulting in Thromboembolism	Encourage ROM exercises in unaffected extremities q 2 hr; encourage ankle flexion exercises and pushing against the footboard q 2 hr; apply antiembolic stockings (if ordered); encourage self-care (which encourages active movement of the extremities) to extent patient is able to assume these tasks; check for calf tenderness or pain and inspect legs for signs of swelling or redness q 2–4 hr; check peripheral pulses, color, and temperature of extremities, q 2–4 hr	No evidence of development of thromboembolism; patient performs ROM exercises and other activities as instructed
Respiratory Problems (Pneumonia, Atelectasis, etc.) *Ineffective breathing pattern related to postanesthesia state, postoperative immobility, and pain*	Encourage deep breathing and coughing q 2 hr; monitor temperature q 4 hr; auscultate lungs q 4 hr; encourage fluids	Lungs remain clear on auscultation; deep breathing and coughing are performed q 2 hr; patient increases fluid intake
Constipation *Constipation related to decreased peristalsis secondary to effects of anesthesia, immobility, and pain medication*	Encourage fluid intake; obtain dietary consult regarding dietary change (prune juice, bran, high-fiber foods); administer stool softener if ordered; check for bowel movement and consistency of stool daily	Constipation relieved or avoided
Urinary Tract Problems (Urinary Retention, Urinary Tract Infection) *Altered patterns of urinary elimination: urinary retention secondary to surgery and immobility*	Increase fluid intake; monitor intake and output; cleanse anal and perineal area after each bowel movement (especially important in female patients to prevent lower urinary tract contamination with *Escherichia coli*); observe urine for evidence of infection (cloudiness, sediment, odor)	Maintains adequate fluid intake and urinary output; no evidence of urinary tract infection
Limited Range of Motion in Joints (Other Than Hip) of Affected Side *Impaired physical mobility related to pain and activity restriction*	Perform passive exercises to knee and ankle q 2–4 hr	No evidence of joint restriction

Continued

Nursing Care Plan 55-1
Postoperative Management of the Patient With a Fractured Hip Continued

Potential Problem and Potential Nursing Diagnosis	Nursing Intervention	Outcome Criteria
Surgical Wound Infection *Potential for wound infection related to prolonged immobility, contact with contagious agents, loss of defense against bacterial invasion*	Take vital signs q 4 hr; inspect incision at time of each dressing change; use aseptic technique for all dressing changes; inspect dressing for evidence of drainage each time patient is repositioned	No evidence of wound infection
Decreased Muscle Strength When Ambulatory; Muscle Contractures *Impaired physical mobility: contractures related to loss of motion secondary to pain, bedrest*	Encourage ROM exercises, quadriceps and gluteal exercises q 2–4 hr; encourage participation in self-care; encourage use of upper extremities for movement in bed; collaborate with physical and occupational therapists for exercise and muscle-strengthening programs; assist patient out of bed into chair as ordered	Ambulates with aid (walker, cane, crutches, nursing personnel) without apparent loss of muscle strength and ambulates at optimum level of ability
Mental Changes (Confusion, Depression); Dependency on Others *Ineffective individual coping in response to identifiable stressors*	Orient as necessary; converse with patient; provide diversional activities; offer encouragement regarding progress; encourage communication with others (visitors, other patients, hospital personnel); encourage participation in decisions regarding own care; encourage independence by having patient participate in own care	Remains oriented; no depression or withdrawal apparent

ROM, range-of-motion.

Anxiety. Pain produces anxiety. Because pain is most severe during the first postoperative days, narcotic analgesics should be administered as ordered.

Discomfort also results in anxiety. Those who are immobilized and require extended hospitalization often have a problem dealing with minor discomforts that other patients tend to ignore. Wrinkled sheets, cold coffee, or inability to reach the television remote control can create anxiety. The nurse must make every attempt to control or eliminate those situations that appear to upset the patient.

There may be other causes of anxiety related to hospitalization and the results of surgery. Patients should be given time to discuss their concerns. If a problem warrants referral to a social service worker or community agency, this should be discussed with the physician.

Colonic Constipation. Immobility can result in colonic constipation. A record of bowel movements

should be kept. If constipation occurs, this should be brought to the attention of the physician. Some physicians routinely prescribe a stool softener as well as a high-fiber diet for these patients. The patient also should be encouraged to drink fluids.

Respiratory Function. Coughing and deep-breathing exercises should be encouraged every 2 hours until the patient is able to be out of bed and ambulate. The lungs should be auscultated at least daily. The physician should be informed if chills, fever, or productive cough occurs or if abnormal breath sounds are noted.

Impaired Skin Integrity. Although some orthopedic surgeries confine the patient to bed or limit movement for only a few days, other surgeries require prolonged immobility. General skin care, keeping the skin clean and dry, and keeping the bottom sheet free of wrinkles are important in helping prevent skin problems.

Pressure areas should be inspected daily for early signs of skin breakdown. When noted, immediate steps should be taken to relieve pressure on the affected areas. Various methods can be used to do this, such as an air or egg crate mattress or sheepskin pad. A silicone and zinc oxide mixture or tincture of benzoin applied to susceptible areas may be of value but should never replace good skin care. There also are a variety of beds on the market, such as the Clinitron bed, that help relieve pressure on the bony prominences.

Self-Care Deficit.   One or two days after surgery, the patient may be able to participate in some self-care activities. The nurse must evaluate the patient's ability to participate in these activities and then determine how much assistance is needed. Self-care is encouraged because movement of the unaffected extremities is a form of active exercise.

Knowledge Deficit.   The discharge teaching plan depends on the type of surgery performed and the physician's specific orders. The prescribed rehabilitation plan should be reviewed with the patient or a family member. The importance of rehabilitation should be stressed.

The following information may be incorporated in a patient teaching plan:

1. Eat a well-balanced and nutritious diet and drink plenty of fluids.
2. Follow the physician's instructions regarding care of the incision.
3. Perform the exercises prescribed by the physician and physical therapist.
4. Take the prescribed medications as directed on the container.
5. Notify the physician if fever, chills, sudden onset of pain, or redness, swelling, or drainage from the incision occur. The physician also should be notified if any other problem occurs, such as nausea, vomiting, difficulty urinating, constipation, or productive cough.

Evaluation

- Pain and discomfort are relieved
- Vital signs are normal
- No evidence of infection
- Physical mobility is improved
- Anxiety is reduced
- Bowel elimination is normal
- Patient coughs and deep breathes every 2 hours; lungs are clear to auscultation
- Skin is clean and dry with no evidence of decubitus formation
- Patient assumes most or all responsibility for own care
- Patient demonstrates understanding of home care

management, rehabilitation exercises, wound care, problems requiring notifying the physician

RHEUMATIC DISORDERS

A *rheumatic disorder* involves bones, joints, and muscles. The various types of rheumatic disorders, taken as a group, are the most common connective tissue diseases. There are more than 100 different types of rheumatic disorders.

Rheumatoid Arthritis

Arthritis means inflammation of a joint. Along with degenerative joint disease, rheumatoid arthritis is one of the major causes of arthritic disability in adults.

Rheumatoid arthritis is a systemic inflammatory disorder of connective tissue characterized by chronicity, remissions, and exacerbations. Its nature is not fully understood, and its cause is unknown. This crippling disease strikes during the most productive years of adulthood, usually in the 20- to 40-year-old group; however, the disorder also can be found in older individuals. Women appear to be affected more than men in the younger age groups, but the incidence in older individuals is about equal.

Synovitis (inflammation of the synovial membrane surrounding a joint) is the earliest pathologic change and causes congestion and edema. Pathophysiologic changes follow, leading to the formation of a tissue that adheres to the opposite joint surface, inhibiting motion. This is the stage of *fibrous ankylosis* (abnormal immobility of a joint).

When the restricting band of tissue becomes calcified, as it may, the stage of *osseous ankylosis* has occurred, and the joint no longer exists. This process —from nonspecific synovitis to complete ossification of the joint—may take years, and it may occur at different rates in different joints in the same patient.

Constitutional symptoms and joint changes, which may become permanent deformities, are part of the disease (Fig. 55-10).

Symptoms

In most patients, the onset of rheumatoid arthritis is insidious. Over a period of time, patients notice that a joint or two is stiff when they wake up in the morning, or there may be momentary discomfort in a joint. Slowly, some joints, usually the fingers, become moderately sore, red, and swollen. Over a period of weeks, other joints become involved. Swelling and pain may come and go. In the meantime, patients find that they tire easily. They lose weight and may develop fever and malaise. Tolerance for any kind of stress is lessened, and temperature changes are tolerated poorly. Although the diet may be adequate in iron, patients

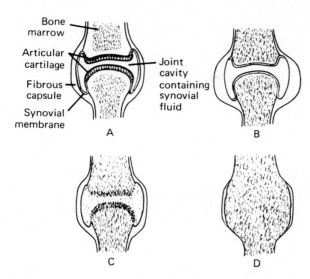

Figure 55–10. Pathologic changes in rheumatoid arthritis. (*A*) Normal ball-and-socket joint. (*B*) Same joint, showing progression of pannus formation, destruction of cartilage, and acute inflammation. (*C*) Inflammation subsided; fibrous ankylosis. (*D*) Bony ankylosis; the joint is immobile.

characteristically have a persistent anemia because of the effect of this disorder on the blood-forming organs.

The local effects on joints is due to the disease itself as well as the body's reactions against the inflammatory process. For example, the replacement of damaged tissue by fibrosis is a defense mechanism of the body; however, scars due to fibrosis can lead to crippling contractures.

Some patients develop subcutaneous nodules. These appear over pressure points, such as the elbow or the base of the spine. Though usually painless, they may be painful if continuous pressure is put on them, as in a chair-bound patient with nodules at the base of the spine.

Muscles become weak and atrophy, partially from disuse. Because of connective tissue and neurovascular changes, the extremities often have a smooth, glossy appearance, and they may be cold and clammy.

As the disease progresses, muscle wasting around affected joints accentuates the appearance of swelling. The proximal finger joints swell the most, and as deformity develops, the fingers may point toward the lateral aspect of the hand (Fig. 55-11). Extremities often become cold and moist. Patients in this stage of the disease have considerable pain at rest as well as when moving.

The symptoms may vanish suddenly for no apparent reason. Inflammation leaves joints that were sore and red; the patient is not stiff, has no fever, and the pain is gone. Yet the symptoms almost invariably return after the patient has had a symptom-free period. Inflammation causes more joint damage, followed by another

remission. The pattern of remissions and exacerbations can continue for years.

Without treatment—and sometimes with it—the joint may be totally destroyed. As the synovial space is replaced with bony growth, motion is lost. When the joint becomes immobile, the pain of the inflammation is lessened, but there still is discomfort because of contractures and immobility.

Diagnosis

Diagnosis is based on symptoms and physical examination of the affected joints. Radiographs may be taken to determine the extent of joint damage. Aspiration of the synovial fluid under local anesthesia may be done for microscopic examination. In rheumatoid arthritis, the synovial fluid usually appears cloudy and dark yellow and may contain white blood cells. Arthroscopic examination also may be carried out to visualize the extent of joint damage as well as to obtain a sample of synovial fluid.

Laboratory tests that may be ordered include a C-reactive protein (which may be positive), complete blood count (CBC; which may show anemia), and a rheumatoid factor (RF; which may be positive).

Treatment

Although rheumatoid arthritis cannot be cured, much can be done to lessen its damage. One of the aims of treatment should be to decrease the inflammation of the joint before it has become one bone. Early treatment before the onset of fibrous or bony ankylosis gives the best results. Treatment should be designed to make the patient more comfortable, to prevent or cor-

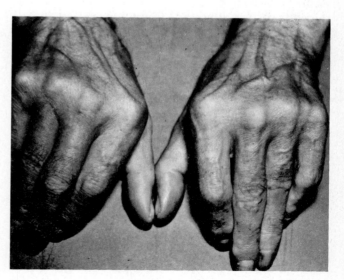

Figure 55–11. Appearance typical of arthritic hands. The joints become sore, swollen, and deformed. (Medichrome, Clay-Adams, Inc, New York, NY)

rect deformities, and to maintain or restore function of the affected parts of the musculoskeletal system.

Optimal health conditions should be maintained because supporting the resistance of the body to the inflammation is one of the few truly therapeutic steps that medicine has to offer. Rest, both systemic and local, should be balanced carefully with exercise. Even during an acute phase of the illness, some movement of the affected parts is usually prescribed to help lessen the possibility of bony ankylosis, muscle wasting, osteoporosis, and the debilitating effects of prolonged rest. Deep-breathing and prescribed exercises, graded to the condition of the patient, strengthen general body tone and keep specific muscle groups from atrophy. The patient should be encouraged to eat a nutritious, well-balanced diet, even though anorexia may be present. Unless there are other medical complications, such as diabetes or hypertension, this diet need not be modified from that of a normal individual.

Drug therapy in rheumatoid arthritis is not curative, but it helps relieve pain, and in some instances, it depresses the inflammatory process. Because of the long-term nature of this disorder, relief of pain by the use of narcotics should be avoided.

SALICYLATES. Aspirin (acetylsalicylic acid) is the major drug in this group. In early rheumatoid arthritis, it has an antiinflammatory action and relieves joint pain. In chronic rheumatoid arthritis, the relief appears less dramatic, but still it is present and probably is related more to the general analgesic properties of aspirin than to any specific action.

CORTICOSTEROIDS. Corticosteroids do not cure arthritis, but they do give the patient prompt relief from pain and stiffness. Both physical and mental well-being are improved. Long-term use of a corticosteroid may result in adverse effects that are more disabling than the disease being treated. Close supervision by the physician is imperative.

OTHER DRUGS. Phenylbutazone (Butazolidin) and oxyphenbutazone are drugs with analgesic and antiinflammatory activity. Because both drugs can cause serious adverse effects, particularly to the bone marrow and kidneys, patients must be under close medical supervision while taking either of these drugs.

Another group of drugs used in the treatment of rheumatoid arthritis are the nonsteroidal antiinflammatory drugs (NSAIDs). Like aspirin, these drugs are used in the treatment of osteoarthritis and for the relief of minor pain. They possess antiinflammatory, analgesic, and antipyretic activities. Examples of drugs in this group include fenoprofen (Nalfon), ibuprofen (Motrin), indomethacin (Indocin), meclofenamate (Meclomen), ketoprofen (Orudis), sulindac (Clinoril), and flurbiprofen (Ansaid).

The gold salts auranofin (Ridaura), aurothioglucose (Solganal), and sodium thiomalate (Myochrysine) produce less dramatic results in treatment because 2 or 3 months may elapse between the start of gold therapy and the therapeutic results of decreased inflammation and pain. The time lapse may be discouraging to the patient. Therapy with gold is not always effective. The use of gold can result in serious adverse effects, including jaundice, blood dyscrasias, hepatitis, hematuria, toxic nephritis, and severe gastrointestinal disorders. The patient should be observed carefully by blood counts and urinalysis and questioned about skin manifestations to detect early the more severe toxic effects. Aurothioglucose and sodium thiomalate are given intramuscularly; auranofin is given orally.

Hydroxychloroquine sulfate (Plaquenil) also may be prescribed for patients not responding to aspirin and the NSAIDs. Penicillamine (Cuprimine) may be prescribed for those not responding to other less toxic therapies. Response to this drug is slow (2 or 3 months), and the adverse effects are severe.

Azathioprine, an immunosuppressive drug, is used in severe cases of patients not responding to other therapies. Methotrexate, an antineoplastic agent and captopril (Capoten), an antihypertensive drug, are being used investigatively in those not responding to other therapies.

Degenerative Joint Disease (Osteoarthritis)

Osteoarthritis is a disease of the joints characterized by a slow and steady progression of destructive changes. Unlike rheumatoid arthritis, degenerative joint disease has no remissions and no systemic symptoms, such as malaise and fever. It is a wear-and-tear disease that may start as early as the middle 30s, but it is mainly an affliction of later middle life and old age. Repeated trauma may lead to degenerative changes. Obese people, whose joints must bear heavy weight, are more likely to develop early symptoms than are lean people. Genetic predisposition to arthritis also may be a factor in the occurrence of the disease.

Osteoarthritis is a reflection of generalized aging. The cartilage that covers the bone edge becomes thin and ragged and no longer springs back into shape after normal use. Finally, the bone end is bare. The synovial membrane, which at first is normal, becomes thickened. The fibrous tissue around the joint ossifies. These changes, which occur slowly, give the patient pain and limited motion of the joint. Ankylosis does not occur.

Symptoms

Osteoarthritis is a progressive disease. Early symptoms are stiffness—usually at night or in the morning—and pain that may be noted after exercise. Later, symptoms are more prominent: marked joint enlargement, pronounced stiffness, and pain after exercise. Heberden's nodes, or enlargement of the distal interphalangeal joints of the fingers, is a common symptom.

Diagnosis

Diagnosis is made on the basis of symptoms and examination of the affected joints. Radiographs also demonstrate joint changes.

Treatment

Proper local rest of the affected joints is more important than total body rest. Short periods of moderate exercise are helpful. Repeated five or six times a day, exercises should be regulated by the feeling of the joint. Postural defects that add to the strain on a joint theoretically should be corrected; but since posture is the result of the habit of a lifetime, it probably will not change after middle age. Heat to the part may afford some relief of pain. Obese patients should lose weight. Anything that helps to relieve strain on the sore joints helps to prevent further joint destruction. Support may be given with strapping, belts, braces, canes, or crutches.

Aspirin and the NSAIDs should be used for the relief of pain and the control of inflammation (see previous section on Rheumatoid Arthritis). Although these drugs do not prevent or cure this disorder, they may decrease the severity of joint destruction. Corticosteroids may be injected into areas of acute inflammation during the acute stage; however, when possible, long-term use of these agents should be avoided. Narcotics should be avoided because the disease is chronic in nature.

Gout

Gout is a metabolic disorder in which the body is unable to properly metabolize purines, which are end products of the digestion of certain proteins. This inability results in an accumulation of uric acid in the bloodstream (hyperuricemia). Deposits of urate (a salt of uric acid) crystals occur in body tissues, chiefly in and around joints, causing local inflammation and irritation. Gout is more common in men than in women.

Symptoms

An attack of gout is characterized by a sudden onset of acute pain and tenderness in a joint. The skin turns red and the part swells and is warm. Fever may be present. The attack may subside in 1 to 2 weeks, but moderate swelling and tenderness may persist beyond that time. There is usually a symptom-free period followed by another attack, which may occur at any time.

Diagnosis

Diagnosis is made by examination of the affected joint, a thorough patient history, serum uric acid levels (which may or may not be elevated), finding of urate crystals in synovial fluid obtained by aspiration of the affected joint, radiographic examination, and the finding of *tophi*, which are subcutaneous deposits of uric acid crystals. Tophi usually are found on the outer ear (pinna) and at affected joints.

Treatment

Although gout cannot be cured in the sense of removing the basic metabolic difficulty of constant or recurrent hyperuricemia, the attacks usually can be controlled to the point that they no longer occur. The regimen must be individualized for each patient and may need to be changed from time to time in response to the changes in the course of the disease. For treatment to succeed, the patient must understand the nature of gout and adhere to the prescribed treatment regimen.

The aim of treatment is to decrease the amount of sodium urate in the extracellular fluid so that deposits do not form. This is attempted in two major ways: (1) by decreasing the amount of purine ingested and (2) by using uricosuric drugs, which promote the renal excretion of urates by inhibiting the tubular resorption of urates. Excess uric acid in the body of a patient with gout is derived from a process of internal biosynthesis; consequently, except for severe forms of gout, there is less emphasis on strict diet restriction than on uricosuric drugs. Most patients are not placed on rigid diets, although they may be instructed not to eat foods extremely high in purine. The reaction to food and alcoholic drinks is extremely individual.

The prescribed diet should be adequate in proteins —with concentration on low-purine proteins—low in fat, and rich in carbohydrates. Large fluid intake and no alcohol usually are recommended.

Pain during a severe acute attack may require the short-term use of narcotics. Acute attacks of gout may be treated with colchicine or phenylbutazone (Butazolidin). Colchicine may be prescribed to be given every 1 or 2 hours until the pain subsides or nausea, vomiting, intestinal cramping, and diarrhea develop. When one or more of these symptoms occurs, the drug should be temporarily stopped. Drugs used in the long-term management of gout include colchicine, allopurinol (Zyloprim), probenecid (Benemid), indomethacin (Indocin), and sulfinpyrazone (Anturane). To prevent future attacks, drug therapy should be continued after the acute attack subsides. Treatment also should be aimed at preventing permanent joint damage. Increased fluid intake should be recommended to reduce the possibility of urate stone formation in the kidney. If the patient is obese, a weight-reduction diet should be planned to reduce strain on the involved joints.

Other treatment of advanced gout includes surgery to remove large tophi. Surgery also may be employed in an attempt to correct crippling deformities that may result when treatment is delayed and to fuse unstable joints to increase their function.

Ankylosing Spondylitis

Ankylosing spondylitis, or Marie-Strumpell disease, is a chronic, progressive disease of unknown etiology. This connective tissue disorder almost always begins in early adulthood and is more common in men.

Ankylosing spondylitis affects the spine and the surrounding cartilaginous joints, such as the sacroiliac joints and soft tissues around the vertebrae. It is a chronic and progressive disease that results in immobility and fixation (ankylosis) of the affected areas.

Symptoms

The most common symptoms are pain and stiffness in the lower back. As the disease progresses, the spine becomes more immobile, thus restricting normal movement. Other manifestations of this disorder are *aortitis* (inflammation of the aorta) and *iridocyclitis* (inflammation of the iris and ciliary body of the eye).

Diagnosis

Diagnosis is made by physical examination and radiographs of the spine and affected joints.

Treatment

Treatment of this disorder is supportive, the major goal being the maintenance of functional posture. Aspirin, indomethacin (Indocin), phenylbutazone (Butazolidin), or NSAIDs usually are prescribed for the relief of pain and inflammation. Sleeping on a firm mattress (preferably without a pillow) and following a prescribed exercise program may help prevent spinal deformity, especially in the early stages of the disease. Severe hip involvement may be treated with a total hip replacement. A back brace also may be prescribed for some patients.

Lupus Erythematosus

There are two major types of lupus erythematosus: systemic lupus erythematosus (SLE) and discoid lupus erythematosus (DLE). *Systemic* lupus erythematosus, as the name implies, affects multiple body systems such as the skin, joints, kidney, serous membranes of the heart and lungs, lymph nodes, and gastrointestinal tract. *Discoid* lupus erythematosus affects only the skin. The most common type of lupus erythematosus is

SLE, but patients with DLE may ultimately develop the systemic form of the disease.

Lupus erythematosus is more common in women than in men. Most patients have this disorder in the third or fourth decade of life, but it may be seen in young children as well as in middle-aged and elderly adults.

Symptoms

The earlier signs and symptoms of SLE may include fever, weight loss, pain in the joints (arthralgia), malaise, muscle pain, and extreme fatigue. These symptoms are vague and may persist for several months to 2 years before more prominent symptoms develop and the patient seeks medical advice. The more prominent symptoms of this disorder include a butterfly-shaped rash on the face (over the bridge of the nose and the cheeks), behavioral disturbances (confusion, hallucinations, irritability), chest pain (due to involvement of the pleura or pericarditis), fluid retention and hematuria (due to renal involvement), progressive weight loss, nausea and vomiting, and in women, irregular and/or heavy menses.

Other signs of the disease include nonspecific electrocardiographic changes, a pericardial friction rub, pulmonary ragiographic changes, enlargement of the spleen and lymph nodes, Raynaud's phenomenon (vasospasm of the smaller vessels of the hands and feet resulting in blanching of the skin, and at times pain and cyanosis of the extremities) and proteinuria and hematuria.

The symptoms of DLE are related only to the skin, the most prominent symptom being the appearance of a butterfly-shaped rash. Skin manifestations of the disorder also may be found on the forehead, ear lobes, and scalp. Scalp involvement usually results in patchy loss of hair (alopecia). These symptoms also may be seen in people with SLE.

Diagnosis

Diagnosis is based on symptoms and on laboratory tests, which may include a CBC, antinuclear antibody (ANA), urinalysis, lupus erythematosus cell preparation (LE prep), and the antideoxyribonucleic acid antibody test. The ANA is positive in almost all patients with SLE. The antideoxyribonucleic acid antibody test may be ordered after a positive ANA for confirmation of the diagnosis. The diagnosis of DLE is based primarily on the appearance of the skin manifestations of the disorder. Additional tests, such as a renal biopsy, may be performed to determine the effect of the disorder on other body systems.

Treatment

There is no specific treatment for this disorder, and medical management is aimed at the prevention and treatment of acute exacerbations of the disorder. The patient should be instructed to avoid sunlight and ultraviolet radiation. Immunizations, blood transfusions, and certain drugs, such as the sulfonamides and penicillin, should be avoided when possible. Drugs used in treatment may include aspirin or an NSAID for fever and joint discomfort and corticosteroids. Topical corticosteroids may be used for skin manifestations. Use of sunscreens should be advised whenever the patient goes out of doors. Bed rest and planned periods of exercise should be recommended when the disease is active. Other symptoms, such as vomiting, renal involvement, and cardiac or pulmonary symptoms should be treated as the need arises.

NURSING PROCESS —THE PATIENT WHO HAS A RHEUMATIC DISORDER

Assessment
Most patients with rheumatic disorders are treated on an outpatient basis. A few may require hospitalization for treatment of the acute phase of the disorder, for surgery on a degenerative joint, or for other medical or surgical disorders.

A complete medical, drug, and allergy history should be obtained, vital signs should be taken, and the patient should be weighed. If previous drug or other type of therapy was prescribed, a complete description of the therapy, dosage, and results of treatment should be obtained.

Physical assessment should include an evaluation of the patient's physical mobility, the joints or areas involved, the degree and amount of pain or discomfort, the location of joint deformities, and the ability or inability to perform physical activities such as walking, bathing, and eating.

Nursing Diagnosis
Depending on the degree of involvement and other factors, one or more of the following nursing diagnoses may apply. For patients scheduled for orthopedic surgery, refer to the nursing process for the patient having orthopedic surgery.

- Pain and discomfort (specify acute or chronic) related to joint inflammation or deformity
- Impaired physical mobility related to joint deformity or pain
- Total or partial (specify areas) self-care deficit related to joint inflammation or deformity
- Anxiety related to pain, discomfort, other factors (specify)
- Ineffective individual coping related to change in appearance (joint deformities, side effects of corticosteroid therapy)

- Colonic constipation related to immobility
- Diarrhea related to drug therapy
- Potential for disuse syndrome related to rheumatic disease
- Impaired skin integrity related to immobility
- Altered nutrition: less than body requirements related to inadequate food intake
- Knowledge deficit of home care management, treatment regimen

Planning and Implementation
The major goals of the patient may include relief of pain and discomfort, improved physical mobility, improved ability to care for self, reduction in anxiety, normal bowel elimination, improved ability to cope with symptoms of the disorder, improved nutrition, and understanding of the prescribed treatment regimen.

The major goals of nursing management may include relief of pain and discomfort, meeting the patient's physical and emotional needs, improved nutrition, normal bowel elimination, and preparation of an effective teaching plan for management of the disorder.

During the acute phase of the disorder, some patients appear seriously ill. Vital signs should be monitored every 4 hours. Intake and output should be measured, especially when there are gastrointestinal or renal symptoms, which may be seen in those with lupus erythematosus or colchicine therapy for acute gout. Behavioral changes caused by the disorder or corticosteroid therapy may require extra safety precautions.

Pain, Discomfort. Analgesic and antiinflammatory drugs should be ordered for pain. Management of acute pain should involve keeping the patient as comfortable as possible. A bed cradle may be placed over the affected joint to protect it from the pressure of the bed linen. The involved joints should be inspected frequently for redness and warmth during an acute attack. Because joints may be extremely painful, it is necessary to inquire whether the pain is being reduced by medication. Elevation of the joint also may make the patient more comfortable.

Joint inflammation and pain, which may result in limitation of motion, joint deformity, and muscle atrophy, should be managed by good body alignment, gentleness in the performance of nursing activities, and, when ordered, passive exercises.

Impaired Physical Mobility, Self-Care Deficit. Because of pain and joint deformity, some patients have difficulty walking, getting out of bed, bathing, grooming, and so forth. In addition, the amount of allowed physical mobility may be prescribed by the physician. The patient should be encouraged to move and use the extremities within the confines of the physician's recommendations. Physical therapy may be prescribed for some patients, depending on the treatment regimen.

An evaluation of the patient's physical abilities and limitations should be made during the initial assessment, including the ability to eat (holding a fork, cutting food, holding cups or glasses), the ability to bathe and groom self (shaving, dressing, combing the hair), the ability to walk, and the ability to get out of bed with or without assistance.

Once abilities and limitations are documented, management should include tasks or solutions that help the patient be as self-sufficient as possible within the limitations of the disorder. For example, evaluation may reveal that the patient can eat without help but needs containers opened, liquids poured, and a straw for drinking fluids.

Those with acute gout are usually allowed to exercise the joint after the pain and redness disappear. Early ambulation is necessary to ensure good joint function.

Anxiety, Ineffective Individual Coping. Pain, discomfort, the uncertainty of the future, and the inability to perform certain tasks may result in varying degrees of anxiety. Those having had the disease for a long time may be accustomed to having tasks performed for them, they may understand and accept the physical limitations imposed by the disease, and they may know what the future most probably will bring. Others never become accustomed to the problems associated with the disorder.

The patient must be allowed time to discuss feelings and concerns. An understanding and empathic attitude may help relieve some anxiety and may help the patient begin to cope with the many problems associated with the disorder.

Colonic Constipation, Diarrhea. Prolonged immobility may result in constipation. On the other hand, the patient may experience diarrhea as a result of drug therapy. A record of bowel movements should be kept. If constipation occurs, the physician should be informed because a stool softener, a laxative, or a high-fiber diet may be necessary. Unless contraindicated for other reasons, such as renal involvement in those with lupus erythematosus, fluids should be encouraged.

If sudden diarrhea occurs, the physician must be informed immediately because this may be an adverse reaction to drug therapy. Those receiving colchicine every 1 or 2 hours for acute gout may experience diarrhea. An explanation about the hourly administration of colchicine should include the ne-

cessity of giving the drug until gastrointestinal symptoms develop or the pain is relieved. This can be the starting point in discharge teaching because it involves the patient in the management of the disease. Knowing *what* to expect and *why* the gastrointestinal symptoms may have to be tolerated for a short time also reduces anxiety created by the occurrence of this problem.

Potential for Disuse Syndrome. Many body systems are affected when mobility is severely impaired. The skin, respiratory, cardiovascular, musculoskeletal, and gastrointestinal are examples of systems that may be affected. Nursing management depends on the degree of the effect as well as on the physician's orders. Although not applicable in all patients or situations, the following nursing interventions help reduce problems associated with disuse:

1. Change patient's position every 2 hours.
2. Encourage fluid intake.
3. Encourage coughing and deep breathing every 2 hours.
4. Encourage use and movement of the extremities.
5. Help prevent skin breakdown.
6. Help promote good body alignment.
7. Encourage adequate food intake.
8. Set realistic goals.
9. Encourage the patient when a goal is attained.
10. Promote patient and family participation in care.

Impaired Skin Integrity. Any immobilized patient requires special skin care. Changing the patient's position, massaging areas prone to excess pressure, keeping the skin clean and dry, and, sometimes, using special mattresses or protective devices are necessary for these patients.

Altered Nutrition. Small, frequent meals may be better tolerated than three large meals per day. The patient should be weighed weekly or as ordered, and any weight loss should be brought to the attention of the physician.

Knowledge Deficit. Education is important in helping the patient and family manage the disease during its chronic phase and in preventing, when possible, acute exacerbations of the illness. The drug regimen and adverse drug effects should be reviewed with the patient and family. The following general areas may be included in a teaching plan for the patient with a rheumatic disorder:

1. Rest frequently during the day. Do not exceed the physical limitations recommended by the physician. Avoid those activities that cause severe pain or discomfort.

2. Take the prescribed or recommended medications exactly as ordered. Do not stop taking the medication if symptoms are relieved unless advised to do so by the physician. If symptoms become worse, do not increase the dosage of the drug unless advised to do so by the physician.
3. Eat a well-balanced diet; drink extra fluids.
4. Do not use other nonprescription drugs unless their use is approved by the physician.
5. Avoid exposure to infection.
6. Inform other physicians and dentists of current therapy before any treatment, surgery, or drugs are prescribed.
7. For those with lupus erythematosus: Avoid exposure to sunlight and ultraviolet radiation whenever possible, since such exposure can result in an acute relapse of the disease. Effective sunscreens (preferably those recommended by the physician), clothing that covers the arms and legs, and wide-brimmed sunhats are recommended whenever it is necessary to go out of doors. Sunlamps and tanning booths must be avoided.
8. Notify the physician if any of the following should occur: adverse drug effects, an increase in the severity of symptoms, involvement in other joints, weight loss, prolonged anorexia, nausea, vomiting, fever, cough, dyspnea, difficult urination, infection, or any other unusual occurrence.

Evaluation

- Pain and discomfort are relieved or controlled
- Patient demonstrates improvement in physical mobility
- Patient assumes increasing responsibility for own care
- Anxiety is reduced
- Bowel elimination is normal
- Patient demonstrates improvement in ability to cope with problems related to the disorder
- Symptoms related to disuse syndrome are improved or corrected
- Skin remains intact; no evidence of skin breakdown
- Diet intake is adequate; weight remains stable
- Patient demonstrates understanding of treatment regimen, importance of medication, things to avoid, and events that require notifying the physician

LOW BACK PAIN

Pain in the lower back is a common disorder. Examples of causes of low back pain include muscle strain, osteoarthritis involving the spine, metastatic bone lesions, obesity, poor posture, lack of exercise, and some uterine or menstrual disorders. Low back pain may subside in a short time or become chronic in nature.

Symptoms

Intermittent or continuous pain in the lower back is the predominate symptom.

Diagnosis

Diagnosis is based on symptoms and radiograph of the area. A CT scan also may be done. Additional tests or examinations may be performed to rule out physical disorders that may cause back pain, such as uterine disorders, metastatic carcinoma, or vertebral fractures.

Treatment

Treatment depends on the cause (if known) and the severity of the disorder. Mild symptoms usually respond to the application of heat and analgesics or muscle relaxants. The patient should be encouraged to avoid those activities that cause further discomfort until pain is relieved.

Other therapies may include an exercise program, physical therapy, weight loss, and back braces. Pelvic traction may be necessary for those who do not respond to other methods of treatment. In this type of traction, a canvas belt is placed around the waist and hips. The belt has two canvas straps attached to a spreader bar and a pulley, and weights are added to the end of the pulley. This type of traction may be used at home, provided that the individual has a bed frame that can support the apparatus. The effectiveness of this method of treatment varies.

OSTEOPOROSIS

Normally, in osteoporosis, there is a slow, continuous turnover of bone. *Osteoblasts*, which are bone-building cells, secrete substances necessary for the formation of bone. *Osteoclasts*, another type of bone cell, continually reabsorb and break down bone. In the normal individual, this process of bone formation and bone breakdown occurs at an even rate. *Osteoporosis* is an increase in the porosity of bone. In this disorder, a loss of bone substance exceeds the rate of bone formation.

Osteoporosis occurs principally in older individuals and affects women more often than men. Women appear to have a higher incidence of the disease because of the decrease in estrogen production after menopause. Decreased estrogen levels appear to cause an increase in bone resorption by the osteoclasts, resulting in a general porosity of bone structure and ultimate weakening of the bone. Other causes of osteoporosis include Cushing's syndrome, prolonged use of high doses of corticosteroids, prolonged periods of immobility, hyperparathyroidism, and dietary deficiency of vitamin D and calcium. These causes of osteoporosis may be seen in any age group of both sexes.

Symptoms

Most individuals have few if any symptoms. Some individuals may complain of varying degrees of bone pain or tenderness. The bone pain or tenderness that may occur in some individuals is often in the lower back and is probably due to microscopic fractures occurring in the vertebrae. These fractures are commonly referred to as compression fractures. Bone deformities (especially in the spine) and pathologic fractures also may be seen.

Diagnosis

Radiographic examination of the bones shows a loss of bone, especially in the vertebrae. Laboratory studies are usually normal but may be performed to rule out other disorders such as multiple myeloma, hyperparathyroidism, or metastatic bone lesions. Single-photon absorptiometry may be used to periodically monitor bone loss in the wrist and to serve as a guide to therapy.

Treatment

Osteoporosis cannot be treated directly, but the rate of bone resorption may be slowed by medical management. Bone pain or tenderness may respond to the use of mild analgesics such as aspirin. A nutritious, well-balanced diet that is high in calcium, vitamin D, and protein should be recommended. Oral calcium preparations, (calcium gluconate, calcium lactate, calcium carbonate, or dibasic calcium phosphate) may be taken to supplement the dietary intake of calcium. Some of these preparations also contain vitamin D, which is necessary for the absorption of calcium in the intestine. Adequate periods of rest and exercise and estrogen replacement therapy or androgen therapy for postmenopausal women also may be part of medical management.

BURSITIS

Bursitis is an inflammation of the bursa. Trauma is the most common cause of acute bursitis.

Symptoms

Painful movement of a joint such as the elbow or shoulder is the most common symptom.

Diagnosis

Diagnosis is based on the patient's symptoms. A radiograph of the area may reveal a calcified bursa.

Treatment

Rest of the joint is usually recommended. Salicylates or NSAIDs may be recommended or prescribed. If the problem persists, a corticosteroid preparation may be injected into the areas to reduce inflammation. After a reduction of pain and inflammation, the patient should be instructed to begin mild ROM exercises but

advised to avoid traumatizing or overusing the joint. Failure to use the joint after pain and inflammation is controlled may result in partial limitation of joint motion.

RECONSTRUCTIVE JOINT SURGERY

Arthroplasty

Arthroplasty, the reconstruction of a joint destroyed by disease or injury, may be performed to restore adequate joint function. When all hope of salvaging the joint is gone, and it is still painful or troublesome to the patient, an arthrodesis (fusion of the joint surfaces) may be performed, eliminating movement in the joint but relieving the pain that had accompanied movement.

Total Joint Replacement

The two joints most frequently replaced are the knee and the hip. Other joints that may be replaced are the elbow, ankle, wrist, and finger joints. Joint replacement is considered when severe pain and disability of a joint cannot be corrected or controlled by other means. The most common conditions requiring total joint replacement are rheumatoid arthritis and os-

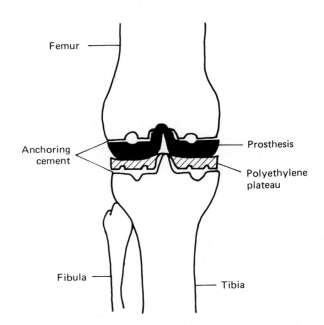

Figure 55–12.   A total knee replacement showing the insertion of the prosthesis and the polyethylene plateau. The prosthesis allows for full movement of the knee.

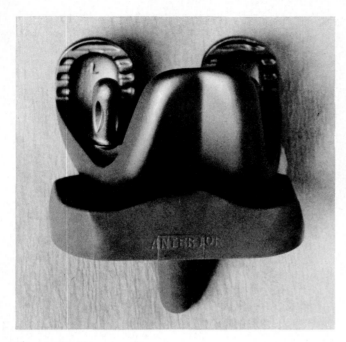

Figure 55–13. A total knee replacement prosthesis using an RMC (Richard's maximum contact) total knee system. (Photograph by D. Atkinson)

teoarthritis. Other conditions that may require total joint replacement are trauma and congenital deformity.

The materials used for manufacture of a joint prosthesis are metal, silastic, and high-density polyethylene (Figs. 55-12 through 55-14). The joint replacements are cemented to the bone with a bonding agent.

NURSING PROCESS —THE PATIENT UNDERGOING JOINT SURGERY

Preoperative Period

Assessment

A complete medical, drug, and allergy history should be taken. The patient's mobility should be evaluated if joint replacement or reconstruction involves the hip or knee. A list of all drugs currently taken should be recorded. Vital signs and weight should be obtained.

Nursing Diagnosis

Depending on the patient and the area of surgery, one or more of the following nursing diagnoses may apply:

- Anxiety related to surgery, results of surgery, discomfort, other factors (specify).
- Chronic pain related to joint disease.
- Impaired physical mobility related to joint disease.
- Knowledge deficit of preoperative preparations, postoperative management.

Planning and Implementation

The major goals of the patient may include reduction in anxiety, relief of pain, and understanding of preoperative preparations and postoperative management.

The major goals of nursing management may include preparing the patient physically and emotionally for surgery.

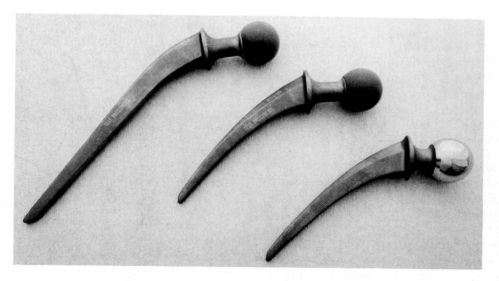

Figure 55–14. Total hip replacement prosthetic devices. Two trial prostheses are on the left; the prosthesis that is finally inserted in the patient is on the right. Trial prostheses are used during surgery to determine correct fitting prior to inserting the real prosthesis. (Photographs by D. Atkinson)

Preoperative preparation for total joint replacement depends on what joint is being replaced and the age and physical condition of the patient. The patient scheduled for a total hip replacement is often elderly and therefore must be in the best physical condition possible before surgery. The arthritic patient who has been taking aspirin or other antiarthritic agents should have laboratory tests, such as a CBC, prothrombin time, and bleeding and clotting time, to determine the effect of the drugs on the blood clotting mechanism or blood cell production. Normally, an antiarthritic agent is discontinued until laboratory tests are within normal limits, because surgery cannot be scheduled if the patient has a bleeding problem or if the red or white blood cell count is below normal.

The day before surgery, the skin over and adjacent to the operative site should be shaved. The surgeon also may order a scrubbing of the operative skin site with an antiseptic or germicidal solution one or more times the evening before surgery.

Because one of the most potentially serious postoperative complications is infection, a prophylactic antibiotic may be prescribed before surgery. Although laminar air flow rooms in the operating room suite have reduced the incidence of postoperative infection, there still remains the potential for infection in every orthopedic surgery.

Anxiety. In addition to normal preoperative anxiety, the patient may be concerned about the return of joint function and relief of pain once the area has healed. The physician discusses the anticipated results of surgery with the patient before surgery. The nurse should reassure the patient that every effort will be made to restore joint function and relieve pain.

Pain, Impaired Physical Mobility. Depending on the degree of pain and discomfort, an analgesic may or may not be ordered before surgery. The physician may order bed rest to reduce preoperative discomfort and pain. If the patient scheduled for a hip or knee replacement is allowed to get out of bed, assistance may be necessary.

Knowledge Deficit. All preoperative preparations should be explained to the patient. Postoperative management also should be discussed, including the possible use of splints, traction, or other immobilizing devices. Coughing and deep-breathing exercises should be demonstrated, and the patient should be allowed to practice these maneuvers the evening before surgery. An incentive spirometer also may be used after surgery to encourage deep breathing. Directions for use and practice time are best given during the preoperative period.

Evaluation

- Anxiety is reduced
- Pain and discomfort are controlled
- Patient ambulates with assistance (when needed)
- Patient demonstrates understanding of preoperative preparations and postoperative management
- Patient practices effective deep-breathing and coughing exercises

Postoperative Period

Assessment
Special preparations for the postoperative period are ordered by the physician and may include a special mattress, overhead bars or frame, and trapeze.

When the patient returns from surgery, vital signs should be taken and the chart reviewed for orders regarding immobilization, allowed movement or turning, position of the extremities, and so on. It is extremely important that these orders are fully understood because incorrect movement or placement of a limb may result in displacement of the prosthesis or irreparable damage to the reconstructed joint.

Nursing Diagnosis
Depending on the operative site, the type of surgery, and other factors, one or more of the following nursing diagnoses may apply. Additional diagnoses pertaining to any surgical patient also may be added.

- Pain related to surgery.
- Impaired physical mobility related to surgery, immobilization devices.
- Potential for infection related to surgery.
- Colonic constipation related to immobility.
- Potential for disuse syndrome related to surgery, immobilization, other factors (specify).
- Self-care deficit related to surgery, immobility.
- Potential impaired home management related to difficulty in maintaining self and home after surgery.
- Knowledge deficit of home care management.

Planning and Implementation
The major goals of the patient may include relief of pain, absence of infection, continued intact skin, maximum pulmonary function, normal bowel function, improved physical mobility, improved ability to care for self, and understanding of home care management.

The major goals of nursing management may include relief of pain and discomfort, absence of infection, prevention of skin breakdown, maximum pulmonary function, normal bowel function, identification of factors that may impair optimal home care, and development of an effective postdischarge teaching plan.

Because techniques for total joint replacement or reconstruction vary, the surgeon's orders are usually detailed. If there is any question about the meaning of an order or what can and cannot be done, the nurse should consult the surgeon before instituting any nursing task.

Vital signs should be monitored as ordered and intake and output measured until the patient is able to take oral fluids and is voiding. The voiding pattern should be monitored, and the physician should be informed if the patient complains of dysuria or is voiding in frequent, small amounts.

Postoperative management of the patient having a hip or knee arthroplasty is summarized in Chart 55-3. In general, care of the patient with a knee or hip replacement is the same as that for a standard arthroplasty.

Chart 55–3. Postoperative Management of the Patient Who Has a Hip or Knee Arthroplasty

Hip Arthroplasty
- The leg *must* be maintained in a position of *abduction*.
- Balanced suspension traction should be used for about 3 weeks.
- A pillow should be placed between the knees to prevent accidental adduction.
- A trochanter roll should be used for the unoperated leg to prevent external rotation.
- Isometric exercises should be instituted.
- Deep-breathing exercises should be performed hourly for the first 1 or 2 days after surgery, then every 2 or 3 hr while awake.
- The head of the bed should be kept flat until orders are written to raise the head of the bed. Increase in height should be gradual.
- Blood pressure, pulse, and respirations should be taken every 1 to 2 hr for the first 24 hr, then every 4 hr. Nursing judgment or the physician's instructions may alter the frequency of these measurements.
- Temperature should be taken every 4 hr for 5 or more days.
- The dressing should be checked for drainage and reinforced if necessary.
- Voiding and intake and output should be checked.
- The color and temperature of the extremity should be checked and any changes reported immediately.

Knee Arthroplasty
- The leg should be elevated to prevent edema.
- Vital signs and temperature should be checked as for the patient with a hip arthroplasty.
- Voiding and intake and output should be checked.
- The color and temperature of the extremity should be checked and any changes reported immediately.
- Leg exercises, which usually begin the first or second postoperative day, should be supervised.

Pain. Narcotic analgesics are necessary for several days after surgery and should be administered as ordered. Each time the patient requests an analgesic, the location and type of pain should be evaluated. Parenteral injections should be avoided in the hip or thigh of the operative side. Pain in an area other than the operative site should be reported immediately to the physician. Gentleness should be used when moving the patient or adjusting pillows or immobilization devices.

Impaired Physical Mobility. When the patient has a total hip replacement or hip arthroplasty, turning the patient and raising the head of the bed may or may not be allowed. If turning is allowed, pillows should be placed between the patient's legs before he or she is turned. *The leg must be kept in an abducted position at all times,* or the prosthetic or repaired femoral head may become dislocated from the acetabulum. Those having hip surgery are usually not turned on the operative side.

Buck's traction may be ordered for approximately 48 hours after surgery for total hip replacement. An immobilizing device such as a cast or commercial knee immobilizer may be ordered when the patient has a total knee replacement.

Potential for Infection. Vital signs should be monitored and the dressing checked for drainage every 4 hours. Any gradual or sudden increase in temperature or purulent drainage on the dressing should be reported immediately.

Some physicians insert a drain into the wound and order it connected to a specific type of suction. The amount and type of drainage from the wound should be noted.

Most patients receive prophylactic antibiotics for 7 to 10 days after surgery. Unfortunately, infection may occur weeks, months, or even several years after surgery and require removal of the prosthesis as well as prolonged and intensive therapy.

Colonic Constipation. Constipation may be seen once the patient is able to eat. A record of bowel movements should be kept, and fluids should be encouraged. If constipation does occur, the physician should be informed. Many physicians prescribe a stool softener to prevent constipation once the patient is eating.

Potential for Disuse Syndrome. Many patients are allowed out of bed the second or third day after a total hip replacement. Care must be exercised that full assistance is given, preferably by two people, and that the leg on the operative side is moved according to the physician's instructions. The amount of weight or the avoidance of weight bearing on the operative extremity also is prescribed by the physician. The use and placement of pillows or trochanter rolls and the institution of isometric exercises are prescribed by the physician. Usually, exercises begin the day after surgery and are given by the physical therapist. Exercises are necessary to maintain muscle tone and prevent muscle atrophy.

When the patient has a knee arthroplasty or replacement, the extremity may be ordered elevated while the patient is in bed. Ice packs also may be ordered to reduce edema. A continuous passive motion device may be ordered immediately after surgery. This machine provides automatic ROM exercises that promote healing of the knee joint as well as increase circulation to the operative area. The physician orders the amount of extension and flexion produced by the machine as well as the frequency of use.

Those with a knee arthroplasty or replacement may be allowed out of bed the day after surgery. Initially, no weight bearing is allowed on the extremity, and the patient should be instructed to place all weight on the unoperated side. For safety reasons, two individuals should assist the patient out of bed for the first few postoperative days.

Coughing and deep-breathing exercises every 2 hours while awake are necessary to promote maximum lung function. The lungs should be auscultated daily and the physician notified if abnormal lung sounds are heard, if chills and fever occur, or if the patient fails to deep breathe adequately.

The extremity of the operative side should be inspected every 2 to 4 hours for circulation impairment. The color and temperature of the knee, leg, and toes should be noted and peripheral pulses monitored. Any deviation from normal may indicate circulation impairment as a result of thrombus formation and must be reported to the physician *immediately*.

Most patients having hip or knee replacement or repair are allowed to ambulate using a walker (hip, knee) or crutches (knee). The physician determines the type of device to be used. The physical therapist works with the patient and gives instructions for the use of the prescribed device. The patient must always be assisted when using the device to walk.

Self-Care Deficit. Many patients are able to participate in some self-care activities the day after surgery. The ability of the patient to engage in self-care activities is evaluated on a daily basis. The patient is encouraged to use the upper extremities, use the trapeze (if one is ordered) to move or lift the hips (when

this is allowed), and participate as much as possible in his or her own care.

Potential Impaired Home Management. Because activities are limited until full healing has taken place, the patient will require a support system when at home. The availability of assistance at home is best discussed with the patient or a family member before surgery but also may be further explored during the postoperative period. The patient will require assistance with moving and walking as well as help with meals, transportation to the physician's office, and other household tasks. Certain physical aspects of the home (stairs, location of bathroom, etc.) may be a problem during the recovery period. Once these problems are known, the nurse may be able to offer suggestions. If the patient lives alone, or if a family member is not available to assist the patient during the day, other arrangements should be discussed with the family.

Knowledge Deficit. The physician discusses with the patient what must or must not be done when at home. Some physicians give printed instructions to the patient. The nurse should review these instructions with the patient or family member to be sure they are correctly understood. The following general points can be included in the patient teaching plan:

1. Follow the directions of the physician. Do not resume any activity that has been restricted until told to do so.
2. Exercise the operative extremity as directed by the physician. Perform the prescribed exercises faithfully. Use the recommended device (walker, cane, crutches) for walking. Observe safety when walking.
3. Avoid crossing the legs, sleeping on the operative side until permitted to do so, prolonged sitting, low chairs, lifting, and excessive bending or twisting.
4. Assistance will be required in dressing (especially putting on pants, socks, or shoes). Wear good support shoes when walking; avoid loose-fitting footwear when walking.
5. Keep all physical therapy appointments. Follow the directions of the therapist regarding exercises and movement.
6. Avoid constipation by drinking plenty of fluids and eating a high-fiber diet. If constipation occurs, contact the physician before using a laxative or other method of relieving constipation.
7. Do not use or take any nonprescription drug unless it has been approved by the physician. Do not apply any ointment or cream to the incision unless it has been approved by the physician.
8. Continue to cough and deep breathe at 2- to 3-hour intervals until fully ambulatory.
9. Contact the physician if any of the following should occur: sudden pain, redness or swelling in the operative area, chills, fever, difficulty in or pain when urinating, chest pain, or cough.

Evaluation

- Pain is controlled
- Physical mobility is improved; patient ambulates with recommended device
- No apparent infection; vital signs are normal
- Bowel function is normal
- Patient coughs and deep breathes at recommended intervals; lungs are clear to auscultation
- Extremity is normal in color and temperature; peripheral pulses are palpable
- No evidence of injury or slipping of prosthesis
- Patient executes prescribed exercises
- Problems regarding home management are identified and resolved
- Patient assumes responsibility for most or all of self-care
- Patient demonstrates understanding of home care management, things to avoid, exercises, importance of physical therapy, events requiring contacting the physician

OSTEOMYELITIS

Osteomyelitis is an infection of the bone, most commonly caused by the organisms *Staphylococcus aureus* and *Streptococcus pyogenes*. *Acute osteomyelitis* is most often caused by bacteria reaching the bone by way of the bloodstream. *Acute localized osteomyelitis* is most often caused by direct contamination of the bone due to trauma, for example, penetrating wounds or compound fractures. Occasionally, surgical contamination or direct extension of bacteria from an infected area adjacent to the bone, such as the pin sites of skeletal traction, can cause osteomyelitis.

Symptoms

Symptoms occur suddenly: high fever, chills, rapid pulse, tenderness or pain over the affected area, redness, and swelling. After several days, necrosis of the bone may occur.

Diagnosis

Diagnosis may be made by radiographic examination; radiographic evidence may not be apparent, however, during the early stages of infection, and diagnosis may depend on symptoms as well as physical examination. Laboratory tests usually show a rise in the leukocyte count, an elevated erythrocyte sedimentation rate, and possibly a positive blood culture.

Treatment

There are three weapons to combat osteomyelitis: the patient's own defenses, aided by rest and good nutrition; antibiotics; and surgical drainage.

In the early stage of treatment, the antibiotic may be given by continuous intravenous infusion. Some physicians make a series of drill holes in the bone to evacuate pus and relieve pressure. Antibiotics or sterile normal saline are put directly into the wound, and a catheter may be left in place for periodic irrigation or continuous drip of antibiotic or sterile normal saline solution. The patient may be placed in isolation until the infection is controlled. Later, a bone graft or internal fixation using pins or screws may be necessary to stabilize the weakened bone.

Complications

The diseased bone may lengthen as bone growth is stimulated, or it may shorten because of the destruction of the epiphyseal plate. Perhaps the most discouraging complication is the tendency of osteomyelitis to become chronic, requiring rehospitalization and repeated courses of antibiotic therapy. Chart 55-4 summarizes nursing management of the patient with osteomyelitis.

BONE TUMORS

Bone tumors may be malignant or benign. Malignant tumors may be primary, that is, originating in the bone, or secondary, that is, originating elsewhere in the body and traveling to the bone (metastasized). Primary malignant tumors are called *sarcomas* (eg, osteogenic sarcoma, Ewing's sarcoma, and osteochondrosarcoma), are highly malignant, and metastasize early, usually to the lungs.

Chart 55–4. Management of the Patient With Osteomyelitis

- Isolation techniques should be instituted if drainage is present.
- A deodorizer should be used if the drainage has an unpleasant odor.
- Pillows, trochanter rolls, sandbags, and so on should be used to support and keep the unaffected extremity in proper alignment.
- The affected side should be kept in proper alignment if a splint has not been applied. This may be difficult because of severe pain.
- The affected parts should be handled gently and with great care.
- Sheepskin boots or pads, or sponge rubber, should be used to protect elbows and heels.
- A footboard should be used to prevent footdrop.
- An alternating pressure mattress should be used if there is early evidence of decubitus ulcer formation.
- Fluids should be encouraged; intake and output should be measured.
- A good dietary intake is important. A high-protein high-vitamin diet is essential to healing.
- Signs of recurrent infection should be looked for: chills, fever, rapid pulse, pain, redness, tenderness.

Symptoms

Symptoms of malignant tumors of the bone are persistent pain, swelling, and difficulty in moving the involved extremity.

Diagnosis

Diagnosis is made by radiographic examination, radioisotope bone scan, and an open or closed biopsy of the tumor. The serum alkaline phosphatase may be elevated.

Treatment

Treatment of primary malignant bone tumors involves surgical removal of the tumor by amputation of the extremity or by wide local resection. Radiation therapy and chemotherapy may be used in addition to surgery. Chemotherapy after surgery may destroy tumor cells that have escaped from the original tumor site.

Metastatic bone tumors are usually found in the pelvis, spine, and ribs. These tumors are inoperable but may be controlled (but not cured) with radiation, antineoplastic drugs, or hormone therapy.

Benign tumors are removed by curettage (scraping) or by local excision. If the patient has surgery for removal of a benign tumor, refer to the nursing process for the patient undergoing orthopedic surgery. If the patient has a malignant tumor and amputation is necessary, refer to the nursing process for the patient undergoing an amputation (later in this chapter) and to Chapter 19.

PAGET'S DISEASE

Paget's disease (osteitis deformans) is a disorder characterized by abnormal bone remodeling. Normally, bone is constantly being formed and resorbed (broken down). In Paget's disease, the resorbed bone is high in mineral content but poorly constructed. The most common areas of involvement are the long bones and the skull. The cause of Paget's disease is unknown, but a family history of the disorder is not uncommon.

Symptoms

Some patients are asymptomatic, and Paget's disease is not discovered until a radiograph for another problem reveals the disorder. The asymptomatic patient may have some mild skeletal deformity due to the disorder but disregarded the occurrence.

Other patients have marked skeletal deformities, which may include enlargement of the skull, bowing of the long bones, and kyphosis (hunchback). Bone pain and tenderness on pressure may be seen.

Diagnosis

Radiographs and a bone scan may be used to identify the affected areas. The bone scan often detects Paget's disease in its earlier stages. The serum alkaline phosphatase is usually elevated, and the urinary hydroxyproline (an amino acid found in collagen) excretion increased. Hypercalcemia (increased calcium in the blood), hypercalcinuria, (increased calcium in the urine), and the formation of kidney stones (nephrolithiasis) may occur after fracture or immobilization of the affected bones. Occasionally, the lesions undergo malignant changes.

Treatment

If the patient has no symptoms, treatment is usually not necessary. Those with symptoms may require several treatment approaches. Pain usually can be controlled with analgesics such as aspirin or the NSAIDs. Those with moderate to severe pain may require treatment with calcitonin (Calcimar), a drug that appears to block the resorption of bone and decrease the rate of bone turnover.

Treatment with calcitonin usually results in a fall in the serum alkaline phosphatase and urinary excretion of hydroxyproline, followed by regression of the lesions. Calcitonin is not an analgesic, but reduces pain because the lesions tend to regress. The patient may still require analgesics until bone pain is relieved.

Another drug used for those in the more advanced stage of the disease is EHDP or etidronate disodium (Didronel, Didronel IV), which may be given by the oral or intravenous routes. This drug reduces normal and abnormal bone resorption and secondarily reduces bone formation that is coupled to bone resorption.

AMPUTATION

The following are reasons for amputation:

- Accidental and extensive trauma to extremities
- Death of tissues from peripheral vascular insufficiency or from peripheral vasospastic diseases such as Buerger's disease and Raynaud's disease
- Malignant tumors
- Longstanding infections of bone and tissue that prohibit restoration of function
- Thermal injuries
- Deformation of a limb rendering it useless and a hindrance
- Conditions that may endanger the life of the patient, such as vascular accidents and gas bacillus infections

The decision to amputate is made when all other methods of therapy have failed. The physician decides how much of the limb must be amputated to maintain circulation and healthy structures in the remainder of the limb. Young patients often recover better from an amputation than elderly patients for reasons such as motivation to return to as near normal as possible, general good health, and the physical ability to participate in a rehabilitation program.

Amputation can be performed at any level in the lower extremity, but there are preferred levels above and below the knee to facilitate fitting with available prostheses. A stump that is too long or too short creates fitting problems and discomfort. More than 90% of amputations in the lower extremities are at the standard above- or below-knee levels. The ideal level above the knee (AK amputation) is in the middle third of the thigh, the longest preferred stump being one that is within 4 inches above the knee. The standard below-knee (BK amputation) level of choice is in the middle third of the leg, but not lower than the musculocutaneous junction of the calf muscles. Knee disarticulations (amputation through a joint), disarticulation at the ankle joint, and partial foot amputations are occasionally performed.

When the surgeon decides that amputation is inevitable, the first decision made involves the level of amputation. Although a number of tests are available, including arteriography, often the final decision can be made only by observing the vascularity of the tissues on the operating table.

Amputation of an Upper Extremity

The arms are highly specialized in function. Loss of an arm or any part of an arm—especially the dominant arm—often requires great physical and emotional adjustment during the preoperative as well as the postoperative periods.

In the upper extremity, the principle followed is to save all possible length and tissue, with the exception of partial hand amputations. An amputation through any part of the hand that does not leave functioning elements is obstructive to the use of a prosthesis. The surgical objective is to create a gently tapering stump with muscular padding over the end. The upper extremity amputation stump moves more within the socket and is subject to more variations in friction than the lower extremity stump.

A soft dressing anchored with an elastic bandage may be applied to the stump after surgery. In some cases, a rigid plaster dressing is attached immediately after surgery. Most patients with upper extremity amputations can be measured for a prosthesis shortly after the surgical scar heals. Various types of prostheses are available for upper extremity amputees.

Not *all* upper extremity amputees can be fitted with or learn how to use a prosthesis. Some find it difficult to accept the hook-type of extremity and prefer no prosthesis; this occurs most frequently in cases in which the nondominant limb was amputated. New prostheses, however, use microcircuits. The fingers are covered with a realistic-appearing "skin" and may be opened and closed by muscle activation of the microcircuit. For many, this more natural-looking type of prosthesis is preferable to the hook-type prosthesis.

Amputation of a Lower Extremity

Amputation of a lower extremity is more common than amputation of an upper extremity. Because a lower limb prosthesis is sometimes less conspicuous and has a more natural appearance than an upper limb prosthesis, it may be accepted more readily.

Unless evidence suggests that the knee cannot be saved, an attempt is made to amputate below the knee. Amputation above the knee is more disabling than amputation below the knee. Because function is achieved in relation to agility, older people do not do as well with an amputation above the knee, but most of them can be fitted with prostheses.

Some patients have an immediate fitting of a temporary prosthesis in the operating room, which is intended to get the patient up as soon as possible (Fig. 55-15). A pylon with a foot and ankle attachment is fitted to the cast, and the patient is allowed to stand with a limited amount of weight placed on the amputated extremity. As the stump heals and edema disappears, a second cast may be fitted. Ultimately, a conventional prosthesis is fitted and must be custom made to conform to the stump as well as to the patient's needs.

The advancement made in lower extremity prostheses allows for good movement in the knee and ankle so

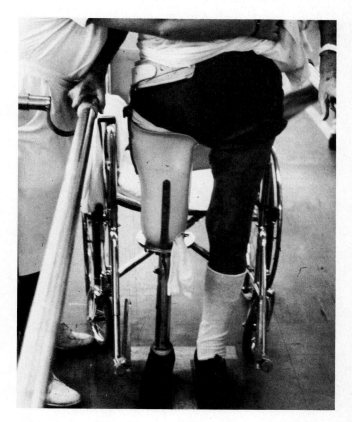

Figure 55-15. Temporary, removable above-knee socket and walking pylon. (Institute of Rehabilitation Medicine, New York University Medical Center, New York, NY)

that walking is close to normal and does not require the use of a cane or other supporting device once the final prosthesis has been fitted.

NURSING PROCESS —THE PATIENT UNDERGOING AN AMPUTATION

Preoperative Period

Assessment

Before surgery, the physician evaluates the patient's general health, motivation and ability to use a prosthesis, and the type of prosthesis that will best fit and give the best results. In an emergency, a complete evaluation is not possible.

A complete medical, drug, and allergy history should be obtained and the patient evaluated for mental and emotional acceptance of the surgical procedure. In some instances, the patient may be acutely ill, such as a patient with a gangrenous extremity accompanied by severe symptoms that include fever, disorientation, and electrolyte imbalances.

Unless surgery is an emergency, the patient should be treated for any disorder that may influence healing, for example, uncontrolled diabetes mellitus, dehydration, infection, electrolyte imbalances, poor nutrition, and chronic respiratory disorders.

Nursing Diagnosis

Depending on many factors, including the age and physical condition of the patient, one or more of the following nursing diagnoses may apply. If the patient has concurrent problems, such as dehydration, fever, or severe trauma to the extremity, additional diagnoses will need to be added.

- Anxiety related to surgery, loss (whole, part) of an extremity
- Anticipatory grieving related to loss (whole, part) of an extremity
- Ineffective individual coping related to scheduled amputation
- Pain related to trauma, malignancy, lack of blood supply to the extremity, other factors (specify)
- Knowledge deficit of the procedure, preoperative and postoperative management

Planning and Implementation

The major goals of the patient may include reduction in anxiety, acceptance of the necessity for surgery, reduction of pain, and understanding of preoperative preparations and postoperative management.

The major goals of nursing management may include preparing the patient physically and emotionally for surgery. The physical preparations for surgery depend on many factors, such as the patient's age and condition and the surgeon's preferences. If the operation is not an emergency, there is time to prepare the patient for some of the things that will be required after surgery. A good diet, including plenty of fluids, helps the patient withstand the shock of surgery. If the patient's condition permits, postoperative exercises should be started and practiced before surgery. An overhead bar and trapeze should be put on the bed so that the patient with either an upper or lower extremity amputation can practice using this device.

Anxiety. Unless the patient is acutely ill, anxiety most likely is a factor before surgery. This is especially so in the young patient. The patient must be allowed time to talk to family members and to discuss the surgery and what will happen after surgery and at home.

Patients vary in their reactions to the impending loss of a limb. These reactions are based on variables such as age, education, and the intellectual, economic, and emotional status of the individual. Other factors include what the loss of the part means to the individual and how well the individual has dealt with previous losses. In general, a gradual state of depression and a degree of hopelessness are common. The patient with diabetes, for example, may be angry because despite the extra care given to the legs and the dietary deprivation that was endured, it still becomes necessary to lose a limb.

Anticipatory Grieving, Ineffective Individual Coping. Grieving may begin during the preoperative period if the patient is reasonably aware of the diagnosis and has had time to consider the impact of an amputation. The amount of grief is thought to be proportional to the symbolic significance of the part and the resultant degree of disability and deformity.

When amputation is inevitable, the physician discusses with the patient and family the extent of physical disability, the psychological, aesthetic, social, and vocational implications, and the realistic possibilities for prosthetic restoration. An attempt should be made to reduce anxieties and misunderstandings because radical surgery constitutes a severe threat to most people. Although still faced with a crisis, this approach establishes the groundwork for assisting the patient to accept and to adjust to the realities of the situation. Not all amputees can benefit from a prosthesis, and the surgeon should be careful not to make casual promises to soothe a patient before surgery.

Pain. Those with severe pain in the extremity may require a narcotic analgesic before surgery. The limb should be watched closely for changes, such as spread of gangrene or increased loss of circulation evidenced by symptoms such as severe pain, color changes, and lack of peripheral pulses. The physician should be kept informed of any problems as they occur because surgery may become an emergency. It should be remembered that most of these patients also are suffering emotional pain. If extreme anxiety or depression is noted, the physician should be informed.

Knowledge Deficit. All preoperative preparations should be explained to the patient. Questions raised by the patient or family should be answered by the physician or nurse. Care should be exercised in answering questions about prosthetic devices and their use because it is always possible that the amputation may need to involve more of the limb than originally anticipated.

Postoperative maneuvers, such as coughing and deep-breathing exercises and exercises of the extremities, should be reviewed with the patient. If time and the patient's condition permit, these should be practiced before surgery.

Evaluation

- Anxiety is reduced
- Patient expresses grief but begins to show acceptance of reason for surgery
- Pain is controlled
- Patient demonstrates a beginning ability to cope with the scheduled amputation
- Patient demonstrates understanding of the surgery, expected results, and preoperative and postoperative management

Postoperative Period

Assessment
Vital signs should be taken and the chart reviewed for the type and level of amputation. The type of dressing or prosthesis applied to the stump should be noted and the patient's general condition evaluated.

Nursing Diagnosis
Depending on the type of and reason for amputation, the age and condition of the patient, and other factors, one or more of the following nursing diagnoses may apply:

- Pain related to surgery, infection, stump neuroma, phantom limb sensation
- Anxiety related to pain, use of a prosthesis, change in self-image, other factors (specify)
- Potential for infection related to surgery

- Hyperthermia related to infection
- Impaired skin integrity related to surgical amputation, immobility
- Total or partial (specify areas) self-care deficit related to upper extremity amputation of dominant arm or hand, surgery
- Ineffective individual coping related to change in body image
- Dysfunctional grieving related to loss of body part
- Impaired physical mobility related to loss of extremity
- Ineffective breathing pattern related to immobility
- Knowledge deficit of stump care, prosthesis use, home management

Planning and Implementation
The major goals of the patient may include relief of pain and discomfort, reduction in anxiety, absence of infection, maintenance of skin integrity, improved ability to care for self, improved coping ability, movement through the grieving process, improvement in self-concept, improvement in mobility, effective breathing pattern, and understanding of stump care or prosthesis management.

The major goals of nursing management may include relief of pain and discomfort, reduction in anxiety, absence of infection, maintenance of skin integrity, assistance with physical needs, emotional support, absence of pulmonary complications, and development of an effective discharge teaching plan.

Postoperative care may vary, depending on the type of amputation, the surgeon's preference for immediate postoperative care of an amputation, and whether the prosthetic device was fitted at the time of surgery or later. Postoperative management of a patient with an amputation of an upper or lower extremity is summarized in Chart 55-5.

PHANTOM-LIMB SENSATION AND PHANTOM PAIN. The surgeon may inform the patient of the phenomenon of phantom-limb sensation. This is the patient's sensation of the presence of the amputated limb. It is a normal, frequently occurring, physiologic response after amputation.

On the other hand, phantom-limb pain is the presence of pain or other abnormal sensations, such as burning, tingling, throbbing, or itching, in the amputated extremity. Pain felt from the phantom limb can be an extremely serious problem in relation to the emotional status of the patient and the ability to use a prosthesis. Severe, prolonged phantom-limb pain may require surgical removal of nerve endings at the end of the stump. The sensation of a phantom limb should be explained as a normal phenomenon so that the patient is not disturbed by an awareness of the amputated part.

After patients learn to use a prosthesis, although still aware of the phantom, they usually learn to ignore its presence. The patient merely may feel that

Chart 55–5.   Nursing Management of the Patient After an Amputation

No Prosthesis Fitted at the Time of Surgery

☐ Bed boards or a firm mattress must be in place before the patient returns from the operating room.

☐ Skin traction apparatus should be affixed to the bed if a *guillotine*, or *open amputation* (ie, no skin covering the stump) is performed. The physician usually orders the equipment to be put on the bed before surgery.

☐ Any overhead frame with a trapeze may be added to the bed to aid in moving the patient.

☐ To prevent edema, elevation of the stump on pillows, or elevation of the foot of the bed for the first 24 to 48 hr after surgery may be necessary.

☐ A footboard should be used to support the unoperated extremity.

☐ Isolation technique is usually necessary if control of infection was the reason for amputation.

☐ The stump should be checked for drainage and the color and amount recorded on the patient's chart.

☐ A plastic-backed drainage pad should be placed beneath or on top of the stump to reduce linen changes due to drainage.

☐ A tourniquet must be kept *in plain sight.* If severe hemorrhage occurs, the tourniquet should be applied and the physician called immediately.

☐ Range-of-motion exercises should be begun as soon as movement is tolerated.

Prosthesis Fitted at the Time of or Immediately After Surgery

☐ The stump must remain in the plaster cast.

☐ If the cast becomes dislodged from the stump, the stump should be wrapped immediately with an elastic bandage and the physician called.

☐ If dressings covering the operative area also become dislodged, sterile nonadhesive dressings (such as Telfa pads) should be placed over the incision before the elastic bandage is applied. Several rolls of elastic bandages and sterile nonadhesive dressings should be kept at the bedside and in plain view.

☐ A suspension harness, fitted around the waist, should be attached to the cast to keep it secure and in place. The harness should be slightly tightened when the patient is ambulatory and slightly loosened when the patient is in bed.

☐ A drain covered with a small dressing may be inserted in the incision and may protrude through the end of the cast. The color and amount of drainage (if any) should be noted and recorded on the patient's chart.

the foot or the hand is still there. The experience of phantom limb sensation after amputation consists of somesthetic and kinesthetic sensations that feel as real as those in the opposite limb or as in the limb before amputation. Amputation phantoms can persist for months or decades, or they can come and go. CARING FOR THE STUMP.   In a *closed amputation (flap amputation)* skin flaps cover the bone end. In an *open amputation (guillotine amputation)*, the end of the stump is open with no skin covering the stump. Open amputations are usually performed in the presence of infection. Skin traction is applied, and the infected area is allowed to drain. The traction must be continuous. The surgeon may arrange the traction so that the patient can turn over in bed. If the patient is incontinent, waterproof material should be secured around the outside of the bandage to prevent soiling of the wound.

Closed amputations usually are covered with pressure dressings. Drains may or may not be inserted in the incision. The stump may be elevated on a pillow for the first 24 to 48 hours to prevent edema of the stump. Many physicians prefer elevation of the foot of the bed because stump elevation promotes contracture of the remaining leg muscles. A bed board or a firm mattress provides support under the

hips, thus preventing flexion and contraction of the hip joint.

Although some drainage is usually considered normal, hemorrhage is a complication of amputations. Oozing around the incision may be seen, and the dressing should be reinforced as needed. Plastic-backed drainage pads can be placed under the stump. If drainage is near the top, a smaller pad may be placed between the stump and the top sheet. This protects the linen, reduces linen changes, and also prevents unsightly drainage from staining the top sheet. Stains, odors, and the sight of blood are upsetting to the patient and visitors. If a top sheet directly over the stump is uncomfortable, a drainage pad should be laid lightly over the stump and the top sheet secured around the groin and the unoperated side.

The type of surgery performed influences the length of time for stump conditioning, shrinking, and shaping. Some general principles, however, must be observed. Only when there no longer is the possibility of infection and the scar is well on the way to healing should shrinking bandaging be done. To help the stump shrink and shape properly for a prosthesis, elastic bandages may be applied to the stump. The physician generally determines the method for applying the bandages as well as other tasks to be carried out when caring for the stump. Upper extremity stumps do not need as massive a shrinkage over a long period as do those of the lower extremity. They are not subjected to supporting the great forces of body weight, even when a prosthesis is used, and they usually stabilize in about 6 months.

The stump is usually bandaged first with an over-and-under motion and then with a spiral motion (Fig. 55-16). All parts of the wrapped limb should be equally compressed. Proximal compression should be achieved by spirals and doubling back the bandage to avoid circular constriction. If the proximal part of the stump is compressed more tightly than the rest of the limb, edema results in the end of the stump. When a bandage is applied to an AK amputation, the spirals should be continued as high as possible to avoid a roll of flesh above the bandage. The bandage should be changed at least twice dur-

ing the day and before the patient retires for the night, at which time the underlying skin should be inspected for signs of infection, excessive drainage, or separation of wound edges.

EXERCISES AND POSITIONING.   Exercises and positioning of the patient in bed are important. With the rigid dressing, there is no danger of the patient developing flexion contractures of the stump. When a rigid dressing is not used, bed positioning to prevent contractures after a lower extremity amputation is important. The nurse may assist in the prevention of contractures in the following ways:

1. Assist and teach the patient to roll both from side to side and in the prone position to create extension for the amputation stump. Because the patient may experience a great deal of pain in the immediate postoperative period, a good time for using the prone position is about 30 minutes after administration of an analgesic.

    The patient should be instructed to, while lying on

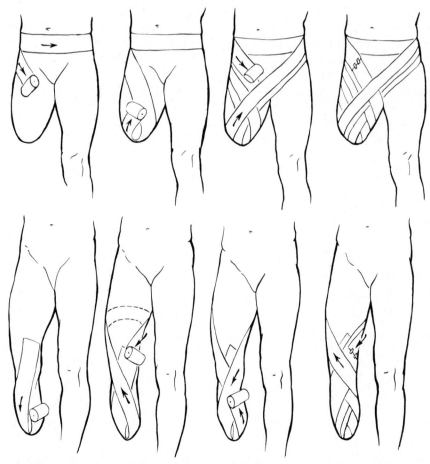

Figure 55–16.   In bandaging a stump of the upper leg, the bandage is anchored at the waist. Apply the bandage while the patient is standing on the unaffected leg. A criss-cross (rather than a circular) pattern is followed around the leg, starting at the stump end. Each loop overlaps the previous one by at least half its width. The same principles apply to bandaging a stump of the lower leg. Anchoring is accomplished without a circular turn around the leg.

the abdomen, adduct the stump so it presses against the other leg. The toes should extend over the end of the mattress so they are not pressed down into the mattress. When lying on the unaffected side, the patient should flex gently and extend the stump. When a patient with a BK amputation is in the supine position, and a pillow has been placed momentarily under the knee on the operative side, the knee gently can be flexed and extended. The patient should be taught to use the trapeze to change position in bed, using the arms and the trapeze rather than pushing with the heel.

2. Be sure that the patient is lying on a firm mattress. A sagging mattress can cause a flexion contracture.

3. Work with the physical therapist to implement a program of exercises for the patient to prevent contractures.

COMPLICATIONS. Hematoma, hemorrhage, and infection are complications that may be seen during the immediate postoperative period. Complications that may occur late in the postoperative course include chronic osteomyelitis (after persistent infection) and, rarely, a burning pain (causalgia), the cause of which is not known. Pain also may be caused by a stump neuroma, which is formed when the cut ends of nerves become entangled in the healing scar. A neuroma may be treated with injections of procaine, or reamputation may be necessary.

Some oozing may occur that will stain the rigid plaster dressing. The stain should be marked with a pen and periodically observed to determine whether excessive bleeding is taking place. If oozing occurs, the physician should be notified immediately. When a rigid dressing is not applied, the same principle should be used in observing the compressive dressing with the elastic bandages.

There is the possibility of hemorrhage in an amputation stump when a rigid plaster dressing is not applied. A tourniquet should be kept at the bedside where it can be seen and used. If hemorrhage occurs, the tourniquet should be applied, and the physician should be contacted immediately.

REHABILITATION. Rehabilitation may be a long process, and long-range planning requires teamwork. Each team member—physician, nurse, therapist, and prosthetist—has an important role in rehabilitation of the patient. Assessment of the patient by all members of the team is necessary throughout the entire rehabilitation process. Complications may occur and require additional treatment or surgery. The patient may face obstacles weeks and months after discharge from the hospital, and vocational and psychiatric counseling may be needed, especially for the younger patient.

A prosthesis is not designed to replace the lost part, its functions, or its appearance. Therefore, the function achieved should not be compared with normal function but should be evaluated against the patient's best potential. The amputee's potential depends on variables such as age, type of amputation, condition of the amputation stump, physical status, condition of the remaining limb, concurrent debilitating illness, visual motor coordination, motivation, acceptance, cooperation, and insight. Patients vary greatly in learning capacity and in their ability to achieve function with a prosthesis. The period allotted for their training also varies and is affected by factors such as the speed with which the patient learns and the potential for rehabilitation.

A person who loses the dominant hand has the choice of learning to do everything with the other hand or of learning to use a prosthesis. Because the loss of a hand is a devastating disability, it is important to restore the sense of purposeful use as soon as possible. The physician, physical therapist, and prosthetist should work with the patient in an attempt to restore the best function possible.

The training of an upper extremity amputee should consist of teaching the patient to apply and operate the prosthesis. The patient should be taught procedures to bend and lock the elbow and proper use of the harness. The patient then should be given increasingly difficult operations to perform with the terminal device, whether it is the hook or the hand. All the operations of the elbow and terminal devices are controlled by the shoulder on the amputated side. Training for use of some of the newer microcircuit devices should be carried out in the same manner.

The purpose of a lower extremity prosthesis is to provide weight support and comfort as well as the capacity to ambulate with safety, with or without mechanical aids. The process should be begun by teaching the patient to apply the prosthesis properly without assistance. Training usually starts with standing and weight-shifting between parallel bars to get the feel of weight support and balance. The next step usually involves heel and toe balance and rocking and hip hiking to get the prosthesis off the ground. Early steps begin by advancing the prosthesis first and bringing up the other leg to the standing position. With practice, alternate steps and increasing weight bearing are progressively accomplished. Initially, crutches, a walker, or canes should be used until the patient has sufficient confidence and stability to discard them. Any discomfort caused by the prosthesis should be corrected as soon as possible.

Rehabilitation means assessing strengths and liabilities and helping the patient to make the most of what remains. It is equally vital that the physician, the nurse, the physical and occupational therapists, the family, and the patient be realistic about what is expected. The nurse can also help these patients realize that they have assets as well as problems. When people are discouraged, they sometimes fail to see that they have strengths with which to work. The nurse who can help a patient see both sides of the ledger is better able to help him or her become self-directing.

Pain. Narcotic analgesics are required for several days after surgery, after which time pain may be controlled with an oral narcotic or nonnarcotic analgesic. Pain must always be evaluated before the administration of an analgesic. Pain in an area other than the operative area requires investigation and notification of the physician.

Anxiety. These patients usually experience frequent bouts and varying degrees of anxiety during the postoperative and rehabilitative periods. Each new problem should be dealt with as it arises, and the patient should be helped to accept and understand the situation. Examples of anxiety-provoking events are the phantom-limb sensation, phantom-limb pain, standing for the first time (lower extremity amputation), and seeing and using a prosthesis. The nurse should provide encouragement, emotional support, and understanding. Questions should be answered or referred to the physician or therapist. The family also should be encouraged to emotionally support the patient because a good support system often helps the patient face each new problem, accept failure, and develop a determination to overcome obstacles.

Potential for Infection. Infection is a serious complication of surgery. Any excessive drainage or signs of infection should be reported immediately. Vital signs should be taken at the prescribed intervals. Any sudden or slow rise in temperature or chills must be brought to the immediate attention of the physician. Most patients receive prophylactic antibiotics during the first 5 to 10 days after surgery.

Impaired Skin Integrity. Although some patients may be out of bed 1 or 2 days after surgery, elderly patients may require a longer period of immobility, especially if other medical disorders are present. The skin over pressure areas, such as the hips, heels, and sacral areas of the elderly as well as the young, should be inspected each time the patient is repositioned, turned, or requires care of the stump. Early signs of skin breakdown should be identified and steps should be taken to prevent further impairment of skin integrity.

Self-Care Deficit. Patients with a lower extremity amputation often can assume some of their own care

1 or 2 days after surgery. Those with an upper extremity amputation, especially an amputation of the dominant side, may require assistance until they are able to learn to use the opposite extremity.

Ineffective Individual Coping. The attitude of family members has great bearing on how the patient accepts and copes with the surgery and cooperates in postoperative care and rehabilitation. Some patients require an extended period of time to cope with an amputation and may require psychological counseling. Other patients accept the amputation and are determined to use a prosthesis. All members of the medical team may help the patient cope by listening, understanding, and giving encouragement each time a new task is accomplished.

Dysfunctional Grieving. Many of the serious psychological problems resulting from the thought of amputation are lessened by recently improved surgical procedures, making it possible for amputees to ambulate almost immediately after surgery. Despite immediate postsurgical fitting and early ambulation, the patient cannot be hurried through the stages of grieving and acceptance. Patients need support to proceed at their own pace to fully integrate the experience. These patients must be allowed time to express their feelings and to talk about their loss. Praise when a task is accomplished improves confidence and helps patients begin to adapt to the change and to move through the grieving process.

Some patients are unable to accept amputation and refuse to wear and use a prosthesis. If the reason for refusal is known, it may be possible for the physician, physical therapist, prosthetist, or nurse to help the patient accept a prosthesis. Sometimes, a simple adjustment, surgical revision of the stump, or practice and encouragement is all that is needed. The patient cannot be forced to use a prosthesis; the patient must make his or her own decision.

Impaired Physical Mobility. Exercises should be encouraged during the early postoperative period. Physical therapy is usually started early, with the therapist instructing the patient in the type of exercises to be performed. The patient should be encouraged to use the trapeze to assist movement in bed. Exercises of the operated as well as unoperated side prevent muscle weakness and atrophy, shorten the recovery period, and enhance the use of the prosthesis and other supporting devices, such as a walker, crutches, or a cane.

During the healing period, the patient may become ambulatory and should be made aware of the importance of good posture. In amputations above the elbow and higher, there is a tendency for the trunk to tilt away from the side of the amputation and for the head to tilt toward it. Eventual foreshortening of the shoulder girdle can result in scoliosis (curvature of the spine). This is of greater importance in growing children. For this reason, deep breathing, bilateral adduction and abduction exercises for the scapulae, and shoulder shrugging should be shown to the patient by the physical therapist and should be practiced several times daily. The nurse should be give the patient support and supervision as necessary.

The patient with a temporary prosthesis may be allowed to sit on the edge of the bed and dangle the unaffected leg on the day of surgery. On the first or second postoperative day, the patient may be permitted to stand and regain a sense of balance. Stepping on the floor with the temporary prosthesis and weight bearing of about 10% of body weight usually is permitted at this time.

The patient can progress to walking with crutches or a walker or in parallel bars 2 to 4 days after the amputation, with a high degree of safety, if a temporary prosthesis has been applied. Full weight bearing on the stump may not be permitted until 6 weeks after amputation because although the skin may heal in 2 weeks, at least 6 weeks are required for deep tissue scars to mature sufficiently to withstand the forces of full weight-bearing.

It is necessary to maintain a full range of motion in the remaining joints and build up strength in the muscles by the time the prosthesis is finally fitted. This is accomplished by passive exercises and by encouraging the patient to perform active exercises within tolerance. The nurse should work with the physical therapist by positioning the patient properly in bed, by encouraging exercises, and by supervising the patient as attempts are made to stand, to transfer weight, and to maintain balance.

When an amputation is performed on an older patient, there may be coexisting debilitating and degenerative diseases, many of which are disabling in themselves. The quality of physical mobility and performance with a prosthesis may fall far short of normal, both for upper and lower extremity amputations.

Respiratory Function. Although many patients with a temporary prosthesis are ambulated as soon as possible, those with a stump dressing may be kept in bed for a longer period of time. All amputees should be encouraged to deep breathe and cough every 2 hours while awake until they are fully ambulatory. The lungs should be auscultated daily, and the physician should be informed if abnormal breathing sounds are heard or if the patient experiences fever, cough, chills, or other signs of a respiratory problem.

Knowledge Deficit. The discharge teaching plan depends on many factors, including the length of hospitalization, the type and location of the amputation, the age and physical condition of the patient, and the type of dressing or prosthesis the patient wears.

The home atmosphere and physical plan should be determined before discharge. Modifications in living arrangements, the use of a wheelchair, or other accommodations or changes may need to be made for some individuals.

If the patient has to bandage the stump at home, both the patient and the family should be taught how to apply the bandage and how to care for the stump. The patient also should be advised to wash the bandages, to rinse them well, and to lay them flat to dry because hanging tends to decrease the elasticity. When the bandages are dry, they should be rolled without stretching.

The following general points may be included in the patient teaching plan:

1. Follow the physician's recommendations regarding caring for the stump, applying a stump dressing, washing the stump, and elevating the stump when sitting.
2. Do not apply nonprescription drugs (ointments, creams, topical pain relievers) to the stump unless use of a specific product has been approved by the physician.
3. Physical therapy and exercises are an important part of rehabilitation and wearing a prosthesis. Adhere to the plan of scheduled exercises and complete each group of exercises as outlined by the physical therapist.
4. Do not exceed the physician's recommendations regarding weight-bearing and joint flexion.
5. Eat a well-balanced and nutritious diet or follow the diet recommended by the physician. Gaining excess weight must be avoided during the recovery period because weight gain may interfere with use of a lower extremity prosthesis.
6. A phantom-limb sensation may persist for a period of time; this is normal.
7. Avoid injury to the stump, even though it appears to be healed.
8. Continue deep-breathing exercises until fully mobile.
9. Contact the physician if fever, chills, productive cough, bleeding or oozing from the stump, purulent drainage from the incision, new or different pain in the stump, or any change in the appearance in the stump occur.

Evaluation

- Pain and discomfort are controlled
- Anxiety is reduced
- Vital signs are normal
- No evidence of infection or other complications
- Skin remains intact
- Patient assumes most or all responsibility for own care
- Patient demonstrates an ability to cope with change in body image

- Patient demonstrates movement through the grieving process
- Patient demonstrates improved physical mobility
- Lungs are clear to auscultation; patient performs deep-breathing exercises
- Patient demonstrates knowledge and understanding of stump care, prosthesis use, home management

DISORDERS OF THE FEET
Hallux Valgus

Hallux valgus, also called bunions, is a deformity of the great (large) toe. Causes of hallux valgus are heredity, arthritis, or tight or improperly fitting shoes.

Symptoms
The toe deviates toward the next toe. Severe deformity may result in an overlapping of the great toe with the adjacent toe. Pain on walking or flexing the foot, tenderness, and redness of the joint are usually present.

Diagnosis
Diagnosis is made by physical examination. A radiograph of the foot is done to determine the degree of joint deformity.

Treatment
No treatment is necessary if pain is not severe and the patient has little or no difficulty. Low-heeled, properly fitted shoes should be recommended. Surgery (bunionectomy), which involves removal of the bunion and correction of the deformity, may be performed when the individual has pain and difficulty walking. This surgery is often performed on an outpatient or short-term admission basis, with the patient discharged in the late afternoon or the following morning. Rest, elevation of the foot, and analgesics should be prescribed.

Corns and Calluses

A *corn* is an overgrowth of the epidermis resulting from excessive pressure or rubbing. Tight or incorrectly fitted shoes and arthritic foot deformities are two causes of corns.

A *callus* is a thickened layer of skin resulting from pressure, friction, or use. Calluses are usually found on the hands and feet, although other areas of the body subject to excessive pressure or use also may develop a callus.

Treatment
Self-treatment involving soaking the area in warm water until the corn is softened usually causes no problem. This can be followed by application of a protective pad to reduce pressure on the area. Self-treatment involving scraping or application of liquids to remove the corn can result in infection. Corns not cured by softening and the wearing of a protective pad are best treated by a podiatrist.

Calluses of the feet can be treated by soaking and then using a rough cloth to remove the moist skin. Deep calluses or calluses causing a problem are best treated by a podiatrist.

DISORDERS OF THE HAND
Carpal Tunnel Syndrome

Carpal tunnel syndrome occurs when a nerve in the hand (the median nerve) is compressed by a tendon. The syndrome may be seen in those using their hands at occupations such as typing.

Symptoms
Pain, numbness, loss of feeling, and weakness of the thumb and first and second fingers are common complaints.

Diagnosis
Diagnosis is based on physical examination and symptoms.

Treatment
Rest of the hands (when possible) is advised. A splint may be applied to the hand and wrist, and injection of a corticosteroid preparation may relieve the discomfort. If conservative treatment is not successful, surgery to release the pressure of the ligament on the median nerve may be performed.

General Nutritional Considerations

☐ Rehabilitative efforts for the patient with an amputation of the arm include use of the prosthesis while eating and selection of foods and utensils that the patient can easily manage.

☐ A diet high in proteins, vitamins, and minerals may be ordered for the patient who is immobilized for a long period of time.

☐ Calcium is needed for the repair of bone. A diet high in calcium and restricted in foods that inhibit the absorption of calcium (such as fats and certain breakfast cereals) may be ordered. Phosphorus, which also is needed for the repair of bone, is usually present in adequate amounts in the average diet.

☐ Fluids should be forced to prevent formation of kidney stones, one of the hazards of immobility. Additional fluids can be supplied between meals in the form of milk shakes, gelatin, and other foods as well as water.

☐ Patients with arthritic deformities of the hands, arms, and shoulders may need assistance in cutting their food and opening cartons or covers on the hospital tray.

☐ Occasionally, patients with gout may need to restrict their intake of foods high in purine, for example, liver, kidney, and meat extracts.

☐ Overweight patients with osteoarthritis should be encouraged to lose weight and may need a reduction diet prescribed by the physician and tailored to their needs.

General Pharmacologic Considerations

☐ Stool softeners, such as docusate sodium (Colace) or docusate calcium (Surfak), may be necessary to prevent constipation in the patient immobilized for a long period of time.

☐ Vitamin and mineral supplements may be ordered for patients immobilized in traction, especially if dietary intake is poor.

☐ Patients receiving calcium as a mineral supplement also require additional vitamin D. An adequate amount of this vitamin must be present for calcium to be absorbed from the wall of the intestine.

☐ Arthritic patients should be warned about drugs, health foods, and certain food substances available in drug form and promoted as cures for arthritis.

☐ Patients taking large doses of salicylates should be told of the signs of gastrointestinal bleeding, salicylism, and the possibility of easy bruising and other bleeding tendencies.

☐ Signs of salicylism include headache, nausea, vomiting, tinnitus, increased pulse and respiratory rates, fever, mental confusion, drowsiness.

☐ Large doses of salicylates can interfere with the clotting mechanism of the blood. Patients taking these drugs are instructed to inform their physicians and dentists of their prolonged and high-dose ingestion of salicylates.

☐ Patients with gout need detailed instructions about their medical regimens in relation to the drugs to be taken and the importance of increasing their fluid intake to reduce the possibility of urate stone formation in the urinary tract.

☐ Patients with diseases of the bones and joints should be cautioned against discontinuing their drugs if and when they begin to feel improved.

☐ Patients taking aspirin for arthritis should be instructed *not* to substitute buffered aspirin or enteric-coated aspirin for regular aspirin unless the physician approves the change. Aspirin cannot be used in patients with ulcers, history of ulcers, or bleeding disorders.

☐ The most common adverse effects of NSAIDs are related to the gastrointestinal tract: nausea, vomiting, diarrhea, and constipation. Gastrointestinal bleeding, which in some cases is severe, has been reported with the use of these drugs.

☐ Calcitonin may be used in the treatment of Paget's disease and is administered subcutaneously. Some of the adverse effects associated with calcitonin include nausea (with or without vomiting), inflammation at the injection site, increased urinary frequency, anorexia, diarrhea, and abdominal pain.

General Gerontologic Considerations

☐ Fractures take longer to heal in elderly patients and thus may require a longer period of immobilization, which leads to an increase in the incidence of postfracture complications.

☐ Various degrees of arteriovenous insufficiency are present in elderly patients, increasing the possibility of thrombus formation and embolization. Arteriovenous insufficiency also can lead to delayed healing of the fracture and ischemia of the immobilized extremity, with the possibility of the development of gangrene.

☐ An adequate fluid intake is essential for any patient on prolonged bed rest. Elderly patients may need frequent reminders to drink fluids.

☐ Elderly patients often have poor muscle tone. After a fracture of the hip or a bone in the extremity, active and passive exercises of all the extremities are essential if adequate muscle tone is to be restored. Prolonged physical therapy also may be required to restore adequate muscle tone.

☐ Arthritis, especially osteoarthritis, is a common problem in most elderly patients. Depending on the degree of severity and deformity, these patients often require additional assistance with and time for the activities of daily living.

☐ After a hip arthroplasty or total hip replacement procedure, a confused elderly patient may fail to keep the operative leg in a position of abduction. Sand bags or other devices may be necessary to maintain correct leg alignment until such time as the patient is able to follow the physician's orders regarding leg alignment.

☐ When an elderly patient accepts the wearing of a prosthesis, additional time must be spent in explaining the care and application of the prosthetic device as well as care of the stump.

☐ Because muscle strength is often decreased, elderly patients require additional physical support when learning to ambulate with a prosthesis.

☐ Elderly patients are more likely to have a concomitant disease that may hinder adaptation to the use of a prosthesis.

Suggested Readings

☐ Ceccio CM, Horosz JE. Teaching the elderly amputee to meet the world. RN September 1988;51:70. *(Additional coverage of subject matter)*

☐ Dunajcik LM. When the hip joint must be replaced. RN April 1989;52:62. *(Additional coverage and illustrations that reinforce subject matter)*

☐ Farrell J. Illustrated guide to orthopedic nursing. 3rd ed. Philadelphia: JB Lippincott, 1986. *(Additional and in-depth coverage of subject matter)*

☐ Frazier D. Advances in prostheses. RN September 1988;51:73. *(Additional coverage of subject matter)*

☐ Krug BM. The hip: nursing fracture patients to full recovery. RN April 1989;52:56. *(Additional coverage and illustrations that reinforce subject matter)*

☐ Miller RA, Evans WE. Nurse and patient: allies preventing amputation. RN July 1988;51:38. *(Additional coverage of subject matter)*

☐ Peters VJ, Fox JM. Knee surgery clears a hurdle. RN July 1988;51:20. *(Additional coverage and illustrations that reinforce subject matter)*

☐ Redheffer GM, Bailey M. Assessing and splinting fractures. Nursing '89 June 1989;19:51. *(Additional coverage and photos that reinforce subject matter)*

- Introduction to the Integumentary System
- Integumentary Disorders

The Integumentary System

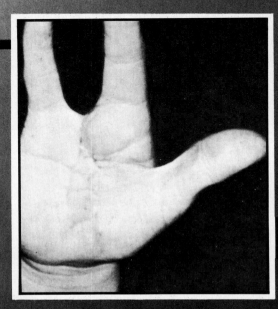

Unit 15

Chapter 56

Introduction to the Integumentary System

On completion of this chapter the student will:

- Be familiar with the basic anatomy and physiology of the skin and accessory structures

- Know the basic principles of the physical assessment of the patient with a skin disorder

The skin, the largest body organ, is a protective barrier between the body's internal and external environments. Because the skin is in constant contact with the environment, it is often subject to injury and irritation.

ANATOMY

The skin is composed of two layers: the *epidermis*, which is the outermost layer; and the *dermis*, which lies below the epidermis. The cells that compose the epidermis are constantly shed, and renewed epithelial cells originating in the dermis move upward to the epidermis. The dermis consists of connective tissue that is directly beneath the epidermis. It also consists of elastic fibers, blood vessels, sensory and motor nerve fibers, sweat and sebaceous (oil) glands, and hair follicles (roots). The dermis is attached to muscles and bones by subcutaneous tissue, which is composed of connective tissue and fat cells.

The color of the skin is determined by a pigment called *melanin*, which is manufactured by *melanocytes* located in the epidermis. The production of melanin is under the control of the middle or intermediate lobe (pars intermedia) of the pituitary gland, which secretes melanocyte-stimulating hormone. The more melanin in the epidermis, the darker the skin color.

ACCESSORY SKIN STRUCTURES

The hair and nails are accessory skin structures. Hair is present over most body areas. The exceptions are the soles of the feet and palms of the hands. In some areas, the hair is extremely fine and barely visible, with individual hairs widely spaced. In other areas, the hair is dense, thick, and more visible. In some areas, the hair serves a specific function; for example, the eyelashes and eyebrows keep dust and dirt particles out of the eyes. The nails consist of *keratin*, a tough protein substance that also is present in hair. Nails protect the ends of the fingers and toes.

FUNCTIONS OF THE SKIN
Protection

A primary function of the skin is the formation of a protective barrier between the outside world and underlying organs and structures of the body. This barrier prevents microorganisms and other foreign substances from coming in contact with the structures below the epidermis and prevents a loss of water from the structures below the surface of the skin.

Temperature Regulation

Heat is continuously produced inside the body. To maintain an even body temperature, the skin, by several methods, heats or cools the structures below. The heat produced by the body is dissipated primarily through the skin. The respiratory passages also aid in dissipating heat.

Heat is lost by any warm object, including the body, by three methods: radiation, conduction, and convection. *Radiation* is the ability of a warm object to transfer heat to a distant object of lower temperature. An example of radiation is heat moving from an object into the surrounding air. *Conduction* is the transfer of heat from a warm object to a cooler object. An example of conduction is placing a cool cloth on warm skin. The evaporation of moisture from the skin (eg, perspiration, water placed on the skin) is another example of heat loss by conduction. The heat of the body below the skin (the warmer object) is transferred to the water (the cooler object) on the skin. The water then evaporates. *Convection* is the transfer of heat by means of currents of liquids or gasses in which the warm air molecules move away from the body. An example of convection is a cool breeze that moves the warm molecules that are close to the body surface away from the body surface.

When the temperature outside the body is warm (close to or higher than the temperature inside the body), radiation and convection are ineffective. The only way heat can then be transferred from the body is by conduction. This is why exposure to warm temperatures can raise the body temperature and result in heatstroke (see Chapter 17).

Sensory

The skin serves as a means of monitoring the outside environment as well as warning of danger. Specialized nerve endings in the skin respond to pressure, pain, heat, and cold.

ASSESSMENT OF THE PATIENT WHO HAS A SKIN DISORDER

A skin lesion may appear suddenly or develop over a period of time. Some skin lesions can result in severe physical discomfort; some can be life-threatening. Other skin lesions cause minor discomfort or none at all. Some skin lesions can be difficult to diagnose. Others are readily diagnosed, but the cause may be obscure. A detailed patient history may aid in determining the diagnosis, cause, and treatment of certain types of skin disorders. Initial assessment of the patient with a disorder of the skin should include a thorough patient history as well as visual inspection of the skin. The nurse should base the patient history on the pa-

tient's symptoms or complaints. The patient with a sudden onset of urticaria (hives) accompanied by intense itching is different from the patient with a skin rash of 6 weeks' duration who is seeking medical attention only now. The latter individual has a disorder that is not an apparent emergency, and a detailed history is indicated. The other patient may be experiencing a severe drug reaction, and the nurse should quickly assess the patient and immediately contact a physician.

History

The following areas may be included in a thorough history of the individual with a dermatologic disorder:

History of the Disorder
- When and where the disorder began or first appeared
- Where the lesions are now
- Any changes in the disorder since it first appeared, including an increase or decrease in symptoms, changes in appearance or color, change in location, or spread to other areas

Physical Symptoms (Patient's Description)
- Physical sensations pertaining to the disorder: type (pain, itching, burning, etc.) and intensity
- Other physical or emotional problems that appear to be associated with the disorder
- Factors that appear to make the condition better or worse

Allergy History
- Known or suspected allergies
- *All* medications taken or used recently
- Recent changes in the use of personal products, such as soaps, deodorants, and cosmetics

Environmental Changes
- Present and past occupations
- Recent changes in the physical location of work or living areas
- Recent additions to work or living areas, such as pets, plants, sprays, dust, and pollutants

Emotional/Hormonal Changes
- Presence of added stress in occupation or personal life
- Changes in the lesions before, during, or after menstruation

Other
- Previous illnesses diagnosed and treated
- Previous or present problems not brought to the attention of the physician

Inspection

Visual inspection of the skin, including the scalp, hair, and nails, is the second part of the assessment. The mucous membranes of the mouth also should be examined, particularly when the lesions are on the face, head, or neck. Skin lesions and surrounding areas should be described as accurately as possible. Chart 56-1 gives for descriptions of various types of skin

Chart 56-1. Terminology Used in Describing Various Types of Skin Lesions

- **Atheroma** a fatty plaque
- **Bleb** a blister filled with fluid
- **Bulla** a large blister filled with fluid
- **Comedo** (pl. *comedones*) blackhead
- **Cyst** a sac or capsule containing fluid or semisolid material
- **Excoriation** an abrasion of the outer layer of the skin
- **Exfoliated cells** dead cells shed from the skin, mucous membrane, or bone
- **Exudate** fluid usually containing pus, bacteria, dead cells
- **Fissure** a groove, crack, or slit
- **Hyperplasia** extra growth of normal tissue
- **Macule** a discolored area that is neither raised nor depressed
- **Maculopapular** multiple lesions consisting of both macules and papules
- **Nodule** a small node
- **Papule** a small, solid, red elevation on the skin
- **Petechiae** tiny hemorrhagic spots on the skin
- **Pustule** a small elevation on the skin containing pus or lymph
- **Ulcer** a depression or defect
- **Vesicle** a small sac containing serous, seropurulent, or bloody fluid
- **Wheal** a raised lesion often accompanied by severe itching; a hive

lesions. The sites of the lesions (chin, left hand, anterior chest wall) also are listed.

As with any nursing assessment, judgment dictates the extent of the physical examination. In some dermatologic disorders, it may be necessary to examine other body organs or structures because some systemic disorders can produce dermatologic symptoms (Table 56-1).

Ongoing assessments depend on the treatments selected by the physician. Data from the initial assessment should be referred to as a baseline for recording response to treatment. Any new lesions, as well as changes in those lesions initially present, should be accurately described on the patient's record.

DIAGNOSTIC TESTS

The diagnosis of a skin disorder is made chiefly by visual inspection. Some disorders may require additional testing, including the following:

Biopsy—A biopsy may be performed to identify malignant or premalignant lesions. A biopsy also may be of value in helping to identify some skin disorders.

Culture and sensitivity tests—Culture and sensitivity tests may be taken of lesions that are suspected or known to contain microorganisms.

Allergy tests—Patch and intradermal testing may be done to determine an allergy to an offending substance (see also Chapter 10).

METHODS OF TREATING SKIN DISORDERS

Both topical and systemic treatment may be used in skin disorders. Topical preparations for the skin often are combinations of several ingredients carefully chosen by the dermatologist for their specific effects. Even patients who have similar skin disorders may respond differently to a particular preparation.

Table 56-1. Systemic Disorders With Dermatologic Symptoms

Condition	Cause	Description and Course	Treatment
Periarteritis nodosa (polyarteritis nodosa)	Unknown	Nodules appear along the course of arteries. There may be muscle and joint pain, nausea, vomiting, diarrhea, abdominal pain, fever, and weight loss.	Corticosteroids
Systemic lupus erythematosus	Believed to be autoimmune disorder; affects collagen	Red butterfly pattern over the cheeks and bridge of the nose; painful joints; edema; fever, and anemia. Kidneys, heart, and lungs may be affected.	Corticosteroids, salicylates, and other antiinflammatory agents, hydroxychloroquine (Plaquenil)
Scleroderma (progressive systemic sclerosis)	Unknown; some evidence suggests autoimmune cause	Hardening of collagen in many organs. Skin becomes tight and smooth; movement becomes difficult. The heart and lungs may be affected, causing dyspnea, cyanosis, and edema. The esophagus and intestines are often involved.	Symptomatic treatment including heat, physical therapy, salicylates, corticosteroids

Many skin disorders grow worse when the patient is tired or under emotional stress. Therefore, rest and sleep are an important part of treatment. Diet also may be an important part of treatment because certain foods may cause skin disorders in some individuals and therefore must be eliminated from the diet.

Drugs

Drugs may be used as single agents or combined in one product with other agents. Examples of drugs used in the treatment of skin disorders include the following:

1. *Corticosteroids*—Corticosteroids may be applied topically or administered systemically (orally, intramuscularly, intravenously). They may relieve symptoms, but they do not effect a cure. When used systemically, corticosteroids can have serious toxic effects; therefore, they should be used primarily to relieve acute problems. Continued use in long-term conditions brings greater risk and is justified only when the disease itself is serious and cannot be relieved by other treatments. Used as directed, topical application of a corticosteroid does not result in the pronounced adverse effects seen with systemic administration.
2. *Antihistamines*—Antihistamines are frequently prescribed when allergy is a factor in causing the skin disorder. They also are useful in relieving itching.
3. *Antibiotic, antifungal, and antiviral agents*—These drugs are used to treat infectious disorders and may be applied topically or administered systemically.
4. *Scabicides and pediculicides*—These agents are used in the treatment of infestations with the scabies mite and lice.
5. *Local anesthetics*—Topical application of a local anesthetic may be used to relieve minor pain and itching.
6. *Emollients, ointments, powders, and lotions*—These agents, which may be combined with other agents, soothe, protect, and soften the skin.
7. *Antiseborrheic agents*—Antiseborrheic shampoo agents are used in the control of dandruff.
8. *Antiseptics*—Antiseptics are used to reduce the number of bacteria on the skin.
9. *Keratolytics*—Keratolytics dissolve thickened, cornified skin such as that seen with warts, corns, and calluses. Their action causes the treated area to soften and swell, facilitating removal.

Wet Dressings

Wet dressings may be used to apply a solution to certain types of skin lesions. Dressings should be applied loosely, and those applied to open, denuded areas should be sterile. Cotton should not be placed next to the skin because of its tendency to stick to moist surfaces. When necessary, dressings can be anchored with nonallergenic tape or gauze.

When a wet dressing is applied, the physician determines whether the procedure is to be clean or sterile. The nature of the lesion (acute or chronic; open, weeping, or dry) helps to determine whether sterile techniques must be used. Medication in the form of a cream, lotion, or ointment may be applied to the skin before or after the wet dressing. It is most important that the medication be applied exactly as prescribed, such as a thin layer evenly spread over the area, or a thick layer dabbed on the area. Care must be taken in applying medication so that lesions are not broken or the skin surfaces abraded.

Wet dressings have a cooling and soothing effect, produced by the evaporation of the moisture from the dressing. They may be applied by either the open or the closed method.

Open method—Moist compresses are applied and are left open to the air. The affected part should not be covered with bedclothes. The bed linen beneath the patient should be protected by a plastic sheet or by disposable plastic-backed incontinence pads.

Closed method—Moist compresses are applied and then covered with waterproof material, such as plastic sheeting.

Baths

Various solutions, powders, and oils may be added to water to relieve inflammation and itching and to aid in the removal of crusts and scales. Examples of products that may be prescribed are starch, sodium bicarbonate (baking soda), oatmeal colloid bath preparations, and oils. A bath may involve the entire body or a part of the body, such as an arm or hand.

The tub or container is filled with lukewarm water. The drug or product is then added and the water stirred so that the preparation thoroughly mixes. The whole body or a body part is immersed in the water. A washcloth or a compress may be used to apply the solution to the face and any other parts not covered by the solution. The cloth or compress should be applied gently, without rubbing the skin. Soap is not used during this type of bath. Although the primary purpose of the bath is to soothe, it also helps to cleanse the skin.

Suggested Readings

☐ Fuller J, Schaller-Ayers J. Health assessment: a nursing approach. Philadelphia: JB Lippincott, 1990. *(Additional coverage of subject matter)*

Chapter 57

Integumentary Disorders

- Use the nursing process in the management of a patient with a skin disorder

- List and discuss the types, symptoms, diagnoses, and treatment of benign, premalignant, and malignant skin lesions

- Use the nursing process in the management of a patient with a malignant or benign skin lesion

- List the symptoms, diagnosis, and treatment of stasis ulcers

- Use the nursing process in the management of a patient with a stasis ulcer

- List the symptoms, diagnosis, and treatment of pemphigus and exfoliative dermatitis

- Use the nursing process in the management of a patient with a severe skin disorder

- List and discuss the classifications of burns, the physiologic changes after a burn, and the initial treatment of burns

- Use the nursing process in the management of the burned patient

COMMON DISORDERS OF THE SKIN AND RELATED STRUCTURES

Dryness

The sebaceous glands, which surround the hair follicles, secrete sebum, an oily substance that protects the hair and skin from becoming excessively dry. Some people, however, produce less sebum than is desirable for keeping the skin soft. This is particularly common during later life.

Heredity is important in determining the type of skin that a person has. Dry or oily skins are most common among individuals with a family history of these conditions.

Creams help to keep the skin soft and smooth by reducing the loss of moisture from the skin. Creams and lotions help to prevent dryness and chapping, particularly during cold weather, when moisture is lost more quickly. Wearing rubber gloves when using soaps and detergents for laundry and dish washing also is helpful in preventing dryness. These simple measures can greatly reduce chapping and cracking, which make the skin not only unattractive and uncomfortable but also vulnerable to infection and rashes.

Pruritus

Although pruritus (itching) is a common and distressing symptom of many skin diseases, the mechanism of itching is still somewhat obscure. The itch impulse probably has a lower frequency and intensity than does the pain impulse, thus differentiating the feeling of pain from the sensation of itching. Pruritus also may be a symptom of another disorder, such as diabetes mellitus, jaundice due to biliary obstruction, or drug allergy. The elderly patient, whose skin is often dry and scaly, may have pruritus.

Treatment is aimed at eliminating the cause, if known or suspected, as well as providing as much relief as possible. Oils, such as Alpha-Keri, may be added to bath water to aid in relieving dryness. Additional aids in relieving pruritus include starch baths, creams, lotions, or ointments. Antihistamines, administered systemically, may be prescribed, especially if the pruritus is due to an allergy.

Exposure to Sunlight

Tanning is the skin's response to exposure to sunlight, helping to protect it against the damaging effects of excessive ultraviolet light. Prolonged and excessive exposure to sunlight is believed to cause premature aging of the skin. Prolonged exposure, particularly of fair-skinned people who tend not to tan effectively, can cause a painful sunburn. Adolescents and young adults tolerate exposure to sunlight better than do older people because the skin becomes thinner, drier, and less protective with increasing age. Skin cancer is more common among those whose skin has had excessive exposure to sun and wind. The use of sunlamps or repeated exposure to the sun to develop a tanned and supposedly healthy look is not recommended because this method of tanning also may result in premature aging and skin cancer. Also, if the eyes are not protected, cataracts may form.

Sebaceous Cysts

Sebaceous cysts are caused by obstruction of the duct of a sebaceous gland. The gland continues to secrete sebum despite the obstruction, causing accumulation of an oily secretion in the blocked duct. A small swelling appears that can grow large and unsightly. Treatment of the condition is surgical excision of the cyst. If the lesion is small, it may be removed in a physician's office; larger cysts may need to be removed in a hospital operating room.

Herpes Simplex

Herpes simplex is caused by the herpes simplex virus type 1 (HSV1). Herpes simplex virus type 2 (HSV2), the causative agent of herpes genitalis (see Chapter 9), is related to HSV1. Generally, HSV1 causes infection above the waist, and HSV2 causes infection below the waist; however, either virus can be the cause of an infection above or below the waist.

It is believed that many individuals harbor the HSV1 virus, probably starting in childhood. It also appears that a variety of factors, including colds, fever, emotional upsets, and menses may precipitate the appearance of herpes.

Symptoms
A group of blisters occurs on reddened, inflamed skin, usually near the mouth or on the genitals. Pain and burning usually accompany the lesion. Herpes simplex around the mouth is often called a *cold sore* or a *fever blister*. The lesions subside in about a week. Some people are especially susceptible to herpes simplex and have frequent recurrence of the lesions.

Diagnosis
Diagnosis is made by visual examination.

Treatment
The symptoms are usually mild, and the condition subsides without treatment. No specific treatment can shorten the duration of the lesion; however, some physicians prescribe topical acyclovir (Zovirax) for those with severe, widespread lesions or for immunocompromised patients (those having an ineffective immune system) who develop a herpes simplex infection.

Pediculosis

An infestation with pediculi (lice) results in *pediculosis*. The following terms are used to describe pediculosis:

Pediculosis capitis—Infestation of the hair or the scalp
Pediculosis corporis—Infestation of the body surfaces with a louse larger than the one that affects the scalp and the hair. This parasite and its eggs also may be found in the patient's clothing, particularly within cuffs and seams
Pediculosis pubis—Infestation of the pubic area with a tiny louse shaped like a crab, hence the lay term *crabs*. Although this condition occurs primarily in the pubic area, it may occur in the hairy areas of the axillae

Symptoms
Symptoms include itching and irritation of the skin. Scratching denudes the skin, making it susceptible to infection.

Diagnosis
Diagnosis is made by visual inspection. In pediculosis capitis, the eggs are deposited on the hair near the scalp, cannot be brushed out as dandruff can, and are attached firmly to the hair. The lice are tiny, grayish-brown creatures that can be seen when they move on the scalp, body, or pubic area.

Treatment
Benzyl benzoate and γ-benzene hexachloride can be found in a variety of ointments, powders, shampoos, and lotions that are effective in killing pediculi. Although the pediculi can be promptly killed by these agents, repeated infestations are likely if the individual continues to have close contact with others who harbor the parasites and if personal hygiene is poor. Pediculosis capitis can be spread by shared toilet articles, like combs, and by close personal contact, such as that occurring in crowded places. Pediculosis pubis can be transmitted during sexual intercourse.

Scabies

Scabies is caused by infestation with the itch mite (*Sarcoptes scabiei*).

Symptoms
Symptoms include intense itching, which is usually worse at night, accompanied by excoriation and burrows (the lesion caused when the female itch mite

invades the skin, burrowing underneath and leaving a dark line). The lesions most often occur between the fingers and on the forearms, the axillae, the waistline, women's nipples, men's genitals, the umbilicus, and the lower back.

Diagnosis
Diagnosis is made by examining the affected areas.

Treatment
γ-Benzene hexachloride and crotamiton cream or lotion may be prescribed. The medication should be applied to the entire body (from the neck down) in a thin layer, left on for 8 to 12 hours, and then removed by washing. Thorough bathing, clean clothing, and the avoidance of contact with others who have scabies are essential in preventing recurrence. Before any treatment is started, the patient must have a thorough bath. After medication has been applied, a complete change of clothing is necessary because the itch mite can be transmitted readily from one person to another by close personal contact and by sharing towels and clothing.

Bedbug Infestation

The bites are caused by tiny, dark brown insects that infest mattresses and wooden bed frames. In heavily infested dwellings, bedbugs may live in crevices of the woodwork or in upholstered furniture. Although they are more common in crowded, unsanitary homes, bedbugs may be brought into any home on clothing or even on newspapers.

Symptoms
The symptoms of bedbug bites include the appearance of wheals (hives) with central points or dots. These lesions may appear on any part of the body, but they most commonly are found on the wrists, ankles, and buttocks.

Diagnosis
Diagnosis is made by examination of the bites and patient history.

Treatment
Usually the bites require little local treatment. Sometimes calamine lotion or another type of soothing lotion is applied to relieve discomfort. The services of an exterminator are frequently required to get rid of the bugs.

Seborrheic Dermatitis

The common term for mild seborrheic dermatitis is *dandruff*.

Symptoms
The familiar symptoms are oily scalp, formation of oily scales, itching, and irritation. Severe cases are characterized by inflammation with redness, swelling, and, sometimes, exudation and infection. Seborrheic dermatitis frequently accompanies acne, but, unlike acne, it is not limited typically to adolescence. Often it persists throughout adulthood. It primarily affects the scalp, but it may spread to the eyebrows, the skin around the ears, the forehead near the hairline, and other areas of the body where there are large numbers of sebaceous glands, causing the skin in these areas to be red, oily, and scaly.

Diagnosis
Diagnosis is based on visual examination of affected areas.

Treatment
Treatment includes regular cleansing and application of local medication between shampoos. When the oiliness is severe, daily shampoos may be needed. Although the scales are removed by washing, they promptly accumulate again until the condition is controlled. The physician usually advises the use of an antiseborrheic shampoo. When the condition is unresponsive, mildly antiseptic lotions or medicated ointments may be prescribed for use between shampoos. Seborrheic dermatitis of areas other than the scalp may be treated with corticosteroid or antibiotic ointments.

Prompt and persistent treatment often results in great improvement, to the degree that only good scalp hygiene is required to avoid a return of the condition. Many people, however, continue to require regular medical treatment to control the symptoms. These individuals have chronically overactive sebaceous glands.

Contact Dermatitis

The skin is one of the organs most frequently affected by allergy. There are two types of contact dermatitis: allergic contact dermatitis and primary irritant dermatitis. *Allergic contact dermatitis* develops after contact with one or more substances, such as cosmetics, drugs, clothing, detergents, and dyes. On *skin* contact, the sensitive individual develops an inflammatory reaction. *Primary irritant dermatitis* results from contact with substances such as solvents and strong detergents. It is not caused by an allergy and appears, in many instances, to be due to the irritating quality of the substance.

Symptoms
The skin response is characterized by dilatation of the blood vessels, causing redness and swelling, and some-

times by vesiculation (blister formation) and oozing. Itching is a prominent symptom.

Diagnosis

Diagnosis is made by visual examination of the area. A detailed and thorough patient history is usually necessary to identify the offending substances.

Treatment

If the contact dermatitis is thought to be an allergic reaction, patch tests may identify the responsible substances. Treatment of both types of contact dermatitis is to remove the substances causing the reaction. Repeated episodes can result in a leathery thickening of the skin. The patient may be instructed to apply a lotion, ointment, or cream to the affected areas. Systemic drugs to relieve itching and treat infection may be necessary. In more severe cases, wet dressings may be prescribed, possibly followed by the application of a topical medication.

Acne Vulgaris

Acne vulgaris is one of the most common skin conditions. The cause is not fully understood, but acne characteristically occurs during adolescence; it is believed to be related to the hormonal changes that occur when secondary sex characteristics are developing. Other factors, such as a genetic disposition to acne and bacterial infection of the sebaceous glands and hair follicles, also may play a role.

Symptoms

The skin of the affected areas (usually face, chest, and back) is excessively oily. The lesions consist of comedones (blackheads, whiteheads), papules (pimples), and pustules (pimples filled with pus). In severe cases, cysts sometimes occur, appearing as large, reddish swellings. The severity of the condition ranges from an occasional pimple to a large number of bright red pimples and blackheads. Severe acne, if neglected, can lead to the formation of deep, pitted scars that leave the skin permanently pockmarked. Oiliness of the scalp and the shedding of oily scales (seborrhea) often accompany acne. Infection and the formation of pustules are fostered by picking and squeezing the lesions.

The possibility of scarring from severe acne is too often overlooked. These scars are *not* outgrown, and they can spoil a complexion for life. The emotional scars are just as important. For some young people, these matters mean only temporary distress; for others, severe or unusually prolonged acne can interfere seriously with their developing into poised, confident adults. Acne that is pronounced or unsightly should be

treated—the more prompt the treatment, the less likelihood of scars, physical or emotional.

Diagnosis

Diagnosis is made by visual examination of the affected areas. On occasion, a culture and sensitivity test may be done if the lesions appear infected.

Treatment

Drug therapy may include the topical application of tretinoin (Retin-A) or oral administration of isotretinoin (Accutane). Topical and systemic antibiotics, in low doses, also are used in some instances of severe acne and have produced good results.

Women who are pregnant or who may become pregnant are not prescribed and must not take oral isotretinoin because there is a high risk of birth defects associated with its use. It is recommended that this drug only be used for those who (1) have severe cystic acne that does not respond to other therapies, (2) are reliable in understanding and carrying out the treatment regimen, (3) are capable of complying with mandatory contraceptive measures, and (4) have a negative pregnancy test 2 weeks before beginning therapy.

The physician can remove the blackheads and drain the pustules with special instruments. This process should never be attempted by the patient because infection and scarring can be caused by unskilled manipulation.

The physician also may recommend any one or more of the following: keeping the nails short and clean (to prevent spreading infection); washing the skin with an antibacterial soap; using an abrasive soap to remove dead skin; avoiding the use of perfumed soaps and skin cosmetics; keeping the hands away from the face; keeping the hair away from the face (this is especially important in those with long hair); and keeping the hair clean by washing and avoiding the use of cosmetic hair products (sprays, gels, and so forth).

The patient should be instructed to wash the hands thoroughly before applying medication or carrying out any other treatment of the lesions. Medicated preparations should be used only with the physician's advice. Topical ointments and creams prescribed by the physician must be applied as directed.

Dermatophytosis

Dermatophytoses (tinea) are superficial fungus infections. *Dermatophytes* (also called tinea) are fungi that are parasitic on the skin. The terms *tinea pedis, tinea capitis,* and *tinea corporis* identify the areas of infection, namely, feet, head, and body. Another common term for this infection is *ringworm*, a misnomer because the infection is not caused by a worm; it is fungal in origin.

Symptoms

In tinea pedis (also known as athlete's foot), the infection usually begins in the toes, and particularly in the skin between them. The affected skin becomes red, scaly, cracked, and sore. Sometimes the condition also affects the sides of the toes and the soles of the feet. It may spread to the hands, axillae, and groin. The nails also may become involved and are characteristically yellow, friable, and opaque.

Tinea capitis (ringworm of the scalp) is more common in children. The fungus invades the hair shaft below the scalp. This is followed by breaking off of the hair, usually close to the scalp. The areas of infection are rounded, and one or more patches of infection may be found.

Tinea corporis, or ringworm of the body, usually involves nonhairy areas of the skin.

Diagnosis

Diagnosis is made by visual examination of the affected areas. Early diagnosis and treatment are important in preventing spread.

Treatment

Treatment of tinea pedis includes the topical use of antifungal agents, such as benzoic and salicylic acids ointment (Whitfield's ointment), undecylenic acid, and tolnaftate. Griseofulvin (Grisactin) also is useful in treatment and is given orally. The drug may be required for many weeks to eradicate the infection.

Tinea pedis may be transmitted from person to person through towels, locker rooms, and bathroom floors. Towels and slippers should not be shared, and people using locker rooms or community bathrooms in dormitories should avoid going barefoot. Keeping the feet (particularly the area between the toes) dry increases resistance to the infection. People whose feet perspire freely often find that powdering between the toes helps to keep the area dry. Washing and drying the feet, and putting on clean, dry socks and a different pair of shoes after coming home from work is another aspect of personal hygiene that helps to keep the skin of the feet healthy.

Treatment of tinea capitis includes the use of the systemic antifungal agent griseofulvin, which is taken with meals. A local antifungal agent also may be prescribed to destroy fungus present on the hair shafts above the surface of the scalp.

Treatment of tinea corporis includes the use of topical antifungal agents for less severe infections. Griseofulvin, taken orally, is prescribed for more severe infections.

Impetigo Contagiosa

More common in children than adults, impetigo is usually caused by a streptococcal or a staphylococcal infection of the skin.

Symptoms

Symptoms include erythema and vesicles that rupture and are covered with a sticky yellow crust. Face and hands are common sites.

Diagnosis

Diagnosis is made by visual inspection of the lesions.

Treatment

Impetigo is highly contagious, and contact with other people with the lesions or exudate should be avoided. The patient should never share towels or bed linen. Meticulous hand washing after application of medication is important. The patient must avoid touching the lesions unnecessarily. Because the condition can be spread from one part of the body to another, as well as to other people, the hands must be thoroughly washed immediately after touching the lesions. The infected individual should keep away from other family members as much as possible. Children should be kept out of school until the lesions clear.

The crusts can be removed with soap and water before any local medications are applied. Gloves should be worn, and the applicators or gauze used for this purpose must be wrapped carefully and immediately discarded. Systemic and topical antibiotics may be ordered.

Usually the condition is cured in a week. It can be especially severe in the newborn, however, and it can even cause death.

Psoriasis

Both men and women are affected by psoriasis, usually during young adulthood and middle life.

Symptoms

The disorder is characterized by patches of erythema (redness) covered with silvery scales, usually on the extensor surfaces of the elbows and the knees, the lower back, and the scalp. Itching is usually absent or slight, but occasionally it is severe. The lesions are obvious and unsightly; the scales tend to shed.

Diagnosis

Diagnosis is made by visual examination of the lesions.

Treatment

There is no cure for psoriasis. Treatment is aimed at the control of scaling and itching. Some factors that apparently cause a flare-up of the disorder are stress, alcoholism, infection, and trauma. The patient must understand that treatment is usually for a lifetime and the plan of therapy must be followed.

Treatment is individualized and may include the use of topical agents such as coal tar extract, corticosteroids, or anthralin. Anthralin, a distillate of crude coal tar, may be used on thick plaques but may irritate the unaffected skin areas. Corticosteroids applied topically have proved beneficial. Methotrexate, an antimetabolite used in the treatment of cancer, may be prescribed in cases that are severe and do not respond to other forms of therapy. This drug inhibits the production of cells that divide rapidly (cancer cells, cells composing the skin and mucous membranes, and so on) and is capable of decreasing plaque formation. Dosage must be carefully regulated because such drugs can cause serious adverse effects.

Etretinate (Tegison) is related to retinoic acid and retinol (vitamin A) and may be used to treat psoriasis not responding to other therapies. The use of this drug is recommended only for those who are reliable in understanding and carrying out the treatment regimen, are capable of complying with mandatory contraceptive measures, and do not intend to become pregnant.

Another method of treatment is the injection of triamcinolone acetonide into isolated psoriatic plaques. This method of treatment has been successful in some cases. Photochemotherapy has also been used for severe, disabling psoriasis that has not responded to other methods of treatment. The patient is be instructed to take oral methoxsalen 1 or 2 hours before exposure to ultraviolet light. This form of treatment is most often given in a physician's office or clinic. The extent of exposure is based on the patient's skin tolerance. Treatments are not given more often than once every other day, since phototoxic reactions may not be apparent until 48 hours after each exposure. Once the psoriasis clears, the patient should be placed on a maintenance treatment program.

Some patients respond well to treatment; others receive only minor relief. However, the condition tends to recur. Patients with psoriasis should be wary of a variety of widely advertised remedies that promise quick relief but rarely give it.

Furuncle, Carbuncle, Furunculosis

Streptococci, staphylococci, and other pathogenic organisms often exist harmlessly on the surface of the skin, but when the normal protective functions of the skin are impaired, these pathogens may cause infection. Often, an injury such as that caused by squeezing a pimple is the immediate cause because it allows infection to enter through a break in the skin. Furunculosis can occur as a result of lowered resistance, poor general health, and poor diet. Sometimes virulent strains of hospital-type staphylococci are the cause.

Symptoms
The descriptive symptoms of these conditions are as follows:

Furuncle (boil)—A furuncle is a whitish, raised, painful lesion, surrounded by erythema. The area feels hard to the touch. After a few days, the lesion exudes pus, and later a core. It heals, leaving a tiny scar. Neglect or mismanagement can cause a larger, obvious scar.
Carbuncle—A carbuncle is a large swollen lesion, often on the back of the neck, surrounded by erythema. It is acutely painful; it has several openings through which pus drains.
Furunculosis—The patient with furunculosis has multiple furuncles and also may have fever, anorexia, weakness, and malaise.

Diagnosis
Diagnosis is made by examining the lesion. Culture and sensitivity tests may be ordered if antibiotic therapy is planned.

Treatment
Hot wet soaks are used to localize the infection. For a single boil, this usually is the only treatment necessary. Antibiotics may be ordered to control the infection. Often, large doses are prescribed when fever is present, or if the lesion is a carbuncle. Incision and drainage may be necessary.

The patient should never pick or squeeze a boil because this practice favors spread of the infection to surrounding tissues or even to the bloodstream, resulting in septicemia. Drainage from a boil is infectious; strict aseptic technique is essential when applying or changing a dressing to prevent the spread of the infection to other parts of the patient's body or to other people.

NURSING PROCESS —THE PATIENT WHO HAS A SKIN DISORDER

Assessment
The involved areas should be inspected, and a complete and thorough medical, drug, and allergy history should be obtained (see Chapter 56).

Nursing Diagnosis
Depending on the type of lesion and the symptoms, one or more of the following nursing diagnoses may apply:

■ Anxiety related to symptoms, treatment regimen, other factors (specify)
■ Pain related to infection or type of skin disorder
■ Pruritus related to dryness, systemic disease, other factors (specify)
■ Potential for infection related to scratching, poor hand-washing techniques, poor physical condition, other factors (specify)

- Impaired skin integrity related to symptoms of disorder, scratching, other factors (specify)
- Body image disturbance related to disfigurement
- Knowledge deficit of treatment regimen, techniques of drug administration

Planning and Implementation

The major goals of the patient may include reduction in anxiety, relief of symptoms, absence of infection, intact skin, improved self-image, and understanding of the prescribed treatment regimen.

The major goals of nursing management may include relief of symptoms, reduction in anxiety, prevention of infection and skin breakdown, and preparation of an effective patient teaching plan.

Pain.   Although not all disorders are painful, some patients may require analgesics. Gentleness is essential in caring for patients with a painful skin disorder.

Pruritus.   Certain factors tend to make itching worse, including excessive warmth, rough fabrics, emotional stress, and idleness. Itching usually is worse at night, probably because the patient's attention is not occupied and therefore the patient is more aware of the sensation. Every effort must be made to determine what substances or events may cause itching and, when possible, to remove or correct them.

Severe itching is agony. Scratching leads to trauma and excoriation, often to infection. Helping the patient with severe pruritus to obtain some degree of comfort and to avoid scratching is a challenge. It is an even greater challenge when the patient is unable to cooperate because of mental confusion or disorientation. Measures that may reduce itching or prevent the patient from breaking the skin by repeated scratching include the following:

- Keeping the nails short and clean
- Providing light cotton bedding and clothing that allow normal evaporation of moisture from the skin (the use of wool, synthetics, and other dense fibers should be avoided)
- Having the patient wear white cotton gloves if scratching occurs during sleep
- Avoiding the use of regular soap for bathing; hypoallergenic or glycerin soaps often can be used without causing skin irritation or itching
- Using tepid bath water and patting rather than rubbing the skin dry

The results of the prescribed oral or topical agent should be noted. If the drug fails to relieve itching, the physician should be informed.

Potential for Infection.   Some skin disorders are of themselves infectious. There also are situations in which infection is introduced because of scratching, poor hand-washing techniques (patient and nurse), or *autoinnoculation* (the patient spreads the infection to other parts of the body by touching the unaffected areas after touching the infected areas). The patient should be instructed to wash the hands thoroughly with soap and water and to avoid touching other areas of the body after touching an infected area.

Impaired Skin Integrity.   A wet dressing should not be allowed to become completely dry. The nurse may be the first to discover a dressing that needs attention and should never moisten it by pouring solution over the dry, outer layers of the gauze. The solution may not penetrate to the gauze next to the patient's skin, and can carry dirt inward from the surface of the dressing. The dressing must be completely removed, and the treatment resumed. If the dressing is dry and has stuck to the skin, it is necessary to first remove the outer layers of gauze, then moisten the inner layer with solution, using an Asepto syringe. After at least 20 minutes, an attempt should be made to remove the adherent dressing. If the dressing does not come loose, additional solution can be added and allowed to soak into the area. A dressing that is stuck must never be pulled at roughly because this causes pain as well as trauma to the skin.

Open wet dressings are usually applied at intervals, for example, for 15 minutes every 2 hours. These dressings must be removed and discarded at the end of each treatment because the compresses dry out quickly. Adherence of dry compresses to the skin, followed by difficult removal, defeats the purpose of this type of dressing.

One problem associated with continuous closed wet dressings is the absorption of water through the skin. This may result in skin softening and, ultimately, in *maceration* (softening and wrinkling of the skin). It is most important that compresses used in wet dressings be removed as prescribed. If there is no written order about dressing changes, the nurse should remove and reapply the compresses at least once a day and preferably every 8 hours. The skin should be inspected at this time, and any softening or severe wrinkling should be reported immediately.

When tub baths are prescribed, the bathroom should be comfortably warm, and small amounts of hot water should be added at periodic intervals to prevent the water from becoming cold and the patient chilly. When the treatment is over, the skin should be patted dry. Rubbing the skin can cause irritation and may open skin lesions. If a topical drug is to be applied after the bath, it should be applied immediately after the patient's skin has been dried.

Irritation and increased itching may result if the application of a local medication is delayed after the bath. Anyone using a bath oil additive must take special care in getting in and out of the tub because oil leaves a slippery residue on the tub surface.

Body Image Disturbance, Anxiety. Because the skin is visible, skin lesions can result in a disturbance in body image and self-esteem. It is not difficult to understand why people who suffer severe facial disfigurement or have pronounced skin disorders on exposed parts of the body often undergo personality changes and at times varying degrees of anxiety. They become acutely and painfully aware of the stares, the avoidance, and even the revulsion of other people, and they tend to withdraw from social and business contacts.

It is important to show acceptance of patients with a disfigurement or a skin disorder. They need a great deal of understanding and emotional support from all members of the health team.

Knowledge Deficit. Many skin disorders are treated on an outpatient basis. The patient must have a full understanding of the complete treatment regimen.

The following general information can be included in the patient teaching plan. The points to be included should depend on the type of skin disorder and the method of treatment.

1. Follow the directions of the physician regarding the prescribed medications.
2. Apply topical drugs exactly as prescribed. Prepare the skin before application precisely as directed by the physician..
3. Take the prescribed oral drugs in the dose and at the intervals printed on the container.
4. Do not increase or decrease the dose or intervals of topical or oral drugs.
5. Do not use any nonprescription oral or topical drugs unless their use has been approved by the physician.
6. Keep the skin clean. Use a mild soap for cleansing the skin. Avoid using perfumes, perfumed soaps or lotions, or soaps that contain deodorants unless their use is approved by the physician. Avoid using any facial cosmetics unless their use is approved by the physician.
7. Keep the hair short, clean, and away from the face and forehead. Wash the hair at the intervals suggested by the physician. Avoid the use of dyes, rinses, sprays, and other styling products unless their use is approved by the physician.
8. Wash the hands thoroughly before as well as after applying topical medications. Keep the hands away from the affected areas. If the area must be touched, the hands must be thoroughly washed before as well as after touching the area.
9. If an infection is present, follow the advice of the physician to prevent the spread of the infection to other individuals and to other parts of the body. Soak towels and washcloths in bleach and wash in hot water separate from other laundry. Clothing also should be washed in hot water separate from the laundry of other family members.
10. Never try to remove, squeeze, or prick a pimple, boil, or any other type of skin lesion because a serious infection can occur.

Evaluation

- Anxiety is reduced
- Pain is controlled
- Pruritus is relieved
- No evidence of infection
- Skin remains intact
- Patient demonstrates evidence of accepting changes in body image
- Patient demonstrates understanding of treatment regimen, method of applying or taking the prescribed agents, methods of preventing the spread of infection

BENIGN AND POTENTIALLY MALIGNANT SKIN LESIONS

For early diagnosis and treatment to be possible, it is important to be aware that some common benign skin lesions have the potential to become malignant. Skin lesions usually are readily observable, and this facilitates prompt action.

Angiomas and Pigmented Nevi

Angiomas (birthmarks) are vascular tumors that may be found anywhere on the body and are almost always visible at birth. *Pigmented nevi* (moles) also are usually present at birth. In some cases, the beginnings of the nevi are present at birth but may not be visible until later in life. Angiomas and pigmented nevi are benign lesions, but nevi can become malignant.

Symptoms
Angiomas and pigmented nevi are not painful. The color of angiomas may vary from deep red or violet to bright red. The lesion may be either flat or raised, and the surface and edges are usually irregular. A pigmented nevus may be found in various shades of brown as well as black. The surface is usually irregular and soft.

Diagnosis
Diagnosis is made by visual inspection. If the tissue is removed, it should be examined microscopically to be sure that there are no malignant changes.

Treatment

Angiomas sometimes can be disguised by the use of special masking cosmetics. The argon laser may be used to remove angiomas. Most often, several treatments are necessary. Most angiomas can be made to be almost invisible after laser therapy.

Any pigmented nevus that becomes irritated, bleeds, or begins to grow larger should have prompt medical attention because these changes may indicate a malignant process. Black, smooth moles are the most likely to become malignant and therefore should be removed and microscopically examined. Light brown moles that are not located where irritation from clothing is a problem usually do not have to be removed unless it is desirable for cosmetic reasons.

Senile Keratoses

Senile keratoses are usually seen on the skin of older people. They are most likely to occur on exposed portions of the skin, such as the face, the ears, or the hands.

Symptoms

Senile keratoses are brownish, raised, scaly spots. They are not painful.

Diagnosis

Diagnosis is made by visual inspection.

Treatment

Those who develop senile keratoses should be advised to seek medical attention. Because the lesions are common and seem to be insignificant, they are often disregarded. They may become malignant, however, and their removal usually is recommended.

Warts (Verrucae)

Warts are caused by the papilloma virus and may be found anywhere on the skin.

Symptoms

Their appearance varies depending on their location. Some may appear flat, others cauliflowerlike. Warts are usually painful. Warts on the soles of the feet (plantar warts) are often painful and require treatment.

Diagnosis

Diagnosis is made by visual inspection.

Treatment

Unless located in an area that causes problems, treatment is often unnecessary. Plantar warts may be re-moved by *electrodesiccation* (use of electricity to destroy tissue) or by the application of keratolytic agents, such as canthracin and salicylic acid.

MALIGNANT SKIN LESIONS

Several factors predispose to malignant changes in the skin:

- Prolonged, repeated exposure to ultraviolet rays
- Exposure to radiation
- Ulcerations of long duration and scar tissue (both are prone to malignant changes)

Malignant growths of the skin are usually primary lesions. Their spread to other parts of the body or the tissues below may be prevented by prompt removal of the malignant tissue.

The following are the more common types of malignant skin lesions:

Malignant melanoma—Malignant melanoma is a highly malignant, rapidly spreading lesion. Usually it is coal black (Fig. 56-1). Wide surgical excision may be attempted to save the patient's life; however, because of the rapid spread, the prognosis is poor.

Squamous cell carcinoma—Squamous cell carcinoma is another dangerous type of lesion because it tends to metastasize to the internal organs. This type of cancer often occurs on the tongue or the lower lip and is more dangerous because it can invade deeper tissues and metastasize in its late stages.

Basal cell carcinoma—These carcinomas arise from the epidermal basal cells and are the most common type of skin cancer. Basal cell carcinomas do not tend to spread unless they are not removed.

Symptoms

Symptoms vary, but usually the new appearance of a growth or a change in color of the skin is the first

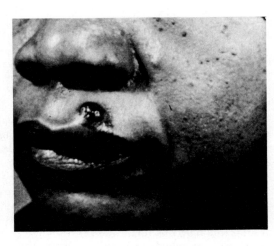

Figure 57–1.   Melanoma. (Medichrome, Clay-Adams, Inc, New York, NY)

symptom the patient notices. Squamous cell carcinomas appear as rough, scaly tumors, whereas basal cell carcinomas appear waxy and have a raised, pearly border.

Malignant melanoma may be first detected when the patient notes a change in the color, size, or general appearance of a mole or pigmented area.

Diagnosis
Diagnosis is made by visual inspection and confirmed by biopsy.

Treatment
Depending on the size and the location of the lesion, treatment of squamous cell and basal cell carcinomas may involve electrodesiccation, surgical excision, *cryosurgery* (the application of liquid nitrogen—a deep-freezing substance—to the tumor), or radiation therapy. The patient should be followed at regular intervals for at least 3 to 5 years to be sure regrowth has not occurred.

The treatment of multiple myeloma usually involves radical excision of the tumor and adjacent tissues, followed by chemotherapy.

NURSING PROCESS —THE PATIENT WHO HAS A MALIGNANT OR BENIGN SKIN LESION

Assessment
A complete medical, drug, and allergy history should be obtained, and the skin lesion should be examined and described in the patient's record. It is important to determine facts about the lesion, including: when the lesion first was noticed; whether the lesion has undergone any recent changes and, if so, what kind of changes; and what prescribed or patient-initiated treatments, if any, have been used.

Nursing Diagnosis
Depending on the type of lesion, one or more of the following nursing diagnoses may apply. Most of these lesions are treated on an outpatient basis. Those with a suspected or known malignant melanoma are admitted for radical surgery and intensive therapy. These patients require many additional diagnoses pertaining to chemotherapy and radical surgery.

- Anxiety related to diagnosis, symptoms, treatment regimen, other factors (specify)
- Pain following removal of the lesion
- Knowledge deficit of treatment regimen, posttreatment management

Planning and Implementation
The major goals of the patient may include reduction in anxiety, relief of pain or discomfort, and understanding of the treatment regimen and posttreatment management.

The major goals of nursing management may include reduction in anxiety, relief of pain, and thorough explanation of the treatment and posttreatment management.

Anxiety. The procedure for removal or treatment of the lesion is explained by the physician. The patient may still exhibit anxiety over having a local anesthetic injected. The nurse can instruct the patient to look away from the area. Staying with the patient until the removal or treatment is completed also may lessen anxiety.

Pain. Most lesions (with the exception being malignant melanoma) are removed or treated under local anesthesia. Pain may be experienced after the effects of the anesthetic have worn off. The physician may recommend an analgesic, such as acetaminophen (Tylenol), or prescribe a narcotic analgesic, such as codeine.

Knowledge Deficit. The physician gives the patient posttreatment instructions. The nurse should review these instructions with the patient. The following may be included in a patient teaching plan:

1. Do not remove the scab by pulling at it or soaking it. The scab must be allowed to dry and fall off.
2. Do not put any nonprescription medication on the area.
3. If a drug has been prescribed, take or use it exactly as directed.
4. Follow the directions of the physician regarding removing or changing the bandage or dressing or keeping the area uncovered.
5. Contact the physician if there is continued bleeding, if the scab comes off and the area bleeds, or if fever and chills occur.
6. Keep all follow-up appointments.

Evaluation
- Anxiety is reduced
- Pain is relieved
- Patient demonstrates understanding of posttreatment management and events that require contacting the physician

STASIS ULCERS

The word *stasis* means stagnation or standing still. *Stasis ulcers* are skin manifestations resulting from inadequate or poor circulation in the legs. Ulceration of the tissues of the legs most commonly is due to an inadequate arterial or venous blood supply to an extremity, resulting in ischemia and ultimately necrosis of tissues. Arteriosclerosis and chronic thrombophlebitis are the most common causes of stasis ulcers.

Symptoms

Symptoms usually include a feeling of heaviness and fatigue in the legs, pain, swelling and one or more ulcerated areas. Infection and poor healing are common.

Diagnosis

Diagnosis is made by visual examination of the affected extremity and by patient history of symptoms.

Treatment

The primary objectives of treatment are to control infection and promote healing of the ulcerated area. Culture and sensitivity studies may be done to identify the microorganisms present in the wound and to aid in the selection of appropriate antibiotic therapy. Healing is encouraged by complete bed rest and treatment of the infection. Additional treatment modalities may have to be employed to encourage healing. These treatment methods include skin grafting, wound debridement, topical application of enzyme preparations that aid in the removal of necrotic tissue and purulent exudates, and application of a Dome-paste bandage. In some cases, surgical procedures, such as arterial grafts or bypasses, may be used to correct arterial insufficiency.

NURSING PROCESS —THE PATIENT WHO HAS A STASIS ULCER

Assessment

A complete medical, drug, and allergy history should be obtained. The affected areas should be inspected and described on the patient's chart. Vital signs should be taken and the patient weighed. An evaluation of the patient's physical condition should be made. Many of these patients are older, and therefore, one or more physical problems may be present, such as severe arthritis and a poor nutritional status.

Nursing Diagnosis

Depending on the extent of the ulcer, one or more of the following nursing diagnoses may apply. Concurrent medical disorders may require additional nursing diagnoses.

- Pain related to necrosis of tissue
- Impaired tissue integrity related to peripheral vascular alterations (insufficiency)
- Impaired physical mobility related to enforced bed rest
- Potential for infection related to break in the skin
- Knowledge deficit of home care management

Planning and Implementation

The major goals of the patient may include relief of pain, improved wound healing, improved physical mobility, absence of infection, and understanding of home care.

The major goals of nursing management may include relief of pain or discomfort, healing of the ulcer, absence of infection, and preparation of an effective and thorough plan of patient teaching.

Because these ulcers tend to heal slowly, the patient may become discouraged. Meticulous technique is especially important when carrying out prescribed care, such as the application of ointments and dressings. A diet high in proteins and vitamins is usually ordered. The patient should be encouraged to eat the prescribed diet because food intake is a part of the treatment regimen.

Some treatments are performed only by the physician, such as the removal of dead tissue from the wound (débridement) and the application of a Dome-paste bandage. Other treatments, such as wound irrigations or the application of a topical enzyme, are usually performed by the nurse.

Pain. Narcotics usually should be avoided, if possible, because of the long-term nature of the condition and the consequent danger of addiction. Nonnarcotic analgesics may give relief, particularly when they are used in combination with measures to improve circulation, such as changes in position, exercise, warmth, and vasodilators.

Care should be exercised when applying the prescribed medications to the ulcer because the area is usually painful. Pain can sometimes be lessened by avoiding chilling of the extremities. Warm socks and slippers should be worn if the patient is allowed out of bed. A bed cradle may be ordered to keep covers off the feet. An extra blanket over the cradle may prevent chilling of the legs and feet.

Impaired Tissue Integrity, Impaired Physical Mobility. Depending on the type of vascular insufficiency, the physician may order the extremity elevated (venous insufficiency) or elevation of the head of the bed (arterial insufficiency).

When the patient is on complete bed rest, skin breakdown may occur in other areas, especially over bony prominences. The patient's position should be changed every 2 hours, and bony prominences should be inspected for signs of skin breakdown. If signs of breakdown are apparent, it is most important that immediate measures are taken to prevent further impairment of skin integrity. A lamb's wool pad under the heels or lamb's wool boots can be used to prevent skin breakdown and necrosis of the heels. An alternating pressure mattress or other device can be used to reduce pressure on the sacral area and hips.

The patient should be encouraged to exercise and use the upper extremities every two hours. Once healing has begun, the patient may be allowed out of bed and ambulatory for short periods. Care should be taken to prevent any trauma to the legs, such as bumping into chairs or stools. If skin grafting is done, the area must be protected until the graft heals.

Potential for Infection. Antibiotics may be ordered to prevent or treat an infection. The affected area should be inspected daily for signs of infection, namely, purulent wound drainage and redness beyond the affected area. Vital signs should be monitored every 4 hours or as ordered. A rise in temperature, chills, and any increase in the amount or change in the type drainage should be reported to the physician.

Knowledge Deficit. The teaching plan depends on the physician's recommendations for home care. The following general points can be included in a patient teaching plan:

1. Eat a well-balanced and nutritious diet.
2. Avoid injury to the area; exercise care when walking.
3. Do *not* put dressings, salves, or ointments on the area unless their use has been prescribed or recommended by the physician.
4. Take or use the prescribed medications exactly as ordered.
5. Follow the recommendations of the physician regarding physical activity, position of the leg when sitting, and so forth. These recommendations are extremely important because they help increase the blood supply to the legs.
6. Contact the physician if any of the following should occur: chills, fever, drainage (blood, pus) from the area, sudden onset of pain, the ulcer recurs, a new ulcer forms, or any change in the color of the leg or area around the healed ulcer.

Evaluation

- Pain is controlled
- Ulcer is healed; skin around the ulcer is normal or near normal in appearance
- Physical mobility is improved; patient is able to ambulate with assistance
- No evidence of infection; vital signs are normal

- Patient demonstrates understanding of home management, things to avoid, events that require contacting the physician

SEVERE SKIN DISORDERS

Pemphigus

There are several types of this uncommon dermatologic disorder, but the type most often seen is pemphigus vulgaris.

Symptoms

The disorder is characterized by blisters—also called *bullae*—that are filled with fluid. The sizes of the bullae vary, and they are randomly distributed on the body surface. They also may be found on mucous membranes of the mouth, throat, nose, and vagina. The fluid in the blisters contains water, electrolytes, and protein, and they are easily ruptured. Following rupture of a bulla, bleeding, oozing, and infection may occur.

Diagnosis

Diagnosis is made by visual examination of the lesions. A biopsy of a blister wall also may be performed to note microscopic tissue changes associated with pemphigus.

Treatment

Treatment is directed toward preventing formation of new lesions and protecting the lesions already formed. This latter aspect of treatment is not always effective because the bullae rupture easily. An attempt should be made to prevent the rupture of many bullae at one time because the loss of fluid, protein, and electrolytes and the danger of infection of the open areas can be serious.

Corticosteroid therapy is used in the treatment of pemphigus. Often, large doses are required until the disease appears to be under control or in remission. The dosage is then slowly decreased over time. Despite treatment, the prognosis is poor in many, though not all, patients. Death is usually due to an acute infection and other complications brought on by prolonged inactivity.

Exfoliative Dermatitis

Exfoliative dermatitis is a severe condition that may be caused by allergy to a drug or that may be a secondary reaction to an underlying skin disorder or other disease, such as a lymphoma.

Symptoms

The upper layers of the skin are red and peel or scale off over fairly large areas of the body. Chills, fever, malaise, and pruritus also may be seen.

Diagnosis

Diagnosis is made by patient history and visual inspection of the affected areas. Culture and sensitivity studies may be done if an infection is present.

Treatment

Antibiotics may be administered to prevent or treat an infection. Fluid and electrolyte imbalances, when present, should be corrected. Measures should be taken to correct the cause, if known. All drugs should be stopped immediately, with the exception of initiating antibiotic therapy. Vital signs and electrolyte and fluid balance should be closely monitored since the skin does not have the ability to regulate body temperature (*thermoregulation*) and provide protection for underlying tissues. Excessive water may be lost through the skin of these patients, because loss of the dermis also increases water loss through the skin. Emollients, soothing baths, and cool compresses may be prescribed to relieve discomfort and itching. Corticosteroids also may be prescribed.

NURSING PROCESS —THE PATIENT WHO HAS A SEVERE SKIN DISORDER

Assessment

Although pemphigus and exfoliative dermatitis are severe skin disorders, even relatively mild skin disorders can become severe under certain circumstances.

A complete medical, drug, and allergy history should be obtained. Vital signs should be taken and the patient weighed. A general evaluation of the patient's physical and mental status and ability to carry out any type of activity (walking, grooming, eating) should be made.

Nursing Diagnosis

Depending on the symptoms, degree of severity, and type of disorder, one or more of the following nursing diagnoses may apply:

- Pain related to infection, open skin lesions
- Anxiety related to pain, discomfort, disfigurement, other factors (specify)
- Impaired skin integrity related to damage to dermal or epidermal tissue
- Potential for infection related to open skin lesions
- Hypothermia related to open skin lesions, loss of der-

mal layer of skin (large area), lack of effective thermoregulation
- Fluid volume deficit related to excessive loss of water through open skin lesions, loss of dermis
- Altered oral mucous membranes related to blistering and erosions (pemphigus)
- Ineffective individual coping related to chronic disease condition, appearance of skin, slow response to treatment, other factors (specify)
- Knowledge deficit of home care management

Planning and Evaluation

The major goals of the patient may include relief of pain and discomfort, reduction in anxiety, improved skin and oral mucous membrane integrity, absence of infection, normal body temperature, absence of fluid and electrolyte imbalances, ability to accept condition, and understanding of home care.

The major goals of nursing management may include relief of pain and discomfort, preservation of skin and oral mucous membrane integrity, prevention of hypothermia, prevention of a fluid volume deficit, helping the patient effectively cope with the disorder, and development of an effective patient teaching plan.

Pain.   Some patients may experience severe pain when moved. When it is necessary to turn or move the patient, great care must be exercised, and it may be necessary to plan these tasks carefully before the patient is touched or moved. Cool, wet dressings may be used to soothe the areas, but the dressings must be applied with great care because pain may result from even the lightest touch or pressure.

Depending on the type of disorder, analgesics may be ordered for pain. Narcotics should be avoided, when possible, because many severe skin disorders are chronic in nature and require an extended period of time to heal.

Anxiety.   Anxiety can be caused by many factors, such as the presence of severe symptoms (pain, itching) that respond poorly to medications or treatments. Treatment often must be carried out over an extended period of time, and the lesions may be disfiguring or difficult for the family or other visitors to look at. The patient easily can become discouraged and depressed. These patients must be allowed time to talk about their problems because talking may be the only way of relieving their concerns.

Impaired Skin Integrity, Potential for Infection.   Every effort must be made to prevent infection, further injury to the skin, or reopening of skin lesions. Dressings always should be applied and removed gently. When wet dressings are ordered, they should be kept moist and *never* be allowed to become dry and affixed to the skin. The patient should be moved with great care so that the affected areas do not rub against the bottom sheet.

The skin should be inspected at least daily for new areas of involvement, abrasions, opening of lesions, purulent drainage or other signs of infection, and any change in the appearance of the skin.

Hypothermia. The room must be kept warm because the patient may be a candidate for hypothermia when large areas of the skin are involved. Vital signs should be monitored, and any decrease in body temperature should be discussed with the physician. Nursing methods that may be used to correct hypothermia include increasing room temperature and covering areas not affected with extra blankets. Unless contraindicated, solutions applied to wet dressings should be at body temperature because cool solutions lower body temperature. This problem also should be discussed with the physician because other methods may need to be tried.

Fluids Volume Deficit. The patient should be observed for signs of fluid volume deficit and electrolyte imbalances (see Chapter 12). Intake and output should be measured, and the physician should be informed if the urinary output falls below 500 mL/day or the urine appears concentrated. Unless ordered otherwise, extra fluids should be encouraged. If the patient fails to take oral fluids, the physician should be informed because intravenous therapy may be necessary.

Altered Oral Mucous Membranes. If the oral mucous membranes are involved, the patient will find it difficult to eat and drink. Liquid, nonirritating, high-calorie fluids may be ordered. Meticulous oral care is necessary. Parenteral nutrition may be necessary if the patient is unable to maintain an adequate nutrition intake.

Ineffective Individual Coping. Many patients become discouraged because of their slow response to treatment, pain, and the chronic status of their disorder. The nurse must listen to the patient and show concern when giving care. Nursing tasks must not be rushed because this gives the patient the feeling that the caregiver is disinterested or repulsed by the appearance of the skin lesions.

Knowledge Deficit. The physician gives the patient or family instructions regarding home care. The nurse should determine if specific instructions or demonstrations, such as how to apply dressings or wet soaks, are needed.

The following may be included in a patient teaching plan:

1. Take or apply the prescribed medications exactly as ordered.
2. Follow the treatment outlined by the physician. Do not take or apply any nonprescription drug unless its use is approved by the physician. Do not apply dressings to the affected areas unless the use of dressings is recommended by the physician. If dressings are recommended, they must be sterile.
3. Avoid injury to the affected areas.
4. Contact the physician if any of the following occur: fever, chills, new lesions, or infection or drainage from old lesions.

Evaluation

- Pain is relieved
- Anxiety is reduced
- Skin remains intact; healing of the dermis is evident
- No evidence of infection; vital signs are normal
- No evidence of fluid volume deficit or electrolyte imbalance
- Oral mucous membranes are intact; affected areas show signs of healing
- Patient demonstrates evidence of coping with the disorder and openly discusses problems and concerns
- Patient demonstrates understanding of home care management, treatment regimen, events requiring contacting the physician

COSMETIC AND RECONSTRUCTIVE SURGERY

The terms *plastic surgery* and *reconstructive surgery* are often used interchangeably to refer to the repair of defects that may be congenital or acquired through injury or radical surgery. The repair surgery may be performed for cosmetic purposes or to improve function. For example, a crooked nose may be straightened, or contracted scar tissue in the axilla may be freed to restore normal motion to the arm. A deformed hand may be totally reconstructed by the repair of tendon, bone, nerve, or skin. An eyelid that has been damaged by trauma may be repaired by a pedicle graft or advancement flaps.

The following are the four main types of conditions treated by plastic surgery:

- Congenital deformities, such as harelip and protruding ears
- Deformities resulting from trauma, such as burns and automobile accidents
- Conditions for which the patient seeks cosmetic surgery, such as face-lifting
- Disfigurement resulting from malignant disease, such as cancer of the mouth

Plastic surgery holds the promise of a more normal appearance and improved function for many patients. Both appearance and function are important considerations; however, their relative importance varies with the part of the body involved. Surgical treatment that produces the greatest functional improvement may not be the same as that which leads to the most satisfactory cosmetic result. Examples of plastic surgery performed for cosmetic purposes follow.

Face-Lifting and Blepharoplasty

Most of the incision for face-lifting is made in the hairline. Wrinkles are removed by tightening the fascia and skin and removing excess skin. Most of the fine scar resulting from surgery is concealed by the hair.

Frequently, *blepharoplasty* (eyelid reconstruction) is carried out as part of the surgical procedure in an effort to remove the appearance that frequently sets in at about the age of 50, when the elastic fibers of the dermis relax and some of the subcutaneous fat that produces a youthful look becomes absorbed. In eyelid reconstruction, incisions are made that are hidden in normal crease lines. The excessive eyelid skin and orbital fat (if necessary) are removed.

Rhinoplasty

Rhinoplasty is reconstructive surgery of the nose. Because the nose is the most exposed part of the face, it is frequently injured, often without the individual's remembering the accident. Improvements in appearance, breathing, and the senses of smell and taste—as well as improvements in poise, assurance, and morale —usually are apparent within 2 or 3 weeks after reconstructive surgery.

Dermabrasion

Dermabrasion is a technique for removing surface layers of scarred skin. It is useful in lessening scars such as the pitting from severe acne. The outermost layers of the skin are removed by sandpaper, a rotating wire brush, chemicals (chemical face peeling), or a diamond wheel. A local anesthetic, such as an ethyl chloride and Freon mixture, may be used during the procedure. Afterward, the skin feels raw and sore, and some crusting from serous exudate occurs. Patients frequently say that the discomfort is much like that from a burn. The patient should be instructed not to wash the area until sufficient healing has occurred. Picking and touching the area must be avoided because this contact might cause infection or produce marking of the tissues.

Tattooing

Tattooing is used to change the color of the skin. Pigments are blended to just the right shade for the patient's skin and then are implanted into it. The treatment is useful in matching the color of grafted skin to the surrounding skin more exactly. The pigments may shift position beneath the skin, however, so that they are no longer effective in covering up the blemish. Also, the pigments sometimes look different in environments of various temperatures. Tattooing and dermabrasion are usually carried out in a physician's office or in a clinic.

Artificial Parts

Artificial parts may be used to camouflage defects. For instance, part of a nose or an ear may be made of plastic to match the patient's features so exactly that it is hard to tell which is the prosthetic part and which is natural. Plastic materials also are used as a framework or as supporting structures over which the patient's tissues grow. For instance, a plastic material may be used beneath the skin to correct an underdeveloped chin.

Mammoplasty

Mammoplasty may be performed to change the size and shape of the breasts. Very large breasts may make a woman self-conscious, contribute to poor posture, and interfere with breathing. Excess skin and subcutaneous tissue is removed surgically under general anesthesia. Afterward, the patient must wear a firm-support brassiere for several months until healing is complete and the tissues are firm.

Surgery is sometimes undertaken to enlarge small breasts; this is called *augmentation mammoplasty*. Tissues from the patient's own body, such as from the buttocks, or plastic materials, such as silicone gel within a Silastic bag, are used as an implant between the chest wall and the breast. Placing the material here, rather than inside the breast, has two advantages: (1) the function of the breast is unimpaired and the woman can lactate normally; and (2) the possibility of carcinogenesis from introduction of foreign materials in breast tissue is reduced.

SKIN GRAFTING

There are several types of skin grafting, depending on the tissue used in the graft. An *autograft* uses the patient's own skin, which is transplanted from one part of the body to another. Only autograft or skin transplanted from one identical twin to another can become a permanent part of the patient's own skin. A second method is obtaining skin from another individual, usually a cadaver. This is called an *allograft* or *homograft*. Allografts are useful in temporarily closing large defects, thus preventing further loss of tissue fluid. Although allografts slough away after 1 or more weeks and must be replaced by autografts, they tide the patient over the critical period of illness until the patient's own skin can be used for skin grafting. A third method of skin grafting is the use of animal skins, principally pig skin. This is called a *heterograft* or *xenograft*. Like allografts, this is a temporary method of closing large skin defects as are seen in burns or other injuries in which a large area of skin has been damaged. Some newer types of heterografts are made of synthetic and biosynthetic materials.

Other body tissues, such as bone and cartilage, also may be used as grafts. Skin grafting is done in surgery, under general anesthesia. Refer to the section on skin grafting under the section on burn treatment methods later in this chapter for information on how skin grafts are used to treat the burned patient.

Types of Skin Grafts

Split-thickness and *full-thickness* grafts are the two basic types of skin grafts. Split-thickness autografts vary in thickness (from 0.008- to 0.024-inch grafts), size, and shape, and are usually obtained from the buttocks or thighs. The skin is removed from the donor site by the use of a dermatome, a scalpel, or another special instrument. A *pinch graft* is a small piece of skin cut from the patient's donor site and placed on the recipient site. A *postage stamp graft* is a piece of skin about the size of a stamp and, like the pinch graft, is cut from the donor site and placed on the recipient site. A *full cover graft* is a large piece of skin removed by means of a dermatome or another special instrument. Sutures are usually necessary to anchor this type of graft in place. A *slit graft* (also called a *lace* or an *expansile* graft) is used when the area available as a donor site is limited, as in patients with extensive burns. The skin is removed from the donor site and passed through an instrument that puts slits in it; thus, a smaller piece of skin is stretched to cover a larger area (Fig. 57-2).

Full-thickness grafts usually are used to restore function to and improve the cosmetic appearance of a burned area. When the recipient site is the face or neck, the skin from the donor site is matched as closely as possible to the skin of the recipient site. Although split-thickness grafts cover the area, they do not give as good a cosmetic appearance as full-thickness grafts.

Free full-thickness grafts, which may be 0.035-inch thick, are skin grafts that include subcutaneous tissue.

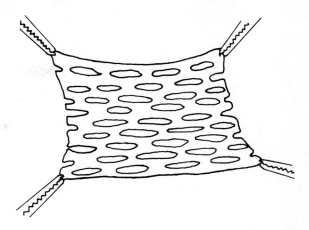

Figure 57–2. The slit or lace graft. The slits allow for stretching of the graft.

This type of graft may be used in burns during the management stage when the burned area is fairly small or when the hands, face, and neck are involved. *Pedicle flaps* (Fig. 57-3) are full-thickness grafts that include skin and subcutaneous fat with a tube formed from the piece of skin. This tube is then moved to another site and anchored.

For grafts to take, there must be sufficient blood supply to the part and an absence of infection. The graft must stick close to the tissues on which it is to grow; excess blood or serous fluid can cause the graft to become separated from the tissues and fail to grow. Sometimes warm, moist saline compresses are placed on pedicle grafts. The skin being transplanted by a pedicle has blood supplied from the donor site. The warmth transmitted to the recipient bed through the graft is believed to favor the development of blood circulation in the graft.

Surgeons use various methods of grafting, depending on the size and location of the recipient site, the available areas of donor sites, the condition of donor sites, and the patient's age. When grafts are planned during the treatment and rehabilitation stages, the surgeon carefully evaluates present and future needs. Serious problems that may occur after skin grafting involve infection or failure of the graft to take properly; repeated grafts may be necessary if the autograft is rejected. These factors, as well as others pertinent to a specific patient, must be taken into account when plans are made for skin grafting.

Patients with skin grafts have two sites to be cared for before and after surgery—the donor site and the recipient site. Care must be taken to avoid excessive pressure on the recipient site. This area also should be kept immobile because movement of the graft can interrupt *vascularization* (the development of new blood vessels) between the graft and the recipient bed. If adequate vascularization does not occur, the

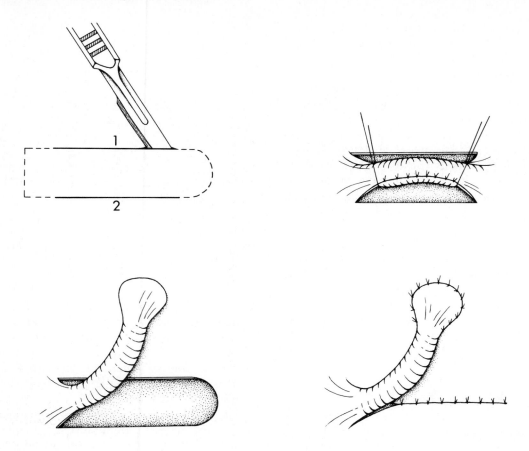

Figure 57–3.   Tube pedicle graft. (*A*) Area of skin selected (*dotted lines*) and area of incision to form tube (*solid lines 1 and 2*). (*B*) Tube formed by suturing edges 1 and 2 of A on underside. (*C*) One end of pedicle is cut free and raised, ready to be sutured to recipient site. (*D*) End of pedicle sutured to recipient site. Donor bed edges (*dotted lines*) are approximated and closed with suture.

graft will not take—that is, the graft will slough off of the recipient bed. Extreme care should be taken in changing bed linen and repositioning or moving the patient in any way because the graft must remain undisturbed until healing has occurred.

Dressings over the donor and recipient sites are changed by the physician. Both sites should be watched for evidence of bleeding or purulent exudate on the dressing. Tube pedicle grafts should be watched closely for any signs of skin color changes. In tube pedicle grafts, the donor end supplies blood vessels (and therefore nourishment) by means of the tube to the recipient site. If any area of the graft (donor end, tube pedicle, recipient site) becomes pale or cyanotic, this may indicate a lack of proper circulation through the graft. The donor and recipient sites also should be inspected for signs of infection, namely, redness or presence of a purulent exudate. Donor and recipient sites may need to be immobilized, for example, when the donor site is the abdomen and the recipient site is the forearm. The type of immobilization necessary depends on the donor and recipient sites of the pedicle

graft. There are variations of pedicle grafts, but the management is similar.

BURN INJURIES

A person who sustains serious burns is confronted with problems resulting from pain, mutilation, fear of death, disfigurement, separation, immobilization, helplessness, and possible abandonment.

Classification of Burns

Burns may be classified as *first-, second-, third-,* or *fourth-degree* burns. Another classification is *partial-thickness* or *full-thickness* burns. The relative depth of each is shown in Figure 57-4 and explained in Table 57-1. Determining the depth of a burn is often difficult because there may be a combination of all degrees of burn. Both locally and systemically, the deeper the burn, the greater the damage. Burns caused by electricity are characteristically deep, involving not only the

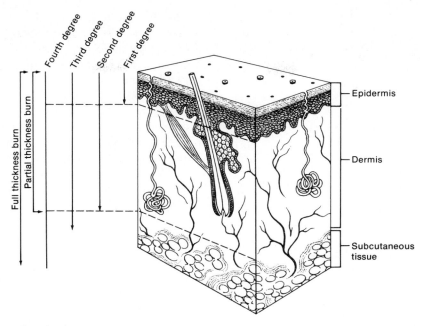

Figure 57–4. A cross-section of the skin showing the relative depths of the types of burn injury.

skin but also blood vessels, muscles, tendons, and bones.

The second measure of damage is the extent of the area: the larger the burn area, the greater the damage to the body. Severe sunburn (first-degree) over 85% of the body causes a much greater disturbance of fluid and electrolyte regulation than a third-degree burn on the tip of a forefinger. Because physicians base their prescriptions for fluid replacement therapy on both the degree and the extent of the body surface injured, the diagnosis includes both these factors. The "rule of nines" (Fig. 57-5) is one method of estimating how much of the patient's skin surface is involved. Special charts and graphs, such as the Berkow chart, also are used to estimate the extent of involvement.

Physiologic Changes After a Burn Injury

Many physiologic changes occur almost immediately after a severe burn injury. Deep and widespread burns almost always result in more drastic changes than do those that are less severe or widespread (Table 57-2). It also should be noted that even small areas of injury can result in moderately severe to severe physiologic changes in the very young and the very old.

Table 57–1. Degree, Depth, and Characteristics of Burn Injuries

Degree of Burn	Depth	Characteristics
First-degree (partial-thickness)	Epidermis	Red or pink in color; pain is present; edema may be present but subsides quickly; no scarring occurs.
Second-degree (partial-thickness)	Epidermis and dermis	Color may vary from mottled pink to red, white, dull white, tan (depending on depth); blistering, pain, some scarring occurs.
Third-degree (full-thickness)	Epidermis, dermis, subcutaneous tissues	Color may vary: white, tan, black, brown, bright red; surface may be wet or dry; leathery covering (eschar) is present; no pain; scarring occurs.
Fourth-degree (full-thickness)	Epidermis, dermis, subcutaneous tissue; may include subcutaneous fat, fascia, muscle and bone	Surface is blackened, depressed; no pain; scarring occurs.

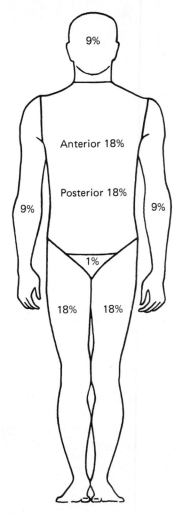

9%

Anterior 18%

Posterior 18%

9%   9%

1%

18%   18%

Figure 57–5. The "rule of nines," a simplified method for estimating the percentage of the body surface covered by burns. According to this method, the entire head is 9% of the body surface area; each entire arm is 9%; each entire leg is 18%; the genital region is 1%; the front torso is 18%; and the back torso is 18%. Physicians often sketch the burned area on a diagram such as this to facilitate the calculation of the percent of the body burned.

The extent of physiologic change is determined by laboratory studies—arterial blood gas studies and serum and urine electrolytes. After a burn, fluid from the body moves toward the burned area, accounting for the edema at the burn site. Some of the fluid is then trapped in this area, is unavailable for use by the body, and therefore becomes fluid loss. Fluid also is lost from the burned area, often in extremely large amounts, in the forms of water vapor and seepage.

Potassium levels increase as the ions move from the burned area into the bloodstream. Once diuresis begins, potassium levels decrease and must be closely monitored. Decreased levels are as serious as increased levels. Sodium levels may decrease initially as the ion

leaves the body along with the fluid lost from the burned area. Protein also is lost.

Initial hemoglobin level and *hematocrit* (the volume, expressed as a percentage of erythrocytes that are packed by centrifugation in a given volume of blood) may be reported as normal or above normal. Plasma, the liquid component of the blood, escapes from the bloodstream, resulting in a decrease in the plasma volume (the total amount of plasma in all blood vessels). Parts *A* and *B* of Figure 57-6, illustrate normal plasma volume and reduced plasma volume. There are the same number of cells in *B* as in *A*, but there is less plasma in which the cells are suspended. When comparing the number of cells in a given amount of fluid, there are more cells per mL of solution in *B* than in *A*. This is an illustration of *hemoconcentration*. The patient could be anemic, but because of plasma loss with resulting hemoconcentration, some blood studies may appear normal. Hemoconcentration presents another problem, namely, the sluggish flow of blood through blood vessels. This may result in inadequate nutrition of healthy body cells and organs; a fall in blood pressure usually follows. If physiologic changes are not *immediately* recognized and corrected, irreversible shock can occur. These changes usually happen rapidly and may change from hour to hour, which is one reason that burned patients require intensive care by skilled personnel.

Initial First Aid Treatment

At the scene of a fire, the first priority is to prevent further injury to the victim. If the clothing is on fire,

Table 57–2.   Initial Fluid, Electrolyte, and Blood Disturbances in the Burned Patient

Problem	*Rationale*
Fluid loss (dehydration)	Fluid moves toward the burned area, resulting in localized edema.
	Fluid seeps from the burn area.
Electrolyte disturbances	Potassium (K⁺) levels are initially increased (hyperkalemia) as the ion moves *from* damaged cells *to* the bloodstream.
	Sodium (Na⁺) levels may initially decrease (hyponatremia) as the ion leaves the body along with fluids lost from the wounds.
Anemia	Anemia due to destruction of red blood cells at the site of the injury.

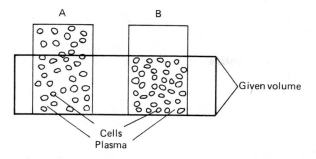

Figure 57-6. (*A*) Normal plasma volume. (*B*) Loss of plasma volume.

the victim should be placed in a *horizontal* position and rolled in a blanket to smother the fire. Laying the victim flat prevents the fire, hot air, and smoke from rising toward the head and entering the respiratory passages. The victim must be immediately taken to a hospital for examination. During transport, it is important that individuals who have been burned around the face and neck or who may have inhaled smoke, chemicals, steam, or flames be observed *closely* for respiratory difficulty. When these substances are inhaled, the mucous membrane lining the respiratory passages may be damaged or extremely irritated, resulting in edema of the respiratory passages that decreases the amount of air reaching the lungs. In addition, there may be excessive mucus secretion, which also makes breathing difficult. The hospital should be made aware, if possible, that a burned patient will arrive shortly. Estimations of the extent of the burn and any problems the victim appears to have aid in the mobilization and preparation of emergency personnel.

As soon as the patient arrives at the hospital, the physician assesses the extent of injury and the immediate problems and needs of the patient. Along with the burn, the patient may have incurred other body injuries—fractures, head injury, lacerations, and so on.

The primary focus of the immediate treatment phase is to determine the respiratory status and then to meet the patient's fluid needs. Intravenous fluids should be administered, including plasma expanders, such as dextran (Gentran), if blood or excessive fluid is lost. A cutdown may be necessary, and a central venous pressure line may be inserted at this time or later to monitor the patient's fluid requirements. The patient is usually weighed with a bed scale to determine fluid gain and loss. Analgesics also are given, often intravenously, to relieve pain and apprehension.

Initial Hospital Treatment

Once the patient is admitted, the medical team must work quickly to assess the extent of injury and to formulate an immediate plan of care (Charts 57-1 and 57-2). In many hospital emergency departments, materials necessary to manage the burned patient are kept ready for immediate use, and written procedure on the initial management of the patient may be provided as well. *One of the most important initial steps in management of these patients is establishing and maintaining a patent airway.*

Chart 57-1. Initial Management of the Burned Patient

- Establish and maintain an adequate airway.
- Begin intravenous fluids. A cutdown may be necessary.
- Administer intravenous analgesics for relief of pain.
- Withhold oral fluids.
- Insert indwelling urethral catheter.
- Give tetanus immune globulin, toxoid, or antitoxin and antibiotics as ordered.
- Draw blood for laboratory studies.
- Give burned areas initial care.

Chart 57-2. Nursing Management of the Burned Patient

- Check blood pressure, pulse, respirations:
  Hourly (or oftener) during the acute stage, which may last 3 or 4 days.
  Every 2 to 4 hr thereafter or according to the physician's order, unit policy, or nurse's judgment.
- Check temperature every 1 or 4 hr or as ordered.
- Record daily weights by use of a bed scale.
- Monitor intake and output:
  Urine output may be measured hourly during the acute phase.
  Urine is tested for specific gravity, glucose, ketones, and protein hourly during the acute phase.
  Output and other urine tests may be measured at less frequent intervals after the acute phase.
- Nursing observations:
  Describe burned areas accurately, noting any signs of crust or eschar formation, infection, cracking of crusts or eschar, oozing, bleeding.
  Describe the patient's mental state: oriented, disoriented, confused, depressed, withdrawn, and so on.
- Assure proper positioning of burned extremities, which is important in preventing contractures.
- Assist with active or passive exercises as ordered by the physician. The physical therapist may do some of the exercises with nursing personnel repeating the movements at specified intervals.

The first step in management of the burned area is removal of all clothing. Some pieces of clothing may have adhered to the injured area, and care must be taken in separating cloth fibers from the wound. The body hair around the perimeter of the burns usually should be shaved as soon as possible because hair is a source of bacterial wound contamination. When the head, neck, and upper chest are burned, singed eyebrows and eyelashes should be clipped, head hair shaved, the lips and mouth cleansed, and the lips lubricated. Eye ointments or irrigations should be used to remove dirt and to lubricate the lid margins.

The burned areas should be cleansed to remove debris. This may be done in the emergency department or after the patient is transferred to the burn unit or general hospital unit. After cleansing, topical medications may be applied. Hospital procedures on initial management may vary, depending on the extent of treatment given in the emergency department. Personnel should observe clean technique (*clean* cap, gown, mask, gloves) during initial treatment, although some hospitals use sterile technique.

If the patient has difficulty breathing or if there is edema of the face and neck, an endotracheal tube may be inserted or a tracheostomy performed. A tracheostomy is rarely done if there are severe burns on the anterior neck. In this case, an endotracheal tube is inserted. It is *extremely important* that the respiratory rate be *closely* monitored and the patient observed for *any* sign of respiratory distress.

Intravenous fluids should be started immediately. The physician determines which extremity to use and what type of fluid to administer. Blood samples are usually drawn at this time. An indwelling urethral catheter is inserted and attached to a closed drainage system because the urinary output must be measured frequently during the first few days.

The physician may order intravenous analgesics for pain, which often is severe. Because pain can cause a drop in blood pressure, analgesics are important at this time. Laboratory studies, such as serum electrolytes, also are ordered. Blood pressure, pulse, and respirations should be taken immediately and frequently thereafter. If both arms are burned, the blood pressure may be taken on the leg by wrapping the cuff around the thigh and placing the stethoscope over the popliteal artery behind the knee. This technique is not always possible because the popliteal artery is not close to the surface of the body. Electronic devices, such as a Doppler or Dynamapp device, may be necessary to accurately monitor the blood pressure since edema and burns of the extremities may make use of a blood pressure cuff difficult. Tetanus and antibiotics also may be administered at this time or after the burned areas have been cleansed.

Burn Treatment Methods

When the emergency is over, the body must repair itself. The energy required to meet the emergency was greatly in excess of normal. Because large areas of fat deposits have been used, and the caloric intake over the past several days has been low, patients often are emaciated. As much as 10 kg (22 lb) may be lost, even if the loss of edema is not considered. Debilitation is dangerous because it reduces the patient's resistance to infection, delays the healing of the skin, and impedes the growth of new granulation tissue and the progress of skin grafts.

Open Method.   The *open* or *exposure method* exposes the burned areas to air, allowing the formation of a hard crust on top of the burn. Over areas of a third-degree or full-thickness burn, *eschar*, a hard leathery crust made of dehydrated dead skin, forms. The crust over a second-degree or partial-thickness burn forms in 2 or 3 days, and *epithelialization* (regrowth of skin) is completed in about 2 or 3 weeks. At this time, the crust falls off. Eschar also forms in 2 or 3 days, gradually begins to loosen, and is debrided or further loosened by whirlpool baths. A dressing may be used to cover the exposed areas as the eschar is removed. If the eschar constricts the area and impairs circulation, an *escharotomy* (an excision into the eschar) is done to relieve pressure on the affected area. New skin cannot grow beneath eschar.

With the open method of treatment, the patient is placed in isolation, sterile linen is used, and personnel and visitors wear sterile gowns and masks. The skin of the burned patient is sensitive to drafts and temperature changes; therefore, a bed cradle or sheets may be placed over the patient for protection from drafts and temperature changes.

Occlusive Dressings (Closed Method).   Occlusive dressings are used most often when the arms, hands, feet, or legs are burned. Although there are variations, the burned area is covered with an ointment and gauze. Gauze impregnated with a drug ointment also is used. Additional gauze, or a fluff dressing and gauze, is applied to cover the dressing adjacent to the skin.

Drug Therapy

Drugs used in the treatment of burns are mafenide (Sulfamylon), silver nitrate ($AgNO_3$) 0.5% solution, povidone-iodine (Betadine), gentamicin (Garamycin) 0.1% cream, nitrofurazone (Furacin), and silver sulfadiazine (Silvadene) 1% ointment. The solutions may be applied in the form of wet dressings or dabbed on the areas. The ointments are dabbed on the area or impregnated in gauze that is laid on the burn. Drugs have various advantages and disadvantages, and no one preparation appears to be superior to another. All drugs should be applied using sterile technique.

Silver Nitrate. Silver nitrate 0.5% is a solution applied by the continuous wet-dressing technique. The burned surface must be free of grease or oil film before gauze dressings are applied. The gauze should be wet with the silver nitrate solution before application, anchored with stretch bandages, and kept continuously wet. Unusually thick dressings may have a catheter inserted in one of the middle layers to aid in the wetting of all layers of gauze. A blanket may be placed over the patient to slow down evaporation of the solution. One disadvantage in the use of silver nitrate is the loss of electrolytes—sodium and potassium—from body fluids. Silver nitrate is hypotonic and draws fluid from a wound. Serum electrolyte levels must be monitored—usually three or four times a day—and oral or intravenous supplements given as needed. *Anything* coming in contact with the silver nitrate solution becomes stained dark brown or black, including bed linen, floors, metal, and skin. Skin stains eventually wear off, but stains on inanimate objects are usually permanent.

The dressings should be changed one to three times a day, at which time a tub bath usually is given. Because dressing changes are painful, analgesics should be administered 20 to 30 minutes before the procedure to be fully effective.

Mafenide. Mafenide (Sulfamylon) is a cream that is dabbed on the injured area, with the area left uncovered or covered with a single layer of fine mesh gauze. A generous amount of mafenide should be applied by hand once or twice a day, using a sterile glove or a sterile tongue blade. The cream should be reapplied if rubbed off between applications. A tub bath—usually in a Hubbard tank—should be used to remove previously applied cream.

Patients usually complain of a stinging or burning sensation when mafenide is first applied. They may require an analgesic 20 to 30 minutes before the tub bath and application of the drug. Mafenide has carbonic anhydrase inhibitor properties, and with continued use, acidosis can occur. The respiratory system usually compensates for acidosis, but the physician may order oral sodium bicarbonate ($NaHCO_3$) to counteract this drug action, especially in patients who have had damage to the lining of the respiratory tract.

Silver Sulfadiazine. Silver sulfadiazine 1% is a water-soluble ointment applied in the same manner as mafenide. It does not sting when applied, nor does it disturb electrolyte or acid-base balances as do the pre-

viously mentioned drugs. This drug is particularly effective in controlling *Pseudomonas* infections, one of the most common burn wound infections.

Other Drugs. Nitrofurazone and gentamicin may be prescribed for application to burned areas. Nitrofurazone is used with caution in those with known or suspected renal impairment. Gentamicin is useful for short periods of time for treatment of infections not responding to other agents. It also may be necessary to administer antibiotics systemically to those patients with overwhelming infections.

Skin Grafting

First- and second-degree burns (partial-thickness burns) heal without grafting; full-thickness burns require grafting because the skin layers capable of regeneration have been destroyed. Skin grafting is necessary during the management and rehabilitation stages of third-degree burns, and the management stage of many second-degree burns. Some second-degree burns may require grafting for cosmetic reasons. The purpose of a skin graft during the management stage is to lessen the possibility of infection, minimize fluid loss by evaporation, and prevent loss of function.

Bacteria present in the air, on the skin, and on objects in the environment cause no problem to others but *can* cause serious infections in burn wounds. The control of infection is of *primary* importance because infection is one of the major causes of death in these patients.

Unassisted healing, that is, healing without the use of temporary grafts, in second-degree burns can result in an overgrowth of granulation tissue. Good granulation tissue without excessive overgrowth is necessary for successful skin grafting during the rehabilitation stage. The purpose of skin grafting during the rehabilitation stage is the restoration of cosmetic appearance and function.

Other Treatment Modalities

Temporary skin grafting has problems. The patient may not have enough skin from which to obtain a graft, grafts from cadavers are often difficult to obtain, and grafts using animal skin have drawbacks, such as rapid rejection (in some patients). Newer synthetic and biosynthetic products that are being used for some patients. These grafts are reasonably priced, easy to obtain, have a long shelf-life, and are often effective. Some of these products are knitted, elastic fabric that can be formed or fitted to areas to which it is often difficult to attach a temporary graft, and they remain in place about 2 weeks or more.

Pressure garments made of elasticized cloth or plastic may be applied over the burned area once healing has begun. These garments prevent scars and wound contractures. The patient may need to wear a pressure garment for up to 2 years after the burn injury.

Prognosis

In recent years, such large strides have been made in the treatment of burn shock that patients who would have died several years ago are saved today. This is especially true of patients who are not very young or very old and who have no preexisting disease. Patients saved from dying in shock, however, may later succumb to other complications, such as septicemia and renal failure.

NURSING PROCESS —THE BURNED PATIENT

Assessment

The initial assessment covers the extent and depth of injury and usually is made by the physician with assistance from the nurse. The materials necessary for immediate treatment should be made quickly available. Depending on hospital policy, clean or sterile technique should be used during the initial examination.

Assessment focuses on the major priorities, namely respiratory and cardiac status. Vital signs should be taken either with a blood pressure cuff or a Doppler or Dynamapp device. Shock may be present in any patient, and this, along with other problems, must be quickly recognized and efficiently treated.

Nursing Diagnosis

Depending on the extent and degree of burns, some or all of the following nursing diagnoses may apply. The relation to the nursing diagnosis also may change as the patient progresses through treatment and the stages of healing.

- Anxiety related to pain, injury, treatment modalities, other factors (specify)
- Fear related to pain, treatment modalities, possible death
- Acute pain related to burn injury, treatments
- Fluid volume deficit related to fluid loss from burn wound
- Potential for infection related to loss of epidermis, dermis
- Hyperthermia related to infection
- Hypothermia related to loss of body heat through open skin wounds
- Constipation related to immobility, effect of narcotics on peristalsis
- Altered nutrition: less than body requirements related

to increased caloric requirements secondary to burn injury, inability to take oral fluids and food
- Ineffective individual coping related to disfigurement
- Grieving related to disfigurement, impact of injury on future
- Sensory/perceptual alterations related to electrolyte and fluid imbalances, sleep deprivation, isolation
- Social isolation related to infection control measures
- Impaired verbal communication related to burns around the mouth, edema of respiratory passages
- Impaired physical mobility (specify upper or lower limbs or both) related to burn injury, contractures
- Sleep pattern disturbance related to pain, treatments, physical restrictions
- Impaired skin integrity related to immobility, infection, other factors (specify)
- Ineffective airway clearance related to edema of respiratory passages, inability to remove airway secretions
- Total self-care deficit related to burn injury
- Ineffective family coping related to patient's recovery, appearance, future medical care, psychological and financial problems
- Knowledge deficit of home care management

Planning and Implementation

The major goals of the patient may include reduction in fear, anxiety, and pain; a clear airway; absence of fluid and electrolyte imbalances, infection, and constipation; normal vital signs; adequate nutrition; improved communication; improved ability to cope; improved physical mobility and ability to care for self; improved sleep patterns; absence of decubitus; and understanding of home care management.

The major goals of nursing management may include relieving pain, anxiety, and fear; meeting the patient's immediate and long-term needs; recognizing and preventing complications; and helping the patient return to his or her fullest potential.

The major complications associated with severe burns are infection, fluid and electrolyte imbalances, renal failure, respiratory distress, and shock. The major focus of initial management is on airway clearance, breathing, and circulation. Patients who suffer severe burns require skilled and specialized management throughout hospitalization. The nursing process may vary and may be more detailed than presented here because the degree and extent of injury varies and because many coexisting factors may alter nursing management.

Methods of treatment may vary; therefore, the nurse must be familiar with the policies and procedures outlined in the hospital procedure manual. Any order that seems unclear should be questioned, and no procedure should be undertaken unless the nurse is thoroughly familiar with equipment or methods of performance.

Once emergency care is given, the following objectives of immediate and long-term management must be met: (1) the patient's needs must be met now and in the future, (2) the patient must undergo rehabilitation, and (3) infection must be kept to a minimum.

When the patient arrives in the hospital unit, he or she may be placed on a regular bed, CircOlectric bed, or other type of turning frame. Sterile or clean linen should be be used, depending on the method of treatment or hospital policy. Nonadherent absorbent pads should be placed under the burned areas to absorb excess moisture. Personnel and visitors must wear sterile or clean caps, gowns, and masks. Hospitals may use a special record sheet for recording nursing tasks and observations. If none is available, certain nursing tasks should be included in a plan of care (see Chart 57-2). These may be modified according to specific policies of the unit, the extent of burns, and the patient's condition.

GASTROINTESTINAL ULCERS. For unknown reasons, burned patients sometimes develop a gastrointestinal ulcer (Curling's ulcer). Ulcers are more common in patients with extensive burns but may be seen in any burned patient. The symptom most suggestive of an ulcer is onset or increase in anorexia, associated with abdominal distention due to gastric dilatation. The stool may be positive for occult blood. Severe bleeding of the ulcer may result in tarry stools.

As the patient recovers physiologic balance from the widespread disturbances caused by the burn, his or her appetite should slowly improve. If there is a reversal of this trend, it should be reported to the physician. The nurse also should observe for blood in the stool and in the nasogastric tube (if one has been inserted) or for hematemesis. Some patients have no symptoms until there is sudden gastrointestinal hemorrhage.

GASTROINTESTINAL DISTURBANCES, CONSTIPATION. Dilatation of the stomach may occur, characterized by regurgitation of fluid, discomfort, anorexia, and nausea. The patient may be dyspneic because the distended stomach is pressing on the diaphragm, interfering with respiration. In addition, fecal impaction may follow paralytic ileus and administration of narcotic analgesics, as well as be related to immobility.

Bowel sounds should be auscultated every 2 to 4 hours or as ordered, and a record of bowel movements should be kept. A change in the frequency of bowel sounds, absence of bowel movements, or abdominal distention should be brought to the attention of the physician.

ANEMIA. A number of factors contribute to the burned patient's anemia. Heat causes red blood cell destruction or makes the cells abnormally fragile, which shortens their life. Red blood cells are trapped in dilated capillaries. Infection depresses the function of hematopoietic tissue. Blood is lost from granulating wounds at dressing changes. Treatment includes blood transfusions and a high-protein, iron-rich diet, with iron supplements.

Anxiety, Fear, and Pain.   Pain following a burn injury is often severe and must be controlled with the administration of narcotic analgesics. Because pain also can be an indication of other problems such as a gastrointestinal ulcer (discussed earlier), pneumonia, and embolus or thrombus formation, the type and location of pain should be carefully evaluated.

Every effort should be made to reduce the anxiety and fear related to a severe burn injury. The nurse must identify those factors or situations that are causing anxiety or fear and attempt to solve the immediate problem. Explaining treatments, administering the prescribed narcotic 20 to 30 minutes before treatments, and practicing gentleness when giving care often help reduce the emotions associated with severe trauma.

Fluid Volume Deficit.   Fluid intake and urinary output should be monitored *closely*. Oliguria or anuria is usual, but occasionally there is diuresis. If this complication is going to occur, it usually does so by the 10th to the 12th day after the patient is burned. The physician should be kept informed of the patient's urinary output.

Intravenous fluids should be carefully balanced to meet the patient's needs and must be closely monitored to prevent fluid overload or a fluid volume deficit.

Potential for Infection, Body Temperature.   Wound infection and septicemia are responsible for a large number of the deaths of burned patients who survive the shock period. In addition to the overall lowered resistance of the burned patient, edema and thrombosis in the traumatized subcutaneous tissue obstruct bacteria-fighting mechanisms. There is always some infection in third-degree burns.

Vital signs should be monitored at frequent intervals. The physician may order a rectal temperature probe inserted in the rectum to closely monitor the patient's temperature as well as to decrease the amount of movement necessary to insert a rectal thermometer. The physician should be kept informed of any changes in the body temperature.

Hyperthermia may be the first indication of infection, and the body temperature characteristically mounts rapidly, rarely staying below 102°F. The pulse is rapid and yet regular. The odor or the appearance of the burn (if it is exposed) may change. The odor of infection is different from that of burn exudate. A dry-appearing crust may harbor copious amounts of pus beneath its surface. Through close and frequent contact with the patient, the nurse is in an excellent position to be the first observer of infection and should remain alert to its possible existence.

Treatment of infection may include continuous saline soaks warmed to about normal body temperature and systemic or topical antibiotics. The physician may order dressing changes every 4 hours with removal of the dead tissue loosened by the soaks.

Septicemia may result in oliguria, hypotension, tachypnea, paralytic ileus, disorientation (related to the degree of the fever), and cardiac failure. The patient may need oxygen, nasogastric suction, and blood; and intravenous fluid therapy may have to be resumed or increased.

Administering aspirin and sponging the unburned areas may be ordered for fever. Only those portions of the patient's body that are covered by unbroken skin should be sponged. If there is a high fever, the patient may be placed on a hypothermic blanket.

Even when the patient has a fever, every effort should be made to avoid drastic changes in the body temperature. The conservation of body heat depends on the circumstances. If the patient has a high fever, the physician may order exposure of body areas to room temperature (as well as other hypothermic measures) for a period of time or until the temperature drops to a certain level. On the other hand, a slight elevation in body temperature may not require cooling measures, and body heat should be conserved. In this instance, the room should be kept warm, all dressings and bath solutions should be warmed to body temperature, and uninjured areas should be covered with blankets or sheets.

Altered Nutrition.   The nutritional needs of the patient first should be met with intravenous fluids, followed by total parenteral nutrition. The administration of parenteral fluids or nutritional formulas should be closely monitored because excessive or rapid fluid administration places an added strain on the heart. Once the patient begins to recover, oral fluids and a soft diet may be ordered. The patient's food and fluid intake should be closely monitored. Persistent anorexia should be discussed with the physician because a well-balanced diet is important during the recovery phase.

Emotional Support.   Throughout the long hospitalization and rehabilitation period, the patient re-

quires a great deal of emotional support as he or she begins to cope with the severity and extent of the trauma. During the acute phase, mental changes may be due to electrolyte and fluid imbalances, lack of oxygen, or severe pain. Some burned patients may be alcoholics, drug addicts, or elderly people who are senile. Senility or withdrawal from alcohol or narcotics can add to the behavior changes caused by physiologic problems such as electrolyte imbalances, which further compound the problem of identifying the underlying causes of the behavior disorder.

Depression may occur after the acute phase has passed. The seriousness and the extent of the injury, pain and discomfort, the long recovery period, repeated surgery for skin grafts, the monotony of hospital routine, financial needs, and concern about disfigurement can influence the patient's mental outlook. Coupled with this is the patient's previous emotional makeup and stability.

Social Isolation, Impaired Verbal Communication.   Since patients have little to occupy their minds except hospital routine, treatments, and their personal welfare, communication with the patient becomes an essential component in a plan of care. Television or radio is invaluable, but if not available, nursing personnel must try to provide contact with the outside world. Discussion of what is happening —the weather, sports, special news events, and so on—must be relayed to the patient, and visitors should be allowed if possible.

Some patients may have difficulty communicating their needs because of facial burns or respiratory involvement requiring a tracheostomy. The nurse should make every effort to help the patient communicate by nodding or using hand signals.

Impaired Physical Mobility.   Because of the pull of tightening scar tissue, patients with third-degree burns may develop contractures that are both disfiguring and crippling. If contractures develop, plastic surgery is indicated. Every effort is made to prevent contractures, but this is a difficult problem when mobility must be limited because certain areas of the body are being treated with dressings and later skin grafting. To minimize contractures in extremities with third-degree burns, the physician may order extension and immobilization of the extremity with splints, sandbags, or pressure garments made of elasticized cloth or plastic.

As soon as healing has advanced sufficiently so that movement does not crack the eschar, a program of physical therapy should be started. Both passive and active whirlpool baths and exercises, carried out first underwater and then outside the tank, may be ordered.

Sleep Pattern Disturbance. When possible, treatments should be arranged so that the patient has adequate periods of rest and time to sleep. Noise should be kept to a minimum and the room darkened as much as possible during the nighttime hours.

Impaired Skin Integrity. Decubitus ulcers can occur on unburned areas because the patient is immobilized and has lost much body protein. Frequent turning and position changing and good skin care to unburned areas help prevent decubitus ulcers. Any signs of impairment of the unaffected areas of the body must be dealt with immediately.

Ineffective Airway Clearance. Pneumonia can follow immobilization and debilitation. A patient with burns of the chest finds it painful to cough up secretions but must be encouraged to do so. The physician may order the use of an incentive spirometer to encourage deep breathing. The lungs should be auscultated every 8 hours and abnormal breath sounds, a productive cough, chills, or fever should be reported to the physician.

Atelectasis may be caused by the aspiration of gastric contents after tube feedings or vomiting, as well as by mucous plugs retained in the respiratory passages. Great care should be exercised in the administration of tube feedings.

Self-Care Deficit. All the patient's physical needs should be met until such time as some of the responsibility for these needs can be assumed by the patient. During rehabilitation, the performance of tasks such as brushing the teeth and eating are part of physical, occupational, and emotional therapies.

Ineffective Family Coping. Families need emotional support because of the seriousness of the injury, and the long hospitalization affects them as well as the patient. When possible, the methods of and reasons for treatment should be thoroughly explained to the patient and family members to help them adjust to this difficult situation. Thoughts uppermost in their minds are disfigurement and what can be done to correct this problem, the costs of a long hospitalization and repeated operations, and the patient's future. Families need ample opportunity to discuss these problems with the physician. If it is noted that a particular problem is worrying the family or the patient, the nurse should report this to the physician.

Knowledge Deficit. Discharge planning should begin as soon as the acute phase is over. The scope of planning depends on the patient and family, the extent of burns, and the success of treatment. Patients with minimal injuries may require only basic discharge preparation, whereas those with extensive injuries require thorough planning by means of a team approach. In addition to the physician, nurse, physical therapist, and social service worker, discharge planning may require community resources. The patient may require counseling (psychiatric, vocational), the supervision of a community health nurse, and financial assistance. There is no rigid guideline for long-range planning because patients must be evaluated according to their specific needs. The points included in discharge planning depend on the physician's orders, the patient's physical condition, and the patient or family's ability to carry out these orders.

Long-range planning may need to include future surgery for cosmetic effects, for revision of scar tissue, or for restoration of function. Vocational rehabilitation may be necessary for patients who are unable to return to their previous work. Because some patients incur severe functional limitation and disfigurement, discharge planning must be thorough, with *all* members of the health team making a concentrated effort to return the patient to as normal a life as possible.

Evaluation

- Anxiety and fear are reduced
- Pain is controlled
- Airway is clear; lungs are clear to auscultation
- No evidence of fluid or electrolyte imbalances
- Vital signs are normal
- No evidence of infection
- Patient maintains adequate food and fluid intake
- Bowel elimination is normal
- Patient is able to communicate with others
- Patient demonstrates evidence of coping with problems related to injury
- Social contacts are provided; patient appears interested in topical events
- Patient shows improvement in physical mobility
- Sleep pattern is normal
- Patient remains mentally clear
- Patient shows evidence of moving through the grieving process
- Skin of areas not burned remain intact; no evidence of decubitus formation
- Self-care needs are met
- Patient demonstrates understanding of home care management

General Nutritional Considerations

☐ The burned patient has lost massive amounts of fluid as well as serum proteins and electrolytes. Initially, these losses are replaced by intravenous or nasogastric feedings.

☐ Diet therapy for the burned patient must be focused on providing foods that the patient will consume. If the patient does not eat an adequate diet, tube feedings may be necessary because a high-protein, high-calorie, high-vitamin, and high-mineral diet is absolutely essential in the healing of burns.

General Pharmacologic Considerations

☐ Ointments, creams, and lotions prescribed for dermatologic disorders must be applied *exactly* as the physician directs (eg, sparingly or thick or thin coat covering the lesion). The patient should be reminded that unless the drug is applied exactly as ordered, it may not be of therapeutic value, and if an excessive amount is used, the drug is being wasted.

☐ Drugs prescribed for dermatologic conditions may relieve symptoms but do not necessarily cure the disease. Skin disorders may require long-term therapy, often with a periodic change in prescriptions. This can be discouraging to the patient. The nurse should encourage persistence in following the physician's instructions.

☐ Individuals using acne preparations containing benzoyl peroxide should be warned that this ingredient is an oxidizing agent and may remove the color from clothing, rugs, furniture, and so on. Thorough washing of the hands following use may not remove all the drug, and permanent fabric discoloration may still occur. Users of products containing benzoyl peroxide should wear disposable plastic gloves when applying the drug.

☐ Patients receiving photochemotherapy for severe psoriasis must follow the physician's directions regarding the timing of taking the drug methoxsalen, which is usually taken 1 or 2 hours before exposure to ultraviolet light.

☐ Isotretinoin (Accutane) is used in the treatment of severe acne. Dosage is determined by the patient's weight. This drug is capable of causing *severe* birth defects. In sexually active individuals, effective contraception *must* be used for at least 1 month before starting therapy, during therapy, and for 1 month after therapy is discontinued. Patients who take isotretinoin should be warned not to increase the dosage of the drug if the acne becomes worse or does not respond to treatment.

☐ To be effective, each drug used in the treatment of burns must be applied exactly as ordered by the physician.

☐ When used for the treatment of burns, silver nitrate soaks must be continuous. The dressings must not be allowed to dry out because a concentrated silver nitrate solution can harm tissue.

☐ Sterile technique should be used in the application of topical drugs for the treatment of burns.

General Gerontologic Considerations

☐ Elderly patients requiring medicated tub baths for a skin disorder must be carefully supervised when getting into and out of the tub, since some of these preparations leave a slippery residue on the tub surface.

☐ The elderly patient with any type of skin lesion should be advised to seek medical attention and cautioned against self-medication.

☐ Excessive drying of the skin may result in pruritus and infection. Elderly patients should be encouraged to apply creams and lotions to the skin, especially during winter or when living in a hot, dry climate.

☐ Burns can result in serious complications in the elderly patient because of diminished renal, cardiac, and respiratory functions associated with the aging process.

☐ Elderly patients with extensive burns have a high mortality rate, and even small burned areas can produce serious complications.

Suggested Readings

☐ Coleman DA, Bennett ML, Young D. A worse-case guide for any case of psoriasis. RN March 1988;51:39. *(Additional coverage of subject matter)*

☐ Cuzzel JZ. Clues: itching and burning in skin folds. Am J Nurs January 1990;90:23. *(Additional coverage of subject matter)*

☐ Dunn ML, Cockerline EB, Rice MR. Treatment options for psoriasis. Am J Nurs August 1988;88:1082. *(Additional coverage of subject matter)*

☐ Farrell J. Nursing care of the older person. Philadelphia: JB Lippincott, 1990. *(In-depth coverage of subject matter)*

☐ Fischbach FT. A manual of laboratory diagnostic tests. 3rd ed. Philadelphia: JB Lippincott, 1988. *(Additional coverage of subject matter)*

☐ Fuller J, Schaller-Ayers J. Health assessment: a nursing approach. Philadelphia: JB Lippincott, 1990. *(Additional coverage of subject matter)*

☐ Gruendemann BJ, Meeker MH. Alexander's care of the patient in surgery. 8th ed. St Louis: CV Mosby, 1987. *(In-depth coverage of subject matter)*

☐ Horne MM, Swearingen PL. Pocket guide to fluids and electrolytes. St Louis: CV Mosby, 1988. *(Additional coverage of subject matter)*

☐ Hudak CM, Gallo BM, Benz JJ. Critical care nursing: a holistic approach. 5th ed. Philadelphia: JB Lippincott, 1990. *(In-depth coverage of subject matter)*

☐ Johnson GE, Hannah KJ. Pharmacology and the nursing process. Philadelphia: WB Saunders, 1987. *(Additional coverage of subject matter)*

☐ Lombardo B, Cave LA, Naso S, Bernadina D. Group support for derm patients. Am J Nurs August 1988;88:1088. *(Additional coverage of subject matter)*

☐ Martin LM. Nursing implications of today's burn care techniques. RN May 1989;52:26. *(Additional coverage and illustrations that reinforce subject matter)*

☐ Prigel CL. How to spot melanoma. Nursing '87 June 1987;17:60. *(Additional coverage of subject matter)*

☐ Stern C. Melanoma: the most lethal skin cancer. RN July 1987;50:53. *(Additional coverage of subject matter)*

☐ Vargo N. The skin cancer success story. RN July 1987;50:50. *(Additional coverage of subject matter)*

Appendix A

Abbreviations

ACTH adrenocorticotropic hormone
ADL activities of daily living
ALS amyotrophic lateral sclerosis
ARDS adult respiratory distress syndrome
BPH benign prostatic hypertrophy
BSE breast self-examination
BUN blood urea nitrogen
CAPD continuous ambulatory peritoneal dialysis
CBC complete blood count
CHF congestive heart failure
COPD chronic obstructive pulmonary disease
CPAP continuous positive airway pressure
CPPV continuous positive pressure ventilation
CPR cardiopulmonary resuscitation
CSF cerebrospinal fluid
CT scan computed (computerized) tomography scan
cu cubic
CVA cerebrovascular accident, costovertebral angle
CVP central venous pressure
D and C dilatation and curettage
DKA diabetic ketoacidosis
dL 100 mL
DVT deep vein thrombosis
ECG (also **EKG**) electrocardiogram
EEG electroencephalogram
ESWL extracorporeal shock wave lithotripsy
FBS fasting blood sugar (glucose)
FSH follicle-stimulating hormone
g gram
GH growth hormone
GI gastrointestinal
GU genitourinary
GYN gynecology, gynecologic
HCG human chorionic gonadotropin
HCl chemical abbreviation for hydrochloride
HPF high-power field (refers to magnification power of a microscope)
IABP intraaortic balloon pump
ICP intracranial pressure
IOP intraocular pressure
IU international unit
IUD intrauterine device

IPPB intermittent positive-pressure breathing
IVF in vitro fertilization
IVP intravenous pyelogram
kg kilogram
L liter
laser light amplification by stimulated emission of radiation
LH luteinizing hormone
LOC level of consciousness
LP lumbar puncture
LPF low-power field
mEq milliequivalent
mg milligram
mm millimeter
mmHg millimeters of mercury
mU milliunit
MRI magnetic resonance imaging
μg microgram
μL microliter; also used for cubic millimeter
μm micrometer
μU microunit
NPO nothing by mouth
NSU nonspecific urethritis
OTC over-the-counter (nonprescription) drugs
PCNL percutaneous nephrostolithotomy
PCP *Pneumocystis carinii* pneumonia
PEEP positive end-expiratory pressure
PEG pneumoencephalogram
PET positron emission tomography
PID pelvic inflammatory disease
PMS premenstrual syndrome
PUL percutaneous ultrasonic lithotripsy
PVC premature ventricular contraction
RBCs red blood cells
ROM range-of-motion (exercises)
SMR submucous resection
SPECT single-photon emission computed tomography
STD sexually transmitted disease
TPN total parenteral nutrition
TSH thyroid-stimulating hormone
TUR transurethral resection
TURP transurethral resection of the prostate
URI upper respiratory tract infection
UTI urinary tract infection
WBCs white blood cells

Appendix B

Laboratory Values

Laboratory values vary somewhat in different references. Laboratory technique also may alter values.

Blood Coagulation Tests (Normal Values)

Bleeding time (Ivy or Duke)	3–10 minutes
Partial thromboplastin time (PTT)	30–45 seconds
Coagulation time (Lee-White)	5–10 minutes (glass tubes)
Prothrombin time (one-stage)	12–16 seconds; 70%–100% of control

Hematology (Normal Values)

Platelet count	150,000–400,000/μL
Reticulocyte count	0.5%–2.5%
Sedimentation rate (ESR)	
Male	0–15 mm/hr
Female	0–20 mm/hr
Complete blood count (CBC)	
Hematocrit	
Male	42%–52%
Female	38%–47%
Hemoglobin	
Male	14–16 g/dL
Female	12–14 g/dL
Red cell count	
Male	4.6–6.2 million/μL
Female	4.2–5.4 million/μL
White cell count	5,000–10,000
Segmented neutrophils	60%–70%
Eosinophils	1%–4%
Basophils	0%–0.5%
Lymphocytes	20%–30%
Monocytes	2%–6%
Erythrocyte indices	
Mean corpuscular volume (MCV)	82–98 μm^3
Mean corpuscular hemoglobin (MCH)	27–32 pg per cell
Mean corpuscular hemoglobin concentration (MCHC)	32%–36%

Blood Volume

Erythrocyte (RBC) mass	28–32 mL/kg body weight
Plasma volume	36–45 mL/kg body weight

Whole Blood, Serum, and Plasma Chemistries (Normal Values)

Ammonia	to 100 μg/dL
Amylase	80–150 Somogyi units/dL
Bilirubin, total direct (conjugated)	0.1–1.0 mg/dL 0.1–0.2 mg/dL
Indirect (unconjugated)	0.1–0.8 mg/dL
Anion gap (or R factor)	±12 mEq/L
Blood gases	
pH	7.35–7.45
Paco$_2$	35–45 mmHg
Pao$_2$	80–100 mmHg
HCO$^-_3$ (bicarbonate)	22–26 mEq/L
SO$_2$	95%–98% arterial blood 70%–75% mixed venous blood
Calcium	9–11 mg/dL
Carbon dioxide (CO$_2$ content)	24–32 mEq/L
Carcinoembryonic antigen (CEA)	0–2.5 ng/mL
Cephalin flocculation	negative to 1+
Chloride	95–105 mEq/L
Cholesterol	150–300 mg/dL
Copper	65–170 μg/dL
Creatine phosphokinase (CPK)	0–20 units*
Creatinine	0.5–1.2 mg/dL
Glucose (fasting)	80–120 mg/dL
Icterus index	1–6 units
Insulin	4–24 μU/mL
Iodine, protein bound (PBI)	4.0–8.0 μg/dL
Iron, total	60–150 μg/dL
Ketone bodies	negative
Lactic dehydrogenase (LDH)	200–500 mU/mL
Lactic dehydrogenase, isoenzymes	
LDH-1	25%–33%
LDH-2	37%–41%
LDH-3	15%–21%
LDH-4	7%–10%
LDH-5	3%–7%
Lipase	4–24 U/L
Lipids (total)	400–1000 mg/dL
Magnesium	1.5–2.5 mEq/L
Nonprotein nitrogen (NPN)	16–35 mg/dL
Phosphatase, acid	1.0–5.0 King-Armstrong units
Phosphatase, alkaline	3–13 King-Armstrong units

* Varies widely depending on method used.

Potassium	3.5–5.5 mEq/L
Proteins, total	6.0–8.0 g/dL
Albumin	3.5–5.0 g/dL
Globulin	1.5–3.0 g/dL
Sodium	135–145 mEq/L
T$_4$ (thyroxine)	5.0–11.0 µg/dL (T$_4$ by column)
	6.0–11.8 µg/dL (Murphy-Pattee)
Transaminase	
SGOT	8–28 units
SGPT	5–25 units
Triglycerides	10–190 mg/mL
Urea nitrogen (BUN)	8–20 mg/mL
Uric acid	2.5–8.0 mg/dL

Urine

Acetoacetic acid	negative
Acetone	negative
Albumin (qualitative)	negative
Aldosterone (24-hr specimen)	2–20 µg/24 hr
Color	pale yellow to dark amber
Creatinine clearance	600–1,800 mg/24 hr
Estrogens (24-hr specimen	
Ovulation	28–100 µg/24 hr
Luteal peak	22–105 µg/24 hr
At menses	4–25 µg/24 hr
Postmenopause	less than 10 µg/24 hr
Male	4–24 µg/24 hr
Glucose	negative to trace
17-hydroxycorticosteroids (as 17-ketogenic steroids or 17-KGS)	male—9–22 mg/24 hr female—6–15 mg/24 hr
17-ketosteroids	male—9–22 mg/24 hr female—6–15 mg/24 hr
Microscopic examination	RBC 0–3/hpf WBC 0–4/hpf casts rare/hpf
pH	4.5–8.0
Protein	0–trace
Protein (24-hr)	50–80 mg/24 hr
Specific gravity	1.005–1.035
Turbidity	usually clear (cloudiness not always abnormal)
Volume	600–1,600 mL/24 hr

Cerebrospinal Fluid

Cell count	0–8 cells/µL
Chloride	1.2 × fasting blood level
Colloidal gold curve	not more than 1 in any tube
Color	clear, colorless
Glucose	⅔ fasting blood glucose
Protein	15–45 mg/dL

Serology

Antistreptolysin-O titer (ASLO)	less than 160 Todd units
Cold agglutinins	less than 1:32
C-reactive protein (CRP)	0
Fluorescent treponemal antibodies (FTA)	negative
Hepatitis-associated antigen (HAA or HBAg)	negative
Heterophile antibodies	less than 1:56
Latex fixation	negative
VDRL	nonreactive

Drugs

Barbiturates: coma level phenobarbital	approximately 11 mg/dL
most other barbiturates	2–4 mg/100 mL
Ethanol	0.3%–0.4% marked intoxication
	0.4%–0.5% alcoholic stupor
	over 0.5% coma
Salicylates	20–25 mg/dL therapeutic range
	over 30 mg/dL toxic range
Digitoxin	14–26 ng/mL therapeutic range
	over 35 ng/mL toxic range
Digoxin	0.5–2.0 ng/mL therapeutic range
	over 2.5 ng/mL toxic range
Lidocaine	1.5–6.0 µg/ml therapeutic range
	over 7 µg/mL toxic range

Glossary

abduction. movement of the extremities away from the midline

abscess. a localized collection of pus

accommodation. the ability of the eye to focus at different distances

acetone bodies. *see* ketone bodies

acetylcholine. a neurohormone concerned with the transmission of nerve impulses

acidosis. disturbance in acid–base balance with an accumulation of acid

addiction. a state of periodic or chronic intoxication produced by repeated consumption of a drug

adduction. movement of the extremities toward the midline

adrenergic drugs. drugs that act like or mimic the action of the sympathetic nervous system

aerobic. needing oxygen to live

afferent. to or toward

albuminuria. presence of albumin in the urine

alkalosis. disturbance in acid–base balance with an accumulation of alkali

alkylating agent. an antineoplastic drug that interferes with cell division

allergens. substances that are inhaled or ingested or that come in contact with the skin and cause an allergy

allograft. a graft obtained from the same species (syn., homograft)

alopecia. abnormal loss of hair; baldness

amenorrhea. absence of the menstrual flow

anabolism. building up of body tissue; opposite of catabolism (adj., anabolic)

anaerobe. a microorganism that can survive and grow in the absence of oxygen

anaerobic. unable to survive in the presence of oxygen

analgesic. a drug that relieves pain

anastomosis. a joining, communication, or union (adj., anastomotic)

anemia. a decrease in the number of red blood cells and a lower than normal hemoglobin (adj., anemic)

aneurysm. abnormal dilatation of a blood vessel caused by a defect or weakness in the vessel wall

angina pectoris. chest pain caused by a decrease in blood supply to the myocardium

anorectal. pertaining to the anus and rectum

anorexia. loss of appetite (adj., anorectic)

anoxia. lack of oxygen (adj., anoxic)

antibody. protein substance manufactured by the body in response to the presence of a specific antigen

anticoagulant. a drug that interferes with the blood-clotting mechanism

antiemetic. a drug used to treat or prevent nausea

antigen. a substance that induces the manufacture of antibodies

antihistamine. a drug that appears to compete with histamine receptor sites and is used in the treatment of allergy and motion sickness

antiinfective. against infection; an agent used to treat an infection

antimetabolite. an antineoplastic drug that interferes with cell growth by preventing use of necessary materials

antimicrobial. an agent that destroys or stops the multiplication of microorganisms

antineoplastic. a drug used in the treatment of neoplasms, more specifically malignant diseases

antipyretic. a drug that lowers an elevated body temperature

antiseptic. an agent that slows the multiplication of microorganisms

antitoxin. a substance formed in the body after exposure to a toxin

antivenin. a substance used to neutralize the venom of a poisonous animal

anuria. suppression of urine output

aortitis. inflammation of the aorta

aphasia. inability to use or understand spoken and written language

arterioles. the smallest arteries

arteriosclerosis. loss of elasticity of an artery and thickening of the intima

arthralgia. pain in a joint

arthrodesis. surgical fusion of the joint surfaces

arthroplasty. surgical repair of a joint

ascites. fluid in the abdomen

asthma. paroxysms of dyspnea, wheezing, and coughing, with production of thick, tenacious sputum

astigmatism. visual defect resulting from unequal curvature in the cornea or lens, usually correctable with glasses

asymptomatic. without symptoms

ataxia. motor incoordination

atelectasis. partial or total collapse of the lung

atheroma. fatty plaque

atherosclerosis. a deposit of fatty plaques in the intima of the artery that causes the lumen to become narrowed

atrophy. a wasting with a decrease in size

attenuate. weaken

autograft. a graft taken from one part of the body for another part of the body

aura. in epilepsy, a warning preceding an epileptic seizure

axilla. the armpit

azotemia. an excess accumulation of nitrogens, creatinine, and uric acid in the blood

Babinski. an abnormal response (also called a positive Babinski) that consists of dorsiflexion of the great toe and fanning of the other toes

bacteremia. bacteria in the bloodstream

bactericidal. an agent that kills bacteria

bacteriostatic. an agent that slows the duplication of bacteria

barbiturates. a group of drugs used as sedatives, hypnotics, and anesthetic agents; these drugs have addiction potential

benign. nonmalignant; not serious

bifurcate. to branch, having two branches

biliary. pertaining to bile, liver, and gallbladder

biosynthesis. manufacture of substances by living organisms

blanch. to become pale

bleb. a blister filled with fluid

brachial plexus. a group of nerves in the lower part of the neck and axilla

bradycardia. slowing of the pulse

bronchiectasis. chronic dilatation of bronchi and bronchioles in one or both lungs

bronchiole. a smaller subdivision of the bronchus

bronchiolitis. inflammation of the bronchioles

bronchitis. inflammation of the bronchi

bronchodilator. a drug that dilates the bronchi

bronchography. radiographic visualization of the bronchi after injection of a radiopaque substance into the bronchi

bronchoscopy. direct visual examination of the trachea, two major bronchi, and multiple smaller bronchi

bronchus. one of two branches of the trachea leading to the lungs (pl., bronchi)

bulla. a bleb filled with fluid and sometimes air when located in the lung (pl., bullae)

cachexia. a state of wasting, emaciation (adj., cachectic)

calculus. stone (pl., calculi)

callus. fibrous tissue formed at ends of fractured bone

cancellous bone. the reticular tissue of bone

cannula. a tube inserted into the body; the lumen of the cannula is obstructed with a trocar to facilitate insertion

canthus. the angle formed by the upper and lower eyelids; "corner of the eye"

carbon dioxide. a colorless gas composed of carbon and oxygen; chemical symbol CO_2

carcinogens. agents capable of causing cancer (adj., carcinogenic)

carcinoma. a malignant tumor (syn., cancer)

cardiogenic shock. shock caused by failure of the heart to act as an efficient pump

cardiopulmonary resuscitation. emergency measures taken to restore heart-lung function

carpopedal spasm. spasm of the hands and feet

cartilage. fibrous connective tissue attached to articular surfaces of bone

catabolism. breaking down of body tissue; opposite of anabolism (adj., catabolic)

catalyst. a substance capable of producing change in other substances without being changed itself

cataract. an opacity of the lens of the eye, reducing the amount of light reaching the retina

catecholamine. organic compound normally found in the sympathetic nervous system (eg, epinephrine)

cathartic. a drug that produces bowel movements

catheterization. insertion of a catheter

causalgia. burning pain

cephalgia. headache

cerebration. mental activity, thinking

cerebrovascular accident. lay term, "stroke"; bleeding in or loss of blood supply to part of the brain (abbr., CVA)

cerumen. waxlike secretion in the outer ear canal

cervicitis. inflammation of the cervix

chancre. a round, painless lesion on the genitalia

chemotherapy. therapy by means of chemicals or drugs

Cheyne-Stokes respiration. shallow, rapid breathing that builds in intensity and depth and then decreases, followed by a period of apnea

cholecystectomy. removal of the gallbladder

cholecystitis. inflammation of the gallbladder

cholecystostomy. surgical opening into the gallbladder

choledochotomy. surgical opening into the common bile duct

cholesterol. a sterol contained in animal tissues

cholinergic blocking agent. a drug that inhibits the action of acetylcholine (eg, atropine)

chorea. involuntary muscle twitching

chronic disease. a disease that extends over a long period

Chvostek's sign. when positive, there is spasm of the muscles innervated by the facial nerve when the nerve is tapped at a point anterior to the earlobe

cilia. hairlike projections of some types of epithelial cells that propel mucus, dust, and other foreign particles out of a structure

ciliated. having cilia

circumoral paresthesia. numbness around the mouth

cisternal puncture. insertion of a needle between the cervical vertebrae into the cisterna at the base of the brain to withdraw cerebrospinal fluid

clonus. alternate contraction and relaxation of muscles that results in jerking movements and excessive thrashing of the arms and legs (adj., clonic)

colectomy. removal of all or part of the colon

colic. spasm that causes pain; may be intestinal, uterine, renal, or biliary

collagen. fibrous protein found in connective tissue

collateral circulation. circulation in smaller blood vessels when a large vessel is occluded

colostomy. an opening in the colon; usually one end of the colon is brought to the abdominal wall for the purpose of diverting the fecal stream

coma. a deep, stuporous, unresponsive state

comedo. blackhead (pl., comedones)

commensals. microorganisms that live in a host and do not cause disease

commissurotomy. a surgical breaking or splitting of adherent tissue

concha. one of three bones that protrude from the lateral wall of the nasal cavity (pl., conchae)

concussion. loss of consciousness caused by a blow to the head

congenital. present at birth

conjunctivitis. inflammation of the conjunctiva of the eye

connective tissue. fibrous tissue that supports and connects internal organs and bones

contracture. an abnormal shortening of muscles that usually results in a deformity of the part and renders it resistant to movement

contusion. an injury in which the skin is not broken; a bruise

convulsion. involuntary muscle relaxation and contraction

cordotomy. surgical interruption of sensory pathways in the spinal cord

cortex. outer portion of an organ

corticosteroid. any of the steroids manufactured by the cortex of the adrenal gland

cranium. the skull

crepitation. a crackling or grating sensation or sound

cryosurgery. use of extreme cold to produce cell destruction

cryptorchidism. undescended testicle

crystalluria. crystals in the urine

curettage. scraping

cutaneous. pertaining to the skin

cyanosis. a blue discoloration to the skin, nail beds, or mucous membranes caused by oxygen deficiency

cyst. a sac or capsule that contains fluid or semisolid material

cystectomy. surgical removal of a cyst or the urinary bladder

cystitis. inflammation of the bladder

cystocele. herniation of the urinary bladder into the anterior vagina

cystoscope. an instrument that consists of a light and lens used to visualize the bladder and urethra

cystoscopy. visual examination of the inside of the bladder by use of a cystoscope

debridement. removal of foreign material or dead tissue from a wound

decalcification. loss of calcium from bone

decortication. removal of the cortex or outer layer

decubitus. a bedsore (pl., decubiti)

defibrillation. to stop fibrillation of the heart through use of electric current or drugs

defibrillator. a machine that delivers a specific amount of electric current to the heart

dehiscence. separation of wound edges without protrusion of organs

dehydration. excessive loss of water from the body not compensated by intake

delirium. a state of disorientation and confusion caused by interference with the metabolic processes of the brain

depolarization. transfer of positive ions to the inside of the cell membrane

dermatitis. inflammation of the skin

desensitization. subcutaneous administration of gradually increasing doses of an antigen

dialysis. removal of certain metabolic end products or other substances from the blood when the kidneys are nonfunctioning

diaphoresis. profuse perspiration (adj., diaphoretic)

diastole. relaxation of the atria and ventricles (adj., diastolic)

digitalization. administration of digitalis preparations to achieve a therapeutic blood level

diplopia. double vision

distal. farthest from a point of reference; opposite of proximal

diuresis. secretion of large amounts of urine

diuretic. a drug capable of causing diuresis

dyscrasias. a large group of blood disorders

dysmenorrhea. painful menstruation

dysphagia. difficulty in swallowing

dysphasia. impairment in speech usually caused by a lesion of the brain

dyspnea. difficult breathing; air hunger (adj., dyspneic)

dysrhythmia. abnormal heart rate or rhythm (syn., arrhythmia) *dysuria.* difficult or painful urination

ecchymosis. bleeding into skin or mucous membrane that produces blue-black discolorations

ectopic. out of place; not in correct position

edema. swelling caused by the collection of fluid in the tissues

edentulous. without teeth

efferent. away from

electrocardiogram. the electrical activity of the heart recorded on heat-sensitive paper

electroencephalogram. a record of the electrical activity of the brain

electrolyte. any compound that separates into charged particles (ions) when dissolved in water

element. a chemical subtance, existing free or in combination with other elements, that cannot be further divided into substances different from itself (eg, oxygen, hydrogen, radium)

embolectomy. surgical removal of an embolus

embolism. obstruction of a blood vessel with an embolus

embolus. a mass of undissolved particles, either solid, liquid, or gas, present in blood vessels or lymphatic tissue (pl., emboli)

embryonal. pertaining to an embryo

emollient. skin softener

emphysema. specific morphologic changes in the lung characterized by overdistention of alveolar sacs, rupture of alveolar walls, and destruction of the alveolar capillary bed

empyema. collection of pus in the pleural cavity

encephalitis. an infectious disease of the central nervous system

endarterectomy. removal of the lining of an artery

endocardium. a layer of endothelial tissue lining the interior wall of the heart

endocrine gland. a gland that regulates body activity by the secretion of hormones released directly into the bloodstream

endogenous. arising or coming from within

endometriosis. a condition in which endometrial tissue is located outside the uterus and in various other structures of the pelvis or abdominal wall

endoscope. a tube that contains an optical system, often fiber optics, and a method of illumination; the diameter is small enough to allow insertion into a body cavity

endoscopy. inspection of body cavities or organs by use of an endoscope

endotoxin. a toxin present in a bacterial cell

endotracheal. in the trachea

enema. introduction of fluid into the rectum to remove fecal material

enteritis. inflammation of the intestines

enterostomal therapist. a nurse specifically trained in the care and teaching of ostomy patients

enzyme. a complex protein produced by living cells that functions as a catalyst

epidermis. the outer layer of skin

epistaxis. nosebleed

epithelium. a type of cell that covers internal and external body surfaces

erythema. redness of the skin

erythrocytes. red blood cells

erythropoiesis. the manufacture of red blood cells

eschar. a hard, leathery crust made up of dehydrated dead skin that forms over a full-thickness burn

esophagoscopy. visualization of the esophagus with an endoscope

estrogen. female sex hormone manufactured by the ovaries

etiology. the science that studies the causes of disease

evisceration. separation of wound edges with protrusion of organs

exacerbation. an increase in intensity of symptoms or severity of a disease

excoriation. an abrasion of the outer layer of the skin

exfoliate. the shedding of dead cells

exfoliated cells. dead cells shed from the skin, mucous membrane, or bone

exocrine gland. a gland that secretes externally; opposite of endocrine gland

exogenous. coming or arising from outside the organism

exophthalmos. abnormal bulging or protrusion of the eyes

expectorant. a drug that encourages raising of secretions from the lungs

extracorporeal. outside of the body

extrasystole. *see* premature ventricular contraction

extravasation. the escape of fluid from a blood vessel into surrounding tissues while the needle or catheter is in the vein

exudate. fluid that usually contains pus, bacteria, and dead cells

fasciculation. involuntary contraction of independent muscle fibers

fibrillation. a quivering of muscle fibers

fibrils. small fibers

fibroblast. a cell from which connective tissue is developed

fibrosis. formation of fibrous tissue

fibrous. containing fibers

fissure. a groove, crack, or slit

fistula. a passageway or connection from one area to another

flaccid. relaxed, weak, limp

flatulence. excessive intestinal gas

flatus. gas in the intestinal tract

fluoroscopy. visualization by use of x-rays and a fluorescent screen

footdrop. inability to maintain the foot in a normal position; a dragging of the foot

fungus. a microorganism that belongs to the vegetable family that lives on organic matter (pl., fungi)

τ-globulin. a protein found in the blood and manufactured by lymphoid tissue and reticuloendothelial cells in response to infection

τ-rays. one of three emissions from radioactive substances; similar to x-rays

ganglion. a mass of nerve tissue

gangrene. necrosis of tissue almost always caused by a lack of blood supply to the affected part

gastrectomy. surgical removal of the stomach; may be total (all) or subtotal (part)

gastritis. inflammation of the stomach

gastroscopy. visualization of the stomach by means of an endoscope

gastrostomy. surgical opening into the stomach, usually for the purpose of feeding

gingiva. the gums

gingivitis. inflammation of the gums

glaucoma. a condition that results from increased intraocular pressure owing to a disturbance of the normal balance between the production and drainage of the aqueous humor that fills the anterior chamber

glomerulonephritis. inflammation of the glomeruli; a form of nephritis

glomerulosclerosis. hardening and degeneration of the glomeruli and the renal arterioles

glucagon. manufactured by the pancreas; stimulates release of glucose by the liver

glucocorticoid. one of the adrenal cortical hormones

glycogen. a polysaccharide; starch

glycosuria. presence of glucose in the urine

goiter. enlargement of the thyroid gland

gonads. sex glands; ovaries in the female, testicles in the male

gram positive. a retention of the color of a Gram stain; opposite of gram negative, which does not retain the Gram stain

granulation tissue. tissue formed during the repair and healing of wounds

granulocyte. a type of white blood cell

gumma. a well-defined local lesion of tertiary syphilis

habituation. a condition that results from the repeated consumption of a drug

hallucination. subjective sensory experiences that occur without stimulation from the environment

helminth. a parasitic worm or wormlike organism

hematemesis. vomiting of blood

hematocrit. a measurement of the volume of red blood cells in a given amount of blood

hematogenic shock. shock caused by blood loss

hematoma. a swelling that contains blood

hematopoiesis. the production or development of blood cells

hematopoietic. blood cell–producing

hematuria. blood in the urine

hemianopia. vision in only one half of the normal visual field

hemiplegia. paralysis of one side or one half of the body

hemodialysis. the removal of chemical substances from the blood by passing the blood through a system of tubes surrounded by a dialysate

hemoglobin. the red blood cell pigment that contains iron

hemolysis. destruction of red blood cells

hemoptysis. spitting up of blood from the respiratory tract

hemostasis. stopping of bleeding; stagnation of blood in one area

hemothorax. blood in the pleural cavity

hepatitis. inflammation of the liver

hepatomegaly. enlargement of the liver

hepatotoxic. toxic to the liver

herniorrhaphy. surgical repair of a hernia

heterogeneous. unlike

heterogenous. from another species

heterograft. a graft taken from another person

Homans' sign. pain in the calf on dorsiflexion of the foot

homeostasis. term used to describe a dynamic state of equilibrium of the body

homogeneous. of uniform or like characteristics

homograft. a graft taken from another person (syn., allograft)

hormone. a chemical substance secreted by an endocrine gland and carried to another area by way of the bloodstream

hydrocele. a collection of fluid in the testicles

hydronephrosis. swelling of the kidney pelvis with backflow of urine

hyperaldosteronism. excess production of aldosterone, an adrenal hormone

hypercalcemia. an excess of calcium in the blood

hypercalciuria. an excess of calcium in the urine

hypercapnia. increased carbon dioxide in the blood

hypercholesterolemia. excessive amount of cholesterol in the blood

hyperextension. extreme extension of a part

hyperglycemia. an excess of glucose in the blood

hyperinsulinism. excessive secretion of insulin

hyperkalemia. an excess of potassium in the blood

hypermagnesemia. an excess of magnesium in the blood

hypernatremia. an excess of sodium in the blood

hyperopia.   farsightedness

hyperparathyroidism.   overproduction of parathormone

hyperplasia.   extra growth of normal tissue; increase in the number of cells

hypertension.   sustained elevation of arterial pressure

hyperthermia.   elevation of body temperature; fever

hyperthyroidism.   excessive secretion of thyroid hormone resulting in an increased rate of all metabolic processes

hypertonia.   increased tone of muscles or arteries (adj., hypertonic)

hypertonic solution.   a solution with a greater osmotic pressure than another solution

hypertrophy.   increase in size of an organ or structure (adj., hypertrophied)

hyperuricemia.   accumulation of uric acid in the blood

hypervolemia.   increased volume of circulating blood; opposite of hypovolemia (adj., hypervolemic)

hypnotic.   a drug used to produce sleep

hypocalcemia.   decrease in blood calcium below normal level

hypocapnia.   decrease in carbon dioxide in the blood

hypochloremia.   decrease in the chloride content of the blood below normal level

hypochromic.   lighter than normal in color; less color than normal

hypoglycemia.   decrease in blood glucose below normal level

hypokalemia.   decrease in potassium in the blood below normal level

hypomagnesemia.   decrease in magnesium in the blood below normal level

hyponatremia.   decrease in sodium in the blood below normal level

hypoparathyroidism.   decreased production of parathormone

hypoproteinemia.   decrease in the amount of protein in the blood

hypostatic pneumonia.   pneumonia that results from prolonged immobility with failure to cough, move, and breathe deeply

hypotension.   low blood pressure

hypothermia.   below normal body temperature

hypothyroidism.   a deficiency of thyroid hormones causing a lowered rate of all metabolic processes

hypotonia.   loss of or decrease in muscle tone (adj., hypotonic)

hypotonic solution.   a solution with less osmotic pressure than another solution

hypovolemia.   diminished volume of circulating blood; opposite of hypervolemia (adj., hypovolemic)

hypoxemia.   reduced oxygen in the blood

hypoxia.   reduced oxygen in inspired air (adj., hypoxic)

hysterectomy.   surgical removal of the uterus

iatrogenic.   adverse results caused by medical personnel that could have been avoided by proper care

idiopathic.   cause unknown

illusion.   an inaccurate interpretation of stimuli within the environment

immunocompromised.   a state of being unable to develop immunity to one or more specific antigens

immunodeficient.   decreased ability to develop immunity to one or more specific antigens

immunogen.   another term for antigen

infarction.   area of necrosis, death of tissue

infiltration.   the collection of fluid into tissues (usually subcutaneous tissue) when the needle or catheter is out of the vein

infusate.   an intravenous solution

intercostal.   between the ribs

intracerebral.   within the brain

intractable pain.   pain that cannot be controlled by analgesic medications or good nursing management

intradermal.   within the skin; between the epidermis and the dermis

intraocular.   within the eyeball

intrathecal.   injection into the subarachnoid space of the spinal cord; a lumbar puncture must be performed

intrathoracic.   within the thorax

intravenous.   injection or infusion into the vein

intrinsic factor.   a substance manufactured in the stomach, necessary for the assimilation of vitamin B_{12}; absence produces pernicious anemia

ion.   one or more atoms carrying a positive or negative electrical charge (eg, Na^+, OH^-)

ionization.   the breaking up of molecules into their constituent ions

iridectomy.   removal of a segment of the iris

iridencleisis.   surgical creation of a fistula in the iris for treatment of glaucoma

ischemia.   reduction of blood supply to a part

isolated perfusion.   introduction of an antineoplastic drug to a tumor area after the blood supply is isolated from the rest of the circulation

isotonic.   having the same tone; also, a solution having the same osmotic pressure as the solution being compared with it

isotope.   any one of a series of chemical elements that has the same atomic number but a different atomic weight

jaundice.   a yellowish color to the skin or sclera of eyes caused by excess bile pigment

keratoconjunctivitis.   inflammation of the cornea and conjunctiva

ketone bodies.   chemical intermediate products in

the metabolism of fat; betahydroxybutyric acid, aceto-acetic acid, acetone

ketonemia. presence of ketone bodies in the blood

ketonuria. presence of ketone bodies in the urine

ketosis. an accumulation of ketone bodies in the body

Kussmaul breathing. deep, rasping respirations; air hunger

lamina. the flattened part of the vertebral arch

laminectomy. removal of the posterior arch of the vertebra to expose the spinal cord

laryngectomy. removal of the larynx

laryngofissure. removal of part of the larynx

laser. see abbreviations

latent. hidden

lavage. to wash out

lethargy. sluggishness, stupor (adj., lethargic)

leukemia. a malignant disease of the bone marrow characterized by an abnormal production of white blood cells

leukocyte. a white blood cell

leukocytosis. an increase in the number of leukocytes

leukopenia. a decrease in the number of leukocytes

leukoplakia. patches of white, thickened tissue in the mouth or mucous membrane often considered to be a forerunner of cancer

leukorrhea. a white or yellow-white vaginal discharge

ligation. tying off; application of a ligature (suture) to a part

lithiasis. formation of stones

lobectomy. removal of a lobe

lumbar puncture. insertion of a needle into the subarachnoid space of the spinal cord in the lumbar region

lumen. the inner space or diameter of a tube or tubular organ

lymphadenitis. inflammation of lymph glands

lymphedema. massive edema caused by an obstruction of lymph channels

lymphocytes. white blood cells

lymphoid tissue. lymph tissue; resembling lymph tissue

lymphoma. a tumor of lymphoid tissue

macula. a small, colored spot

macule. a small, colored spot on the skin

malaise. a feeling of discomfort or uneasiness

malignant. harmful; capable of producing death

mastectomy. removal of the breast

mastoiditis. infection of the mastoid process

maximum breathing capacity. the most air a person can voluntarily move in and out of the lungs within 1 minute

meatus. opening

medulla. inner portion of a gland or organ; also, a portion of the upper spinal cord

melena. tarry stools

menarche. the start of menstruation; usually occurs between ages 10 and 14

meninges. collectively, the three coverings of the brain and spinal cord: pia mater, arachnoid membrane, dura mater

meningitis. inflammation of the membranes that surround the brain and spinal cord

menopause. the period when menstruation begins to wane and finally ceases

menorrhagia. excessive bleeding at the time of normal menstruation

metabolism. the sum total of the physical and chemical changes and reactions that take place in the body

metastasis. spread; the spread of disease from one part of the body to another (adj., metastatic; verb, metastasize)

metrorrhagia. bleeding at a time other than a menstrual period

microcytic. smaller than normal cell

mineralocorticoid. hormone produced by the adrenal gland

miotic. a drug that constricts the pupil

Monilia. same as *Candida,* a genus of fungus

monocyte. a type of white blood cell

morbidity. sickness expressed as a rate in relation to population

moribund. dying, near death

morphology. study of shape without regard to function

mortality. death rate

mucolytic. a drug that thins mucus

mucopurulent. consisting of pus and mucus

mucus. fluid secreted by mucous membrane

mydriatic. a drug used to dilate the pupil; usually applied topically

myocardial infarction. lay term, ''heart attack''; infarct of the muscle layer (myocardium) of the heart (abbr., MI)

myocardium. muscle layer of the heart

myopia. nearsightedness

myringoplasty. plastic surgery on the eardrum

myringotomy. incision of the eardrum

myxedema. hypothyroidism in the adult

narcotic. a drug capable of producing stupor and sleep, usually used to relieve pain

nares. nostrils

nasogastric tube. a tube passed through the nose into the stomach

nasopharynx. the section of the pharynx above the soft palate

nebulizer. an atomizer or sprayer that produces a fine mist used for the delivery of medication to the upper respiratory passages *necrosis.*   death of tissue (adj., necrotic)

neoplasm.   new growth (adj., neoplastic)

nephrectomy.   removal of the kidney

nephritis.   inflammation of the kidney

nephron.   structural unit of the kidney

nephrosclerosis.   hardening of renal arteries and arterioles

nephrostomy.   an opening into the kidney

nephrotoxic.   toxic to the kidney

neuralgia.   pain in a nerve

neurohormone.   a chemical substance found in the nervous system that affects nervous system function

neuroma.   a tumor growing from a nerve

neuromuscular.   nerve–muscle

nocturia.   excessive urination during the night

nodule.   a small node

nodular.   having or resembling nodules

norepinephrine.   a neurohormone produced by the adrenal medulla

normotensive.   normal blood pressure

normovolemia.   a normal blood volume (adj., normovolemic)

nosocomial.   hospital-acquired

nuchal rigidity.   pain and stiffness of the neck

nystagmus.   involuntary movement of the eyeball

occlusion.   blockage of a passage

oculogyric crisis.   a rolling downward or upward of the eyes against the patient's will

olfactory.   pertaining to smell

oligomenorrhea.   infrequent menses

oliguria.   decrease in the amount of urine secretion

oophorectomy.   removal of an ovary

ophthalmoscope.   an instrument used to examine the structures of the eye

orchiectomy.   surgical removal of the testicle

orchitis.   inflammation of the testicles

orifice.   entrance; opening

oropharyngeal airway.   an airway inserted in the mouth and extending as far as the oropharynx

orthopnea.   difficulty breathing when lying flat or almost flat

osmotic pressure.   pressure that occurs when two solutions are separated by a semipermeable membrane

ossification.   formation of bone

osteoarthritis.   a chronic arthritic disease of the joints, especially the weight-bearing joints

osteoblast.   a cell concerned with the formation of bone

osteolytic.   bone destruction

osteomyelitis.   infection of the bone

osteoporosis.   loss of calcium from bone

osteotomy.   artificial angling of the bone through a surgical fracture

ostomate.   a person with an ileostomy or colostomy

ostomy.   a surgical opening (eg, colostomy, ileostomy)

otitis.   inflammation of the ear

otosclerosis.   hearing loss resulting from ankylosis of the stapes

otoscope.   an instrument used for examining the external auditory canal and eardrum (tympanic membrane)

ovulation.   release of an ovum (egg) from the mature graafian follicle of the ovary

oxidation.   the process of combining with oxygen

oxygen.   chemical symbol O_2

pacemaker.   the SA (sinoatrial) node; an artificial pacemaker is an electrical device that substitutes for the heart's own pacemaker

pain.   the sensation of physical or mental suffering or hurt that usually causes distress or agony to the one suffering it

palliative.   relieving symptoms without curing the disease

pancreatitis.   inflammation of the pancreas

panhysterectomy.   removal of the entire uterus

Papanicolaou smear (test).   cytologic examination of exfoliated cells

papilledema.   swelling of the optic nerve at its point of entrance into the eye

papule.   a red, elevated area on the skin

paracentesis.   removal of fluid from a cavity

paradoxical pulse.   a pulse that weakens on deep inspiration

paralytic ileus.   paralysis of the intestines and absence of peristalsis

paraplegia.   paralysis of both lower extremities

parathormone.   parathyroid hormone

parenchyma.   the essential parts of an organ (adj., parenchymal)

parenteral nutrition, total.   providing essential nutrients by the intravenous route by means of a catheter in the superior vena cava or an external arteriovenous fistula; also called hyperalimentation

parenteral therapy.   the giving of food, fluids, or other substances by routes other than the alimentary canal

paresthesia.   numbness, prickling, tingling

paroxysm.   a sudden spasm; a sudden recurrence of symptoms

patent.   open (n., patency)

pathogen.   a microorganism that produces harm or disease (adj., pathogenic)

pathophysiology.   the physiology of disordered function

peptic ulcer.   an ulcer in the lower esophagus, stomach, or duodenum

percutaneous.   through the skin

perfusion.   a specialized method of giving a drug

with administration of the maximum dose to an isolated part of the body

pericarditis.   inflammation of the pericardium

pericardium.   the covering of the myocardium

perineum.   the area between the vulva and anus of the female and the scrotum and anus of the male (adj., perineal)

periosteum.   the fibrous covering of bones

peripheral.   to the periphery or the outside edge

peristalsis.   wavelike movements of hollow organs such as the intestine, esophagus, ureter

peritonitis.   inflammation of the peritoneum

petechiae.   tiny hemorrhagic spots on the skin (adj., petechial)

pH.   the degree of alkalinity or acidity. A pH of 7.0 is neutral (eg, neither acidic nor alkaline); a pH below 7.0 is acidic and a pH above 7.0 is alkaline

phlebitis.   inflammation of a vein

phlebography.   injection of contrast media into a vein to visualize the venous system

phlebothrombosis.   presence of clots in a vein with little or no inflammation

phlebotomy.   an opening into a vein

photocoagulation.   use of a laser beam for surgical coagulation

photophobia.   aversion to light

pigmentation.   coloration caused by a deposit of pigments (colored material)

plasma.   the liquid part of blood

plasmapheresis.   a technique for separating the elements of the blood

platelet.   a blood cell concerned with the clotting of blood; also called thrombocyte

pleural effusion.   escape of fluid into the pleural cavity

plexus.   a network of blood vessels or nerves

pneumoencephalography.   an air contrast study performed when there is a suspected abnormality in the brain

pneumonectomy.   removal of a lung

pneumothorax.   air in the pleural cavity

polyarthritis.   inflammation of more than one joint

polycythemia vera.   an abnormal increase in red blood cells

polydipsia.   drinking a great deal of water; excessive thirst

polyp.   a tumor or growth attached by a pedicle to a surface

polyphagia.   increase in the intake of food

polyuria.   excessive secretion of urine; increased urination

postictal state.   the period after a convulsive seizure

postpartum.   after childbirth

postural hypotension.   a feeling of weakness, dizziness, or faintness when suddenly changing position

precordial.   over the heart

premature ventricular contraction.   a ventricular ectopic beat that occurs before depolarization of the ventricles followed by a long pause; the patient may complain of a fluttering sensation in the chest (abbr., PVC)

presbycusis.   loss of hearing as a result of aging

presbyopia.   loss of visual accommodation as a result of aging

proctitis.   inflammation of the anus or rectum

proctoscopy.   visualization of the rectum and anus

prodromal phase.   the early stage of a disease

prognosis.   the outcome or prediction of the course of disease

prolapse.   a dropping of an organ out of its original place or position

prophylactic.   anything used to prevent infection or disease

prostate.   a gland that surrounds the neck of the bladder and urethra in the male

prosthesis.   an artificial substitute for a part (pl., prostheses)

prosthetist.   a person who makes and fits artificial limbs

prothrombin.   a chemical substance in the blood that is converted into thrombin during blood clotting

protozoa.   microorganisms that are members of the animal kingdom, usually one-celled

proximal.   nearest to a point of reference; opposite of distal

pruritus.   itching

psoriasis.   a dermatitis with dull red lesions surrounded by silver scales

psychosomatic symptoms.   bodily symptoms that are psychic or emotional in origin

ptosis.   drooping

pulse pressure.   the numerical difference between the systolic and diastolic blood pressures

purines.   end products of the digestion of certain proteins

purpura.   hemorrhage into the skin and mucous membrane

purulent.   containing pus

pustule.   a small elevation on the skin that contains pus or lymph

pyelitis.   inflammation of the pelvis of the kidney

pyelogram.   an x-ray film of the kidney and ureter

pyuria.   presence of pus in the urine

quadriplegia.   paralysis of all four extremities

quiescent.   inactive, dormant

radiation.   the emission or giving off of rays

radioactive isotope.   an isotope capable of giving off rays

radioactivity.   the ability of a substance to emit alpha, beta, and gamma rays

radioisotope.   an isotope that is radioactive

radiopaque.   not penetrable by x-rays

radiosensitive. sensitive to radiation; easily affected by radiation

rale. abnormal sound heard in chest caused by air passing over secretions or exudate in the bronchi

refractory. resistant to treatment; in the cardiac cycle, resistant to electrical stimulation

repolarization. realignment of ions after depolarization

respirator. a mechanical device that substitutes for or assists with respirations

reticuloendothelial system. cells throughout the body that ingest matter such as bacteria

retinoblastoma. malignant tumor of the retina

rheumatic fever. an inflammatory disease frequently followed by damage to the heart or kidney

rheumatoid arthritis. an inflammatory disease of connective tissue characterized by chronicity, remissions, and exacerbations

rhinitis. a reaction of the nasal mucosa to various allergens

rhizotomy. a sectioning of the posterior nerve root just before it enters the spinal cord, for the relief of pain

rhythmicity. rhythmic activity

rickettsia. parasitic microorganisms that are between bacteria and viruses that require living cells for growth

roentgenography. the obtaining of a film by use of roentgen rays (x-rays)

rubella. German measles

salicylism. a set of symptoms resulting from excessive ingestion of a salicylate

salpingectomy. removal of a fallopian tube

salpingitis. inflammation of the fallopian tubes

saphenous vein. a vein in the leg

sarcoma. a malignant tumor that arises from connective tissue

sclerectomy. removal of a portion of the sclera

sedative. an agent that exerts a calming effect

seizure. another term for a convulsion or an epileptic attack

sensorineural hearing loss. nerve deafness

septicemia. the presence of infective microorganisms in the bloodstream

sigmoidoscopy. visualization of the sigmoid colon, rectum, anus

sinusitis. inflammation of the sinuses

specific gravity. weight of a substance compared with water, which has a specific gravity of 1.000, measured with a hydrometer

sphincter. a circular muscle around an opening

sphygmomanometer. blood pressure apparatus

splenectomy. removal of the spleen

splenomegaly. enlargement of the spleen

sputum. fluid raised from the respiratory passage

stasis. stagnation

stenosis. constriction, narrowing

stertorous. labored breathing that produces a snoring sound

stoma. opening; mouth; artificially created opening

stomatitis. inflammation of the mouth

stool softener. a drug that softens the stool, thereby easing passage

stress incontinence. incontinence of urine when sneezing or coughing

stressor. an incident or condition capable of causing stress

subcutaneous. below or beneath the skin

supine. lying on the back

suprapubic. above the pubic bone

sympathectomy. excision of a portion of the sympathetic nervous system, usually of a nerve, ganglion, or plexus

syncope. fainting

syndrome. a group of signs and symptoms

synovectomy. removal of a synovial membrane

synovial membrane. the membrane lining the capsule of a joint

systole. contraction of the atria and ventricles (adj., systolic)

tachycardia. elevated pulse rate

tachypnea. rapid respiratory rate

tamponade, cardiac. fluid in the pericardial space that compresses the heart

tenacious. clinging, adhesive

tepid. lukewarm

teratoma. a congenital tumor that contains embryonic elements

tetany. tonic spasms

thoracotomy. an opening into the thorax

thrombectomy. surgical removal of a thrombus

thrombocytopenia. decreased number of platelets

thrombolytic. an agent capable of breaking up a thrombus

thrombophlebitis. development of inflammation with the formation of clots within the vein

thrombosis. development of a thrombus

thrombus. a clot obstructing the lumen of a blood vessel

thyroidectomy. removal of the thyroid gland

thyrotoxicosis. a toxic condition caused by hyperactivity of the thyroid gland

tinnitus. ringing in the ears

tonic. characterized by rigid contraction of the muscles

toxigenicity. virulence of a microorganism that produces a toxin

toxin. a poisonous substance

toxoid. a weakened toxin

trabeculae. (carneae cordis) cords or bands attached to the inner walls of the ventricles forming a meshlike network

tracheostomy. an opening into the trachea

tranquilizer. a drug that calms and reduces tension without interfering with normal mental activity

transcutaneous. through the skin

transvenous. through the vein

trephination. the cutting of a piece of bone from the skull

Trichomonas. a parasitic protozoa

trochanter roll. a roll placed parallel to the upper thigh

Trousseau's sign. muscle spasm of the arm and hand produced by application of pressure to the nerves and vessels of the upper arm

ulcer. a depression or defect

ulcerative colitis. inflammation and ulceration of the colon

ultraviolet light. light beyond the violet end of the visible spectrum

unilateral. on one side

urea. end product of protein metabolism

uremia. accumulation of nitrogenous substances in the blood (adj., uremic)

ureter. hollow tube that transports urine from the kidney to the bladder

urethra. hollow tube that transports urine from the bladder to the outside

urethritis. inflammation of the urethra

uricosuric drug. a drug that promotes the excretion of urates

urinalysis. laboratory examination of the urine

urobilinogen. ''conjugated'' bilirubin formed by the liver enters the bile ducts, reaches the intestine, and is changed into urobilinogen that is changed into urobilin, the brown pigment of stool

urticaria. hives

vaccine. a specific infectious agent given for establishing resistance to an infectious disease

vaginitis. inflammation of the vagina

vagotomy. surgical interruption of the vagus nerve

to terminate the transmission of impulses along the nerve fiber

vagus nerve. tenth cranial nerve; innervates structures in the chest, abdomen, head, neck

Valsalva's maneuver. pinching the nostrils while at the same time trying to blow air through the nose

varicella. chicken pox

varicosities. varicose veins

vascular compartment. inside blood vessels

vasoconstriction. constriction or narrowing of a blood vessel

vasodilatation. dilatation or enlargement of the diameter of a blood vessel

vasomotor nerves. nerves that control the size of blood vessels

vasopressor. a drug capable of constricting blood vessels, particularly arteries and arterioles

venostasis. the trapping of blood in an extremity by compression of a vein

venous stasis. interruption in the normal flow of venous blood, stagnation of venous blood

ventilation. the movement of air in and out of the lungs

venules. the smallest veins

vertigo. sensation of moving or sensing that objects are moving; may be used as a synonym for dizziness

vesicle. a small sac that contains fluid

virulence. degree of ability to cause disease

virus. a microorganism covered by a protein coat; a parasite that lives in and is dependent on cells for nutrition, growth, and reproduction

vital capacity. a measure of the amount of air a person can expire after maximal inspiration

vulvovaginitis. inflammation of the vulva and vagina

wheal. a raised lesion often accompanied by severe itching; a hive

xerostomia. dry mouth

yeast. a member of the fungus family

Index

Page numbers followed by f indicate illustrations; those followed by t indicate tabular material.